Paediatric Pathology

Springer

London
Berlin
Heidelberg
New York
Barcelona
Budapest
Hong Kong
Milan
Paris
Santa Clara
Singapore
Tokyo

Colin L. Berry (Ed.)

Paediatric Pathology

Third Edition

With 851 Figures

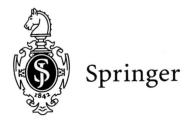

Springer

Sir Colin Berry, DSc, MD, PhD, FRCPath, FRCP
Department of Morbid Anatomy,
The Royal London Hospital,
Whitechapel,
London E1 1 BB, UK.

ISBN 3-540-19936-5 3rd edition. Springer-Verlag Berlin Heidelberg New York

ISBN 3-540-19536-X 2nd edition. Springer-Verlag Berlin Heidelberg New York

ISBN 3-540-10507-7 1st edition. Springer-Verlag Berlin Heidelberg New York

British Library Cataloguing in Publication Data
Paediatric Pathology. – 3Rev. ed
I. Berry, Colin L.
618.92007
ISBN 3-540-19936-5

Library of Congress Cataloging-in-Publication Data
Paediatric pathology / Colin L. Berry (ed.). — 3rd ed
    p.   cm.
  Includes bibliographical references and index.
  ISBN 3-540-19936-5 (hardback: alk. paper)
  1. Pediatric pathology.   I. Berry, Colin Leonard, 1937–   .
  [DNLM: 1. Pediatrics.   2. Pathology.   WS 200 P1255 1995]
RJ49.P3 1995
618.92′007—dc20
DNLM/DCL
for Library of Congress   95–33587

Typesetting: Expo Holdings, Malaysia
Printed and bound at Cambridge University Press, Cambridge UK
28/3830-543210 Printed on acid-free paper

Preface to the First Edition

The increased provision of facilities for neonatal and paediatric care in the last 25 years has been accompanied only in part by appropriate developments in pathology. Specialist pathologists are many fewer than paediatric departments, and details of the advances in knowledge of the pathogenesis of diseases in childhood and of ways of investigating them are not uniformly available. In many institutions an individual with a special interest rather than a special training will be responsible for paediatric pathology and it is to this group of histopathologists that this text is addressed. For this reason it is not written as a comprehensive text and is not intended for use as a reference volume. Areas which may produce particular difficulties for the individual with little specialist knowledge of the very young (e.g. the lung) are dealt with in more detail and, in general, entities in which the histopathology does not differ greatly from that of the adult disease are considered briefly. A brief account of developmental processes is included where prenatal considerations are helpful in understanding a particular entity. A number of specialist topics which are known to trouble those who work in non-specialist departments are described fully (diseases of muscle) or with guides to investigation (metabolic disease). The value of investigation and careful description of abnormalities of development is also emphasized.

The authors are from different backgrounds, paediatric pathologists (J.W. Keeling, J. Cox), pathologists in general departments with extensive experience in paediatric pathology (C.L. Berry, R.A. Risdon, M. Becker, J. Smith) or specialists with an interest in the manifestation of diseases of which they have expert knowledge in the young (P.A. Revell, R.H. Anderson, C.L. Brown, M. Swash, A.E. Becker, B.D. Lake). All are valued and respected friends, who have been asked to contribute in a particular way; any errors or "design" faults are my own.

Acknowledgements

It is a pleasure to thank Professor A.E. Claireaux, a mentor of five of the authors, for his generosity in allowing us to use illustrations of many cases seen at The Hospital for Sick Children, Gt. Ormond Street. Our collective thanks are owed to Miss L. Singer who has made sense of many difficult manuscripts.

Mr Michael Jackson and Mrs J. Dodsworth of Springer-Verlag have been unfailingly generous with help and advice in the preparation of the text.

London   Colin L. Berry
1981

Preface to the Second Edition

Eight years have passed since the first edition of this book was published. It continues to be true that most autopsies in the paediatric age group are done by those who are not full-time paediatric pathologists, but rather individuals with a particular interest in the pattern of disease in the young. Neonatal pathology is achieving deserved recognition as a speciality, but the provision of specialist posts lags behind the development of the subject

For these reasons it is hoped that a text for the interested non-specialist histopathologist will still be useful. This edition has been modified in a number of ways: firstly by a simple updating – with change in knowledge more evident in some fields than others: secondly, by the addition of areas identified as deficient by kind (and critical) reviewers, notably in a new chapter on Infection by Professor R.O.C. Kaschula, but also in other fields, including the provision of more data helpful in estimating age in infants and children at autopsy: thirdly, by modifying the structure of some chapters. Finally, the chapter on the placenta has been omitted as an Editorial decision; the text makes clear that detailed morphometric studies of the placenta are necessary to provide useful data with regard to the infant. These are beyond the scope of this book and detailed texts of placental changes *per se* are available elsewhere. A further Editorial decision has been made in citing only the first page of references.

I am happy that all of the previous contributors agreed to revise their texts and glad to welcome R.O.C. Kaschula to their number. Professor R.A. Risdon is now Head of Department at Great Ormond Street, the pathological "base" of many of us. I thank Dr Mies Becker for her previous contributions and am glad that her careful studies will be published elsewhere. As before, design faults in the volume are my own.

Acknowledgements

Miss L. Singer has again made a valuable contribution to the production of the volume. I am grateful to Mr Michael Jackson and to Mr Roger Dobbing and the Production Department of Springer-Verlag for their help.

London   Colin L. Berry
1989

Preface to the Third Edition

A shorter interval between the second and third editions of this book than between the first and second indicates both the rapid pace of change in pathology and the increasing requirement for all of us to involve ourselves in continuing education – a mandatory requirement for many. This is facilitated by better information and production systems, which now allow shorter intervals between editions, but it is important to note that this book is still intended to provide support for those who carry out paediatric pathology as part of their general duties in histopathology. However, no apologies are made for introducing new scientific concepts into the chapters on malformations and embryonic tumours and elsewhere; these concepts may underlie therapeutic and other interventions in the immediate future.

The chapter on the central nervous system has been completely revised by a new author, Dr Jennian Geddes, and Professor Kaschula has written a new chapter on AIDS in this age group. The singular features of bone marrow disease in childhood are considered by Professor van den Tweel in more new text. New entities have been identified since 1989, and new data which help in dating fetuses are now available. As an example of changes in viewpoint, the pathogenesis of cystic fibrosis is becoming clearer as our knowledge of genetics increases, and this new understanding will modify the book more radically in the future. I hope it will help pathologists to understand disease processes better and inform their own careful studies, which have helped to define phenotypes accurately enough to facilitate good genetic work.

I am glad to welcome new authors and to be able to thank my long-term supporters. The radical changes in hospital and university organization which envelop all of us have not made writing or revising text an easy task, but almost everyone produced their text on time and the publishers have worked very effectively.

Acknowledgements

I am glad to be able to thank Miss Lorraine Singer once again for her help in establishing order where there was chaos and in identifyng areas where expected sections of text had failed to arrive, or where illustrations had disappeared. The Production Department at Springer-Verlag have worked very hard and I would like to thank Roger Dobbing who heads the team. It is with regret that I remember the former contributions of Mr Michael Jackson to the success of earlier editions of this book; medical publishing has lost a great deal by his untimely death.

London   Colin L. Berry
1995

Contents

Contributors

Professor R.H. Anderson
Department of Paediatrics, National Heart and Lung Institute, Dovehouse Street, London SW3 6LY, UK

Professor A.E. Becker
Department of Cardiovascular Pathology, Academic Medical Center, University of Amsterdam, Meilbergdreef 9, 1105 AZ Amsterdam ZO, The Netherlands

Professor Sir Colin Berry
Department of Morbid Anatomy, The Royal London Hospital, Whitechapel, London E1 1BB, UK

Dr C.L. Brown
Department of Morbid Anatomy, The Royal London Hospital, Whitechapel, London E1 1BB, UK

Dr J.N. Cox
Département de pathologie, Hôpital Cantonal Universitaire, 1 rue Michel Servet, CH-1211 Genève 4, Switzerland

Dr J.F. Geddes
Department of Morbid Anatomy, The Royal London Hospital, Whitechapel, London E1 1BB, UK

Professor R.O.C. Kaschula
Department of Pathology, Red Cross Memorial Children's Hospital, Klipfontein Road, Rondebosch, Cape Town, 7700 South Africa

Dr J.W. Keeling
Paediatric Pathology, Royal Hospital for Sick Children, 2 Rillbank Crescent, Edinburgh EH9 1LF, UK

Dr B.D. Lake
Department of Histopathology, Hospital for Sick Children, Great Ormond Street, London WC1N 3JH, UK

Professor P.A. Revell
Department of Histopathology, Royal Free Hospital, Pond Street, London NW3 2QG, UK

Professor R.A. Risdon
Department of Histopathology, Hospital for Sick Children, Great Ormond Street, London
WC1N 3JH, UK

Dr W.G.M. Spliet
University Hospital Utrecht, Department of Pathology, Heidelberglaan 100, 3584 CX Utrecht,
The Netherlands

Dr M. Swash
Department of Neurology, The Royal London Hospital, Whitechapel, London E1 1BB, UK

Professor J.G.M. van den Tweel
University Hospital Utrecht, Department of Pathology, Heidelberglaan 100, 3584 CX Utrecht,
The Netherlands

1 · Examination of the Fetus and the Neonatal Autopsy

Colin L. Berry

Increasing attention is now paid to the examination of the products of conception, fetuses and neonatal deaths in pathology departments as more extensive use is made of the developing processes of genetic investigation and of non-invasive imaging and as demands for genetic counselling increase. The use in the neonatal period of surgical procedures that require accurate antenatal data, interventions of various kinds in metabolic disease and even the advent of intrauterine surgery have all contributed to this trend. The basic methodology of examination of the fetus remains the same for the non-specialist department, but newer data are available to support the importance of this aspect of pathology. The view of Benson et al. (1979) that specialized techniques (such as cell culture and the establishment of cell lines) are best carried out in specialized centres remains valid; recent events in the UK have emphasized the importance of adequate experience and quality control in specialized areas of pathology.

All histopathology laboratories dealing with material from obstetric and gynaecological services in general will receive a significant number of abnormal fetuses and infants each year. Spontaneous abortions, defined as the involuntary expulsion of a child with a birth weight of less than 500 g before the end of the 20th–22nd week of gestation (WHO 1977), have particular characteristics; of the 3472 abortuses studied by Byrne et al. (1985) only 21% contained normal fetuses and 28% contained no fetal tissues. Of these "membrane only" cases there were many with chromosomal anomalies and in complete specimens around 16% of the fetuses over 10 mm long were malformed. Of these types of abortion, 75% occur between weeks 8 and 13 of gestation, and it is thought that this incidence may rise as women postpone their first pregnancy: by 1988, 24% of primiparous women in the Netherlands were over 30 years of age, and the average age at which women have their first child has moved up from 24.3 in 1970 to 27.4 in 1990 (Varmunt 1992).

It is worth emphasizing that simple inspection may be informative in looking at these early specimens (Fig. 1.1). Simple morbid anatomy and histopathology will provide useful data on embryonic and fetal materials, and require only a dissecting microscope and radiographic facilities. Specimens are often received incomplete, fragmented, with or without the placenta, and usually fixed. The techniques recommended take note of these constraints.

Detailed accounts of abnormalities are not given here (they can be found in the relevant chapters), but generalized anomalies are known to occur with certain groups of chromosomal abnormalities, a fact only appreciated following the increased attention paid to these specimens. Thus, in trisomic fetuses, cardiac and renal abnormalities and hypoplasia of lungs, adrenals, ovaries and thymus have been reported in more than 50% of cases (Doshi et al. 1983). Certain trisomies abort within a circumscribed gestational period (trisomy 16 at the end of the first trimester, for example), but there is no temporal constraint for most that permit organogenesis. Trisomy 13, 18 and 21 make up around 20% of all trisomic spontaneous abortions (Warburton et al. 1987).

Further technical details can be found in Berry (1980).

History

As with all surgical specimens, a good history is important but not always provided. The date of the last menstrual period is an essential piece of information if findings are to be properly interpreted. Knowledge of previous reproductive performance is

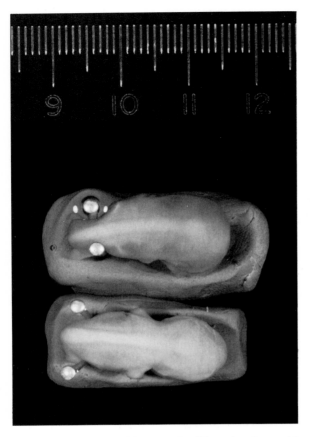

Fig 1.1. Webbed "neck" in an early (34 mm) embryo with Turner's syndrome (45 XO). A control embryo is also shown. (Courtesy of Dr M.J. Seller)

valuable, and the mode of induction of abortion should be stated, if it is not spontaneous.

Table 1.1. Change in crown–rump (CR) length with age

Day	CR (mm)	Day	CR (mm)
21	2–3	127	134.5
28	4–5	134	146.0
35	8	141	156.5
42	15	148	167.0
49	22	155	177.5
56	29.5	162	188.0
63	40.0	169	198.5
70	50.5	176	209.0
77	61.0	183	219.5
84	71.5	190	230.0
91	81.5	197	240.5
98	92.0	204	251.0
105	103.0		
113	113.5		
120	124.0		

crown–heel measurements, but for a pathological laboratory the measurement of foot length is simpler and provides comparable data. Foot length is not affected significantly by fixation or maceration, and an intact foot is often found where the fetus is received in fragments. Data relating foot length to CR length and gestational age, based on the work of Streeter (1920) and Trolle (1948), are shown in Table 1.2; figures for later pregnancy from Usher and McLean (1969) are incorporated. Foot length has the additional advantage that it is seldom directly affected by malformation; for example, anencephalic fetuses have normal foot lengths (Nañagus 1925) although they are otherwise difficult to measure.

The careful studies of Moscoso (see, for example, Moscoso et al. 1987) have established a number of important morphological markers of early human development. From his data (Fig. 1.2), Table 1.3 on tracheal length has been constructed; it is a further useful datum in establishing the gestational age of disrupted specimens.

Dimensions

Many measurements can be made on fetal and embryonic specimens, but there are considerable difficulties with a number of them. Crown–heel lengths measured by different observers under normal laboratory conditions vary considerably, as do crown–rump (CR) measurements. Table 1.1 provides average values for the latter variable, based on a number of series. There is wide variation, however, which depends largely on the reproducibility of the position of the fetus and its degree of maceration. Careful studies such as those of Bagnall et al. (1975) and Birkbeck et al. (1975a) show the value of CR and

Weights

The weights of the placenta and fetus should be determined. Determination of fetal age by weight alone is always imprecise (see Birkbeck et al. 1975b), but marked disproportion between placental and fetal weight may be informative.

There is no doubt that accurate measurement of placental weight is very difficult; different authors have trimmed different parts of the membranes, cut off the cord, drained blood from the organ before weighing etc. The most accurate measurement of the weight of placental tissue is obtained after homoge-

Table 1.2. Foot length of the fetus

End of week	Mean sitting height (mm)	Mean foot length (mm)	Minimum foot length (mm)	Maximum foot length (mm)
$8\frac{1}{2}$	27	4.2	3.8	4.6
9	31	4.6	4.2	5.0
10	40	5.5	5.0	6.0
11	50	6.9	6.0	7.8
12	61	9.1	7.5	10.8
13	74	11.4	9.8	13.0
14	87	14.0	12.5	15.5
15	101	16.8	15.2	18.5
16	116	19.9	18.2	21.6
17	130	23.0	21.0	25.0
18	142	26.8	24.8	28.8
19	153	30.7	28.5	33.0
20	164	33.3	31.0	35.7
21	175	35.2	32.5	38.0
22	186	39.5	36.0	43.0
23	197	42.2	39.0	45.5
24	208	45.2	42.0	48.5
25	218	47.7	44.5	51.0
26	228	50.2	47.0	53.5
27	238	52.7	49.0	56.5
28	247	55.2	51.5	59.0
29	256	57.0	61.0	61.0
30	265	59.2	55.5	63.0
31	274	61.2	57.5	65.0
32	283	63.0	59.0	67.0
33	293	65.0	61.0	69.0
34	302	68.2	64.0	72.5
35	311	70.5	66.0	75.0
36	321	73.5	69.0	78.0
37	331	76.5	72.0	81.0
38	341	78.5	74.0	83.0
39	352	81.0	76.0	86.0
40	362	82.5	77.5	87.5

Table 1.3. Mean, minimal and maximal tracheal measurements related to gestational age

GA (weeks)	Mean (mm)	Min. (mm)	Max. (mm)	SD
5–5.9	1.87	1.6	2.2	0.21
6.5	2.42	2.1	2.7	0.23
7	3.26	3	3.6	0.26
8	3.54	3.4	3.8	0.16
9	3.87	3.7	4	0.12
10	4.91	4	5.5	0.54
11	6.17	5.4	6.9	0.53
12	7.48	6.8	8.2	0.49
13	9.07	8.3	9.8	0.51
14	10.9	10	11.6	0.5
15	12.2	11.4	13.5	0.68
16	13.4	12	13.9	0.37
17	15	14	16	0.7
18	17.1	16	17.9	0.61

GA, gestational age; SD, standard deviation.

nization of the organ and estimation of the haemoglobin in the homogenate; if the value of haemoglobin in cord blood is assumed to be the same as that in the placenta a correction for weight of the contained blood can be made.

This is clearly impracticable as a routine technique. In general, the determination of placental weight in early pregnancy is unhelpful. Fetal weight is exceeded by placental weight until week 14–15 (100 mm CR length, 17 mm foot length), when the placental growth rate falls and that of the fetus increases rapidly. The data of Boyd and Hamilton (1970) are often cited for relative weight, and tables have been constructed from arithmetic regression

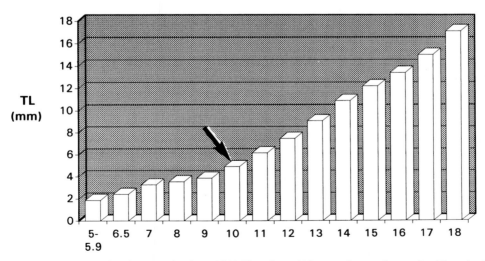

Fig 1.2. Tracheal length (TL) plotted against gestational age (GA). Note the rapid increase in growth rate after 10 weeks. (Courtesy of Dr G. Moscoso)

based on their data. The scatter in the original observations is enormous and, in the author's view, permits only limited statements. At 200 g fetal weight the placenta usually weighs 120 ± 20 g, and at a fetal weight of 1000 g the placenta weighs 250 ± 50 g. For figures for later pregnancy (32 weeks onward) the data of Thomson et al. (1969) for gross placental weight, in which the placenta has not been manipulated or trimmed in any way, are preferred. Fetal and placental weights in early pregnancy are shown in Table 1.4.

Table 1.4. Fetal and placental weight

Weeks	CR length (mm)	Fetal weight (g)	Placental weight (g)
4–8	5–30	0.5–2.9	5.0–27.0
8–12	31–60	2.7–25.0	10.0–80.0
12–16	61–100	11.0–135.0	28.0–134.0
16–20	101–155	57.0–350.0	55.0–198.0

Data from Boyd and Hamilton (1970).

Dating

External examination, careful measurement, infinite technical resources (serial sectioning) and precise historical details will allow most embryos and fetuses to be dated with accuracy. This is neither possible nor necessary in routine practice, and the markers given here are those that any laboratory can determine readily. Dating should be carried out on the basis of several sources of data (history, external form, size, weight, morbid anatomy and histological development).

Chronology of Early Pregnancy

If day 1 is considered to be the day on which a fertilized egg is present in the Fallopian tube, on day 2 there will be a 2- or 4-celled mass present. On day 2, 8- to 12-celled mass is found, on day 4 the blastocele begins to develop, and on day 5 a free blastocyst is found in the uterus. The blastocyst begins to implant on day 6 and implantation is not complete until day 13–14.

Morphological developmental indicators found by certain times are shown in Tables 1.5 and 1.6. These are readily identifiable in selected blocks and demonstration of them does not require serial sectioning. Between 12 and 20 weeks axial skeletal development provides a useful guide (see Fig. 1.3). Embryos can seldom be examined in sufficient detail in routine laboratories, although our knowledge of the morphology of early human malformations is scanty and such studies would be valuable. Serial sectioning is clearly impracticable, and if abnormal embryos are found they are often best examined in a laboratory with a special interest. What follows is a description of how best to deal with fetuses with CR lengths between approximately 30 and 200 mm.

Table 1.5. Morphological markers of development

Time (days)	Central nervous system	Cardiovascular system	Urogenital system	Gastrointestinal system	Respiratory system	Other markers
28	Anterior neuropore closed Cerebral vesicles present Lens placode reaches optic cup	Septum primum present	Metanephros forming	Oesophagus separated from trachea Liver bud present Dorsal pancreatic component present	Lung primordium established Trachea and primitive bronchi present	Thyroid in midline
35	Lens pocket closes	Ventricular septum and semilunar valves forming	Ureteric buds develop Germ cells in genital ridges			Spleen in dorsal mesogastrium
42	Semicircular canals Neurohypophysis develops	Truncus divides, septum secundum appears	Major calyces appear	Hepatic haematopoiesis begins Hernia of umbilical loop	Capillaries in lung parenchyma	Thymus and parathyroids arise from branchial pouches Paddle-shaped hand
50	Lens vesicle a "full" sphere Eyelids developing	Ventricular septum complete	Paramesonephric duct Seminiferous tubules as solid strands	Palatal shelves and salivary glands develop		Thymus invaded by lymphocytes Separate digits

Table 1.6. Later morphological markers

Age (weeks)	Finding
10	Fingerprints present
11	Gut loops return to abdomen
20	Bronchi cease budding
22–25	Three layers of primitive glomeruli present
	Alveoli appear
25–28	Two layers of primitive glomeruli present
	Eyelids open
28–30	One layer of primitive glomeruli present
31	Occasional primitive glomeruli seen
36	No further glomerulogenesis
	Ears flat
	Breast ≃ 3 mm diameter
40	Ears show cartilage ridges
	Breast ≃ 7 mm diameter
	Testes in scrotum
	Full foot creases present
	Ossification centres in lower femoral epiphysis, calcaneus, talus

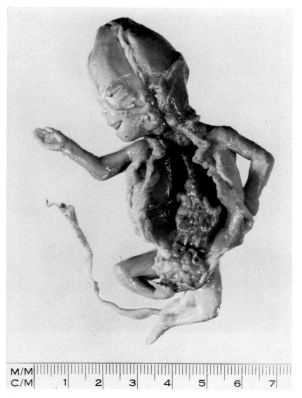

Fig. 1.4. Fetus affected by Meckel's syndrome. Encephalocele is present and horseshoe kidneys, shown to be dysplastic, are also seen. The liver showed cystic bile ducts in histological sections.

External Examination

Abnormal facies may yield useful information, which can either be specific, as in Potter's syndrome (p. 451), or indicative of the presence of possible visceral abnormality (Fig. 1.4). Fetuses are sometimes sent to the laboratory in very small jars, which

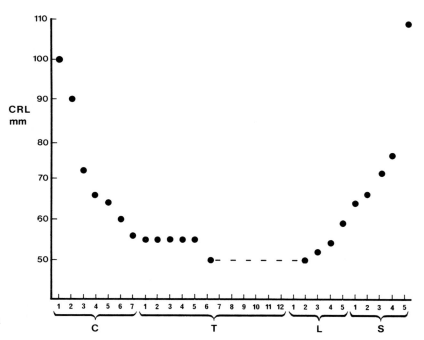

Fig 1.3. Scheme of appearance of vertebral body ossification centres. These are first evident in the lower thoracic region, and spread up and down the spinal column as shown.

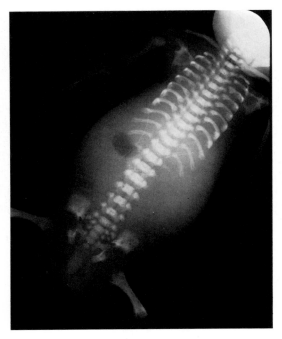

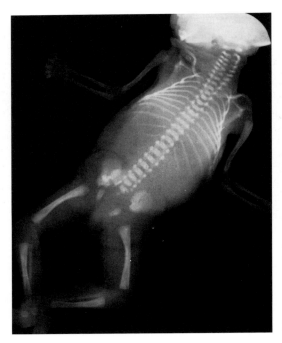

Fig. 1.5. Abnormal rib development in asphyxiating thoracic dystrophy. (Courtesy of the late Dr A.B. Bain)

Fig. 1.6. Bell-shaped thorax in pulmonary hypoplasia – a change seen in several conditions, including Potter's syndrome.

produce interesting facial changes; this artefact should be excluded. Early in the external examination it is helpful to pass a probe into the nose to check the patency of the posterior nares, and to examine the palate.

It is then customary to radiograph the fetus, using a Faxitron cabinet. This simple device permits rapid radiographic pictures to be provided promptly within the department (a Polaroid attachment is available), and will identify bony anomalies, which are usually better examined by further radiography after removal of the viscera (Figs. 1.5, 1.6).

Increasing use of facial photographs have proved valuable in dysmorphic cases (see also pp. 53–55). Resemblance between facial appearances in recurrent reproductive failure may be evident even where no recognizable syndrome can be identified.

Internal Examination

For all fetuses with CR length over 100 mm a mini-autopsy is probably the best procedure. However the use of a modified Rokitansky technique is desirable, the kidneys, ureters and bladder being left in situ while all other viscera are removed "en bloc" after examination of the reflections of the mesentery. This block can then be examined with the aid of the dissecting microscope when necessary.

For smaller fetuses a modification of the Wilson freehand sectioning method (Wilson 1965) used extensively on rodents in teratological studies should be employed. This involves cutting the trunk of the embryo into slices approximately 2–3 mm thick, which are examined from above and below by dissecting microscopy. This technique is simple and thorough (Figs. 1.7, 1.8).

Following removal of the viscera, the skeleton is again radiographed. This gives a good picture of the axial skeleton, which apart from specific abnormalities provides useful information on dating.

Where any tissue appears abnormal, or any organ seems to be too large or too small, a block should be taken.

Abnormalities of Specific Systems

When macroscopic anomalies are found the standard technique is often abandoned.

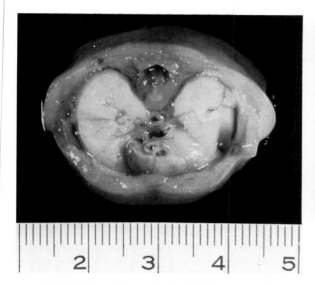

Fig. 1.7. Slice of fetus at the level of the great vessels.

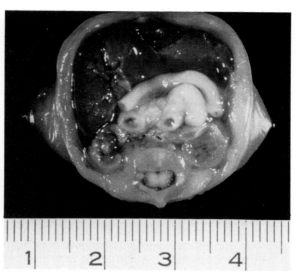

Fig. 1.8. Upper abdominal slice showing kidneys and liver, viewed from below.

Central Nervous System

In general, anomalous portions of the central nervous system should not be dissected as wet specimens. The cerebrospinal axis may be preserved as a unit, and cut in large sections or transversely in a number of blocks (Fig. 1.9). Reports (Granchrow and Ornoy 1979) have emphasized the value of histopathological examination of this type of specimen, which has rarely been performed. Insights into or alternative suggestions for pathogenesis may follow accurate documentation of the changes found (Bell 1979). It must be remembered that examination of neurospinal malformations at term will illustrate the effects of

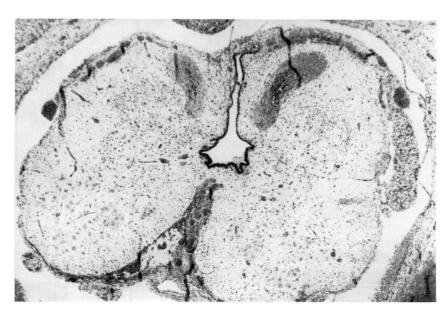

Fig. 1.9. Section of spinal cord above lumbosacral meningomyelocele. The abnormal central canal and partial division of the cord extend dorsally for several vertebral bodies above the defect. From a fetus terminated at 20 weeks for dysraphism. (Methacrylate section; trichrome stain, × 40)

injury or abnormality followed by up to 8 months of attempted repair and further growth. This type of examination, where only the "late" stage of lesion is studied, would yield little information about the pathogenesis of a contracted kidney, for example.

Cardiovascular System

Even without an extensive knowledge of the vastly complex field of congenital heart disease a useful assessment of anomalies can be made if the system of Tynan et al. (1979) is used (see Chapter 3, where the method is described in detail). If the heart is classified in this way a description may be of considerable value to those expert in the field or for later checking, in a place where photography is difficult and where the heart may not always be kept.

Musculoskeletal System

Musculoskeletal abnormalities are well illustrated by radiography, but valuable data can be obtained by section. For example, extra digits can be defined by checking muscle insertions to see whether a "thumb" is really a finger. Abnormalities of the digits have not often been described so carefully, but the information obtained from this type of examination would permit more critical analysis of limb defects. Animal studies suggest that this would be valuable in humans. (See, for example, the work of Theisen et al. 1979 with thalidomide.)

Urogenital System

After removal of other viscera, the kidneys and ureters should be freed from the posterior abdominal wall. The pubes are then split and the pelvic viscera removed. Dissection, or fine probing, will then reveal where aberrant ureters drain, or whether fistulae exist. Fine polythene catheters, heat-sealed at their ends, make good probes.

Metabolic Abnormalities

Prenatal diagnoses are usually made in selected groups. These include women over 35 years of age being screened for chromosomal abnormalities and women who have previously given birth to an infant affected by a malformation, e.g. neurospinal dysraphism. Metabolic disorders are usually sought only after an affected child has been diagnosed,

which emphasizes the value of examining abortion material. It is clearly absurd to suggest, however, that all abortuses are examined for possible metabolic disease, so the role of the pathologist is to look out for abnormalities that might be associated with metabolic disease. Foam cells in the placenta or central nervous system suggest lipidosis, while some of the skeletal anomalies of the mucopolysaccharidoses are recognizable in fetal material, as are some features of the glycogenoses.

Alerting a clinical colleague to the possibility of the presence of such a disorder is a major importance in preventive terms.

Blighted Ova

Examination of spontaneous abortuses reveals an intact or ruptured gestation sac without an embryo or fetus or with a stunted embryo or fusiform fetal mass in approximately 50% of cases. These "blighted ova" indicate massive failure of early development. Microscopic examination of the placenta may show predominantly hydatidiform change or stromal fibrosis and vascular obliteration, two ends of a spectrum suggesting failure of establishment of an adequate maternal or villous circulation, respectively with intermediate mixed findings being common (Rushton 1978). Chromosomal abnormalities are common in this group (see Byrne et al. 1985), but history of recurrent abortion is not found at an enhanced frequency within it. Other placental features that accompany intrauterine death include collapse of the vasculature of the villi, obliterative endarteritis of the arteries of the stem villi, sclerosis of the villous stroma, increased perivillous and intervillous fibrin deposition, increased syncytial knotting and calcification.

Normal Organ Weights in the Fetus

For those who wish to assess growth critically in smaller fetuses the papers of Tanimura et al. (1971) and McBride et al. (1984) will be of great value, each containing much data. In general the liver, kidney, heart, brain and thyroid are a constant proportion of body weight up to a gross weight of 500 g, whereas the thymus, adrenal and spleen increase in weight progressively in this period. The lungs increase and then decrease as a proportion of the body weight.

Table 1.7. Correlation coefficients of organ weights and linear measurements with total femur length

Measurement	Body weight	Femur length
Body weight	1.0000	0.9547
Brain weight	0.9740	0.9526
Liver weight	0.9632	0.9214
Lung weight	0.9468	0.9069
Kidney weight	0.9562	0.9069
Heart weight	0.9504	0.9205
Thymus weight	0.6930	0.6711
Adrenal weight	0.3917	0.4020
Spleen weight	0.6550	0.6276
Foot length	0.8993	0.8828

Table 1.7 is from data in McBride et al. (1984) and relates certain weights to femoral length. This is a reproducible and useful measurement if simple radiographic facilities are available.

Some Normal Histological Appearances During Development

Changes in histological appearance in various tissues or organs with time are illustrated in this section. This is not an attempt to provide an atlas of normal development, but rather a guide that any pathologist can use, taking only a few sections. The appearances are those found by a certain time in pregnancy, although in some instances the changes illustrated may be apparent earlier.

I   *External Form of the Brain*
(see also Table 4.1, p. 134)

The progressive expansion of the cerebral hemispheres and their subsequent convolution occurs over a long period. The hemisphere expands caudally and, ventrolaterally to form the temporal lobe (beginning at *10–11 weeks*). By *20 weeks*, frontal and parietal lobes, separated by the central sulcus, are seen and the occipital lobe is demarcated medially. Further sulci appear (*24 weeks*) and at *36 weeks* the process of cerebral convolution is well advanced.

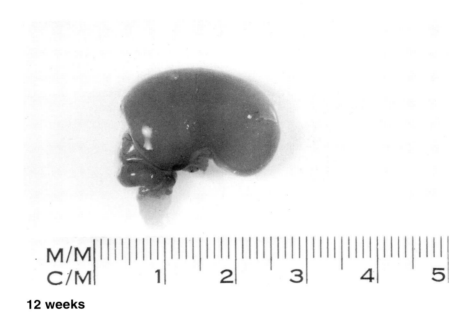

12 weeks

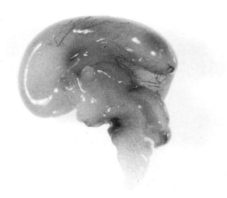

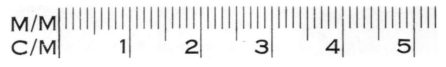

12 weeks

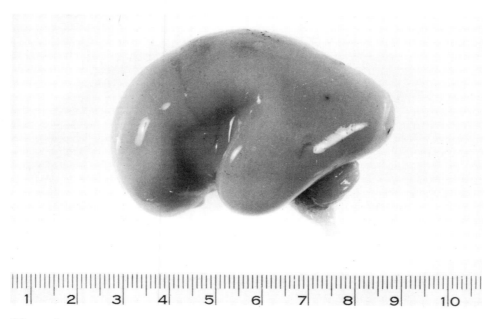

20 weeks

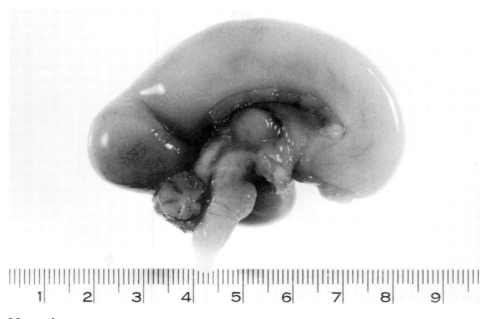

20 weeks

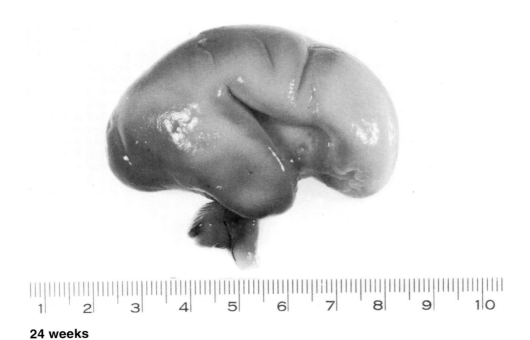

24 weeks

24 weeks

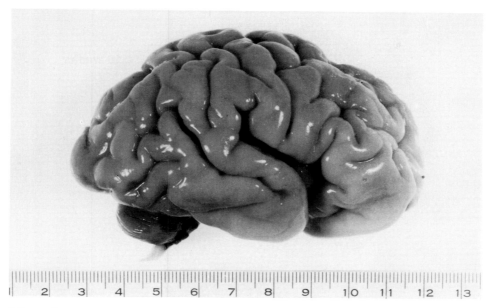

36 weeks

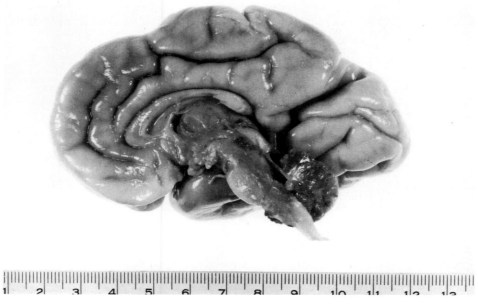

36 weeks

II *Lung*

(see also p. 314)

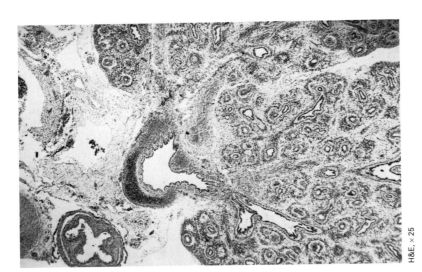

10 weeks

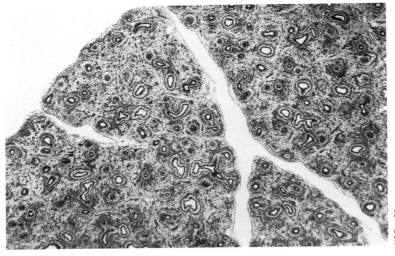

10 weeks

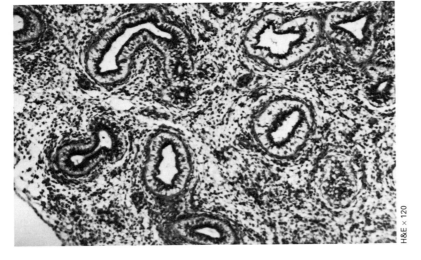

10 weeks

At *10 weeks* development is entirely bronchial, with large amounts of interbronchial mesenchyme. Cartilages have begun to form from pre-cartilage. The bronchi are lined by non-ciliated columnar epithelium, which may be pseudostratified.

10 weeks

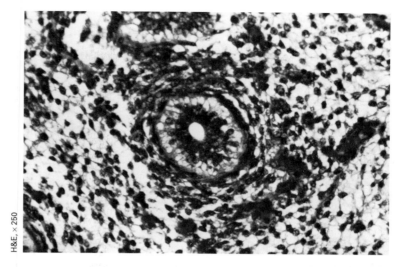

H&E, × 250

14 weeks

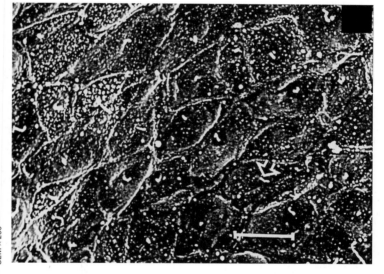

SEM × 260

Terminal air ducts and air sacs.

14 weeks

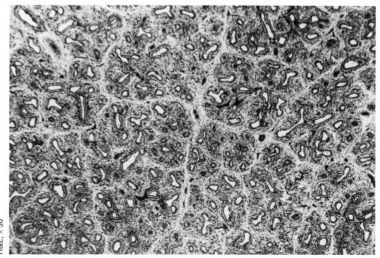

By *14 weeks* the interbronchial mesenchyme is diminishing in extent.

H&E × 30

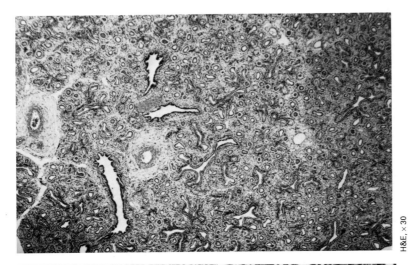

H&E, × 30

16 weeks

By *16 weeks* bronchial development is advanced; the epithelium has lost its pseudostratification and is ciliated.

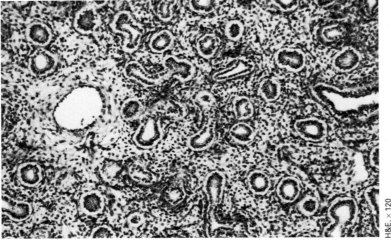

H&E, × 120

16 weeks

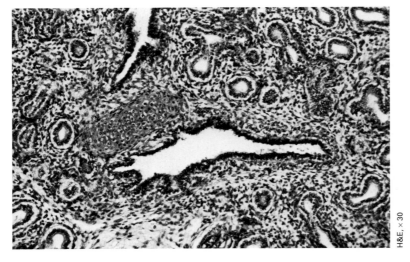

H&E, × 30

16 weeks

22 weeks

At *22–26 weeks* development of the terminal airways begins, with terminal bronchioles giving rise to non-alveolated bronchioles, which will form terminal respiratory bronchioles. Rudimentary alveolar development occurs, but the lining epithelium is prominent.

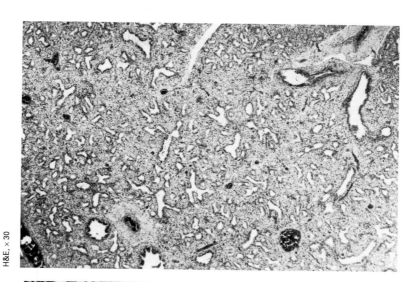

H&E, × 30

22 weeks

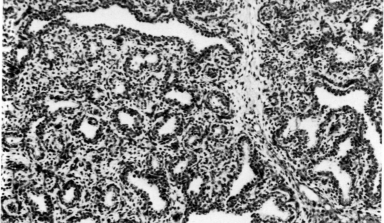

H&E, × 120

26 weeks

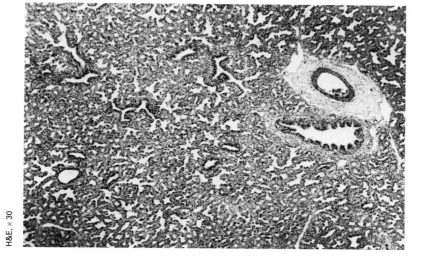

H&E, × 30

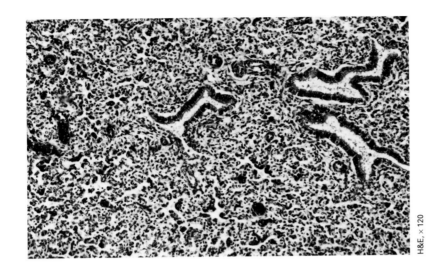

26 weeks

H&E, × 120

III *Kidney*

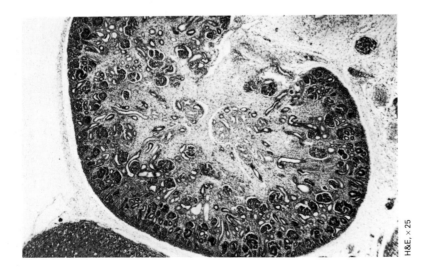

12 weeks

H&E, × 25

12 weeks

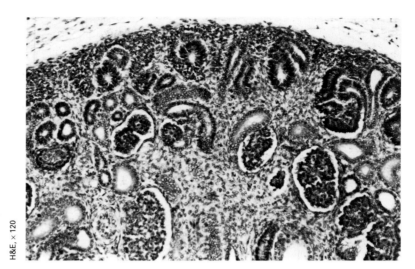

H&E, × 120

16 weeks

The kidney has some corticomedullary demarcation by *12 weeks*, with fetal glomeruli and S-form tubules present. By *16–20* weeks the development of the pyramids is advanced, and cortical, and papillary development encroach on the loose mesenchyme in the central part of the kidney.

H&E, × 25

20 weeks

H&E, × 25

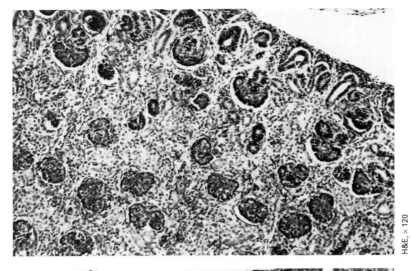

22 weeks

H&E, × 120

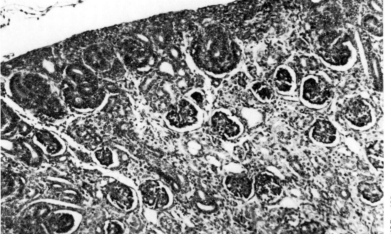

26 weeks

Between *22–36 weeks* the number of layers of primitive glomeruli diminishes from three to two (*26 weeks*) and subsequently to one (*34 weeks*) and finally to zero. Glomerulogenesis ceases at *36 weeks*. It must be emphasized that a wide expanse of cortex should be scanned to allow an impression of how many layers are present.

H&E, × 120

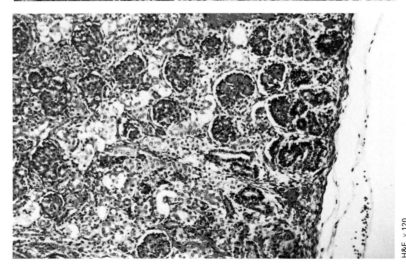

34 weeks

H&E, × 120

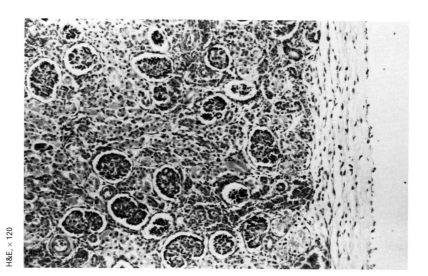

36 weeks

H&E, × 120

IV *Gonads (Testis)*

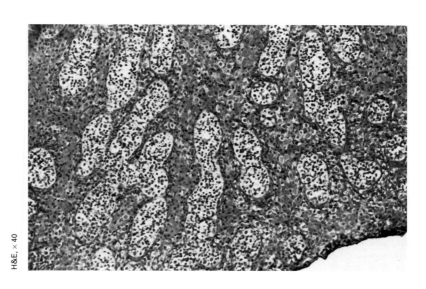

10 weeks

H&E, × 40

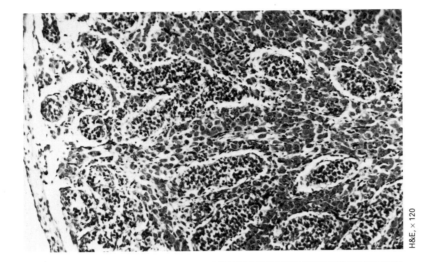

16 weeks

H&E, × 120

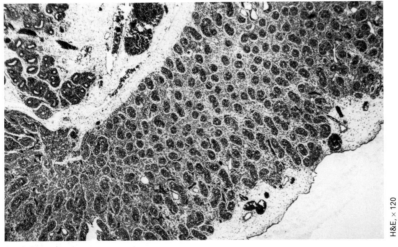

20 weeks

It is often not possible to distinguish
between the two gonads before *10
weeks* of age. The cords of germ cells
are then said to be continuous in
males and interrupted in females, but
this may be difficult to assess. By *16
weeks* this change is obvious and
Leydig cells are present in large
numbers in the developing testis,
where the tubules are canalized.
Stromal development in both gonads
occurs later.

H&E, × 120

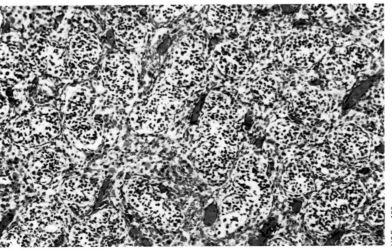

22 weeks

H&E, × 120

Gonads (Ovary)

10 weeks

18 weeks

20 weeks

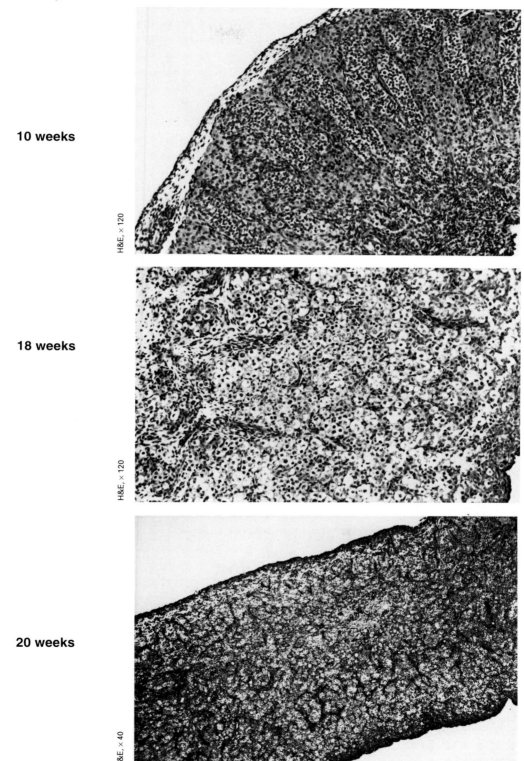

H&E, × 120

H&E, × 120

H&E, × 40

V   *Stomach*

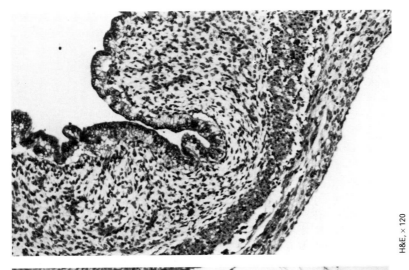

H&E, × 120

10 weeks

At *10 weeks* the stomach has well
defined muscle coats and a broad
loose submucosa. Mucosal folding
and early gland formation are seen by
14–16 weeks and a more organized
mucosal pattern by *20 weeks*.

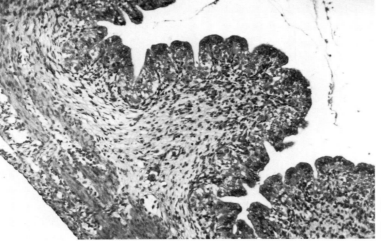

H&E, × 120

14 weeks

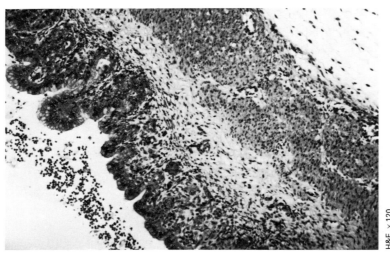

H&E, × 120

16 weeks

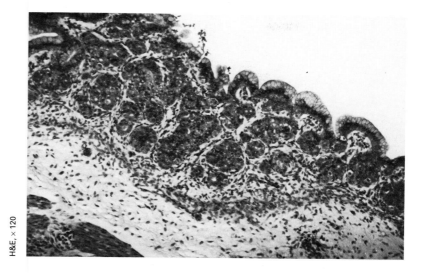

20 weeks

H&E, × 120

VI *Colon*

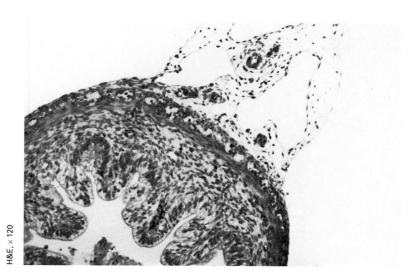

10 weeks

H&E, × 120

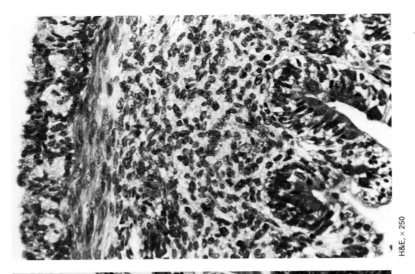

H&E, × 250

14 weeks

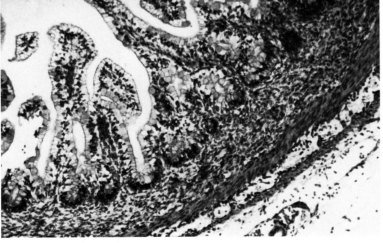

H&E, × 120

18 weeks

At *10 weeks* ganglia are readily seen in the myenteric plexus, being apparently more numerous on the mesenteric border. At *14 weeks* the submucosa is still cellular and broad, but by *18 weeks* this appearance is changing fast. Muscle coats thicken by *20–22 weeks*.

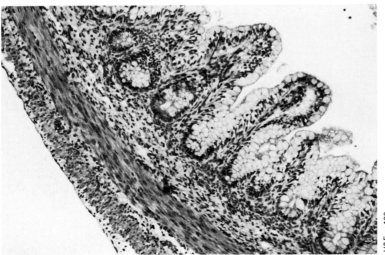

H&E, × 120

22 weeks

VII *Pancreas*

10 weeks

Initially composed of ducts (*10 weeks*), acinar structures begin to form relatively early (*12–14 weeks*). The gland has an abundant stroma at this stage. In the author's experience later development is very variable, an islet tissue, although visible from *16 weeks* on, may vary considerably in amount.

H&E, × 120

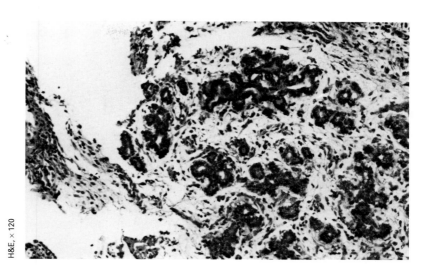

H&E, × 40

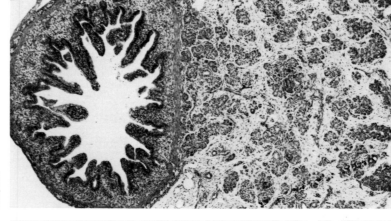

12 weeks

12 weeks

H&E, × 120

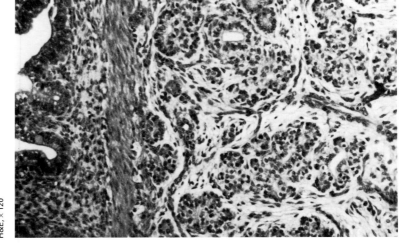

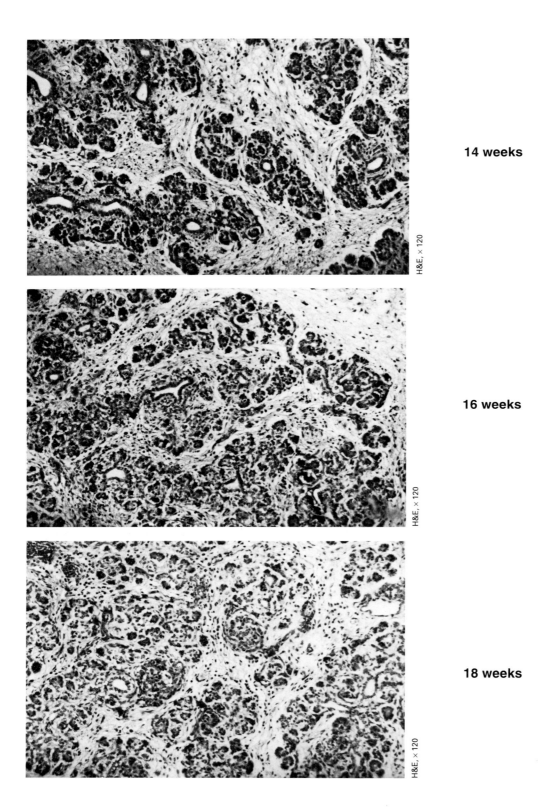

14 weeks

H&E, × 120

16 weeks

H&E, × 120

18 weeks

H&E, × 120

20 weeks

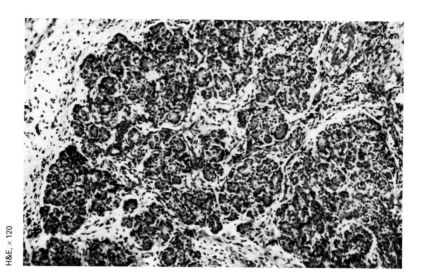

H&E, × 120

VIII *Liver*

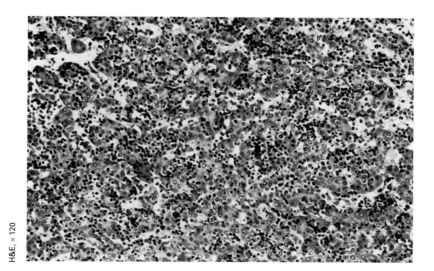

H&E, × 120

Haematopoiesis is established in the liver from *8 weeks*. By *10 weeks* the appearance (shown here) resembles that found at term.

IX *Trachea and Oesophagus*

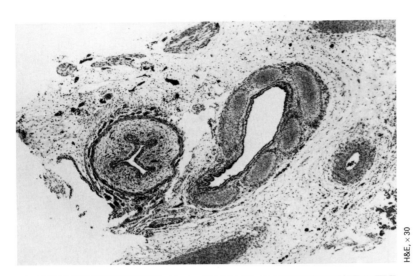

H&E, × 30

10 weeks

By *10 weeks* the trachea and oesophagus are distinct but the muscle coats of the latter are thin. Complete tracheal rings are found.

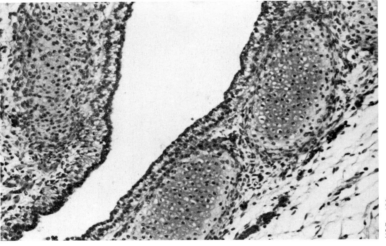

H&E, × 120

10 weeks

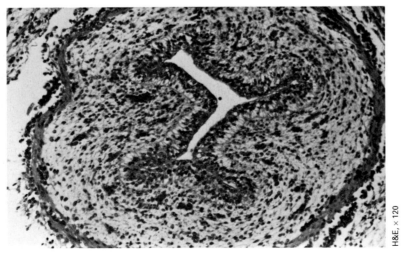

H&E, × 120

10 weeks

12 weeks

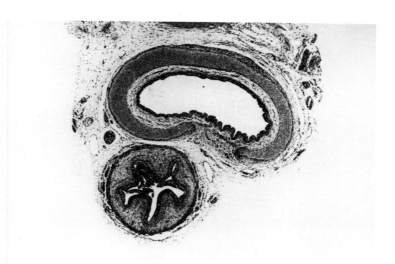

H&E, × 30

At *12 weeks*, both structures have well defined wall components and epithelia are maturing.

X   *Skin*

12 weeks

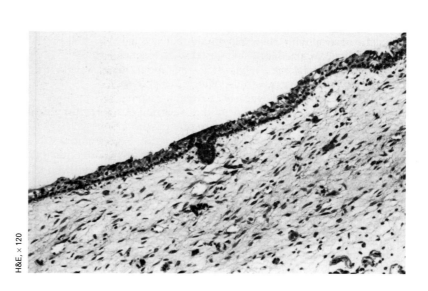

H&E, × 120

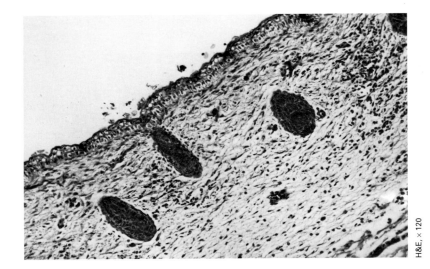

18 weeks

H&E, ×120

Hair follicles are seen in the skin by *12 weeks*, and are more abundant at *18 weeks*.

The Neonatal Autopsy

There are few pathologists who would dispute the assertion that autopsy data are an essential component of the body of knowledge that enables a clinician to assess the sequence of events leading to death. Such an assessment is usually made in an attempt to learn useful lessons in clinical management as well as to determine, for example, whether therapy was effective, staging of a tumour accurate or investigative methods correctly used. A neonatal death is a clinical catastrophy of such magnitude that it is not surprising that our paediatric and obstetric colleagues are anxious to discover what they can about it. Unhappily, their investigations, which depend on autopsy findings to a considerable extent, are sometimes hindered by inadequate procedures carried out by inexperienced junior staff, who are often asked to do these autopsies.

An experienced pathologist has the necessary skills to conduct a satisfactory neonatal autopsy and can almost always answer two important questions: what is the probable gestational age of the infant, and is development normal for this age? This section of the chapter will seek to emphasize the procedures that should be followed in preference to methods more conventionally used for adults. There is no doubt that adequate, simple autopsies on infants will provide badly needed epidemiological data. Although very detailed sections with the use of many additional techniques are important in specialist units, the large number of neonatal autopsies done in general departments should be a valuable source of information.

A major problem is that few pathologists will do more than 15 such autopsies a year. It may therefore be useful to have a checklist like that shown at the end of this chapter (see p. 40) to remind the operator of the data worth recording in these infrequent cases. The two parts of the list differ: the first draws attention to essential clinical data that should be noted; the second is intended to remind the operator of points that might be forgotten when the bulk of normal practice is with adults.

History and Clinical Involvement

Pathologists make only a ritual obeisance in the direction of the notes with some adult autopsies; indeed, in sudden death there may be no real data to be examined. This can never be justified in a neonatal autopsy. There is almost invariably a great deal of information available, beginning with the maternal set (age, height, parity, marital status, menstrual history for pregnancy dating, blood pressure readings – all factors known to affect pregnancy outcome). Details of the history of the baby can then be studied, but it is often necessary to ensure a clinical presence at this stage, in particular to determine that a proper account of the many invasive and sometimes destructive procedures carried out in this age group is available. These historical data are vital, and it is not uncommon to find much in them to assist in an explanation of the mode of death.

Placenta and Cord

In practice it is very difficult to ensure that the placenta and cord of all neonatal deaths reach the laboratory. If death occurs at or around birth these may be available; in later deaths they will usually have been discarded with the more numerous specimens from the normal cases. Schema in which all placentae are kept for 1 month can be devised, but it is remarkable how often material from the "relevant" case is missing.

A number of clearly defined but relatively uncommon conditions of clinical significance may be identified by placental examination, but it is the author's view that unless studies as detailed as those described by Boyd and Scott (1985) and Boyd et al. (1986) are made little useful information is obtained. Placental weights are unreliable as an index of functional capacity (Fox 1978).

External Inspection of the Infant

Photography

Increasingly in clinical paediatrics and in the counselling of parents whose baby is stillborn, photographs of the infant are taken. Copies of these photographs should be obtained for the pathology notes whenever possible. If the appearance of the infant is strange and there is no photographic record, frontal and lateral views of the face and an overall view including the hands should be taken. The value of these photographs is not so much in removing the subjective element from the assessment of "low-set" ears or the degree of prominence of epicanthic folds, although this is useful, but in having a record of abnormalities which are not categorizable at present but which may become so, and in comparing appearances in siblings in those sad cases in which recurrent reproductive failure occurs.

If an attempt is to be made to "syndrome-spot" on the basis of external appearances (and later findings) useful texts are those of Salmon and Lindenbaum (1978), Bergsma (1979) and, perhaps the best, Smith (1982). The massive tome *"Birth defects encyclopedia"* (Buyse 1990) is literally encyclopaedic and

contains valuable photographs and references but is difficult to find your way around.

Measurements

To be useful, measurements must be reliably and reproducibly made in normal mortuary conditions. Weight is such a measurement, as is foot length, but CR and crown–heel lengths are not (see Bagnall et al. 1975). Data from the notes on biparietal diameters (see Table 1.8) and femur length measured by ultrasound are useful and these data together with histological assessments (see pp. 11–31) will usually enable a distinction to be made between the prematurely born and light-for-dates infant. Other measurements are best made from radiographs in cases of special interest.

Table 1.8. Ultrasonic measurements and gestational age

Biparietal diameter (cm)	Length of femur (cm)	Gestation (weeks)
2.0	0.8	12
2.4	1.2	13
2.5	1.4	14
3.0	1.8	15
3.3	2.1	16
3.6	2.4	17
4.0	2.8	18
4.2	3.0	19
4.5	3.3	20

Approximations from the data of Sanders and James (1985).

Campbell (1976) has published data on biparietal diameters, and there are numerous data on individual organ weights in singleton births in the text by Larroche (1977).

Radiography

In an ideal world each neonatal death would be radiographed, for it cannot be doubted that much useful information can be obtained in this way. Radiographics are vital if there is any suggestion of unnatural death. Conditions in which diagnosis is facilitated by radiography, or in which radiographic examination is essential, include:

1. Short-limbed dwarfism
2. Osteogenesis imperfecta
3. Birth trauma
4. Meconium peritonitis
5. Interstitial emphysema (mediastinal, retroperitoneal)
6. Foreign bodies (catheters, needles, etc.)

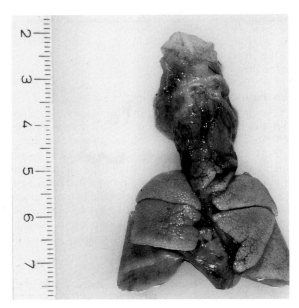

Fig. 1.10. Bilateral right trilobed lungs in a fetus with an unbalanced translocation, at 18 weeks gestation.

It should be noted that radiographic assessment of maturity by the appearance of ossification centres is unreliable, because ossification is affected by many variables, including growth rate, and varies in different races. However, some authors find these centres useful (Russel 1981).

Dissection

Good descriptions of thorough autopsy techniques are given by Barson (1981), Wigglesworth (1984) and Keeling (1993). Some descriptions of neonatal autopsies include manoeuvres such as manometric determination of intrathoracic pressures, which are, in the author's view, neither necessary nor capable of providing data of real biophysical validity. This section will concentrate on manipulations that are unusual in an adult autopsy but will avoid suggesting rituals that are not usually productive.

Incision

An inverted Y is the best incision as it allows preservation of the umbilical vessels and a better exposure of the lower genital tract. This provides the opportunity to split the pubic symphysis and remove the bladder, rectum and genitalia as a block when atresias, fistulae, valves or other anomalies are suspected.

Inspection

Time should be taken to inspect the visceral situs after the anterior chest wall has been removed. The lungs should be checked for their lobar pattern, the hepatic and splenic situs determined and rotation of the mesentery noted.

Gastrointestinal System and Abdominal Cavity

The next step should be to confirm the patency of the rectum and urethra before cutting through the former and removing the gut as far as the duodenum. This allows the liver to be pushed down in order to examine the hepatic veins and to look for aberrant trunks or caval anomalies. The biliary tract should be inspected before removing the liver. The stomach, pancreas and duodenum are now clearly visible, as are the great vessels in the abdomen, the kidneys and adrenals, and the ureters.

Genitourinary System

The kidneys, ureters and bladder can be removed as a block. Splitting the symphysis is rarely necessary.

Thorax

The thymus should be removed, taking care not to damage the brachiocephalic vein. The great arteries should be inspected when the pericardium is opened. After mobilization of the tongue and structures of the neck and deliberate inspection of the palate and choanae (clefts and atresia are easily missed) and following inspection of the inferior vena cava and hepatic veins, the contents of the thorax are removed for further dissection (see Chapter 3), checking the position of the aortic arch as this is done. The cardiac examination should be completed before what follows. In the author's view the liver may usefully be left attached to the heart.

Respiratory Tract

The oesophagus is dissected off the trachea after probing. The larynx is then opened posteriorly and the trachea for a short distance. Then comes a major departure from adult practice: a syringe filled with formol saline is tied in and the lungs inflated before being placed in a container of this fixative. This simple manoeuvre will prevent much agonizing about the significance of certain histological changes (collapse, consolidation) when the lungs are examined later. The weight of the lungs is sometimes used in evaluating pulmonary hypoplasia but, in the view of the author, it is seldom helpful. The diagnosis probably requires morphometric confirmation, and it is necessary to distinguish the type of hypoplasia which occurs with reduction in the number of bronchial divisions (as in diaphragmatic hernia) from that with loss of peripheral lung development (as in oligohydramnios). True hypoplasia of the entire lung is rare.

Central Nervous System

If a pathologist wishes to be confident of the presence of blood in the cerebrospinal fluid as an ante-mortem finding, the only certain procedure to follow is to needle the cisterna magna, preferably via an incision which has exposed the atlanto-occipital space. The skull can then be opened by cutting around the edges of the partly ossified frontal and parietal bones. This is best done on one side at a time, folding the bone flaps outwards so that the cerebral hemisphere on that side can be inspected and the brain moved gently to permit the inspection of the falx cerebri and the venous sinuses. The hemisphere can then be removed by cutting through the cerebral peduncle on that side. The procedure is then repeated and the tentorium cerebelli examined before the cerebellum is removed. Fixation of the neonatal brain does not make it much firmer, and it is usually better to cut it immediately to resolve clinical difficulties – usually about intraventricular haemorrhage.

If there is a history of difficult delivery (e.g. with the after-coming head of a breech), it is necessary to examine the upper part of the spinal cord for evidence of haemorrhage or bony dislocation.

Weighing of Organs

There is no doubt that the weighing of organs and the expression of their size relative to body weight is a useful exercise in assessing intrauterine growth and maturity. However, the balance used must be calibrated and of appropriate scale; a suitable digital balance capable of measurement to 1 g accuracy should be used; rather than buying special scales, laboratory balances may be used. Some normal values for defined populations are given in Tables 1.9, and other relevant data on growth and development in Fig. 1.11 and Table 1.10.

Recently, a most valuable study has been reported by Barr et al. (1994). They have reviewed a large collection of fetuses to establish values in somatic and visceral morphometry, using curve-fitting techniques to minimize scatter. The limited data presented are very valuable.

Post-mortem Microbiology

Although many pathologists can cite occasions when post-mortem microbiology has been useful, these are rare and the taking of routine swabs or other specimens at autopsy represents a waste of resources. If evidence of infection is to be sought, it should be via techniques whereby microbiological components or products are detected at the site of pathological change. Immunofluorescence has been largely superseded by immunocytochemistry, but DNA hybridization and the polymerase chain reaction are of increasing value as commercial preparations become available. The advantages are that non-viable organisms and gene products can be detected in specimens in which there has been considerable overgrowth by post-mortem proliferation of symbionts or contaminants.

Histopathology

If a pathologist wishes to acquire a good idea of the range of appearances seen in neonatal post-mortem material, an extensive set of blocks taken from each case will provide a useful source of reference. If there is a special interest, blocks can be chosen appropriately; for example, many fistulae are best examined histologically. Cerebral changes in anoxia may be evaluated using a modification of the technique described by Gruenwald and Lawrence (1968). Points relating to specific systems are dealt with in the relevant chapters.

Macerated Infants

Contrary to the views of many pathologists, it is worth examining the macerated stillbirth. About 15% of such cases are due to malformation, and this datum alone justifies the procedure in terms of its value in genetic counselling.

Wrinkling of the skin with slipping and easily rubbed away epidermis occurs within about 12 h of intrauterine death. Within another 12 h blisters appear and rupture, leaving brownish-red areas, a colour which the whole baby and the cord adopt. Autolysis, with effusions in the serous cavities which are stained by haemolysis, overlapping of the skull bones and distortion of the limbs are present by 48 h.

Table 1.9. Weight of newborn infants and their organs by groups of body weights

Body weight (g)	Number of cases	Heart (g)	Lungs, combined (g)	Spleen (g)	Liver (g)	Adrenal glands, combined (g)	Kidneys, combined (g)	Thymus (g)	Brain (g)	Gestational age (weeks; days)
500	317	5.0 ±1.6	12 ±5	1.3 ±0.8	26 ±10	2.6 ±1.7	5.4 ±2.1	2.2 ±0.8	70 ±18	23, 5 ± 2, 3
750	311	6.3 ±1.8	19 ±6	2.0 ±1.2	39 ±12	3.2 ±1.5	7.8 ±2.6	2.8 ±1.3	107 ±27	26, 0 ± 2, 6
1000	295	7.7 ±2.0	4 ±8	2.6 ±1.5	47 ±12	3.5 ±1.6	10.4 ±3.4	3.7 ±2.0	143 ±34	27, 5 ± 3, 1
1250	217	9.6 ±3.3	30 ±9	3.4 ±1.8	56 ±21	4.0 ±1.7	12.9 ±3.9	4.9 ±2.1	174 ±38	29, 0 ± 3, 0
1500	167	11.5 ±3.3	34 ±11	4.3 ±2.0	65 ±18	4.5 ±1.8	14.9 ±4.2	6.1 ±2.7	219 ±52	31, 3 ± 2, 3
1750	148	12.8 ±3.2	40 ±13	5.0 ±2.5	74 ±20	5.3 ±2.0	17.4 ±4.7	6.8 ±3.0	247 ±51	32, 4 ± 2, 6
2000	140	14.9 ±4.2	44 ±13	6.0 ±2.7	82 ±23	5.3 ±2.0	18.8 ±5.0	7.9 ±3.4	281 ±56	34, 6 ± 3, 2
2250	124	16.0 ±4.3	48 ±15	7.0 ±3.3	88 ±24	6.0 ±2.3	20.2 ±4.9	8.2 ±3.4	308 ±49	36, 4 ± 3, 0
2500	120	17.7 ±4.2	48 ±14	8.5 ±3.5	105 ±21	7.1 ±2.8	22.6 ±5.5	8.3 ±4.4	339 ±50	38, 0 ± 3, 2
2750	138	19.1 ±3.8	51 ±51	9.1 ±3.6	117 ±26	7.5 ±2.7	24.0 ±5.4	9.6 ±3.8	362 ±48	39, 2 ± 2, 2
3000	144	20.7 ±5.3	53 ±13	10.1 ±3.3	127 ±30	8.3 ±2.9	24.7 ±5.3	10.2 ±4.3	380 ±55	40, 0 ± 2, 1
3250	133	21.5 ±4.3	59 ±18	11.0 ±4.0	145 ±33	9.2 ±3.4	27.3 ±6.6	11.6 ±4.4	395 ±53	40, 4 ± 1, 6
3500	106	22.8 ±5.9	63 ±17	11.3 ±3.6	153 ±33	9.8 ±3.5	28.0 ±6.5	12.8 ±5.1	411 ±55	40, 4 ± 1, 5
3750	57	23.8 ±5.1	65 ±15	12.5 ±4.1	159 ±40	10.2 ±3.3	29.5 ±6.8	13.0 ±4.8	413 ±55	40, 6 ± 2, 3
4000	31	25.8 ±5.3	67 ±20	14.1 ±4.0	180 ±39	10.8 ±3.4	30 ±6.2	11.4 ±3.2	420 ±62	41, 4 ± 1, 3
4250	15	26.5 ±5.3	68 ±16	13.0 ±2.5	197 ±42	12.0 ±3.7	30.7 ±5.8	11.7 ±3.7	415 ±38	41, 2 ± 2, 1

Data from Gruenwald and Minh (1960).

Table 1.10. Chronology of the human dentition[a]

Tooth	Hard tissue formation begins[b] (fertilization age in utero, weeks)		Amount of enamel formed at birth	Enamel completed (after birth)	Root completed (years)	Eruption	Exfoliation (years)
Primary Dentition							
Maxillary							
Central incisor	14	(13–16)	Five-sixths	$1\frac{1}{2}$ mo.	$1\frac{1}{2}$	$7\frac{1}{2}$ mo.	6–7
Lateral incisor	16	$(14\frac{2}{3}-16\frac{1}{2})$[c]	Two-thirds	$2\frac{1}{2}$ mo.	2	9 mo.	7–8
Canine	17	(15–18)[c]	One-third	9 mo.	$3\frac{1}{4}$	18 mo.	10–12
First molar	$15\frac{1}{2}$	$(14\frac{1}{2}-17)$	Cusps united; occlusal completely calcified plus a half to three-fourths crown height[b]	6 mo.	$2\frac{1}{2}$	14 mo.	9–11
Second molar	19	$(16-23\frac{1}{2})$	Cusps united; occlusal incompletely calcified; calcified tissue covers a fifth to a fourth crown height[b]	11 mo.	3	24 mo.	10–12
Mandibular							
Central incisor	14	(13–16)	Three-fifths	$2\frac{1}{2}$ mo.	$1\frac{1}{2}$	6 mo.	6–7
Lateral incisor	16	$(14\frac{2}{3}-)$[c]	Three-fifths	3 mo.	$1\frac{1}{2}$	7 mo.	7–8
Canine	17	(16–)[c]	One-third	9 mo.	$3\frac{1}{4}$	16 mo.	9–12
First molar	$15\frac{1}{2}$	$(14\frac{1}{2}-17)$	Cusps united; occlusal completely calcified[b]	$5\frac{1}{2}$ mo.	$2\frac{1}{4}$	12 mo.	9–11
Second molar	18	$(17-19\frac{1}{2})$	Cusps united; occlusal incompletely calcified[b]	10 mo.	3	20 mo.	10–12
Permanent Dentition							
Maxillary							
Central		3–4 mo.		4–5 yr.	10	7–8 yr.	
Lateral		10–12 mo.		4–5 yr.	11	8–9 yr.	
Cuspid		4–5 mo.		6–7 yr.	13–15	11–12 yr.	
First premolar		$1\frac{1}{2}-1\frac{3}{4}$ yr.		5–6 yr.	12–13	10–11 yr.	
Second premolar		$2-2\frac{1}{4}$ yr.		6–7 yr.	12–14	10–12 yr.	
First molar		At birth	Sometimes a trace	$2\frac{1}{2}-3$ yr.	9–10	6–7 yr.	
Second molar		$2\frac{1}{2}-3$ yr.		7–8 yr.	14–16	12–13 yr.	
Third molar		7–9 yr.		12–16 yr.	18–25	17–21 yr.	
Mandibular							
Central		3–4 mo.		4–5 yr.	9	6–7 yr.	
Lateral		3–4 mo.		4–5 yr.	10	7–8 yr.	
Cuspid		4–5 mo.		6–7 yr.	12–14	9–10 yr.	
First premolar		$1\frac{3}{4}-2$ yr.		5–6 yr.	12–13	10–12 yr.	
Second premolar		$2\frac{1}{4}-2\frac{1}{2}$ yr.		6–7 yr.	13–14	11–12 yr.	
First molar		At birth	Sometimes a trace	$2\frac{1}{2}-3$ yr.	9–10	6–7 yr.	
Second molar		$2\frac{1}{2}-3$ yr.		7–8 yr.	14–15	11–13 yr.	
Third molar		8–10 yr.		12–16 yr.	18–25	17–21 yr.	

[a]After Logan and Kronfeld (1933).

[b]Data from Kraus and Jordan (1965).

[c]Variation ranges of lateral incisors and canines from data by Nomata (1964). Fetal length-to-age conversions were made; no values are available for late onset in mandibular, lateral incisors and canines because all values from Nomata's data are earlier than the mean values from Kraus and Jordan (1965). Fetal length–age data from Patten (1946).

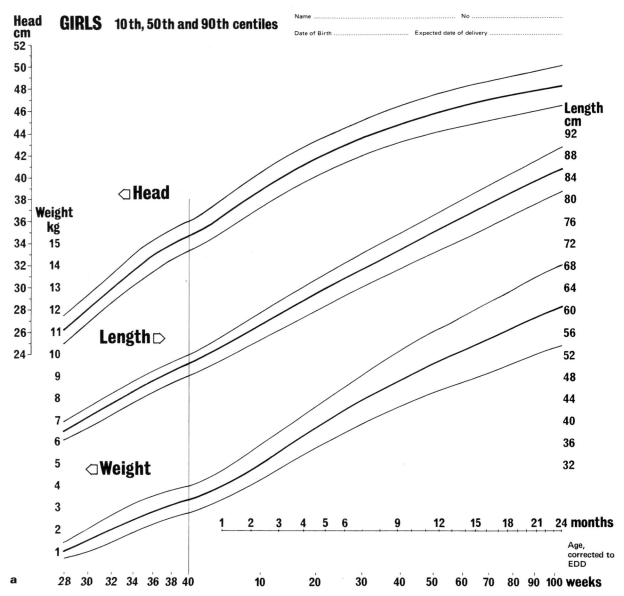

Fig. 1.11. Growth charts: **a** girls; **b** boys. (Prepared by Drs D. Gairdner and J. Pearson. First published in *Archives of Disease in Childhood*, 1971. Reproduced by permission of the publisher, Castlemead Publications)

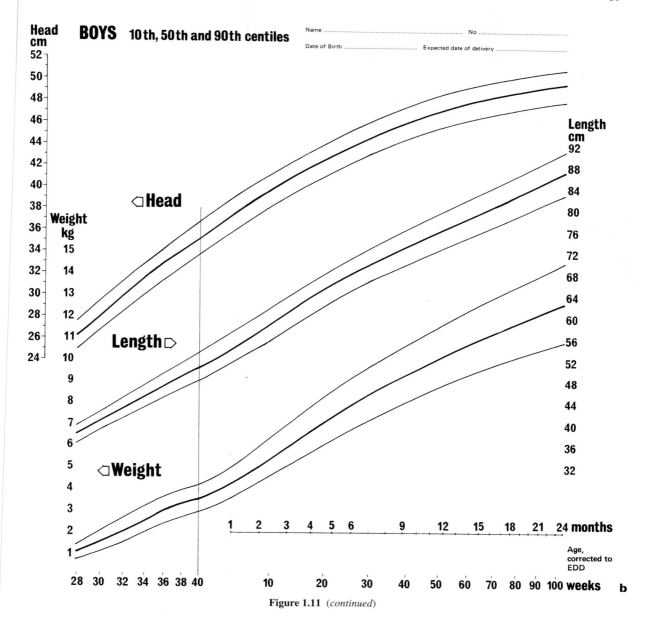

Figure 1.11 (*continued*)

Checklist for Paediatric Autopsy

1. Clinical Details

Name	PM No.	Delivery Date / /
		Date of Death / /
Sex M/F		

Mother's name	Hospital No.	Date of birth / /
Civil state		
Previous pregnancies	Date	Outcome
	1.	
	2.	
	3.	
	4.	
	5.	
	6.	

LMP / /
EDD / /

Height	Weight	Blood group
Highest diastolic blood pressure		Date / /
Albuminuria		Date / /
		/ /
		/ /
		/ /

Previous		
Hypertension	Yes/No	
Diabetes	Yes/No	
Epilepsy	Yes/No	
Other Disease	Yes/No	Specify

Labour and Delivery
Onset	Spontaneous/induced/not known/Caesar
Time/(24 h clock)	Date / /
Delivery (24 h clock)	Date / /
Duration	Hours
Fetal monitoring	Yes/No	Heart
		Electrode

Signs of distress (tick)	None
	Meconium-stained liquor
	Abnormal heart rate
	Reduced movements
	Other (specify)

Mode of delivery (tick)	Spontaneous
	Section
	Forceps
	Breech extraction
	Other (specify)

Birth weight (g)
Singleton/twin/triplet/other

Neonate
Therapy	Ventilation	Yes/No	IPP
			CPAP
			Other
	Resuscitation	Yes/No	
	Transfusion	Yes/No	Exchange
			Conventional
	Other	Yes/No	Specify

Clinical summary

2. Autopsy Checklist

Placenta	Weight
Cord	Length
	No. of vessels
Membranes	Check fetal and maternal surface.
Haemorrhage	?Maternal surface concavity

Baby
Face	Photograph	Yes/No
External anomalies	Ears Size
	Position
	No. of digits Hands
	Feet
	Palmar creases
	Patency of orifices Mouth
	Ears
	Nose
	Anus
	Urethra
	Vagina
	Back (palpate spine)
	Note incisions, drains, needle punctures
Internal	Free tongue and pharynx
	Check palate and choanae
	Examine larynx (intubation)
	Note visceral situs
	Check fixation of mesentary
	Check diaphragm
	Remove gut (duodenum to rectum)
	Probe oesophagus
	Check inferior vena cava and superior vena cava
	Note lobulation of lungs
	Remove thoracic contents (see p. 71)
	Remove genitourinary tract
	Examine skull and central nervous system

References

Bagnall KM, Jones PRM, Harris PF (1975) Estimating the age of human foetus from crown rump measurements. Ann Hum Biol 2: 387

Barr M, Blackburn WR, Cooley NR, (1994) Human fetal somatic and visceral morphometrics. Teratology 49: 487

Barson AJ (ed)(1981) The perinatal postmortem. In: Laboratory investigation of fetal disease. Wright, Bristol, p 476

Bell JE (1979) Fused suprarenal glands in association with central nervous system defects in the first half of fetal life. J Pathol 127: 191

Benson PF, Fensom AH, Polani PE (1979) Prenatal diagnosis of metabolic errors. Lancet i: 161

Bergsma D (1979) Birth defects compendium, 2nd edn. Macmillan, London

Berry CL (1980) The examination of embryonic and fetal material in diagnostic histopathology laboratories. J Clin Pathol 33: 317

Birkbeck JA, Billewicz WZ, Thomson AM (1975a) Human foetal

measurements between 50 and 150 days of gestation, in relation to crown–heel length. Ann Hum Biol 2: 173

Birkbeck JA, Billewicz WZ, Thomson AM (1975b) Foetal growth from 50 to 150 days of gestation. Ann Hum Biol 2: 319

Boyd JD, Hamilton WJ (1970) The human placenta. Heffer, Cambridge

Boyd PA, Scott A (1985) Quantitative structural studies on human placentas associated with pre-eclampsia, essential hypertension and intrauterine growth retardation. Br J Obstet Gynaecol 92: 721

Boyd PA, Scott A, Keeling Jean W (1986) Quantitative structural studies on placentas from pregnancies complicated by diabetes melitus. Br J Obstet Gynaecol 93: 31

Buyse ML (ed) (1990) Birth defects encyclopedia. Blackwell Scientific, Oxford

Byrne J, Warburton D, Kline J, Blanc W, Stein Z (1985) Morphology of early fetal deaths and their chromosomal characteristics. Teratology 32: 297

Campbell S (1976) Fetal growth. In: Beardf RW, Nathanielsz PW (eds) Fetal physiology and medicine. Saunders, London, pp 271–301

Doshi N, Surti U, Szulnan A (1983) Morphologic anomalies in triploid liveborn fetuses. Hum Pathol 14: 716

Fox H (1978) Pathology of the placenta. Saunders, London

Granchrow D, Ornoy A (1979) Possible evidence for secondary degeneration of central nervous system in the etiology of anencephaly and brain dysraphia. A study in the young human fetuses. Virchows Arch (Pathol Anat) 384: 285

Gruenwald P, Lawrence KL (1968) A method of examining the brain of the newborn. Dev Med Child Neurol 10: 64

Gruenwald P, Minh HN (1960) Evaluation of body and organ weights in perinatal pathology. Am J Clin Pathol 34: 247

Keeling JW (1993) The perinatal necropsy. In: Keeling JW (ed) Fetal and neonatal pathology. Springer-Verlag, London pp 1–32

Kraus BS, Jordon RE (1965) The human dentition before birth. Lea and Febiger, Philadelphia, pp 107, 109, 127

Larroche JC (1977) Developmental pathology of neonate. Excerpta Medica, Amsterdam

Logan WHG, Kronfeld R (1933) Development of the human jaws and surrounding structures from birth to the age of fifteen years. Am Dent Assoc 20: 379

McBride M, Baillie J, Poland BJ (1984) Growth parameters in normal fetuses. Teratology 29: 185

Moscoso GJ, Driver M, Whimster WF (1987) Ciliogenesis of the human respiratory epithelium during the pre-natal period. Pediatr Pathol 3: 341

Nañagus JC (1925) A comparison of the growth of the body dimensions of anencephalic human fetuses with normal fetal growth as determined by graphic analysis and empirical formulae. Am J Anat 35: 455

Nomata N (1964) Chronological study on the crown formation of the human deciduous dentition. Bull Tokyo Med Dent Univ 11: 55

Patten B (1946) Human embryology. Blakiston, Philadelphia, p 184

Rushton DI (1978) Simplified classification of spontaneous abortions. J. Med Genet 15: 1

Russel JGB (1981) Radiological assessment of age, retardation and death. In: Barson AJ (ed) Laboratory investigation of fetal disease. Wright, Bristol, pp 3–16

Salmon MA, Lindenbaum RH (1978) Developmental defects and syndromes. HM & M Publishers, Aylesbury

Sanders RC, James AE Jr (1985) The principles and practice of ultrasonography in obstetrics and gynaecology, 3rd ed. Appleton-Century-Crofts, Norwalk

Smith DW (1982) Recognisable patterns of human malformation. Saunders, Philadelphia

Streeter GL (1920) Weight, sitting height, head size, foot length and menstrual age of the human embryo. Carnegie Institute Contributions to Embryology 11: 143

Tanimura T, Nelson T, Hollingsworth RR, Shepard TH (1971) Weight standards for organs from early human fetuses. Anat Rec 171: 227

Theisen CT, Bodin JD, Svododa JA, Pettinelli MW (1979) Unusual muscle abnormalities associated with thalidomide treatment in a Rhesus monkey: a case report. Teratology 19: 313

Thomson AM, Billewicz WZ, Hytten FE (1969) The weight of the placenta in relation to birthweight. J Obstet Gynaecol Br Cwlth 76: 865

Trolle D (1948) Age of foetus determined from its measures. Acta Obstet Gynecol Scand 27: 327

Tynan MJ, Becker AE, Macartney FJ, Jimenez MQ, Shinebourne EA, Anderson RH (1979) Nomenclature and classification of congenital heart disease. Br Heart J 41: 544

Usher R, McLean F (1969) Intrauterine growth of liveborn caucasian infants at sea level: standards obtained from measurements in 7 dimensions of infants born between 25 and 44 weeks of gestation. J Pediatr 74: 901

Varmunt J (1992) Geboort: ontwikkelingen in het verleden en toekomstverwachtingen. Maandstatistiek van de bevolkig. (CBS) 92: 18

Warburton D, Kline J, Stein Z, Hutzler M, Chin A, Hassold T (1987) Does the karyotype of a spontaneous abortion predict the karyotype of a subsequent abortion? Evidence from 273 women with two karyotyped spontaneous abortions. J Hum Genet 41: 465

WHO (1977) Recommended definitions, terminology and format for statistical tables related to the perinatal period and use of a new certificate for cause of perinatal deaths. Acta Obstet Gynaecol Scand 56: 247

Wigglesworth JS (1984) Perinatal pathology. Saunders, Philadelphia

Wilson JG (1965) Methods for administrating agents and detecting malformations in experimental animals. In: Wilson JG, Warkany J (ed) Teratology–Principles and techniques. University of Chicago Press, Chicago

2 · Congenital Malformations

Colin L. Berry

Our understanding of development has increased immeasurably in the past 10 years. Mechanisms of growth control, morphogenesis and differentiation are now sufficiently well understood for serious attempts at mechanistic explanations of certain malformation syndromes, and the data accumulating from the human genome project and similar projects on mice and the nematode *C. elegans* indicate how genes may influence these processes (see Berry 1992, 1994[a,b]).

Vertebrate development is now seen to be a process driven mainly by cellular interaction rather than direct genetic instruction; there is no slavish following of a construction blueprint. The processes involved in development have been conserved over an enormous time-scale, are limited in their variety, are identical or closely related to those processes disturbed in neoplasia, and are capable of disturbance by environmental factors. All of these characteristics make them of significance to pathologists. (For those who wish to brush up their embryology an excellent general account is that of Gilbert 1992. A number of the basic cellular processes involved are described in the text of Alberts et al. 1989)

In general it is true to say that many growth control and cell signalling mechanisms are used repeatedly in development, often in different ways at different stages. Members of the fibroblast growth factor (FGF), transforming growth factor β (TGF-β) and ^{Wnt} gene families – acting as signalling factors over short distances – are effective in causing the undifferentiated ectoderm of the animal hemisphere to form mesoderm. The TGF-β family of polypeptides is used not only in this phase but also later in development in the phase of branchial arch differentiation, formation of the lung and formation of the bones of the face. A further example of varied use is seen in the many factors of critical importance in development of organs that act by mechanisms which are not direct in terms of an effect on the lineage or genealogy of their anlage. These effects may be mediated via the extracellular matrix, the cytoskeleton or cell junctions. The extracellular matrix (ECM) may differ significantly in composition at different locations in ways that are permissive or restrictive to cell adhesion, division or mobility; cell surface receptors for different components of the matrix may be the regulating factors in these functions and are clearly expressed differentially in different cell groups. Growth factors may bind to the matrix selectively, affecting local concentrations and thus affecting the production of local matrix components or the controlled release of the factors by, say, variable rates of degradation (see Adams and Watt 1993).

An important characteristic of developmental mechanisms is that there often appears to be considerable redundancy in the operating systems – a point pathologists should recognize when they identify particular gene products as "characteristic" of particular cell types. In a number of cases of apparent redundancy the additional mechanism may be effective in increasing the specificity of a process, acting as a form of "fine tuning" of a regulatory process (Wolpert 1992) – an analogy would be the differing processes that contribute to the effective monitoring of the fidelity of DNA reproduction. Disturbance of a "vital" process may thus be remarkably ineffective in disturbing development.

It is possible in some instances to note the effects of direct intervention with pattern formation on the phenotype. Where this is so, the subject is discussed in the relevant chapter.

This chapter confines itself to dealing with congenital abnormalities as defined by McKeown and Record (1960): "macroscopic abnormalities of structures attributable to faulty development and present at birth". This definition excludes metabolic defects such as glycogen storage disease and the haemoglobinopathies; these abnormalities, which are caused by single genes of large effect, inherited according to Mendelian patterns, collectively account for less than 1% of human malformations and are not described in this account, although many are described elsewhere in the book. We shall consider here the larger groups of malformations and, in particular, the ways in which various epidemiological and other studies have contributed to knowledge of their pathogenesis. It should be emphasized that accurate pathological identification of malformation and malformation syndromes is an essential step in identifying aetiological factors, and one where the pathologist has a large part to play.

Better understanding of many of the processes of development has transformed our understanding of dysmorphogenesis in recent years. The careful characterization of defects commented on above has provided a ready base in human medicine from which a number of intuitive leaps can be made. Before considering some of these new discoveries it is still important to emphasize that, for the pathologist, the variation in incidence of malformations at different times in pregnancy must be considered in determining the nature of his or her response to requests for examination of material. The classical studies of Nishimura on abortions have shown that in Japan, where the incidence of neural tube defects is low (around 1 per 1000 births), such abnormalities occur in over 13 per 1000 aborted embryos (see Nishimura 1970). Many of these abnormal embryos have an abnormal karyotype, a finding confirmed in other studies. Up to 28 weeks' gestation about 40% of abortions are chromosomally abnormal (Warburton et al. 1980). Of these, about half are trisomic, 15% are triploid, the extra set of chromosomes being of paternal origin in 75% of cases, and 20% are monosomy X. The rest are structural anomalies and a variety of post-fertilization errors (tetraploidy, mosaicism, hypertriploidy, etc.).

These findings have been verified by more recent studies using newer techniques (see, for example, Eiben et al. 1990 for a study using direct preparations from chorionic villi) and do not appear to be changing with time – Shepard et al. (1989) have found no evidence of change in a 20 year period.

Monosomic conceptuses probably cease development earlier than those with extra chromosomes (Gropp 1973). However, chromosomally abnormal conceptuses clearly survive to term, and such abnormality is often associated with malformation (Machin 1974). The figures of Witschi (1969) and of Roberts and Lowe (1975) suggesting that around 80% of human conceptuses abort were based on estimates; the development of the methodology of in vivo fertilization has provided the stimulus both for advances in endocrinology and the direct observations that show how good the estimates were. In four studies sera or urine from women were tested for the presence of human chorionic gonadotrophin (HCG) from the date of the last menstrual period (LMP). The studies include more than 1200 cycles in women attempting to conceive, and collectively they suggest a survival rate of around 60% of postimplantation embryos (see Klein and Stein 1985 for a review). In vitro studies suggest that earlier losses between fertilization and implantation may be as high as 78% but are probably around 60% in most groups. Table 2.1 shows the estimates of the date of loss arrived at by Klein and Stein, based on recent data. It seems likely that the normal outcome of human pregnancy is abortion, and that this represents an effective mechanism for the prevention of defects.

Shiota et al. (1987) have found a high prevalence of defective human embryos in the early postimplantation period, examining a large number of embryos by serial sectioning. Embryos from induced abortions between 14 and 28 days after fertilization showed gross abnormality in 13.5% of cases, and a further 19% were degenerating. These data, from a different type of material, confirm the conclusions outlined above.

The frequency of specific defects varies considerably from country to country. Within countries it varies from region to region and among different social classes. Thus, central nervous system defects are much commoner in England and Wales than in the West Indies or Japan; they are three times commoner in infants of social class V than in infants of social classes I and II; and they are three times commoner in the valleys of South Wales than along its coastal plain (Lowe 1972; Richards et al. 1972). These are important variations and may give valuable clues to aetiology but, as previously emphasized, the figures must be regarded with some caution in terms of the *incidence* of defects.

It is important to realize, in spite of what follows in terms of pathogenesis of defects, that these variations, which are based on variations in the genetics of populations, are not set in stone. The Medical Research Council study of folic acid supplementation of high-risk groups for neurospinal dysraphism indicates clearly how environmental factors may interact with genotype to determine phenotype (MRC 1991).

In contrast to the variability in the incidence of specific defects, total malformation rates for differing

Table 2.1. Probability of spontaneous abortion for 100 fertilized ova: a speculation based on the current literature

Time from ovulation	Pregnancies at beginning of interval	No. of fetal deaths	No. of births	Probability (%) of fetal death in gestation interval or later	Probability (%) of fetal death in gestation interval
1–6 days	100	54.55	0	75	54.55
7–13	45.45	11.21	0	45	24.66
14–20	34.25	2.80	0	27	8.18
3–5 weeks	31.45	2.38	0	20.50	7.56
6–9	29.07	1.90	0	14.00	6.52
10–13	27.17	1.20	0	8.00	4.42
14–17	25.97	0.35	0	3.74	1.33
18–21	25.63	0.22	0.01	2.44	0.85
22–25	25.40	0.08	0.04	1.61	0.31
26–29	25.28	0.08	0.24	1.31	0.30
30–33	24.97	0.08	0.66	1.02	0.30
34–37	24.22	0.08	9.72	0.74	0.34
38 +	14.42	0.10	14.33	0.68	0.68

Data from Klein and Stein (1985).

groups *at birth* appear to be roughly comparable (Table 2.2). This finding even applies to primitive South American Indian groups (Neel 1974). Neel has suggested that this general consistency supports the concept that the malformed represent that percentage of individuals in every generation that falls below the threshold of the obligate proportion of loci needed, in a heterozygous state, to ensure normal development.

Deaths due to congenital malformations in 1975, 1983 and 1992 are shown in Table 2.3. The considerable drop in incidence commented on previously is now more obvious, reflecting, at least in part, the tendency to more frequent intervention in early pregnancy as diagnostic techniques improve. Surgical treatment in early life is also more effective, and this combination is reducing the size of this important problem in health care. However, Fig. 2.1 shows a different perspective, based on data from the USA. As other causes of infant mortality diminish, the percentage of deaths due to malformation increases (after Sever et al. 1993).

The approximate frequency of the various types of defect and their sex ratio are given by Carter (1976), and Table 2.4 is based on this information.

Table 2.2. Prevalence of some external malformations in 3000 embryos and fetuses compared with prevalence at birth

Malformation	Prevalence per 1000		Loss
	Abortions	Birth	(%)
Neural tube	13.1	1.0	92
Cleft lip and palate	24.4	2.7	98
Polydactyly	9.0	0.9	90
Cyclopia and cebocephalia	6.2	0.1	98

Data from several sources, including Nishimura (1970).

Table 2.3. Deaths resulting from congenital malformations in England and Wales in 1975, and 1992

Deaths due to	All ages			Under 1 year			1–4 years			5–9 years			10–14 years		
	1975	1983	1992	1975	1983	1992	1975	1983	1992	1975	1983	1992	1975	1983	1992
All causes	582 841	579 608	558 313	9488	6381	4539	4699	1093	874	1140	660	516	1046	846	521
All malformations	3804	2944	1565	2303	1699	370	319	241	163	163	60	58	102	69	43
All CNS malformations (excluding neurofibromatosis)	1025	888	158	826	633	77	66	72	44	53	25	17	27	42	20
All malformations of the heart and great vessels	1693	1407	833	885	845	208	200	251	98	192	58	79	56	50	29
All malformations of the genitourinary system	331	229	215	108	79	2	9	3	1	3	1	2	6	1	–
All gastrointestinal malformations	195	175	123	109	95	26	22	23	11	7	3	5	1	1	–

Data from Mortality Statistics (cause), Series DH2 No. 2 (1975), No. 10 (1983) and No. 19 (1992) and Mortality Statistics (childhood), Series DH3 No. 12 (1983), Office of Population Censuses and Surveys.

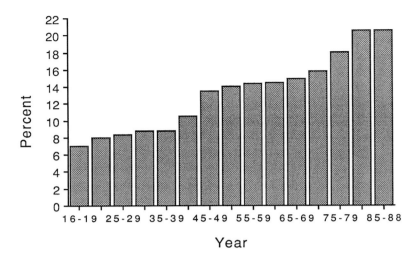

Fig. 2.1. Percentage of infant deaths attributed to birth defects in the USA, 1916–1988.

Table 2.4. Approximate frequency and sex ratio of the more common major congenital malformations in Great Britain

Malformation	Frequency/1000 live and stillbirths	Approximate sex ratio (M : F)
Spina bifida cystica	2.5	0.6
Anencephaly	2.0	0.3
Congenital heart defects	6.0	1.0
Pyloric stenosis	3.0	4.0
Cleft lip (± cleft palate)	1.0	1.8
Congenital dislocation of the hip	1.0	0.14

Genetics of Common Malformations

The largest groups of defects in humans (those of the central nervous system, musculoskeletal system and cardiovascular system) are found to have a number of characteristics in common when studied epidemiologically. The defects are common; familial aggregates are found; there is variation in prevalence with birth rank and parental age; and variation occurs with season of birth and with geographical localization. The recurrence rate in siblings is of the order of 1%–5%, much higher than the prevalence in the general population but too low for any simple Mendelian explanation. Finally, the recurrence rate in dizygotic twins is the same as that in siblings, whereas that in monozygotic twins is 20%–50%. These findings suggest that both genetic and environmental factors affect the prevalence of the anomalies.

The data have been used to construct a model of polygenic or multifactorial inheritance of congenital abnormality, described by Carter (1965, 1969) and subsequently modified by Falconer (1965) and Edwards (1969). The hypothesis can best be explained as follows. Where two or more alleles are present at a gene locus with a frequency of more than 1%, genetic polymorphism is said to exist. If the character to be studied is several steps away from the primary product of gene activity, it is likely that the different products of many genes are involved in the observed variation of the character. If there is polymorphism at several of these gene loci, the character is likely to be continuously and normally distributed (Fig. 2.2). If the expression of the gene is further modified by local factors acting via the environment, these will provide a further source of variation of the character concerned. Height, intelligence, blood pressure and fingerprint ridge count (Fig. 2.3) all show continuous variation with normal distribution. Although the degree of polymorphism necessary under the hypothesis is high, biochemical studies have shown that it exists in humans. This polymorphism is central to the hypothesis presented and enables it to be tested in a number of ways.

In characters on which environmental factors have little influence, it is possible to predict the degree to which the relatives of index cases will resemble them. A monozygotic twin with all genes in common with the index patient will have a regression coefficient of 1.0 (complete resemblance). A parent passes on half his or her genes to a child, with a resultant regression coefficient of 0.5 (child on parent). Siblings will inherit the same member of a gene pair from one parent in half the possible instances on average, so that their regression on the index patient will also be 0.5. Uncles, nephews and grandparents (second-degree relatives) have an average of a quarter of their genes in common with

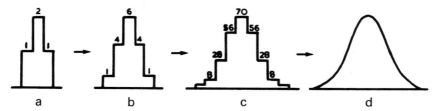

Fig. 2.2. The effect of increasing the number of additive alleles at two loci on the phenotype. Where more than four genes are involved the character is likely to be normally distributed. **a** Two alleles at one locus; **b** two alleles at each of two loci; **c** three alleles at each of two loci; **d** normal curve from alleles at many gene loci.

the index patient, so that their regression coefficients are 0.25. Third-degree relatives (cousins) have an average of 1 in 8 of their genes in common, with a resultant regression coefficient of 0.125.

The original model of polygenic inheritance proposed by Carter separated genetic and environmental factors, using the distribution of genetic predisposition to a defect to indicate a population at risk for the triggering effect of environmental factors (Fig. 2.4). He assumed that the distribution of predisposition in relatives would be "normal" with a scale that gave a normal curve in the general population, and also that the variance in relatives was the same as that in the general population. Neither of these assumptions is true, but they do not introduce large errors.

Malformations are unlike the continuously variable characteristics discussed above in that they are threshold in type, i.e. present or absent. Thus, because first-degree relatives have a genetic correlation of 0.5 with the index patients they will have a curve of distribution about a mean approximately half-way between that of the general population and the index patients beyond the threshold. The position

of the mean for second-degree relatives would be shifted one-quarter of the distance between the general population mean and the index patients; that for third-degree relatives would be shifted one-eighth of the distance from the population mean towards the index patients.

As an example, in a defect occurring at a population frequency of 1 in 100 for which we assume a 100% heritability, the proportion of first-degree relatives beyond the threshold – and thus, in this example, affected – will be 8%. For second-degree relatives the figure is 1.2%, and for third-degree relatives 0.4%. Taking the example of cleft lip with or without cleft palate, we would have calculated correlations of 0.5, 0.25 and 0.125 for first-, second- and third-degree relatives, respectively. The observed figures indicate correlations of about 0.35, 0.19 and 0.085, suggesting a heritability (see below) of about 70%, which is supported by twin studies.

In the improved polygenic model of Falconer (Fig. 2.5), the liability to produce a defect, composed of both genetic and environmental factors, is shown along the x-axis. Because environmental factors are

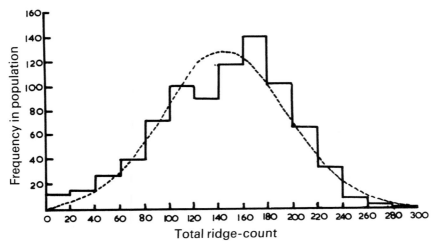

Fig. 2.3. Fingerprint ridge count in a population of 825 British males with the calculated "normal" curve with the same mean and standard deviation. (After Holt 1961)

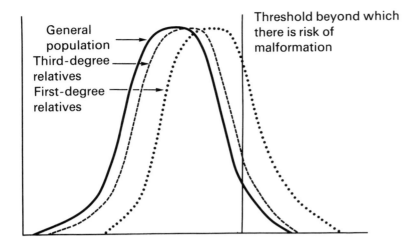

Fig. 2.4. Carter's model. The curve for second-degree relatives is omitted for the sake of clarity.

included it is appropriate to consider all those beyond the threshold as affected and to estimate an upper limit of the heritability of the malformation from the birth frequency in the general population and the proportion of the relatives affected. With this type of model it has been calculated that heritability for pyloric stenosis is about 60%, estimated from the first-degree relatives of male patients, and 90% for female relatives of female patients. For neural tube malformations heritability is about 60%, with similar values for talipes equinovarus.

Extensive studies of polygenically determined defects have shown up certain other characteristics, which are important to the pathologist's role in providing documentation for those involved in genetic counselling. These are:

1. The more severe the malformation in the index patient, the greater the risk to relatives.
2. If there is a preponderance of one sex in affected individuals, the risk will be higher for the relatives of the less frequently affected sex.
3. The risks to relatives are likely to be higher where the index patient already has one near relative affected, because the presence of two patients is an indication of a high-risk family.

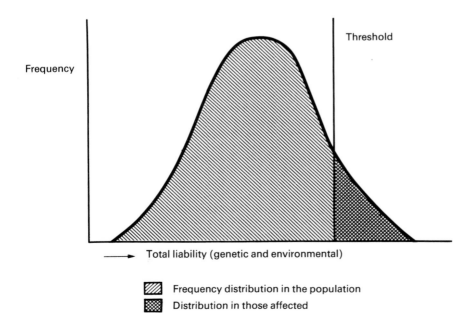

Fig. 2.5. Falconer's model.

Variance and Heritability

The two concepts of variance and heritability are important in consideration of the causation of many human malformations. The familiar concepts of normal distribution and standard deviation will not be considered further here, but the square of the standard deviation, the variance (σ^2), is used in population genetics because it can be partitioned or fractionated into additive components by analysis of variance. The phenotypic variance (σ_P^2) of a particular trait in a population is the result of different genotypic effects and their interaction with environmental influences. From an analysis of variance the genetic (σ_G^2) and environmental (σ_E^2) components can be calculated. From this it is evident that

$$\sigma_P^2 = \sigma_G^2 + \sigma_E^2$$

Both genetic and environmental components can be further fractionated into other specific contributions (e.g. climatic, age-dependent or birth-rank effects, and additive, epistatic (interaction) or dominance-genetic effects).

In attempts to attribute the various causative factors in any malformation to genetic or environmental factors, estimates of heritability are of great importance. Heritability is the ratio of the genetic variance to the phenotypic variance

$$h^2 = \frac{\sigma_G^2}{\sigma_P^2}$$

σ_G^2 includes all types of genetic factors. However, only additive variance has predictive value, and heritability is thus often defined as

$$h^2 = \frac{\sigma_A^2}{\sigma_P^2}$$

The reasons for adopting this narrowed concept are as follows. Additive effects are seen when a gene contributes a constant increment to the phenotype whenever it is present in the genotype and where heterozygotes have a phenotype exactly intermediate between the two homozygotes. If an allele exhibits partial dominance when present in the heterozygote, the extent of this effect can be determined by analysis of variance, which will also identify additive effects in genes showing various degrees of interaction. If, as frequently occurs, there is a multiple allelic series, with varying degrees of dominance,

$$A^1 > A^2 > A^3 > A^4$$

the gene A^3, which will be dominant in one parent (A^3A^4), may be combined with a gene (A^2) that was recessive in the other parent (A^1A^2). In the offspring ($A^2 A^3$), A^2 now appears as a dominant allele. In other words, when dominance or complex interactions are involved, one cannot predict the contribution a parent will make to the phenotype of its offspring.

Heritability is valuable in the study of large populations. If all the phenotypic variability for a given trait is attributable to environmental factors the heritability will be zero. If all the variability is of genetic origin (e.g. blood groups) it is 100%. Most traits in outbred populations have intermediate values.

Heritability in metric traits can be calculated from correlations between offspring and the mid-parent value (the mean of the two parents) because the progeny receive half their genes from each parent: alternatively, it can be calculated from twice the correlation between offspring and one parent ($h^2 = 2r$). The same relationship is valid for siblings (sharing half their genes). Half-sibs have only a 25% genetic relationship; therefore $h^2 = 4r$.

Accurate determination of regression coefficients in monozygotic and dizygotic twins can be used to estimate the heritability of a defect. The use of twin studies to calculate heritabilities depends on the fact that the variance within dizygotic twin pairs is caused by half the additive genetic variation in the population, plus the variation attributable to environmental differences between the two members of the twin pair, whereas the variance within monozygotic twins is caused entirely by environmental differences.

As an example of such a study, Table 2.5 shows the results of examination of fingerprint ridge count, which, of the characters showing a normal distribution, shows the highest value for calculated heritability in humans: 92%.

Table 2.5. Observed correlations of relatives for total fingerprint ridge count compared with the theoretical correlations expected with simple additive inheritance

Type of relationship	Observed correlation	Theoretical correlation
Husband–wife	0.05±0.007	0.00
Monozygotic twins	0.95±0.07	1.00
Dizygotic twins	0.49±0.08	0.50
Sib–sib	0.50±0.04	0.50
Parent–child	0.48±0.03	0.50

After Holt (1961).

Abnormalities of Neural Tube Closure

A vast descriptive literature exists on defects of the development of the neural tube (their terminology is discussed in detail in Chapter 5). In most epidemiological studies two large groups are considered, "anencephaly", including craniorachischisis (combined anencephaly and spina bifida), and "spina bifida", which includes meningocele, myelocele and encephalocele.

Variations in reported incidence in various countries are extreme (Table 2.6). In the UK the prevalence varies from around 1.4–1.5 per 1000 total births, for the two groups of defects in London, to rates approximately three times as high in Belfast. Few rates higher than about 1 per 1000 have been reported except from the British Isles, north-eastern North America and the Middle East. Some Sikh communities have frequencies of about 3 per 1000 (see Leck 1974).

Table 2.6. Range of highest to lowest frequencies in congenital defects of the central nervous system in single births in various countries

Malformation	Frequency per 1000 total births		Centre	
	Lowest	Highest	Lowest	Highest
Anencephalus	0.11	4.09	Bogota	Belfast
Anencephalus and spina bifida	0.03	0.61	Santiago	Alexandria
Hydrocephalus	0.05	1.99	Calcutta	Alexandria
Hydrocephalus and spina bifida	0.03	1.64	Manila Bogota	Belfast
Spina bifida	0.03	2.59	Manila	Belfast
All neural tube defects	0.62	10.21	Medellin	Belfast

Data from Lilienfeld (1969).

From studies of the epidemiology of these two groups of defects it is evident that they must have related causes, because they show such similar variations in incidence. Furthermore, these causes must be partly environmental, since in children of the same genetic background there is marked variation with place, time, maternal age and parity, and socioeconomic status. The relatively low incidence in the offspring of Jewish women born in Israel after their parents had migrated there from other Middle Eastern countries, while high rates were seen in the children of mothers who were themselves born elsewhere in the Middle East (Naggan 1971), supports the suggestion that both environmental and genetic influences may be important in pathogenesis. Leck suggests that the stability of the rates for Sikhs and Ashkenazim could also be of environmental origin. The low rates for blacks may also be related to maternal factors rather than fetal genes, because the rates for children of black fathers and European mothers may be as

high as those for Europeans (Leck 1972). Where detailed studies of the incidence of anencephalus have been made, some interesting trends have developed with time. In two investigations, Edwards (1958) and Fedrick (1976) examined the incidence of anencephalus in Scotland. A considerable variation in differing geographical locations had persisted, although relative frequencies had changed and there was an overall decline in the incidence of the lesion, most marked in those under 20 years of age and in the lower social classes. There was little seasonal variation in the time of delivery, but years with excessive numbers of cases have occurred (1961, 1971). Similar episodes have occurred in New England, Berlin and Birmingham (see Leck 1974). In Great Britain a prolonged "epidemic" may have lasted from 1920 to the late 1940s, and in recent years there is evidence of a decline, beginning in 1974 (Owens et al. 1981). Thus in 1961 neural tube defects comprised 26.4% of all anomalies; by 1979 this had reduced to 12.32%, a change not explicable by termination of affected pregnancies detected by screening. However, pregnancies in women under 20 and over 35 years, the two high-risk groups, have decreased markedly in this period, although this is an apparently numerically insufficient explanation of the phenomenon.

Seasonal variation in prevalence presents a very confused picture. For spina bifida there is a peak in children conceived in mid-spring and a trough in early autumn conceptions, but anencephalus may show this or other patterns. The picture is more clear-cut when variation in maternal age and parity is considered. Associations between these variables are found whenever large series are studied (see Leck 1974 for a bibliography). In all instances there is agreement that the defects are least common in second births. Among births after the second, the tendency for most countries is for the prevalence to increase with parity, and there is a tendency for increasing prevalence with increasing maternal age. Variations with social class are less clear-cut and the higher prevalence in lower social classes has been found to be less marked in recent studies and to be very variable in extent.

The sex ratio (male to female) for the defects is around 0.7:1 and 0.8:1 for spina bifida and 0.45:1 for anencephaly in Great Britain, rising to unity in oriental populations. The female anencephalic rate appears to be both higher and more variable than the male rate (Rogers and Morris 1973).

Family studies show that concordance is less common in twins than is recurrence in sibships. Apart from this hazard the sibs of index cases are particularly liable to be aborted, and may have spina bifida occulta more often than other children (Carter et al.

1968; Carter and Evans 1973). It seems that both parental and maternal effects can affect prevalence, and in areas of high prevalence consanguinity can more than double the risk.

Various estimates suggest that about half of all embryos for fetuses with CNS defects are aborted. This may account for the paradox that neural tube defects are less common in the twins of children with those defects than in other sibs.

Possible environmental factors of significance had been debated for years, but the therapeutic initiative of vitamin supplementation in neural tube defects taken by Smithells et al. (1981) was highly controversial. Despite the difficulties in establishing proper trials in this context (see Anonymous 1982a), a successful trial of one aspect of this problem has been completed, with great potential health benefit (see p. 44).

Cleft Lip and Palate

Cleft lip and palate combined (CL + P) and cleft lip alone (CL) are closer to each other, in aetiological terms, than to cleft palate alone (CP) (see review by Leck 1976). Approximately 20% of children with facial clefts have associated major malformations, the proportion of individuals with CP and associated defects being the highest in the group.

The lips develop during the 4th to 7th weeks of intrauterine life, the palate from the 4th to 8th weeks – these dates depending a little on the starting point assumed. Genetic data suggest that a mechanism altering lip development may have a secondary effect on palatal development, but that the latter may be affected independently of the former (Woolf 1971), and that both these processes increase in frequency with parental age.

All studies in which data are adequate show between 0.6 and 1.35 per 1000 total births for Caucasoids, but Mongoloids have higher rates and Negroids considerably lower. Hawaiian studies show that children of mixed genetic background have an intermediate liability to CL±P (Ching and Chung 1974). Fraser and Pashayan (1970) suggested that differences in facial shape were important in determining this malformation, as has been shown for the mouse – a suggestion supported by more recent work in human (see Kurisu et al. 1974).

The frequency of CL alone varies considerably in different regions of England and Wales (25%–33% in most studies, but up to 47% in North East England: Knox and Braithwaite 1962), a variability also seen in Mongoloid races. In both groups unilateral clefts of the lip are commoner than bilateral ones, and about two-thirds are left-sided. In addition, CL shows

some evidence of clustering (see Leck 1976 for a bibliography), although investigation of seasonal variations does not suggest a specific pattern or provide evidence for specific aetiological factors, e.g. influenza.

There is a marked trend for the prevalence of CL + P to rise with maternal age; in CL alone this effect is much less marked (Hay and Barbano 1972). Parity appears to have little effect regardless of age.

Cleft Palate Alone

Rates for CP range from 0.4 to 0.8 per 1000 in Caucasians (see Leck 1976 for a bibliography). Face shape is also probably important in this defect; in Finland Saxen (1975) has shown that the prevalence is highest in the east of the country, where faces are wider. The prevalence of CL increases with maternal age, as does that of CL + P, but there is some evidence to suggest that an independent paternal effect may also be important.

Family Patterns of Occurrence

For CL + P, if we assume a general population incidence of 1 per 1000, the concurrence rate for monozygotic twins is 400 times the population figure, and the rates for first-, second- and third-degree relatives are 40, 7 and 3 times this figure respectively.

Congenital Heart Defects

The problem of the prevalence of defects is nowhere more difficult to resolve than in the large group of abnormalities that affect the heart and great vessels. Prolonged follow-up and sophisticated study is necessary for proper ascertainment, and investigations that satisfy these major criteria are few. Rates of 6–8 per 1000 births are generally found (e.g. Yerushalmy 1970; Fedrick et al. 1971). The prevalence at birth of all defects increases with maternal age and is high in monozygotic twin pairs (Mitchell et al. 1971; Kenna et al. 1975). The increased incidence with high maternal age persists even when allowance is made for the well documented association of Down's syndrome with congenital heart disease. The eight commonest lesions (ventricular septal defect, patent ductus arteriosus, aortic stenosis, atrial septal defect, coarctation of the aorta, Fallot's tetralogy, pulmonary stenosis, and the transposition complexes) account for about 80% of all defects. Defects of the ventricular septum are the commonest single group (approximately 30% of the total in most series). From a number of studies patent ductus arteriosus appears to be more common in females, whereas transposition, coarctation of the aorta and aortic stenosis are commoner in males.

A possible aetiological factor, hypoxia, has been identified from surveys of patent ductus arteriosus. This defect has been shown to increase with altitude, and at places over 4500 m high it occurs at 30 times the frequency observed at sea level (Peñaloza et al. 1964). It seems likely, however, that other factors, perhaps involving hypoxia, are involved. Short gestation, low birth weight and fetal or neonatal asphyxia are also associated with increased frequency of the diagnosis.

Other cardiac defects show no convincing seasonal or geographical associations.

In a large survey (1494 cases and 1572 controls), Ferencz et al. (1987) found a strong association of congenital heart defects with chromosomal abnormalities, mainly affecting chromosomes 13, 18 and 21 (93% of the cytogenetic defects found), and an association with CNS, eye, anterior abdominal wall, and alimentary and urinary tract anomalies. There was no association with cleft lip and palate, inguinal hernia or lower limb anomalies.

Infantile Hypertrophic Pyloric Stenosis

Rates of between 2 and 4 per 1000 births have been recorded for infantile hypertrophic pyloric stenosis in Great Britain, significantly higher than the 1–3 or less per 1000 recorded for other countries (see Leck 1976 for a bibliography). Again, there are diagnostic difficulties, particularly in establishing the relationship of true hypertrophic pyloric stenosis, treated surgically, to "pylorospasm", which can be conservatively managed. The male:female ratio is 4:1 or 5:1 in all studies, and there is a significant excess of first-born children. In a recent report, Bear (1978) has shown that an excess of male births over females is also found among unaffected members of sibships in which more than one case of pyloric stenosis has occurred.

Tumour size in pyloric stenosis tends to increase with age, suggesting postnatal development of the muscular hypertrophy. Dodge (1971, 1973) considers that feeding frequency and habits may affect the development of the anomaly, and that gastrin, which can produce pyloric hypertrophy in puppies, may play an important role. Some cases of pyloric stenosis have apparently had their origin at birth and have required operative intervention in the first weeks of life (Powell 1962; Laurence 1963; Lloyd-Davies 1963), but this is uncommon, the mean age at opera-

tion being 7 weeks. More recently, involvement of nerves in which NO acts as a neurotransmitter have been implicated in the pathogenesis of the defect.

The disease shows the characteristics of polygenic inheritance (Carter 1969), with heritability of 68% (sons–fathers), 54% (brothers–brothers) or 90% (daughters–mothers). This illustrates the general point that, when one sex is seldom affected, individuals of that sex who do express the defect have a higher genetic "load" tending to produce the abnormality.

Musculoskeletal System Defects

Club Foot

In abnormalities of the club foot type it is extremely difficult to obtain accurate data, because many apparent defects disappear in the first weeks of life. If these infants are disregarded, and cases of talipes equinovarus (TEV) with other defects are excluded, the prevalence in Caucasoid races is between 2–4 per 1000 with TEV and 1 per 1000 each for talipes calcaneovalgus (TCV) and metatarsus virus (MV) (Wynne-Davies 1964; Chung and Myrianthopolus 1968). Within-series comparisons suggest that TEV is half as common in children of Oriental origin and six times as common in Polynesian children as in Caucasoids (Ching et al. 1969).

Significant trends have been reported with season of birth, multiple births, and maternal age and parity (Hay and Wehring 1970; Dunn 1976). Dunn has suggested that this defect may be a manifestation of postural moulding in utero, and that multiple births will enhance this tendency.

Congenital Dislocation of the Hip

In recent years there have been wide swings in the supposed frequency of occurrence of congenital dislocation of the hip, owing in part to difficulties in diagnosis and variation in the diagnostic criteria used. However, both unstable hip and congenital dislocation show similar epidemiological trends, namely a four- to six-fold excess of females over males, a preponderance of bilateral cases, relatively high rates in first-born children and among those born in winter, a frequent history of breech delivery, and an association between the defect and high social class (see Leck 1976 for a bibliography). Dunn (1976) also considers moulding important in this defect, suggesting that breech delivery following oligohydramnios may be an important aetiological factor. The female excess is thought to be the result of hormone-induced joint laxity.

Carter and Wilkinson (1964) first emphasized the role of both acetabular dysplasia (inherited polygenically) and dominantly inherited persistent joint laxity in the genesis of the defect. The importance of these factors was confirmed by the later studies of Wynne-Davies (1970a, b). In her work she found a higher proportion of affected individuals in first-degree than in second- and third-degree relatives and also showed that patients with the highest degree of acetabular dyplasia had the highest proportion of affected children. These individuals tended to be in the last diagnostic group; patients diagnosed early were more likely to show persistent joint laxity. However, in most cases both causative factors were thought to be important.

Chromosomal Abnormality and Malformations

It has already been emphasized that the bulk of embryos with chromosomal abnormalities are aborted. Between three and five liveborn infants per 100 are chromosomally abnormal, with Down's syndrome (47, +21), Klinefelter's syndrome (47 XXY), and 47 XYY and 47 XXX all having frequencies greater than 1 per 1000. The predominance of sex chromosome anomalies in these syndromes is probably related to the relative paucity of genetic information in them, loss or duplication of an autosome having much more serious effects on development.

The general effects of chromosome anomalies are growth retardation, mental retardation, and impaired fertility. Phenotypically, generalizations of this kind are impossible.

The classic study on the incidence of chromosomal defects is that of Boué et al. (1975), who carried out retrospective and prospective studies on 1500 karyotyped spontaneous human abortions. Concentrating on abortuses of less than 12 weeks' gestational age, they found 577 normal and 921 abnormal karyotypes. In the normal group they found morphological abnormalities, which suggested undetected zygotic causes. Structural chromosomal anomalies were rare (3.8% of defects), the bulk of the abnormalities being numerical and the result of errors at the time of gametogenesis (non-disjunction at meiosis), at the time of fertilization (triploidy caused by digyny or dispermy), or during the early division of the fertilized ovum (tetraploidy or mosaicism). The incidence of chromosome anomalies remained stable over the 6 years studied. There was no evidence of a collective or singular tendency for anomalies to show evidence of seasonal variation.

From this work it appears that 61.5% of spontaneous abortions have chromosomal defects, a figure in good general agreement with those given in the studies of Therkelsen et al. (1974) (54.7%) and Kajii et al. (1973) (59%), and which appears not to be changing (see Eiben et al. 1990).

As reported by other groups, almost all monosomies were monosomy X (about 15% of the anomalies studied). Trisomy 16 was the most frequent autosomal trisomy. It must be emphasized that even studies of this type are selected and demonstrate only some of the total errors that may occur in early development. The blighted ovum familiar to pathologists examining abortuses is a manifestation of massive developmental failure. The accompanying placental changes can give useful indicators of possible anomalies (Boué et al. 1976), but van Lijnschoten et al. (1993) have shown that many of the indicators claimed to be related to an abnormal karyotype do not predict accurately when studies attempting to predict the genotype from villous phenotype are carried out.

The numbers of chromosomal abnormalities at term have been demonstrated by Machin (1974). He found that 9% of macerated stillbirths, 4% of fresh stillbirths and 6% of early neonatal deaths had an abnormal karyotype – this despite the fact that adequate cultures were obtained from only 18% of macerated stillbirths, 76% of fresh stillbirths (intrapartum death), and 90% of early neonatal deaths. Again a striking maternal age effect was found, with mothers over 40 having a much greater risk of bearing a chromosomally abnormal child. Further effects of age are documented in the massive collaborative study of 52 965 pregnancies in women over 34 years of age (Fergusson-Smith and Yates 1984). Chromosome aberrations were found in 1200 pregnancies and age-specific incidence rates were derived. For trisomy 21 the rate rose from 0.38% at 35 years to 5.75% at 46 years. Rates for trisomy 18 rose from 0.05% to 0.76% at 43 years and for trisomy 16 from 0.02% to 0.21% at 42 years. With older mothers the capacity to sustain a trisomic fetus is apparently impaired.

Some Common Syndromes

Those who wish to find a detailed description of the anomalies found in various chromosomal defects should consult the excellent review of Gilbert and Opitz (1982), which is valuable if sometimes a little uncritical. Some basic data are given below for common syndromes.

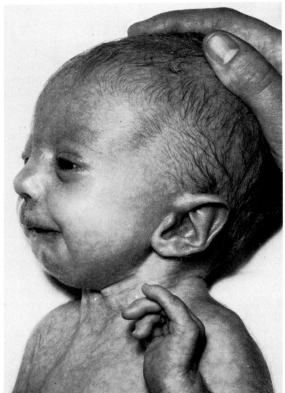

a

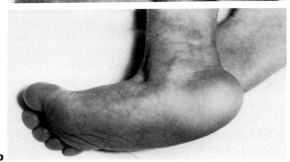

b

Fig. 2.6. Trisomy 18. **a** Micrognathia and the pinched face are evident; **b** rocker-bottom foot. (Courtesy of Professor P. Polani)

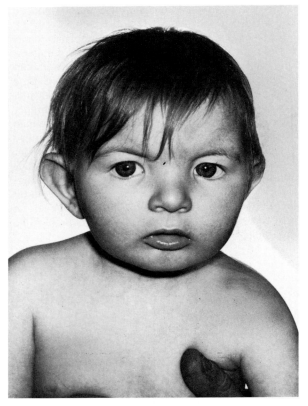

Fig. 2.7. Cri-du-chat syndrome with marked hypertelorism. (Courtesy of Professor P. Polani)

Trisomy 18 (Trisomy D, Edwards' Syndrome)

Trisomy 18 usually occurs *de novo*, although a few instances are due to familial balanced translocations. It is commoner in females (3:1), with a greatly increased frequency with advancing maternal age. The frequency of occurrence has been variously calculated at 1 per 3086 and 1 per 7000 births (see Kinoshita et al. 1989 for a bibliography). Affected infants are small with a narrow pinched face, protruding occiput, low-set ears and marked micrognathia.

The hands are often clenched, with digits II and V overriding III and IV. Rocker-bottom feet are seen. Dermatoglyphic changes include the presence of arches on all fingertips. Most affected infants die within 6 months of birth (Fig. 2.6; see also pp. 140, 290).

Congenital heart disease, Meckel's diverticulum and horseshoe kidney are commonly found (see pp. 128, 235) and Nakamura et al. (1986) have suggested that cerebellar and pontine hypoplasia are characteristic.

5p– (Cri-du-chat Syndrome)

In the cri-du-chat syndrome a variable amount of material is lost from the short arm of chromosome 5. There is microcephaly and gross hypertelorism. The name is derived from a peculiar mewing cry, which is gradually lost if the child survives and which is due to laryngeal hypoplasia. Preauricular skin tags are sometimes found. There is severe growth failure and mental retardation in survivors (Fig. 2.7).

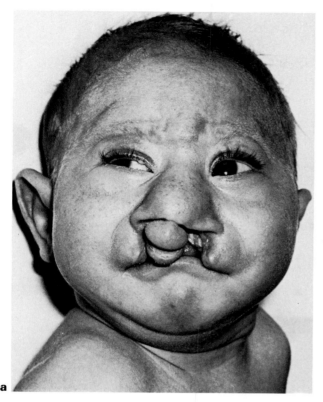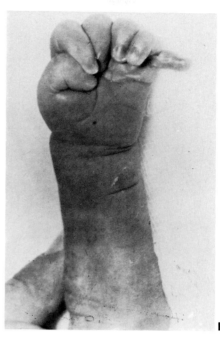

Fig. 2.8. a Facial defects in Patau's syndrome. **b** Polydactyly. (Courtesy of Professor P. Polani)

Trisomy 13 (Trisomy E, Patau's Syndrome)

The infants are small for gestational age. About one-third of cases have a scalp defect in the region of the vertex. Midline facial defects, microphthalmia, and anophthalmia or cyclops are found; the nose is often large and bulbous. Holoprosencephaly may occur. Polydactyly is common and the individuals are usually profoundly mentally retarded (Fig. 2.8; see also p. 140).

Trisomy 21 (Down's Syndrome)

Classically, trisomy 21 is characterized by a small head with flattened occiput, low-set ears with rolled-over helix, flattened nasal bridge, slanting eyes, and prominent epicanthic folds. The mouth is open, with the tongue protruding. Hands are short and spatulate, a transverse palmar crease is present with an incurved fourth finger, and dermatoglyphic abnormalities are seen. Wide separation of the great and second toes is found in some cases (Fig. 2.9). Congenital heart disease is common, with endocardial cushion defects and ventricular septal defects the most frequently occurring anomalies (see p. 92).

Human Teratogens

In view of the complex genetic and environmental factors involved in the causation of malformations it is evident that establishing the role of potential teratogens is difficult. Heritability for the large groups of human defects is in excess of 60%, and maternal age, birth rank, season, altitude, etc., all add some loading, providing a background against which teratogens must be assessed. Undoubted teratogens exist for humans; these will be considered briefly below. Despite extensive testing of compounds, it is likely that unknown teratogens of possibly cumulative effect are introduced into the environment from time to time. We may console ourselves with the fact that the prevalence of malformation has changed very little with time, so that such effects are probably not large. Nevertheless, the approach of Smithells and

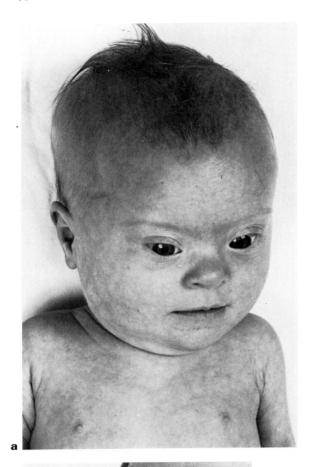

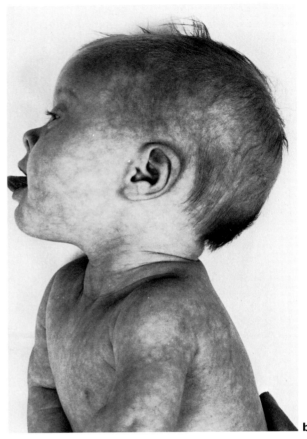

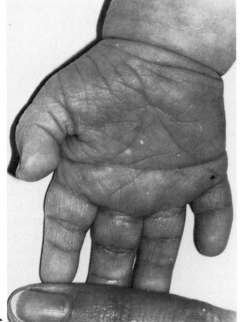

Fig. 2.9. Down's syndrome. **a** Typical facies; **b** prominent tongue; **c** spatulate hand with transverse palmar crease and incurved fourth finger. (Courtesy of Professor P. Polani)

Sheppard (1978) is eminently sensible. They point out that avoidance of unnecessary medication in pregnancy, particularly in the first trimester, is prudent but that there will always be occasions where the health of the mother (and hence the fetus) requires drug administration. The safety of pharmacologically active compounds can be tested by examining centralized prescription records and following up births to mothers taking a particular medicine in a particular period. Smithells and Sheppard have described this technique and discussed its merits clearly, in demonstrating the absence of a teratogenic effect from Bendectin. Direct human observation suggests that the relevant period of exposure for the production of particular malformations can be precisely determined, a factor which greatly strengthens the technique. As an example, Terrible and Pertile

(1975) have shown that more than 80% of congenital heart disease surviving to term is induced in the 5th to 6th week of pregnancy. Sensitive periods for particular systems are shown in Table 2.7.

Table 2.7. Sensitive periods for human development

No. of days after conception	System(s) at risk
19–21	Eye, brian, spinal cord, heart, aortic arch
22–26	Eye, brain, aortic arch, heart, jaw, limbs
26–28	Limbs, palate, urogenital system, heart, eye
28–37	Palate, urogenital system, limbs, heart
38–41	Palate, urogenital system, limbs, heart
42–46	Urogenital system, palate, fingers
46–50	Fingers, genital system
90–260	External genitalia, weight

Established human teratogens are few. Since the first edition of this book new compounds that appear to be dangerous have been identified, but extensive reviews have "cleared" others, for example the contraceptive sex steroids (WHO 1981; Wiseman and Dodds-Smith 1984). It should be remembered that pharmacological effects will occur in the fetus after drug exhibition to the mother. Effects such as virilization of female fetuses by progestagens may be expected.

Radiation

Murphy (1929) reported on the outcome of the 625 pregnancies in which women were exposed to "pelvic radium therapy" or roentgen irradiation either before or after conception, collecting his data from a review and a questionnaire sent to 1700 gynaecologists and radiologists. Radiation was therapeutic rather than diagnostic and in some cases it had been used in a direct attempt to induce sterility. Approximately a quarter of 625 pregnancies ended in abortion; in this respect preconception irradiation was less likely to induce abortion than postconception treatment. Neither the stillbirth rate nor the infant mortality rate was increased by preconception irradiation. Malformations in 402 term infants in this group included one case each of microcephaly, anencephaly, phocomelia, tracheal stenosis and congenital heart disease. A parietal bony defect was noted and one child was recorded as "deformed", with no further description provided. These figures suggest little real effect on the incidence of major malformation.

There were no stillbirths after postconception irradiation. Of the 74 full-term infants born after this treatment 17 had microcephaly, two had hydrocephalus, one was blind and growth-retarded, one had spina bifida and club feet, one had a "malformation of the head", and one had deformed upper extremities. A divergent squint was seen in one further child, and a case of Down's syndrome was recorded in a child whose mother had had only a diagnostic radiograph.

Although there are faults in this early study, it clearly established the importance of high-dose irradiation in the production of microcephaly and mental retardation, an association unhappily confirmed at Hiroshima and Nagasaki, where Blot and Miller (1973) found that children irradiated in utero had an increased chance of being microcephalic or retarded, or both. Many isolated reports have been well reviewed by Brent (1977).

It will be evident that therapeutic radiation has usually been given in ignorance of pregnancy (e.g. in ankylosing spondylitis) and reports of this are now, happily, rare. There appears to be no evidence to suggest that present levels of diagnostic irradiation are associated with an increased frequency of congenital defects (see Anonymous 1981), and its role in oncogenesis in childhood is also uncertain (see p. 900).

Cytotoxic Drugs

Following the early reports of abnormalities induced by a folic acid antagonist (Thiersch 1952), a number of experimental studies have confirmed the expected teratogenicity of cytotoxic compounds. These studies have been ably reviewed by Connors (1975). Methotrexate, azathioprine and cyclophosphamide are all teratogenic in animals and might be administered to pregnant women. In general, however, such compounds are not given in pregnancy unless for compelling clinical reasons such as malignant disease in the mother. The few data available suggest that early treatment at high doses usually results in abortion rather than the production of a live child with malformations. A report of myeloschisis in a leukaemic woman treated with busulphan was published by Abramovici et al. (1978). Studies of a group of young people successfully treated for lymphoma by mustine, vinblastine, procarbazine and prednisolone have been reported (King et al. 1985). Men were rendered permanently azoospermic, but about half the women were fertile after therapy. From this and other studies it is likely that infertility in males will be the major human reproductive problem associated with cytotoxic drug therapy, although other regimens may be less destructive. Men with testicular cancer may produce normal children after chemotherapy: 30 were reported born to 25 such men in the report of Senturia et al. (1985).

Thalidomide

The details of the Thalidomide incident are now well documented. The general morphological features are shown in Table 2.8 and the compound will not be considered in detail here. Later reports of the affected children (Stephenson 1976) suggest that a greater degree of central nervous system damage may have occurred than was first thought. A review by Quibell (1981) outlines the difficulties experienced after 20 years by 389 survivors of the Thalidomide Trust's beneficiaries, and an up-to-date and comprehensive account of the syndrome is found in Newman (1985).

Table 2.8. Abnormalities in thalidomide-affected children

Defects of the upper limbs
1. Amelia – arm absent
2. Short phocomelia – flipper only present
3. Long phocomelia – humerus and ulna both present but short
4. Short forearm – upper arm normal
5. Radial aplasia – normal ulna or hypoplasia
6. Absence of radial digits
7. Hypoplasia of thumb or thenar muscles or both
8. Triphalangeal thumb

Defects of the lower limbs
1. Phocomelia– rudimentary bone present between pelvis and foot
2. Femoral hypoplasia – lower limb normal
3. Deformities of tibia and/or fibula
4. Deformities of feet only
5. Congenital dislocation of the hip

Defects of internal organs
1. Congenital heart disease
2. Anomalies of the kidneys
3. Anomalies of the alimentary tract
4. Choanal atresia

Defects of the eyes and ears
1. Anotia – absence of the pinna
2. Microtia – small deformed pinna
3. Facial palsy – may be associated with 1 and 2.
4. External ophthalmoplegia – may be associated with 3
5. Anophthalmos
6. Microphthalmos
7. Coloboma

Thalidomide is perhaps the best example to date of the effects of chirality on toxicity: only the L form is teratogenic.

Warfarin

In 1966 Di Saia described a female infant with bilateral optic atrophy, mental retardation and nasal malformation, born to a mother with a history of ingestion of several drugs during pregnancy, includ-ing warfarin. Further reports (Kerber et al. 1968), including a follow-up of the original case (Becker et al. 1975), resulted in the identification of further characteristics of the syndrome and retrospective reviews of many cases (see Warkany 1976 for a bibliography).

In general, the anticoagulant has been given to women with prosthetic heart valves during pregnancy or to those suffering from deep vein thrombosis. The majority of infants born to women treated in this way are normal, but abnormalities found include nasal malformations (hypoplasia of the nasal bridge, choanal stenosis), optic atrophy, microcephaly and mental retardation, hypotonia, and, in one instance, agenesis of the corpus callosum (Holzgreve et al. 1976). A distinctive finding is the so-called stippled epiphysis, a change resembling Conradi–Hünermann disease or chondrodystrophia congenita calcificans. Discrete punctate areas of calcification are seen in the epiphyses of long bones, and are thought to be the result of local haemorrhage.

Hall et al. (1980) suggest that heparin also has serious effects and that it should not be simply regarded as a reassuring alternative. However, the adverse outcomes of pregnancy associated with heparin are not related to maldevelopment; adverse pregnancy outcome is common in this group of patients and is compounded by a haemorrhagic tendency.

Alcohol

Warnings about the effects of alcohol on development have been given since biblical times (Judges 13:7), but despite an interesting description of the offspring of alcoholic mothers in a report of a Select Committee of the House of Commons (Select Committee on Drunkenness 1834) the syndrome now associated with excessive alcohol intake in pregnancy was not recognized until the observations of Lemoine et al. (1968) and Jones et al. (1973). The specific syndrome is well documented, and various studies have shown that the frequent abuse of other drugs by alcoholics are not central to its production. The various estimates of the frequency of the condition vary widely, as do the criteria used to define the syndrome. A study in Belfast suggests an incidence of 1.7 per 1000 births there (Halliday et al. 1982).

The features of the syndrome are as shown in Table 2.9. In addition to these features, the babies are light and their linear growth rate and average weight gain are both greatly reduced despite adequate caloric intakes. Catch-up growth does not occur. Histopathological study of the brain shows altered neuronal and glial migration with cerebellar dysplasia and heterotopic cell clusters on the surface of the brain (Clarren et al. 1978).

Table 2.9. Fetal and alcohol syndrome

Growth	Below 2 SD from mean, adipose tissue disproportionally affected
Central nervous system	Microcephaly, hypotonia, mental retardation
	May be irritable or hyperactive infants
Heart	Atrial septal defects common
Facies	Short palpebral fissures – may be ptosis, epicanthic folds prominent
Nose	Short and up-turned
Mouth	Thinned vermillion border of upper lip, diminished philtrum

The effects of non-alcoholic patterns of alcohol ingestion on the outcome of pregnancy have not yet been shown to be harmful, although a vigorous debate continues (Anonymous 1983; English and Bower 1983).

There is also controversy about the effect of binge or sporadic drinking, which appears to be dangerous experimentally if high blood levels are reached (Berry and Stuckey 1984). The same work suggests that considerable variation in the response to alcohol of different human populations may be expected.

Anticonvulsants

Meadow's report (1968) was the first to associate congenital abnormalities and anticonvulsants when he described six infants with cleft lip and palate and certain other anomalies born to mothers taking these compounds during pregnancy. Janz and Fuchs (1964) had previously reported five malformations (including three cases of cleft lip and palate) in 225 epileptic mothers taking anticonvulsants, but concluded that the difference between their study group and controls was not significant. Smithells (1976), in reviewing the many studies that have followed these observations, concluded that there is a real association between the drugs and malformation, that it is drug ingestion rather than the epileptic condition that is critical, that phenytoin is more teratogenic than phenobarbitone, and that the two combined are more teratogenic than either alone. Individuals developing malformations are more likely to have a defect in arene oxide detoxification; these compounds are reactive intermediates in phenytoin metabolism (see Strickler et al. 1985). Primidone is largely metabolized to phenobarbitone in the body, and probably has similar effects. In infants born to treated epileptic

mothers the incidence of cleft lip and palate is about 12 times, and that of congenital heart disease about three times, that in the general population. Phalangeal hypoplasia (mainly the terminal phalanx) and hypoplasia of the fingernails and toenails may also occur. Facial abnormalities, including a short nose with a broad depressed bridge and prominent epicanthic folds, have also been described (Hanson 1976).

Speidel and Meadow (1974) pointed out that defects have been reported in association with other anticonvulsants, but a specific trimethadione syndrome has been identified by Goldman and Yaffe (1978), which differs from that described above in the presence of V-shaped eyebrows and low-set ears with an anteriorly folded helix. Phalangeal hypoplasia does not occur. Sodium valproate (valproic acid) has been found to be associated with an increase in the incidence of spina bifida in children whose mothers had used the compound during pregnancy (see reports summarized in Anonymous 1982b).

The data are affected by many of the common problems that affect human studies; for example, two of the nine cases reported from France had family histories of neural tube defects and there is the problem of multiple anticonvulsant drug use (features of other anticonvulsant drug syndromes have been included in the reports). An Italian group has questioned the strength of the association (Mastroiacovo et al. 1983) on the basis of a birth defect registry study. However, a careful review by Lammer et al. (1987) confirmed an association of valproate exposure and spina bifida; they gave figures of a 1%–2% absolute risk (around the spontaneous occurrence rate). No increase in malformations of other systems was found.

Vitamin A and Analogues

Although there is a good deal of data showing teratogenic effects of retinol in animals, at doses that are high in terms of human equivalents, it is only comparatively recently that human anomalies have been reported in women taking these compounds for skin disease. Relevant compounds are vitamin A alcohol (retinol), retinoic acid (tretinoin when in the all-*trans* form), a synthetic aromatic derivative of the acid (Tigason) and isotretinoin (13-*cis*-retinoic acid).

These compounds may be prescribed by dermatologists for acne and psoriasis, and warnings are given about their use when pregnancy is possible.

A review of human data is given by Lammer et al. (1985). Of 154 exposed pregnancies, 95 were electively terminated. There were 12 abortions in the remaining 59 pregnancies and, of the 47 continuing, three ended in stillbirths with anomalies, 18 in abnormal live births and 26 in normal live births. Microtia and/or microphthalmia, external auditory meatus atresia and microcephaly occur as specific associations, and dilatation of the ventricular system was also found.

As with most other human teratogens, however, there are clear instances of exposure without effect. Kassis et al. (1985) report a normal child born after exposure of the mother to isotretinoin (Accutane) for 6 months before conception and for the first 8 weeks of pregnancy. A useful review is that of Rosa et al. (1986).

In 1993 the Department of Health in the United Kingdom issued advice to pregnant women on the consumption of Vitamin A in pregnancy, warning of the dangers of over-provision from supplements and liver.

Penicillamine

Other compounds may act in a similar fashion to warfarin, i.e. having a predictable effect on the fetus from the pharmacological effects on the maternofetal unit as a whole. This chelating agent is used in Wilson's disease, scleroderma, rheumatoid disease and autoimmune disorders. Many normal pregnancies have been reported after penicillamine use, but also five cases of cutis laxa with skin laxity, hyperextensible joints and reduction of elastic tissue in skin biopsies (see Rosa 1986 for a review).

Methylmercury Compounds

The effects of the release of organic mercury compounds into Minamata Bay in the 1960s were manifest in the subsequent birth of children with cerebral palsy and mental retardation to mothers who had ingested heavily contaminated shellfish from the bay. Following a disastrous outbreak of methylmercury poisoning in rural Iraq in 1972 due to the ingestion of home-made bread made from wheat treated with a methylmercury fungicide, it has been found that methylmercury passes readily from mother to fetus and may also be transmitted via breast milk. Gross impairment of motor and mental development has occurred in some individuals (Amin-Zaki et al. 1974).

Although methylmercury is not teratogenic in the sense of producing congenital anomalies of the type formally defined at the beginning of this chapter, neuropathological changes have been found to occur in affected individuals (Matsumoto et al. 1965).

Hyperthermia

From the experimental work of a number of authors, notably Edwards (see review by Edwards and Wanner 1977), it is evident that short periods of hyperthermia are teratogenic in animals. Other studies have suggested that this may also be true in humans (Miller et al. 1978), although serious reservations have been expressed about most of the reported observations (Leck 1978).

The Operating Room Environment

There is evidence to support the contention that spontaneous abortion rates are higher than normal in women working in surgical theatres (see Smithells 1976 for a bibliography). Data for malformation rates are not convincing, however; skin naevi, malabsorption syndrome and hernias have been included as malformations in some series (Corbett et al. 1974). No prospective study has been reported to date.

Smoking

Simpson (1957) first drew attention to the problems of smoking in pregnancy in a preliminary report. The general conclusions that can be drawn from the many publications on the subject since are that smokers' babies weigh between 150 and 250 g less than those of non-smokers, and that twice as many infants under 2500 g are born to smokers. There is a direct relationship between the number of cigarettes smoked and the reduction in weight, and this reduction is independent of other infant and maternal factors known to influence birth weight (Meyer et al. 1976).

These effects have been accompanied by an increasing awareness of the effects of smoking in early pregnancy, where in the study of Boué et al. (1975) it was found that 50% of the fetuses aborted by mothers who smoked and inhaled had normal karyotypes, suggesting an enhanced loss of normal conceptuses in these individuals. From the large Ontario Perinatal Mortality Study (1967) it is evident that after controlling for a number of variables (maternal height, weight, birthplace, age, parity, etc.) smoking less than one packet of cigarettes a day increased perinatal mortality by 20%; this increase rose to 35% for those smoking more than one packet. Increased risk of in utero death in the 20- to 28-week period and deaths in premature infants born in this period were associated with increases in the rate of placenta praevia and abruptio placentae. (See Fielding 1978 for a bibliography.)

A detailed and comprehensive review of the literature has been made by Sidle and published by the Spastics Society (Sidle 1982).

Diabetes Mellitus and Malformation

There have been a number of large studies on the outcome of diabetic pregnancies, and a generally accepted view is that malformations involving all systems occur more frequently in the children of diabetic mothers (see Mills et al. 1979), probably at around twice the normal frequency. The defects are of the type that develop in the first 7 weeks of gestation, which is interesting in view of the poor early growth of the diabetic conceptus (Pedersen and Molsted-Pedersen 1981), which may be an important factor in pathogenesis. A number of positive assertions can be made: diabetic fathers do not have an increased incidence of abnormal offspring; prediabetic women are not at increased risk of producing abnormal infants; and women with gestational diabetes and those controlled by oral hypoglycaemic agents also appear to follow natural population trends for abnormality.

A specific association is found in the caudal regression syndrome (agenesis or hypoplasia of the femorae with agenesis of lower vertebrae), for which the relative risk for infants of diabetic mothers is over 200. No other specific findings occur.

Insulin is not involved in the pathogenesis per se: it does not cross the placenta until well after the sensitive developmental period and is not produced by the fetus in the first 8 weeks of gestation (Like and Orci 1972). Metabolic disturbances of complex growth patterns are a possible cause of the increase in a wide spectrum of anomalies.

Using modern non-invasive techniques, the Pedersens have confirmed their earlier suggestion that early growth retardation is critical in the causation of malformations in diabetic conceptuses (Pedersen and Molsted-Pedersen 1991; Pedersen 1992).

Infectious Causes of Abnormal Development

Rubella

Maternal rubella infection has been associated with fetal infection rates of approximately 90% in the first 8–10 weeks in some series (Rawles et al. 1968), and on the basis of this fact and other data the number of abnormal fetuses produced suggests that some are infected without damage. Fetal infection may not occur when the mother is affected, although this pattern of events probably does not occur until after 16 weeks' gestation. In a study of 1016 women with confirmed rubella infection at different stages of pregnancy, Miller et al. (1982) found that congenital infection rates were 80% in the first 12 weeks, 54% at 13–14 weeks and 25% at the end of the second trimester.

In most developed countries where there is no programme of mass immunization 5%–20% of the population between 15 and 35 years is at risk of infection. This figure varies from 25% to 70% in developing countries, despite the endemic nature of the disease. This unexpected pattern is not seen in South America, where figures for susceptibles are similar to or lower than those found in the USA, owing to a high rate of prepubertal infection.

Fetal rubella may be associated both with congenital malformations and with chronic infection that persists for months or years after birth. Rubella virus may be isolated from an abortus, from the placenta or amniotic fluid, and from most viscera. In the live-born child the virus can be recovered from the throat, urine, meconium, and conjunctival and cerebrospinal fluids. Reports of positive culture from cataract material, liver biopsies and ductal tissue have also been made.

The features of congenital rubella include a general failure of growth (manifest both before and after birth), eye changes (cataracts, usually bilateral, microphthalmia, pigmentary retinopathy), central nervous system changes (microcephaly, retardation, progressive panencephalitis), congenital heart disease (patent ductus arteriosus, pulmonary artery lesions including localized stenosis and hypoplasia, aortic stenosis, ventricular septal defects, Fallot's tetralogy, myocarditis), defects of hearing, hepatitis, interstitial pneumonitis, a chronic rash and persistent lymphadenopathy. Bone changes may also occur.

The pathological findings have been described in detail by Singer et al. (1967) and Driscoll (1969). (See also pp. 171, 737).

Congenital Syphilis

Although adequate antenatal care should prevent congenital syphilis, recent increases in its frequency in several countries should alert pathologists to the possibility of the diagnosis. The risk to the fetus depends on the stage of the disease in the mother. If primary or secondary syphilis is untreated, half of the infants are stillborn, premature or die as neonates, and survivors are almost invariably affected. In early latent syphilis 20%–60% of infants are normal, 20% premature and 16% stillborn, 4% die as neonates and 40% have congenital syphilis (Fiumara et al. 1952). The manifestations are protean, and range from hydrops with hepatosplenomegaly and haemolytic anaemia, periostitis, and meningitis to those defects identified in childhood, namely interstitial keratitis, eighth-nerve deafness, bony defects (abnormal teeth, saddle nose, frontal bossing), cutaneous lesions and hepatic fibrosis.

Toxoplasmosis

Infection with *Toxoplasma gondii* is said to occur in half the population of the USA (Krick and Remington 1978), and may be responsible for up to 3000 abnormal births per year there. The infection is a zoonosis, members of the cat family being the definitive hosts.

Congenital toxoplasmosis occurs when a previously uninfected woman is infected during pregnancy. The protozoans are then transmitted across the placenta to the fetus, where they cause multiple lesions in many organs. Early reports emphasized the importance of central nervous system involvement with the production of microcephalus, hydrocephalus, microphthalmus and chorioretinitis. Periventricular calcification was considered to be a specific feature (see p. 172). More recently it has been realized that newborn infants with active disease may have fever, convulsions, maculopapular skin rash, lymphadenopathy, hepatosplenomegaly, icterus and thrombocytopenia. Such symptoms are associated with a 40% mortality rate. As with other infections, early (first-trimester) infections are associated with the most tissue damage. An immunohistochemical method exists for the identification of the organism in sections (Conley et al. 1981).

Cytomegalovirus Infection

Infection by cytomegalovirus (CMV) (see also pp. 739–741) is probably the commonest viral infection of the human fetus, occurring in 4–10 infants per 1000 births (Dudgeon 1976). Congenital abnormalities occur less frequently in this disease than in rubella, with central nervous system involvement a major feature. A classic presentation in the newborn is with hepatosplenomegaly, jaundice and petechial haemorrhages (often with thrombocytopenia). This picture is not incompatible with recovery, but if respiratory or central nervous system involvement is evident the prognosis is worsened. A destructive

encephalitis with calcification may occur; microcephaly is sometimes evident, and fits and spasticity may develop.

It is generally assumed that infection occurs following maternal infection in early pregnancy, but this is uncertain and many women carry the virus in the cervix. It has been shown that placental infection without involvement of the fetus may occur.

Other Virus Infections

Isolated cases of malformation associated with herpes simplex virus have been reported, usually involving the central nervous system. In one instance HSV has been isolated from the cerebrospinal fluid. Microcephaly, cerebral calcification, microphthalmia and skin rashes have all been reported (South et al. 1969).

Evidence for the association of mumps or enterovirus infections is not good. Similarly, despite extensive studies, no convincing association of influenza and subsequent malformation has been demonstrated (Dudgeon 1976). A detailed account of other fetal viral infections is found in Remington and Klein (1983).

Paternal Effects of Teratogens

Despite concern expressed mainly on the basis of animal experiments, the data for men are reassuring from the point of view of teratogenesis as opposed to fertility (see p. 57). There are no compounds which produce transmissible genetic changes responsible for congenital defects in humans.

References

Abramovici A, Shaklai M, Pinkhas J (1978) Myeloschisis in a six weeks embryo of a leukaemic woman treated by busulphan. Teratology 18: 241

Adams JC, Watt FM (1993) Regulation of development and differentiation by the extracellular matrix. Development 117: 1183

Alberts B, Bray D, Lewis J, Raff M, Roberts K, Watson JD (1989) Molecular biology and the cell, 2nd edn. Garland Publishing, London

Amin-Zaki L, Elhassani S. Majeed MA, Clarkson TW, Doherty RA, Greenwood M (1974) Intrauterine methylmercury poisoning in Iraq. Pediatrics 54: 587

Anonymous (1981) Imaging techniques in obstetrics. Lancet i: 923

Anonymous (1982a) Vitamins to prevent neural tube defects. Lancet ii: 1255

Anonymous (1982b) Valproate and malformations. Lancet ii: 1313

Anonymous (1983) Alcohol and the fetus: is zero the only option? Lancet i: 682

Bear JC (1978) The association of sex ratio anomalies with pyeloric stenosis. Teratology 17: 19

Becker MH, Genieser NB, Finegold M, Miranda D, Spackman T (1975) Chondrodysplasia punctata: is maternal warfarin therapy a factor? Am J Dis Child 129: 356

Berry CL (1992) What's in a homebox? The development of pattern during embryonic growth. Virchows Arch [A] 420: 291

Berry CL (1994a) The molecular basis of development. In: Kirkham N, Hall P (eds) Progress in pathology. Churchill Livingstone, Edinburgh, Madrid, Melbourne, New York, Tokyo, pp 121–132

Berry CL (1994b) Building an embryo with limited resources. In: Anichkov N (ed) Current topics in histology and pathology: scientific papers. Russian Division of Internal Academy of Pathology, St Petersburg pp 9–25

Berry CL, Stuckey E (1984) The effects of high dose sporadic (binge) alcohol intake in mice. J Pathol 142: 175

Blot WJ, Miller RW (1973) Mental retardation following in utero exposure to the atomic bombs of Hiroshima and Nagasaki. Radiology 106: 617

Boué J, Boué A, Lazar P (1975) Retrospective epidemiological studies of 1500 karyotyped spontaneous human abortions. Teratology 12: 11

Boué J, Phillipe E, Giroud A, Boué A (1976) Phenotypic expression of lethal chromosome anomalies in human abortuses. Teratology 14: 3

Brent RL (1977) Radiation and other physical agents. In: Wilson JG, Clarke Fraser F (eds) General principles and etiology. Plenum Press, New York (Handbook of teratology, vol I, p 153)

Carter CO (1965) The inheritance of common congenital malformations. Prog Med Genet 4: 59

Carter CO (1969) Genetics of common disorders. Br Med Bull 25: 52

Carter CO (1976) Genetics of common single malformations. Br Med Bull 32: 21

Carter CO, Evans K (1973) Spina bifida and anencephalus in Greater London. J Med Genet 10: 209

Carter CO, Wilkinson JA (1964) Genetic and environmental factors in the aetiology of congenital dislocation of the hip. Clin Orthop 33: 119

Carter CO, David PA, Laurence KM (1968) A family study of major central nervous system malformations in South Wales. J Med Genet 5: 81

Ching GHS, Chung CS (1974) A genetic study of cleft lip and palate in Hawaii. I. Interracial crosses. Am J Hum Genet 26: 162

Ching GHS, Chung CS, Nemechek RW (1969) Genetic and epidemiological studies of clubfoot in Hawaii: ascertainment and incidence. Am J Hum Genet 21: 566

Chung CS, Myrianthopolus NC (1968) Racial and prenatal factors in major congenital malformations. Am J Hum Genet 20: 44

Clarren SK, Alvord EC, Sumi SM (1978) Brain malformations related to prenatal exposure to ethanol. J Pediatr 92: 64

Conley FK, Jenkins Kay A, Remington JS (1981) Toxoplasma gondii infection of the central nervous system. Use of the peroxidase – antiperoxidase method to demonstrate Toxoplasma in formalin fixed, paraffin embedded tissue sections. Hum Pathol 12: 690

Connors TA (1975) Cylotoxic agents in teratogenic research. In: Berry CL, Poswillo DE (eds) Teratology: trends and applications. Springer, New York, p 49

Corbett TH, Cornell RG, Endres JL, Weding K (1974) Birth defects among children of nurse – anesthetists. Anesthesiology 41: 341

Di Saia J (1966) Pregnancy and delivery of a patient with a Starr – Edwards mitral valve prosthesis. Report of a case. Obstet Gynecol 28: 469

Dodge JA (1971) Abnormal distribution of ABO blood groups in infantile pyloric stenosis. J Med Genet 8: 468

Dodge JA (1973) Infantile pyloric stenosis. Inheritance, psyche and soma. Ir J Med Sci 142: 6

Driscoll SG (1969) Histopathology of gestational rubella. Am J Dis Child 118: 49

Dudgeon JA (1976) Infective causes of human malformations. Br Med Bull 32: 77

Dunn PM (1976) Congenital postural deformities. Br Med Bull 32: 71

Edwards JH (1958) Congenital malformations of the central nervous system in Scotland. Br J Prev Soc Med 12: 115

Edwards JH (1969) Familial predisposition in man. Br Med Bull 25: 58

Edwards MJ, Wanner RA (1977) Extremes of temperature. In: Wilson JG, Clarke Fraser F (eds) General principles and etiology, Plenum Press, New York (Handbook of teratology, vol I, p 421)

Eiben I, Bartels I, Barr-Porsch S, Borgmann S, Gatz G, Gellert G, Gobel R, Hammans W, Hentemann M, Osmers R, Raauskolb R, Hasmann I (1990) Cytogenic analysis of 750 spontaneous abortions with the direct preparation method of chorionic villi and its implications for studying genetic causes of pregnancy wastage. Am J Hum Genet 47: 656

English D, Bower C (1983) Alcohol consumption, pregnancy, and low birth weight. Lancet i: 1111

Falconer DS (1965) The inheritance of liability to certain diseases, estimated from the incidence among relatives. Ann Hum Genet 29: 51

Fedrick J (1976) Anencephalus in Scotland 1961–1972. Br J Prev Soc Med 30: 132

Fedrick J, Alberman ED, Goldstein H (1971) Possible teratogenic effect of cigarette smoking. Nature 231: 529

Ferencz C, Rubin JD, McCarter RJ, Boughman JA, Wilson PD, Brenner JI, Neill CA, Perry LW, Hepner SI, Downing JW (1987) Cardiac and non-cardiac malformations: observations in a population based study. Teratology 35: 367

Fergusson-Smith MA, Yates JRW (1984) Maternal age specific rates for chromosome aberrations and factors influencing them: report of a collaborative European study on 52,965 amniocenteses. Prenat Diagn 4: 5

Fielding JE (1978) Smoking and pregnancy. N Engl J Med 298: 337

Fiumara NJ, Flemming WL, Downing JG, Good FL (1952) The incidence of prenatal syphilis at the Boston City Hospital. N Engl J Med 247: 48

Fraser FC, Pashayan H (1970) Relation of face shape to susceptibility to congenital cleft lip. A preliminary case report. J Med Genet 7: 112

Gilbert SF (1992) Developmental biology, 3rd edn. Sinauer Associates, Sunderland, Massachusetts

Gilbert EF, Opitz JM (1982) Developmental and other pathologic changes in syndromes caused by chromosome abnormalities. Perspect Pediatr Pathol 7: 1

Goldman AS, Yaffe SJ (1978) Fetal trimethadione syndrome. Teratology 17:103

Gropp A (1973) Fetal mortality due to aneuploidy and irregular meiotic segregation in the mouse. In: Boué A, Thibault C (eds) Les accidents chromosomiques de la reproduction. INSERM, Paris, p 255

Hall JG, Pauli RM, Wilson KM (1980) Maternal and fetal sequelae of anticoagulation during pregnancy. Am J Med 68: 122

Halliday H, Reid MMc, McClure G (1982) Results of heavy drinking in pregnancy. Br J Obstet Gynaecol 89: 892

Hanson JWM (1976) Fetal hydantoin syndrome. Teratology 13: 185

Hay S, Barbano SH (1972) Independent effects of maternal age and birth order on the incidence of selected congenital malformations. Teratology 6: 271

Hay S, Wehring DA (1970) Congenital malformations in twins. Am J Hum Genet 22: 622

Holt SB (1961) Quantitative genetics of finger-print patterns. Br Med Bull 17(3): 247

Holzgreve W, Garey JC, Hall BD (1976) Warfarin-induced fetal abnormalities. Lancet ii: 914

Janz D, Fuchs U (1964) Sind antiepileptische Medikamente während der Schwangerschaft schädlich? Dtsch Med Wochenschr 89: 241

Jones KL, Smith DW, Ulleland CB, Streissguth AP (1973) Pattern of malformation in offspring of chronic alcoholic mothers. Lancet i: 1267

Kajii T, Chama K, Nukawa N, Ferrier A, Avirachan S (1973) Banding analysis of chromosomal karyotpyes in spontaneous abortion. Am J Hum Genet 25: 539

Kassis I, Sunderji S, Abdul-Karim R (1985) Isotretinoin (Accutane) and pregnancy. Teratology 32: 145

Kenna AP, Smithells RW, Fielding DW (1975) Congenital heart disease in Liverpool 1960–1969. Q J Med 44 (173): 17

Kerber IJ, Warr OS, Richardson CJ (1968) Pregnancy in a patient with a prosthetic mitral valve. Association with a fetal anomaly attributed to warfarin sodium. JAMA 203: 223

King DJ, Ratcliffe MA, Dawson AA, Bennett JE, Klopper AL (1985) Fertility in young men and women after treatment for lymphoma: a study of a population. J Clin Pathol 38: 1247

Kinoshita M, Nakamura Y, Nakano R, Morimatsu M, Fukuda S, Nishimi Y, Hashimoto T (1989) Thirty-one autopsy cases of trisomy 18: clinical features and pathological findings. Pediatr Pathol 9: 445

Klein J, Stein Z (1985) Very early pregnancy. In: Dixon R (ed) Reproductive toxicology. Raven Press, New York, p 251

Knox G, Braithwaite F (1962) Cleft lip and palates in Northumberland and Durham. Arch Dis Child 38: 66

Krick JA, Remington JS (1978) Toxoplasmosis in the adult, an overview. JAMA 298: 550

Kurisu K, Niswander JD, Johnston MC, Maxaheri M (1974) Facial morphology as an indicator of genetic predisposition to cleft lip and palate. Am J Hum Genet 26: 703

Lammer EJ, Chen DT, Hoar RM, Agnish ND, Benke PJ, Braun JT, Curry CJ, Fernhoff PM, Grix AW, Lott IT, Richard JM, Sun SC (1985) Retinoic acid embryopathy. N Engl J Med 313: 837

Lammer EJ, Sever LE, Oakley GP (1987) Teratogen update: valproic acid. Teratology 35: 465

Laurence KM (1963) Hypertrophic pyloric stenosis. Lancet i: 224

Leck I (1972) The etiology of human malformations. Insights from epidemiology. Teratology 5: 303

Leck I (1974) Causation of neural tube defects: clues from epidemiology. Br Med Bull 30: 158

Leck I (1976) Descriptive epidemiology of common malformations (excluding central nervous system defects). Br Med Bull 32: 45

Leck I (1978) Maternal hyperthermia and anencephaly. Lancet i: 671

Lemoine P, Harousseau H, Borteyni JP (1968) Les enfants de parents alcooliques: anomalies observées. Quest Med 25: 476

Like A, Orci L (1972) Embryogenesis of the human pancreatic islets. A light and electronmicroscopic study. Diabetes 21: 511

Lilienfeld AM (1969) Population differences in frequency of malformation at birth. In: Fraser FC, McKusick VA (eds) Congenital malformations. Proceedings of the Third International Congress. Exerpta Medica, Amsterdam, p 251

Lloyd-Davies RW (1963) Hypertrophic pyloric stenosis. Lancet i: 110

Lowe CR (1972) Congenital malformations and the problems of their control. Br Med J 3: 515

Machin GA (1974) Chromosome abnormality and perinatal death. Lancet i: 594

Mastroiacovo P, Bertollini R, Morandini S, Segni G (1983) Maternal epilepsy, valproate exposure, and birth defects. Lancet ii: 1499

Matsumoto H, Koya G, Takeuchi T (1965) Fetal minamata disease. A neuropathological study of two cases of intrauterine intoxication by a methylmercury compound. J Neuropathol Exp Neurol 24: 563

McKeown T, Record RC (1960) Malformations in a population observed for five years after birth. In: Wolstenholme GEW, O'Connor CM (eds) Ciba Foundation Symposium on Congenital Malformations. Churchill, London, p 2

Meadow SR (1968) Anticonvulsant drugs and congenital abnormalities. Lancet ii: 1269

Meyer MB, Jonas BS, Tonascia JA (1976) Perinatal events associated with maternal smoking during pregnancy. Am J Epidemiol 103: 464

Miller P, Smith DW, Shepard TH (1978) Maternal hyperthermia as a possible cause of anencephaly. Lancet i: 519

Miller EM, Cradock-Wilson JE, Pollock TM (1982) Consequences of confirmed maternal rubella at successive stages of pregnancy. Lancet ii: 781

Mills JL, Baker L, Goldman AS (1979) Malformations in the children of diabetic mothers occur before the seventh gestational week. Diabetes 28: 292

Mitchell SC, Sellman AH, Westphal MC, Park J (1971) Etiologic correlates in a study of congenital heart disease in 56,109 births. Am J Cardiol 28: 653

MRC Vitamin Study Research Group (1991) Prevention of neural tube defects: results of the Medical Research Council vitamin study. Lancet 338: 131

Murphy DP (1929) The outcome of 625 pregnancies in women subjected to pelvic radium or roentgen irradiation. Am J Obstet Gynecol 18: 179

Naggan L (1971) Anencephaly and spina bifida in Israel. Pediatrics 47: 577

Nakamura Y, Hashimoto T, Sasaguri Y (1986) Brain anomalies found in 18 trisomy: CT scanning, morphologic and morphometric study. Clin Neuropathol 5: 47

Neel JV (1974) A note on congenital defects in two unacculturated Indian tribes. In: Janerick DT, Skalko RG, Porter IH (eds) Congenital defects, new directions in research. Academic Press, New York, p 3

Newman CGH (1985) Clinical aspects of thalidomide embryopathy – a continuing preoccupation. Teratology 32: 133

Nishimura H (1970) Incidence of malformations in abortions. In: Fraser FC, McKusick A (eds) Congenital malformations. Proceedings of the Third International Congress. Exerpta Medica, Amsterdam, p 275

Ontario Perinatal Study Committee (1967) Second report of the perinatal mortality study in ten university teaching hospitals, vol I. Ontario Department of Health, Toronto

Owens JR, McAllister E, Harris F. West L (1981) 19 year incidence of neural tube defects in an area under constant surveillance. Lancet ii: 1032

Pedersen JF (1992) Fetal crown–rump length measurement by ultrasound in normal pregnancy. Br J Obstet Gynaecol 89: 926

Pedersen JF, Molsted-Pedersen L (1991) Early fetal growth delay detected by ultrasound marks increased risk of congenital malformation in diabetic pregnancy. Br Med J 238: 269

Peñaloza D, Arias-Stella J, Sime F, Recavarren S, Marticorena E (1964) The heart and pulmonary circulation in children at high altitudes: physiological, anatomical and clinical observations. Pediatrics 34: 568

Powell BW (1962) Hypertrophic pyloric stenosis. Lancet ii: 1326

Quibell EP (1981) The thalidomide embryopathy. Practioner 225: 721

Rawles WE, Desmyter J, Melnick JL (1968) Serological diagnosis and fetal involvement in maternal rubella. Criteria for abortions. JAMA 203: 627

Remington JS, Klein JO (1983) Infectious diseases of the fetus and newborn infant. Saunders, Philadelphia

Richards IDG, Roberts CJ, Lloyd S (1972) Dolichol phosphates as acceptors of manrose from guanosine diphosphate manrose in liver systems. Br J Prev Soc Med 26: 89

Roberts CJ, Lowe CR (1975) Where have all the conceptions gone? Lancet i: 498

Rogers SC, Morris M (1973) Anencephalus: a changing sex ratio. Br J Prev Soc Med 27: 81

Rosa FW (1986) Teratogen update: penicillamine. Teratology 33: 127

Rosa FW, Wilk AL, Kelsey FO (1986) Teratogen update: vitamin A congeners. Teratology 33: 355

Saxen I (1975) Epidemiology of cleft lip and palate. An attempt to rule out chance correlations. Br J Prev Soc Med 29: 103

Select Committee on Drunkenness (1834) Report on drunkenness presented to the House of Commons

Senturia YD, Peckham CS, Peckham MJ (1985) Children fathered by men treated for testicular cancer. Lancet ii: 766

Sever L, Lynberg MC, Edmonds LD (1993) The impact of congenital malformations on public health. Teratology 48: 547

Shepard TH, Fantel AG, Fitzsimmonds J (1989) Congenital defect rates among spontaneous abortuses: twenty years of monitoring. 39: 325

Shiota K, Uwabe C, Nishimura H (1987) High prevalence of defective human embryos at the early post-implantation period. Teratology 35: 309

Sidle N (1982) Smoking and pregnancy – a review.Spastics Society, London

Simpson WJA (1957) A preliminary report on cigarette smoking and the incidence of prematurity. Am J Obstet Gynecol 73: 808

Singer DB, Rudolph AJ, Rosenberg HS, Rawles WE, Noniuk M (1967) Pathology of the congenital rubella syndrome. J Pediatr 71: 665

Smithells RW (1973) Defects and disabilities of thalidomide children. Br Med J i: 269

Smithells RW (1976) Environmental teratogens of man. Br Med Bull 32: 27

Smithells RW, Sheppard S (1978) Teratogenicity testing in humans. A method demonstrating safety of Bendectin. Teratology 17: 31

Smithells RW, Sheppard S. Schorah CJ, Seller MJ, Nevin CN, Harris R, Read AP, Fielding DW (1981) Apparent prevention of neural tube defects by periconceptional vitamin supplementation. Arch Dis Child 56: 911

South MA, Tompkins WAF, Morris CR, Rawles WE (1969) Congenital malformation of the central nervous system associated with genital type (type 2) herpesvirus. J Pediatr 75: 13

Speidel BD, Meadow SR (1974) Epilepsy, anticonvulsants and congenital malformations. Drugs 8: 354

Stephenson JBP (1976) Epilepsy: a neurological complication of thalidomide embryopathy. Dev Med Child Neurol 18: 189

Strickler SM, Miller MA, Andermann E, Dansky LV, Seni M-H, Spielberg SP (1985) Genetic predisposition to phenytoin-induced birth defects. Lancet ii: 746

Terrible V, Pertile G (1975) Congenital heart disease risk during pregnancy. Lancet ii: 1981

Therkelsen AJ, Grunnet N, Hjort T, Myhre O, Jensen J, Jonasson J, Lauritson JG, Lindsten B, Petersen B (1974) Studies on spontaneous abortions. In: Boué A, Thibault C (eds) Chromosomal errors in relation to reproductive failure. INSERM, Paris

Thiersch JB (1952) Therapeutic abortions with a folic acid antagonist, 4-aminopterolyglutamic acid (4-amino-PGA). Am J Obstet Gynecol 63: 1298

van Lijnschoten G, Arends JW, Leffers P, de la Fuente AA, van der Looij HJ, Geraedts JP (1993) The value of histomorphological features of chorionic villi in early spontaneous abortion for the prediction of karyotype. Histopathology 22: 557

Warburton D, Stein Z, Kline J, Susser M (1980) Chromosomal abnormalities in spontaneous abortions: data from the New York study. In: Porter IH, Hook EB (eds) Human embryonic and fetal death. Academic, New York, p 261

Warkany J (1976) Warfarin embryopathology. Teratology 14: 205

WHO Scientific Group (1981) WHO Technical Report Series No. 657. World Health Organization, Geneva

Wiseman RA, Dodds-Smith IC (1984) Cardiovascular birth defects and antenatal exposure to female sex hormones: a re-evaluation of some base data. Teratology 30: 359

Witschi E (1969) Teratogenic effects from overripeness of the egg. In: Fraser FC, McKusick A (eds) Congenital malformations. Proceedings of the Third International Conference. Exerpta Medica, Amsterdam, p 157

Wolpert L (1992) Gastrulation and the evolution of development. Development, Supplement: Gastrulation, pp 7–13

Woolf CM (1971) Congenital cleft lip. A genetic study of 496 propositi. J Med Genet 8: 65

Wynne-Davies R (1964) Family studies and the cause of congenital club foot. Talipes equinovarus, talipes calcaneovalgus and metatarsus varus. J Bone Joint Surg [Br] 46: 445

Wynne-Davies R (1970a) A family study of neonatal and late-diagnosis congenital dislocation of the hip. J Med Genet 7: 315

Wynne-Davies R (1970b) Acetabular dysplasia and familial joint laxity: two etiological factors in congenital dislocation of the hip. A review of 589 patients and their families. J Bone Joint Surg [Br] 52: 704

Yerushalmy J (1970) The California Child Health and Development Studies. Study design and some illustrative findings on congenital heart disease. In: Fraser FC, McKusick A (eds) Congenital malformations. Proceedings of the Third International Conference. Exerpta Medica, Amsterdam, p 199

3 · Cardiac Pathology

Anton E. Becker and Robert H. Anderson

The pathology of the heart in the paediatric age group can be divided into that of congenital lesions and of postnatally acquired heart disease.

The first category is by far the larger, but experience has shown that many pathologists consider a congenitally malformed heart a mystery, a notion based on the misconception that profound knowledge of embryology is a prerequisite for its understanding. In this chapter we will show how, without any knowledge of cardiac embryogenesis, it is possible to classify a congenitally malformed heart and to understand the pathophysiology from the anatomy observed (Becker and Anderson 1981).

In recent years, interest in congenital disease has revived, mainly as the result of the surgeon's urge for a detailed and unambiguous description of congenital cardiac malformations. This renaissance has led to the development of sequential segmental analysis of the congenitally malformed heart. Being a purely descriptive system, such analysis avoids all matters of controversial interpretation.

Postnatally acquired heart disease in the paediatric age group is of minor importance in the West. Acquired disease in the setting of congenital heart disease, in contrast, is achieving increasing significance.

Autopsy Technique

It is not our purpose to describe a full autopsy technique in detail, but simply to point out some steps that are of particular significance in patients with congenital heart disease.

Examination of the Arrangement of the Organs (Situs)

Particular attention should be given to the arrangement of the abdominal and thoracic organs, because important information can immediately be obtained. Thus, a jumbled arrangement of the abdominal organs is almost always associated with an abnormal arrangement of the lungs and abnormalities within the heart. The finding of *absence of the spleen*, therefore, should immediately alert the pathologist to the likelihood of an abnormal thoracic arrangement. Nearly always, asplenia is accompanied by bilateral symmetry of the tracheobronchial tree resulting in the presence of paired eparterial (morphologically right) bronchi and, usually, of paired trilobed lungs (Fig. 3.1; see also p. 76). In turn, the presence of bilateral eparterial bronchi (dextroisomerism of the bronchi) is nearly always associated with an abnormal atrial arrangement in which both atrial appendages show anatomical features of the morphologically right appendage. One can then anticipate severe abnormalities in the cardiovascular system.

Identification of *polysplenia* is also of significance. In this condition, multiple spleens are present, located on both sides of the mesogastrium (Fig. 3.2a). This finding must be distinguished from accessory spleens, which are always present on the left side of the mesogastrium, as is the normal spleen. Polysplenia has a tendency to be associated with symmetrical development of left-sided structures, so that the lungs show two lobes on either side, with bilateral hyparterial bronchi (Fig. 3.2b). As with right isomerism, this left isomerism is usually accompanied by symmetrical development of the atrial appendages, both of which

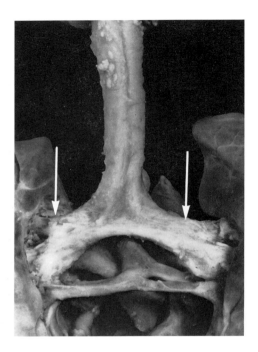

Fig. 3.1. The presence of paired eparterial bronchi (*arrows*) in a patient with absence of the spleen. Heart–lung preparation viewed from behind, showing in detail the artery to the lower lobes on both sides passing beneath the upper lobe bronchus. (Compare Fig. 3.2b)

◄─────────────────────────────────────

show morphologically left characteristics. Recognition of this condition will again serve as an indicator of the presence of cardiovascular abnormalities.

The pathophysiological consequences of symmetrical development of the organs reach far beyond the splenic abnormalities themselves. For this reason, the term "visceral symmetry syndrome" has been introduced (see p. 76), which is preferred to "asplenia syndrome" and "polysplenia syndrome". The syndrome describes a specific arrangement of the body, namely an isomeric arrangement which can be of morphologically right or left pattern (Macartney et al. 1980). Recognition of an isomeric arrangement at autopsy makes in situ preparation of the systemic and pulmonary venous systems mandatory.

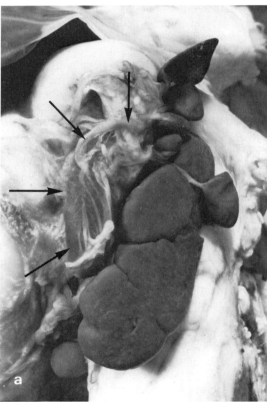

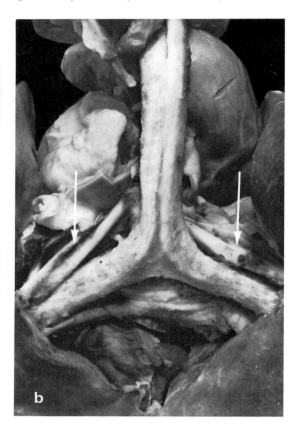

Fig. 3.2. Patient with multiple spleens. **a** Shows the splenic mass on both sides of the mesogastrium in detail. It is made up of multiple spleens, the ones on the right (*arrows*) being covered by the mesentery. **b** Lungs of the same patient. The lower lobe pulmonary arteries on both sides cross over the upper lobe bronchi (*arrows*). (Compare Fig. 3.1)

Examination of the Heart

An abnormal location of the cardiac apex can give clues to the likelihood of intracardiac malformations, but in itself does not constitute a cardiac anomaly. A midline heart with its apex pointing downwards should suggest the possibility of some sort of rotational disturbance, particularly when associated with an isomeric arrangement of the organs. The heart can be in the right side of the chest with the apex pointing to the right with any atrial arrangement. In the presence of the usual arrangement of the thoracic organs and atria, it is often associated with discordant atrioventricular connections and abnormal connections of the great arteries, such as discordant ventriculoarterial connections (see also p. 79). The finding of a left-sided heart with mirror-image atrial arrangement should alert the pathologist to similar possibilities (see p. 82).

Proceeding to the systemic and pulmonary venous systems, two points can be made. Firstly, the finding of a suprahepatic segment of the inferior caval vein does not always indicate the presence of normal drainage of the abdominal venous return. Indeed, drainage of the infrahepatic inferior caval vein via the azygous venous system into the superior caval vein frequently occurs in the presence of a normal suprahepatic. This arrangement, if found, should raise suspicion of the visceral symmetry syndrome. The second point relates to the type of pulmonary venous connection. When normally connected, the heart is restricted in its mobility after the pericardium has been opened. In most instances of abnormal pulmonary venous connections, the heart can easily be lifted out of its posterior pericardial bed, immediately alerting the pathologist to the presence of this condition (Fig. 3.3).

As already discussed, the morphology of the atrial appendages is of particular significance, raising the suspicion of the presence of an abnormal abdominothoracic arrangement when bilaterally symmetrical (see p. 80). Juxtaposition of atrial appendages, defined as the positioning of both appendages at the same side of the arterial pedicle,

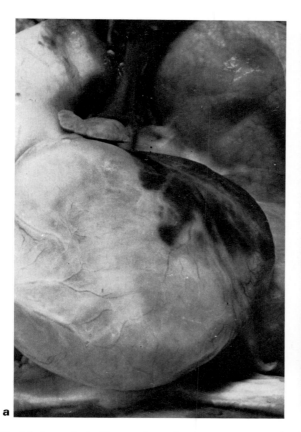 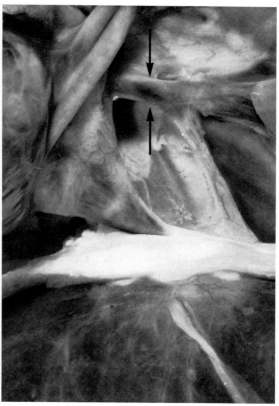

Fig. 3.3. In a patient with anomalous pulmonary venous connection, it is an easy matter to lift the heart from its pericardial bed because the left atrium is no longer anchored by normally connected pulmonary veins. **a** The heart in situ. **b** The heart tilted ventrally and to the right. Note the anomalous common channel (*arrows*) draining the left lung.

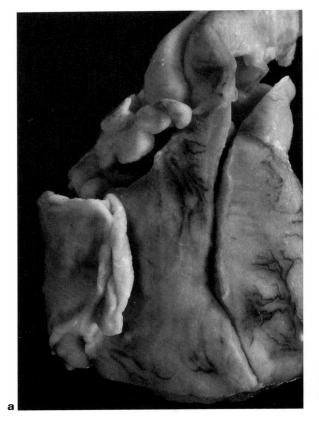

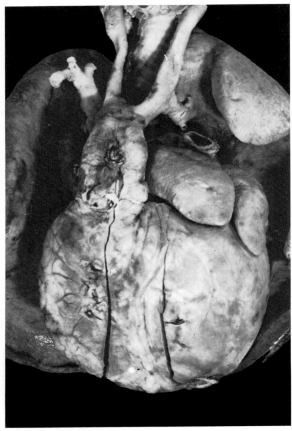

Fig. 3.4. Juxtaposition of the atrial appendages. **a** Both appendages are located to the right of the arterial pedicle; right juxtaposition. **b** Left juxtaposition.

whether right or left (Fig. 3.4), is an important feature indicating serious additional cardiac malformations in most instances (Melhuish and Van Praagh 1968).

The epicardial course of the coronary arteries is particularly useful in determining the position and size of the ventricles. In hearts with marked underdevelopment of one or other ventricles, the anterior and posterior descending coronary arteries clearly indicate the plane of the interventricular septum and the position of the diminutive ventricle. Similarly, in other complicated cardiac malformations, such as hearts with straddling atrioventricular valves or hearts with a univentricular atrioventricular connection with one dominant and one rudimentary ventricle, the surface anatomy of the coronary arteries is an excellent guide to the position of the septum.

Examination of the heart should also focus on the great arteries. An abnormal relationship between the aorta and pulmonary trunk tends to indicate abnormal connections between arteries and ventricles, although an abnormal relationship in itself is not indicative of any particular ventriculoarterial connection or of a specific underlying ventricular anatomy.

Dissection of Veins and Arteries

As stated above, an in situ dissection of veins in both thorax and abdomen is desirable in the presence of isomeric bodily arrangement. In situ dissection of the aortic arch and its main branches is also advisable. In this fashion, an aberrant subclavian artery will be identified *before* it is severed. Moreover, careful dissection will reveal the presence or absence of systemic collateral vessels to the lungs. This observation is significant in the pathophysiology of any case, but particularly in the presence of pulmonary atresia. The state of the arterial duct needs careful evaluation. A reliable impression of its functional status can be obtained from inspection of its exterior, particularly its size relative to the pulmonary trunk and aortic arch, and its aortic and pulmonary orifices. In our experience, probing of the duct is not strictly necessary and may give a false impression of its functional significance. Too often a duct is found to be "probe patent", with the connotation of being functionally open, whereas the pathologist has pushed a probe through a constricted lumen. Moreover, probing the duct will damage its interior and may thus hamper histological investigations regarding its state of closure.

Dissection of the Heart

The heart and lungs, together with the great arteries and the trachea, should preferably be removed in one block. This technique has the advantage that the various interrelationships are preserved, and a careful dissection is then possible in more pleasant surroundings than are usually provided by an autopsy room.

The heart should be opened in such a way as to minimize the risk of damaging the internal architecture or the conduction system. To this end, the following guidelines are suggested, although one should always be prepared to adjust the method according to the findings observed on examination and during opening.

The right atrium can be opened through an incision starting in the right atrial appendage and curving down towards the right atrioventricular junctional area, thereby skirting the terminal groove (Fig. 3.5a). Septal structures and the valves of the venous sinus are thus left intact. Moreover, abnormal structures within the right atrial cavity are not directly compromised, while a good display of the interior is obtained. The left atrium is opened by incising the roof of the cavity between the two lower lobe veins (Fig. 3.5b). The incision can be extended into these veins, thereby creating a good view of the rest of the atrium. Ostial stenosis of pulmonary veins or an unexpected division of the atrium (cortriatriatum) can thus be diagnosed before irreversible damage has been inflicted. Such an incision will not open a persistent left superior caval vein. The right-sided ventricle is best opened by incising its anterior wall guided by a probe through an arterial outlet (Fig. 3.5c). Extension of the incision will depend on the architecture encountered. A similar approach is appropriate for the left-sided ventricle (Fig. 3.5d). If no arterial outlet is present, the ventricular cavity can be opened in its inlet part, leaving the atrioventricular junctional area intact. Similarly, the ventriculoarterial junction should be inspected prior to incision.

The Conduction System

In some instances, full pathological examination of the heart may require a study of the conduction system. This is another topic that is shrouded in mystery for many pathologists, but we feel this attitude is unjustified, because the examination is not difficult to perform. In the normal heart, the sinus node is located in the terminal groove lateral to the junction of the superior caval vein and the right atrium. The atrioventricular conduction tissues are located in the atrial septum adjacent to the central fibrous body, and the atrioventricular bundle (of His) is found between the membranous and muscular components of the ventricular septum. Removal of the entire right atrium and the atrioventricular junction in neonatal hearts will permit study of the conduction system by either serial or subserial sectioning (Fig. 3.6). In larger hearts, separate blocks containing the sinus node and the atrioventricular conduction tissues can be removed and sectioned in a similar fashion. It is our opinion that insistence on full serial sectioning in any study of the conduction system deters investigators from this task. Although such a technique is clearly ideal, a considerable amount of information can be obtained by using subserial methods (Davies 1971; Smith et al. 1977; Becker et al. 1978a). Conduction tissue in malformed hearts will be discussed briefly in the appropriate sections. For study in these hearts, it is necessary to examine any union of a ventricular septal structure, if present, with the atrioventricular junctions.

Sequential Segmental Analysis of the Heart

Segmental analysis of the heart (Van Praagh 1972; Shinebourne et al. 1976; Brandt and Calder 1977; Anderson et al. 1984a) is based on the identification of the various building blocks of the heart, and the way in which these segments are connected. In other words, a basic flow pattern through the heart is established through a number of sequential steps. We will discuss these steps in order, beginning with chamber identification, followed by the connections and relations at different junctional levels (Tynan et al. 1979; Anderson and Ho 1986).

Chamber Identification

The identification of cardiac chambers is based on morphological criteria (Figs. 3.7, 3.8).

The fundamental criterion distinguishing between right and left atria is the morphological aspect of the atrial appendages (Fig. 3.9). The right atrial appendage has a broad pedicle and is blunt, while the left atrial appendage has a narrow pedicle and is narrower and hooked (Fig. 3.9). Furthermore, and of greater anatomic significance, the pectinate muscles of the morphologically right appendage extend round

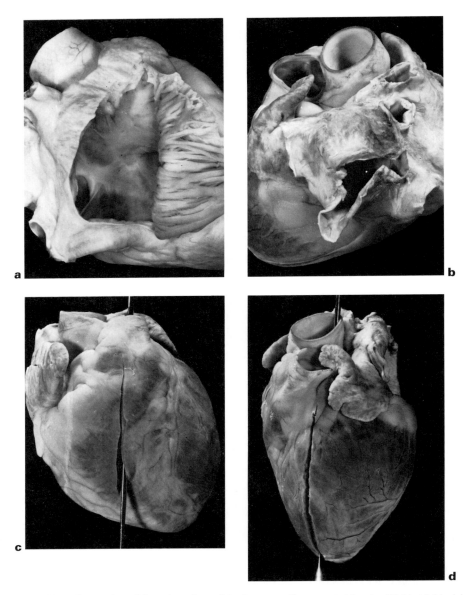

Fig. 3.5. The initial incisions for opening of the atria and ventricles in a normally connected heart. **a** Right atrial incision. **b** Left atrial incision, connecting the ostia of the right and left lower lobe pulmonary veins. Both incisions enable a clear inspection of the interior of the atria and atrioventricular orifices with a minimal chance of damaging important structures. **c** Incision of the right ventricular anterior wall, guided by a probe. **d** A similar left ventricular incision. The initial incision should be made approximately halfway along the right ventricular outflow and close to the apex in the left ventricle. Elongation of the incision should always be accompanied by close inspection.

the entirety of the vestibule of the atrioventricular valve. In contrast, the pectinate muscles of the morphologically left atrium are limited in their extent, and the posterior junction of the venous component and the vestibule is smooth. Other features, such as venous connections and septal characteristics, are highly variable and may not be much help when the anomaly is complex. In such complex cases the clinician generally relies on tracheobronchial anatomy, as visualized by a penetrating chest radiograph or on the arrangement of the abdominal great vessels as revealed by ultrasound to infer atrial arrangement (Deanfield et al. 1980; Huhta et al. 1982).

This approach is based on the premise that tracheobronchial morphology, the arrangement of the abdominal vessels and anatomy of the atrial

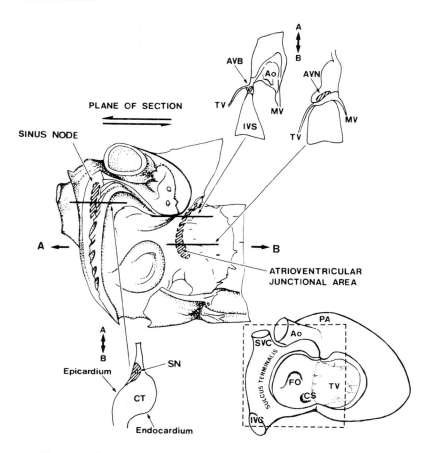

Fig. 3.6. The block removed for study of the conduction tissues from the neonatal heart and representative sections through the sinus node and atrioventricular conduction axis.

appendages are concordant (Macartney et al. 1978). Few exceptions to this rule have been described (Caruso and Becker 1979).

Identification of the morphologically right and left ventricles is based predominantly on the pattern of the ventricular trabeculations and on the architecture of the atrioventricular valvar apparatus. It is important to appreciate that a normal ventricle has *three* anatomical components (Figs. 3.8, 3.10). These are the inlet, (that part related to and supporting the atrioventricular valve), the apical trabecular component and the outlet, (that part supporting the arterial valve). As will be seen, this tripartite ventricular division is of major significance in categorization of hearts with straddling valves or a univentricular atrioventricular connection.

Atrial Arrangement

Once the morphology of the appendages has been identified, the arrangement of the atrial chambers can be established. Usual arrangement (solitus) is present when the morphologically right appendage is on the right and the morphologically left appendage is on the left. The mirror-image situation is described as such (Fig. 3.11). Atrial isomerism characterizes the situation in which both appendages exhibit features of either morphologically right or morphologically left structures. Isomerism can therefore be of right or left types (Fig. 3.12).

When atrial arrangement has been established, additional anomalies need a separate specification, e.g. "persistent left superior caval vein connected to the coronary sinus" or "unilateral total anomalous pulmonary venous connection to right atrium".

Atrioventricular Junction

In the normal heart the atrioventricular connections are *concordant*, i.e. the morphologically right atrium connects to the morphologically right ventricle through the tricuspid valve and the left atrium con-

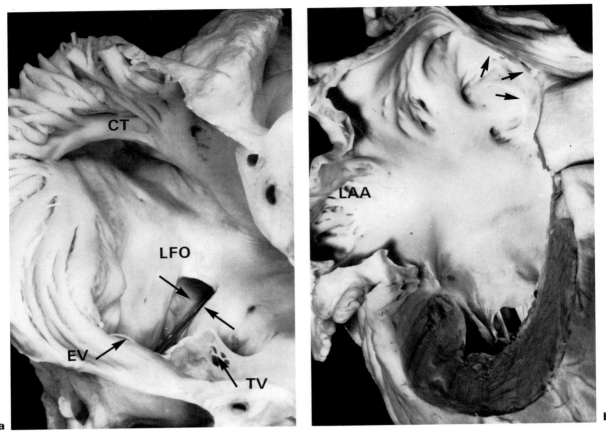

Fig. 3.7. Anatomical characteristics of morphological right and left atria. **a** Opened right atrium with an extensive terminal crest (*CT*) with parallel pectinate muscles. The rim of the oval fossa (*LFO*) delineates the area of the oval foramen through which a probe has been passed (*arrows*). Note also the remnants of the right valve of the embryonic venous sinus, recognizable as the Eustachian (*EV*) and Thebesian (*TV*) valves. **b** Left atrium and left atrial appendage (*LAA*). There is no terminal crest and the flap valve of the oval fossa is seen on the roughened septal surface (*arrows*).

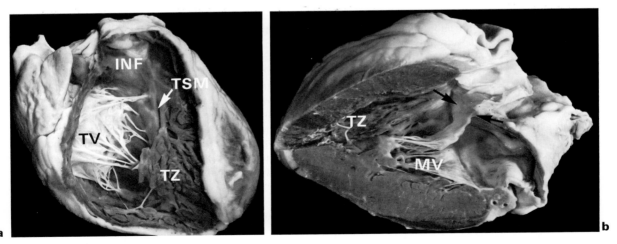

Fig. 3.8. The anatomical characteristics of the right and left ventricles. **a** Opened right ventricle with the tricuspid valve (*TV*) in its inlet position, the coarse trabecular zone (*TZ*), the complete muscular infundibulum (*INF*) and the septomarginal trabeculation (*TSM*) on the septal surface. **b** Opened left ventricle containing the mitral valve (*MV*) in its inlet portion, the fine trabecular zone (*TZ*), the smooth septal surface, and the arterial valve in fibrous continuity with the mitral valve (*arrows*).

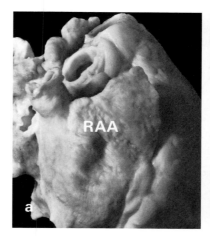
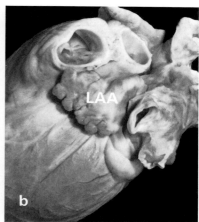

Fig. 3.9. The difference in morphology between the right (*RAA*, **a**) and left (*LAA*, **b**) atrial appendages.

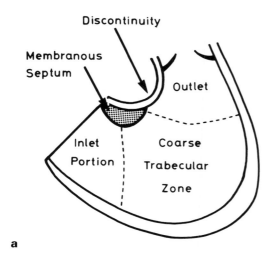

a

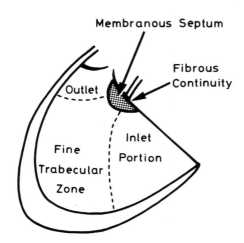

b

Fig. 3.10. The anatomical zones of the right (**a**) and left (**b**) ventricles. (Compare Fig. 3.8.)

nects to the left ventricle through the mitral valve (Fig. 3.13a). In congenital heart malformations, however, one should be prepared for the finding of an abnormal type of atrioventricular connection. If the right atrium connects to a morphologically left ventricle and the left atrium to a morphologically right ventricle the connections are termed "*discordant*" (Fig. 3.13b). Another possibility is that both atria connect to the same ventricle, a situation termed "*double-inlet atrioventricular connection*" (Fig. 3.13d). One of the atrial chambers may have no connection, either actual or potential, with the underlying chambers, a situation defined as "*absence of one atrioventricular connection*" (Fig. 3.13e).

From the above definitions it follows that connections can be classified as either concordant or discordant only when positive identification of *both* atria and ventricles has been established. In atrial isomerism (see p. 73), any connection between the atria and the two underlying ventricles is classified by necessity as an *ambiguous connection* (Fig. 3.13c). When each atrium connects to its own ventricle, the topological pattern of the ventricles is added to give a full account of the situation, for instance "ambiguous atrioventricular connection with right-hand ventricular topology" (Fig. 3.14). Isomeric atria, however, may connect to only one underlying chamber, either via a double inlet connection or because of the absence of one connection (Fig. 3.14). In these circumstances, the appropriate connection can be defined accordingly. Indeed, hearts with usual or mirror-image atrial arrangement and either double-inlet connection or absence of one connection have the additional feature that the atrial chambers connect to only one ventricle (with the exception of hearts with overriding atrioventricular valves). We have used this fact to categorize all such hearts as having a

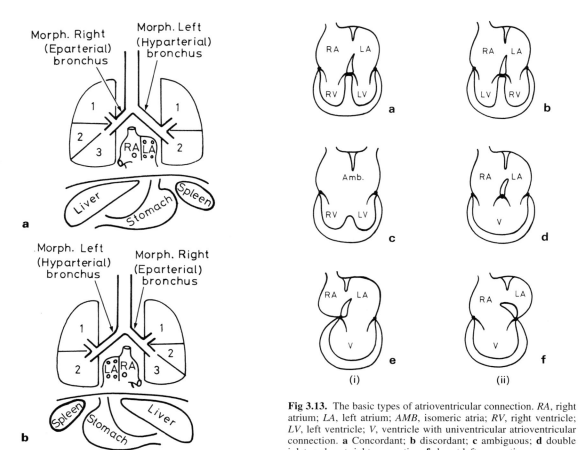

Fig. 3.11. The arrangement of thoracic and abdominal organs in usual (**a**) and mirror-image (**b**) arrangements.

Fig 3.13. The basic types of atrioventricular connection. *RA*, right atrium; *LA*, left atrium; *AMB*, isomeric atria; *RV*, right ventricle; *LV*, left ventricle; *V*, ventricle with univentricular atrioventricular connection. **a** Concordant; **b** discordant; **c** ambiguous; **d** double inlet; **e** absent right connection; **f** absent left connection.

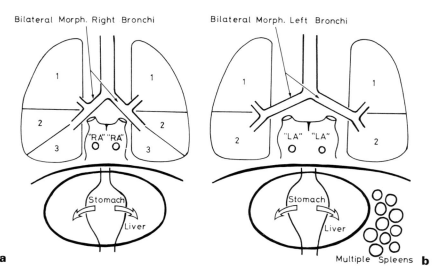

Fig. 3.12. The usual arrangement of thoracoabdominal organs in the two forms of isomerism of the atrial appendages, the right type, usually with asplenia (**a**), and the left pattern, usually with polysplenia (**b**).

univentricular atrioventricular connection (Anderson et al. 1983). Such hearts were previously classified as having "single ventricles" or as being "univentricular hearts". This approach makes little sense, because most possess two ventricles, although one lacks its inlet component and is therefore rudimentary. The rudimentary ventricle, nonetheless, can readily be recognized and described as of right or left morphology according to the pattern of its apical trabecular component (Fig. 3.15) even when it also lacks its outlet component (Anderson et al. 1984b). The relationships of these rudimentary ventricles to the dominant ventricle are best specified in simple descriptive terms.

Very rarely, hearts with a univentricular atrioventricular connection can have a solitary ventricle within their ventricular mass. This may be because the rudimentary ventricle is so small as to be unrecognizable without resort to histology. More usually it is because the solitary ventricle is of indeterminate apical trabecular pattern and is a true single ventricle.

It should be emphasized that, thus far, only the *type* of atrioventricular connection has been considered, together with the consequences it has for ventricular morphology and terminology. As a second step, the *mode* of the connection should be established (Fig. 3.16). In the normal heart the connection is established through two "perforate" atrioventricular junctions. In the malformed heart, one of the two connections may be composed of an imperforate membrane. In this situation the atrium will still be in

potential connection with the underlying ventricle. This situation is therefore basically different, as far as the anatomy is concerned, from an absent connection, in which not even a potential connection is present (Fig. 3.17). An "imperforate" valve may thus coincide with concordant, discordant, ambiguous or double inlet atrioventricular connections. Another mode of connection is that characterized by presence of a "common atrioventricular valve". If such a common valve occurs with concordant atrioventricular connections, the right atrium still connects to the right ventricle and the left atrium to the left ventricle. In more complicated conditions, however, discordant or double inlet connections can be present through a common atrioventricular valve. We would not use the term "common valve" in hearts with an absent atrioventricular connection. This is because, in these hearts, the valve present connects to only one atrium. A third, and more complicated, mode of connection is the one in which the tension apparatus of an atrioventricular valve is attached to both sides of an underlying ventricular septum; a condition called a "straddling atrioventricular valve. Usually such a valve has overriding of its orifice. This arrangement will raise problems in classification of the heart, because the degree of overriding may vary considerably. It is for this reason that a 50% rule has been introduced (Tynan et al. 1979). If an atrioventricular junction overrides a ventricular septum by 50% or more, the orifice is considered to belong to the ventricle receiving the greater part of its circumference, because the degree of overriding determines the type of connection. For instance, if the right atrioventricular valve connects through a straddling valve for the major part to a left ventricle, which also receives the left atrioventricular valve, the connection is a "double inlet with a straddling right atrioventricular valve" (Fig. 3.18a). If, however, a similar architecture is present, but with the straddling right atrioventricular valve committed mainly to the right ventricle, the situation would be "concordant with straddling right atrioventricular valve" (Fig. 3.18b). This approach may seem cumbersome at first glance, but it has the advantage that it accounts for a basic pattern of flow and permits an unequivocal description of the atrioventricular connections. It does not affect the description of the ventricles themselves, because this is determined according to the nature of their apical trabecular component. Thus, in the example of the straddling right atrioventricular valve (Fig. 3.18), the degree of overriding only changes the type of connection and does not alter the morphology of the underlying ventricles (Fig. 3.18).

As indicated above, when the type and mode of atrioventricular connections have been established, attention should be given to the topology and rela-

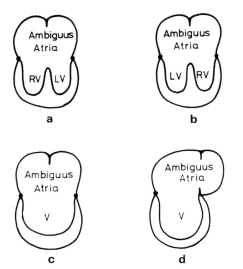

Fig. 3.14. The ventricular relationships and atrioventricular connections possible with isomeric atrial chambers. **a, b** Ambiguous atrioventricular connections; **c** double inlet ventricle; **d** absent left AV connection. It can also exist with absent right atrioventricular correction. Abbreviations as in Fig. 3.13.

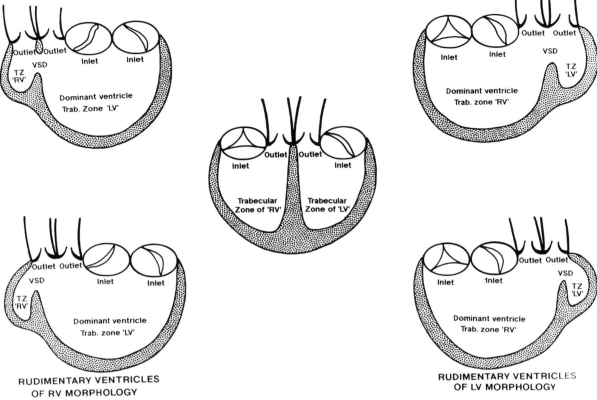

Fig. 3.15. The components of dominant ventricles and rudimentary ventricles and the way they can be arranged to form hearts with double inlet atrioventricular connection. (Reproduced from Tynan et al. 1979, by permission of the editor of the *British Heart Journal*)

tionships of chambers in the ventricular mass. A rotational disturbance during the development of the heart may result in the atrioventricular valves and ventricles acquiring an abnormal spatial position. This may lead to peculiar relative positions, such as the "criss-cross" or "superoinferior" or "upstairs – downstairs" atrioventricular relationships. These conditions can occur with any type and with all modes of atrioventricular connection.

Ventriculoarterial Junctions

In the normal heart, the morphologically right ventricle conveys blood into the pulmonary trunk and the left ventricle into the aorta. The arterial junctions are guarded by arterial valves, each having three leaflets. the pulmonary valve is usually widely separated from the tricuspid valve by a bar of muscle, the supraventricular crest (see Fig. 3.8a), and the aortic valve

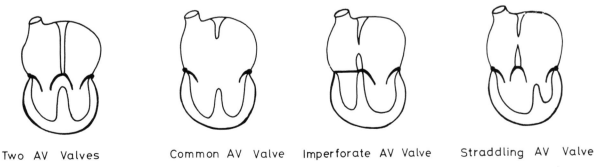

Fig. 3.16. The four different modes of atrioventricular connection that can exist with the various types of connection. Note that the imperforate valve should be distinguished from an absent atrioventricular connection. (Compare Fig. 3.17)

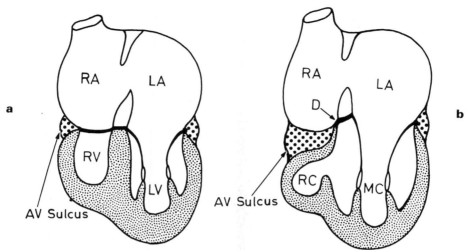

Fig. 3.17. The difference between an imperforate tricuspid valve (mode of connection, **a**) and an absent right atrioventricular connection (type of connection, **b**). In the latter the dimple (*D*) in the right atrial (*RA*) floor points to the main chamber (*MC*). The other chamber is rudimentary (*RC*) and the heart is univentricular.

shows fibrous continuity with the mitral valve (see Fig. 3.8b). The pulmonary orifice is normally anterior and slightly to the left of the aortic one. This type of ventriculoarterial connection is designated as "concordant" (Fig. 3.19a) with normal relationships. In some rare forms of congenital heart disease, concordant ventriculoarterial connections may be present but with an abnormal relationship, e.g. with the pul-

monary trunk posterior and to the right and the aorta anterior and to the left. This condition has been termed "anatomically corrected malposition".

Where the aorta arises from the right ventricle and the pulmonary trunk from the left, the connections are defined as "discordant" (Fig. 3.19b). Usually this is designated "transposition of the great arteries". The term "transposition", however, is highly controversial

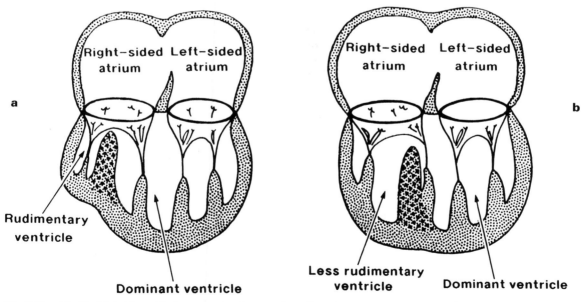

Fig. 3.18. a Double-inlet atrioventricular connection; **b** concordant, discordant or ambiguous atrioventricular connection. Overriding of an atrioventricular valve determines the precise atrioventricular connection but has no effect on the description of ventricles. (Modified from Tynan et al. 1979 by permission of the Editor of the *British Heart Journal*)

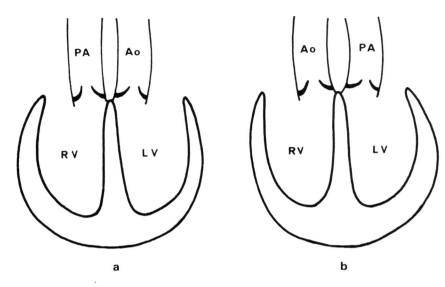

Fig. 3.19. The difference between concordant (**a**) and discordant (**b**) ventriculoarterial connections.

and not unanimously interpreted (Becker 1978). For this reason we will use the term "transposition" only when further qualified by such terms as "complete" or "corrected" (Becker and Anderson 1982; see also p. 101). The relationships of the discordantly connected great arteries also need further specification, like "aorta anterior and to the right" or "to the left" (Fig. 3.20).

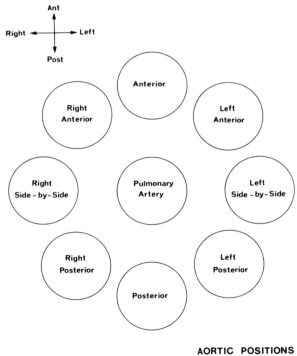

AORTIC POSITIONS

Fig. 3.20. Variability in aortic position relative to the pulmonary artery with any arterial connection.

Other types of arterial connection are "double outlet" (Fig. 3.21) and "single outlet of the heart" (Fig. 3.22). In double outlet, more than half of both great arteries arise from one ventricle, which can be of right, left or indeterminate morphology.

In the single-outlet heart, there is only one arterial trunk connected to the ventricles. The pathologist has an advantage over the clinician in being able, in most instances, to specify this condition further. There are four possibilities (Fig. 3.22):

1. Common arterial trunk
2. Pulmonary atresia with the aorta as the single arterial trunk
3. Aortic atresia with a single pulmonary trunk
4. Solitary arterial trunk with absence of the intrapericardial pulmonary arteries.

As with the atrioventricular connections, each type of ventriculoarterial connection needs further specification according to the mode of connection. Valvar atresia of, for example, a pulmonary valve may coincide with any of the afore-mentioned types of connection except single outlet. The clinician may have classified a cardiac condition as "single outlet, large ventricular septal defect and pulmonary atresia", but the pathologist may be able to show potential concordant, discordant or double-outlet connections. In other instances of single-outlet heart, however, even the pathologist will be unable to find any connection between the atretic trunk and the ventricular mass on examination of the heart, and these are cases of true single outlet of the heart.

An "overriding arterial valve" creates a similar problem with respect to the classification of the type of connections as described for the atrioventricular junction (Ueda and Becker 1985). Again, a 50% rule

double outlet ventriculo-arterial connexions

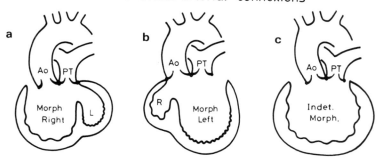

Fig. 3.21 a-c. The three types of double-outlet ventriculoarterial connection: **a** from the right ventricle; **b** from left ventricle; **c** from indeterminate ventricle.

has been advocated (Kirklin et al. 1973). An artery is considered to arise from a ventricle when 50% or more of its circumference is committed to that chamber (Fig. 3.23). In other words, a double-outlet arterial connection could occur with two overriding arterial valves, both committed mainly to the same chamber. Similarly, concordant (Fig. 3.23) and dis- cordant arterial connections may coincide with an overriding arterial valve.

Any description of the arterial junction is incom- plete without identification of any abnormal relation- ships, such as the relative position of the greater arteries (see Fig. 3.20) and the morphology of the ventricular outflow tracts, i.e. the presence or absence

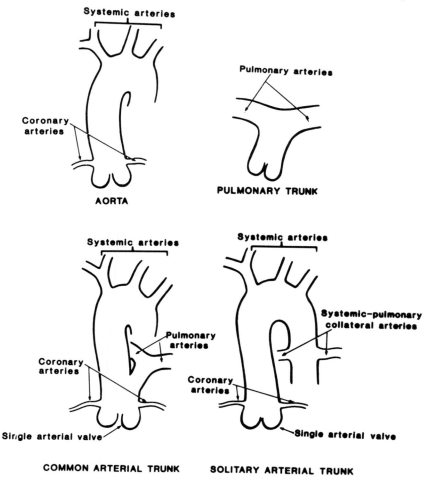

Fig. 3.22. Criteria for definition of an arterial trunk. Each trunk can be found as the sole outlet from the ventricular mass.

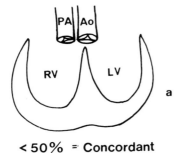

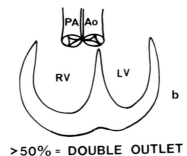

< 50% = Concordant   >50% = DOUBLE OUTLET

Fig. 3.23. The effect of an overriding arterial valve on the ventriculoarterial connections.

of a subaortic infundibulum or subpulmonary infundibulum.

Use of Sequential Segmental Analysis

With the use of the sequential segmental cardiac analysis depicted above, any type of congenitally malformed heart can be described, irrespective of its complexity. Moreover, the approach avoids controversial matters where different schools of opinion collide and where the same term may have different connotations.

It should be emphasized, however, that the method for analysis presently advocated (Tynan et al. 1979) is not put forward as a system for classifying congenital heart diseases or to replace current classifications. It merely facilitates a descriptive approach to the malformed heart, which will enable anyone to discuss a complex case in full knowledge of how the various building blocks have been put together, irrespective of pre-existing detailed knowledge regarding the official name coined for the condition concerned.

Congenital Heart Disease

In the western world, approximately eight newborns per 1000 have congenital heart disease (Campbell 1968; Hoffman and Christianson, 1978). Precise data on the prevalance of congenital heart disease might lead to the identification of some of the environmental and genetic factors involved in its aetiology. For this reason, the study of stillborn and aborted fetuses is importance. Despite the fact that congenital heart defects in only a minority of cases contribute to intrauterine death, its incidence is remarkably high when searched for carefully. In a series of 247 unselected spontaneous abortions, congenital heart disease was detected in 15.7% (Gerlis 1985). Among

stillbirths, the incidence varies from 1.2% to 5.4% (Šamánek et al. 1985).

The most frequent conditions existing in the neonatal period are ventricular septal defect, patent arterial duct, atrial septal defect, aortic coarctation, complete transposition, Fallot's tetralogy, pulmonary stenosis and aortic stenosis, in descending order of frequency (Campbell 1968). The significance of these malformations for mortality varies considerably. It can be said that approximately 30% of babies born with a congenital heart defect will die within the first year of life. The malformations that carry the highest early mortality risk are, in descending order of frequency, aortic coarctation, left heart hypoplasia, complete transposition, extreme forms of Fallot's tetralogy, right heart hypoplasia and double-outlet right ventricle (Rowe and Mehrizi 1968).

The pathological aspects of these and other malformations will be discussed briefly in the sections below. A subdivision is made into conditions with a basically normal segmental arrangement and those with an abnormal arrangement.

Congenital Heart Malformations with Normal Junctional Connections

All defects to be discussed in this section will show concordant atrioventricular and ventriculoarterial connections, with usual arrangement of the atria assumed for the purpose of description. They can, of course, all exist with mirror-image atrial arrangement and concordant atrioventricular and ventriculoarterial connections, but this is exceedingly rare.

Anomalous Systemic Venous Connections

The most common anomalous systemic venous connection is "persistence of the left superior caval vein" (Fig. 3.24), a condition that in itself has no functional significance. The vein runs to the heart anterior to the lung hilus as a continuation of the left brachiocephalic vein and usually connects to the coronary

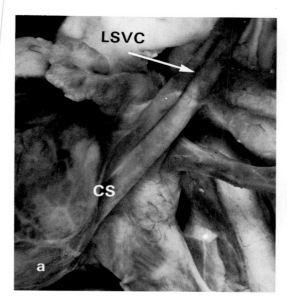
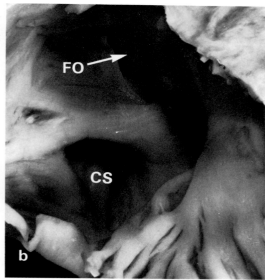

Fig. 3.24. Persistent left superior caval vein. **a** Course of the vein (*LSVC*) as it descends ventral to the hilus of the left lung. The vein continues as the coronary sinus (*CS*). For a good display the heart has been lifted out of its pericardial bed, a procedure facilitated by an anomalous pulmonary venous connection (same case as illustrated in Fig. 3.3). **b** Enlarged ostium of the coronary sinus (*CS*) in the opened right atrium. *FO*, oval foramen.

sinus. The orifice of the coronary sinus is larger than normal (Fig. 3.24b), and this observation may alert the pathologist to the presence of the anomaly if it has been missed during the initial inspection of the exterior of the heart.

More rarely, a persistent left superior caval vein connects directly to the left atrium. In these instances, the coronary sinus is said to be unroofed. As a consequence, the orifice of the coronary sinus functions as an interatrial communication (see p. 86). This particular condition, however, is often part of a more complex malformation. In rare cases, the persistent left superior caval vein, draining into a coronary sinus, can be associated with absence or atresia of the usual right-sided superior caval vein. The persistent left superior caval vein is then the sole channel for the systemic venous return to the heart, the venous system of the neck and upper mediastinum being a mirror image of the normal.

Abnormalities of the connections of the inferior caval vein are rare and almost always accompany a complex cardiac malformation.

At the site of the orifice of the inferior caval vein an extensive remnant of the right valve of the embryonic venous sinus may be present, called the Chiari network (Fig. 3.25). In rare instances, a sail-like membrane is observed, causing an obstruction to the inlet of the right ventricle. The anomaly may be described as a divided right atrium ("*cor triatriatum dexter*") (Doucette and Knoblich 1963).

The orifice of the coronary sinus in the right atrium is occasionally occluded or congenitally narrowed. The functional significance of this condition remains speculative.

Anomalous Pulmonary Venous Connections

There is a vast variety of anatomical arrangements of anomalous pulmonary venous connections. Basically, the anomalies can be divided into bilateral and unilateral types, each of which may display *total* or *partial* involvement of the venous connections. If inspection of the heart has aroused suspicion of an abnormality in the pulmonary venous connections, in situ preparation is mandatory, and the pathologist should be prepared to dissect a complex system of venous connections. "Bilateral totally anomalous pulmonary venous connection" is characterized by total absence of a direct connection to the left atrium. In the usual instance, the pulmonary veins join together behind the left atrium in a confluence. A distinct channel connects the confluence to the systemic venous side of the heart. The most common locations for such an abnormal connection are, in descending order, the left innominate (brachiocephalic) vein, the coronary sinus, the superior caval vein, and the right atrium itself (Fig. 3.26). In rare instances the anomalous connection is established below the diaphragm (Fig. 3.27a). In these cases there is a long venous channel,

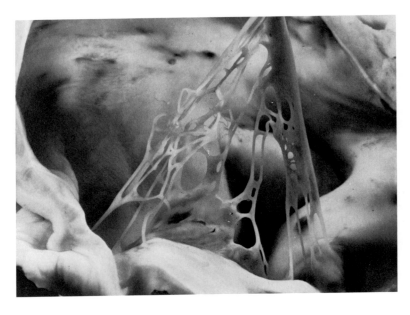

Fig. 3.25. A Chiari network guarding the orifice of the inferior caval vein.

generally accompanying the oesophagus on its way through the diaphragm, which then connects to the portal venous system or the inferior caval vein. Generally, infradiaphragmatic connections have an extremely poor prognosis because they result in a severe obstruction to pulmonary venous drainage. Early mortality, often without proper diagnosis, may occur. The pathologist should therefore be alerted to this arrangement, particularly when examination of

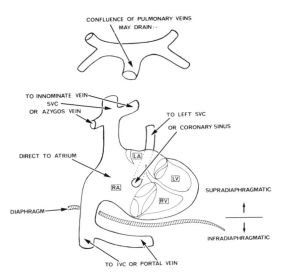

Fig. 3.26. The most common sites for an abnormal connection, in patients with bilateral totally anomalous pulmonary venous connection.

the organs has suggested the presence of isomerism (see p. 74). In the presence of a bilateral (or unilateral) totally anomalous pulmonary venous connection, different sites of drainage of parts of the venous system may be found in the same patient. In particular, in patients with bilateral totally anomalous pulmonary venous connection to the coronary sinus, the left upper lobe of the lung can have a separate venous connection to the left innominate vein with or without additional interconnections with the main pulmonary venous route (Fig. 3.27b).

A particular form of "unilateral anomalous pulmonary venous connection" is the Scimitar syndrome. in this malformation, frequently associated with other anomalies, the pulmonary veins of the right lung, or more frequently of the right lower lobe, connect through a single venous trunk to the inferior caval vein. The right lung itself is often hypoplastic and the heart occupies a right-sided position. There may also be systemic-pulmonary collateral arteries supplying the anomalous lung, which may be sequestrated.

It is important for the pathologist also to realize that the clinical symptomatology and prognosis depend mostly on the presence or absence of obstructed drainage. Such obstructions usually result from intrinsic abnormalities, such as the presence of a long narrow channel conveying blood from the confluence to the systemic venous side or drainage into a relatively high-resistance area, e.g. the portal venous system. Rare instances of obstruction caused by external compression can occur when the connecting vein runs between a pulmonary artery and a main bronchus.

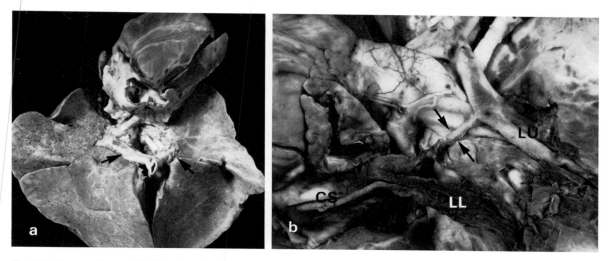

Fig. 3.27. Two specimens with bilateral totally anomalous pulmonary venous connection. **a** The right and left pulmonary veins (*arrows*) join into a common channel which passes through the diaphragm and is connected to the portal vein. The anomalous connection has been divided to the level of the diaphragm. Note the increased mobility of the heart, as the left atrium is no longer anchored posteriorly by pulmonary veins. (Compare Fig. 3.3) **b** Bilateral totally anomalous pulmonary sinus (*CS*). The left upper lobe vein (*LU*) takes a separate route connecting the left innominate vein. A tiny vein interconnects the two systems (*between arrows*).

Divided Left Atrium

When the left atrium is divided ("cor triatriatum sinister"), the pulmonary veins connect to a distinct chamber, located posterior to the left atrium. The venous confluence communicates with the left atrium through an opening, which can vary considerably in size but is usually "pin-hole" size (Fig. 3.28). because of the restriction of pulmonary venous flow, pulmonary congestion occurs with right heart overload and a low cardiac output. The anatomical counterpart of these haemodynamic consequences is expressed in

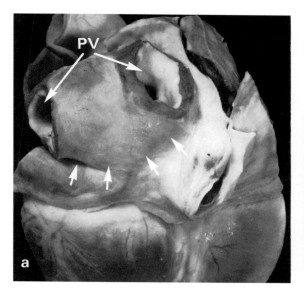

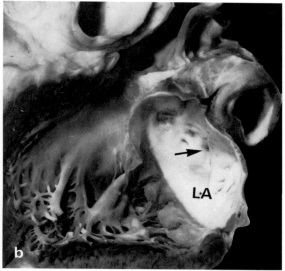

Fig. 3.28. Heart with a divided left atrium. **a** Posterior aspect of the heart. The confluence of the pulmonary veins is vaguely outlined (*arrows*) from the inferior part of the left atrium. Note the marked myocardial hypertrophy at the site where the pulmonary venous connection (*PV*) have been cut. **b** Left side of this heart after removal of the anterolateral wall. A pinhole-size opening (*arrow*) is present between the inferior part of the left atrium (*LA*) and the "extra" atrium. Note the difference in myocardial thickness between the two chambers.

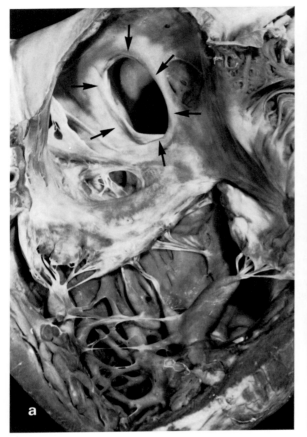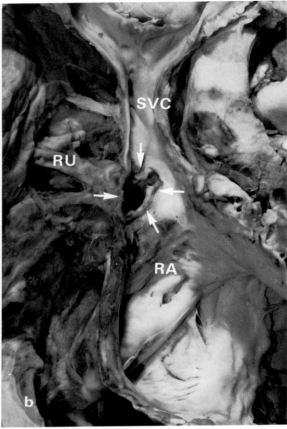

Fig. 3.29. Two different types of atrial septal defect. **a** A large atrial septal defect within the oval fossa (*arrows*). **b** A sinus venosus defect (*arrows*), located at the base of the superior caval vein (*SVC*) where it enters the right atrium (*RA*). The ostium of the right upper lobe vein (*RU*) is intimately related to the defect.

hypertrophy of right heart structures and the wall of the "extra" atrium, while the pulmonary veins reveal "arterialization".

Interatrial Communications

An interatrial communication can occur at different locations within the atrial chambers, although not all involve the atrial septum. The most common type is an "atrial septal defect within the oval fossa" (also called secundum type). This defect is present at the site of the oval fossa and can range in extent from localized small fenestrations in the floor of the fossa, just underneath the rim, to a large defect extending almost down to the level of the atrioventricular valves (Fig. 3.29a). Such defects should not be confused with a probe-patent oval foramen or a defect secondary to atrial stretch. The latter occurs when excessive dilatation of the left atrium stretches the

floor of the fossa (i.e. the embryonic septum primum), creating a functional defect beneath the rim. Conditions accompanied by an excessive left atrial overload can lead to herniation of the free edge of the primary septum into the right atrium. In hearts with aortic or mitral atresia this is a common finding, and right atrial overload, e.g. in tricuspid atresia, may cause aneurysm of the floor of the fossa into the left atrium. A defect of the oval fossa may be associated with anatomical abnormalities of the mitral valvar apparatus or with aortic coarctation.

A rarer type of defect can occur at the site of the anticipated orifice of the coronary sinus, the coronary sinus defect. It is almost always associated with a persistent left superior caval vein draining directly into the left atrium (p. 83). It is questionable whether such a communication should be classified as an atrial septal defect, but in extremely rare circumstances the coronary sinus may have developed in part, so that bidirectional shunting between the atria

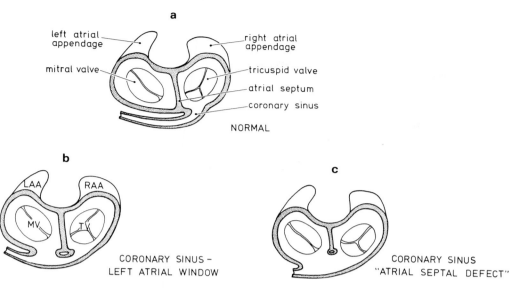

Fig. 3.30. a Normally constructed heart. **b, c** The close relationship between an atrial septal defect of the coronary sinus type (**c**) associated with a persistent left superior caval vein draining into the left atrium, and the situation in which the wall of the coronary sinus has only partially developed, so that bidirectional atrial shunting in a similar anatomical location is possible (**b**).

can occur through its orifice in the right atrium. If the coronary sinus is better developed, windows may be present between coronary sinus and left atrium, permitting similar shunts (Fig. 3.30).

A special form of interatrial communication is the "sinus venosus". In this condition, the defect is situated at the base of the superior caval vein, where it enters the right atrium and is outside the confines of the atrial septum. The orifice of the right upper lobe pulmonary vein is intimately related to the defect and the superior caval vein overrides the floor of the defect (see Fig. 3.29b).

The "primum type of atrial septal defect" will be discussed under the heading of atrioventricular septal defects (p. 90).

An atrial septal defect will lead to an obligatory left-to-right shunt and an augmented pulmonary blood flow. The natural course of the disease will ultimately lead to irreversible pulmonary hypertension due to plexogenic pulmonary arteriopathy.

Ventricular Septal Defects

The terminology of ventricular septal defects is complicated and not uniformly accepted (Becu et al. 1956; Warden et al. 1957; Lev 1959; Goor et al. 1970).

The classification of ventricular septal defects used in this section (Fig. 3.31) was proposed by Soto et al. in 1980. It is based on the premise that the muscular ventricular septum, as with the ventricles, is composed of three parts, i.e. an inlet part, a trabecular part, and an outlet or infundibular part (see Fig. 3.10). The three parts join at the site of the right fibrous trigone, from which the interventricular part of the membranous septum is derived.

Three basic types of septal defect are then recognized (Fig. 3.31).

A "perimembranous defect" is defined as one in which the membranous septum, either its atrioventricular component or a remnant of its interventricular component, forms part of the rim (Fig. 3.32). Perimembranous defects can extend to open into any of the three components of the right ventricle or can be confluent, a feature permitting further subclassification if required. The significance of recognizing a defect as perimembranous in nature is that, irrespective of its main direction of extension, the main axis of the atrioventricular conduction system will be present in its inferior rim – a feature of paramount interest to the surgeon.

"Muscular ventricular septal defects" are defined as those completely surrounded by musculature. Again, the subclassification of this type of defect is based on the localization of the defect according to the three parts of the ventricular septum. In other words, a muscular defect can occur in the inlet, trabecular or outlet septa and should be designated accordingly (see Fig. 3.31). Muscular defects in the inlet septum may have the atrioventricular conduction axis close to their anterosuperior rim. Defects in the outlet part or trabecular part of the ventricular

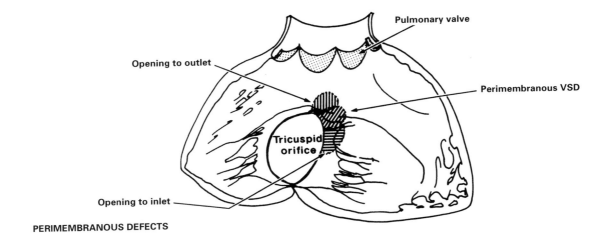

Pulmonary valve

Opening to outlet

Perimembranous VSD

Tricuspid orifice

Opening to inlet

PERIMEMBRANOUS DEFECTS

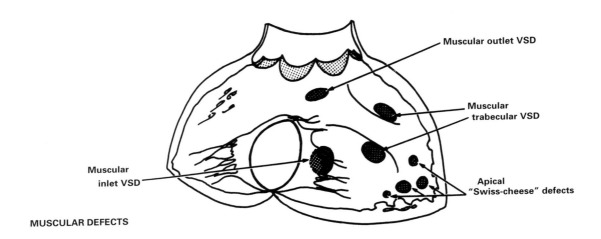

Muscular outlet VSD

Muscular trabecular VSD

Muscular inlet VSD

Apical "Swiss-cheese" defects

MUSCULAR DEFECTS

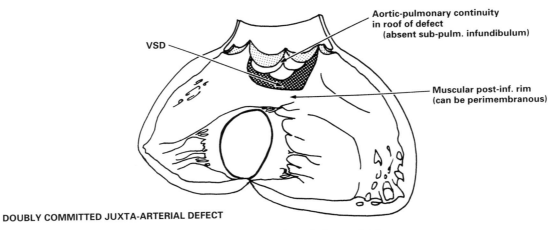

Aortic-pulmonary continuity in roof of defect (absent sub-pulm. infundibulum)

VSD

Muscular post-inf. rim (can be perimembranous)

DOUBLY COMMITTED JUXTA-ARTERIAL DEFECT

Fig. 3.31. The basic types of ventricular septal defects.

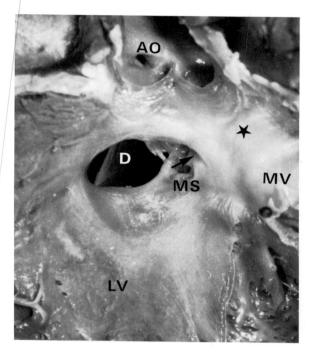

Fig. 3.32. The opened left ventricular (*LV*) outflow revealing a perimembranous defect (*D*) with a remnant of the membranous septum (*MS*) in its posterior rim. Components of the tricuspid valve are visible through the defect. The area of fibrous continuity between the aorta (*AO*) and the mitral valve (*MV*) is indicated by an *asterisk*.

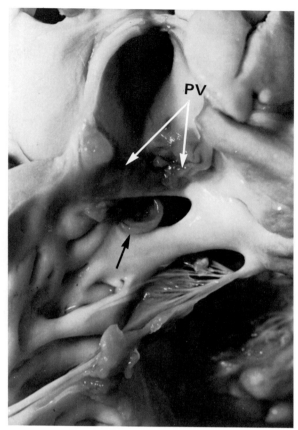

Fig. 3.33. The opened right ventricular outflow revealing a doubly committed subarterial ventricular septal defect and a prolapsed aortic valve cusp (*arrow*). *PV*, pulmonary valve.

septum remain remote from the atrioventricular conduction bundle.

The third category is the doubly committed "subarterial ventricular septal defect" (Fig. 3.33). This defect occurs in the region of the ventricular outlets but borders immediately on the arterial junction, so that the conjoined arterial valves constitute its upper rim. This particular type of defect, when small, is prone to develop early prolapse of the aortic valve. Subarterial defects occur much more frequently in Japan than in any other part of the world and in those areas are often named "subpulmonic" defects. The crest of the septum may be formed by the septomarginal trabeculation, which buttresses the conduction system from the rim, or the defect may expand to become perimembranous.

The frequency of spontaneous closure of a ventricular septal defect is high, as deduced from the marked discrepancy between postnatally, clinically identified ventricular septal defects and those that eventually need surgical repair or come to autopsy.

The small muscular type may close spontaneously with growth of the heart and hypertrophy of muscle cells. In small perimembranous defects, an aneurysm of tricuspid leaflet tissue may form and become adherent to the edges of the defect. The adjacent part of the tricuspid valve may also become involved in this process.

In some patients, a ventricular septal defect is part of a more complicated cardiovascular abnormality. A particular association is seen in patients with a ventricular septal defect, subvalvar aortic stenosis resulting from leftward deviation of the outlet septum, and an interrupted aortic arch (Fig. 3.34). Moreover, aortic coarctation in a symptomatic neonate is often associated with a ventricular septal defect characterized by leftward deviation of the outlet septum. The flow hypothesis to explain the occurrence of aortic coarctation is related in part to this common association (see p. 113).

The presence of a ventricular septal defect will lead to an obligatory left-to-right shunt. The right

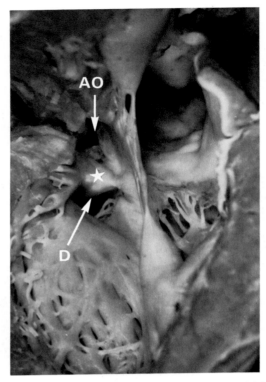

Fig. 3.34. The combined occurrence of a ventricular septal defect (*D*) and subvalvar aortic stenosis, caused by leftward deviation of the outlet septum (*asterisk*), *AO*, aorta.

ventricle will have to accommodate a high pressure and this will be reflected in changes in the pulmonary circulation. The natural history of a patient with such a defect will thus become complicated by plexogenic pulmonary arteriopathy at a much earlier date than in patients with atrial septal defect. In the case of an otherwise uncomplicated ventricular septal defect it is generally accepted that it is unlikely for pulmonary hypertension to become irreversible before the age of 2 years.

Atrioventricular Septal Defects

The group of lesions variously known as "atrioventricular defects", "atrioventricular canal malformations" or "endocardial cushion defects" (Somerville 1978) are unified by absence of the atrioventricular septal structures which, in the normal heart, separate the right atrium from the left ventricle (Becker and Anderson 1982). There are several anatomical consequences of this deficiency. First, there is a common atrioventricular junction, in contrast to the separate junctions guarded by the mitral and tricuspid valves

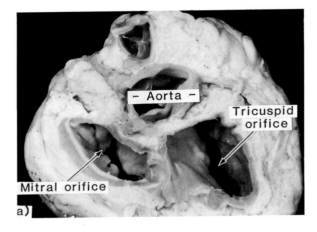

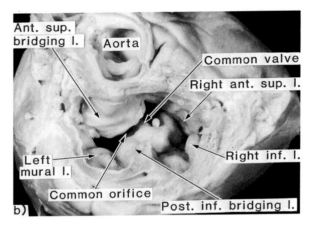

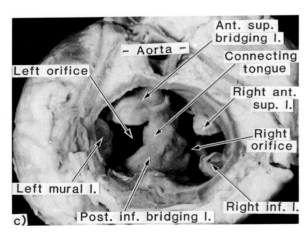

Fig. 3.35. Differences between the atrioventricular junction in the normal heart (**a**), where the aortic valve is wedged deeply between the mitral and tricuspid orifices in "shamrock" fashion, and the arrangements in atrioventricular septal defect with (**b**) common orifice and (**c**) separate orifices, in which the aorta is "unwedged". This produces a "snowman" arrangement relative to the aorta, *ante. sup.*, anterosuperior; *post. inf.*, posteroinferior; *l*, leaflet.

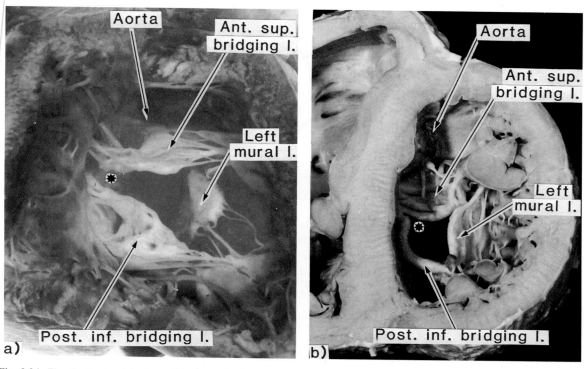

Fig. 3.36. The short axis of the heart from beneath, showing **a** the left atrioventricular valve in atrioventricular septal defect with common orifice and **b** one with separate right and left orifices. Note that the left valve has a three-leaflet arrangement. The cleft (*asterisk*) is simply the space between the left ventricular components of the bridging leaflets. *ant. sup.*, anterosuperior; *post. inf.*, posteroinferior; *l*, leaflet.

in the normal heart (Fig. 3.35). Second, the aortic valve and subaortic outflow tract are no longer wedged between the mitral and tricuspid orifices but are anterosuperiorly located. Third, there is a gross disproportion between the inlet and outlet dimensions of the ventricular mass, this ratio being unity in the normal heart. Finally, almost always, there is a hole at the anticipated site of the atrioventricular septum, hence our preferred term for the group, "atrioventricular septal defects". The anatomy described above is uniform for the whole group of lesions. It is customary, however, to subdivide the group into "complete" and "partial" forms. The artificiality of this convention is then shown by the necessity to describe "transitional" forms to account for those hearts which cannot adequately be described as complete or partial. In reality, there are several anatomical features that enable subcategorizations to be made.

The first division is made according to whether the common atrioventricular junction is guarded by a common valve or separate right and left atrioventricular valves. The basic morphology of the valve or the valves is the same. The junction is guarded by a five-leaflet mechanism. Two of the leaflets are confined to the right ventricle (the anterosuperior and inferior leaflets) and one to the left ventricle (the mural leaflet). The other two leaflets, situated in anterosuperior and posteroinferior position, cross the septum to be tethered in both ventricles. They are the bridging leaflets. The two bridging leaflets are separate and discrete structures when the atrioventricular orifice is common (Fig. 3.35b), but are united by a connecting tongue when there are separate right and left orifices (Fig. 3.35c). The left ventricular component of the valve bears scant resemblance to the normal mitral valve, differing in respect of the annulus, leaflets and papillary muscle arrangement (Carpentier 1978; Penkoske et al. 1985). The so-called cleft is in reality the space between the left ventricular components of the two bridging leaflets, whether there is a common orifice or separate right and left atrioventricular valves (Fig. 3.36).

The second significant anatomical variation determines the potential level of shunting through the atrioventricular septal defect. This depends on the relationship of the bridging leaflets to the septal structures (Fig. 3.37). If the bridging leaflets are firmly adherent to the ventricular septum, the only

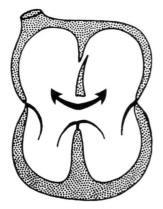

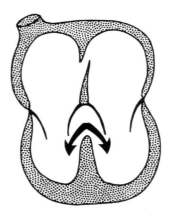

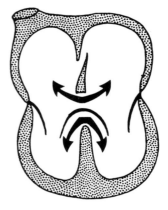

**Bridging leaflets attached
to Interventricular septum –
Interatrial communication
("Ostium primum ASD")**

a

**Bridging leaflets attached
to Interatrial septum
Interventricular communication
("Isolated VSD")**

b

**Floating bridging leaflet(s)
Interatrial and
interventricular communications
(Usually common orifice)**

c

Fig. 3.37. Shunting through the atrioventricular septal defect is conditioned by the attachment of the bridging leaflets to the septal structures. *ASD*, atrioventricular septal defect; *VSD*, ventricular septal defect.

possibility for shunting is at atrial level (unless there is a coexisting muscular ventricular septal defect). If the leaflets are attached to the underside of the atrial septum, the only possibility for shunting is at ventricular level. If, however, the leaflets float free from both septal structures, shunting can occur at both atrial and ventricular levels depending on the pressures in the various chambers. Usually the potential for shunting is restricted to the atrial level where there are separate right and left atrioventricular valves ("partial" defect or "ostium primum atrial septal defect"). Cases with a common orifice, in contrast, usually provide the potential for both atrial and ventricular shunting ("complete" defects). These are by no means universal associations, nevertheless, and it is necessary to account for the arrangement of the orifices separately from the potential level of shunting if all hearts are to be accurately classified.

The third significant feature for anatomical categorization is the relationship of the atrioventricular junction to the ventricular mass. Usually the atrial chambers are equally committed to the ventricles, giving the "balanced" arrangement. Sometimes the right side of the heart is much larger than the left side, usually with obstructive lesions of the aortic outflow tract and arch (right ventricular dominance). Alternatively, the left side of the heart may be dominant, this arrangement tending to occur in association with subpulmonary stenosis or atresia.

An atrioventricular septal defect can also coexist with other lesions elsewhere in the heart. There may be a Fallot-type outflow tract pathology (Lev et al. 1961), in the sense that the aorta overrides the ventricular septum while the pulmonary outflow tract is considerably narrowed. It may also occur with Ebstein's malformation (see p. 93) of the right ventricular (tricuspid) component of the common valve (Caruso et al. 1978). Both associated conditions will dramatically alter the course of the disease.

The abnormality at the level of the atrioventricular junction influences markedly the topography of the atrioventricular conduction tissue axis (Lev 1958; Feldt et al. 1970). The atrioventricular node is displaced posteriorly by virtue of the large septal defect. The atrioventricular (His) bundle, however, is elongated, running along the crest of the ventricular septum. The left bundle branches show an early "take-off", thereby creating a widened gap between them and the final evolution of the right bundle branch. This peculiar anatomy probably underlies the characteristic vectocardiogram, which indicates early activation of the posterior left ventricular wall (Durrer et al. 1966). The course of the bundle, moreover, may explain why early degenerative changes can occur, providing an anatomical basis for the frequent occurrence of "spontaneous" atrioventricular dissociation in the natural course of the disease.

Atrioventricular septal defects with common valve orifice are the most common cardiac conditions occurring with the trisomy 21 syndrome (see p. 54).

Tricuspid Valvar Abnormalities

The right atrioventricular orifice can be diminished in size, a feature which in most cases indicates hypoplasia of the right ventricle, often associated with pulmonary atresia. Frequently the tricuspid valve guarding such a hypoplastic ostium shows features of Ebstein's malformation (see below).

In "tricuspid atresia", the right atrium has no outlet other than the oval foramen or a true atrial septal defect. Two types can be recognized. In the classic form of tricuspid atresia there is no potential communication between the right atrium and the underlying ventricular mass. From an anatomical point of view, this type of malformation belongs to the category of hearts with univentricular atrioventricular connection, and will be discussed under that heading (see p. 108). The second form of tricuspid atresia is extremely rare. It consists of an imperforate valve separating the right atrium from an underlying ventricle (see Fig. 3.17). This imperforate valve may show evidence of Ebstein's malformation. The fundamental difference between this condition and classic tricuspid atresia is that a formed but usually hypoplastic right ventricle is usually present, in proper alignment with the right atrium.

"Ebstein's malformation" of the tricuspid valve is characterized by the combined occurrence of distal displacement of some of the tricuspid valve attachments and dysplasia of the valve leaflets (Fig. 3.38). Both these features vary in extent (Becker et al. 1971). Distal displacement always affects the septal attachment of the valve but may include the posterolateral insertions. The anterosuperior leaflet, however, will always be attached to the atrioventricular junction. The distal displacement of part of the valve creates an "atrialized part" of the right ventricle.

Dysplasia of valve leaflets is characterized by a curtain-like appearance, with valve leaflets having direct insertions into the ventricular wall. Fusion of leaflets may occur, so that a small orifice remains as the only inlet to the right ventricle. As indicated above, some forms of imperforate right valve are basically imperforate Ebstein's malformations. Moreover, the dyplastic valve leaflets can contain bands of myocardium.

Ebstein's malformation of the tricuspid valve is often associated with an atrial septal defect of the oval fossa type, together with pulmonary valve abnormalities. In some instances a ventricular septal defect can coexist. A high incidence of Wolf–Parkinson–White syndrome occurs, usually of the septal right-sided type.

In hearts with discordant atrioventricular connections, such as congenitally corrected transposition

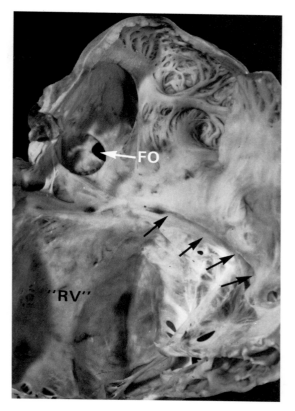

Fig. 3.38. A heart with Ebstein's malformation of the tricuspid valve. There is distal displacement of the basal attachments of the septal and posterior leaflets, creating a large "atrial" part of the right ventricle (*RV*). The anterior leaflet takes origin from the annulus fibrosus (*arrow*), but is curtain-like and has many direct insertions into the ventricular wall. *FO*, oval foramen.

(see p. 101), there is relatively high incidence of Ebstein-like malformation of the morphologically tricuspid valve.

Mitral Valvar Abnormalities

Isolated mitral valvar abnormalities are rare. "Mitral atresia" is the most common form being due in most instances to an imperforate valve. In the majority of cases, however, the atrioventricular junction is characterized by absence of the atrioventricular connection, so that the architecture is similar to that seen in hearts with classic tricuspid atresia (see p. 109). Congenital mitral stenosis can take various forms with underdevelopment of the mitral valve ring and valve apparatus as the most common type (Ruckman and Van Praagh 1978). "Parachute mitral valve" is the condition in which all tendinous cords of the valve insert into one papillary muscle, thereby

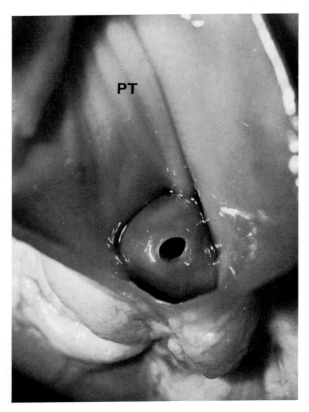

Fig. 3.39. A dome-shaped pulmonary valve stenosis, viewed from above after opening of the pulmonary trunk (*PT*).

creating a funnel-type ventricular inlet. This condition can occur as an isolated lesion but is frequently part of a more complex malformation, which includes additional anomalies like aortic coarctation, muscular subaortic stenosis and supravalvar stenosing ring of the left atrium (Shone et al. 1963). One or both papillary muscles may be extremely hypoplastic, thus mimicking "true" parachute mitral valve. Exceptionally, both papillary muscles may be absent, with cords directly originating from the left ventricular wall.

Abnormal cordal attachments of the mitral valvar apparatus may occur in isolation.

Pulmonary Valvar Abnormalities

Bicuspid and quadricuspid pulmonary valves can occur and are themselves of no or of only limited clinical significance.

Pulmonary Valvar Stenosis. This abnormality is frequent in isolation. The valve in this condition nearly always shows a dome-shaped stenosis (Fig.

3.39). The pulmonary trunk reveals a post-stenotic dilatation. The ventricular septum is mostly intact. At the atrial level, a patent oval foramen or a "true" atrial septal defect may be present, facilitating decompression of right heart chambers. The term "trilogy of Fallot" has been used, inappropriately, for the latter.

The condition leads to colossal right ventricular hypertrophy, particularly in cases without an atrial vent. Hypertrophy may ultimately also affect the left ventricular wall (Harinck et al. 1977).

Pulmonary Valvar Dysplasia. In pulmonary valvar dysplasia, the valve consists of three leaflets, which are thickened and have a gelatinous aspect. The condition can occur in isolation but is more frequently part of Noonan's syndrome.

Pulmonary Atresia with Intact Ventricular Septum. This abnormality takes various forms, the most common being that in which an imperforate valve is present at the level of the arterial junction (Fig. 3.40a); in other cases a muscular segment intervenes between ventricle and pulmonary trunk (Fig. 3.40b). The pulmonary trunk is nearly always small, in contrast to the dilated pulmonary trunk in patients with isolated pulmonary valvar stenosis. The pulmonary blood supply is dependent on the arterial duct, which in these cases is characteristically elongated, taking a curved course from its aortic site to the truncal bifurcation. The intrapulmonary arteries are thin-walled, as in all instances of diminished pulmonary flow. The number of peripheral arteries is probably lower than normal. The right ventricle can be small or of normal size, although occasionally a dilated right ventricular cavity is seen. Fistulous communications may be present, connecting the right ventricular cavity to branches of the coronary arteries and serving as an outlet for the right ventricle. In such instances examination of the heart will reveal tortuous dilated epicardial coronary arteries.

Pulmonary Atresia with Ventricular Septal Defect. In the presence of a septal defect, pulmonary atresia is usually infundibular. The aorta, being the only outlet for the heart, usually overrides the septum to a varying degree, and the situation closely resembles an extreme degree of Fallot's tetralogy, except that the deviation of the outlet septum is complete, producing atresia of the right ventricular outflow tract (Fig. 3.41). The origin and course of the blood vessels supplying the lungs is usually highly complex. There may be an arterial duct connecting the aorta to moderately well developed central pulmonary arteries, but in other instances an intricate system of major aorticopulmonary collateral arteries supplies the pulmonary arteries. The latter supply all

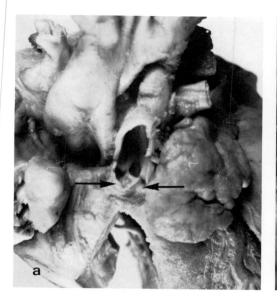
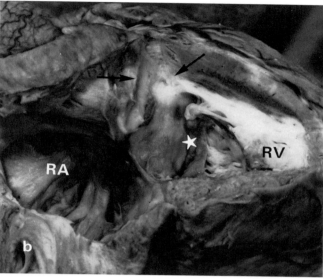

Fig. 3.40. Pulmonary atresia and intact ventricular septum. **a** Imperforate valve at the level of the arterial junction (*arrows*). **b** An intervening muscular segment (*arrows*). The anterior free wall has been removed, revealing a minute, thick-walled right ventricle (*RV*). Note the hypoplastic tricuspid orifice guarded by a valve showing septal displacement (*asterisk*) characteristic for Ebstein's malformation, a frequently associated anomaly in this condition. *RA*, right atrium.

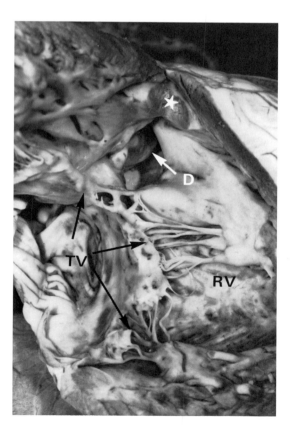

or part of the lungs, either with the central pulmonary arteries or in isolation.

Aortic Valvar Abnormalities

A bicuspid aortic valve usually has no functional significance in children. The pathological consequences of this anomaly may appear later in life. Quadricuspid aortic valve is extremely rare and most probably has no functional significance.

"Aortic stenosis" of valvar origin is nearly always caused by a unicommissural, unicuspid aortic valve (Fig. 3.42a). When viewed from its aortic aspect, the valve has a modified dome-shaped appearance with a keyhole of orifice. From its commissural insertion the valve executes a U-turn without inserting into the aortic wall, and re-inserts at the site of the initial commissure (Fig. 3.42a). In the base of the valve an

Fig. 3.41. The opened right ventricle (*RV*) in a heart with pulmonary atresia and ventricular septal defect (*D*). The outflow part shows a striking similarity with that in classic Fallot's tetralogy (Compare Fig. 3.55b), hence the term "extreme Fallot". The infundibular septum (*asterisk*) shows an extreme anterior deviation producing atresia of the pulmonary outflow tract. The aorta is seen to override the defect. *TV*, tricuspid valve.

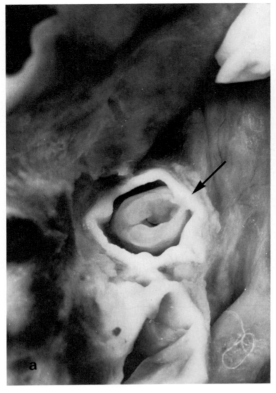
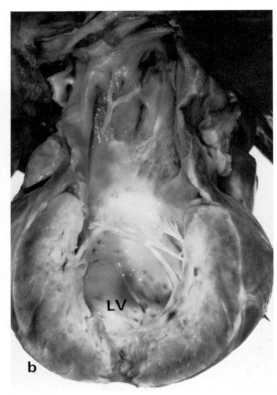

Fig. 3.42. A unicommissural, unicuspid aortic valve. **a** The stenotic unicommissural (*arrow*), viewed from its aortic aspect. **b** Marked left ventricular (*LV*) myocardial hypertrophy with extensive subendocardial fibrosis caused by impaired myocardial perfusion.

occasional shallow raphe can be present. This condition can be associated with either a small or a normal-sized left ventricle. In most instances the ventricular septum is intact, but some degree of ventricular hypertrophy is manifest. At an early age ischaemia will affect the myocardium, so that subendocardial infarction of the left ventricular wall will appear (Fig. 3.42b). Myocardial ischaemia underlies sudden death, which is common in these patients. Moreover, left ventricular scarring will affect the pump function, so that left heart failure can appear early in the disease. Dilated left heart chambers and structural changes in the pulmonary vasculature may underline this sequence of events.

"Aortic valvar dysplasia" is a rare condition which, like pulmonary valvar dysplasia, is often part of Noonan's syndrome.

In "aortic atresia" the ascending aorta is a narrow channel, which conducts blood retrogradely to the coronary arteries. Coronary arterial flow and blood flow to the head and upper body depend on patency of the arterial duct, hence the early high mortality associated with this lesion. Usually aortic artresia is accompanied by hypoplasia of the left heart. This

exists in two discrete forms. In the first the left atrioventricular connection is absent and the left ventricle is represented by its apical trabecular component (see p. 77). In the other form there is mitral stenosis because of a small valvar apparatus, and the ventricular chamber shows considerable endocardial fibroelastosis (Fig. 3.43). In rate instances, aortic atresia is associated with a ventricular septal defect and a normally sized left ventricle and mitral valve.

Supravalvar Aortic Stenosis

Supravalvar aortic stenosis is characterized by an obstruction in the aorta beyond the level of the aortic valve. There are three types of supravalvar aortic stenosis. The most common form is the hourglass type, in which a funnel-shaped stenosis is present (Fig. 3.44). The aortic media in the affected region shows a mosaic pattern, i.e. a disorderly arrangement of the lamellar aortic units. A second form of supravalvar aortic stenosis is the segmental type, which is characterized by a uniform thickening of the wall affecting the greater part of the ascending aorta.

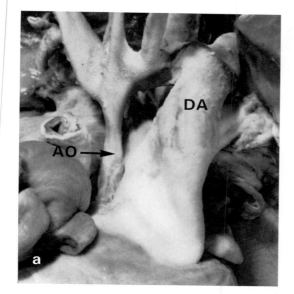

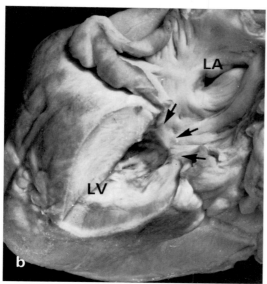

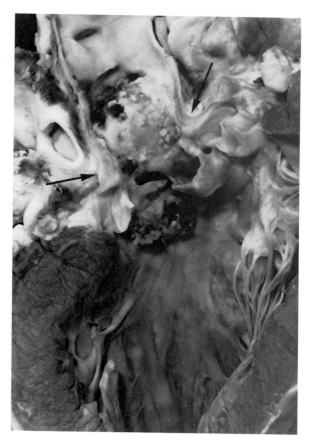

Fig. 3.44. Supravalvar aortic stenosis of the hourglass type.

Fig. 3.43. Aortic atresia. **a** The hypoplastic ascending aorta (*AO*). Systemic flow depends on patency of the arterial duct (*DA*). **b** Extreme hypoplasia of the left ventricle (*LV*) connected to the left atrium (*LA*) through a minute mitral orifice (*arrows*) guarded by a basically normal mitral valve.

In some cases the diseased wall may extend into the innominate (brachiocephalic), carotid and subclavian arteries. The least common type of supravalvar aortic stenosis is that in which a perforate membrane obstructs the ascending aorta.

Location of the obstruction distal to the origin of the coronary arteries, so that the latter originate from a high-pressure chamber, is common to all forms. In rare circumstances supravalvar aortic stenosis may be associated with similar structural changes in the pulmonary trunk and/or central pulmonary arteries. If the latter circumstance prevails, the aortic abnormality is most often part of a non-familial but otherwise complex syndrome, which consists of mental retardation and a particular facies, often in association with a syndrome of hypercalcaemia (William's or Beuren's syndrome). A familial form can occur, which lacks these additional features but in which multiple aortic and pulmonary stenoses can be present.

Subvalvar Aortic Stenosis

Subaortic stenosis can have various substrates. At present the classification advocated is that based on the functional characteristics of the stenotic site. Three major types are distinguished: a dynamic type, a fixed type, and a mixed type. The dynamic type is known also as "hypertrophic cardiomyopathy", considered an autosomal dominant disorder. The disease may become manifest in childhood, but a delayed onset of symptoms and a variable clinical expression are characteristic of the disease. Until recently the anomaly was considered to cause asymmetric septal thickening and, on that basis, left ventricular outflow tract obstruction. Clinical terms, such as ASH. (asymmetric septal hypertrophy), IHSS. (idiopathic hypertrophic subaortic stenosis) and HOCM. (hypertrophic obstructive cardiomyopathy), are all based on this premise. Recently, it has been shown that symmetric hypertrophy occurs in over one-third of patients and that approximately 15% will have apical hypertrophy of the left ventricle (Shapiro and McKenna, 1983).

Unexplained left ventricular hypertrophy is the leading sign, and congestive heart failure due to non-compliant ventricles is the most important symptom in infancy. In older children and young adults the disease may first present as sudden and unexpected death.

The pathological diagnosis is based on the gross recognition of marked myocardial hypertrophy – whether symmetric or asymmetric – associated microscopically with disorderly arranged myocardial tissues. The latter features, collectively known as "disarray" and "disorganization" also occur in the normal heart, but in hypertrophic cardiomyopathy this texture is much more widespread. Furthermore, other features occur, such as distinct hypertrophy of myocytes, bizarre-shaped nuclei often with perinuclear halos, and an increase in interstitial fibrous tissue, particularly in older children and adults. Knowledge of the variable histological expression is important for the interpretation of endomyocardial biopsies. Other causes of secondary and physiological hypertrophy, such as left ventricular hypertrophy in diabetic mothers and Pompe's disease (see p. 839) should be excluded. Hypertrophic cardiomyopathy may coexist with a variety of syndromes, including Noonan's syndrome (see p. 123), lentiginosis and Friedreich's ataxia (see p. 165). Some infants may gradually develop signs of a dynamic subaortic obstruction in the course of various types of congenital heart malformation.

Fixed types of subaortic stenosis can take several forms. The most common type is that in which a discrete subvalvar fibrous ridge is present on the ventricular septal surface, continuing on to the ventricular aspect of the aortic leaflet of the mitral valve. In many instances this fibrous ridge is intimately related to one of the aortic valvar leaflets (Fig. 3.45). This shelf-like type of subaortic stenosis is usually mild and carries a favourable prognosis. In contrast, the "tunnel" type of subaortic stenosis has a more serious outlook. In this condition a fibromuscular tunnel is present underneath the aortic valve. The abnormal

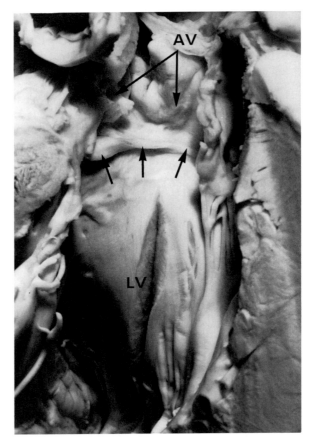

Fig. 3.45. Left ventricular outflow (*LV*), opened from the apex through the anterior mitral leaflet. The outflow tract is obstructed by a fibrous ridge (*arrows*), intimately related to the aortic valve (*AV*).

segment has an intimate relation with the mitral valve and in most instances intervenes between the mitral and aortic valves. Another form of fixed subvulvar aortic stenosis is characterized by abnormal septal attachments of the mitral valvar apparatus, a condition often associated with an atrioventricular septal defect.

The third type of subaortic stenosis is a combination of dynamic and fixed forms. Thus, in many instances of a dynamic outflow tract obstruction, a marked fibrous thickening of the overlying endocardium occurs, contributing to the degree of stenosis.

Aortopulmonary Window

From a pathogenic point of view, the aortopulmonary window is closely related to a common arterial trunk (see p. 81).

The condition is characterized by a window-like communication between adjacent parts of the walls of the pulmonary trunk and the ascending aorta (Fig. 3.46). The window is situated above the level of the arterial valves in the region between the orifices of the right and left coronary arteries. Viewed from the pulmonary trunk, the window is present in the posterolateral area, just underneath and anterior to the origin of the right pulmonary artery.

Both great arteries display separate arterial valves, unlike the situation in the classic common arterial trunk. Moreover, the ventricular septum is usually intact.

An obligatory left-to-right shunt occurs, which usually leads to early plexogenic pulmonary arteriopathy and irreversible pulmonary hypertension.

Abnormalities of the Arterial Duct (Ductus Arteriosus)

Premature closure of the arterial duct has occasionally been reported as a cause of intrauterine death (Becker et al. 1977). Careful inspection of the duct, particularly during an autopsy on a stillborn fetus, may further substantiate the potential significance of this observation.

More commonly, problems arise from persistent patency of the arterial duct. In the mature neonate the duct is usually permanently closed at approximately 3 weeks. In prematurely born neonates, however, it may remain patent for some months after birth. It is generally accepted that a duct that is still patent at 3 months of age will only rarely close spontaneously. The precise mechanisms of closure are not fully understood at present, and neither is the reason for persistent patency. Recent histological studies of patent ducts have revealed an abnormal structural characteristic – an uninterrupted internal elastic lamina at the site of intimal cushions and in some instances "aorticization" of the wall (Gittenberger-de Groot 1977).

In recent years the administration of prostaglandins has been advocated to prevent the duct from closing where the life of the baby depends on its function (e.g. in patients with pulmonary atresia and intact ventricular septum). Prostaglandins decrease the vascular tone of the vessel. Histological studies have shown that the wall becomes oedematous and the danger of intimal tears, dissection, and rupture is real; the pathologist should be aware of this while examining the duct (Gittenberger-de Groot et al. 1978).

A patent arterial duct usually causes an aortic-to-pulmonary shunt with pulmonary hypertension as a result. In time, irreversible pulmonary vascular changes can appear.

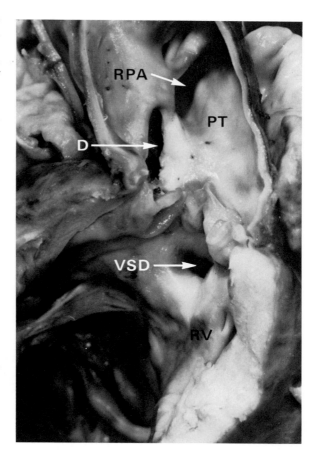

Fig. 3.46. Heart specimen with aorticopulmonary window, viewed through the opened right ventricular outflow (*RV*) and pulmonary trunk (*PT*). The defect (*D*) is located in the postero-lateral area, just underneath and anterior to the origin of the right pulmonary artery (*RPA*). Note the presence of a ventricular septal defect (*VSD*).

Abnormalities of the Coronary Arteries

Congenital abnormalities of the coronary arteries have been divided into minor and major forms. Minor congenital abnormalities consist of reduplication or translocation of orifices, or abnormalities in the proximal course of the coronary arteries. It has been suggested that some of these minor variations are less minor than initially thought (Becker 1981). Translocation of the orifice of the left coronary artery to the right coronary sinus can lead to a situation in which the main stem of the left coronary artery runs between the pulmonary trunk and the aortic root. Cases of sudden death associated with this condition have been reported. Moreover, translocation of an orifice to the side of the commissural attachment may result in a slit-like ostium which in time may become

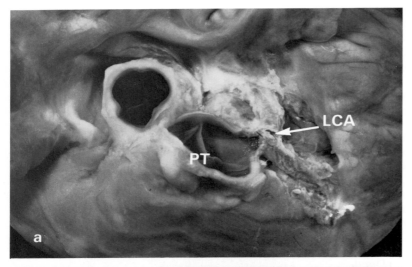

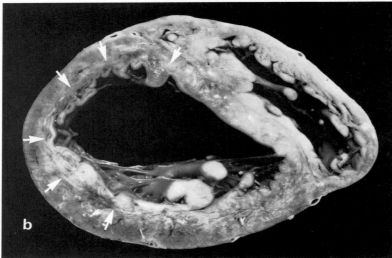

Fig. 3.47. Aberrant origin of the left coronary artery from the pulmonary trunk. **a** Site of origin of the left coronary artery (*LCA*) from the pulmonary trunk (*PT*). **b** Transsection of the left ventricle, showing extensive, mainly subendocardial, myocardial necrosis (*arrows*) of the left ventricle.

compromised by degenerative aortic wall changes leading to stenosis.

The most common abnormal course is that in which the left circumflex artery originates from the proximal segment of the right coronary artery and runs posterior to the aortic root before it takes its usual course in the left atrioventricular groove.

In hearts with abnormal relationships of the great arteries, abnormalities in the course of the coronary arteries are more common. Major forms of congenital coronary arterial abnormalities generally have direct functional consequences.

Aberrant origin of the left coronary artery from the pulmonary trunk (Bland et al. 1933) is of major clinical significance (Fig. 3.47a). Owing to the pressure drop in the pulmonary trunk after birth and the concomitant hypertrophy of the myocardial cells of the left ventricle, a decrease in flow is established in the left coronary artery and ischaemia or left ventricular myocardial infarction occurs often with mitral insufficiency as the leading symptom. If the neonate survives this initial period, recurrent ischaemic attacks may occur at later ages. In these instances abundant collateral arteries will have developed between the right coronary artery, normally originating from the aorta, and the aberrant left coronary artery. These collaterals can result in a preferential shunting of blood from the coronary arterial system to the pulmonary trunk. Large areas of left ventricular myocardium may thus be deprived of an adequate blood supply (Fig. 3.47b). In all instances of sudden death of an adolescent the pathologist should look for this particular congenital abnormality.

Aberrant right coronary artery from the pulmonary trunk is extremely rare and usually has no consequences in the paediatric or adolescent age groups.

Coronary arterial fistula can occur between the right and left ventricular chambers and the epicardial coronary arteries. Such fistula often accompany conditions with increased intracavitary pressures, such as arterial valvar atresia, but occasionally occur as isolated lesions. Usually such fistula have limited functional significance. Examination of the heart may reveal the condition from the presence of dilated and tortuous epicardial coronary arteries.

Congenital Heart Malformations with Abnormal Junctional Connections

The malformations discussed in this section all involve at least one abnormal junctional connection. They can exist with mirror-image atrial arrangement, but such cases are rare. They will therefore be described with usual atrial arrangement assumed.

Congenitally Corrected Transposition

Congenitally corrected transposition is characterized by *dis*cordant atrioventricular connections, in association with *dis*cordant ventriculoarterial connections. In other words, the right atrium connects to the morphologically left ventricle, from which arises the pulmonary trunk, while the left atrium connects to the morphologically right ventricle, from which arises the aorta (Fig. 3.48). This usually occurs with normally arranged atria, but the same configuration may occur with a mirror-image atrial arrangement. The flow pattern is such that system venous blood is conveyed into the pulmonary trunk, albeit by way of the "wrong" ventricle, while pulmonary venous blood is directed into the systemic circulation, again along an abnormal route. The "transposition" of the great arteries, in the sense of discordant ventriculoarterial connections, is thus "corrected" because of "inversion" of ventricles, in the sense of discordant atrioventricular connections; hence the name "congenitally corrected transposition".

The condition is usually complicated by additional anomalies (Losekoot et al. 1983), the most common being ventricular septal defect, subpulmonary outflow obstruction, and Ebstein-like malformation of the (left-sided) morphologically tricuspid valve. The natural course of the disease is greatly influenced by these anomalies.

The condition is further complicated by an abnormal disposition of the atrioventricular conduction tissues (Anderson et al. 1974, 1975). Because of the malalignment between the interatrial septum and the inflow part of the interventricular septum, a regularly positioned posterior node is usually unable to contact the ventricular myocardium. It is known that during development a complete ring of conduction tissue surrounds the tricuspid orifice, with an expansion at the anterolateral margin. In corrected transposition, this anterolateral node takes over as the connecting atrioventricular node, and from it a penetrating atrioventricular bundle descends on to the ventricular septum. This bundle is closely related to the fibrous annulus of the mitral valve and takes an elongated course, encircling the pulmonary outflow tract anteriorly to descend along the anterior rim of a ventricular septal defect if present. The abnormal disposition of the atrioventricular conduction axis is surgically very significant. Moreover, the attenuated course of the bundle, in close contact with the mitral valvar attachment, may explain the high frequency of spontaneous atrioventricular dissociation that occurs in the natural history of this condition.

Complete Transposition

Complete transposition is characterized by *dis*cordant ventriculoarterial connections, while the atrioventricular connections are *con*cordant (Fig. 3.49). Thus, the right atrium connects to a right ventricle, from which the aorta arises, and the left atrium connects to the left ventricle, which gives rise to the pulmonary trunk. This can occur with either usual or mirror-image atrial arrangement.

In the usual case of complete transposition, the aorta is positioned anterior to and to the right of the pulmonary trunk. It is not uncommon, however, to find the aorta either in front or to the left of the pulmonary trunk, although the internal arrangement characterized by the discordant ventriculoarterial connections is not altered. As a consequence of the abnormal aortic position, the left coronary artery will often run anterior to the pulmonary trunk; this can be anticipated in all hearts with an anteriorly positioned aorta.

Basically, the anatomical arrangements in complete transposition result in two separate circulatory pathways. Therefore life can only be sustained if exchange of blood between the two circulations can occur. Most cases of complete transposition will display a shunt possibility at atrial level, either through a patent oval foramen or through a true atrial septal defect. Other sites of possible interchange

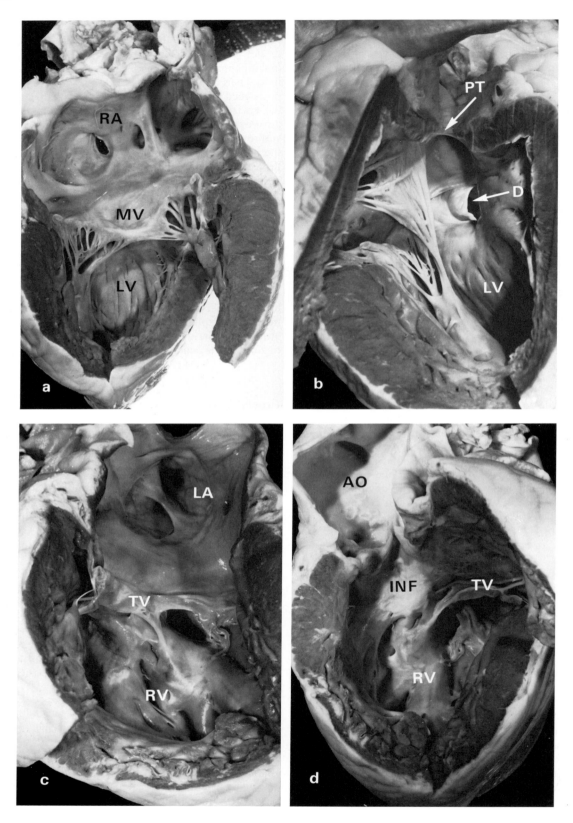

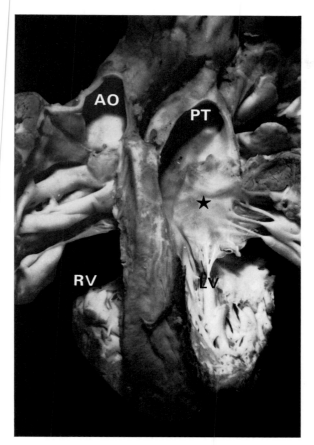

Fig. 3.49. The characteristics of complete transposition. A concordant atrioventricular connection is complicated by a discordant ventriculoarterial connection. The aorta (*AO*) arises from the right ventricle (*RV*), the two being separated by an infundibulum. The pulmonary trunk (*PT*) arises from the left ventricle (*LV*) and there is fibrous continuity (*asterisk*) between pulmonary and mitral valves.

between the two circulations are a ventricular septal defect or a persistent arterial duct.

Complete transposition can be subdivided into three categories: those with an intact ventricular

◀ ──────────────────────

Fig. 3.48. Congenitally corrected transposition in the setting of usual atrial arrangement. **a** Opened right side of the heart. The right atrium (*RA*) connects to the morphologically left ventricle (*LV*). The atrioventricular junction is guarded by the mitral valve (*MV*). **b** Outflow tract of the left ventricle (*LV*) into the pulmonary trunk (*PT*), which is in a posterior location. There is a large ventricular septal defect (*D*). **c** Opened left side of the heart. The left atrium (*LA*) connects to the morphologically right ventricle (*RV*) via the tricuspid valve (*RV*). **d** Outflow tract of the right ventricle (*RV*) leading into an anteriorly positioned aorta (*AO*) separated from the tricuspid valve (*TV*) by the infundibulum (*INF*).

septum; those with a ventricular septal defect; and those with a ventricular septal defect and pulmonary stenosis.

The ventricular septal defects in these hearts can be located in similar sites to those of isolated defects, although malalignment outlet defects are more frequent (Fig. 3.50).

Pulmonary stenosis can be of valvar origin, but a subvalvar outflow tract obstruction is often also present (Fig. 3.51). Pulmonary stenosis can provide protection against the development of pulmonary vascular disease, which is a common and early complication in patients with complete transposition and a ventricular septal defect without pulmonary stenosis.

A brief note should be added on the surgical repair of complete transposition of the great arteries, because it is likely that the pathologist, at least in centres where cardiac surgery is performed, will be confronted with a corrected specimen.

The operative procedure most commonly followed used to be the Mustard operation. The essence of this repair is to convey the venous returns to their appropriate great arteries by redirecting their atrial routes. The atrial septum is removed and a baffle is constructed inside the "common" atrium in such a way that the pulmonary venous return is conveyed into the right ventricle (Fig. 3.52a) while the systemic venous blood is directed into the left ventricle (Fig. 3.52b). In most centres, the baffle was constructed from either pericardium or a synthetic material. A similar procedure is the Senning operation, in which flaps of atrial tissue are used for the rerouting of blood.

More recently an "arterial switch" operation has been advocated, in which the great arteries are divided and switched back to the appropriate ventricles, with relocation of the coronary arteries in the "new aortic root".

Double-Outlet Right Ventricle

In double-outlet right ventricle both great arteries arise mainly from the right ventricle. In most cases the aorta is to the right of the pulmonary trunk, in a side-by-side relationship (Fig. 3.53). When inspected from the interior, the two arterial outlets are separated by a distinct rim of muscle – the outlet (infundibular) septum (Fig. 3.53).

Subclassification is based on the position of the ventricular septal defect, which may be subaortic (Fig. 3.53a), subpulmonary (Fig. 3.53b), doubly committed, or non-committed.

In the double-outlet right ventricle with subpulmonary defect (Fig. 3.53b), the pulmonary trunk is closely related to the ventricular septum and in some instances may straddle the septum. The Taussig –

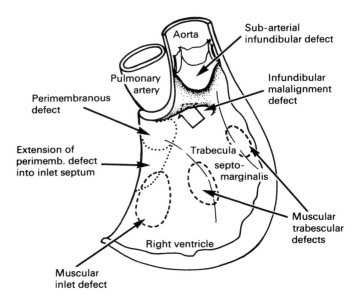

Fig. 3.50. The various sites of a ventricular septal defect in complete transposition. The condition shows a relatively high incidence of malalignment outlet defects.

Bing heart is the classic example in this category (Taussig and Bing 1949). It is also from this particular case that the paradigm of a bilateral infundibulum ("double conus") has been set (Van Praagh 1968). It has long been advocated that, for a heart to be classified as double-outlet right ventricle, the arterial valve should be separated from the mitral valve by a rim of muscle and the two arterial valves should be positioned at the same level. Meanwhile, however, many specimens have been observed that show fibrous continuity between the atrioventricular and arterial valves, but otherwise fulfil all criteria of a

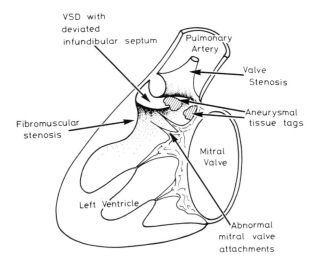

Fig. 3.51. The various types of left ventricular outflow obstruction as they may occur in complete transposition of the great arteries. VSD, Ventricular septal defect.

true double outlet (Lev et al. 1972). The classification of the heart as a double outlet, therefore, to our minds no longer depends on the presence of such a "bilateral infundibulum" but on the ventricular connection of the great arteries.

The clinical significance of double-outlet right ventricle with a subpulmonary defect is that preferential shunting of blood may occur from the left ventricle into the pulmonary trunk. From a functional point of view, this closely resembles the position in complete transposition with ventricular septal defect. In contrast, double-outlet right ventricle with subaortic defect can involve preferential shunting from the left ventricle into the aorta, and clinically the case can thus resemble an ordinary ventricular septal defect or a tetralogy of Fallot.

A doubly committed defect is present underneath both arterial ostia, while a non-committed defect is remote from the arterial outlets.

Double-outlet right ventricle can be complicated by additional anomalies. Thus pulmonary stenosis frequently occurs with a subaortic defect, and narrowing of the subaortic outflow tract is frequent with subpulmonary defect, the latter often being associated with coarctation of the aorta. Straddling mitral valve is also frequent with subpulmonary defects (Kitamura et al. 1974).

Tetralogy of Fallot

Tetralogy of Fallot is characterized by the combined presence of a dextroposed aorta, a malalignment type of outlet ventricular septal defect, pulmonary

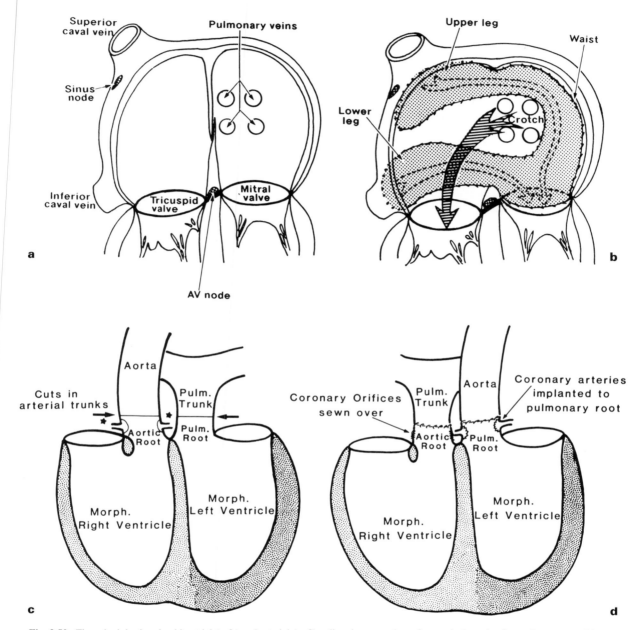

Fig. 3.52. The principles involved in atrial (**a, b**) and arterial (**c, d**) redirection procedures for surgical repair of complete transposition. **a, b** The Mustard operation. **a** Before operation. The atrial septum is removed and a trouser-shaped patch inserted to direct the systemic venous return to the mitral valve and the pulmonary venous return to the tricuspid valve (**b**). **c, d** The principle of the arterial switch procedure. **c** The preoperative arrangement. **d** The situation after the procedure.

infundibular stenosis, and right ventricular hypertrophy. The hallmark of the condition is the abnormal relationship of structures composing the outflow parts of the hearts (Becker et al. 1975; Becker and Anderson 1978). The aorta is dextroposed and has a more anterior position than normal (Fig. 3.54). In

addition, the outlet septum is deviated anteriorly, thereby creating the infundibular outflow tract stenosis of the right ventricle (Fig. 3.55). At the same time, the abnormally positioned outlet septum contributes to the presence of the malalignment type of defect, which is usually but not always perimembranous. The

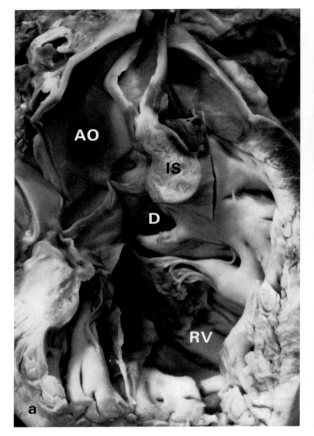 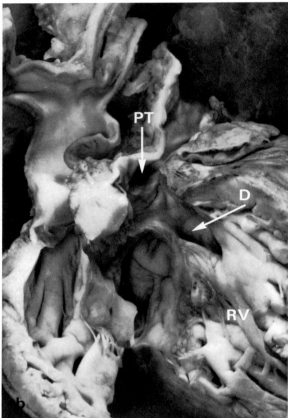

Fig. 3.53. Heart specimens with double outlet right ventricle, in which the right ventricle (*RV*) and arterial outlets have been opened. The two great arteries show a side-by-side relationship, both outlets being separated by the outlet (infundibular) septum (*IS*). **a** Ventricular septal defect (*D*) in a subaortic (*AO*) position. **b** Defect (*D*) underneath the pulmonary trunk (*PT*).

tetralogy of Fallot is therefore characterized by the morphology of the outflow parts of both ventricles. From the point of view of the ventriculoarterial connections, the condition can occur with either concordant or double-outlet connections, depending on the degree of aortic override (Shinebourne and Anderson 1978). In our opinion the term "tetralogy of Fallot" should be restricted to hearts that fulfil the anatomical criteria outlined above. Most cases exhibit fibrous continuity between the mitral valve and the dextroposed aortic valve, but this feature is not crucial to the diagnosis.

From the brief description of the anatomy, it follows that the malformation varies in its degree of severity. The degree of anterior deviation of the outlet (infundibular) septum also differs from one case to another, and induced hypertrophy may in time aggravate the severity of the stenosis. Insight into these anatomical features may explain a clinical spectrum of Fallot's tetralogy, ranging from "pink" Fallots to the classic deeply cyanotic infant.

An understanding of the basic structural abnormality of Fallot's tetralogy will also clarify the association of a "Fallot-type" outflow tract pathology with other cardiac malformations, such as atrioventricular septal defects (see p. 87). In a proportion of cases the ventricular septal defect has an entirely muscular rim on account of the fusion of the septomarginal trabeculum with the right-sided ventriculo-infundibular fold.

In approximately 25% of cases of tetralogy of Fallot, a right-sided aortic arch is present.

Common Arterial Trunk

Common arterial trunk is characterized by a single arterial trunk as the only outlet from the heart. It gives rise to the coronary arteries, at least one of the pulmonary arteries, and the ascending aorta (Crupi et al. 1977). There is one arterial orifice (Fig. 3.56) guarded by an arterial valve, which in the majority of

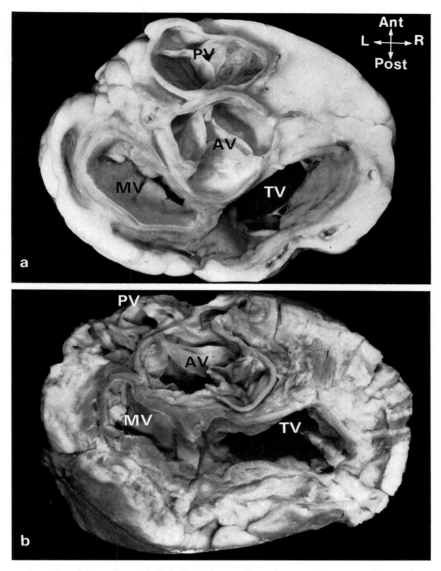

Fig. 3.54. The abnormal position of the aortic root in Fallot's tetralogy. **a** Base of a *normally* constructed heart after removal of both atria and the great arteries. The aortic valve (*AV*) takes a wedge position between the tricuspid (*TV*) and mitral (*MV*) valves. **b** Similar dissection in a heart with Fallot's tetralogy. The aortic valve (*AV*) is slightly dextroposed and displaced anteriorly. Note the position of the aortic valve relative to that of the pulmonary valve (*PV*), compared with that in the normal heart (**a**). (Reproduced from Becker and Anderson 1978, by permission of Churchill Livingstone, Edinburgh)

cases is composed of three leaflets. A truncal valve with a different number of leaflets is encountered in about 30% of cases. Immediately underneath the valve a septal defect is present (Fig. 3.56). The trunk overrides the ventricular septum showing a slight preference for the right ventricle, although its position varies considerably. In the usual case the truncal valve is in direct fibrous continuity with the mitral valve, but is separated from the tricuspid valve by a rim of muscle (the right ventriculoinfundibular fold).

Two major anatomical types of common trunk can be recognized, depending on the origin of the pulmonary arteries. The first type is characterized by a common pulmonary trunk, from which the right and left pulmonary arteries arise (type 1 according to the classification of Collett and Edwards 1949). The second variety shows separate origins of the two pulmonary arteries from the truncus (types II and III in the classification of Collett and Edwards). In rare instances, one of the pulmonary arteries originates

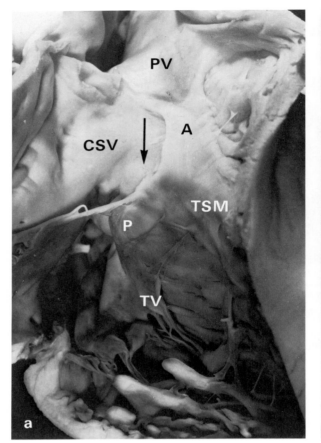 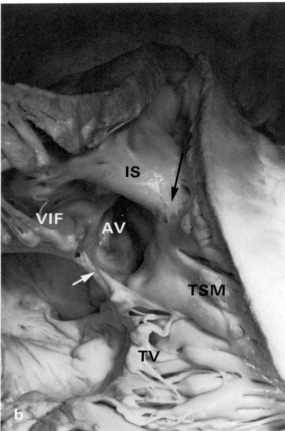

Fig. 3.55. The abnormal right ventricular outflow tract anatomy in Fallot's tetralogy: **a** Outflow tract in a normally constructed heart. The septomarginal trabeculation (*TSM*) shows anterior (*A*) and posterior (*P*) extensions, which embrace (*black arrow*) the supraventricular crest (*CSV*) **b** Anatomy in Fallot's tetralogy. The outlet (infundibular) septum (*IS*) is deviated anteriorly and the relationship with the trabeculation (*TSM*) has altered considerably (compare the *black arrows* in **a** and **b**). The outlet septum (*IS*) has separated from the ventriculoinfundibular folds (*VIF*), both of which merge inconspicuously in the normally constructed heart, forming the supraventricular crest (compare **a**). A large ventricular septal defect is present, through which the aortic valve (*AV*) is readily identified as overriding the ventricular septum. The aortic valve and the triscuspid valve (*TV*) are brought into close proximity (*white arrow*). (Reproduced from Becker and Anderson 1978, by permission of Churchill Livingstone, Edinburgh)

from the aorta after its separation from the common trunk.

A particular type of malformation is that in which the pulmonary blood supply originates from the descending thoracic aorta. This particular anomaly is not uniformly accepted as a true common trunk. At present the discussion around this anomaly is focused on the question as to whether or not central pulmonary arteries (i.e. pulmonary arteries within the pericardial sac) are present (Thiene et al. 1976; Sotomora and Edwards 1978). The pathologist will play a major role in settling the question. Until the argument is settled, the condition is best described as a solitary arterial trunk.

Common arterial trunk shows a distinct tendency to be associated with a right-sided aortic arch, which

occurs in approximately 40% of cases. From a functional point of view, pulmonary hypertension is likely to occur with early development of plexogenic pulmonary arteriopathy.

Hearts with Univentricular Atrioventricular Connection

Hearts with univentricular atrioventricular connection are characterized by the fact that the atrial inlet portions are committed to only one ventricle (Anderson et al. 1984b). Previously we described this group in terms of "univentricular hearts" (Anderson et al. 1979). We now recognize that this term is both illogi-

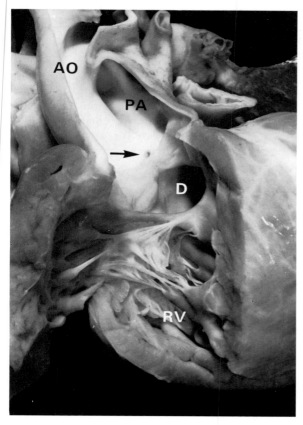

Fig. 3.56. A common arterial trunk. The right ventricle (*RV*) has been opened. The heart has one arterial orifice, which overrides a ventricular septal defect (*D*). A single arterial trunk gives rise to the coronary arteries (*arrow* points to an anomalously located single ostium), the pulmonary trunk and arteries (*PA*), and the aorta (*AO*).

cal and inaccurate, because most hearts possess two ventricles, albeit that one is rudimentary. As outlined earlier, hearts grouped together because of their uni-ventricular atrioventricular connection (a term which is both accurate and logical) can exist with two perfor-ate atrioventricular valves, one perforate and one imperforate atrioventricular valve, a common atrio-ventricular valve, a straddling atrioventricular valve as long as the major circumference of the straddler connects to the dominant ventricle, or with the absence of the right or left atrioventricular connection.

Further classification is based on the morphology of the dominant ventricle, the presence or absence of a rudimentary ventricle within the ventricular mass and the ventriculoarterial connections (Fig. 3.57).

The most common form is the one designated "double-inlet left ventricle with a rudimentary right ventricle" (synonym, single or common ventricle of left ventricular type). In this anomaly, the two atria connect to the dominant ventricle, which displays a trabecular pattern of left ventricular characteristics (Fig. 3.58b). A small rudimentary ventricle not receiving an atrial inlet is positioned anteriorly in the ventricular mass (Fig. 3.58a). This chamber may be located on the right anterior shoulder of the heart, but it can also be positioned directly anterior or on the left shoulder. The rudimentary ventricle connects to the left ventricle via a ventricular septal defect, which may vary in size. In the usual condition, the rudimen-tary ventricle acts as an outlet chamber in the sense that the aorta arises from it. The aorta is thus posi-tioned anterior to the pulmonary trunk, which orig-inates from the dominant ventricle (Fig. 3.58). The relationship between aorta and pulmonary trunk can vary according to the position of the rudimentary right ventricle. Less commonly, the pulmonary trunk or both arteries arise from the right ventricle, or both arteries arise from the left ventricle, in which case the rudimentary ventricle is simply a trabecular pouch. The location of the rudimentary right ventricle is significant for surgical correction. The conduction tissue always arises from an anterior node, as in cor-rected transposition.

The second major type is "double-inlet right ven-tricle with rudimentary left ventricle", characterized by the dominant ventricle having right ventricular tra-becular characteristics (Fig. 3.59a). The rudimentary ventricle is usually positioned posteriorly and dis-plays left ventricular trabecular characteristics (Fig. 3.59b). In most cases the rudimentary ventricle does not act as an outlet chamber, but is a trabecular pouch with both great arteries originating from the dominant right ventricle. The conducting tissue is usually posi-tioned posteriorly because the trabecular septum extends to the crux cordis.

The third major category is "double inlet to a soli-tary and indeterminate ventricle". In this condition the trabecular characteristics of the sole chamber cannot be recognized as either right ventricular or left ventricular. In addition, the heart possesses only one chamber within the ventricular mass, which receives both atrial inputs and supports both great arteries. There is no rudimentary ventricle.

The conduction tissue in these hearts can be any-where, but usually arises from an anterior node.

Tricuspid Atresia. Classic tricuspid atresia is char-acterized by an absent right atrioventricular connec-tion (Anderson et al. 1977). Thus, a deep furrow is present between the right atrium and the underlying ventricular mass, so that there is not even a potential connection between the right atrium and the right ventricular chamber (Fig. 3.60). The only outlet of the right atrium is by way of a patent oval foramen or an atrial septal defect. The left atrium connects to a

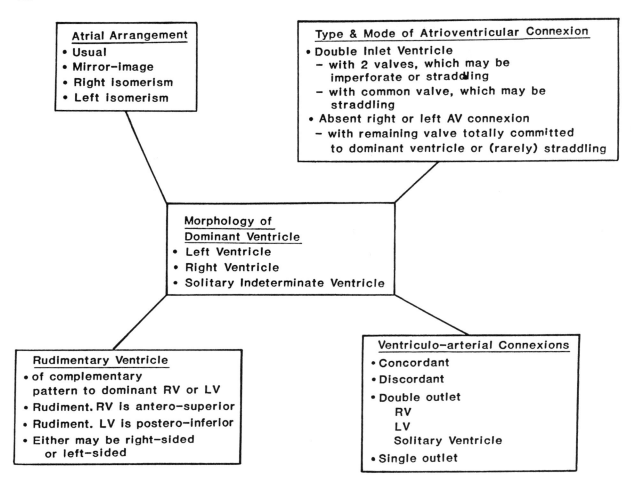

Fig. 3.57. Classification of hearts with univentricular atrioventricular connection based on the morphology of the dominant ventricle, the presence or absence of a rudimentary ventricle, and the ventriculoarterial connections.

dominant left ventricle, which in turn gives rise to a rudimentary right ventricle usually carried on the right anterior shoulder of the heart. The heart therefore exhibits a univentricular atrioventricular connection. An important difference with double-inlet left ventricle concerns the ventriculoarterial connections. In most cases of classic tricuspid atresia the rudimentary right ventricle supports the pulmonary trunk, the aorta arising from the dominant left ventricle (Fig. 3.60). The reverse usually occurs in double-inlet left ventricle (see Fig. 3.58). In a minority of hearts with the arrangement of classic tricuspid atresia, however, discordant ventriculoarterial connections can be present. Very rarely there is a double-outlet or single-outlet connection running from either the rudimentary or the dominant ventricle.

The type of ventriculoarterial connections seen in classic tricuspid atresia largely determines the clinical profile of the case. In patients with concordant

ventriculoarterial connections (the common situation), a diminished pulmonary flow is usually present, whereas patients with discordant ventriculoarterial connections often develop hyperkinetic pulmonary hypertension.

Fig. 3.59. Double-inlet right ventricle with rudimentary left ventricle. **a** Opened dominant right ventricle (*MC"RV"*), receiving almost all of both atrial inlets through a common atrioventricular valve (*CAVV*). Underneath the valve a defect is present (*SD*), through which a probe could be passed into a minute chamber with left ventricular characteristics (see **b**). There is an "ostium primum" (*OP*) atrial septal defect. *RA*, right atrium. **b** The rudimentary left ventricle (*OC"LV"*) from which the aorta (*AO*) arises is shown. The minute portion of the common atrioventricular valve related to this rudimentary ventricle is indicated (*CAVV* to *MC*). (Reproduced from Keeton et al. 1979, by permission of the Editor of *Circulation*)

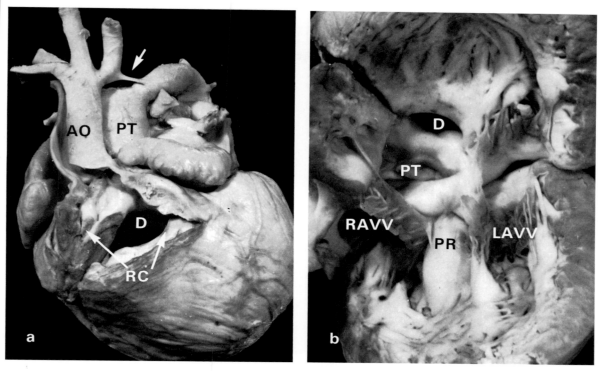

Fig. 3.58. Heart specimen classified as double inlet left ventricle with rudimentary right ventricle. **a** Anterior view of the heart specimen. A rudimentary ventricle (*RC*) is present in the right anterior shoulder of the heart and gives rise to the aorta (*AO*), which is anterior to and to the right of the pulmonary trunk (*PT*). The latter arises from the dominant ventricle (see **b**). The ventricular septal defect is clearly seen (*D*). There is atresia of the aortic arch (*arrows*) in this particular specimen. **b** Interior of the dominant left ventricle after the heart has been opened like a shell. The right (*RAVV*) and left (*LAVV*) atrioventricular valves enter the ventricle from which the pulmonary trunk (*PT*) arises. There is a posterior ridge (*PR*) between the two valves, but the absence of an inlet septum is conspicuous. The septum separating the rudimentary and dominant ventricles is anterior and shows the fine trabeculations reminiscent of a morphological left ventricle. The rudimentary ventricle receives no atrial inlets, as can be seen from the position of the ventricular septal defect (*D*) relative to both atrioventricular valves.

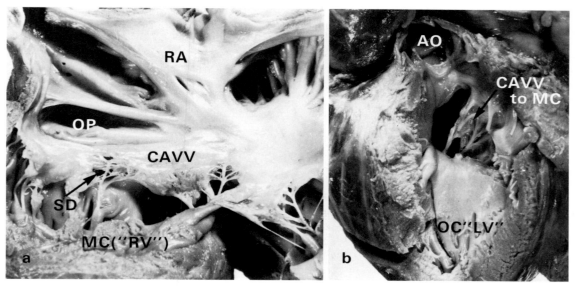

Fig. 3.59

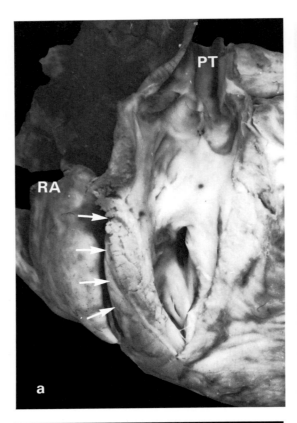

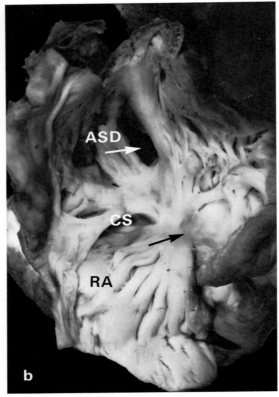

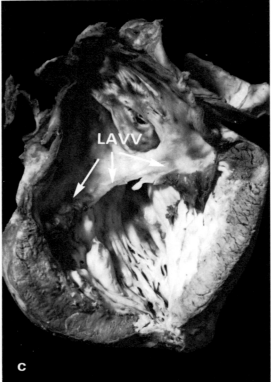

Fig. 3.60. Heart specimen with classic tricuspid atresia. **a** The opened rudimentary right ventricle, which is separated from the right atrium (*RA*) by a deep furrow (*arrows*), so that not even a potential connection is present. The pulmonary trunk (*PT*) arises from the right ventricle, in contrast to the usual discordant ventriculoarterial connection present in double-inlet left ventricle (compare Fig. 3.58a). **b** The opened right atrium (*RA*), revealing the absence of an atrioventricular connection. A dimple is present in the floor of the right atrium (*black arrow*), pointing towards the dominant rather than the rudimentary ventricle. The only outlet of the right atrium is through a large atrial septal defect of the oval fossa type (*ASD*). *CS*, coronary sinus. **c** The opened left side of the heart. The greater part of the left atrioventricular valve (*LAVV*) has been cut away to reveal the left ventricular trabecular pattern present in the dominant ventricle. The site of the ventricular septal defect (*arrow*) is barely visible.

Mitral Atresia. Most examples of atresia of the left atrioventricular orifice are due to absence of the left atrioventricular connection. Such hearts, like those with classic tricuspid atresia, are also examples of univentricular atrioventricular connection. Usually absence of the left connection is associated with aortic atresia and an intact septum, and frequently the atretic aorta cannot be traced to the hypoplastic left ventricle, which is a trabecular pouch. In the presence of a septal defect, the chamber is larger and may be in potential communication with the atretic aorta. This type of mitral atresia therefore represents univentricular connection to a dominant right ventricle. Absence of the left connection also occurs in the setting of univentricular connection to a dominant left ventricle with a left-sided rudimentary right ventricle. It is arguable whether this anomaly is mitral or tricuspid atresia. It is unequivocally absence of the left atrioventricular connection, and underlines the significance of the descriptive approach to sequential segmental analysis.

Mitral atresia can also occur with an imperforate valve. This in itself is extremely rare, but when it occurs it tends to be associated with double-outlet right ventricle.

Congenital Malformations of the Aorta

The principal malformations affecting the aortic arch are aortic coarctation, interrupted aortic arch and vascular rings.

Coarctation of the Thoracic Aorta

In classic coarctation, a shelf-like obstruction is present in the aortic arch, which projects into the lumen from the posterosuperior wall and is situated immediately beyond the origin of the left subclavian artery (Fig. 3.61). Histological examination at the site of obstruction will reveal an infolding of the media (Fig. 3.61b), accentuated on the internal surface by an intimal thickening, which in the infant has a mucoid appearance similar to ductal tissue but in older children and adults is a thick layer of collagen and elastin fibres. In a vast majority of cases the site of obstruction is opposite the aortic orifice of the arterial duct (or ligament) and adjacent to the proximal aortic segment. A coarctation in this position is therefore classified as "juxtaductal", although it is extremely rare for a coarctation to occur distal to the orifice of the duct; in fact the occurrence of coarctation in this particular location is questionable. The terms "preductal" and "postductal" coarctation have previously been used in relation to the site of obstruction relative to the arterial duct. In such a terminology preductal coarctation has often been considered synonymous with "infantile coarctation". In the symptomatic neonate, however, the situation is usually much more complicated. In these instances it is common for a segment of the aortic arch to be underdeveloped: a condition termed "tubular hypoplasia" or "aortic arch hypoplasia" (Fig. 3.62). The hypolastic segment is most commonly present between the origin of the left subclavian artery and the site of insertion of the arterial duct, but other sites can be affected. Tubular hypoplasia frequently coexists with a discrete shelf-like coarctation, and is also frequently associated with a ventricular septal defect and additional left ventricular inlet and/or outlet obstructions. It is this combination of anomalies that underlies the serious prognosis of a symptomatic coarctation in infancy.

The pathogenesis of coarctation is still controversial. The original Skodaic concept that ductal tissue extends into the aortic wall, leading to constriction, may indeed be operative in cases with classic coarctation in the sense of localized shelf-like obstruction. It has been suggested (Rudolph et al. 1972) that reduced flow through the aortic arch during development could lead to insufficient vascular development. This concept, which relates to the common occurrence of additional anomalies, could explain the presence of tubular hypoplasia.

In early infancy, coarctation of the aorta results in biventricular hypertrophy. The secondary effects on the systemic vessels, both proximal and distal to the obstruction, will develop in time.

Interrupted Aortic Arch

This condition is characterized by complete interruption of the arch, most commonly localized immediately distal to the left subclavian artery. Other sites, however, may also be affected. The descending thoracic aorta is fed through a patent arterial duct. The condition is nearly always associated with a ventricular septal defect (see p. 87). In "atresia" of the aortic arch a fibrous strand connects the proximal and distal segments of the aorta, whereas in interrupted aortic arch no such remnant can be identified.

Vascular Rings

"Vascular rings" form a complex group of anomalies of the aortic arch system. The various anomalies can be understood from the developmental scheme of aortic arches (Stewart et al. 1964). The most common type of vascular ring develops when an aberrant subclavian artery originates from the descending aorta beyond the aortic arch. The initial part of this aber-

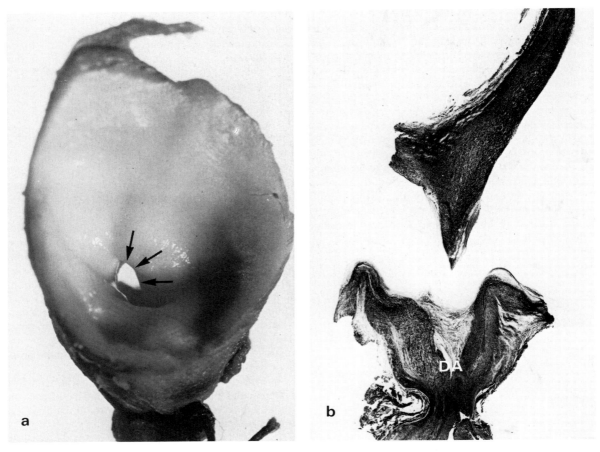

Fig. 3.61. Surgically resected specimen of "classic" aortic coarctation. **a** The gross specimen, viewed from the distal aortic end. A shelf-like infolding projects into the lumen from the posterosuperior wall (*arrows*). **b** Histological section from this specimen. The infolding of the media is opposite the site of insertion of the arterial duct (*DA*). (Elastin tissue stain, x 8)

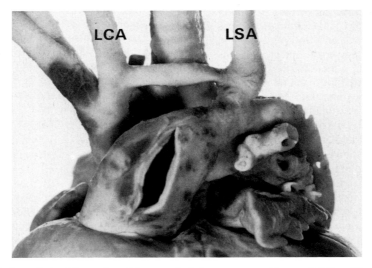

Fig. 3.62. Tubular hypoplasia of the aortic arch between the left common carotid artery (*LCA*) and the left subclavian artery (*LSA*).

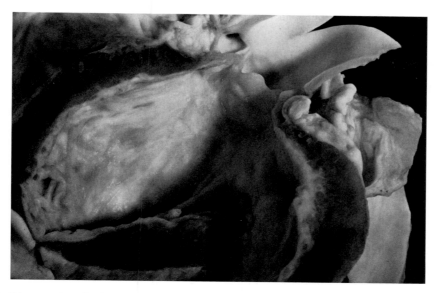

Fig. 3.63. Primary endocardial fibroelastosis. The opened left ventricle exhibits diffuse thickening of the endocardium.

rant artery is formed by the dorsal segment of the contralateral arch system. In most cases the subclavian artery will run behind the oesophagus, leaving a slight impression, but the anomaly has no clinical significance. True "dysphagia lusoria" develops when the aberrant artery connects to the contralateral pulmonary artery by way of an arterial duct or ligament. In these instances the vascular anomaly constitutes a ring compressing the enclosed trachea and oesophagus.

Other types of vascular ring are extremely rare and will not be discussed further.

Congenital Malformations of the Central Pulmonary Arteries

Development anomalies of the central pulmonary arteries are rare. Unilateral absence of a pulmonary artery can occur. In most cases the contralateral lung is supplied through a separate "pulmonary" artery which originates from the aorta.

The term "vascular sling" is reserved for the rare case in which the left pulmonary artery originates from the right pulmonary artery (Lubbers et al. 1975). From this aberrant origin the artery courses to the left lung hilus and passes between the trachea and oesophagus, producing an impression in the anterior wall of the oesophagus.

Isolated Congenital Abnormalities of Endocardium, Myocardium and Pericardium

Isolated congenital abnormalities of the endocardium, myocardium and pericardium are rare lesions, which do not fit any of the previous headings. The lesions appear to be isolated, but further study may show this is not so.

Endocardium

Fibroelastosis of the endocardium is a common finding in hearts exhibiting other congenital anomalies that lead to increased volume or pressure within a cardiac chamber. Primary endocardial fibroelastosis, however, occurs without associated cardiac anomalies. It most commonly affects the left ventricle. The endocardium is greatly thickened, giving the inner surface of the left ventricle a whitish appearance (Fig. 3.63). Histological studies show that the thickening is composed of alternating layers of collagen and elastin. The underlying myocardium reveals no abnormalities. This histological appearance is not pathognomonic for primary endocardial fibroelastosis, because a similar architecture is found in hearts with secondary fibroelastosis, e.g. in hypoplastic left hearts associated with aortic valvar anomalies.

Primary endocardial fibroelastosis is subdidivided into a dilated type, in which the left ventricular chamber is of normal size or enlarged, and a contracted type characterized by a small left ventricular cavity. Differentiation of the latter condition from isolated left ventricular hypoplasia becomes arbitary. Because of the fibroelastic endocardial layer, the papillary muscle groups of the mitral valve apparatus appear to originate at a higher level than usual. This is probably an illusion, but it is undoubtedly true that in a high percentage of cases the mitral valve apparatus has been involved by the endocardial process so that mitral valve insufficiency has occurred.

The nature of the disease remains obscure. Several aetiological factors have been suggested, but a primary myocardial disorder with compensatory endocardial thickening is the most likely cause.

Myocardium

Congenital aneurysms or diverticula of the heart occur. These abnormalities show a predilection for the region of the cardiac apex and the atrioventricular junctional area. Diverticula in the former site have a tendency to be associated with defects in the pericardium and diaphragm.

Uhl's disease (Uhl 1952) is characterized by focal absence of myocardium of the right ventricular wall, so that endocardium and epicardium become adherent.

"Foamy myocardial transformation of infancy" is a rare disease, known also under a variety of names such as "infantile cardiomyopathy with histiocytoid change", "oncocytic cardiomyopathy" and "Purkinje cell tumour" (for a review see Becker and Anderson 1981). The cardiomyopathy manifests clinically with cardiac arrhythmias very early in life, often immediately after birth. The pathology is characterized by a peculiar transformation of myocardial cells into swollen, often rounded or polyhydral cells with a slightly granular eosinophilic and often abundantly vacuolated cytoplasm. Thus, the cells give a foamy appearance. The abnormality may be patchily distributed or diffusely present. Ultrastructural studies reveal an increased number of mitochondria, which in themselves show abnormalities. The pathogenesis remains unclear, but a relationship with the peripheral Purkinje system has been suggested.

Pericardium

Congenital defects of the pericardium can be partial or complete. In the case of total absence of the pericardium, the heart and lung lie together within one serous cavity. In a partial defect, part of the heart may herniate into the defect – a condition that may become symptomatic.

Pericardial cysts and diverticula occur as a form of developmental anomaly showing preference for the cardiophrenic angle.

Epicardial cysts also occur but are extremely rare.

Congenital Heart Block

Proper formation of the atrioventricular conduction axis depends on normal cardiac septation with proper alignment of atrial and ventricular septa and apposition of the different segments of the developing atrioventricular conduction axis with proper differentiation of the enveloping sulcus tissue.

It follows that congenital heart block can occur in hearts with a major developmental anomaly of septation. It can also be found in hearts with a failure of proper apposition of the segments, or in which the sulcus tissue has not disappeared. In these the hearts may be otherwise normal.

The first category includes conditions such as congenitally corrected transposition (see p. 101) and double-inlet ventricle. The second category can be subdivided according to the level of the developmental anomaly. Two basic varieties are recognized: "atrial-axis" discontinuity and "nodoventricular" discontinuity (Becker et al. 1978b) (Fig. 3.64). In the atrial-axis form the proximal part of the conduction axis is poorly developed and devoid of atrial inputs, whereas the distal parts of the atrioventricular conduction axis are well formed and normally located. In nodoventricular discontinuity the proximal and distal segments of the atrioventricular conduction are well formed, but the two are completely separated by dense fibrous tissue of the annulus fibrosus. Histological studies are the only means of distinguishing between these varieties of congenital heart block.

Heart Block and Connective Tissue Disease

The association of congenital complete heart block with maternal connective tissue and collagen disease is well documented (Hull et al. 1966; McCue et al. 1977). Indeed, the presence of maternal anti-Ro (SS-A) antibodies may serve as markers for congenital heart block (Scott et al. 1983). Antibody deposition in infant atrial tissue in one report (Litsey et al. 1985) provides evidence that antibodies transmitted placentally may have direct action on cardiac tissue. Recent studies on a small series show anatomical differences

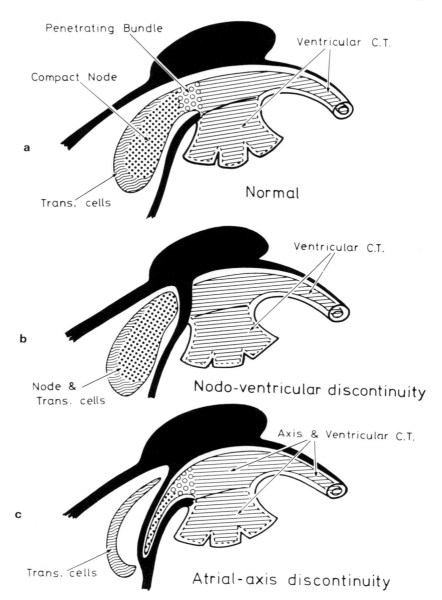

Fig. 3.64. a Normal heart. **b, c** The basic anatomical varieties of congenitally complete heart block in otherwise normal hearts. (Reproduced from Becker et al. 1978c, by permission of Churchill Livingstone, Edinburgh)

in cardiac conduction axis discontinuity in relation to anti-Ro status of maternal serum (Ho et al. 1986).

Complications of Congenital Heart Disease

One of the major hazards of a congenitally malformed heart is that the anomaly may induce further pathological changes both in the heart itself and in other organ systems. These changes relate primarily to abnormal circulatory pathways, e.g. in conditions where systemic venous blood is conveyed directly into the aorta or with left-to-right shunts with an increased pulmonary circulation; to a low cardiac output with insufficient perfusion of such organs as the brain, the kidneys and the heart itself; to compensatory myocardial hypertrophy, which may in some instances aggravate the functional consequences of the malformation; or to sites of laceration within the heart resulting from the underlying malformation, rendering certain structures in the heart susceptible to infectious endocarditis.

In view of all this it is advisable to perform a complete autopsy on any individual who has died of "congenital heart disease" to obtain a full insight into the pathophysiology of the disease.

Systemic Thromboemboli and Thrombosis

Paradoxical thromboemboli are a potential danger in all conditions in which right-to-left shunts exist. Emboli that originate in the systemic venous site of the circulation may cross into the systemic arterial circulation at all levels where mixing of the greater and lesser circulations occurs. Moreover, in the grossly desaturated (cyanotic) patient with a markedly increased haematocrit, "spontaneous" thrombosis can occur, leading to irreversible changes in such vital organs as the brain.

Brain Abscess

The complication of a brain abscess is particularly likely in patients with a right-to-left shunt, whatever the anatomy of the underlying cardiac condition. In most cases the heart itself does not contain an infectious focus. The development of the brain abscess relates to the abnormal circulatory pathways. Infected systemic venous blood is no longer "filtered" in the lungs, but is in part conveyed directly into the systemic arterial circulation. This abnormal flow pattern will also lead to systemic arterial desaturation and hypoxia of the brain, which renders the brain particularly vulnerable to infection with anaerobic microorganisms.

Renal Pathology

Renal insufficiency may appear clinically, particularly in patients suffering from low cardiac output (e.g. aortic stenosis) or in those with diminished perfusion of the kidneys (e.g. coarctation of the aorta). In some instances histological examination of the kidney reveals pathological changes consistent with renal ischaemia. Careful examination of the glomeruli may reveal the existence of a process of intravascular clotting consequent on the cardiac disorder. Severe cyanosis is usually associated with glomerular hypertrophy.

Myocardial Pathology

It has long been known that, in many patients with congenital heart malformations, the myocardium contains areas of necrosis (Berry 1967; Franciosi and Blanc 1968). Both recent necrosis and various stages of repair can also be encountered. In some instances it is evident that the changes must have occurred during intrauterine life, because extensive scarring, often accompanied by calcific deposits, can be present at birth. In such circumstances it is not immediately apparent whether myocardial cell death has been caused by a circulatory insufficiency or by other mechanisms, such as acquired intrauterine toxic or infectious diseases.

In patients who have lived with a congenital heart defect for a variable period, it is sometimes evident that actual myocardial infarction has occurred. This is a particularly frequent finding where coronary perfusion has been minimal, above all when combined with marked myocardial hypertrophy. Long-standing myocardial hypertrophy is nearly always accompanied by focal intramural fibrosis, which is most probably related to these mechanisms.

The significance of secondary degenerative changes in the natural history of patients who have undergone surgical "correction" of their congenital heart defect remains speculative. There is accumulating clinical evidence, however, that myocardial dysfunction in survivors becomes a major problem. In other conditions compensatory myocardial hypertrophy can have a deleterious effect in aggravating the clinical course of the disease. The outflow tract stenosis in tetralogy of Fallot can be cited as an example in this respect. The infundibulum is narrow at birth, owing to an intrinsic abnormality of septal structure (see p. 104). It may become further narrowed because of myocardial hypertrophy and secondary endocardial fibroelastosis. The disease may thus gradually progress towards functional pulmonary atresia. In other conditions, e.g. classic tricuspid atresia or double-inlet left ventricle, the ventricular septal defect may diminish in size because of myocardial hypertrophy and fibroelastosis, and diminished flow in the corresponding great artery will result. In some individuals suffering from various types of congenital heart disease, myocardial hypertrophy may develop to such an extent that hypertrophic (obstructive) cardiomyopathy appears. The precise pathogenetic mechanisms underlying this disorder are still not known.

Similarly, primarily induced right ventricular hypertrophy (e.g. in patients with "isolated" pulmonary valve stenosis and intact ventricular septum) may in time lead to left ventricular myocardial hypertrophy and, rarely, to left ventricular outflow tract

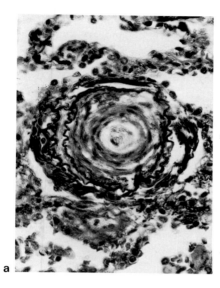 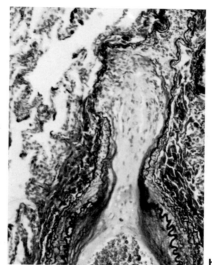

Fig. 3.65. Micrographs showing two stages of plexogenic pulmonary arteriopathy. **a** A pulmonary artery with a concentric lamellar type of intimal fibrosis (x 350). **b** A plexiform lesion (x 140). (Elastin tissue stain)

obstruction. The pathogenetic mechanisms in these cases are probably related to alterations in the geometry of the left ventricular cavity.

Infectious Endocarditis

Infectious endocarditis in congenital heart disease usually affects sites of endothelial damage, these being a direct consequence of the haemodynamic abnormalities resulting from the defect. In ventricular septal defects, the edges of affected sites reveal endocardial thickening. Similarly the tricuspid valve can become involved, as can parts of the right ventricular septum and free wall. Early structural changes are induced within the leaflets of anatomically abnormal valves, rendering them susceptible to infection. Bicuspid aortic valve is a classic example, although complications of this condition are rarely significant in the paediatric age group.

Pulmonary Vascular Pathology

It is important to realize that the pulmonary vascular bed should be considered to be intimately associated with any cardiac abnormality. Indeed, the "success" of most surgical corrections in congenital heart disease depends on the state of the pulmonary vascular bed before operation.

In childhood there are three major categories of induced pulmonary vascular changes to consider. These occur firstly in conditions with an increased pulmonary arterial flow, secondly in those with decreased flow, and finally in situations with primarily pulmonary venous hypertension.

Increased Pulmonary Flow

In these conditions a left-to-right shunt is nearly always present. The pulmonary vascular bed will initially adapt to the increased flow, enabling a large percentage of total cardiac output to pass through the lungs. In time, however, structural changes will occur, the first expression of which is medial hypertrophy of muscular pulmonary arteries. These changes may gradually become complicated by a proliferation of intimal cells, leading to a concentric lamellar type of intimal fibrosis (Fig. 3.65a). The pulmonary arteries may ultimately develop fibrinoid necrosis and plexiform lesions (Fig. 3.65b). The term "plexogenic pulmonary arteriopathy" has been introduced to indicate this morphological pattern (World Health Organization 1975; Wagenvoort and Wagenvoort 1977). In the fully developed state, plexiform lesions will be present, but in less advanced instances the only change indicative of the onset of this train of events is medial hypertrophy, which is considered to be reversible in nature. In contrast, it is generally accepted that fibrinoid necrosis and plexiform lesions represent irreversible damage to pulmonary arteries. There is evidence that pulmonary hypertension with early plexogenic changes, such as cellular intimal proliferation, and with limited intimal fibrosis can still be reversible.

The structural characteristics of plexogenic pulmonary arteriopathy do not depend on the type of shunt. Thus, the structural changes are similar

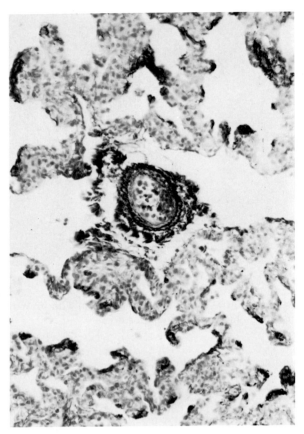

Fig. 3.66. Micrograph showing "arterialization" of a pulmonary vein. (Elastin tissue stain, x 65)

whether the patient has an atrial or a ventricular septal defect, a persistent arterial duct or a common arterial trunk. The major difference is that irreversible arteriopathy will develop much later in patients with an atrial septal defect than in those with a "post-tricuspid" shunt.

Decreased Pulmonary Flow

In patients with pulmonary stenosis, irrespective of the underlying cause, the pulmonary arteries are characteristically thin walled and often dilated. Intravascular thrombosis and subsequent organization may result in cushion-like intimal fibrosis and the formation of intravascular fibrous septa.

Pulmonary Venous Hypertension

A variety of congenital cardiac malformations can lead to pulmonary venous congestion and hyperten-

sion. This in turn leads to medial hypertrophy of pulmonary veins, which in some instances (e.g. aortic atresia) can be present even before birth. The media of these veins may develop a structural rearrangement of elastin fibres, so that distinct internal and external laminae are formed. This process is called "arterialization" and can be regarded as a reliable indicator of elevated pulmonary venous pressure (Fig. 3.66). The main feature of the pulmonary arteries in children with pulmonary venous hypertension is medial hypertrophy and muscularization of small arterioles; these arteries are devoid of easily recognized media under normal circumstances. Plexiform lesions do not develop.

Bronchial Compression

In a minority of patients with a left-to-right shunt, respiratory symptoms may not be caused primarily by the development of pulmonary vascular disease, but by compression of bronchi secondary to dilatation of pulmonary arteries. The anatomy of the pulmonary arterial tree in relation to that of the tracheobronchial tree shows certain sites of predilection for bronchial compression. These are the left main stem bronchus and site of origin of the left upper lobe bronchus, and the right-sided intermediate bronchus and site of origin of the right middle lobe bronchus.

Dilatation of pulmonary arteries with increased intraluminal pressure may lead to external compression of the bronchi at these sites, which may result in either hyperinflation or atelectasis of the corresponding lobes.

Postnatally Acquired Heart Disease

The abnormalities described above are acquired, but still relate directly to the presence of an underlying congenital heart malformation. The heart may also be involved in many other disease processes, none of which is specific to the heart.

The most important group is that of the infectious diseases. Myocarditis and pericarditis can complicate almost any infectious disease, whether acquired in the prenatal or the postnatal period. The inflammatory process in the heart is usually non-specific, and a definitive diagnosis depends on a full autopsy and bacteriological and virological studies. With the early recognition and treatment of most infectious disease, at least in the western world, their significance for cardial pathology has declined. The same applies to rheumatic fever, which in Europe no longer plays an important role in early morbidity and mortality.

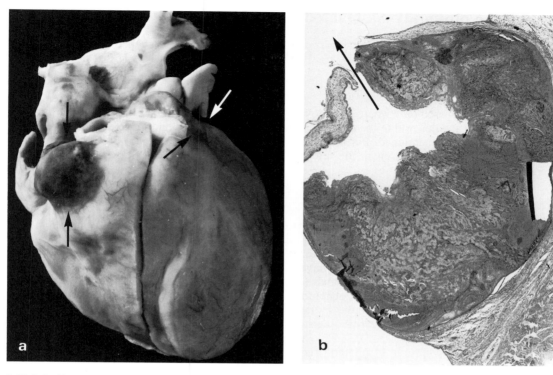

Fig. 3.67. Infantile periarteritis nodosa affecting the coronary arteries. **a** Mycotic aneurysms in the proximal segments of both coronary arteries (*arrows*). The infant died of cardiac tamponade caused by a rupture of the aneurysm in the right coronary artery. **b** Histological section of the aneurysm at the site of rupture (*arrow*). (Elastin tissue stain, x 7)

"Idiopathic dilated cardiomyopathy", also known as congestive cardiomyopathy, is a relatively rare disease in children, but when it occurs it usually follows a grave course. The aetiology and pathogenesis of the disease remains unclear. The histopathological abnormalities are usually limited and not necessarily related to the basic disorder. Active inflammatory disease is usually ruled out when the patient is studied, and endomyocardial biopsies have as yet proved to be of little help in determining the nature of the underlying disorder. A possible relationship with a viral infection has been suggested.

"Infantile periarteritis nodosa" needs a brief discussion. This disease of unknown aetiology has a marked tendency to affect the coronary arteries. In such patients arteritis, with a predominantly mononuclear cellular infiltrate, and thrombosis can lead to myocardial infarction and death. Moreover, the disease may lead to the formation of coronary aneurysms, which may ultimately rupture, causing cardiac tamponade (Fig. 3.67). A positive diagnosis of infantile periarteritis nodosa always depends on histological verification, because the clinical spectrum is complex and is considered non specific.

A "new" disease entity has been reported, called Kawasaki's disease (synonym, mucocutaneous lymph node syndrome) (Kawasaki et al. 1974; Tanaka et al. 1976; Fujiwara and Hamashima 1978), which in Japan appears to be one of the most frequent causes of cardiovascular disease in infancy. The diagnosis of Kawasaki's disease is made primarily on clinical grounds. It is of interest, therefore, that patients who die of the disease (approximately 1%–2% of those affected) show pathological changes that cannot be distinguished from those of infantile periarteritis nodosa. Coronary arteritis with thrombosis and coronary aneurysms are present in nearly all instances. Furthermore, histologically non-specific interstitial myocarditis is also identified in some cases. It is suggested, therefore, that the medium-sized arteries constitute the target organ for an immune disorder, the nature of which remains unclear. Thus, infantile periarteritis nodosa, being a descriptive term, could be regarded as the pathological substrate of Kawasaki's disease (Becker 1976).

Syndromes Commonly Associated with Cardiovascular Malformations

Syndromes will be discussed only where a cardiovascular anomaly plays a major role in the disease. The type of anomaly will be mentioned. Further details regarding the syndromes are given in the relevant chapters.

Visceral Symmetry Syndromes

Syndromes of visceral symmetry constitute a complex developmental disorder, and they have a profound tendency to be associated with anomalies of the cardiovascular system. Recognition of abdominal visceral heterotaxia and isomerism of the thoracic organs should immediately alert the pathologist to these syndromes.

"Visceral symmetry syndrome of bilateral right-sided type" (right isomerism) is nearly always associated with an absent spleen, hence the term "asplenia syndrome" (synonym, Ivemark's syndrome) (Van Mierop et al. 1972).

The abdominal organs in over 50% of cases show a bilaterally symmetrical liver with the gallbladder, stomach, duodenum and pancreas on the right side, accompanied by varying degrees of malrotation of the intestines. There are usually bilateral *tri*lobed lungs, and dissection of the tracheobronchial anatomy will show bilateral eparterial bronchi in nearly all cases. The cardiovascular system is highly abnormal in these instances. Bilateral superior caval veins, both draining to their respective atria, are present in the majority of cases. The abdominal part of the inferior caval vein ascends on either the right of the left side of the spine, in close association with the abdominal aorta, and enters the atrium on its corresponding side. Totally anomalous pulmonary venous connection is the rule. Even in the cases where the pulmonary veins enter an atrium they do so in the intercaval part derived from the embryonic venous sinus, and therefore connect in an anomalous way. The heart in the vast majority of cases shows major abnormalities. The two atria, apart from the anomalous systemic and pulmonary venous connections, show isomeric appendages of the morphologically right type. The coronary sinus is absent, in keeping with the high incidence of a persistent left superior caval vein draining directly into the left-sided atrium. The atrial septum is abnormal and in most cases consists of a

small triangular muscular band, which originates from the posteroinferior atrial wall and inserts with its apex into the anterior atrial wall. This band bridges a common atrioventricular orifice, which is almost invariably present. In the majority of patients there is double-inlet atrioventricular connection, usually through a common valve (see the section on tricuspid atresia, p. 109). Usually the relative positions of the great arteries are abnormal, with the aorta anterior to the pulmonary trunk, and pulmonary stenosis and atresia are commonly associated anomalies.

A high degree of consistency in the pattern of the cardiovascular abnormalities is present in the right atrial isomeric variety of visceral symmetry syndrome.

"Visceral symmetry syndrome of the bilateral left-sided type" (left isomerism) is nearly always associated with multiple spleens located to both sides of the dorsal mesogastrium; hence the name "polysplenia syndrome" (Van Mierop et al. 1972).

The abdominal organs reveal isomerism of the liver in approximately 25% of cases. In the remainder the major lobe is more commonly found on the left than on the right side. The gallbladder has a tendency to be associated with the major lobe, but it can be positioned in the midline or absent. In the majority of cases, the stomach, duodenum and pancreas are found on the right side. Malrotation of the intestines is a frequent condition. There are bilateral *bi*lobed lungs, although bilateral hypartial bronchi are a more consistent finding. In most instances the cardiovascular system will show abnormalities. Bilateral superior caval veins occur in about half the cases. A single superior caval vein is more commonly found on the right than on the left side. In the majority of patients the inferior caval vein connects to the azygous venous system, whether right- or left-sided, and drains by way of it into the superior caval vein. Separate common hepatic veins usually connect the liver to the right- or the left-sided atrium, but a suprahepatic common channel is found in about one-third. Juxtaposition of the abdominal segment of the inferior caval vein and the aorta may occur, albeit less frequently than in cases with right atrial isomerism. In some instances the right and left pulmonary veins connect to their respective sides of the atria, the sites of entrance being widely separated and often indicated by a groove in the posteroinferior atrial wall. In other cases the right and left pulmonary veins connect to one of the atria. In some cases the atrial septum is intact, but the majority of patients have some sort of atrial septal defect. At the level of the atrioventricular junction a common atrioventricular valve will be present in approximately 50% of cases. Two ventricles are almost always present, with a high frequency of double outlet right ventricle. Some type of ventricular septal defect is almost always present. Pulmonary valve anomalies on the other hand, are rare.

In the left isomeric variety of visceral symmetry syndrome, the spectrum of cardiovascular anomalies is much wider than in right isomerism, and includes a higher percentage of potentially correctable lesions.

Syndromes with Autosomal Chromosomal Anomalies

A variety of syndromes involve autosomal chromosomal anomalies, and the majority of them present a complex constellation of malformations. It is rare for cardiovascular anomalies to present as the leading clinical feature.

Trisomy 13–15 (D Syndrome)

The predominant cardiovascular anomaly in trisomy 13–15 is ventricular septal defect, although other malformations, such as tetralogy of Fallot, can be present. The combination of polydactyly with cheilognathopalatoschisis should suggest the possibility of this trisomy.

Trisomy 16–18 (E Syndrome)

The major cardiovascular anomalies that accompany the other malformations present in trisomy 16–18 are ventricular septal defect and patent aterial duct.

Trisomy 21 (Down's Syndrome)

In about 40% of affected patients, trisomy 21 is associated with a congenital malformation of the heart. The most common conditions are atrioventricular septal defects and isolated ventricular septal defects.

Syndromes with Sex Chromosomal Anomalies

Among the various syndromes with sex chromosomal anomalies, Turner's syndrome may involve major cardiovascular anomalies with distinct clinical significance. The most commonly associated conditions are lymphoedema, caused by abnormalities in the development of the lymphatic system, and aortic coarctation and ventricular septal defect.

Noonan's Syndrome

A familiar syndrome with an autosomal dominant trait, Noonan's syndrome is phenotypically closely related to Turner's syndrome, but with a normal karyotype. Cardiac abnormalities are apparent in approximately 50%–60% of patients. The most frequent abnormality is pulmonary stenosis, resulting from valve dysplasia. Other abnormalities may be present, such as dysplasia of the aortic valve, patent arterial duct, anomalous pulmonary venous connection and aortic coarctation. Recent reports emphasize a high frequency of hypertrophic cardiomyopathy underlying a dynamic type of left ventricular outflow tract obstruction (see p. 97).

Glycogen Storage Diseases

The glycogen storage diseases (see also pp. 839 and 853) are characterized by a genetically determined abnormality of the carbohydrate metabolism, which results in an intracellular accumulation of glycogen. Different forms exist, of which type II (Pompe's disease) is the one that primarily affects the heart. The condition is caused by a deficiency of the enzyme acid maltase and is characterized grossly by cardiomegaly. Histological studies reveal massive accumulation of glycogen in all myocardial cells, which on routinely processed sections stained with haematoxylin and eosin exhibit extensive vacuolization of myocytes (Fig. 3.68).

Mucopolysaccharidosis

The various types of mucopolysaccharidosis (see also pp. 841 and 847) are characterized by an abnormal accumulation of mucopolysaccharides present in large vacuolated cells. Different types exist, of which type I (Hurler's disease) and type II (Hunter's disease) affect the heart. Both conditions lead to dwarfism, with a characteristic facial appearance. Type I is transmitted as an autosomal recessive trait, in contrast to type II, which is an X-linked recessive. In both conditions the abnormal products accumulated are chondroitin sulphate B and heparin sulphate.

The cardiac valves are the structures mainly affected. On gross examination they show marked fibrosis, with thickened chordae; in this the condition

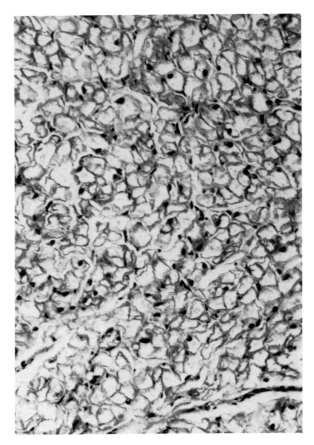

Fig. 3.68. Micrograph showing extensive vacuolization of the myocardial cells in glycogen storage disease. (H&E, x 230)

is reminiscent of rheumatic valve disease, from which it should be differentiated. Histological studies reveal the large vacuolated clear cells. Fresh tissue is needed to demonstrate the accumulated mucopolysaccharides, because the abnormal products are water soluble.

The abnormalities are not restricted to the valves, but can present focally in the myocardium and coronary arteries.

Marfan's Syndrome

Marfan's syndrome is inherited as an autosomal dominant trait in most cases. The fundamental problem is a deficiency of fibrillar fibres, which has been related to a genetic defect on chromosome 15 (Kainulainen et al. 1990). The abnormalities that occur within the cardiovascular system all relate to the disorder of the elastic tissues. An early sign of the disease is dilation of the aortic root. The most characteristic cardiac lesions are "floppy" valves, in the sense of large redundant valve leaflets and attenuated chordae, leading to valve prolapse and insufficiency. The symptoms relate mainly to affected aortic and mitral valves. A common complication is dissecting aneurysm of the aorta. Cardiovascular symptoms rarely occur in children.

Ehlers–Danlos Syndrome

An autosomal dominant disease, Ehlers–Danlos syndrome is characterized by a connective tissue abnormality that can affect the cardiovascular system. The changes, therefore, are like those that occur in Marfan's disease. A specific morphological change is as yet unknown. The coarse fragmented elastin fibres seen with the light microscope are probably an expression of an underlying primary collagen disorder. Clinical manifestations of this disease in childhood are rare.

Holt–Oram Syndrome

Holt–Oram syndrome is an inherited disease showing an autosomal dominant trait. It is characterized by skeletal abnormalities, the most striking of which is an abnormal, often elongated, thumb. The most frequently associated cardiac anomaly is atrial septal defect of the oval fossa type.

Osteogenesis Imperfecta

Similar abnormalities to those in Marfan's syndrome have been described in osteogenesis imperfecta, although the cardiovascular problems in osteogenesis imperfecta rarely dominate the clinical symptomatology.

Neuromuscular Disorders

In some instances a skeletal myopathy is associated with cardiac abnormalities. This is particularly true for Friedreich's ataxia, in which electrocardiographic abnormalities and heart failure can occur at a young age. Histological studies reveal non-specific interstitial fibrosis with regressive changes of myocytes. Similar changes have been reported to occur in the myocardium of patients suffering from dystrophia myotonica and forms of progressive muscular dystrophy.

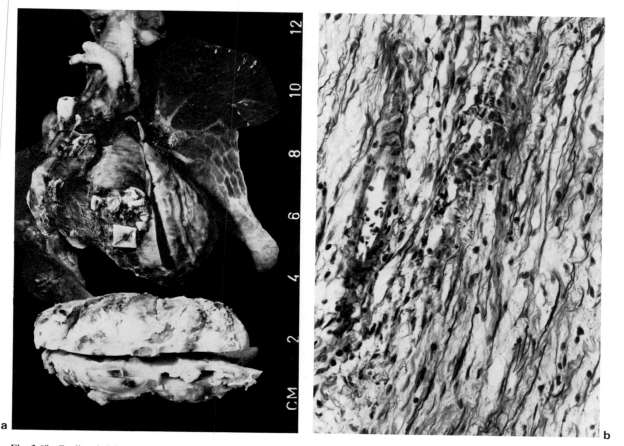

Fig. 3.69. Cardiac rhabdomyoma. **a** Incised left ventricle with the rhabdomyoma located in its anterior wall extending into the ventricular septum, thereby reducing the left ventricular cavity to a slit-like space. **b** Micrograph revealing the spider cell architecture characteristic for rhabdomyoma. (H&E, x 350)

Cardiac Tumours

Primary cardiac tumours are extremely rare. Secondary or metastatic tumours of the heart are also rare in children, malignant lymphoma and neuroblastoma being the least uncommon. Leukaemic deposits are often in the heart if carefully looked for.

The primary cardiac tumours that most frequently become symptomatic in children are rhabdomyomas, fibromas, myxomas and teratomas (McAllister and Fenoglio 1978).

Rhabdomyoma

Rhabdomyomas of the heart occur as circumscribed nodules of a greyish-tan colour within an otherwise normal-appearing myocardium (Fig. 3.69a). On microscopic examination the affected area shows markedly swollen myocytes with an irregular vacuolization. The vacuoles differ in size and are separated by thin strands of cytoplasm in which cross-striations may sometimes be identified. This architecture gives the characteristic appearance of the so-called spider cell (Fig. 3.69b). A diastase-resistant polysaccharide can sometimes be demonstrated within the cells. Microscopic studies of other areas of the myocardium, which grossly appear unaffected, will often reveal additional minute foci of a similar architecture. In symptomatic patients intracavitary extension is frequent.

Cardiac rhabdomyomas are currently regarded as hamartomas, most likely as a result of arrested cardiocyte maturation. It is of interest that cardiac rhabdomyoma has a strong tendency to be associated with tuberous sclerosis.

Spontaneous regression of these lesions may occur and, hence, surgical intervention is not indicated unless cardiac symptoms are life-threatening.

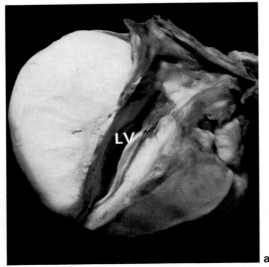

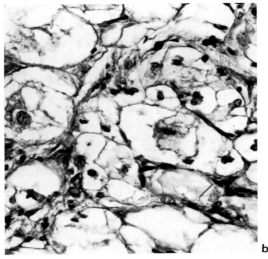

Fig. 3.70. Cardiac fibroma. **a** Autopsy specimen of the heart, in relation to the surgically removed fibroma. The latter was located in the right ventricular free wall and extended into the ventricular septum. At surgery the lesion appeared well delineated. **b** Micrograph exhibiting the characteristic compact arrangement of wavy collagen fibres. (Elastin tissue stain, counterstained with Van Gieson stain, x 350)

Cardiac Fibroma

Cardiac fibroma is the second most common cardiac tumour in children and ranks third in patients of 1 year or younger. There is a distinct tendency for the lesions to occur in the left ventricular free wall or the ventricular septum (Fig. 3.70). Gross examination reveals an apparently circumscribed lesion (Fig. 3.70a), which appears homogeneous and whitish on its cut surface. Microscopic studies reveal a compact

arrangement of wavy collagen fibres with sparse vascularity (Fig. 3.70b). At the periphery the lesion may interdigitate with pre-existent myocardial fibres. The symptomatology is largely related to the size and site of the lesion. Successful extirpation of cardiac fibromas has been reported (Geha et al. 1967). The term "cardiac fibromatosis" has been advocated (Turi et al. 1980).

Cardiac Myxoma

Cardiac myxoma is a relatively rare tumour in children. Of 130 patients with a myxoma, 9% were under 15 years of age, the youngest patient being 4 years of age (McAllister and Fenoglio 1978). The youngest patient seen by us was a boy aged 17 years with a left ventricular myxoma, who died suddenly and unexpectedly during mild exercise (Fig. 3.71).

There is a distinct preference for myxomas to occur in the left atrium, but each cardiac chamber can be affected. The symptomatology largely depends on their position, size and texture. Myxomas that are friable may easily give rise to emboli, either composed of tumour fragments or of thrombotic material.

Their gross and microscopic features are no different from those encountered in adults. Cardiac myxoma is a true neoplasm, showing extensive growth and recurrence if not completely excised.

Cardiac Teratoma

In patients under 1 year of age cardiac teratoma is the second most common primary cardiac tumour. Teratomas by definition contain elements derived from all three germ layers, therefore their classification should be no problem for the pathologist. The majority of teratomas of the heart are extracardiac, although intrapericardial. Their usual location is at the base of the heart and most of these lesions are attached to the root of the great arteries. Intrapericardial teratomas may grow to bizarre dimensions, thus affecting cardiac function.

Miscellaneous Lesions

Other primary cardiac tumours can occur in the paediatric group, but they seldom become symptomatic. All histological types of haemangioma (cavernous, capillary and mixed types) have been incidental findings at autopsy, but occasionally such a vascular anomaly can cause haemopericardium and tamponade.

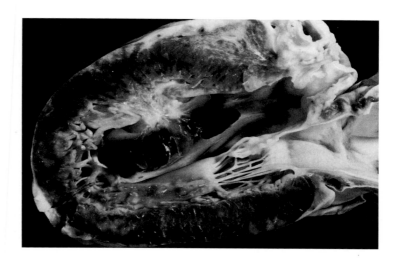

Fig. 3.71. Myxoma from the left ventricle causing obstruction and sudden death in a boy aged 17 years.

The suspicion that a cardiac lesion may be a haemangioma is usually aroused by its gross aspect. Some haemangiomas appear to be circumscribed, but extensive spread is often present between pre-existent myocardial fibres.

Mesothelioma of the atrioventricular node deserves mention because this unique tumour can underlie conduction abnormalities (atrioventricular dissociation) and sudden death. The lesion replaces in part the atrioventricular node and is composed of tubules lined by a single or multiple layer of predominantly flat cuboid cells. The tubules are embedded in a fibrous stroma. The histological appearance is somewhat reminiscent of that seen in mesothelioma. The nature of the lesion, however, remains speculative.

Blood cysts are small red nodules that appear predominantly on the mitral and tricuspid valves in almost any neonatal heart. The "cyst" is formed by crevices in the valve leaflets, filled with "trapped" blood, giving the characteristic appearance. The lesions tend to disappear with time and are completely benign.

There have been isolated reports of primary malignant cardiac tumours, such as malignant teratoma, rhabdomyosarcoma, neurogenic sarcoma and fibrosarcoma, occurring in children.

References

Anderson RH, Ho SY (1986) The diagnosis and naming of congenitally malformed hearts. In: Macartney FJ (ed) Congenital heart disease. MTP Press, Lancaster, p 1

Anderson RH, Becker AE, Arnold R, Wilkinson JL (1974) The conducting tissues in congenitally corrected transposition. Circulation 50: 911

Anderson RH, Becker AE, Gerlis LM (1975) The pulmonary outflow tract in classically corrected transposition. J Thorac Cardiovasc Surg 69: 747

Anderson RH, Wilkinson JL, Gerlis LM, Smith A, Becker AE (1977) Atresia of the right atrioventricular orifice. Br Heart J 39: 414

Anderson RH, Tynan MJ, Freedom RM, Quero-Jimenez M, Macartney FJ, Shinebourne EA, Van Mierop LHS, Wilkinson JL, Becker AE (1979) Ventricular morphology in the univentricular heart. Herz 4: 184

Anderson RH, Macartney FJ, Tynan M, Becker AE, Freedom RM, Godman MJ, Hunter S, Quero-Jimenez M, Rigby ML, Shinebourne EA, Sutherland G, Smallhorn JG, Soto B, Thiene G, Wilkinson JL, Wilcox BR, Zuberbuhler JR (1983) Univentricular atrioventricular connection: the single ventricle trap unsprung. Pediatr Cardiol 4: 273

Anderson RH, Becker AE, Freedom RM, Macartney FJ, Quero-Jimenez M, Shinebourne EA, Wilkinson JL, Tynan M (1984a) Sequential segmental analysis of congenital heart disease. Pediatr Cardiol 5: 281

Anderson RH, Becker AE, Tynan M, Macartney FJ, Rigby ML, Wilkinson JL (1984b) The univentricular atrioventricular connection: getting to the root of a thorny problem. Am J Cardiol 54: 822

Becker AE (1976) Kawasaki disease. Lancet i: 864

Becker AE (1978) Transposition of the great arteries: introductory remarks. In: Van Mierop LHS, Oppenheimer-Dekker A, Bruins CLDC (eds) Embryology and teratology of the heart and the great arteries. Martinus Nijhoff, The Hague, p 91

Becker AE (1981) Congenital malformations of the coronary arteries. In: Becker AE, Losekoot TG, Marcelleti C, Anderson RH (eds) Churchill Livingstone, Edinburgh

Becker AE, Anderson RH (1978) Fallot's tetralogy – developmental aspects, anatomy and conducting tissues. In: Anderson RH, Shinebourne EA (eds) Paediatric cardiology (1977). Churchill-Livingstone, Edingburgh, p. 245

Becker AE, Anderson RH (1981) Pathology of congenital heart disease. Butterworths, London

Becker AE, Anderson RH (1982) Atrioventricular septal defects. What's in a name? J Thorac Cardiovasc Surg 83: 461

Becker AE, Becker MJ, Edwards JE (1971) Pathologic spectrum of dysplasia of the tricuspid valve. Features in common with Ebstein's malformation. Arch Pathol 91: 167

Becker AE, Connon M, Anderson RH (1975) Tetralogy of Fallot. A morphometric and geometric study. Am J Cardiol 35: 402

Becker AE, Becker MJ, Wagenvoort CA (1977) Premature contraction of the ductus arteriosus: a cause of foetal death. J Pathol 121: 187

Becker AE, Lie KI, Anderson RH (1978a) Bundle-branch block in the setting of acute anteroseptal myocardial infarction. Br Heart J 40: 773

Becker AE, Losekoot TG, Anderson RH (1978b) The conducting tissues in congenitally complete heart block. Clinicopathologic correlation in three patients. In: Van Mierop LHS, Oppenheimer-Dekker A, Bruins CLDC (eds) Embryology and teratology of the heart and the great arteries. Martinus Nijhoff, The Hague, p 43

Becker AE, Losekoot TG, Anderson RH (1978c) Congenitally complete heart block. In: Goodman MJ, Marquis RM (eds) Paediatric cardiology, vol 2. Churchill Livingstone, Edinburgh, p 422

Becu LM, Fontana RS, DuShane JW, Kirklin JW, Burchell HB, Edwards JE (1956) Anatomic and pathologic studies in ventricular septal defects. Circulation 14: 349

Berry CL (1967) Myocardial ischemia in infancy and childhood. J Clin Pathol 20: 38

Bland EF, White PD, Garland J (1933) Congenital anomalies of the coronary arteries: report of an unusual case associated with cardiac hypertrophy. Am Heart J 8: 787

Brandt PWT, Calder AL (1977) Cardiac connections: the segmental approach to radiologic diagnosis in congenital heart disease. Current Probs Radiol 7: 1–35

Campbell M (1968) The incidence and later distribution of malformations of the heart. In: Watson H (ed) Paediatric cardiology. Lloyd-Luke, London

Carpentier A (1978) Surgical anatomy and management of the mitral component of atrioventricular caval defects. In: Anderson RH, Shinebourne EA (eds) Paediatric cardiology (1977). Churchill Livingstone, Edinburgh, p 477

Caruso G, Becker AE (1979) How to determine atrial situs? Considerations initiated by three cases of absent spleen with a discordant anatomy between bronchi and atria. Br Heart J 41: 559

Caruso G, Losekoot TG, Becker AE (1978) Ebstein's anomaly in persistent common atrioventricular canal. Br Heart J 40: 1275

Collett RW, Edwards JE (1949) Persistent truncus arteriosus: a classification according to anatomic types. Surg Clin North Am 29: 1245

Crupi G, Macartney FJ, Anderson RH (1977) Persistent truncus arteriosus. A study of 66 autopsy cases with special reference to definition and morphogenesis. Am J Cardiol 40: 569

Davies MJ (1971) Pathology of conducting tissue of the heart. Butterworths, London

Deanfield JE, Leanage R, Stroobant J, Chrispin AR, Taylor JFN, Macartney FJ (1980) Use of high kilovoltage filtered beam radiographs for detection of bronchial situs in infants and young children. Br Heart J 44: 577

Doucette J, Knoblich R (1963) Persistent right valve of the sinus venosus. So-called cor triatriatum dextrum: review of the literature and report of a case. Arch Pathol 75: 105

Durrer D, Roos JR, van Dam RT (1966) The genesis of the electrocardiogram of patients with ostium primum defects (ventral atrial septal defects). Am Heart J 71: 642

Feldt RH, DuShane JW, Titus JL (1970) The atrioventricular conduction system in persistent common atrioventricular canal defect: correlations with electrocardiogram. Circulation 42: 437

Franciosi RA, Blanc WA (1968) Myocardial infarcts in infants and children. I. A necropsy study in congenital heart disease. J Pediatr 73: 309

Fujiwara H, Hamashima Y (1978) Pathology of the heart in Kawasaki disease. Pediatrics 61: 100

Geha AS, Weidman WH, Soule EH, McGoon DC (1967) Intramural ventricular cardiac fibroma. Successful removal in two cases and review of the literature. Circulation 36: 427

Gerlis LM (1985) Cardiac malformations in spontaneous abortions. Int J Cardiol 7: 29

Gittenberger-de Groot AC (1977) Persistent ductus arteriosus: most probably a primary congenital malformation. Br Heart J 39: 610

Gittenberger-de Groot AC, Moulaert AJ, Harinck E, Becker AE (1978) Histopathology of the ductus arteriosus after prostaglandin E₁ administration in ductus dependent cardiac anomalies. Br Heart J 40: 215

Goor DA, Lillehei CW, Rees R, Edwards JE (1970) Isolated ventricular septal defect. Development basis for various types and presentation of classification. Chest 58: 468

Harinck E, Becker AE, Gittenberger-de Groot AC, Oppenheimer-Dekker A, Versprille A (1977) The left ventricle in congenital isolated pulmonary valve stenosis. A morphological study. Br Heart J 39: 429

Ho SY, Escher E, Anderson RH, Michaelsson M (1986) Anatomy of congenital complete heart block and relation to maternal anti-Ro antibodies. Am J Cardiol 58: 291

Hoffman JIE, Christianson E (1978) Congenital heart disease in a cohort of 19 502 births with long term follow up. Am J Cardiol 42: 641

Huhta JC, Smallhorn JF, Macartney FJ (1982) Two-dimensional echocardiographic diagnosis of situs. Br Heart J 48: 97

Hull D, Binns BAO, Joye D (1966) Congenital heart block with widespread fibrosis due to maternal lupus erythematosus. Arch Dis Child 41: 688

Kainulainen K, Pulkkinen L, Savolainen A, Kaitila I, Peltonen L (1990) Location on chromosome 15 of the gene defect causing Marfan syndrome. N Engl J Med 323: 935

Kawasaki T, Kosaki F, Okawa S, Shigematsu I, Yanagawa H (1974) A new infantile acute febrile mucocutaneous lymphnode syndrome (MCLS) prevailing in Japan. Pediatrics 54: 271

Keeton BR, Macartney FJ, Hunter S, Mortera C, Rees P, Shinebourne EA, Tynan M, Wilkinson JL, Anderson RH (1979) Univentricular heart of right ventricular type with double or common inlet. Circulation 59: 403

Kirklin JW, Pacifico AD, Bargeron LM, Soto B (1973) Cardiac repair in anatomically corrected malposition of the great arteries. Circulation 48: 153

Kitamura N, Takao A, Ando M (1974) Taussig–Bing heart with mitral valve straddling: case reports and postmortem study. Circulation 49: 761

Lev M (1958) The architecture of the conduction system in congenital heart disease. I. Common atrioventricular orifice. Arch Pathol 65: 174

Lev M (1959) The pathologic anatomy of ventricular septal defects. Dis Chest 35: 533

Lev M, Agustsson MH, Arcilla R (1961) The pathologic anatomy of common atrioventricular orifice associated with tetralogy of Fallot. J Clin Pathol 36: 408

Lev M, Bharati S, Meng CCL, Liberthson RR, Paul MH, Idriss F (1972) A concept of double outlet right ventricle. J Thorac Cardiovasc Surg 64: 271

Litsey SE, Noonan JA, O'Connor WN, Cottrill CM, Mitchell B (1985) Maternal connective tissue disease and congenital heart block. Demonstration of immunoglobulin in cardiac tissue. N Engl J Med 312: 98

Losekoot TG, Anderson RH, Becker AE, Danielson GK, Soto B (1983) Congenitally connected transposition. Churchill Livingstone, Edinburgh

Lubbers WJ, Tegelaers WHH, Losekoot TG, Becker AE (1975) Aberrant origin of left pulmonary artery (vascular sling). Report of the clinical and anatomic features in three patients. Eur J Cardiol 2: 477

Macartney FJ, Partridge JB, Shinebourne EA, Tynan MJ, Anderson RH (1978) Identification of atrial situs. In: Anderson RH, Shinebourne EA (eds) Paediatric cardiology (1977). Churchill Livingstone, Edinburgh, p 16

Macartney FJ, Zuberbuhler JR, Anderson RH (1980) Morphological considerations pertaining to recognition of atrial isomerism. Consequences for sequential chamber localization Br Heart J 44: 657

McAllister HA, Fenoglio JJ (1978) Tumours of the cardiovascular system. Atlas of tumour pathology

McCue CM, Mantakers ME, Tinglestad JB, Ruddy S (1977) Congenital heart block in newborns of mothers with connective tissue disease. Circulation 56: 82

Melhuish BP, Van Praagh R (1968) Juxtaposition of the atrial appendages: a sign of severe cyanotic congenital heart disease. Br Heart J 30: 269

Penkoske PA, Neches WH, Anderson RH, Zuberbuhler JR (1985) Further observations on the morphology of atrioventricular septal defects. J Thorac Cardiovasc Surg 90: 622

Rowe RD, Mehrizi A (1968) The neonate with congenital heart disease. Saunders, Philadelphia

Ruckman RN, Van Praagh R (1978) Anatomic types of congenital mitral stenosis. Report of 49 autopsy cases with consideration of diagnosis and surgical implications. Am J Cardiol 42: 592

Rudolph AM, Heymann MA, Spitznas U (1972) Hemodynamic considerations in the development of narrowing of the aorta. Am J Cardiol 30: 514

Šamánek M, Goetzova J, Benesova D (1985) Distribution of congenital heart malformations in an autopsied child population. Int J Cardiol 8: 235

Scott JB, Maddison PJ, Taylor PV, Esscher E, Scott O, Skinner RD (1983) Connective tissue disease, antibodies to ribonucleoprotein, and congenital heart block. N Engl J Med 4: 204

Shapiro LM, McKenna WJ (1983) Distribution of left ventricular hypertrophy in hypertrophic cardiomyopathy: a two-dimensional echocardiographic study. J Am Coll Cardiol 2: 437

Shinebourne EA, Anderson RH (1978) Fallot's tetralogy – angiographic–anatomic correlations. In: Anderson RH. Shinebourne EA (eds) Paediatric cardiology (1977). Churchill Livingstone, Edinburgh, p 258

Shinebourne EA, Anderson RH (1979) Concise paediatric cardiology. Oxford University Press, Oxford

Shinebourne EA, Macartney FJ, Anderson RH (1976) Sequential chamber localization – logical approach to diagnosis in congenital heart disease. Br Heart J 38: 327

Shone JD, Sellers RD, Anderson RC, Adams P Jr, Lillehei CW, Edwards JE (1963) The developmental complex of 'parachute mitral valve', supravalvular ring of left atrium, subaortic stenosis, and coarctation of aorta. Am J Cardiol 11: 714

Smith A, Ho SY, Anderson RH (1977) Histological study of the cardiac conducting system as a routine procedure. Med Lab Sci 34: 223

Somerville J (1978) Introduction: atrioventricular canal malformations. In: Anderson RH, Shinebourne EA (eds) Paediatric cardiology (1977). Churchill Livingstone, Edinburgh, p 417

Soto B, Becker AE, Moulaert AJ, Lie JT, Anderson RH (1980) Classification of isolated ventricular septal defects. Br Heart J 43: 332

Sotomora RF, Edwards JE (1978) Anatomic identification of so-called absent pulmonary artery. Circulation 57: 624

Stewart JR, Kincaid OW, Edwards JE (1964) An atlas of vascular rings and related malformation of the aortic arch system. Thomas, Springfield

Tanaka N, Sekimoto K, Naoe S (1976) Kawasaki disease. Relationship with infantile periarteritis nodosa. Arch Pathol Lab Med 100: 81

Taussig HB, Bing RJ (1949) Complete transposition of aorta and levoposition of the pulmonary artery: clinical, physiological and pathological findings. Am Heart J 37: 551

Thiene G, Bortolotti U, Gallucci V, Terribile V, Pellegrino PA (1976) Anatomical study of truncus arteriosus communis with embryological and surgical considerations. Br Heart J 38: 1109

Turi GK, Albala A, Fenoglio JJ (1980) Cardiac fibromatosis: an ultra-structural study. Hum Pathol 11: 577

Tynan MJ, Becker AE, Macartney FJ, Quero-Jimenez M, Shinebourne EA, Anderson RH (1979) The nomenclature and classification of congenital heart disease. Br Heart J 41: 544

Ueda M, Becker AE (1985) Classification of hearts with overriding aortic and pulmonary valves. Int J Cardiol 9: 357

Uhl HSM (1952) A previously congenital malformation of the right ventricle. Bull Johns Hopkins Hospital 91: 197

Van Mierop LHS, Gessner IH, Schiebler GL (1972) Asplenia and polysplenia syndromes. Birth Defects 8: 36

Van Praagh R (1968) What is the Taussig–Bing malformation? Circulation 38: 445

Van Praagh R (1972) The sequential approach to diagnosis in congenital heart disease. Birth Defects 8: 4

Wagenvoort CA, Wagenvoort N (1977) Pathology of pulmonary hypertension. Wiley, New York

Warden HE, DeWall RA, Cohen M, Varco RB, Lillehei CW (1957) A surgical pathologic classification for isolated ventricular septal defects and for those in Fallot's tetralogy based on observations made on 120 patients during repair under direct vision. J Thorac Cardiovasc Surg 33: 21

World Health Organization (1975) Primary pulmonary hypertension. In: Hatano S, Strasser T (eds) Report on a WHO meeting. WHO, Geneva

4 · Central Nervous System

Jennian Geddes

The specialist aspects of neuropathology in the paediatric period may be daunting for the generalist. As the immature brain goes through the various stages of development, it produces correspondingly varying responses to injury, any of which may differ markedly from those seen in the mature brain. In addition, patterns of brain damage are frequently non-specific, so that a single pathological agent acting at different times in gestation may produce different patterns of injury. This can result in a blurring of the border between different types of pathology – for example, malformations and destructive lesions. A further problem is that clinical details that might shed light on the pathogenesis of a given pattern of brain damage are seldom available, except for events occurring late in gestation or after birth. Finally, a vast number of rare conditions affecting the central nervous system (CNS) typically present in childhood and are not seen later in life. These features combine to create the subset of specialized problems within neuropathology that this chapter explores.

Cell Populations in the CNS and their Reactions

Most *neurons* have lost the capacity to divide by the end of gestation, although they may still migrate and mature. They do so at different rates, with the result that some nuclear groups may appear morphologically adult while others still resemble neuroblasts. The appearance of damaged neurons will depend on their degree of development: if they are mature, they

will show reactions to injury similar to those of adult neurons – cytoplasmic eosinophilia and/or shrinkage, and nuclear pyknosis (Fig. 4.1). In immature neuronal groups, which have small round nuclei and little stainable cytoplasm, these changes are not seen, and neuronal death can be detected only from the pres-

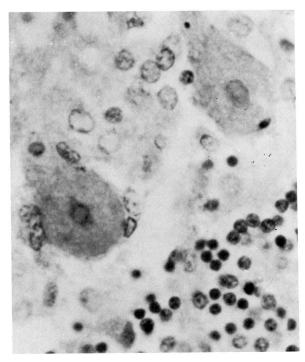

Fig. 4.1. Purkinje cells in the cerebellum, undergoing acute necrosis. The nucleus is shrunken and pyknotic, and the cytoplasm deeply eosinophilic. (H&E ×400)

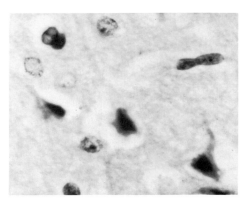

Fig. 4.2. Triangular cells with pyknotic nuclei are neurons showing ischaemic change. The pale nuclei are astrocytic. (H&E ×900)

ence of karyorrhexis – always bearing in mind that karyorrhexis is a normal feature of the continuous cell loss that occurs in development, particularly during the second trimester. When neurons die under pathological conditions, astrocytes and microglia proliferate, and the term neuronophagia describes collections of cells, principally microglial, surrounding a dying neuron (Fig. 4.2). With time, astrocytic proliferation and fibre formation ("gliosis") may be the sole marker of neuronal death, although sometimes

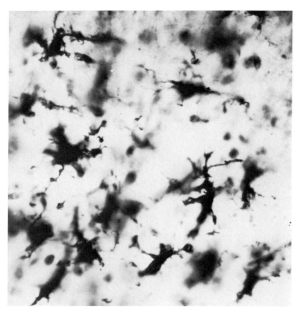

Fig. 4.3. Activated microglia in cerebellar white matter. Although immunoperoxidase stains are now used to demonstrate microglia, their morphology is best demonstrated by traditional silver impregnations such as Weil–Davenport, shown here. (×400)

neurons encrusted with iron and calcium, described as "ferruginated", persist as tombstones at the site of damage. This is a particular feature of hypoxic-ischaemic damage to the basal ganglia in neonates and infants. Neuronal loss is invariably followed by axonal degeneration, which results in loss of myelin as a secondary event.

Microglia, the resident macrophages of the central nervous system, are derived from bone marrow precursor cells (Ling and Wong 1993; Altman 1994), and are not, despite their name, of glial lineage. They can be demonstrated in the fetal brain from around the end of the first trimester (Gilles et al. 1983), some time before astrocytes make their appearance. Resting microglia are inconspicuous in normal brain parenchyma, in which they appear as dark cigar-shaped nuclei, lacking stainable cytoplasm, lying between neurons or axons. Immunostaining of microglial antigens (CD68 is a good marker) reveals a small amount of perinuclear cytoplasm and characteristic branching processes. Microglial activation is a feature of most pathological processes in the CNS, and is characterized by morphological changes (increase in the amount of cytoplasm and the number of cell processes) accompanied by upregulation of the expression of cell surface molecules (Fig. 4.3) (Perry et al. 1993). Hyperplasia also occurs, and nodular aggregates of microglia are typical of some encephalitides and of diffuse traumatic axonal damage. Under certain circumstances microglia in the cerebral cortex may become greatly elongated, and are referred to as "rod" cells. First described in paretic neurosyphilis, rod cells may be found in any slowly progressive encephalopathy – for example, subacute sclerosing panencephalitis or HIV-1 encephalitis. During the first half of gestation, before the brain is capable of mounting an astrocytic response, the tissue response to injury consists solely of microglial and macrophage proliferation, and glial "scar" formation does not occur. As a result, resorption of necrotic tissue early in intrauterine life can produce a lesion that more closely resembles a malformation than the aftermath of a destructive process.

Glial cells comprise astrocytes, oligodendrocytes and ependymal cells and their precursors. The *radial glia*, which guide neuroblast migration, can be demonstrated by glial fibrillary acidic protein (GFAP) from about the age of 12 weeks, and are thought to be tanycytes, a GFAP-expressing subpopulation of ependymal cells. During development, astrocytic and oligodendrocytic precursor cells proliferate in the subventricular zone and migrate into all parts of the CNS, where they differentiate into mature glial cells. *Astrocytes* are not detected until after most neuronal migration has finished, at about 15 weeks' gestational age at the earliest. These are a

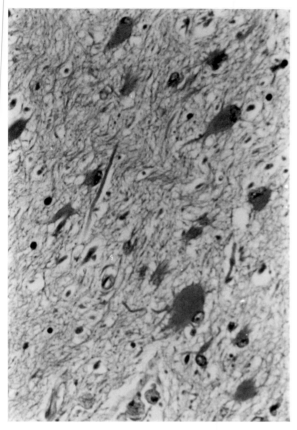

Fig. 4.4. Reactive astrocytes in white matter, showing eccentric nuclei and abundant cytoplasm with processes. Reactive astrocytes tend to be regularly spaced through the neuropil, unlike neoplastic gemistocytes. (H&E, ×330)

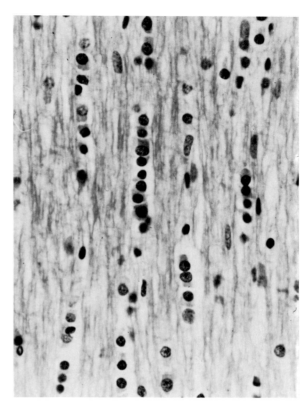

Fig. 4.5. Myelination glia in the internal capsule at 36 weeks. The nuclei are lined up between fibres, and many of them have cytoplasm, not normally seen in mature oligodendroglia. (H&E, ×400)

heterogeneous group of cells which develop from different precursor cells but have a number of features in common, principally the expression of the cytoplasmic intermediate filament GFAP. In the resting state, astrocytic cytoplasm does not stain well with haematoxylin and eosin (H&E), but can be detected with the aid of an immunoperoxidase stain for GFAP. Hypertrophied ("reactive") astrocytes with eosinophilic cytoplasm and stellate processes (Fig. 4.4) proliferate in any almost any pathological process. In the infant brain, one has to be careful not to mistake *myelination glia* for reactive astrocytes. Myelination glia (Fig. 4.5) are oligodendrocyte precursors present in myelinating white matter; their cytoplasm contains large amounts of premyelin lipids. Myelinating white matter is generally much more cellular than white matter in a mature brain, and once again the diagnosis of reactive astrocytosis has to be made with care in an infant brain. As myelination finishes, the cellular density decreases and the

cells increasingly resemble mature oligodendrocytes. *Oligodendrocytes* are small cells, with a round nucleus surrounded by a thin rim of cytoplasm, found in greatest numbers in white matter, lying between myelinated fibres. They are GFAP negative, but can be stained by antisera to carbonic anhydrase C. Occasional oligodendrocytes are seen in grey matter, adjacent to neuronal cell bodies. *Ependymal cells* line the entire ventricular system and the central canal of the spinal cord, forming a continuous layer of cuboidal or columnar ciliated epithelium, which rests directly on the neuropil. In certain areas, notably adjacent to the occipital horns of the lateral ventricles, by the aqueduct and beside the lateral angles of the fourth ventricle, small islands of ectopic ependymal cells and tubules are normally found in the subependymal layers. The *tanycyte*, an ultrastructurally distinct cell in the ependyma, differs from other ependymal cells seen on light microscopy in that it expresses GFAP.

Assessment of Gestational Age

A brief account of the principal events in the normal development of the CNS is given below, in the section on malformations; fuller descriptions of the timing of events during the development of the brain are given by Gilles et al. (1983), Friede (1989) and Larroche (1991a).

Any attempt to evaluate gestational age must of course take into account fetal measurements and weights of all the organs. Anatomical development of the brain, assessed on external examination from the gyration of the cerebral cortex, and microscopically from the anatomical development of cortex and deep grey structures, is also important; the major morphological changes in the hemispheres are illustrated on pp. 9–12. Perhaps the most reliable index of gestational age, however, is the degree of myelination that has taken place in the CNS. Myelination begins in the second half of gestation and occurs in sequence, in general terms in a caudal–rostral direction. It continues during early childhood, and is essentially complete by the age of seven. The spinal cord and its roots begin to acquire myelin during the second trimester of pregnancy, and myelination starts in the brain stem by the beginning of the third

trimester. At full term a few hemispheric tracts have myelinated, although the bulk of the cerebral white matter still lacks myelin, which accounts for the extreme softness of the neonatal brain. The first pathways to myelinate are those involved in relaying sensory information from the periphery, so that structures such as the posterior columns, the lateral and medial lemnisci, the medial longitudinal fascicle, and the superior and inferior cerebellar peduncles, which are all involved in the perception of touch, proprioception, auditory and vestibular stimuli, are myelinated by the end of gestation, while pathways involved in the *integration* of sensory information become myelinated later. The order and timing of myelination of individual anatomical structures is now well established, both during gestation and in postnatal life (Brody et al. 1987; Gilles 1991), and with the use of thick (15 μm) sections stained by a method such as luxol-fast blue one can screen a small number of defined "marker" sites for the presence of myelin. Gilles et al. (1983), have suggested using six blocks of this purpose, three each from the brain stem and the cerebrum: Table 4.1 shows some of their recommended levels, and structures that can be identified at each. Remember that the timing of myelination may vary slightly if a structure is examined at a different part of the brain stem. The dates

Table 4.1 Timing of myelination in selected anatomical regions during gestation

Gestational structure		Structure in which myelin is detected*	Age (weeks)
Cord	gracile fascile	Gracile fascicle in posterior columns (thoracic cord)	25
Medulla	ICP — MLF — ML pyramids	Inferior cerebellar peduncle (ICP) Medial lemniscus (ML) Pyramid	27 27 40
Pons	MLF — SCP LL	Medial longitudinal fascicle (MLF) Lateral lemniscus (LL) Superior cerebellar peduncle (SCP)	25 28 33
Midbrain		Corticospinal tract	40
Hemispheres	corticospinal tract	Optic chiasm Optic tract Posterior limb of internal capsule	41 37 36

* Naked eye detection of myelin on appropriately stained sections. The dates given are the gestational ages at which at least 80% of fetuses showed macroscopic evidence of myelination (Gilles et al. 1983).

given are the gestational ages by which over 80% of fetuses can be expected to have evidence of myelination, detected by naked eye inspection of a section stained for myelin. The medial longitudinal fascicle shows full myelination in over 80% of fetuses at all levels by 28 weeks and in 99% at 36 weeks. A block containing this structure stained, with a control block from the brain of a normal postnatal infant, provides a useful indication of the acquisition of myelin, but for full assessment a range of anatomical structures should be examined.

Malformations

When the CNS is known or suspected to be abnormal, a good clinical history is essential, because the history may influence the way the brain and spinal cord are removed at autopsy. For example, if severe hydrocephalus is present, a modified approach may be necessary (Laurence and Martin 1959; Gilles 1991). The clinical summary should say whether there is any family history of CNS malformations, and whether the pregnancy, and any previous pregnancy, was normal, and should give details of labour (including Apgar scores), postnatal course and acquisition of developmental milestones. For perinatal autopsies, the placenta should be available for inspection and histology, and it should be examined for evidence of infection. The results of investigations including chromosome studies should be known. All anomalies should be described or photographed, including those outside the CNS, in case a recognized pattern of findings can be identified. Fresh material (brain or CSF) may have to be taken for microbiology or metabolic investigations. Standard measurements including head circumference and biparietal diameter should be taken and related to standard growth curves; hand and foot prints may also be taken. Once the head is opened, the relationship of the brain size to the size of the calvarium should be noted. If the brain is found to be smaller than the calvarium, and is not merely a collapsed hydrocephalic brain, tissue destruction has taken place, because the growth of the skull parallels that of the brain. For fetal and young infant brains, which are very soft, it may be advisable to inject a small quantity of formalin under the skull a few hours before the autopsy. The brain can be removed directly into a weighed container of formalin, and can be examined and photographed after fixation, if necessary, under water. Systematic external examination should cover the following points: is there disproportion in the brain? Are the hemispheres normal? Is the gyral pattern normal and appropriate for the gestation age? Are there any cystic lesions? Is the corpus callosum present? Are the olfactory bulbs and tracts present or absent? (It is assumed that they have not been cut off during removal of the brain – an easy thing to do.) The internal appearances of the brain are usually best examined from coronal slices of uniform thickness laid out in order.

A useful way of classifying the principal CNS malformations is to consider the main "critical" periods in the formation of the nervous system and the defects that may result from intereference with that process. These periods are formation of the neural tube, formation of the telencephalic vesicles, and neuronal migration. Essentially, much of the crucial early development of the CNS is complete before pregnancy is likely to be confirmed – that is, during the fifth and sixth weeks after the last menstrual period – and fetuses of this gestational age are rarely available for study. As a result, the precise timing of events in humans is uncertain (O'Rahilly et al. 1984; Muller and O'Rahilly 1987), although much is now known of the process in other species, particularly rodents, which provide useful experimental models – for reviews, see Morriss-Kay (1981) and Copp et al. (1990). The first stage is formation of the neural tube from the neural plate, a process known as *neurulation*. In higher vertebrates, including humans, neurulation can be divided morphologically into two stages. Briefly, *primary* neurulation occurs along most of the neural tube, producing the brain and a large part of the spinal cord. In this process, the two neural folds from opposite sides of the neural plate become progressively more elevated, converge and fuse in the dorsal midline to complete the neural tube. Midline fusion of the neural folds occurs first in what will become the cervical region and continues sequentially in a both cranial and caudal direction. In segments caudal to the posterior neuropore, *secondary* neurulation occurs. Here the neural tube differentiates directly by canalization of the medullary cord, without prior formation of neural folds. In the human embryo, neurulation is believed to start around 22 days gestational age, and the neural tube is believed to be fully formed with anterior and posterior neuropores closed between 24 and 28 days (O'Rahilly et al. 1984). Thus *neural tube defects* such as anencephaly, cephaloceles and spinal lesions such as meningomyelocele result from some disturbance either during the relatively short time during which neurulation takes place or possibly soon after (see below, and Marin-Padilla and Marin-Padilla 1981).

In the second main period of CNS development, after the closure of the neural tube, prosencephalic diverticulation occurs. Regional differences in

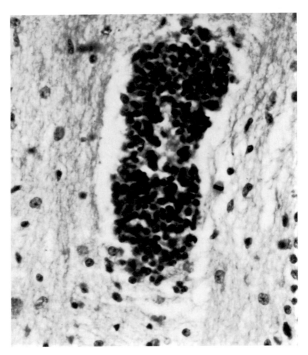

Fig. 4.6. Migrating neuroblasts around vessels in corona radiata at 36 weeks. Note an astrocyte in mitosis. (H&E ×400)

growth rates along the neural tube result in the development of a complex series of forebrain flexures, and the main regions of the brain become distinguishable by 36 days. From the sides of the single prosencephalic cavity, paired telencephalic vesicles grow out to form two rudimentary hemispheres, with the neural tube between them developing into the basal ganglia. This period (approximately 30–35 days) also sees the formation of the early structures and olfactory bulbs. Interference with normal cleavage of the forebrain into hemispheres and diencephalon results in disturbances of structures derived from the anterior telencephalic wall, often with associated facial abnormalities, the morphological spectrum ranging from holoprosencephaly to arhinencephaly.

The third period of brain development is neuronal migration, during which neuronal and glial cells migrate to the cortical plate from the proliferating neuroepithelium in the ventricular wall (Fig. 4.6). Most of the migration of postmitotic neuroblasts to the future neocortex takes place between about 7 and 16 weeks' gestation, and is guided by a network of glial fibres, formed by specialized radial glia. (During the process of migration, neuroblasts may be seen clustered around vessels, and at first sight may resemble perivascular lymphocytic cuffing.) Migration occurs in an orderly fashion, with successive waves of neurons arriving at the cortex to form each neuronal layer. The deepest cortical cell layers are formed first, and each subsequent neuronal layer is formed outside them, having migrated through the previous layer to lie beyond it. The final six-layered cortical structure can be distinguished increasingly clearly from early in the fifth month (Larroche 1962). Once migration is completed, neuronal differentiation takes place, at a rate that varies according to the neuronal groups involved. The deep pyramidal cell layer matures first in the cortex, and most of the rest of the cortical neuronal population differentiate much later. A large number of conditions result from interference with the normal process of neuronal migration, the most important of which are agyria/pachygyria (lissencephaly), polymicrogyria, and neuronal heterotopias of various types.

During the second half of intrauterine life, with the basic cytoarchitecture of the cerebrum established, neurons develop processes and connections, while glial cells and blood vessels proliferate. This is the time of maximum growth of the brain, during which the cortical gyral pattern develops to accommodate increasing cerebral volume. Interference with this period of growth results in destructive lesions, rather than malformations, which include the entities porencephaly, hydranencephaly and multicystic encephalopathy.

Axial-skeletal Dysraphic Disorders

Neural Tube Defects

Neural tube defects (NTD) are the major congenital anomalies of the CNS, and among the most common seen in humans. Their mechanism of production is uncertain, but data from humans and rodents show that both genetic and environmental factors are important in causation. Interactions both between different genes and between genes and a variety of environmental agents can be demonstrated in mutant and "non-mutant" mouse strains (for a review, see Copp et al. 1990). The neural tube defects comprise spina bifida occulta, spina bifida cystica, anencephaly and cephalocele, which together form a spectrum of conditions involving the brain, spinal cord, vertebrae and associated ectodermal and mesodermal structures. The pathogenesis of these malformations is complex, and is now thought to be related to a primary deficiency in the mesoderm, rather than in the neuroepithelium (see below). This hypothesis has lead to the Chiari hindbrain malformations being classified with the neural tube defects as "axial-skeletal dysraphic disorders" (Marin-Padilla 1991; Berry 1992).

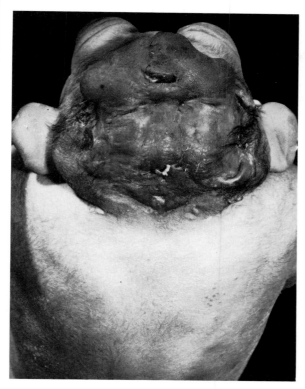

Fig. 4.7. Anencephalic fetus from above and behind. A mass of vascular tissue represents the brain.

Occult spina bifida is the most common of all dysraphic lesions, with a frequency in a large adult autopsy series of 5%; spina bifida cystica, in which the cyst contains either meninges and cord (meningomyelocele) or meninges alone (meningocele), occurs between 1 and 2.5 per 1000 live births, and anencephaly occurs between 0.5 and 2.0 per 1000 live births (Friede 1989). *Anencephaly*, the most extreme form of NTD, is four times as frequent in females than in males. This is true both in human fetuses and in mouse models of anencephaly, whether genetic or environmentally induced. The explanation, which has some support from experimental work, may lie in the fact that neurulation takes longer in females, with the result that there is a longer vulnerable period for the development of NTDs (Copp et al. 1990). Although many anencephalic fetuses may reach term, the anomaly is incompatible with extrauterine life. The cranial vault is hypoplastic or absent, and the skull base is invariably maldeveloped, with markedly shallow cranial fossae. Normal eyes are usually present, although they appear particularly protruberant as a result of the shallow orbits. Because the cranial space is inadequate, the brain becomes wholly or partially extruded as it develops and,

lacking the protection of meninges or calvarium, progressively degenerates (Fig. 4.7). Variable amounts of residual brain form an amorphous mass of highly vascular neuroglial tissue called the "area cerebrovasculosa", in which occasional normal structures such as cranial nerves may be identifiable. The spinal column is always abnormally developed in cases of anencephaly: at the milder end of the spectrum there is failure of fusion of the cervical vertebral spines; in more severe cases, there is a continuous open defect exposing both cord and the residual brain. This last condition is known as *craniorrachischisis*.

Cephalocele is the term used for the herniation of intracranial contents outside the skull. If, as is usual, both meninges and brain tissue are involved, the malformation is known as a meningoencephalocele (Fig. 4.8); if meninges only are present, it is called a meningocele. Cephaloceles, though related to other neural tube defects, are far less frequent, and are seen in 0.8–3.0 per 10 000 live births (Naidich et al. 1992). Most occur in the occipital region, protruding through a defect in the occiput or in the occiput and foramen magnum combined. They are usually covered by atrophic skin, and the cyst contents include meninges and cerebellum, brain stem or cerebrum, depending on the site. Other sites of extracranial herniation of brain or meninges, such as skull base or parietal or frontal bones, are rare. A small number of cephaloceles occur as part of a described syndrome, the most common of which is the Meckel–Gruber syndrome.

Meningomyelocele is the more extreme form of spina bifida cystica, and accounts for between 80% and 90% of cases of spina bifida cystica (Friede 1989). The lumbosacral region is usually affected (Fig. 4.9): the myelocele may be partly covered by a layer of epithelium, but the central region is exposed, resulting in free communication between the cerebrospinal fluid (CSF) space and the amniotic fluid. Further epithelialization may take place after birth. The malformation appears either as a flattened open defect or as a globular cystic mass in the lower back. In either case, it is composed of fibrovascular connective tissue, leptomeninges and disorganized neuroglial tissue. The cord is often abnormal both proximal and distal to the myelocele: hydromyelia (dilation of the central canal) or diastematomyelia (duplication of the spinal cord) may be present, and distally the filum terminale may be tethered by a band of dense fibrous tissue. Occasionally other mesenchymal elements – for example, a lipoma – are included in the anomaly, when the term lipomeningomyelocele is used. Up to 80% of infants with meningomyelocele have hydrocephalus, and in many of these type 2 Chiari malformation is also present. Scoliosis and kyphosis are also often seen: these may either be congenital in origin,

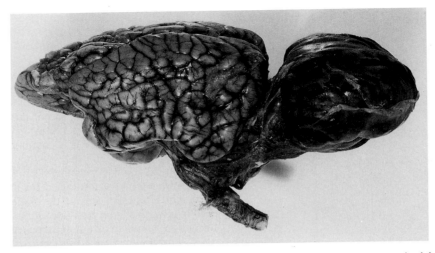

Fig. 4.8. A large occipital encephalocele in a child of 2 months. The brain was asymmetrical, and the sac contained the left posterior temporal, parietal and occipital lobes, and part of the right occipital lobe, together with a rudimentary portion of cerebellum.

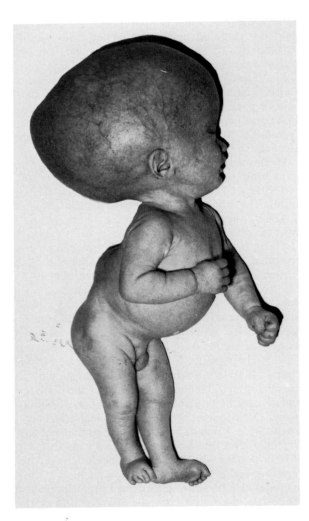

caused by bony malformations such as hemivertebrae or solid bony bars, or develop from muscle imbalance in the absence of bony abnormalities.

In *meningocele* a cystic swelling in the lumbar region overlies a defect in the vertebral arches. The meninges protrude through this defect, covered by skin or an epithelial membrane, which may ulcerate. Hydrocephalus and type 2 Chiari malformation are common. If the spinal cord is open to the air, meningitis resulting from ascending infection is inevitable.

Chiari Malformations

Chiari originally described a number of complex CNS malformations involving the brain stem and cerebellum, the name of Arnold being subsequently linked with his for the type 2 anomaly. The Chiari malformations are of three main types, each describing a different degree of displacement of posterior fossa contents into the cervical canal. Type 3, in which cervical spina bifida and an occupied cephalocele are added to the features of the type 2 anomaly, is rare. Type 1 Chiari malformation, which presents with hydrocephalus in older children or adults, is defined as herniation of the cerebellar tonsils through the foramen magnum. There is usually associated syringomyelia, but not a neural tube defect, and some cases may be the result of chronic tonsillar herniation secondary to raised intracranial pressure. However, many patients with this condition have associated

Fig. 4.9. Lumbar spina bifida cystica and hydrocephalus.

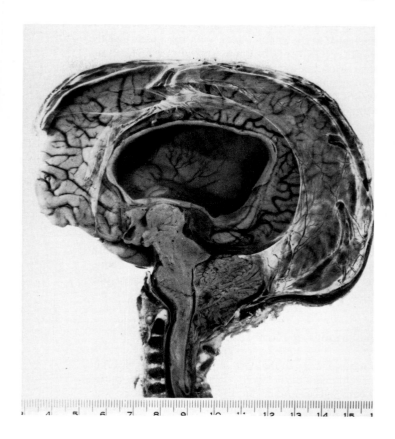

Fig. 4.10. Type 2 Chiari malformation, causing hydrocephalus. The elongated medulla extends into the spinal canal and is covered posteriorly by the cerebellar tonsils. Impaction of posterior fossa structures into the spinal canal obstructs the flow of CSF.

craniovertebral junction abnormalities: occipital dysplasia producing an abnormal posterior fossa has been demonstrated in over two-thirds of a large adult series (Schady et al. 1987).

The type 2 anomaly, the classic "Arnold–Chiari malformation" (Fig. 4.10), is more severe. It is a complex malformation involving the axial skeleton, cervical cord, brain stem and cerebellum, seen to varying degrees in all patients with meningomyelocele, and occasionally in patients who do not have dysraphic disorders. The pathogenesis of the Chiari 2 malformation has been disputed, and the various theories are well reviewed by Friede (1989). Magnetic resonance imaging (MRI), which enables the anatomy of the brain to be seen in great detail, has demonstrated the constant association of abnormal skull development with the neuraxial anomalies. Detailed descriptions of the skull changes have been given by Marin-Padilla (1991) and Muller and O'Rahilly (1991). One plausible explanation of the sequence of events comes from experimental work suggesting that primary mesodermal insufficiency is responsible. Such a defect, acting at different stages of neural fold formation and closure would provide a unifying explanation for both neural tube defects and

the Chiari malformations (Martin-Padilla and Marin-Padilla 1981). Thus, if mesodermal failure occurred before the closure of the neural folds, the most severe open neural tube defects (such as anencephaly and craniorrachischisis) would result; if it interfered with the process of closure, the cephaloceles and spina bifida cystica would be produced; and, finally, mesodermal insufficiency operating after the closure of the neural folds would be responsible for primary malformations of the axial skeleton, which in turn would interfere with *subsequent* growth and development of the nervous system (Muller and O'Rahilly 1991). Chiari malformations would come into the last group, with anomalous development of the chondrocranium resulting in underdevelopment of the occipital bone, which in turn produces an abnormally shaped posterior fossa. Whatever the pathogenic mechanism, the Chiari 2 malformation is best understood as a condition in which the posterior fossa is disproportionately small for cerebellar growth, with the result that the normal contents are squeezed out through the tentorial opening and the foramen magnum, both of which are usually larger than normal. The cerebellum is forced into the foramen magnum, and comes to override the dorsal surface of the cord. The medulla is also forced to grow downwards: it buckles as it is pushed into the spinal canal, with the result that the upper cervical cord becomes kinked in a Z shape and the corresponding roots are stretched. This downward movement also elongates the choroid plexus and fourth ventricle. Above the tentorium, there may be variable hypoplasia of the corpus callosum and beak-like deformity of the quadrigeminal plate. Other associated bony defects include focal erosions of the skull ("craniolacunae"), abnormalities of the occipital bone and atlas, and protrusion of the dens through the anterior rim of the foramen magnum ("basilar invagination"). Hydrocephalus probably occurs because caudal movement of posterior fossa structures into the spinal canal obstructs the flow of CSF, either through the aqueduct or in the cisterna magna. Enlarged lateral ventricles in turn cause further compression of the tentorium and flattening of the aqueduct. Cranial nerve palsies and brain stem signs may follow from the compression.

Anomalies of Forebrain Development

Interference with the normal process of cleavage and development of the early cerebral hemispheres during weeks 4–6 of embryonic life may be partial or complete, and so lead to a spectrum of malformations, ranging from the relatively trivial conditions of olfactory aplasia or fusion of the thalami to severe anomalies associated with craniofacial deformities. The pathology of these forebrain malformations is discussed in detail by Friede (1989) and Harding (1992). *Olfactory aplasia*, which denotes absence of olfactory bulbs and tracts, is the most mild of these conditions. It may be an incidental finding at autopsy, or part of the complex picture seen in *holoprosencephaly* (Fig. 4.11), where major deformities of the cerebrum result from failure of forebrain cleavage. In the most severe cases there is a single globular hemispheric mass, with a single ventricle and abnormal gyration ("alobar" holoprosencephaly). In less extreme examples, a depression or rudimentary fissure posteriorly partially demarcates the two hemispheres ("semilobar" holoprosencephaly). Sometimes the two hemisphere appear to be distinct, but on closer examination are continuous in the midline anteriorly ("lobar" holoprosencephaly). The olfactory bulbs and tracts are invariably absent, accounting for the former name of "arhinencephaly". However, even where the bulbs and tracts are aplastic, the central olfactory structures are always present in these conditions, and so the term arhinencephaly is inappropriate. Skeletal deformities accompany the neuraxial deformities in these conditions, as they do in the neural tube defects, because the development of the

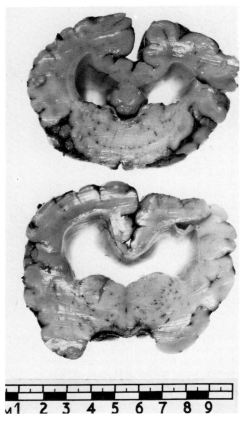

Fig. 4.11. Holoprosencephaly in trisomy 13–15. There is a single ventricle and although the hemispheres appear distinct, the upper (anterior) slice shows fusion of the frontal lobes in the midline.

forebrain is closely linked with the development of the primitive foregut and mesoderm. Some degree of facial malformation is present in all but the relatively rare cases of isolated olfactory aplasia. In severe forms, fusion of the orbits results in cyclopia and the nose is replaced by a proboscis projecting from above the single eye; microphthalmia and flattening of the nose are minor variants of the same process. Holoprosencephaly is closely associated with trisomies 13–15 and 17–18 (Patau and Edwards syndromes).

Abnormalities of Neuronal Migration

A large number of anomalies result from failure of the complex process of neuronal migration. With the use of high-resolution MRI many can be recognized in vivo, and as a group these are now recognized to be a common cause of epilepsy. The reviews of Barth (1987), Friede (1989) and Rorke (1994) are recom-

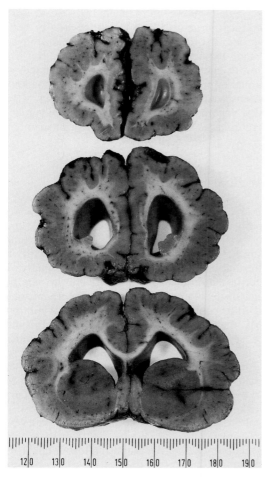

Fig. 4.12. Slices from the brain of a severely subnormal girl who died aged 2 years. The cortical ribbon is grossly abnormal bilaterally, and has the typical "overfolded" appearance of polymicrogyria. There is also marked dilatation of the lateral ventricles.

mended for detailed accounts. The most common malformations resulting from a migration defect are lissencephaly, polymicrogyria and various types of neuronal heterotopias.

Lissencephaly, which means "smooth brain", describes a brain in which there are no sulci (called "agyria") or in which reduced numbers of sulci are present, resulting in abnormally wide and rather flat gyri ("pachygyria"). Both conditions are rare: the brain in both is small, and on slicing the cortex can be seen to be abnormally thick, with correspondingly marked reduction in white matter volume. Basal ganglia are present but may be abnormal. The morphology of the cortex is variable in lissencephaly: it may be ordered into four layers (instead of the usual six) or may lack any organization at all (Barth 1987). The cause is unknown, but is assumed to be interruption of normal migration of neurons from the periventricular region to the cortex – an event that probably occurs around 11–13 weeks of gestation (Friede 1989).

Polymicrogyria (Fig. 4.12), sometimes referred to as "microgyria", has an unpredictable distribution within the brain. It can affect both cerebral hemispheres, one only, or merely part of one hemisphere, and occasionally the distribution corresponds to the territory of a major cerebral artery. It is less common in the cerebellum. Porencephalic defects (see below) often display areas of polymicrogyria round the edge. Polymicrogyric cortex looks abnormal: it may mimic pachygyria with an irregular surface of the gyri, or may have a nodular or cobblestone appearance suggesting too many gyri. Slicing confirms the cortex to be abnormal: it is invariably thicker than it should be, but not nearly as thick as in lissencephaly. Histologically (Fig. 4.13), a polymicrogyric cortex

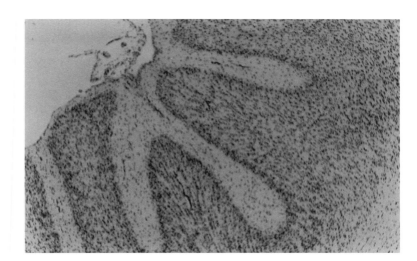

Fig. 4.13. A low-power view of a focus of polymicrogyria. There is abnormal formation of secondary gyri, which appear to share a single molecular (outer) layer of cortex, although a vessel tends to lie between the two adjacent gyri. (Cresyl fast violet ×30)

consists of fewer cell layers than normal – generally only four – with excessive folding that results in fusion or partial fusion of intervening sulci. There is evidence to suggest that some cases of polymicrogyria are caused by laminar ischaemic damage to the cortex, which in turn results in overfolding of the cortex as a consequence of differences in growth rates between outer and inner cortical layers (see review by Barkovich et al. 1992a). Postmigratory hypoxic–ischaemic damage is implicated in reported cases of maternal exposure to carbon monoxide during the second trimester of pregnancy, where the surviving fetuses showed polymicrogria, and in twin-to-twin transfusion syndrome. Placental infection leading of perfusion failure and ischaemic cortical damage is possibly also the underlying mechanism by which polymicrogyria occurs in intrauterine cytomegalovirus infection and toxoplasmosis (Friede and Mikolasek 1978; Marques Dias et al. 1984). However, focal mechanical insults applied to the cortex of newborn rats also produce a variety of migration defects, including polymicrogyria (Barth 1987; Ferrer et al. 1993), and the mechanism whereby polymicrogyria is produced in metabolic disorders such as neonatal adrenoleucodystrophy or Zellweger syndrome must be different again. From isolated cases reports of maternal accidents in which there is accurate timing of the event, polymicrogyria can be dated to a slightly later period in fetal life than lissencephaly, between about 14 and 24 weeks. The clinical effects of polymicrogyria depend on the site and the amount of neocortex affected, and range from mild to severe developmental retardation. Seizures are common (Barkovich et al. 1992a) and neurological development often severely impaired. A related neocortical malformation, described in the older literature as *status verrucosus*, is a relatively common finding in spontaneously aborted fetuses of about 20 weeks; according to Barth (1987), it has been found in between 16% and 26% of routine fetal autopsies. At low power it looks like a mild form of polymicrogyria, but at high magnification may seem to be an artefact or a stage in normal cortical formation, as generally only the upper cortical layers are involved. However, experimental production of status verrucosus in association with other forms of neuronal migration defects in rodents suggests that it is indeed a form of warty cortical dysplasia (Ferrer et al. 1993).

Neuronal heterotopias may be associated with cortical malformations or may be found in otherwise normal brains. Some heterotopias are visible macroscopically; others are recognized only on histology. Large heterotopias typically appear as layers or nodules of aberrant grey matter and may be seen with the naked eye at any site between the periventricular region and the cortex. They are often symmetrical, at first glance giving the appearance of a normal anatomical structure. Smaller collections of heterotopic neurons, recognizable only on histology, are constant features of tuberous sclerosis. Barth has reviewed rare clinical syndromes associated with neuronal migration defects, and discussed the known chromosomal and environmental causes (Barth 1987). Yachnis et al. (1994) have reported cerebellar heterotopias to be present in a significant number of otherwise normal fetal brains.

Miscellaneous Malformations

Agenesis of the corpus callosum (Fig. 4.14) is occasionally seen on its own, as an incidental postmortem finding in a person who was asymptomatic during life, or may occur in combination with other malformations, particularly holoprosencephaly. The defect in the corpus callosum probably results from failure of development of the early interhemispheric glial fibre connections that guide axonal migration across the midline into the opposite hemisphere. Because the axons are unable to cross the midline, they become arranged in abnormal longitudinal "callosal bundles", running parallel with the interhemispheric fissure, which can be detected in life by MRI (Barkovich 1990, 1992b). The defect in the corpus callosum may be partial or complete; however, dilatation of the occipital horns of the lateral ventricles is always present (Friede 1989). If there is any doubt about whether the corpus callosum has formed (for example, in a soft brain), the presence or absence of the cingulate gyrus is helpful, as it is always formed if the corpus callosum is formed.

The *Dandy–Walker malformation*, like agenesis of the corpus callosum, may occur in isolation or in association with a large number of other developmental anomalies of the CNS. The essence of this malformation is absence, or partial absence, of the cerebellar vermis with enormous cyst-like dilatation of the fourth ventricle, enlargement of the posterior cranial fossa, and hydrocephalus. The origin is thought to be an insult to the alar plate, as a result of which the choroid plexus in the roof of the fourth ventricle fails to develop properly, leaving a membranous structure (the area membranacea superior) which balloons progressively to form a thin-walled cyst (Altman et al. 1992). There are a number of variants of the Dandy–Walker anomaly, which are discussed in detail by Norman and Ludwin (1991). Associated systemic malformations in a series of 28 cases reported by Hart et al. (1972) included polydactylism–syndactylism, cleft palate, Klippel–Feil syndrome, Cornelia de Lange syndrome, and the presence of a sixth lumbar vertebra.

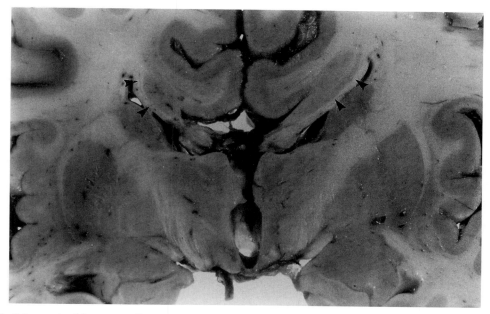

Fig. 4.14. Partial agenesis of the corpus callosum. Abnormal longitudinal white matter bundles, which form in place of the corpus callosum, are indicated by the arrowheads.

Microencephaly, in which the brain is abnormally small, occurs as a secondary phenomenon with a number of cerebral malformations. Primary microencephaly (i.e. without malformations) may have distinct genetic and environmental associations. It may be familial, with cerebral hypoplasia as an isolated finding, or occur as one feature of a non-chromosomal dysgenetic syndrome (listed in detail by Friede 1989), or follow exposure to a number of environmental agents in utero, including irradiation, alcohol (as part of the fetal alcohol syndrome) and infections. Very often there is neither a history of familial microencephaly nor an identifiable cause. Because the growth of the cranium is so closely linked to growth of the brain, the skull also develops abnormally, giving the microencephalic child an abnormal facies. There is usually severe mental retardation. The hemispheres are always small, particularly in relation to the cerebellum, and the brain may appear immature, with a simplified gyral pattern. Anomalies of neuronal migration can be detected on histology.

Spinal Cord Anomalies

Diastematomyelia is duplication of the spinal cord, usually in association with a bony spur or connective tissue septum in the canal. It is often seen with neural tube defects involving the lower cord, but with modern imaging, particularly MRI, asymptomatic diastematomyelia may be found as an isolated finding. A number of types of diastematomyelia are recognized; variants and terminology are discussed by Hori (1982).

Hydromyelia and *syringomyelia* are terms that are often used synonymously, but they are in fact distinct. In hydromyelia the central canal of the cord becomes cystically dilated. This may be an incidental finding at autopsy in an otherwise normal nervous system, or it may accompany a variety of axial-skeletal dysraphic conditions. Because it is merely a dilated central canal, the hydromyelic cavity is lined by ependyma, in contrast to a syringomyelic cavity, which is found in the substance of the cord and has a wall of densely gliotic tissue. Syringomyelia is the result of a variety of different pathological processes in which the common denominator is tissue destruction, and the term merely denotes longitudinal cavitation of the cervical cord substance. Thus secondary cavitation may occur as a sequela of cord necrosis from any cause, or in association with tumours, particularly spinal cord astrocytomas. Rarely, the medulla is also affected ("syringobulbia"). The pathogenesis of syringomyelia as a congenital anomaly is uncertain, but it is seen with obstruction of the foramen magnum, notably Chiari type 1 malformations. It occasionally occurs in the absence of such obstruction.

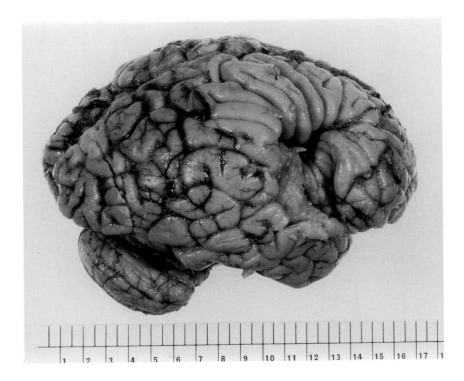

Fig. 4.15. Porencephaly, found at autopsy in a man of 56, who was mentally subnormal and suffered from seizures. The arachnoid has been stripped from around the poros, revealing abnormal gyration with the gyri appearing to radiate into the defect.

Neuropathology of Common Trisomy Syndromes

Neuropathological findings in *Trisomy 21 (Down's syndrome)* are variable. There are no features that are pathognomonic of Down's syndrome on external examination. Most reports describe a brain that is considerably lighter than might be expected for the age, with an abnormal foreshortened shape corresponding to an abnormally shaped skull, and frontal and occipital lobes that are smaller than usual. A number of abnormalities of gyration have been reported, the most usual of which is in the superior temporal gyrus, which is often very markedly angulated and narrowed. A search for microscopic abnormalities is unrewarding: there are no consistent changes in cytoarchitecture of the brain, and children do not demonstrate the neurofibrillary tangles and plaques seen in adults dying of Down's disease.

In *Trisomy 17–18 (Edwards' syndrome)*, the brain may show a number of gross and microscopic abnormalities and, although not all cases in which the brain has been studied report changes, it has been suggested that the yield of lesions is a function of how carefully the brain is examined (Sumi 1970). Reduction in the size of the cerebrum and cerebellum is usual; anomalies of the anterior commissure, hippocampus, pons and inferior olive are among the most common abnormalities described. Cerebral and cerebellar cortical malformations and heterotopias may also be seen, but are more common in trisomy 13–15.

In *Trisomy 13–15 (Patau's syndrome)*, in addition to a large number of somatic abnormalities, the infant shows microencephaly. Holoprosencephaly and arhinencephaly, particularly in association with multiple visceral abnormalities, is relatively common. Neuronal migration defects involving the cerebellum are not uncommon.

Encephaloclastic Lesions

Although resembling malformations, encephaloclastic lesions are in fact the result of brain destruction at different stages of development. In many cases, the original insult is thought to be hypoxic–ischaemic, although there are seldom supporting clinical details, and this assumption is based on the anatomical distribution of lesions, on isolated reports of fetuses surviving documented maternal accidents or infections, and on work in experimental animals. For a full discussion see Friede (1989).

Porencephaly (Fig. 4.15) describes a defect in the cerebrum resulting from hemispheric necrosis in early gestation. This usually corresponds to the terri-

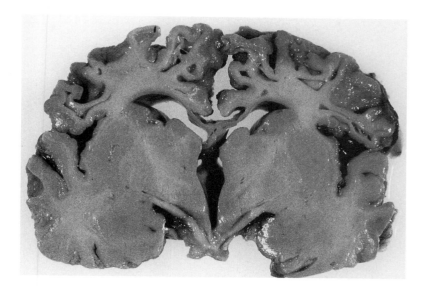

Fig. 4.16. Multicystic encephalopathy in a male who died at the age of 7 months.

tory of the middle cerebral artery, in which a "poros" or hole in the cerebral cortex runs through the white matter to communicate with the ventricles. The defect is often bilateral, although one side may be worse affected than the other. It may be fringed by gyri that appear to radiate out from it in a star shape, and which themselves may show polymicrogyria. The clinical features of porencephaly vary according to the location and extent of the cerebral defect, but commonly include severe mental subnormality and epilepsy.

Essentially, *hydranencephaly* differs from porencephaly only in the extent of the damage produced (Friede and Mikolasek 1978). It is rare and more extensive: a large part of the territory supplied by the internal carotids is destroyed, resulting in dramatically dilated cystic hemispheres with a connective tissue membrane taking the place of destroyed cortex and white matter. Involvement of the corpus striatum and diencephalon varies, but characteristically the posterior fossa contents, particularly the brain stem, are preserved. As a result, the infant survives into postnatal life, but with very severe neurological deficits. The routine use of ultrasound as a prenatal investigation has reduced the frequency of hydranencephaly at term.

Multicystic encephalopathy (Fig. 4.16) results when ischaemic damage occurs late in gestation, often around the time of delivery. As the name suggests, the picture is of multiple cavities in the hemispheres, preferentially involving subcortical white matter and maximal in the territory of the anterior circulation. The pathogenesis of this lesion is clearer, in that there is often a history of twin pregnancy, prolonged labour, or fetal or postpartum respiratory distress. The common denominator is an episode of significant cerebral hypoperfusion. Unlike in porencephaly and hydranencephaly, cavitation in the third trimester excites a mature tissue response and histologically the lesions resemble cystic infarction in older brains.

Hypoxic–ischaemic Brain Damage

Failure of oxygen delivery to the developing brain, whether in utero, during labour or in the immediate postpartum period, results in a spectrum of pathologies, many of which are unique to the immature brain. For a full review of the neuropathology of this complex subject, see Friede (1989), Larroche (1991b) and Rorke (1992a,b). The pathophysiology of perinatal hypoxia-ischaemia is discussed by Greisen (1992), Rorke and Zimmerman (1992), and Vannucci (1992).

Hypoxic–ischaemic brain damage in infants may be either haemorrhagic or ischaemic. *Haemorrhagic* lesions include matrix zone, intraventricular, subarachnoid and subpial haemorrhages. In premature or low birth weight infants, the most common pathology is haemorrhage in the periventricular germinal matrix zone, a collection of neuronal precursor cells situated in the walls of the ventricular system, particularly the lateral ventricles. The germinal matrix lies immediately under the ependymal layer; it is present between about 18 and 34 weeks' gestation and decreases progressively in size as cells migrate to other sites, and as term approaches (Figs. 4.17 and 4.18). It has a characteristic microscopic structure, probably rele-

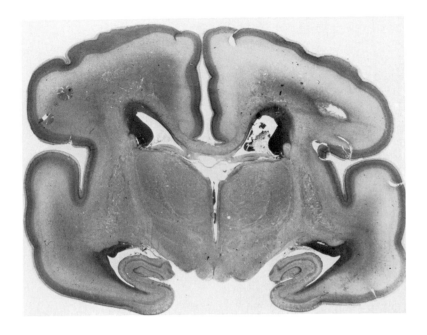

Fig. 4.17. Cross-section of hemispheres at 24 weeks. Note the cellular subependymal germinal matrix region in lateral ventricles and temporal horns.

vant in the production of haemorrhage, in which a network of thin-walled capillaries with very little in the way of connective tissue support runs through a mass of primitive cells. Under adverse conditions such as hypoxia, acidosis, bradycardia, or increases in venous pressure and pCO_2, all of which commonly occur in the premature or low birth weight infant, the capillaries rupture and haemorrhage occurs. The usual site of bleeding is in the germinal matrix near the foramen of Monro; the haemorrhage may track into periventricular white matter, but more commonly ruptures into the ventricles (Fig. 4.19), and extends

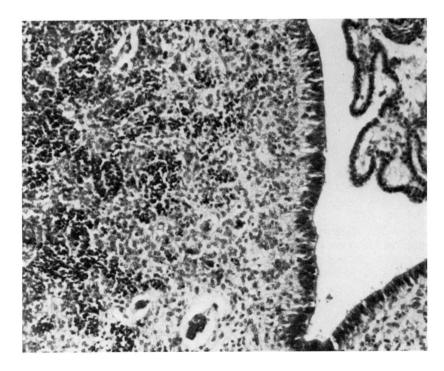

Fig. 4.18. Germinal matrix at 32 weeks. The cells are small neuroblasts, with very little in the way of connective tissue support. (H&E ×100)

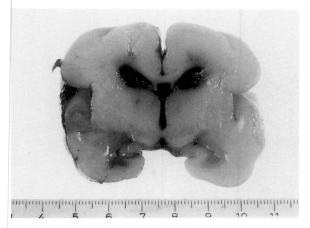

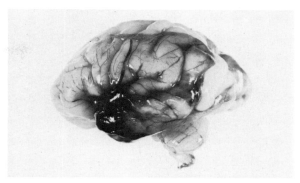

Fig. 4.21. Subarachnoid haematoma over the temporal pole.

Fig. 4.19. Germinal matrix haemorrhage in a fetus born at 26 weeks has ruptured into both lateral ventricles.

through the ventricular system and out from the openings in the roof of the fourth ventricle into the subarachnoid space around the base of the brain. Organization of this haemorrhage is responsible for the obstructive posthaemorrhagic hydrocephalus that is common in survivors of intraventricular haemorrhage. Where the haemorrhage has remained confined to the matrix zone, small haemosiderin-stained periventricular cysts may be the only residua. Rarely, matrix haemorrhage may occur in utero; more commonly it occurs in infants at risk in the first 3 days of postnatal life (see Fig. 4.20). In term infants, the usual source of an intraventricular haemorrhage is not the germinal matrix, which has disappeared by this time, but the choroid plexus: according to Rorke (1992b), cyanotic congenital heart disease is strongly associated with intraventricular haemorrhage at term. Other haemorrhage lesions seen in perinatal asphyxia, but of lesser clinical significance, are subarachnoid haematomas over the lateral temporal lobes (Fig. 4.21) and cerebellar hemispheres, and subpial haematomas, neither of which are seen in adult brains.

A spectrum of ischaemic lesions may also be found in the infant brain. Grey or white matter, either alone or in combination, may be affected; porencephaly, hydranencephaly and multicystic encephalopathy, all of which involve major interruption to

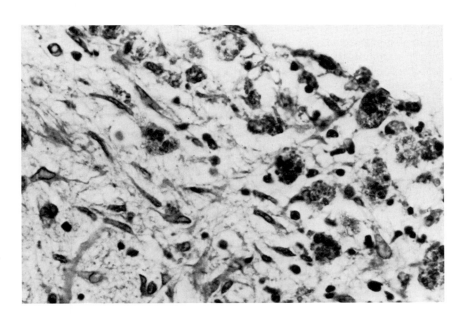

Fig. 4.20. The site of a germinal matrix haemorrhage at 35 days. The haemorrhage has resolved, leaving haemosiderin-laden macrophages.

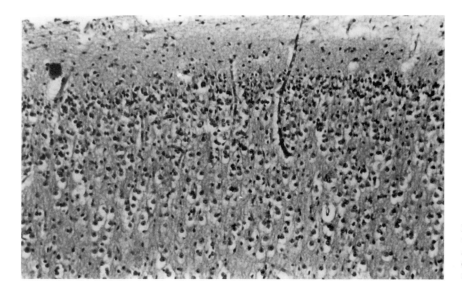

Fig. 4.22. The neocortex at 37 weeks. Most of the neurons appear as round dark nuclei with little cytoplasm: relatively few have a mature phenotype. (H&E ×130)

cerebral perfusion and affect both grey and white matter, have been discussed above. As a general rule, in the developing brain the tissues that are most vulnerable to hypoxic–ischaemic damage are mature neurons and white matter. Neurons throughout the brain vary widely in the rate at which they mature, both morphologically and in terms of function. Cranial nerve nuclei, for example, are fully developed by the second half of gestation, while most of the cortical neurons are morphologically still neuroblasts until late in gestation. In infants of less than 2000 g, most of the neuronal population in the cortex still looks immature (Fig. 4.22), more like oligodendrocytes than neurons, consisting as they do of small round nuclei without a nucleolus or detectable cytoplasm. This variable rate of neuronal maturation largely explains the anatomical patterns of grey matter involvement that are characteristic of hypoxia–ischaemia in infants, and in particular the relative resistance of the infant neocortex to damage. White matter vulnerability results from a number of factors: the relatively high metabolic rate associated with myelination and the fact that, when cerebral perfusion drops, the deep white matter is furthest from the heart and so constitutes the terminal field of supply of the penetrating arteries, which are themselves end-arteries. Failure of autoregulation, which is common is premature infants, aggravates the situation further (see Rorke 1992b).

Hypoxic–ischaemic damage to grey matter in infants may have several patterns, focal or diffuse. Immature neocortical neurons are relatively resistant to hypoxia and the characteristic lesions involve brain stem and cerebellar neuronal groups or the thalamus

and basal ganglia. Both types of injury are unique to the immature brain. However, grey matter injury may be identical to that seen in the mature brain, and lesions such as laminar cortical necrosis, and infarction in boundary zones or in the distribution of a major cerebral artery are not uncommon, particularly in term infants. The term "ulegyria" is a descriptive term, used of the appearance produced when ischaemic cortical damage is maximal in the sulci, resulting in a characteristic pattern of scarring that gives a mushroom-shaped appearance to the gyri. Rarely, the classic patterns of damage to grey matter known as "status marmoratus" is seen: the term describes an unusual but characteristic chalky white appearance of the thalamus and other deep grey structures affected by chronic hypoxia, caused by abnormal myelination of the scarred nuclei. More commonly, neurons in the nuclei of the base of the pons or in brain stem cranial nerve nuclei may show selective necrosis, manifest by nuclear karyorrhexis (Fig. 4.23).

White matter necrosis in the infant has been given a number of names: *periventricular leucomalacia* is the most usual. It describes ischaemic injury to hemispheric white matter (Figs. 4.24–4.26), which may range from frank infarction to diffuse white matter gliosis and disturbance in myelination resulting from partial ischaemic damage. Periventricular leucomalacia is seen in infants of all weights and gestational ages, but is most common in low birth weight, premature infants. The lesions are often bilateral, although not necessarily symmetrical. The damage tends to be maximal around the lateral ventricles, and extends out from the periventricular region, often as

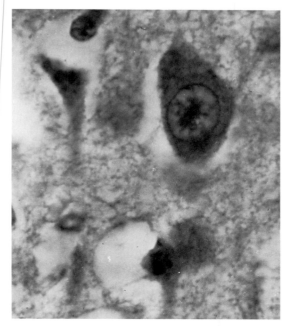

Fig. 4.23. Karyorrhexis of pontine neuronal nuclei in a full-term infant dying at 4 days with hypoxia from congenital heart disease. (H&E, ×1000)

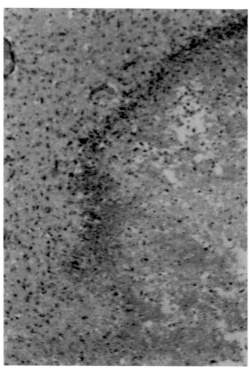

Fig. 4.25. Periventricular leucomalacia: the edge of a necrotic area is well demarcated by a PAS stain. (×350)

far as subcortical white matter. Recent lesions are poorly defined in comparison with surrounding white matter; they are usually slightly discoloured and show characteristic chalky white speckling.

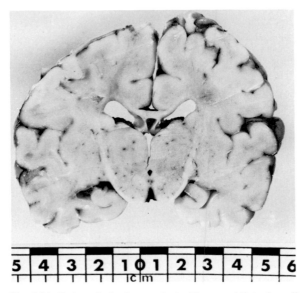

Fig. 4.24. Periventricular leucomalacia. There are bilateral small areas of granular discolouration in the white matter, above and lateral to the angles of the ventricles.

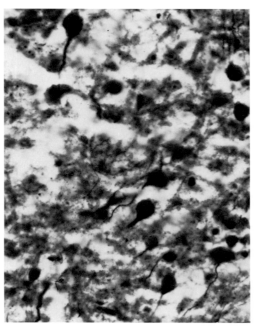

Fig. 4.26. Axonal swellings, here seen round the edge of a focus of periventricular leucomalacia, are a non-specific sign of axonal damage. (Glees, ×400)

Secondary haemorrhage into the lesions may occur, giving the appearance of extensive subependymal haemorrhage. Histologically the changes of periventricular leucomalacia are not very striking: the affected region shows coagulation necrosis, with oedema of the white matter and nuclear pyknosis. A periodic acid–Schiff (PAS) stain delineates the edges of the necrotic zones well. Older lesions become cystic, and are gliotic on microscopy. Larroche, who has made an extensive study of periventricular leucomalacia, reports a significant increase in this condition at autopsy in high-risk infants, attributing it to improved management of small low birth weight infants (Larroche 1991b).

Cerebral Palsy

The term cerebral palsy is applied to congenital nonprogressive neurological disability, resulting from damage to the immature brain. There is a large number of possible underlying aetiologies. Little's early work was instrumental in associating cerebral palsy with perinatal asphyxia (Little 1862), and the belief has persisted that intrapartum anoxic damage is the primary cause of cerebral palsy. Recent work suggests that perinatal factors may be less significant, and *intrauterine* brain injury more important in the aetiology than has been hitherto recognized (Younkin 1992). Magnetic resonance imaging, which enables the anatomical substrates of cerebral palsy to be visualized, has been effectively employed by Truwit and his colleagues, who investigated 40 patients with a clinical diagnosis of cerebral palsy. The principal advantage of this form of neuroimaging lies in the anatomical details revealed, and hence in its ability to demonstrate cortical anomalies, heterotopias, and subtle disease in white matter, as well as large lesions. In the infants who were born prematurely, periventricular leucomalacia was the most common finding in Truwit's series; among children born at term, a wider spectrum of neuropathology was seen, including a high proportion of neuronal migration abnormalities suggesting mid-trimester injury, with perinatal anoxic damage present in only 24% (Truwit et al. 1992).

Table 4.2 Principal causes of hydrocephalus in children

Site of obstruction	Pathology
Extraventricular	
Basal subarachnoid space	Postinflammatory or posthaemorrhagic fibrosis
	Chiari type 2 malformation
	Lissencephaly
	Skull deformities, e.g. achondroplasia, craniosynostosis, Hurler syndrome
Arachnoid granulations	Postinflammatory fibrosis
	Posthaemorrhagic fibrosis
	Superior sagittal sinus thrombosis
	Venous sinus anomalies
	Diffuse spread of tumour, e.g. medulloblastoma
Intraventricular	
Lateral ventricles	Adhesions following ventriculitis
	Obstruction by glioma
Foramen of Monro	Adhesions following ventriculitis
	Ependymoma
	Subependymal giant cell astrocytoma (tuberous sclerosis)
	Teratoma
	Central neurocytoma
Third ventricle	Craniopharyngioma
	Thalamic or hypothalamic glioma
	Pineal tumour
	Vein of Galen aneurysm
Aqueduct	Atresia or stenosis with or without Chiari type 2 malformation
	Tumours of the midbrain
	Postinflammatory gliosis
Fourth ventricle foramina	Dandy–Walker syndrome
	Chiari type 2 malformation
	Postinflammatory gliosis or fibrosis
	Posthaemorrhagic gliosis or fibrosis

Hydrocephalus

Hydrocephalus is defined as dilatation of the ventricular system resulting from absolute or relative overproduction of cerebrospinal fluid (CSF) and, with the rare exception of overproduction of CSF by a choroid plexus papilloma, is always the result of obstruction to the flow of CSF. This may occur at any part of the circulation, from choroid plexus to arachnoid granulations, and some of the most important causes in children are given in Table 4.2. Congenital or infantile hydrocephalus may have a number of causes, of which the most usual are sequelae of haemorrhage (particularly intraventricular haemorrhage) or infection, Chiari type 2 malformation, aqueduct stenosis or atresia, and Dandy–Walker syndrome (Figs. 4.27–4.31). The effects of hydrocephalus are the same, regardless of cause. If the skull sutures are still open, the head expands as a result of progressive enlargement of the ventricles. As the ventricles get bigger, the ependymal lining stretches, and ultimately becomes disrupted; fluid then collects in periventricular white matter. Irreversible tissue damage probably begins during this acute stage of white matter oedema, for, if hydrocephalus is untreated, axonal fragmentation, secondary loss of myelin and cortical damage rapidly occur (Weller and Shulman 1972), as intracranial pressure rises. Distortion and compression of blood vessels by oedema impedes cerebral blood flow, which can be demonstrated by Doppler flow studies. With time, extensive white matter loss and gliosis are seen, the cerebral cortex becomes pro-

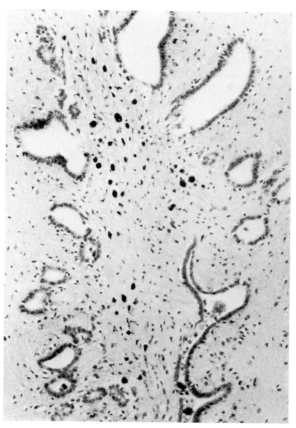

Fig. 4.28. Gliosis of the aqueduct following intraventricular bleeding in fetal life in a case of congenital thrombocytopenic purpura. (PAS, ×100)

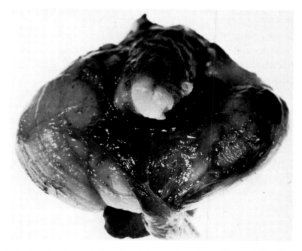

Fig. 4.27. Pigmented and thickened basal meninges following extension of an intraventricular haemorrhage into the basal cisterns. Posthaemorrhagic hydrocephalus is common in such cases (see Fig. 4.29).

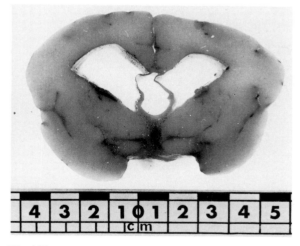

Fig. 4.29. Hydrocephalus following germinal matrix haemorrhage. Residual haematoma is present in the walls of the lateral ventricles.

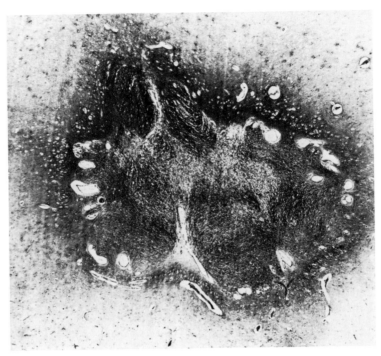

Fig. 4.30. Gliosis of the aqueduct. (Holzer, ×40)

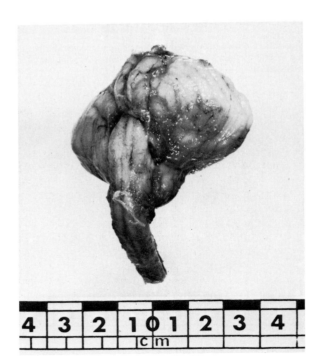

Fig. 4.31. Chiari type 2 malformation. The medulla is elongated and the cerebellar tonsils have been moulded posteriorly by the foramen magnum.

gressively thinned, and secondary long tract degeneration is detectable in the corticospinal tracts in the brain stem and spinal cord. Permanent functional deficits, which in children means impaired motor and intellectual development, are inevitable if tissue damage occurs as a result of delay in treatment. For a full review of the neuropathology of hydrocephalus, see Friede (1989) and Del Bigio (1993).

Abnormalities of the aqueduct of Sylvius, the narrowest and thus the most vulnerable part of the ventricular system, are a relatively common finding in congenital hydrocephalus and are usually due to either stenosis or atresia. True aqueduct stenosis is characterized by a markedly reduced lumen in which there are no histological features that might suggest an acquired cause. This is not as easy to determine as it sounds, because the size and shape of the aqueduct will vary according to the point at which it is measured and the age of the fetus or infant and because, in experimental situations, viral infection such as mumps may produce aqueduct stenosis without gliotic scarring (Johnson and Johnson 1968; Bruni et al. 1985). In humans, mumps is well recognized as a cause of stenosis, particularly in children (for a review, see Ogata et al. 1992). It is possible that in some cases the boundary between malformative and acquired lesions causing hydrocephalus may not be

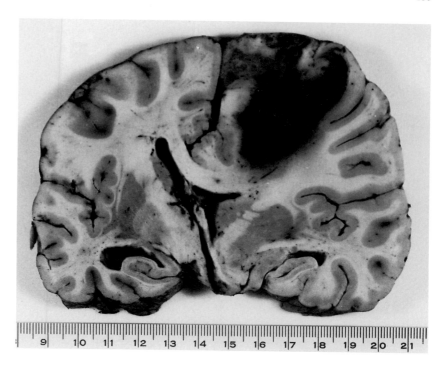

Fig. 4.32. A large haemorrhagic malignant glioma in the frontal white matter of the right hemisphere has produced marked mass effect and shift, both across the midline and downwards, through the tentorial opening.

clearcut. An X-linked form of aqueduct stenosis (Serville et al. 1993) may account for 2% of cases of congenital hydrocephalus (Baraitser 1990). *Atresia* is an anomaly in which the aqueduct lumen is reduplicated: clusters of abnormal small ependymal tubules, some of which may be seen to be blind-ending on serial sections, are present in place of the normal aqueduct. Aqueduct atresia is found in association with the Chiari type 2 malformation, and has also been reported as a sequela of mumps infection; the same is true of obstruction by septum formation.

Raised Intracranial Pressure and Space-occupying Lesions

A rise in systemic blood pressure and vasodilatation of the cerebral arteries and arterioles together normally compensate for any rise in intracranial pressure, but if they fail to do so cerebral perfusion pressure and cerebral blood flow fall, and cerebral hypoxia inevitably follows. A variety of pathological conditions may impede the normal physiological regulation of cerebral blood flow and lead to a rise in intracranial pressure. These include generalized as well as localized processes, and one should not equate the pathology of raised intracranial pressure with the pathology of a mass lesion, although the two

often occur together. The most common generalized causes of raised intracranial pressure in children come under the general categories of traumatic, hypoxic–ischaemic, infective, metabolic and toxic, of which hydrocephalus (see earlier) and diffuse cerebral swelling secondary to head injury, cardiac arrest, meningitis, Reye's syndrome and lead encephalopathy are examples; localized causes include space-occupying lesions of all varieties, e.g. (Fig. 4.32).

Diffuse cerebral swelling is almost invariably due to cerebral oedema (Fig. 4.33) and rarely to expansion of the cerebral blood volume – with the exception of diffuse post-traumatic brain swelling, which is common in children and believed to be of vascular origin (Adams 1992). Cerebral oedema, defined as increase in the brain water content, becomes of significance when it is sufficiently severe to cause ischaemia or brain distortion. It is described as vasogenic, cytotoxic or interstitial, according to the pathogenesis of fluid accumulation. In *vasogenic* oedema, there is an increase in extracellular fluid volume resulting from increased permeability of the brain capillaries, demonstrated by leakage of contrast ("contrast enhancement") on computed tomography (CT) scans. This is seen in association with tumours, infarction, haemorrhage and inflammatory lesions, and is the most common type of oedema, affecting principally white matter. *Cytotoxic* oedema characteristically affects both grey and white matter. It results from cytoplasmic swelling of neurons, glia and

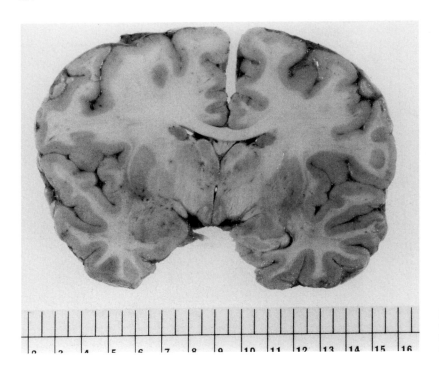

Fig. 4.33. Diffuse cerebral oedema, causing bilateral swelling with compression of the lateral ventricles, in a 14-year-old boy with meningitis.

endothelial cells, and is a particular feature of conditions such as hypoxia–ischaemia and pyogenic meningitis. Hypoxia–ischaemia leads to energy failure and accumulation of intracellular sodium and water, whereas in meningitis diffusion of bacterial cell wall products into the brain produces the same result through a direct toxic action on neuroglial cells. Finally, *interstitial* oedema is accumulation of CSF in the perventricular white matter, as a result of reabsorption of CSF across the ependyma into the neuropil, which occurs in obstructive hydrocephalus.

Many types of cerebral pathology may act as expanding or mass lesions, not only tumours, but also inflammatory foci, haemorrhages, recent infarcts and localized oedema. Significant spatial compensation is possible either if the lesion is benign and expands slowly enough to cause pressure atrophy of adjacent structures or if the fontanelles and cranial sutures are still open, so that the skull can enlarge. In such cases a longer time may elapse before symptoms occur. Once the sutures have fused, however, the cranium is converted into a rigid box divided by folds of dura, the falx and the tentorium cerebelli, into compartments, in which there is very little room for expansion. The cranial cavity contains brain, blood and CSF: brain tissue is effectively incompressible, and the intracranial blood volume relatively small – in a child there is only a small potential reserve to be gained from displacement of CSF from the cranial cavity, after which intracranial pressure starts to rise.

If the lesion is supratentorial, the sequence of events is fairly stereotyped, and unrelated to the nature of the pathological lesion. An expanding mass in one hemisphere gives rise to clinical signs reflecting the anatomical site of the lesion, and causes that hemisphere to swell. The gyri become pressed against the undersurface of the cranial vault, so that at autopsy the dura appears tense and the convexities swollen and flattened. The lateral ventricle on the side of the lesion becomes compressed, and dilatation of the other lateral ventricle may occur as a result of shift of CSF. Pressure on the optic nerve sheath at the base of the brain results in swelling of the optic nerve head, detectable as papilloedema. Pronounced shift of the midline occurs away from the affected side.

These intrinsic compensatory mechanisms exhausted, the expanding hemisphere begins to move out of its compartment, herniating both under the falx and over the edge of the tentorium cerebelli. The cingulate gyrus herniates under the free border of the falx just above the corpus callosum, and may develop a small area of pressure necrosis through being impacted against the falx. Clinically more significant, however, is the herniation of medial temporal lobe structures through the tentorial opening (Fig. 4.34). The uncus (anteriorly) and/or the parahippocampal gyrus (posteriorly) move down through the tentorium, and become deeply grooved by its free margin. Once again, cortical necrosis in the herniating temporal lobe may result from direct compression against

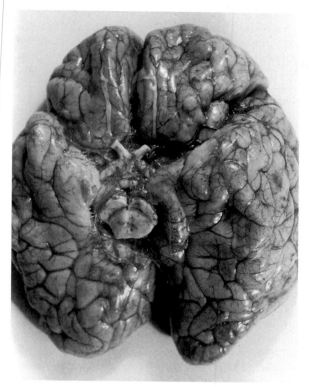

Fig. 4.34. An unfixed brain, photographed at autopsy. The left hemisphere contained an abscess, and was swollen. There is a longitudinal groove on the left medial temporal lobe, caused by herniation through the tentorium cerebelli.

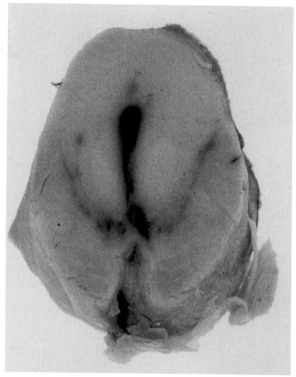

Fig. 4.35. Midline haemorrhage in the midbrain, secondary to a supratentorial mass lesion.

the tentorial edge. It is worth noting that such a focus of medial temporal cortical necrosis, found in a brain that is not swollen at autopsy, may provide useful evidence of a previous episode of raised intracranial pressure.

The movement of the medial temporal lobe through the tentorial opening occurs in a fairly stereotyped sequence. The ipsilateral III nerve is pushed against the medial petroclinoid ligament; this compression preferentially affects the parasympathetic fibres, causing the pupil on that side to dilate. The posterior cerebral artery, lying above the nerve, is also compressed, causing infarction in the inferior temporal and inferomedial occipital cortex, producing a homonymous hemianopia. Downward traction on the abducens nerve by the displaced temporal lobe may additionally produce a VI nerve palsy. Herniation of the temporal lobe through the tentorium also causes the brain stem to be pushed sideways, with the result that the contralateral peduncle becomes pressed against the tentorium. The anterior part of the peduncle contains the corticospinal tracts, damage to which results in an *ipsilateral* hemiplegia (because the corticospinal tracts decussate lower

down in the medulla). With sideways movement of the midbrain, the III nerve and the artery on the other side will become involved, and both pupils eventually become fixed as well as dilated. Diffuse cerebral swelling differs from unilateral swelling only in that there is downward movement of midline structures, principally the diencephalon, through the tentorium, a situation known as central herniation. The ultimate effects on the brain stem are the same as those of a localized supratentorial lesion.

Pressure on the midbrain is responsible for the development of coma; vascular lesions (haemorrhage or infarction) (Fig. 4.35) in the brain stem, resulting from this downward movement, cause death, in combination with rising intracranial pressure. Effacement of the subarachnoid space around the midbrain and lateral flattening of the aqueduct obstruct CSF circulation, and contribute to the rise in intracranial pressure. Although compression of the brain stem by herniation of cerebellar tonsils through the foramen magnum is often described as following transtentorial herniation, in practice true cerebellar tonsillar "coning" is uncommon with a supratentorial lesion, as the combination of rising intracranial pressure and

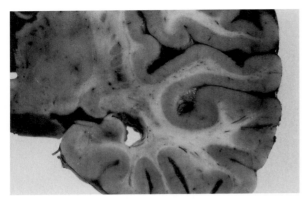

Fig. 4.36. Ammon's horn sclerosis in longstanding epilepsy. The hippocampus is shrunken, causing the temporal horn of the lateral ventricle to dilate.

high brain stem damage is generally sufficient to cause death before this can occur.

Expanding posterior fossa masses may cause direct involvement of cranial nerve nuclei or specific tracts, which means that the site of the lesion can often be diagnosed in life. Some upward movement in the cerebellum may occur into the supratentorial compartment, but more commonly the tonsils become impacted in the foramen magnum and compress the medulla, causing cardiorespiratory arrest. The cerebellar tonsils are moulded by the foramen, and are usually necrotic. The relatively unimpaired conscious level seen in patients with posterior fossa lesions contrasts with the progressive coma accompanied by focal neurological signs typical of the supratentorial mass lesions.

Epilepsy

Epileptic seizures, caused by abnormal electrical discharges from groups of cerebral neurons, are particularly common in children in the first decade. There are many potential underlying causes, but in a high proportion of cases no underlying pathology can be found (Dulac 1994). In the neonate, metabolic disturbances and hypoxic–ischaemic brain damage are common, although serious cerebral malformations may also be responsible. Similar pathologies, particularly brain scarring as a sequela of infection, hypoxia or trauma, may cause infantile seizures; to these may be added inherited metabolic conditions and neurocutaneous syndromes, which tend to present early in childhood. The neuropathological findings in infan-

tile epilepsy have been reviewed by Jellinger (1987). As a generalization, disorders of neuronal migration, including pachygyria, polymicrogyria, neuronal heterotopias and the cortical "tubers" of tuberous sclerosis, probably account for a large proportion of cases of childhood epilepsy, and they can now be seen and diagnosed by MRI. A variety of other focal lesions may on occasion cause seizures: of the neoplasms, slow-growing tumours such gangliogliomas, dysembryoplastic neuroepithelial tumours, pleomorphic xanthoastrocytomas, oligodendrogliomas and pilocytic astrocytomas are all common (Wolf et al. 1993), while glioneuronal hamartomas, abscesses, malignant tumours and vascular malformations may also be responsible. Diffuse lesions associated with fits include infections – encephalitis, meningitis – and a number of biochemical and metabolic disorders, particularly the aminoacidurias. Classic Ammon's horn sclerosis (Figs. 4.36 and 4.37), in which the hippocampus is atrophic and shows segmental neuronal loss and astrocytosis in vulnerable neuronal populations, is common in patients with temporal lobe epilepsy, particularly where there has been a history of febrile seizures in infancy. It was the sole finding in 49% of 249 resected temporal lobes studied by Bruton (1988) and present in association with a second pathology in a further 6%. The hippocampal regions invariably affected are the CA1 (Sommer sector) and CA4 (end folium) segments of the pyramidal cell layer, and to a lesser extent the granule cells of the dentate fascia, all of which display marked cell loss and gliosis. Electroencephalography and electrocorticography show that, when present, Ammon's horn sclerosis is the cause, not the result, of temporal lobe seizures. The pathogenesis of the original lesion is uncertain; the subject is reviewed by Armstrong (1993). Finally, status epilepticus is a more usual complication of epilepsy in children than in adults, and carries a high risk of cerebral damage, and so of residual morbidity.

Lead Poisoning

Lead poisoning results from prolonged or repeated exposure to inorganic lead compounds. The incidence of the condition, which is more common in children, has fallen with the elimination of many former environmental and domestic sources of lead, and the diagnosis is less often made. However, Parry (1991) has drawn attention to the eye cosmetics "surma" and "kohl", which are used widely in Asia, Africa and the Middle East, and which may contain high amounts of lead. According to Brett (1991), in the UK it has been

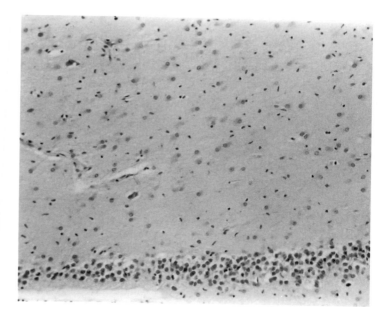

Fig. 4.37. A low-power view of the CA4 region (end folium) of the hippocampus in a case of Ammon's horn sclerosis. The line of dark cells at the bottom is the dentate fascia. Above it there are no neurons to be seen: all the cells in the field are either astrocytes (with faintly distinguishable smudgy cytoplasm) or microglia (elongated nuclei without cytoplasm). (H&E ×140)

traditional among immigrants from such regions to apply surma to the eyelids of neonates, from where lead may enter the nasolacrimal duct and be swallowed and absorbed, causing lead poisoning. Peripheral neuropathy is the most usual manifestation in the adult population, but children suffering from lead toxicity develop an acute encephalopathy (Fig. 4.38), the symptoms of which are varied and non-specific, and include anorexia, vomiting, apathy and seizures. There may be a progressive decline in con-

scious level to coma, accompanied by signs of rising intracranial pressure, and eventually death. The principal findings at autopsy are diffuse brain swelling with transtentorial herniation of the medial temporal lobes and sometimes of the cerebellar tonsils. The brain contains multiple petechial haemorrhages, and vascular damage of various types is the most striking microscopical abnormality (Jacobs and Le Quesne 1992).

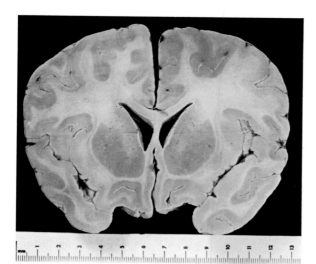

Fig. 4.38. Acute lead encephalopathy. The brain is swollen, the sulci are narrowed and the lateral ventricles compressed. Multiple petechial haemorrhages, not seen in this case, are very common.

Inherited Metabolic Disease

Neurometabolic diseases are individually rare, but together form a group of conditions that are important causes of mental retardation or progressive neurological deterioration. The biochemistry and mode of inheritance of many of the conditions is established, and for these prenatal diagnosis and genetic counselling is now possible. Many of the metabolic disorders affecting the CNS are caused by enzyme defects, which result in accumulation of undigested by-products of metabolism, causing dysfunction and eventually death of the cell. The clinical effects of the biochemical deficiency depend on the cell type involved, and also in some cases on the degree of maturation of the brain. When neurons are principally affected, grey matter disease results (neuronal storage diseases, or *poliodystrophies*), whereas involvement of glia, particularly oligodendroglia, causes white matter pathology, particularly myelin loss, and is characteristic of the *leucodystrophies*.

The classification of inherited metabolic diseases is complex. For comprehensive discussion of the neuropathology and biochemistry, the accounts by Becker and Yates (1990) and Lake (1992) and the reviews edited by Scriver et al. (1989) are recommended. For a non-specialist, it is easiest to approach these conditions from a morphological standpoint – that is, whether they affect primarily grey matter, primarily white matter, or grey and white matter combined. The anatomical distribution dictates the clinical presentation: to generalize, the neuronal storage diseases characteristically produce seizures, mental retardation, myoclonus and retinal lesions, whereas ataxia and major tract signs (pyramidal and sensory tracts, visual and peripheral nerve involvement) are characteristic of a leucodystrophy. In practice, however, the distinction is not always clear cut, especially when both grey and white matter are affected. The clinical picture is more complex in neonates and infants, where any one of a number of non-specific signs, such as feeding difficulties, failure to thrive, seizures or psychomotor retardation, may be the presenting features of an inherited metabolic condition, usually following a period of apparently normal health. A practical point to remember when approaching an autopsy in which there is a possibility of a metabolic disorder is that a piece of the fresh brain (e.g. frontal lobe tip) should be frozen with samples of other tissues in case biochemical studies are found to be necessary later.

Metabolic Diseases Affecting Grey Matter: Neuronal Storage Diseases

Accumulation of by-products of metabolism within lysosomes causes the neuronal cytoplasm to swell; in many of the storage disorders, the neurons are very obviously enlarged, with the nucleus pushed to the periphery of the cell, and cytoplasm that stains with the appropriate techniques (which may include frozen sections) for the stored compounds (see Lake 1992). Sometimes the cells containing the stored material may no longer resemble neurons, and in the endstages of storage diseases there may be few surviving neurons to be seen. When the neurons dies, the ensuing axonal deterioration causes secondary myelin loss, with the result that both the cortex and the white matter become progressively atrophic. On occasion, secondary degeneration and astrocytosis of the white matter may look confusingly like a primary white matter disease, but it is important to realize that the white matter changes are generally secondary to neuronal death, and do not represent primary demyelination.

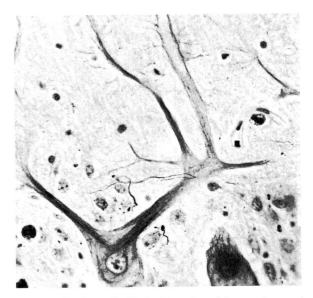

Fig. 4.39. GM-2 gangliosidosis. Distension of the cytoplasm and processes of Purkinje cells of the cerebellar cortex by stored ganglioside. (Glees, ×200)

The majority of the *lipidoses* that affect the central nervous system have their principal effect on neurons, the two exceptions being metachromatic and Krabbe leucodystrophies (discussed below). Each of the neuronal storage diseases has different subtypes, depending on age of onset, organ involved and type of enzyme deficiency, as discussed in detail by Lake, who also describes the staining reactions and ultrastructural appearances of the various stored compounds (Lake 1992). *GM2-gangliosidosis* (Fig. 4.39), which includes the infantile form Tay–Sachs disease, is closely related to *GM1-gangliosidosis*. In both conditions there is a defect in the breakdown of sphingolipids and, as a result, gangliosides accumulate in the central nervous system. This accumulation causes an increase in the volume of cerebral tissue and gives a firm rubbery consistency to the brain, which is often heavier than normal. Histological sections may show reduction in the number of neurons with astrocytosis, which invariably accompanies nerve cells loss in the CNS. Residual neurons and glia have swollen foamy cytoplasm with a nucleus pushed to the periphery of the cell. As in many of the neuronal storage diseases, the white matter shows secondary changes, and there is usually a marked loss of myelinated axons and astrocytosis in the white matter of the cerebral hemispheres and cerebellum. White matter degeneration is to be expected following neuronal loss, but it appears that other mechanisms, particularly storage of gangliosides in the white matter, may also be responsible for myelin breakdown. Some

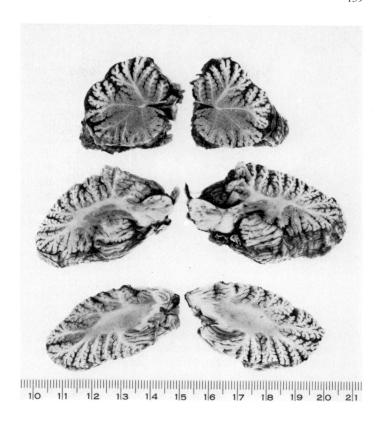

Fig. 4.40. Batten's disease. Atrophic folia of the cerebellar cortex.

of the variants of *Niemann–Pick disease* involve the nervous system, and the pathology is similar to that in the gangliosidoses, with an atrophic brain being found at autopsy. Histologically, the changes are also very similar, with similar anatomical distribution, and a distinction cannot be made between the two groups of diseases on morphological grounds, despite the fact that white matter changes are invariably more marked in Niemann–Pick disease, particularly type A. Neuropathological findings in the neuronopathic form of *Gaucher's disease* are much less marked. The brain may appear normal, and ballooned neurons containing stored material are not seen. Characteristic Gaucher cells – large, rounded, containing fibrillar material in their cytoplasm, and identical to those seen in the spleen and other organs – may sometimes be identified clustered around vessels in the brain. Although there is no obvious storage in neurons, marked neuronal loss in cortex and deep grey nuclei is a feature of CNS involvement in Gaucher's disease, although the distribution is variable.

Batten's disease, or *neuronal ceroid-lipofuscinosis*, is a group of related diseases in which lipopigments accumulate in many tissues of the body, particularly the brain. In late infantile, juvenile and early-juvenile Batten's disease the stored substance is a proteolipid,

but the exact composition of the material in the infantile form is not known, and the underlying defects have not yet been worked out. As in other storage diseases, the brain is firm, and atrophic when disease is longstanding (Fig. 4.40). The histological features are similar to those of the lipidoses, in that there is widespread intracytoplasmic accumulation of lipofuscin-like material in neurons and glial cells. With time, neurons cease to function and are lost, particularly in the cerebral cortex, to be replaced by proliferating astrocytes. Secondary white matter loss occurs, and the white matter is gliotic. A recent review of Batten's disease is given by Rapola (1993).

The *mucopolysaccharidoses* are a group of diseases in which there are deficiencies of enzymes involved in the breakdown of glycosaminoglycans. The resultant accumulation of mucopolysaccharides in the cell cytoplasm further impairs lysosomal function, so that other compounds, such as gangliosides, are also stored in excess. A number of distinct syndromes are recognized (Hurler, Scheie, Hunter, Sanfilippo, Morquio, Maroteaux-Lamy and Sly), each of which has a slightly different phenotype. All of them have a chronic clinical course with multisystem involvement, neurological complications being among the most serious. Mucopolysaccharide deposits in the dura and

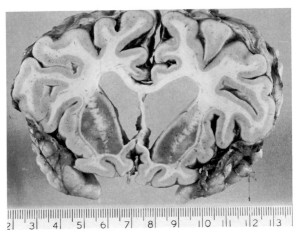

Fig. 4.41. Sanfilippo syndrome (mucopolysaccharidosis III), showing hydrocephalus secondary to leptomeningeal fibrosis.

leptomeninges, both of which can often be markedly thickened, may obstruct the flow of CSF and cause hydrocephalus (Fig. 4.41), and radiculomyelopathies resulting from involvement of nerve roots and/or spinal cord compression by meningeal deposits are not uncommon. The principal effects, however, result from storage of glycosaminoglycans in neurons of the cerebral cortex and deep grey nuclei, which causes profound mental retardation, especially in Hurler, Hunter and Sanfilippo syndromes. The characteristic feature of Morquio syndrome is that there are skeletal anomalies, particularly involving the craniospinal junction and cervical vertebrae, which commonly cause chronic cervical myelopathy, and may result in atlantoaxial instability.

The *mucolipidoses* are rare diseases, the different types now being designated by numbers, which have features resembling both the lipidoses and the mucopolysaccharidoses, but are distinct from them biochemically (see Lake 1992 for details). Most of the *glycogenoses* affect skeletal muscle and liver – less commonly, heart; only the generalized glycogenosis type II (Pompe's disease) in infants or young children also affects the CNS. Astrocytes, ependymal cells, choroid plexus and some neuronal groups all exhibit glycogen accumulation in lysosomes.

Metabolic Diseases Affecting White Matter: Leucodystrophies

The principal metabolic diseases affecting the white matter are the *leucodystrophies*, a heterogeneous group of genetic myelin disorders, in which there is failure either to synthesize or to maintain normal mature myelin. Conventionally, these hereditary (*dys-myelinating*) conditions have been distinguished from acquired non-metabolic *demyelinating* diseases such as multiple sclerosis, but in practice for a pathologist the distinction between dysmyelination and demyelination is not always clear cut, as in practical terms the end result of the leucodystrophies is demyelination – that is, myelin loss with relative axonal preservation. On morphological grounds, the principal difference between the two lies in the anatomical distribution of myelin loss, which in the leucodystrophies tends to be symmetrical in the hemispheres, with remarkably constant sparing of the arcuate or U-fibres that lie immediately under the cortical ribbon, whereas in all the demyelinating diseases myelin loss is asymmetrical and does not spare the U-fibres. Clinically, of course, the two types of disease are entirely distinguishable.

Adrenoleucodystrophy (ALD) is an X-linked peroxisomal disorder in which there is variable but severe neurological disease, associated with adrenocortical failure, and abnormal pigmentation of the skin. The underlying defect is in the metabolism of fatty acids, and results in intracellular accumulation of very long chain fatty acids, the effects of which are most marked in the adrenal cortex and the brain (Fig. 4.42). About half the cases have classical juvenile ALD, which presents between the ages of 3 and 10 years. There is, however, considerable phenotypic variation, even between affected members of the same family (Powers 1985; Moser et al. 1987), and symptoms of adrenal failure are not invariable. Disease in young adults is often a less fulminant process in which symptoms attributable to involvement of the spinal cord rather than the brain predominate, in which case it is known as adrenomyeloneuropathy. The very rare neonatal form of ALD involves multiple peroxisomal defects, and is a different disease (see below).

A common reported finding in autopsy series of ALD is that the severity of the brain involvement correlates poorly with clinical features such as length of disease or degree of adrenal insufficiency (Schaumburg et al. 1975). The brain may appear atrophic externally, but on slicing this can be seen to be due to loss of white matter, rather than to cerebral cortical atrophy. Macroscopically the white matter has a ragged slightly shrunken appearance on slicing, rather than the smooth firm consistency seen in a normal brain. The principal histological feature that distinguishes the disease from other leucodystrophies is the presence of a vigorous mononuclear cell infiltrate around vessels, which gives it a superficial resemblance to acute multiple sclerosis. Unlike multiple sclerosis, however, the inflammation is not confined to the active margins of the lesions, but is

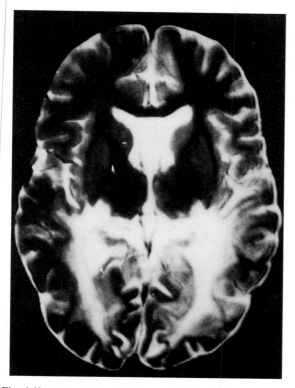

Fig. 4.42. A T$_2$-weighted MRI scan of the brain of a 6-year-old child with X-linked adrenoleucodystrophy shows diffuse abnormality of the posterior white matter which is characteristic of this disease. (Courtesy of Dr W. Taylor, Great Ormond Street Hospital for Sick Children)

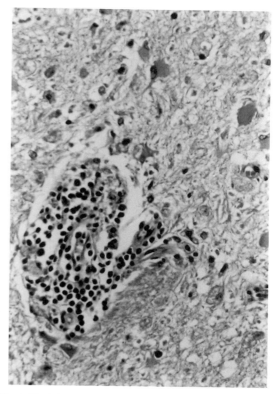

Fig. 4.43. Adrenoleucodystrophy. The hallmark of this disease is pronounced perivascular clustering of lymphocytes and macrophages. Note the reactive astrocytes in the adjacent white matter. (H&E ×280)

present throughout the affected white matter (see Fig. 4.43). PAS-positive macrophages and swollen reactive astrocytes, both of which appear to be involved in phagocytosis of myelin debris and abnormal metabolites, are present in abundance. The macrophages stain positively with Sudan black B, which demonstrates the presence of the lipid degeneration products of myelin. Ultrastructurally, distinctive cytoplasmic inclusions can be identified in brain, adrenals and other tissues (Schaumburg et al. 1975; Takeda et al. 1989).

The mechanism of myelin loss, which in ALD is a form of demyelination, is not understood. It is known that very long chain fatty acids are toxic to cells, but affected tissues outside the CNS do not show the florid inflammatory response seen in the brain. Recent work on the inflammatory component of this disease suggests that there are possibly two stages in the production of the white matter pathology: that the myelin sheath is intrinsically unstable because of accumulation of very long chain fatty acids, and so undergoes spontaneous myelinolysis, and that a process of cytokine-mediated demyelination stimulated by astrocytes and microglial cells follows the liberation of the myelin components (Powers et al. 1992).

It seems likely that the majority of cases described in the literature as "Schilder's disease" were in fact cases of ALD, although it has been suggested that in some the pathology may have been either confluent multiple sclerosis or the predominantly white matter form of subacute sclerosing panencephalitis (SSPE) (Allen and Kirk 1992). Because of the uncertainty about what Schilder originally described, the term has been abandoned (Friede 1989).

Metachromatic leucodystrophy (Fig. 4.44) results from a lysosomal enzyme deficiency that causes accumulation of ceramide sulphatide, a lipid metabolite of myelin breakdown, in cells in many parts of the body, including some neurons (but not those of cerebral cortex). For that reason it could be classed as a lipid storage condition. However, the effects on oligodendroglia are responsible for the clinical features, and it is generally grouped with the white matter diseases.

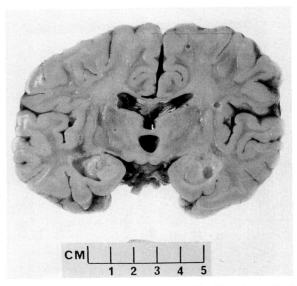

Fig. 4.44. Metachromatic leucodystrophy, involving almost all of the central white matter, which has a shrunken appearance compared with the cortex.

Myelin loss in the cerebral and cerebellar white matter is constant, accompanied by reactive astrocytosis and numerous PAS-positive macrophages. The distinguishing feature, however, is the presence of granular metachromatic deposits in the white matter, both in macrophages and in astrocytes, which can be demonstrated in frozen or cryostat sections, and which are destroyed by routine processing. Because storage of sulphatides also affects the kidneys, the diagnosis may be suspected from the finding of metachromatic granules in urine. As with most leucodystrophies, there are different clinical forms of the disease, with different ages of onset. In *Krabbe disease*, or globoid cell leucodystrophy (Fig. 4.45), the biochemical defect results in accumulation of galactocerebrosides and a toxic related compound psychosine in oligodendroglia, which are progressively destroyed. It is typically a disease of infants. Although the pattern of involvement by the disease is similar to that of other leucodystrophies, Krabbe leucodystrophy differs from them histologically by the presence of pathognomonic globoid cells, multinucleate rounded cells with faintly granular PAS-positive cytoplasm, sitting in clusters in demyelinated white matter. The globoid cells derive from macrophages, and probably represent a specific reaction to the release of large amounts of galactocerebrosides from myelin breakdown (Lake 1992). Fine calcification of the deep grey nuclei may also be seen in Krabbe disease, and may be detectable on a CT scan. In the X-linked condition *Pelizaeus–Merzbacher disease*, one of the constituent proteins of myelin is deficient, causing premature death of oligodendrocytes. Histologically, the pathognomonic feature is a curious pattern in which islands of preserved myelin are to be found, often situated around vessels, in the middle of areas of myelin loss. Despite such disease-specific morphological features, however, in the endstages of any leucodystrophy all that may be left is severe cerebral and cerebellar myelin loss, rarification of axons, dense fibrillary gliosis and small groups of perivascular macrophages.

A number of leucodystrophies are clinically and pathologically well defined, but the relevant biochemical defect has not been identified. These include

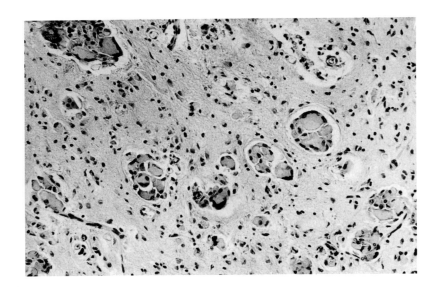

Fig. 4.45. Krabbe disease. Clusters of characteristic multinucleate "globoid" cells in demyelinated white matter.

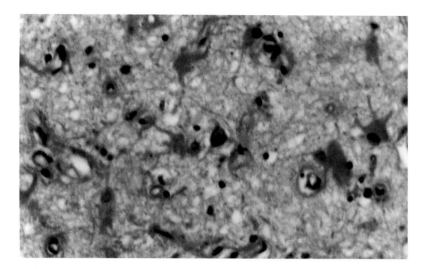

Fig. 4.46. Leigh disease. The neuropil is vacuolated and demyelinated, and there is proliferation of capillaries and astrocytes. Note that neurons are present in the lesion (centre).

Cockayne and *Canavan diseases* and a heterogeneous group of conditions described as *sudanophil leucodystrophy* which lack distinguishing histological features. *Alexander disease*, in which progressive demyelination is accompanied by very marked deposition of Rosenthal fibres throughout the brain, is strikingly different from other leucodystrophies, and is thought to be a primary disease of astroglia. For descriptions, see Allen and Kirk (1992). Finally, a few other metabolic conditions produce non-specific pathology in the white matter: these include some of the *aminoacidurias*, which tend to cause vacuolation and retardation of myelination in neonates, and some demyelination with spongy degneration in those who survive into childhood.

Metabolic Diseases Affecting both Grey and White Matter

The mitochondrial and peroxisomal disorders generally affect both grey and white matter equally, the exception being ALD, which is described under the white matter diseases.

Mitochondrial dysfunction results in impaired ATP production in affected cells, and for that reason tends to involve preferentially tissues that have a high metabolic rate, typically brain, skeletal muscle and liver, and so to produce a wide variety of clinical manifestations. The principal mitochondrial disease that presents in infancy is an autosomal recessive condition known as *subacute necrotizing encephalomyelopathy* or *Leigh disease*, in which the most characteristic clinical features are respiratory difficulties, hypotonia, developmental delay, and a variety of brain stem signs, accompanied by lactic acidosis. There is remarkable consistency in the

anatomical sites involved in the disease, which is usually bilateral and symmetrical: the midbrain, pons and medulla, cerebellum, thalamus, optic nerves and posterior columns of the spinal cord are classically affected (Monpetit et al. 1971; Van Coster et al. 1991). The pathological changes are vacuolation of the neuropil with demyelination, marked capillary proliferation and astrocytosis (Fig. 4.46), but with striking preservation of neurons, which distinguishes the condition from hypoxic–ischaemic brain damage. There may be widespread diffuse myelin loss (Barkovich et al. 1993). A number of underlying biochemical deficiencies are described in Leigh disease, usually either in the pyruvate dehydrogenase complex or in cytochrome oxidase; less commonly other mitochondrial abormalities are found.

Mitochondrial disease presenting in the second decade is more likely to be MELAS syndrome, the acronym being derived from the principal clinical features (*m*itochondrial myopathy, *e*ncephalopathy, *l*actic acidosis and *s*troke-like episodes). Muscle biopsy shows characteristic "ragged-red" fibres with a modified Gomori trichrome stain, an appearance produced by subsarcolemmal accumulation of mitochondria. There is a similar accumulation of mitochondria in the endothelial and smooth muscle cells of cerebral arteries and arterioles (Ohama et al. 1987), which causes the cells to swell and thus probably accounts for the ischaemic episodes. For reviews of the clinical and pathological features of these rare diseases see the accounts by Friede (1989), Duchen and Jacobs (1992) and Barkovich et al. (1993).

The peroxisomal disorders *Zellweger syndrome, neonatal ALD* and *infantile Refsum's disease*, all of which are characterized by abnormalities of hepatic peroxisomes, affect a number of organs, principally the liver and brain. Hepatic pathology is variable in

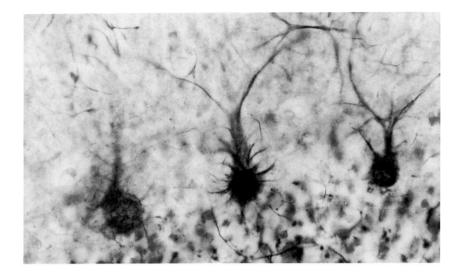

Fig. 4.47. Purkinje cell in Menkes' kinky hair disease showing processes coming directly off the cell body. (×400)

all three conditions; in most severely affected cases established cirrhosis is seen. In Zellweger cerebrohepatorenal syndrome the brain shows multiple neuronal migration defects and myelin breakdown, whereas in neonatal ALD, which is very rare, polymicrogyria is reported as well as white matter demyelination similar to that seen in childhood ALD. Cerebral involvement in infantile Refsum's disease is less marked. A full description of these peroxisomal disorders is given by Lake (1992).

Alper's disease is a familial condition in which, as in the peroxisomal disorders, there is rapidly progressive neurodegeneration associated with variable liver pathology. Preferential sites of involvement in the brain are the neocortex, the thalamus and the caudate nuclei. Changes in the white matter are thought to be secondary to cortical cell loss. Alper's disease has been claimed to be a primary mitochondrial disorder, but this is disputed, and the underlying biochemical abnormality has yet to be established (Harding 1990; Duchen and Jacobs 1992).

Disorders of copper metabolism may have profound effects on the CNS. *Menkes' kinky hair disease* (trichopoliodystrophy), in which there are abnormally low copper and caeruloplasmin levels resulting from impaired absorption of dietary copper, is sometimes classified with the mitochondrial diseases, because the underlying disorder in copper metabolism may lead to *secondary* impairment of mitochondrial metabolism. Menkes' disease is a rare X-linked condition characterized by mental retardation, developmental delay, seizures, and hypopigmented twisted and friable hair. Neuropathologically there is extensive cystic degeneration of cerebral grey and white matter, gliosis and cerebellar cortical abnormalities,

particularly in Purkinje cells (Fig. 4.47). Intracranial vessels may show curious morphological changes, possibly as a result of abnormal elastin in the vessel walls (Becker and Yates 1990). In *Wilson's disease*, another familial disorder of copper metabolism, copper accumulates and is deposited in a number of organs in the body. The effects are clinically most important in the liver, which becomes cirrhotic, and in the brain, which shows neuronal loss and gliosis in the caudate, putamen and globus pallidus, and softening of the central white matter. Onset of neurological disease is usually in late adolescence or during adulthood, and with treatment deaths in childhood are rare. The neuropathological changes are described in detail by Duchen and Jacobs (1992).

Non-inherited Metabolic Encephalopathies

Premature babies and babies born to diabetic mothers are at particular risk of *hypoglycaemia*, which if prolonged may cause widespread cerebral damage. Hypoglycaemia affects neurons in a selective way, the outer cell layers in the cerebral cortex, deep grey nuclei and parts of Ammon's horn being most vulnerable. However, the attribution of pathological changes to hypoglycaemia is not always certain, particularly in neonates and infants, because it almost invariably occurs with seizures and hypoxia–ischaemia, which may themselves cause necrosis in very similar neuronal populations. There are slight differences in the anatomical distribution of lesions, however (Auer et al. 1989), and in older children a distinction may be possible.

In infants the histological features of *hepatic encephalopathy* may be difficult to recognize, but once again in older children the features are similar to those seen in adults, the principal pathology being diffuse astrocytosis of grey matter, particularly cortex and deep grey nuclei. The astrocytes have a characteristic appearance, and are known as Alzheimer type II astrocytes. They can be seen in clusters in the grey matter; their cytoplasm does not stain, and their nuclei are swollen and empty, with a single prominent nucleolus and few chromatin granules.

Unconjugated hyperbilirubinaemia in a neonate carries with it the risk of *kernicterus,* bilirubin staining of the brain accompanied by neuronal necrosis. With the decline in incidence of haemolytic disease of the newborn, this neonatal syndrome is no longer common. In the premature infant, however, kernicterus is occasionally found at autopsy with no history of raised bilirubin levels (Volpe 1987); from animal work, there is considerable evidence now to suggest that this may be because under circumstances such as acidosis or infection the blood–brain barrier opens and allows *conjugated* bilirubin into the tissues (Levine et al. 1982; Larroche 1991b). The bright yellow pigmentation of the brain produced by bilirubin has a characteristic anatomical distribution, and symmetrically involves the globus pallidus, Ammon's horn and subthalamic nucleus. Other structures – inferior olives, substantia nigra, many of the cranial nerve nuclei in the brain stem, the Purkinje cells and dentate nucleus of the cerebellum, and anterior horn cells of the spinal cord – are variably affected. The cortex is usually spared, and unstained areas of the brain appear startlingly white by contrast with affected regions. In sections, some yellow pigment can occasionally be seen, both in neurons, which are shrunken and pyknotic, and free in the neuropil where cells have been lost, but it is mostly lost in routine processing. *Chronic postkernicteric bilirubin encephalopathy* is described in children following hyperbilirubinaemia in the neonatal period. The clinical features of this syndrome do not become evident until the child is a year old, and extrapyramidal abnormalities are the hallmark of the condition, reflecting the degree of damage to the basal ganglia. Gaze palsies and auditory disturbances in turn reflect earlier damage to cranial nerve nuclei in the brain stem. In the few cases reported, there has been intense gliosis marking earlier neuronal loss at sites in the same anatomical distribution as seen in kernicterus.

Findings at autopsy in the acute encephalopathy known as *Reye's syndrome* are non-specific; cerebral swelling due to oedema is usually the only finding in the CNS. However, it is worth remembering not only that a number of toxins and drugs have been associated with Reye's syndrome (Brett 1991), but that some of the inherited metabolic disorders discussed above may also present with an acute encephalopathy that clinically mimics it.

Miscellaneous Neurodegenerative Conditions

Friedreich's ataxia is one of the commonest inherited diseases of the CNS. It shows an autosomal recessive pattern of inheritance, and is slightly more common in males than in females. The disease classically presents in late childhood, with the insidious onset of clumsiness and unsteadiness in a child who was previously healthy. Cerebellar signs – ataxia, intention tremor and dysarthria – become increasingly more marked, and limb weakness develops. Associated musculoskeletal anomalies include kyphoscoliosis and bilateral pes cavus, while hypertrophic cardiomyopathy and diabetes mellitus are also common. The disease is relentlessly progressive; most patients are wheelchair-bound in their teens, and die in their twenties. The changes in the nervous system are seen principally in spinal cord and cerebellum, particularly the former (Fig. 4.48). To look at, the cord appears atrophic. Even on routine stains of transverse sections the degeneration of the white matter of the posterior half of the cord can be seen, but with sections stained for myelin the anatomical distribution of the disease can be appreciated. Long tract degeneration (myelin and axonal loss, and gliosis) is most evident in three separate sensory and motor pathways: the posterior columns, particularly the gracile fascicle, containing sensory fibres from lumbar and sacral segments; the lateral corticospinal pathways; and the dorsal spinocerebellar tracts, which relay proprioceptive information from the upper part of the body. Clarke's nucleus, found in cord segments C8–L2, is the source of the fibres in the dorsal spinocerebellar tracts, and always shows severe neuronal loss. As might be expected, long tract degeneration is most evident distally; corticospinal fibres are most severely affected in the lower part of the cord, and the sensory tracts most affected in proximal segments. Changes in the cerebellum are less marked; the white matter is often gliotic, superior and inferior cerebellar peduncles atrophied, and the dentate nucleus is depleted.

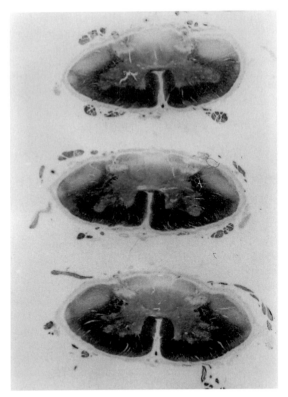

Fig. 4.48. Sections of the cervical cord in a case of Friedreich's ataxia, stained for myelin, show symmetrical long-tract degeneration in the dorsal half of the cord, affecting the posterior columns, dorsal spinocerebellar tracts and part of the corticospinal tracts.

In *juvenile Huntington's disease* the clinical picture is slightly different from that in adults, with epilepsy, dementia, akinesia and rigidity more usual than the chorea seen in older patients. The pathology is, however, similar. The brain shows mild cortical atrophy, and dilatation of the lateral ventricles secondary to atrophy of the striatum (caudate and putamen), which can be seen on slicing; on histology, neuronal loss and gliosis are most marked in the caudate, putamen and cerebral cortex. A full description of the pathological changes in Huntington's disease is given by Richardson (1990).

Werdnig–Hoffmann disease is the most severe of a group of neuromuscular conditions known as spinal muscular atrophy. It is an autosomal recessive disorder, generally diagnosed shortly after birth or in early infancy, caused by progressive degeneration of motor neurons in the brain stem and spinal cord. The only macroscopic finding at autopsy is atrophy of the ventral roots of the spinal cord, which is seen in all conditions where there is loss of anterior horn cells.

Microscopically, there is invariably marked neuronal loss in the brain stem nuclei of cranial nerves VII, IX, X, XI and XII and in the motor nucleus of V nerve, while in the cord anterior horn cell depletion may be dramatic. Residual neurons show degenerative changes, and there is often evidence of neuronophagia, with microglial cells clustered round a dying neuron. Glial stains reveal a marked reactive astrocytosis in the depleted neuronal groups.

Neurocutaneous Syndromes

Neurocutaneous syndromes (or "phakomatoses") are a group of fascinating conditions that are related only in that they all have features that could be considered maldevelopmental. Multiple ectodermal, particularly neuroectodermal, lesions are associated with mesodermal abnormalities, and in most cases there is an established pattern of inheritance. The principal diseases are the tuberous sclerosis, neurofibromatoses, Sturge–Weber syndrome, von Hippel–Lindau syndrome, ataxia–telangiectasia, and neurocutaneous melanosis.

Tuberous Sclerosis

Tuberous sclerosis (TS) is an autosomal dominant disorder with an extremely variable expression, both from one affected family to another and between members of the same family. In its classic form, cutaneous and CNS lesions are present, with lesions in the retina and kidneys. The spinal cord and peripheral nerves are invariably spared – a finding that distinguishes the condition from forms of neurofibromatosis (Richardson 1991). The most common systemic manifestations of the disease, often referred to as the tuberous sclerosis complex, are principally hamartomatous, and include facial angiofibromas (adenoma sebaceum), ungual fibromas and fibrous scalp plaques, together with retinal hamartomas and multiple renal angiomyolipomas, although a number of other lesions may be associated with the disease. In addition to the systemic pathology, there are characteristic central nervous system lesions, which are responsible for most of the clinical problems in these patients: cortical "tubers", white matter heterotopias, and subependymal nodules and giant cell astrocytomas. The classic neurological features of tuberous sclerosis are seizures and mental retardation, but since the advent of improved neuroimaging techniques, particularly MRI, it has been possible to detect lesions in relatively unaffected cases, and

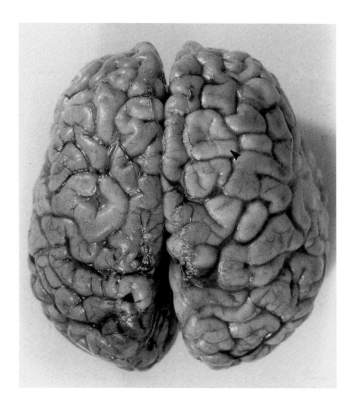

Fig. 4.49. Umbilicated expanded gyri, with the typical appearance of "tubers" (the cortical lesions of tuberous sclerosis) present in both hemispheres. One tuber is marked (arrowhead).

undoubtedly formes frustes of the condition do exist. Small isolated tubers have been detected on MRI in the brains of children of normal intelligence who have seizures (Fryer 1991).

The cortical tubers are nodular umbilicated lesions seen on the surface of the cerebral gyri (Fig. 4.49). Markedly firm or rubbery to palpation, they may be extremely variable in size, often bilateral and sometimes roughly symmetrical. On slicing, the abnormality shows as expansion of affected gyri, with loss of the normal grey–white matter demarcation. Histologically the tubers are quite remarkable. They commonly show marked overlying gliosis, with subpial glial fibres forming a felt-like carpet over the surface of the tuber. Normal cortical cytoarchitecture is lost, and the lesion is composed of haphazardly arranged cells, some with neuronal morphology, some resembling astrocytes and some with features which cannot be confidently identified as either one cell type or the other. Many are exceptionally large and bizarre in form, with prominent nucleoli and abundant pale eosinophilic cytoplasm, and both immunocytochemically and ultrastructurally they may possess glioneuronal features. The cells are separated by parenchyma which tends to be extremely gliotic. (As in multiple *sclerosis*, it is gliosis that gives a firm texture to the lesions.) Relatively normal looking glial and pyramidal cells may be interspersed between the cellular components of the tuber, although neuronal apical dendrites are often abnormally orientated. The lower margins of the tubers are indistinct histologically, and abnormal cells can be found extending into the subjacent white matter. White matter neuronal heterotopias, although frequently widespread, are not usually large enough to be evident macroscopically. They can be picked up especially well with myelin stains, when small islands of abnormal glioneuronal cells can be found dotted at random through the white matter. Subependymal nodules, characteristic of the disease, project into the ventricular system, usually the lateral or third ventricles. They are traditionally described as "candle gutterings", small firm lesions with a characteristic distribution along the thalamostriate groove, or, as Richardson (1991) has pointed out, in the region of the fetal germinal matrix. These nodules are usually heavily calcified, composed of large abnormal cells very similar to the indeterminate cells that occur elsewhere in the brain in TS. In the periventricular nodules they tend to be arranged in sheets. Subependymal nodules do grow slowly with time, and may develop into subependymal giant cell astrocytomas (Fig. 4.50) (Morimoto and Mogami 1986; Scheithauer 1992), which are described below. The tubers, on the other hand, show no tendency to enlarge.

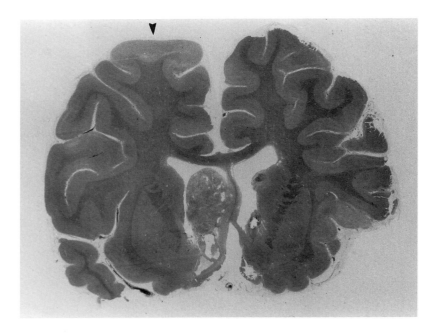

Fig. 4.50. Tuberous sclerosis. A whole brain section, showing a large subependymal giant cell astrocytoma filling the left lateral ventricle. Two calcified subependymal nodules are present in the wall of the other lateral ventricle, and a cortical tuber is indicated.

The anatomical localization of the periventricular and white lesions matter suggests that cellular migration may be deranged in some way in TS: one recent suggestion is that the mutant cells are unable to interact with matrix cell surface molecules in the usual way, resulting in aberrantly sited cells or cells that differentiate abnormally (Lallier 1991).

Neurofibromatosis

Neurofibromatosis is now recognized to have two major forms, referred to as neurofibromatosis types 1 and 2 (NF-1 and NF-2), with possibly a number of other less well characterized variants (Riccardi and Eichner 1986). NF-1 and NF-2 are two distinct conditions, with different inheritance. NF-1, formerly known as von Recklinghausen's disease or "peripheral" neurofibromatosis, is common, occurring in approximately 1 in 4000 live births (Evans et al. 1992b; WHO 1992). It is a potentially serious disorder of the nervous system, but one that is phenotypically extremely variable, even within affected families. The inheritance is autosomal dominant, with a high degree of penetrance, linked to a gene situated on the long arm of chromosome 17. Many cases are presumed to be spontaneous mutations. Manifestations of the disease may be found in any tissues of ectodermal, mesodermal or neural tube origin, and diagnostic criteria for the disease have been carefully defined (Riccardi 1987; Obringer et al. 1989; Evans et al. 1992a). In the central nervous system, patients

may present with intracranial lesions, of which gliomas are potentially the most serious. CNS tumours occur in around 2% of NF-1 patients, and in children with NF-1 comprise nearly half the tumours seen (Sørensen et al. 1986). About 10% of patients develop a glioma, often a cerebellar or hypothalamic astrocytoma, and less commonly both diffuse astrocytic infiltration of the subarachnoid space and gliomatosis cerebri occur (Koszyca et al. 1993). A much larger number, possibly up to 40%, have a low-grade optic nerve glioma, the majority being children under 12 years old. Histologically these are usually pilocytic astrocytomas and are biologically indolent (Lund and Skovby 1991). Neurofibromas are the characteristic tumour of NF-1, however, and are seen not only in the spinal canal but also in the orbit and subcutaneous tissues, and the plexiform variety is pathognomonic of NF-1. Malignant change in peripheral neurofibromas is well recognized in NF-1, being rare in solitary tumours unassociated with the disease. Neuronal heterotopias in the condition are becoming better recognized with increasing use of MRI.

The hallmark of neurofibromatosis 2 ("central" neurofibromatosis) is the production of multiple CNS tumours, particularly nerve sheath tumours, which are always *schwannomas* (Fig. 4.51), not neurofibromas, and for that reason it has been argued that NF-2 is not really a neurofibromatosis at all. The disease is associated with a locus on chromosome 22. Phenotypic variability is less marked than in NF-1, and bilateral acoustic neuromas – or, more correctly, vestibular nerve schwannomas – are the classic mani-

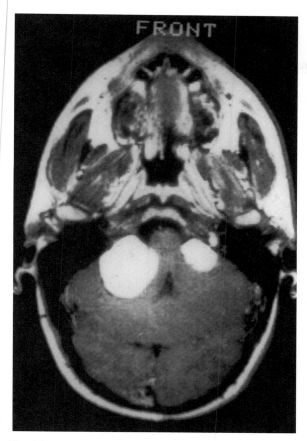

Fig. 4.51. Bilateral acoustic schwannomas in a 19-year-old with NF-2, shown in a T_1-weighted MRI scan of the posterior fossa. (Courtesy of Mr T.T. King)

there may be multiple vascular malformations of the face, eye and meninges, and which manifests as focal or generalized seizures in a child with a facial port-wine naevus, generally in the first year of life. The classic skin lesion lies within the territory of the fifth cranial nerve, and is associated with a vascular malformation in the leptomeninges on the same side. The mass of abnormal vessels lies in the subarachnoid space, and the underlying cortex becomes progressively more atrophic, gliotic and calcified (Fig. 4.52). Chronic partial or incomplete cortical ischaemia resulting from deranged circulation through the leptomeninges (Fig. 4.53) is believed to be the mechanism of pathological progression. Mineralization occurs in and around dying neurons. The process may involve a large portion of the hemisphere, to such an extent that hemiatrophy of the contralateral side of the body may be present; progressive hemiplegia on the contralateral side is common. The inheritance of the condition is not entirely certain, as both autosomal dominant and recessive patterns have been described in families and the genetic defect responsible has not been identified.

Von Hippel–Lindau Syndrome

This is an autosomal dominant disorder in which there is an inherited tendency to develop benign vascular tumours in the cerebellum (Lindau's tumour) and retina (von Hippel's disease), as well as phaeochromocytomas, renal cell carcinoma, and adenomas and cysts in a number of visceral organs. The CNS tumours are always haemangioblastomas and do not usually present until adulthood.

Ataxia–Telangiectasia

An autosomal recessive disorder of both immune and nervous systems, in which progressive ataxia, presenting in infancy, is associated with symmetrical telangiectases in the conjunctiva and skin. Absence or maldevelopment of the thymus, and marked hypoplasia of lymphoid tissue and gonads are also constant findings, associated with a number of immunological abormalities. With progression of the disease, eye movement and pyramidal signs develop. Children are particularly prone to respiratory tract infections, and death usually results from chronic lung disease or malignancy, particularly lymphoma. The most prominent neuropathological findings are in the cerebellum and spinal cord. The cerebellar cortex shows widespread loss of Purkinje cells, with gliosis

festation of the disease. If bilateral eighth nerve tumours are not present, a combination of a family history of NF-2 and other CNS tumours (schwannoma, meningioma, ependymoma, and less commonly astrocytoma) is accepted as diagnostic. Meningiomas in childhood, which are normally rare, are highly suggestive of NF-2. The manifestations of NF-2 occasionally include subcutaneous tumours, but these are schwannomas rather than neurofibromas. The classification of the various types of neurofibromatosis is not fully worked out, and undoubtedly there are patients in whom overlap between the phenotypes does occur.

Sturge–Weber Syndrome

Also known as encephalofacial or encephalotrigeminal angiomatosis, this is a variable disorder in which

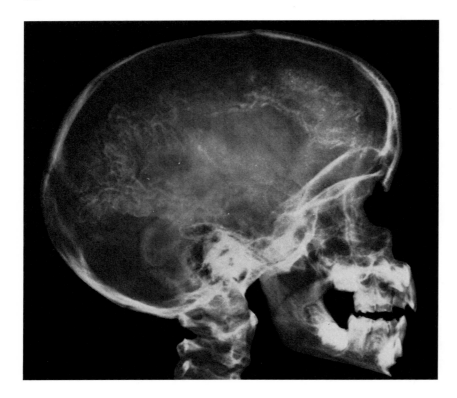

Fig 4.52. Sturge–Weber syndrome. A lateral plain skull radiograph shows cortical calcification in a 15-year-old boy.

of the white matter, while in the cord long tract degeneration in the spinocerebellar pathways and posterior columns, and cell loss in the anterior horns are both marked. Abnormal vessels in the meninges and cerebrum have occasionally been reported (Russell and Rubinstein 1989).

Infections

Any organism that enters the CNS can cause infection. The type of inflammation and damage caused by any one organism depends not only on the type of

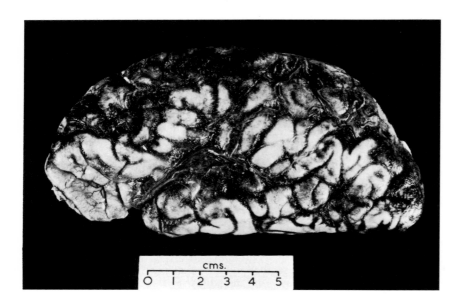

Fig. 4.53. Leptomeningeal angiomatosis in the same case as in Fig. 4.50.

agent involved and its selectivity, but also on the host's ability to react to the antigen. Bacteria, fungi and parasites tend to produce non-selective cerebral necrosis, whereas viruses may infect specific cell populations (the papovavirus that causes progressive multifocal leucoencephalopathy principally infects oligodendrocytes, enteroviruses infect motor neurons, human immunodeficiency virus infects only monocyte-derived cells, etc.). Such selectivity may result in characteristic patterns of pathology.

Fetal Infections

Infections that occur in utero are very frequently destructive. In a child who survives intrauterine infection, a number of non-specific abnormalities may be found. These range from lesions that grossly resemble "primary" malformations (porencephaly, polymicrogyria), lesions that are clearly the result of destructive processes (hydranencephaly, periventricular necrosis), and lesions that can only be detected on histological examination of the brain (neuronal heterotopias). Dystrophic calcification, and hydrocephalus caused by basal meningitis or aqueduct stenosis are features common to a number of infections. Microencephaly following fetal infection may have a number of causes. Widespread destruction of tissue will result in an abnormally small brain, but on occasion there may be little or no obvious pathology and the principal changes will be microscopic. Many of these sequelae of infection may be as important as the infection itself, and in some cases their effect may not present until later in postnatal life or even in infancy and childhood.

Cytomegalovirus (CMV)

A proportion of fetuses infected with CMV during the course of an asymptomatic maternal infection will develop severe CMV disease, which frequently involves the CNS, particularly when infection occurs during the first two trimesters of pregnancy. Lesions in the CNS are widespread and destructive with a characteristic tendency to involve periventricular regions, particularly the germinal matrix in walls of the lateral ventricles, and to calcify. Thus ependymal lesions, often necrotizing, are common, and postinflammatory mineralization may be seen around the ventricles and also in basal ganglia. The intranuclear and cytoplasmic inclusions typical of CMV are found in glia, endothelial and leptomeningeal cells, although rarely in neurons. Cytomegalovirus may cause cerebral malformations such as porencephaly and polymicrogyria (Friede and Mikolasek 1978),

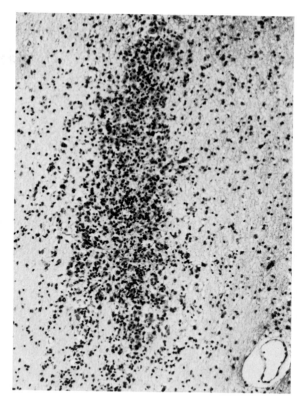

Fig. 4.54. Congenital rubella encephalitis in an 11-day-old baby. The cellular infiltration consists mainly of lymphocytes and plasma cells. (H&E, ×100)

probably as a result of hypoxic damage to the developing cortex (Richman et al. 1974; Barkovich et al. 1992a). The exact mechanism is not clear, but placental infection leading to hypoperfusion has been suggested (Marques Dias et al. 1984).

Rubella

Congenital rubella is now rare, both because of active immunization programmes and as the result of screening of mothers early in pregnancy. Maximum damage to the fetal brain occurs with infection in early gestation (Fucillo and Sever 1973; Friede 1989). A child born with congenital rubella syndrome may have a wide spectrum of abnormalities outside the nervous system, but in the CNS the usual findings are of microencephaly, leptomeningeal thickening and necrotic parenchymal lesions (Fig. 4.54). The mechanism of action of rubella virus on developing fetal tissue is not clear. The virus causes little cellular destruction in human fetal cell cultures, but produces marked inhibition of mitotic activity (Rawls and

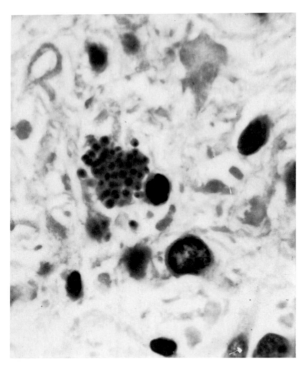

Fig. 4.55. Toxoplasmosis. Organisms in pseudocyst. (H&E, ×1400)

Melnick 1966), and it has been suggested that this action explains the small size of infants with congenital rubella syndrome (Naeye and Blanc 1965). According to Friede (1989), the virus preferentially infects vascular endothelial cells in both placenta and fetus. Certainly vasculopathy is a constant feature of congenital rubella: vessels in the subarachnoid space are involved, as well as parenchymal vessels. The normal architecture of the wall is often destroyed, or partially destroyed, and intimal proliferation and mineralization is common. Perivascular necrosis in both white matter and deep grey nuclei is also seen, although these may be the result of coexistent perinatal asphyxia.

Toxoplasmosis

Like rubella, the effects of infection with toxoplasma in utero are more catastrophic when they occur early in gestation. In the first trimester, the clinical features are very similar to those of severe congenital CMV infection, namely, microencephaly, hydrocephalus, cerebral calcification and chorioretinitis. The destructive lesions of toxoplasmosis calcify with time, as they do in CMV disease, although the distribution of both lesions and calcification tends in toxoplasmosis

to be more randomly distributed and less restricted to periventricular areas. Hydrocephalus, secondary to inflammatory obliteration of the aqueduct, is common. The necrotizing infection is granulomatous, associated with giant cells and chronic inflammatory cells, and both encysted (Fig. 4.55) and free forms of the trophozoite can be found. Isolated encysted organisms found adjacent to a malformation or cavity may represent secondary colonization of the lesion (Friede 1989; Scaravilli 1992), and not the underlying pathology.

Other Infections

Listeria monocytogenes is characteristically transmitted to the fetus during an asymptomatic or mild maternal infection, and in early gestation may result in abortion or stillbirth. Infection in the second half of pregnancy, however, can cause widespread disease, including severe meningoencephalitis with multiple necrotizing microabscesses and granulomata, in which the gram-positive intracellular rod-shaped organisms are found.

Human immunodeficiency virus (HIV) infection in utero may lead to fetal death. Although viral sequences may be isolated from the brain, the only pathological change recorded to date is mild microglial proliferation (Kure et al. 1991). There are, however, few series of fetal brains. At birth, the infection is usually asymptomatic, with early symptoms appearing in the first 6 months of postnatal life.

Postnatal Infections

Neonatal Bacterial Meningitis

Neonatal meningitis caused by bacteria from the flora of the birth canal may be due to a number of organisms, of which group B streptococcus, *Escherichia coli* and *Listeria monocytogenes* are the most important. Although the organisms causing neonatal pyogenic meningitis are radically different from those responsible for the disease later in infancy and childhood, the pathophysiology is essentially the same (see below). The pathological findings differ slightly: if anything, the purulent exudate is even more florid than in older children and, as a result, ventriculitis is more common. Neonatal leptomeningitis tends to cause destruction of cerebral tissue. There is commonly widespread infarction, and abscess formation resulting from superinfection of the infarcts, both of which lead to extensive cavitation of the cerebral hemispheres, producing in survivors a multicystic postmeningitic encephalopathy, often with microen-

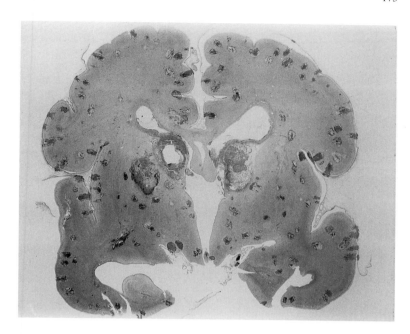

Fig. 4.56. Disseminated cerebral candidiasis in a premature infant. There are multiple microabscesses and granulomata throughout the brain.

cephaly. The cavities tend to be situated adjacent to or communicating with the ventricular system, often as a result of previous ventriculitis. Older infants, by contrast, commonly develop postinflammatory leptomeningeal fibrosis with or without hydrocephalus, but show relatively little in the way of cavitation.

Herpes Simplex Encephalitis

Infection with herpes simplex virus (HSV) type 2, commonly transmitted via the genital tract, is the most usual cause of viral encephalitis in newborn infants, in whom it produces a severe encephalitis which is often fatal. The brain is generally swollen and congested. The pathological changes tend to be diffusely spread through the brain rather than showing the localized lesions typical of acute HSV 1 encephalitis in older children or adults. On histology, pronounced perivascular inflammatory cuffing is found, with mononuclear cells, microglial nodules and intranuclear viral inclusions in neurons, astrocytes and endothelial cells. Vascular thrombosis and infarction may occur, but HSV2 infection tends to be less necrotizing than HSV1.

Other Viruses

A number of other viruses, notably the enteroviruses, may cause acute encephalitis in newborn infants. Poliovirus infection has been reduced by the widespread use of effective immunization, and it is cox-sackie virus type B that may affect neonates, usually in the first month of life. The features are those of an acute viral encephalitis: perivascular inflammatory cuffing, microglial nodules which are often accompanied by polymorphonuclear leucocytes, and reactive astrocytosis. There may be an associated meningitis. Grey matter is characteristically affected and the brain stem and cord are particularly vulnerable. Viral inclusions are not generally found, and there is little tissue necrosis.

Fungi

Candidiasis, infection by *Candida albicans*, is the most common fungal infection of neonates. Infection arises either following transmission from the birth canal, or in the postnatal period, premature children being more vulnerable. The usual manifestation of the disease is a purulent meningitis with involvement of the ventricles, but the brain parenchyma may be involved (Fig. 4.56), characteristically with multiple necrotic lesions, many of them granulomatous, in which the organism can be found in abundance as pseudohyphal or yeast forms.

Childhood Infections

Bacteria

Acute Pyogenic Meningitis. The bacteria that cause pyogenic meningitis vary according to the child's age

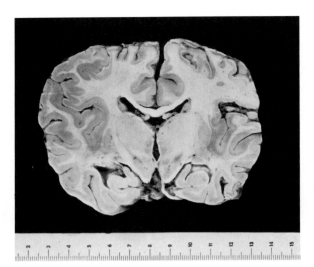

Fig. 4.57. Pyogenic meningitis. Exudate can be seen in the sub-arachnoid space over the convexities; the underlying frontal lobes on both sides are infarcted – note the thinning of the cortex in the affected areas. There is also diffuse brain swelling.

and immune status. In immune-suppressed patients, there are a large number of potential causative organisms, not normally considered pathogenic. In immunologically normal children, the main predisposing factors are congenital anatomical defects, head injury and neurosurgery, but in most cases of pyogenic meningitis no such predisposing conditions can be found.

Haemophilus influenzae is most usually responsible in infants and young children, although this organism should largely disappear, now that an effective vaccine has been introduced.

Neisseria meningitidis is the bacterium that typically causes acute meningitis in children and adolescents, whereas *Streptococcus pneumoniae* is more commonly seen in adults. The effects are the same whatever the causative organism. Once bacteria reach the CNS – usually via the choroid plexus, during the course of a bacteraemia – acute inflammation, which spreads rapidly, results. Macroscopically, the brain is generally swollen and the cortical vessels intensely congested. A subdural effusion is not an uncommon finding in infants (Snedeker et al. 1990). In the early stages, the leptomeninges may merely be cloudy with mild accentuation of perivascular pial sleeves, but the dense layer of pus characteristic of the condition may not have formed. In an established case, however, a creamy layer of pus in the subarachnoid space obscures the cortical gyral pattern and fills the cisterns at the base of the brain. On slicing, the impression of brain swelling may be confirmed, with compression of the sulci and obliteration of the

lateral ventricles, or there may be ventricular dilatation indicating acute hydrocephalus. Pus may be present in the ventricles (ventriculitis), and foci of cerebral infarction may be seen. Microscopically, the subarachnoid space rapidly becomes filled with an acute inflammatory exudate (Fig. 4.57) because there is little resistance to spread through the CSF pathways. Migration of polymorphs leads to the formation of pus which, possibly because of the direction of flow of CSF (Kirkpatrick 1990), is particularly marked over the convexity of the hemispheres. Obstruction of the arachnoid villi by fibrin and polymorphs can cause acute hydrocephalus. Within a few hours, macrophages principally derived from monocytes in the peripheral blood are also to be found. Blood vessels may become damaged and leaky; they become inflamed and/or filled with fibrin. This, in turn, leads to thrombosis (Fig. 4.58) and endarteritis obliterans, both of which are commonly seen with longer survival. The pia generally prevents spread into the brain parenchyma, although small foci or cerebritis may develop, and a pronounced astrocytosis is usually seen in the outer (molecular) layer of the cortex. With time, the composition of the exudate changes, and mononuclear cells – macrophages, lymphocytes and plasma cells – predominate. Organization of the exudate often results in a degree of leptomeningeal fibrosis.

The pathophysiology of acute pyogenic meningitis in children is complex and has been comprehensively reviewed by Ashwal et al. (1992) and Bell (1992). Antibiotic therapy exacerbates the clinical picture because bacterial cell wall lysis promotes the release not only of bacterial endotoxin, but also of a variety of potentially injurious inflammatory mediators from macrophages and endothelial cells, and activation of the complement cascade. Cerebral oedema is probably the most important event affecting outcome, and arises by a number of mechanisms. *Cytotoxic oedema* (cell swelling) develops as a result of release of bacterial cell wall products, which diffuse into the underlying cortex and are directly toxic to neurons and glia. Changes in endothelial cells caused by products of the inflammatory process result in alterations in blood–brain barrier permeability (shown by contrast leakage on CT scan) and thus *vasogenic oedema*. Hydrocephalus resulting from impaired resorption of of CSF leads to ventricular dilatation and *interstitial oedema*. Cerebral swelling occurs, and raised intracranial pressure, reduction in cerebral blood flow and hypoxia are the inevitable consequences. Focal arterial or venous infarction may also occur, and will contribute to the generalized rise in intracranial pressure. The principal causes of death in this disease are generalized septicaemia and cerebral oedema, the latter causing raised intracranial pressure and consid-

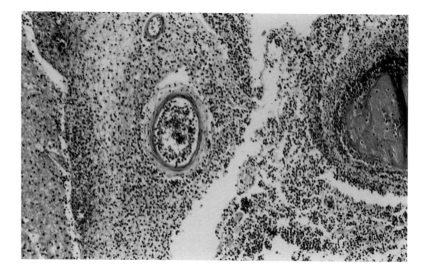

Fig. 4.58. Acute bacterial meningitis. The cortex is on the left. The subarachnoid space is filled with acute inflammatory exudate, and there is a thrombus in the vessel on the right. (H&E, ×135)

erable mass effect, and leading to cardiorespiratory arrest secondary to brain stem compression and ischaemia.

Two important sequelae of bacterial meningitis are chronic hydrocephalus and focal neurological deficits. Hydrocephalus results from organization rather than resolution of the inflammatory exudate, when fibrosis and/or gliosis interferes with the normal flow of CSF at some point along the CSF pathways. The pathological substrate of focal neurological deficits is usually infarction in the brain and spinal cord, caused by vascular thrombosis or spasm. Infarcts are usually arterial, but venous infarction from dural sinus thrombosis is not uncommon. Damage to cranial and spinal nerves may be ischaemic in origin, or the result of fibrous organization of exudate around the nerve roots. Postmeningitic sensorineural hearing impairment, commonly seen in children (Fortnum 1992), may be due to ischaemia or fibrosis affecting the VIII nerve. The particular vulnerability of this nerve to damage in meningitis may be explained by the fact that it has the longest extracranial glial segment of the cranial nerves (Tarlow 1937). Equally, it is possible that infection may spread directly from the subarachnoid space to involve the labyrinth.

Bacterial Abscess. As with pyogenic meningitis, there are a number of conditions that predispose to the development of cerebral abscess. Local suppuration and haematogenous spread from foci elsewhere in the body are both important, chronic ear infection and cyanotic congenital heart disease being the most common underlying factors in children. Blood-borne abscesses are often multiple and are characteristically

sited in the white matter immediately below the cortex, although they may occur anywhere in the brain. Before they become encapsulated, there is a tendency for them to enlarge through the white matter and to rupture into the ventricles (Fig. 4.59). At the very earliest stage, the abscess appears as an

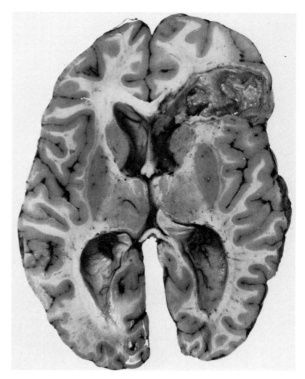

Fig. 4.59. Frontal lobe abscess extending to the ventricle in a case of congenital heart disease.

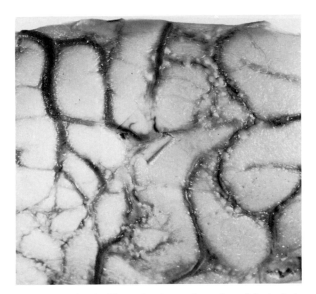

Fig. 4.60. Pinhead miliary tubercles on the surface of the brain in tuberculous meningitis.

ill-defined area of softening or frank necrosis, but as time progresses a capsule slowly forms. Invariably there is much oedema around the lesion, and the brain may show evidence of mass effect, with shift of midline structures and transtentorial herniation. Microscopically, the early lesion is a small focus of organisms and neutrophils resulting from bacterial

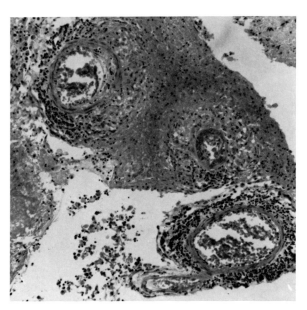

Fig. 4.61. Fibrinoid necrosis of an artery in tuberculous meningitis with surrounding epithelioid cells. (H&E, ×400)

seeding of the brain. This lesion rapidly becomes necrotic, and expands as a result of progressive necrosis of surrounding cells. A layer of granulation tissue surrounds the central necrotic area. Vascular proliferation at the edge of the lesion is intense and it is probably the presence of these new leaky vessels that accounts for the associated oedema. Fibroblasts derived from the reactive vasculature proliferate and produce collagen, with the result that dense fibrous tissue is laid down around the lesion as a capsule. (Fibrosis is unusual in the CNS, except where there is extensive necrosis, and tends to be established at a slower rate than in abscesses in other parts of the body.) A rim of chronic inflammatory cells – lymphocytes and plasma cells – mixed with reactive fibrous astrocytes is characteristic in the surrounding neuropil.

Tuberculosis. Mycobacterium tuberculosis infection of the CNS occurs either during the course of the initial infection as a result of haematogenous dissemination or as part of secondary tuberculosis in a previously sensitized patient. Pathologically, *M. tuberculosis* may produce either meningitis or a parenchymal tuberculoma, the former being more common in western countries. In India, by contrast, the tuberculoma is the most common paediatric intracranial mass lesion (Dastur and Lalitha 1972).

Generalized dissemination of bacilli through the bloodstream results in colonization of the CNS, with tuberculous foci forming in the leptomeninges and subjacent parenchyma. These generally remain dormant until a later date they rupture into the CSF, evoking an inflammatory reaction. The exudate that results is viscous, and tends to collect over the base of the brain, where it may involve cranial nerves. Vessels commonly become secondarily inflamed and thrombosis occurs. (See Figs. 4.60 and 4.61.) With time, organization of the basal exudate, fibrosis and occasionally calcification of the meninges is seen. As in pyogenic bacterial meningitis, obstructive hydrocephalus, cranial nerve damage, cerebral and spinal cord infarction and spinal block may all follow tuberculous meningitis. A tuberculoma behaves principally as a space-occupying lesion.

Neuroborreliosis. Lyme disease is now recognized to be a common infection in children, contracted during the summer and autumn months, following bites by ticks infested with *Borrelia burgdorferi*. It is a not uncommon cause of acute inflammatory CNS disease, of which acute peripheral facial nerve palsy (often bilateral) and aseptic meningitis are the two most usual manifestations. The condition responds to penicillin, and deaths or sequelae of infection are rare (Hansen and Lebech 1992).

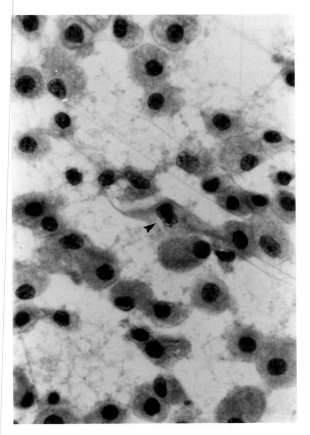

Fig. 4.62. Smear of a biopsy from a case of herpes encephalitis. A single inclusion-bearing cell (*arrowhead*) is present in the middle, among the macrophages.

Viruses

The reaction of the CNS to viral infection is fairly stereotyped, and there are a number of pathological features common to many of the fatal viral encephalitides, although these may vary slightly according to the length of illness and the pathogen. The histological changes typical of viral encephalitis include necrosis, inclusion bodies (for some viruses) and astrocytosis. Perivascular lymphocytic cuffing is a common feature, as is hyperplasia and proliferation of microglia, which can be found both in engulfing dying neurons (neuronophagia) and as small nodules scattered in the white matter. A lymphocytic meningeal infiltrate and secondary hypoxic changes are also frequently present. The anatomical distribution of lesions varies from virus to virus, and may be helpful for diagnosis. In temperate regions, acute viral encephalitis is most usually caused by *herpes simplex* virus, although occasionally other viruses such as varicella–zoster and Epstein–Barr virus,

which characteristically cause a cerebellar syndrome, may be implicated. In other parts of the world viruses transmitted by arthropod vectors are important pathogens, often responsible for epidemics of viral encephalitis. For a full discussion of these encephalitides, see Leestma (1991).

Herpes Simplex Encephalitis. In children, this is almost invariably caused by HSV type 1, which has been latent in peripheral sensory ganglia following a primary infection. The virus is believed to reach the brain as a result of reactivation of infection in the trigeminal ganglia, but the precise route is uncertain. Spread to the nasal mucosa and thence along olfactory pathways would partly explain the characteristic distribution of herpes simplex encephalitis in the basal, frontal and temporal regions, but evidence for this is lacking (Esiri and Kennedy 1992). At autopsy, the brain is swollen, leptomeningeal vessels are congested and a variable degree of softening may be felt. On slicing, there are classically necrotic lesions, involving one or both temporal lobes, with some involvement of insulae, cingulate gyrus and orbital gyri of the frontal lobe. With longer survival, irregular cystic cavitation is seen in these sites. Typical histological findings in the acute illness are those of an acute necrotizing encephalitis. They include perivascular lymphocytic cuffing, microglial nodules and much tissue necrosis with lipid phagocytes. Hypoxic changes in neurons are also usual. Intranuclear viral inclusions (Fig. 4.62) are not easy to find, but the presence of HSV antigen may be demonstrated by immunocytochemistry or in situ hybridization.

Measles. Acute measles encephalitis is now rare, as a result of mass infant vaccination programmes, although with pneumonia it was formerly the most serious, often fatal, complication of measles (Rantala and Uhari 1989; Koskiniemi et al. 1991). It remains so in countries where vaccination rates are low (Raote and Bhave 1992).

Postviral (acute disseminated or *perivenous) encephalomyelitis* is a rare acute neurological illness which classically occurs in a patient recovering from the acute phase of one of the exanthematous viral infections, measles virus being the most common cause. It is occasionally seen as a sequela of vaccination. Virus is not usually isolated from the brain and the condition is believed to be an allergic postinfective phenomenon, but because of its almost invariable association with a preceding viral illness it is included here. Children aged between 6 and 11 years are particularly vulnerable. In a few cases there is no obvious antecedent illness. Between about 5 days and 2–3 weeks after the initial illness, the patient develops signs of an acute encephalopathy: headache,

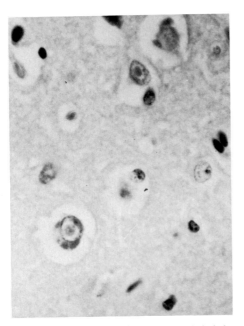

Fig. 4.63. Intranuclear inclusions with characteristic halo seen in cortical neurons in SSPE. (H&E, ×400)

vomiting, meningism, drowsiness, paraplegia, and in severe cases coma and convulsions. Although many patients recover with no residua, others have permanent neurological deficits and up to 20% die in the acute phase (Allen and Kirk 1992). Macroscopically, the brain may look normal, or may be swollen and congested. On slicing, one may detect small grey areas scattered through the white matter: these are foci of demyelination, which is the hallmark of the condition. On microscopy, there is variable mild diffuse inflammation, which may also involve the meninges, and the characteristic perivenous destruction of myelin. Other features are those of acute demyelination, and include activation of migrolia, proliferation of lipid macrophages containing myelin debris, and a reactive astrocytosis. The lesions are widespread through the white matter of the cerebrum, cerebellum and brain stem. A more virulent, and less common, variant is the fulminating condition *acute haemorrhagic leucoencephalitis.* Two recent cases illustrating this spectrum of postinfective CNS complications of measles are described by Pearl et al. (1990).

As well as being a significant cause of acute postinfectious encephalomyelitis, measles is also responsible for an unrelated progressive neurological disease, *subacute sclerosing panencephalitis (SSPE).* Some years after an attack of uncomplicated measles, a child develops insidious behavioural disturbances, with progressive neurological signs including cerebel-

lar ataxia, movement disorders, seizures and progressive decline of cognitive function. The usual course of the disease is over 1–3 years, although more fulminant and more protracted clinical courses have been reported. The macroscopic appearance of the brain will vary according to the length of the disease: it may appear normal, or there may be cerebral atrophy. Brains from patients who have died after a prolonged disease course will show generalized atrophy and may feel hard or rubbery on slicing, a change in texture imparted by intense white matter gliosis. Histologically, mild chronic leptomeningitis with encephalitis is usual, although there is very seldom much in the way of lymphocytic cuffing. Microglial activation is seen early, especially in the cortex, and astrocytosis increases in amount as the disease progresses. Characteristic hard-edged inclusions (Fig. 4.63) are present in abundance in the early stages in neurons and oligodendroglia but become less prominent with time. The degree of neuronal loss is variable, but in a typical end-stage case the cortex is devastated, shrunken and gliotic. Although the disease process is usually a panencephalitis, involving all regions of the brain, in some cases the pathology is principally found in the white matter, when the term "subacute sclerosing leucoencephalitis" has been used. Demyelination, accompanied by macrophages containing sudanophil material is common, although the outstanding feature in the white matter is pronounced reactive astrocytosis with dense glial scarring, which again becomes more prominent with longer disease duration. The diagnosis may be confirmed either by immunocytochemistry, using measles antiserum, or by electron microscopy to show tubular paramyxovirus nucleocapsids.

While measles is now a very rare cause of CNS infection in normal children, it is still an important cause of acute or subacute *inclusion body encephalitis* in children who are immune-suppressed, commonly as a result of underlying acute lymphoblastic leukaemia. Macroscopically, the brain appears normal, although the cortex may appear focally swollen. Histologically there is little in the way of inflammation or astrocytic reaction, but typical intranuclear inclusions may be seen in both cortical neurons and white matter. The severe demyelination and white matter gliosis seen in SSPE are not a feature of this variant of measles encephalitis. As in SSPE, immunocytochemistry or electron microscopy may be used to confirm the diagnosis. A discussion of presentation and diagnosis, and a review of all previously reported cases are given in the papers by Hughes et al. (1993) and Mustafa et al. (1993).

Enteroviruses. In countries in which effective immunization programmes are in operation, the inci-

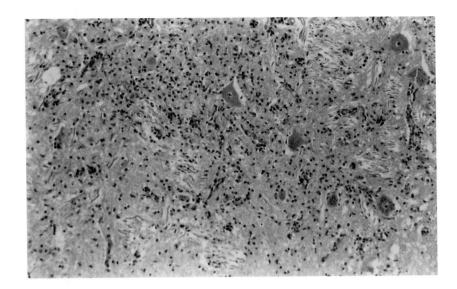

Fig. 4.64. Acute poliomyelitis. The anterior horn of the spinal cord is infiltrated by inflammatory cells. Many of the cells are undergoing neuronophagia. (H&E, ×125)

dence of neurological disease caused by *poliovirus* infection has sharply declined. The virus normally enters the alimentary tract and establishes itself in the lymphoid tissue of the gut. In a very few patients, it spreads into the bloodstream and enters the CNS, probably via the sites at which the blood–brain barrier is deficient, although it is possible that intra-axonal transport into the brain or cord also occurs (Esiri and Kennedy 1992). Once in the nervous system, the virus shows a striking predilection for motor neurons, particularly in the brain stem and spinal cord, but also a number of other neuronal groups in the cerebrum and cerebellum (Leestma 1991). In the acute stage, individual neurons may be engulfed by polymorphs (Fig. 4.64); later, clusters of microglia surround the dying cells, and there is pronounced perivascular lymphocytic cuffing. In long-standing cases, spinal root atrophy and anterior horn cell loss and gliosis may be the only pathological findings. Rarely, other enteroviruses may produce poliomyelitis clinically and pathologically indistinguishable from that caused by the poliovirus. Finally, ECHO and polio viruses are important causes of encephalitis and encephalomyelitis in children with hypogammaglobulinaemia. Both fatal acute encephalitis and persistent chronic infection have been reported (McKinney et al. 1987; Misbah et al. 1992).

Rabies. Rabies provides an example of viral spread by intraneuronal pathways. Following a bite by an infected animal, the virus may be transported up both motor and sensory nerves to the dorsal root ganglia or the spinal cord. Encephalitis or encephalomyelitis develops after a variable latent period. The brain may be swollen but otherwise unremarkable. Histologically, the features are those of a viral infection principally affecting grey matter (a *polio*-encephalomyelitis), with much neuronal destruction, lymphocytic infiltration, microglial proliferation and astrocytosis. The pathognomonic feature is the presence of neuronal cytoplasmic inclusions known as Negri bodies, characteristically seen in cerebellar Purkinje cells and pyramidal neurons of the hippocampus (Fig. 4.65).

HIV-1. Children infected by HIV-1, whether acquired in utero or after birth, show clinical syndromes of CNS involvement different from those seen in adult disease. Progressive decline in intellectual and motor function, loss of developmental milestones, fits, microencephaly and cerebral atrophy are all common. Encephalopathy is one of the most important complications of HIV-1 infection in children and, although the clinical course of HIV-1 encephalopathy may vary enormously from child to child, progressive neurological deterioration is inevitable. Sharer's neuropathological series of children with HIV-1 infection and acquired immune deficiency syndrome (AIDS) is the most recent (Sharer 1992; Sharer and Mintz 1993). Deposition of calcium, iron and other minerals, principally in the lentiform nucleus, in vessel walls and in adjacent neuropil, is characteristic, being found in 92% of the brains in this series; white matter pallor and/or gliosis (present in 78%), collections of lymphocytes, astrocytes and microglia in loose inflammatory nodules (in 75%) and multinucleate cells (Fig. 4.66) (in 61%) were the next most common pathologies.

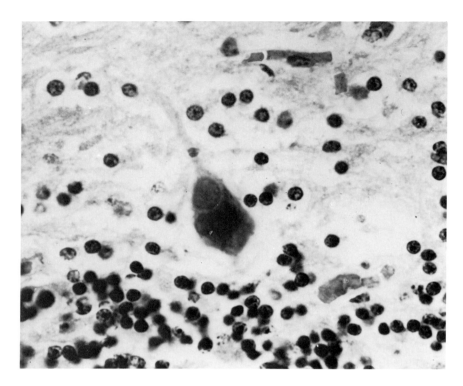

Fig. 4.65. Rabies. Cytoplasmic inclusion. Negri body in Purkinje cell. (H&E, ×400)

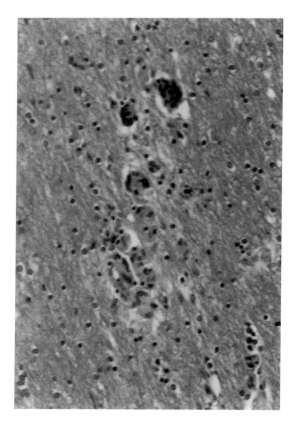

Interestingly, unlike in adult HIV-1 infection, opportunistic infections are rare in children (Kozlowski et al. 1990; Kure et al. 1991), possibly because children dying of AIDS have not lived long enough to be exposed to primary infection by the organisms that tend to colonize the brain in adults. As a result, the neuropathological findings in children are believed to represent relatively "pure" HIV-1 infection (Burns 1992; Scaravilli 1993).

Protozoa

Malaria. In children, malaria is commonly complicated by hypoglycaemia (Taylor et al. 1988; Brewster et al. 1990), probably the result of a combination of factors including limited liver glycogen stores, reduced food intake and intestinal malabsorption (Phillips and Solomon 1990). Added to this, parasitized red cells have a very much greater glucose metabolism than normal cells. The drop in blood

Fig. 4.66. A cluster of typical multinucleate giant cells seen in the white matter in a case of HIV encephalitis. These cells are extremely variable, and although true giant cells with a ring of peripheral nuclei may be seen, some appear to be merely a cluster of nuclei with very little cytoplasm. (H&E, ×140)

glucose may not be recognized and may be prolonged, itself aggravating the brain damage that results from the underlying disease. Involvement of the brain in severe *Plasmodium malariae* infection is manifest clinically by diffuse encephalopathy, seizures and coma. In fatal cases, there is marked cerebral oedema and petechial haemorrhages, principally in the white matter. The cortex may be grey in colour, an appearance probably produced by deposition of malarial "pigment" in the perivascular spaces. Microscopically, these are ring haemorrhages with a central vessel packed with red cells containing organisms. Where there is a glial–microglial reaction to haemorrhage, the lesion is traditionally called a "Durck granuloma", although these are not granulomas according to a modern definition. If the patient survives, these lesions resolve, leaving residual glial scars.

Demyelination

Multiple sclerosis (MS) is not common in children and may present with an atypical clinical picture (Hanefield et al. 1991). Current theories of pathogenesis have been recently reviewed by Allen and Brankin (1993). The pathology of MS in childhood is identical to that in other age groups: acute lesions will show perivenular inflammatory cuffing, oedema and myelin loss with preservation of axons. Sheets of macrophages containing myelin debris, and many reactive astrocytes are usual. The areas of myelin loss characteristically show sharp demarcation from surrounding white matter, and the lesions are haphazardly distributed through the CNS, with a predilection for periventricular sites. Chronic lesions show little inflammation, marked myelin loss with relative axonal preservation, and intense fibrillary gliosis, traditionally demonstrated by the rather toxic Holzer stain, nowadays more safely by a modified phosphotungstic acid haematoxylin stain (Manlow and Munoz 1992).

The other principal demyelinating disease seen in children is a condition known as acute disseminated perivenous encephalomyelitis, which occasionally follows one of the acute childhood viral illnesses, particularly measles. It is clearly a postviral immune-mediated demyelinating disease, and not directly due to the presence of virus in the brain, but because of its close association with measles infection it is described with the diseases caused by that virus (p. 771).

Demyelination is a feature of many of the inherited white matter diseases that are most commonly seen in children, the *leucodystrophies*. Traditionally a distinction has been made between primary demyelin-ation such as that seen in MS and the myelinolysis that results from a metabolic defect, but in practice the distinction is not always easy to make. The leucodystrophies are discussed above.

Cerebrovascular Disease

Stroke in childhood is a rare event, and the pattern of pathology is different from that seen in the adult population. Transient attacks are uncommon in children, except in moyamoya disease (see below); spontaneous intracranial haemorrhage is slightly more common than occlusive vascular disease, unlike in the adult population, where ischaemic strokes are four times as common as haemorrhagic ones (Caplan 1993). Equally, the causes of paediatric stroke tend to be more heterogeneous than in older age groups. Bleeding from an occult vascular malformation, usually an arteriovenous malformation (AVM), is the most common cause of haemorrhagic stroke in children (Toffol et al. 1987; Byard et al. 1991), usually presenting as subarachnoid haemorrhage. Bleeding into a tumour, and haematological causes such as coagulopathies, leukaemia or aplastic anaemia, are also significant causes of intracerebral haemorrhage in children. Occasionally, an apparently trivial head injury may be responsible for dissection of intracranial arteries, and subsequent focal neurological signs. Saccular ("berry") aneurysms are not common in young children, but may occur when there is a co-existent predisposing condition such as coarctation of the aorta, Ehlers–Danlos syndrome or polycystic kidneys. Ischaemic stroke resulting from embolism in association with congenital heart disease is common in very young children (Trescher 1992; Caplan 1993). Infection, particularly meningitis, may cause thrombosis or vasospasm of meningeal vessels at any age. Other important causes of arterial occlusion in children include migraine, sickle cell anaemia, moyamoya disease and fibromuscular dysplasia. Venous infarction resulting from venous thrombosis (Fig. 4.67) is usually as a result of spontaneous superior sagittal sinus occlusion in a setting of dehydration, congenital heart disease, leukaemia or hypercoagulopathy. Any of the venous sinuses may develop thrombosis in pyogenic meningitis or subdural empyema.

The macroscopic appearances and histology of infarction in a child are the same as those seen in the adult brain. Within the first 18–24 h, the infarcted tissue becomes clearly demarcated from surrounding brain. If blood flow is re-established through the area or the cause of infarction is venous occlusion, the

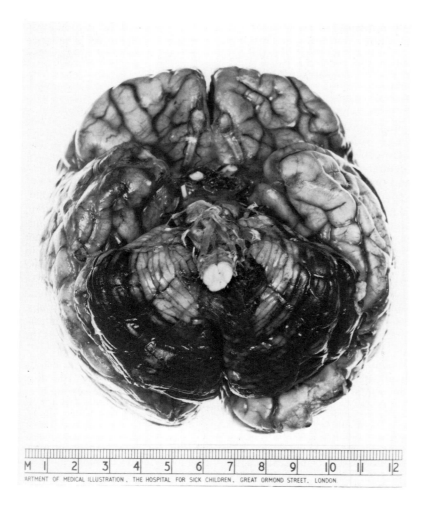

M 1 2 3 4 5 6 7 8 9 10 11 12

ARTMENT OF MEDICAL ILLUSTRATION , THE HOSPITAL FOR SICK CHILDREN , GREAT ORMOND STREET , LONDON.

Fig. 4.67. Haemorrhagic infarction of the cerebellum due to venous thrombosis in a child with congenital heart disease. (Female aged 20 months with transposition of the great arteries).

tissue will be haemorrhagic, rather than pale. Demarcation between grey matter and white matter is very commonly blurred. The infarcted area is initially swollen, and may show considerable mass effect. Even a relatively recent infarct will be different in consistency from surrounding univolved brain, and become progressively softer with time. Artefactual "cracking", or separation of the devitalized tissue from unaffected adjacent tissue, may been seen in fixed tissue at 48–72 h, and liquefaction subsequently becomes visible at about 3–4 days. Microscopically, oedema and pallor of myelin staining are two of the earliest histological alterations, followed by ischaemic neuronal changes (shrinkage of the cell body, pyknosis of the nucleus, and marked eosinophilia of the cytoplasm on routine staining). The acute inflammatory cell infiltrate is never as pronounced in cerebral infarction as in infarction elsewhere in the body, although macrophages are present in abundance after about 24 h, and the gliomesoder-

mal response at the edge of the infarcted area after about a week can be florid.

Moyamoya disease may be responsible for both ischaemic and haemorrhagic stroke, and tends to affect children under 10 years of age. Originally reported from Japan, but now well recognized to occur in non-Japanese populations, this is a rare cerebrovascular disease, diagnosed angiographically (Fig. 4.68), in which there is progressive stenosis or spontaneous occlusion of basal arteries in the circle of Willis, accompanied by development of a compensatory collateral network of vessels in the subarachnoid space. There are reports of familial cases, which suggests a hereditary factor, but there is also strong association with a previous history of chronic respiratory tract infection (Suzuki and Kodama 1983). There is no specific clinical picture, but classically children suffer from repeated transient ischaemic attacks, usually recurrent episodes of hemiplegia (Caplan 1993).

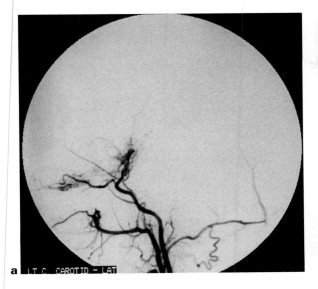

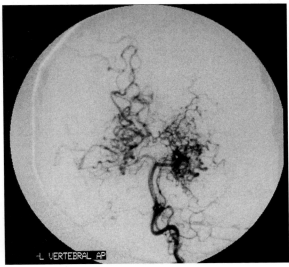

Fig. 4.68. Moyamoya disease in a 7-year-old child: **a** In the carotid angiogram, the only branch of the internal carotid that is fully patent is the ophthalmic artery. The middle cerebral artery is completely blocked, and the anterior so stenosed that it is only shown by later films. **b** In the vertebral angiogram, the typical "puff of smoke" appearance is produced by hypertrophied lenticulostriate and thalamostriate perforating vessels. (Courtesy of Dr W. Taylor, Great Ormond Street Hospital for Sick Children)

Of the *vascular malformations*, arteriovenous malformations and malformations of the great cerebral vein (of Galen) are most common in children. Haemorrhage is the most frequent clinical manifestation of childhood AVMs (Kondziolka et al. 1992);

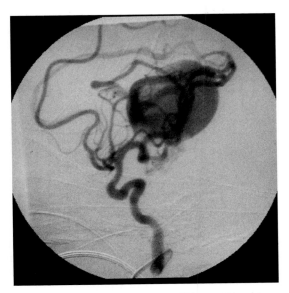

Fig. 4.69. Vein of Galen aneurysm. This carotid angiogram demonstrates that these are complex vascular malformations; besides the dramatically dilated great cerebral vein, multiple feeder arteries and several anomalous vessels are shown. (Courtesy of Dr W. Taylor, Great Ormond Street Hospital for Sick Children)

this is usually into the subarachnoid space, because the lesions tend to abut the cortical surface, but bleeding into the brain parenchyma or the ventricular system may also occur. An arteriovenous fistula involving the great cerebral vein, which is very markedly dilatated, is the usual finding in cases of aneurysms of the vein of Galen (Fig. 4.69). Clinical signs typically develop soon after birth. High-output cardiac failure is a common presentation, and may lead to a diagnosis of congenital heart disease. Compression of the aqueduct or adjacent arteries by the enormously dilated vessels can cause hydrocephalus or local infarction.

Trauma

Birth Injury

When attempting to assess whether damage can be attributed to birth trauma, it may be difficult to distinguish between mechanical birth injury and the effects of concurrent perinatal asphyxia. However, a number of lesions are obviously traumatic in origin. Subcutaneous haemorrhage is common over the vertex, when there is marked moulding of the head during labour and delivery, but extracranial bleeding into other planes (subgaleal and subperiosteal haemorrhage) is less common, and none have direct effects on the CNS. Skull fractures are rare as a result of improved obstetric management. Subdural haemorrhage over the convexities is generally trivial, but in the posterior fossa may be more serious and result from tears of the falx or tentorium, or separation of the lateral and squamous parts of the occipital bone (occipital osteodiastasis). In such cases, laceration of the cerebellum may also occur, and the prognosis is less good (Volpe 1987). Other injuries resulting from birth trauma, such as fractures and high cervical cord damage, are rare.

Accidental Injury

Traumatic injury to the nervous system in the older child produces very similar pathology to that seen in the adult – skull fractures, membrane haemorrhages (extradural and subdural), contusions, intracerebral haemorrhage, diffuse axonal injury, hypoxic brain damage – and for a full account the reader is referred to comprehensive reviews such as that of Adams (1992). In the infant, there are some differences, principally because the skull is capable of greater deformation and because of the immaturity of the nervous system. A peculiar feature of head trauma in young children is the so-called growing fracture, produced by progressive herniation of tissue – granulation tissue, fibrous tissue, leptomeninges – through the fracture site, preventing healing. White matter ("contusional") tears are deceleration injuries particular to infants, slit-like cavities characteristically situated in the frontal lobes in the parasagittal white matter. Although these are generally reported in a setting of deliberate injury (Leestma 1988), where a full neuropathological examination is carried out, it is likely that they also occur in severe deceleration injuries from accidental causes. Finally, severe head injury in children of all ages may result in diffuse brain swelling, which may prove fatal. The actual mechanism is uncertain (Adams 1992), but impaired autoregulation resulting in increased blood volume probably contributes.

Non-accidental Injury (NAI)

Head injury is the most common cause of death in NAI, either in combination with other injuries or on its own. The pattern of skull injury seen in non-accidental paediatric trauma tends to be slightly different from that seen in accidents: complex, depressed fractures are more common than the simple linear variety (Hobbs 1984; Leestma 1988; Friede 1989). Note that the absence of a fracture does *not*

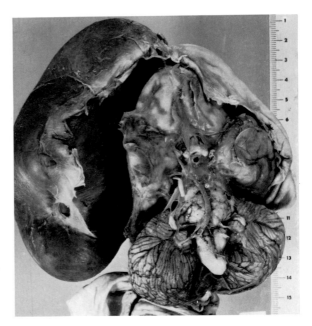

Fig. 4.70. Chronic subdural haematoma.

mean that there is no underlying pathology in the brain.

Subdural haemorrhage is the most common lesion, particularly in children under 2 years of age; its presence in an infant or young child who has no history of accidental trauma should be assumed to be due to NAI, until proved otherwise. The aetiology is often severe shaking, which leads to tearing of veins bridging the subarachnoid space. While the acute subdural presents as a mass lesion, the chronic haematoma (Fig. 4.70) may be clinically silent, with disproportionately increasing head circumference as the only sign of the subdural collection. The signs may be non-specific, such as delay in growth and development, with feeding problems. Macroscopically, the acute subdural is a collection of fresh clotted blood lying between the dura and the arachnoid, with no organizing fibrous membrane over the surface of the haematoma. Neomembrane formation results from proliferation of dural cells around a subdural haemorrhage. It occurs later in children than in adults, and is not usually seen in haematomas less than a month old, but is invariably present around chronic lesions, and may be equal to the dura in thickness. In many cases there is evidence of bleeding on two or more occasions – for example, fresh bleeding into a chronic haematoma containing liquefied blood clot, or separate lesions of different ages. Extradural and intracerebral haemorrhages may also be a feature of NAI.

A characteristic lesion, especially in babies, is the contusional tear, small slit-like white matter lesions, often present at a grey–white matter junction or within large white matter bundles. Contusional tears may be haemorrhagic but frequently are not, and for that reason in a soft infant brain may be confused with artefactual damage. They are probably caused by shearing forces, tend to be associated with severe brain damage, and may be picked up in life on MRI. Other brain damage that may be caused by non-accidental trauma includes diffuse damage to axons and widespread cerebral ischaemia, both of which are common and important causes of severe neurological disability in survivors. Preretinal or subhyaloid haemorrhages are often seen in NAI, but are not pathognomonic, as they can be produced by almost anything that causes a severe rise in intracranial pressure.

Long-term sequelae are common; a combination of significant, often repeated, acceleration–deceleration injuries from shaking, and delay in seeking medical attention contribute significantly to the poor neurological outcome that is usual in victims of non-accidental trauma. The long-term effects may range from vegetative state to mild developmental delay; cerebral atrophy with marked compensatory ventricular dilatation is commonly seen in such children on cerebral imaging (Harwood-Nash 1992).

Sudden Infant Death Syndrome (SIDS)

Sudden infant death characteristically occurs during sleep, and both neurophysiological and neuropathological studies suggest that in infants who die of SIDS there are subtle brain abnormalities causing either defective respiratory control or apnoea of central origin (Kinney et al. 1992). To date, however, no single lethal CNS lesion has been consistently identified. Current neuropathological effort is directed at examination of anatomical regions thought to regulate autonomic and respiratory function, much of the analysis being quantitative (Filiano and Kinney 1992).

Tumours

Virtually all the tumours seen in the adult CNS are also encountered in children. However, the relative prevalence of the different tumour types differs, and there are a few variants that are seen only in infants and very young children. Congenital brain tumours are well recognized: the series of 45 cases diagnosed before 6 months of age reviewed by Buetow et al. (1990) was typical in that the most common tumours were teratomas (12), astrocytomas (9), primitive neuroectodermal tumours (8), medulloblastomas (4), glioblastomas (4), choroid plexus papillomas (3), and a single case each of ependymoma, medulloepithelioma, germinoma, ganglioglioma and haemangiopericytoma. In an international multicentre survey of 886 children with brain tumours in the first year of life, Di Rocco et al. (1991) found astrocytomas (28.6%), medulloblastomas (11.5%), ependymomas (11.4%), choroid plexus papillomas (10.6%), primitive neuroepithelial tumours (6.2%) and teratomas (4.9%) to be most common. With the addition of craniopharyngiomas and epidermoid cysts, the same tumours are seen in older children, whereas meningiomas, pituitary adenomas, schwannomas and metastatic tumours are all rare throughout childhood. In general terms, infratentorial tumours are slightly more common in children, and there is a distinct tendency for them to occur close to the midline (Jellinger and Machacek 1982; Luo et al. 1992). The relative frequency of different types of neoplasm throughout childhood has been reviewed by Schreiber et al. (1982), whose findings have been supported by other large series (Farwell et al. 1977; Jellinger and Machacek 1982; Zülch 1982; Luo et al. 1992). The findings of Luo et al. who report a neurosurgical series of 2000 intracranial tumours in Chinese children under 16, and of Jellinger and Machacek, who reviewed 810 cases of intracranial tumour in the same age group referred to the Vienna Brain Tumour Registry, are summarized and compared in Table 4.3. The frequency of the principal types of tumour are similar, except for craniopharyngioma, germ cell tumours and meningiomas, and it is suggested that these differences reflect geographical factors (Luo et al. 1992). Detailed information about pathology and biology of CNS tumours is given in the comprehensive works by Zülch (1986), Russell and Rubinstein (1989), Burger et al. (1991), Burger and Scheithauer (1994) and Schiffer (1993).

The most widely used classification of brain tumours is that of the World Health Organization (WHO), originally published in 1979 and recently revised (Kleihues et al. 1993a). The classification of the neuroepithelial tumours, which is the largest group, is given in a simplified form in Table 4.4. (Note that a few of these tumours are only seen in adults, and are not described here.) In many cases CNS tumours in children are identical to their adult counterparts, but there are a number of entities unique to or characteristic of children, some of which

Table 4.3 Principal types of intracranial tumour in children under 16 years: results of two large series

	Luo, Beijing, 1992 (2000 cases) %	Jellinger, Vienna, 1982 (810 cases) %
Pilocytic astrocytoma	21.7	
Astrocytoma	21.3[a]	14.3
Glioblastoma	5.3	3.1
Ependymoma	13.1	10.1
Oligodendroglioma	2.5	1.6
Mixed glioma	3.2	1.2
Total gliomas	45.4	52.0
Medulloblastoma	18.5	21.0
Craniopharyngioma	16.6	6.2
Germinoma	3.7	0.9
Meningioma	3.0	1.5
Teratoma	1.7	0.7
Choroid plexus papilloma	1.2	1.1
Epidermoid/dermoid	1.0	2.0
Others	8.9[b]	14.6[c]
Total	100	100

[a] Grade I - II.
[b] Mainly tuberculoma.
[c] Mainly regional tumours and metastases.

Table 4.4 World Health Organization classification of neuroepithelial tumours

Astrocytic tumours
  Astrocytoma
  Malignant astrocytoma
  Glioblastoma

Oligodendroglial tumours
  Oligodendroglioma
  Malignant oligodendroglioma

Ependymal tumours
  Ependymoma
  Malignant ependymoma
  Myxopapillary ependymoma
  Subependymoma

Mixed gliomas
  Oligoastrocytoma
  Malignant oligoastrocytoma

Choroid plexus tumours
  Choroid plexus papilloma
  Choroid plexus carcinoma

Neuronal and neuronal–glial tumours
  Gangliocytoma
  Dysplastic gangliocytoma of the cerebellum
  Desmoplastic infantile ganglioglioma
  Dysembryoplastic neuroepithelial tumour
  Ganglioglioma
  Malignant ganglioglioma
  Central neurocytoma
  Paraganglioma of the filum terminale
  Olfactory neuroblastoma

Pineal parenchymal tumours
  Pineocytoma
  Pineoblastoma[a]

Embryonal tumours
  Medulloepithelioma
  Neuroblastoma
  Ependymoblastoma
  Primitive neuroectodermal tumours
  Medulloblastoma

Simplified from Kleihues et al. (1993a).
[a] Also included with the embryonal tumours.

have a benign clinical course despite worrying histological features. Modern classifications aim to incorporate information gained by advances in immunocytochemistry and molecular biology, precisely because the morphology does not correlate well with prognosis in many of the childhood tumours. The need for accurate prognostic information is vital, because new forms of neuroimaging, image-guided stereotactic biopsy and advances in radiotherapy means that diagnosis and treatment are possible at an early stage. Long survivals are not uncommon with some tumours. However, success achieved by aggressive therapies implies the possibility of long-term side-effects on the CNS; these are discussed below (p. 201).

Neuroepithelial Tumours

Gliomas and Choroid Plexus Tumours

All varieties of gliomas are found in children. The relative frequency of the various types is different from that in adults; ependymomas are more common, oligodendrogliomas rather less so. Diffuse fibrillary astrocytomas may occur, have the same propensity as in adults to undergo anaplasia and progress to glioblastoma, and are therefore graded in the same way (see below). A number of more benign varieties, notably pilocytic astrocytomas and pleomorphic xan-

thoastrocytomas, are typically seen in children or adolescents. The topographical distribution of gliomas is different from that seen in older age groups, and brain stem tumours form a much larger proportion in children; published series suggest that they account for between 10% and 25% of all intracranial tumours in childhood (Epstein and Farmer 1993).

There are a number of inherited disorders that predispose to the development of a glioma, of which the most common are the neurofibromatoses NF-1 (Fig. 4.71) and NF-2 (p. 168). Although gliomas may be seen in both, optic nerve gliomas of the pilocytic variety are particularly common in children with NF-1 (Lund and Skovby 1991; Jenkin et al. 1993). The benign subependymal giant cell astrocytoma is asso-

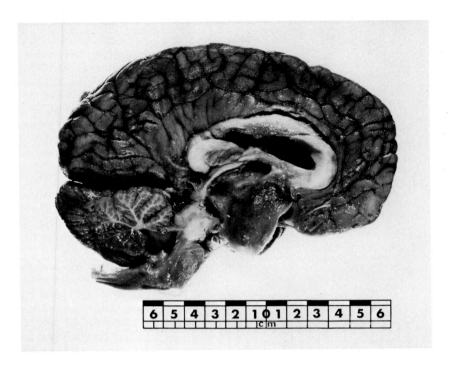

Fig. 4.71. Third ventricle astrocytoma in a patient with NF-1.

ciated almost exclusively with tuberous sclerosis (p. 166). Sufferers from rare inherited disorders such as Li–Fraumeni (Li et al. 1988; Birch 1990) and Turcot syndromes (Mastronardi et al. 1991; Tops et al. 1992) carry a greatly increased risk of developing a range of neuroepithelial tumours – gliomas, glioblastomas and medulloblastomas – and there are clearly a number of other families who have a tendency to develop primary CNS tumours (Vieregge et al. 1987; Bondy et al. 1991; Sieb et al. 1992).

Pilocytic Astrocytoma. This term principally describes a benign astrocytoma with characteristic morphology and behaviour, found predominantly in children and young adults, in whom it represents about 25% of all brain neoplasms (Zülch 1982). Historically, pilocytic astrocytomas have been classified by growth pattern into "juvenile" pilocytic astrocytoma and "diffuse" pilocytic astrocytoma (Russell and Rubinstein 1989). The latter is very much less common and is essentially a tumour of adolescents and adults, occurring in similar sites, but more akin to the infiltrative fibrillary cerebral astrocytomas, with a tendency to anaplastic transformation. The term "pilocytic" is now usually reserved for the juvenile pilocytic astrocytoma: biologically the most benign of the gliomas, it has a very slow growth rate, and long survivals are reported after surgical resection. In a personal (unpublished) case, a patient was entirely well and symptom-free 45 years after resection of a hemispheric pilocytic astrocytoma during childhood.

Classically described in the cerebellum, pilocytic astrocytomas are also to be found in the optic nerves (Fig. 4.72), chiasm and tracts, the region of the third ventricle and thalamus, and occasionally in the cerebral hemispheres and brain stem. In the optic pathways these astrocytomas are very closely associated with NF-1 (Lund and Skovby 1991), and if such a tumour is found NF-1 should be excluded by further investigation. Macroscopically, they appear well circumscribed and often present a clear plane of cleavage to the surgeon. They are commonly cystic, and may contain only a small mural nodule of tumour, the rest of the cyst wall being compressed neuropil. Considerable mass effect with displacement of adjacent structures may result from the size of the cyst.

In keeping with the biological behaviour of pilocytic astrocytoma, the histology is benign. The classical morphology (Fig. 4.73) is biphasic, compact bundles of bipolar fibrillated astrocytes interspersed between loser reticular areas populated by astrocytes with rounded nuclei possessing few fibrils. There are often large numbers of microcysts, which may coalesce to form much larger cysts, particularly in the cerebellum (Ilgren and Stiller 1987). Although the mixed pattern described above is most usual, on occasion the tumour is more homogeneous, with one of the two typical tissue types predominating over the other. Nuclei are almost invariably uniform, although

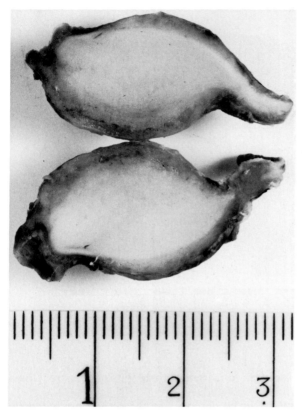

Fig. 4.72. A bisected resection specimen of optic nerve, diffusely swollen by infiltrating glioma.

not infrequently one may see atypical or even multi-nucleate forms, of no prognosfiic significance and presumed to be degenerative. Mitoses in tumour cells are not usual, and if they do occur are suggestive of anaplastic change. Blood vessels are variable: they may have markedly hyalinized walls or may demonstrate florid endothelial cell hyperplasia, in which case mitoses may be seen in proliferating vascular tissue. Active vascular proliferation appears to have no adverse significance, in contrast to its import in diffuse fibrillary astrocytomas. Additional features characteristic of, although not exclusive to, pilocytic tumours are "granular bodies" (rounded eosinophilic granular structures) and Rosenthal fibres (irregular sausage-shaped structures that appear bright red on routine haematoxylin and eosin staining, and are most common in the piloid areas). Although typically seen in both juvenile and diffuse pilocytic tumours, Rosenthal fibres may be found in a variety of other situations. They are common in areas of longstanding gliosis, for example, around syringomyelic cavities or slow-growing tumours such as craniopharyngiomas. Ultrastructural and tissue culture

studies confirm that they are astrocytic products. Granular eosinophilic bodies are also degenerative in origin, and are also thought to be produced by astrocytes. The cell of origin of the pilocytic astrocytoma is obscure. It is assumed to arise from an astrocytic population that is not normally identifiable in the CNS, because of its distinctive behaviour and cytology and the presence of Rosenthal fibres (Burger et al. 1991; VandenBerg 1992).

Astrocytomas are normally inhibited by the glial limitans externa, and do not invade the subarachnoid space (Rutka 1991). However, local invasion of the leptomeninges is very common in pilocytic astrocytomas, particularly in the cerebellum (Ilgren and Stiller 1987). Even so, spread is only local, and seeding through the CSF pathways does not occur.

Diffuse Astrocytomas. These tumours are the same as those seen in adults, occur at the same sites, and have the same tendency to undergo anaplastic change. Cytological atypia, mitoses, vascular endothelial proliferation and necrosis are all poor prognostic signs, and are the histological features that appear to bear the closest relationship to ultimate prognosis. These criteria form the basis of the Daumas-Duport (Ste Anne–Mayo) system, probably the simplest and most reliable system of grading astrocytomas currently in use, with relatively little room for interobserver variability (Daumas-Duport et al. 1988b; Kim et al. 1991). It is important, however, to understand that the use of numerical grading systems in paediatric neuro-oncology is limited, and that grading is probably of prognostic significance only when applied to diffuse hemispheric astrocytomas. Many of the other childhood brain tumours have a relatively good prognosis despite apparently worrying microscopic features, and for these tumours numerical grading is inappropriate because it would lead to overdiagnosis of anaplasia or malignancy.

Brain stem astrocytomas are extremely common in paediatric practice and largely because of their site have been assumed to have a uniformly dismal prognosis. The histology is usually that of a diffuse fibrillary astrocytoma, although pilocytic astrocytomas may occur. The pons is one of the most usual sites, where they gave rise to "pontine hypertrophy". Radiological studies, particularly MRI, have confirmed the painstaking studies of Scherer (1940), who used large whole-brain sections to show that astrocytomas preferentially invade along the anatomical pathways formed by fibre tracts, pia and ependyma, rather than by tissue destruction, at least in the early stages. It is now possible to demonstrate such growth patterns in the brain stem by neuroimaging (Epstein and Farmer 1993), and so identify lower grade astrocytomas.

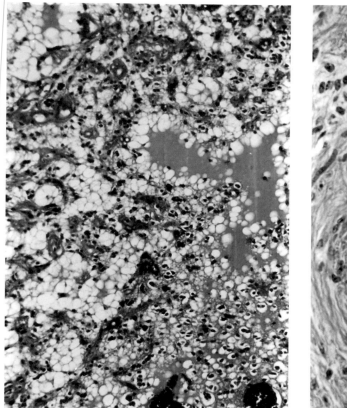
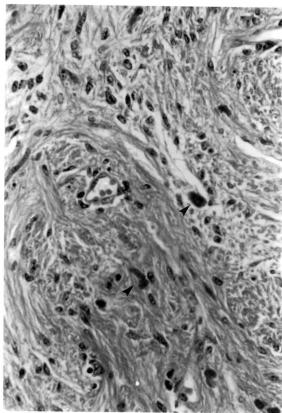

Fig. 4.73. The pilocytic astrocytoma characteristically has two histological patterns: loose cystic areas with microcysts (**a**) are interspersed with densely fibrillated tissue composed of bipolar astrocytic cells (**b**). Rosenthal bodies (*arrowheads*) are a typical feature.

Subependymal Giant Cell Astrocytoma. This is a highly distinctive entity, almost invariably seen in young patients with the tuberous sclerosis complex (Shepherd et al. 1991), which has features of both a hamartoma and a neoplasm. It is thought to arise from the subependymal nodules that typically occur in large numbers in the walls of the lateral ventricle in TS and, unlike the cortical lesions, grow steadily (Morimoto and Mogami 1986) until they become symptomatic by producing raised intracranial pressure or hydrocephalus. Calcification is common. Microscopically, the subependymal giant cell astrocytoma is identical in appearance to the subependymal nodules; its cells are usually gemistocytic, interspersed with fibrillated spindle forms and large ganglioid cells. There is variable expression GFAP. Mitoses and necrosis are not common, but if they are present appear to be of no prognostic significance (Bonnin et al. 1984; Chow et al. 1988; Shepherd et al. 1991). The tumour is entirely benign, and if it is symptomatic requires no treatment apart from

surgery, the usual cause of death being related to raised intracranial pressure. Although it has been reported as occurring infrequently in patients who have no evidence of TS (Bonnin et al. 1984), it seems likely that subependymal giant cell astrocytoma is restricted to TS (Shepherd et al. 1991; Altermatt and Scheithauer 1992) because, with increasing use of MRI, asymptomatic forms of the condition are being recognized, and it is clear that in some patients the condition may show extremely variable expression (Fryer 1991).

Pleomorphic Xanthoastrocytoma. Like the pilocytic astrocytoma, the pleomorphic xanthoastrocytoma is a distinct clinicopathological entity, with a benign course, associated in many instances with prolonged survival after surgery. First described by Kepes et al. (1979), the pleomorphic xanthoastrocytoma is an uncommon tumour seen in adolescents or young adults with a long history of seizures (Kepes 1993). It classically occurs superficially in the temporoparietal

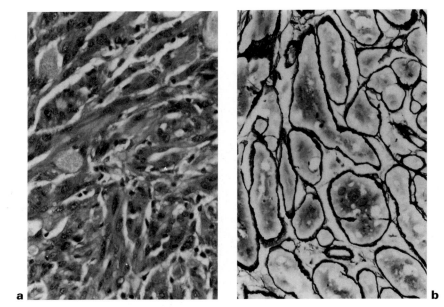

desmoplastic

Fig. 4.74. Pleomorphic xanthoastrocytoma may have a bizarre cytology (**a**), but mitoses are rare. Note the foamy cytoplasm of some of the cells. A very marked reticulin network, not normally seen in astrocytomas, is characteristic (**b**).

region, involving the leptomeninges, and may be cystic. Histologically, as the name suggests, many of the neoplastic cells show lipidization of their cytoplasm, but the characteristic of this tumour is that it displays features which in other tumours might indicate an ominous prognosis (cellular atypia and pleomorphism, with hyperchromatic, often multinucleate and giant forms), and which are curiously at variance with its characteristically benign behaviour. Mitoses are rarely seen, and if coupled with necrosis – again rare – are associated with a malignant course. Also characteristic of the tumour are a dense reticulin pattern, either pericellular or around groups of cells, and scattered collections of perivascular lymphocytes (Fig. 4.74). The tumour may in areas resemble a malignant fibrous histiocytoma, but GFAP staining confirms its astrocytic origin (Burger et al. 1991; Kros et al. 1991; Kawano 1992).

Desmoplastic Tumours of Childhood. In recent years, a number of apparently related tumours have been described, all superficial hemispheric tumours in infants, which are characterized by involvement of both dura and cortex, and which are remarkably fibrous. On histology, they are seen to be composed of dense mesenchymal tissue and a variable admixture of neuroepithelial elements, usually astrocytic, but occasionally also neurons (Taratuto et al. 1984; VandenBerg et al. 1987; Louis et al. 1992). These tumours are rare, and despite their size appear to have

a good prognosis. As more similar cases are reported, it is clear that there is a spectrum of appearances in such tumours: names like "desmoplastic superficial cerebral astrocytoma", "desmoplastic infantile ganglioglioma" and "gliofibroma" probably all describe variants of the same tumour (Paulus et al. 1992; Rushing et al. 1993; VandenBerg 1993).

Glioblastoma. Formerly grouped with the embryonal tumours, glioblastomas are now classified as the most malignant grade of diffuse fibrillary astrocytoma, most often arising as the result of anaplastic change in a lower grade tumour. Clinically and pathologically, however, there have long been grounds for suspecting that there are various subtypes of glioblastoma, including tumours that arise de novo (Russell and Rubinstein 1989), rather than from a pre-existing astrocytoma. Recent studies using techniques of molecular genetic analysis have appeared to confirm this (Kleihues et al. 1993b; von Deimling et al. 1993), and it may soon be possible to define clinically significant subtypes of glioblastoma. Although these highly malignant gliomas are common in adults, they are rare in children, accounting for only 5.3% of intracranial tumours in Luo's series of 2000 children (Luo et al. 1992). The morphological features are the same as those seen in the adult tumours: they are obviously malignant neoplasms which, despite being poorly differentiated, betray their astrocytic origins, and are at least partly

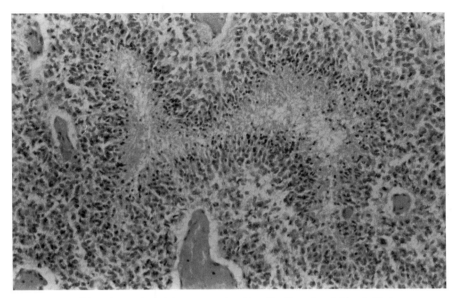

Fig. 4.75. A focus of serpiginous necrosis with palisading of nuclei in glioblastoma.

GFAP positive. Rarely, there is evidence of oligodendroglial differentiation. Cellular atypia, high mitotic rate (although mitoses are never as frequent as in epithelial tumours), proliferation and heaping up of endothelial cells in tumour vessels, and necrosis – classically described as "serpiginous" with palisading of nuclei around the edge of necrotic foci (Fig. 4.75) – are characteristic. Often, however, the necrosis is extensive, and a reticulin stain is helpful in demonstrating the underlying glioma architecture where viable cells are few in number and difficult to identify. Childhood glioblastoma has the same extremely poor prognosis as in adults.

Ependymal Tumours. Ependymomas (Fig. 4.76) are tumours composed predominantly of neoplastic

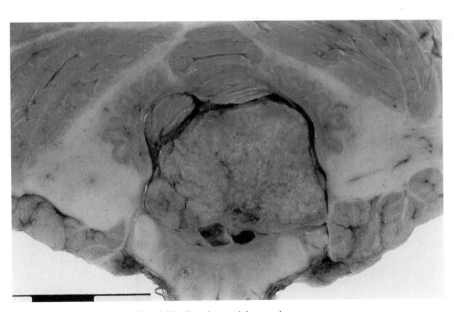

Fig. 4.76. Fourth ventricle ependymoma.

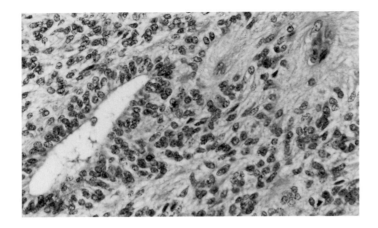

Fig. 4.77. Ependymoma displaying both epithelial and glial features: on the left a tubule, on the right a fibrillated stroma, with two typical perivascular "pseudo-rosettes".

ependyma, the neuroectodermal lining of the ventricular system and the central canal of the spinal cord. They occur at all ages of life, although they are particularly frequent in children, when they tend to present in the posterior fossa and produce hydrocephalus. In a recent review of a series of 298 ependymomas and subependymomas, Schiffer et al. (1991) found that infratentorial tumours, anaplastic variants and subependymomas predominated in children under 4 years of age, spinal tumours were most common in adults, and supratentorial tumours were to be found in all age groups. Although ependymomas are generally histologically benign, the prognosis is not always good (Sutton et al. 1990–91; Schiffer et al. 1991; Chiu et al. 1992), partly because of the site at which they arise, and partly because of their tendency to seed through the neuraxis.

Intriguingly, there appears to be little correlation between histological features and biological behaviour, and the criteria used for diagnosing anaplasia in astrocytomas may not be applicable to ependymomas (Ross and Rubinstein 1989; Sutton et al. 1990–91; Schiffer et al. 1991). The morphological classification of ependymomas currently divides them into ependymoma (which may be cellular, papillary or clear cell), anaplastic ependymoma, myxopapillary ependymoma and subependymoma (Kleihues et al. 1993a). The myxopapillary variant, being almost exclusively found in the region of the cauda equina, is rare in children (Schiffer et al. 1991). Histologically ependymomas express both glial and epithelial features, although most have a strongly glial appearance with variable GFAP expression. There is a tendency in most tumours for the cells to have a perivascular arrangement; the fibrillated cell processes converge on the vessels, thereby creating an eosinophilic cell-free perivascular zone, or "pseudo-rosette", which is particularly striking at low power (Fig. 4.77). True rosettes, in the form of

epithelial acini and tubules in which luminal cells bear cilia, are less commonly seen, but are characteristic, and can be helpful when found in what appears to be a mainly glial tumour. *Subependymomas*, often thought to be hamartomatous rather than neoplastic, are a distinctive variant. They project into ventricles as nodules, often multiple, that show little invasive tendency. Larger symptomatic lesions tend to be more common in childhood, and tumours that appear to be transitional between ependymoma and subependymoma are frequent. Classically, the subependymoma is a fibrillated but poorly cellular tumour, strongly GFAP positive, with a characteristic appearance at low power in which small collections of ependymal cells are randomly scattered through a dense network of fibres. Degenerative changes include haemorrhage and cyst formation. As in juvenile pilocytic astrocytomas, occasional "degenerative" atypical nuclei may be encountered, but mitoses are not usual in subependymomas. Both the general appearances and the tumour cells are reminiscent of the ependymal granulations ("granular ependymitis"), proliferation of subependymal glial cells that characteristically results from ventricular inflammation or chronic hydrocephalus (Nag 1991).

An ependymoma is termed malignant when it shows features of glial anaplasia: increased cellularity, nuclear atypia and pleomorphism, marked mitotic activity, necrosis and endothelial proliferation (Kleihues et al. 1993a). Recent reports, however, have suggested that these histological parameters do not always identify the clinically aggressive tumours (Schiffer et al. 1991), and that correlation with survival is not clear cut (Ross and Rubinstein 1989). Ependymomas do not appear to progress to glioblastoma very commonly (Zülch 1986). Recent pathological reviews of ependymal tumours include those of Schiffer et al. (1991), Chiu et al. (1992), Schofield (1992) and Geyer (1992). The term "ependymoblastoma" is reserved for a primitive neuroectodermal tumour showing some ependymal differentiation, and should not be given to ependymomas showing malignant features.

Oligodendrogliomas. These are essentially tumours of adults, although they are occasionally seen in children, when deep structures such as the thalamus tend to be involved. Posterior fossa or spinal cord oligodendrogliomas are unusual at any age. Calcification is very common, as is spontaneous haemorrhage into the tumour, which may cause sudden coma or a stroke-like picture. Histologically, sheets of round cells with little cytoplasm and nuclei with two or three condensations of chromatin are characteristic. There may be a perinuclear clear space which is an artefact of processing and which gives the tumour cells the well-known "fried egg" appearance. The vascular pattern of the oligodendroglioma is typically one of delicate branching capillaries, and so a reticulin stain on these tumours may be diagnostically helpful, especially when the cells lack perinuclear vacuolation. Note that some oligodendrogliomas contain cells with red cytoplasm which are GFAP positive, but the nuclei still have the characteristic appearances of oligodendroglia rather than of astrocytes. Equally, it is increasingly realized that few oligodendrogliomas are "pure" – that is to say, that there may be an admixture of reactive astrocytes, and some tumours may contain significant numbers of neoplastic astrocytes, either intermingled with the oligodendrocytes or as frank foci of astrocytoma. The most recent edition of the WHO classification of brain tumours (Kleihues et al. 1993a) has recognized the *mixed gliomas*, principally the *oligoastrocytoma*, as a separate tumour type, although the clinical significance of this diagnostic distinction is not yet certain. Oligodendrogliomas have generally been believed to be more slow growing than diffuse cerebral astrocytomas, with a more benign clinical course, although modern analyses of survival data from such patients suggests that this may not be the case (Mørk et al. 1985; Ludwig et al. 1986). It is not entirely established which histological criteria best predict clinical course: the presence of features such as nuclear atypia, mitoses and endothelial proliferation was not of prognostic significance in the study of 208 oligodendroglial tumours from the Cancer Registry of Norway (Mørk et al. 1986), although others have found the Daumas-Duport criteria (Daumas-Duport et al. 1988b) for diffuse astrocytomas, which use precisely these features combined with necrosis, to be helpful in relation to prediction of outcome (Shaw et al. 1992). Ludwig et al. (1986) graded 323 oligodendrogliomas according to the presence or absence of high cell density, pleomor-

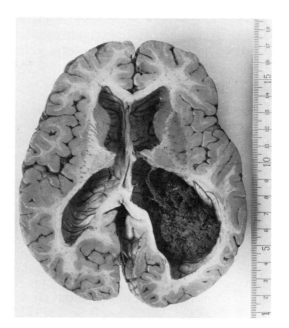

Fig. 4.78. Choroid plexus papilloma.

phism, high nuclear/cytoplasmic ratio, endothelial proliferation and necrosis, and were able to define a grading system that related to prognosis.

Choroid Plexus Tumours. These arise wherever choroid plexus is to be found, the lateral ventricles being the most usual site in children. They are usually papillomas (Fig. 4.78), and are characteristically paediatric tumours, 48% occurring under the age of 10 years in Matson and Crofton's large series (1960). They are large and soft, and are often described as having a cauliflower appearance. Initially they expand within the ventricle and tend to compress adjacent structures in the brain, rather than genuinely invade. Microscopically, their structure recalls that of the normal choroid plexus, and diagnosis is not usually difficult. The papillae are formed of single-layered columnar non-ciliated epithelium, surrounding a fibrovascular core quite different from the glial stroma seen in a papillary ependymoma, which is the main differential diagnosis. Mitoses are not common and are generally a sign of aggressive behaviour. The tumours may express both GFAP and epithelial markers. Their malignant equivalent, the choroid plexus carcinoma, is extremely rare. It is exclusively a tumour of children, and the diagnosis of choroid plexus carcinoma should not be made in adults (Okazaki and Scheithauer 1988; Russell and Rubinstein 1989). Carcinomatous change in a papilloma is recognized by obviously malignant histological features such as loss of papillary architecture, heaping up of the epithelium, nuclear pleomorphism, increased numbers of mitoses and invasion of brain tissue.

Embryonal, Neuronal, Neuronal–Glial and Pineal Tumours

Many of these tumours, though by no means all, are densely cellular embryonal tumours of the CNS, which may or may not show focal evidence of differentiation. Much controversy has been generated by the suggestion that all small blue-celled tumours in children should be classified as "primitive neuroectodermal tumours" (PNETs) (Rorke 1983; Rorke et al. 1985), thereby creating a large diagnostic ragbag of more or less undiagnosable malignant small-cell tumours, into which well recognized entities such as medulloblastoma, cerebral neuroblastoma and so on would be subsumed (Burger and Fuller 1991). The consensus expressed in the latest WHO classification is that the term PNET should be used in a highly restricted sense: that of "primitive neuroectodermal tumour with divergent differentiation" – in other words, a poorly differentiated tumour that shows differentiation along a number of unrelated cell lines.

Medulloblastoma. Although belonging to the embryonal tumours, medulloblastoma is a well recognized entity with highly characteristic clinicopathological features (Tomlinson et al. 1992a, b). For this reason, despite the fact that a cell corresponding to the "medulloblast" has not been identified, the name persists and the tumour is considered to be distinct from other PNETs (Kleihues et al. 1993a). After the astrocytoma, it is the most common CNS tumour in children, accounting for around 20% of intracranial neoplasms (see Table 4.3). A recent population study of 532 cases (Roberts et al. 1991) showed that 77% of patients with medulloblastoma were less than 19 years old at diagnosis; the mean age at presentation was 7.3 years. Males are more commonly affected than females in virtually all studies published. A number of inherited conditions have been identified in which medulloblastoma commonly occurs: these include ataxia–telangiectasia, xeroderma pigmentosum, Turcot and Li–Fraumeni syndromes, and the multiple basal cell naevi syndrome of Gorlin. The question of familial medulloblastoma, including twins concordant for the tumour, has been reviewed by Tijssen (1986).

In children, the medulloblastoma is typically found posteriorly in the midline of the cerebellar vermis, whereas in adults there is a tendency for it to be more

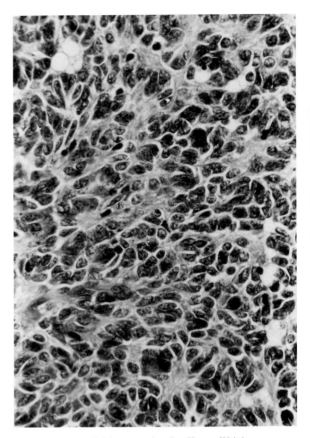

Fig. 4.79. Medulloblastoma, showing Homer Wright rosettes.

laterally sited in the hemispheres. Macroscopically, the tumour is often apparently demarcated from the brain. Except for the hemispheric tumours, which tend to be hard because they contain fibrous tissue which derives from meningeal involvement, medulloblastomas are usually soft. They may show areas of haemorrhage, but not usually calcification. Tumour spread through the subarachnoid space over the surface of cerebellum is common, and may obscure the normal folial pattern, giving a smooth appearance to the folia. Microscopically, this is classically an undifferentiated tumour, composed of sheets of small cells with hyperchromatic round, elongated or carrot-shaped nuclei, usually with very little cytoplasm. Mitoses vary in frequency. Medulloblastomas show a marked capacity for divergent differentiation, usually along neuroblastic or glial lines, rarely towards striated muscle or pigmented neuroepithelium. Neuroblastic differentiation is evident in the characteristic Homer Wright rosettes (Fig. 4.79), in which cell nuclei are grouped round a central fibrillary area which lacks a lumen and may show positivity for

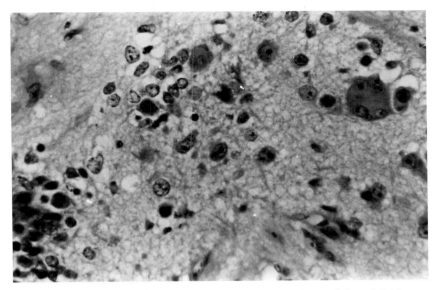

Fig. 4.80. Rarely, a medulloblastoma shows advanced neuronal differentiation: at the bottom left, medulloblastoma cells; left of centre, cells with larger vesicular nuclei have the appearance of neuroblasts; to the right, a number of ganglion cells, including one multinucleate form.

neuronal markers, and neurofibrils can sometimes be demonstrated with classic silver stains. On occasion, more advanced neuronal differentiation is seen, and the cells resemble neuroblasts, with large round pale nuclei and a single nucleolus, set in a fibrillated background. Rarely, differentiation of neuroblasts into recognizable if abnormal ganglion cells is seen (Fig. 4.80), and then the term "cerebellar ganglioneuroblastoma" may be appropriate. A histological variant of medulloblastoma, more common in adults, is the desmoplastic variety, again composed of small dark cells interspersed with nodules of paler cells, which at low power resemble lymphoid follicles. Between the nodules there is a rich intercellular reticulin pattern. Both glial and more usually neuronal markers have been found to be expressed in the islands or nodules. Astrocytic differentiation may be found in medulloblastomas and confirmed by GFAP immunostaining, when the distinction between entrapped reactive astrocytes and genuine maturation of tumour cells into astrocytes can usually be appreciated on morphological grounds.

Medulloblastomas show a marked propensity to seed through CSF pathways, which means that it is one of the few intrinsic CNS tumours in which cytology of the CSF may produce a dignosis. Spread through the cerebrospinal pathways results in "drop metastases" throughout the CSF, and tumour may eventually ensheath the spinal cord completely. Treatment is always given to the entire neuroaxis because of this tendency to CSF dissemination. Unlike other nervous system tumours, medulloblastomas may metastasize outside the CNS, spreading to bone, lymph nodes and soft tissues, usually after surgery or shunting procedures rather than spontaneously.

The histogenesis of medulloblastoma is uncertain. The most likely, but unproven, origin is the external granular cell layer of the cerebellum, which is formed in the fetus from primitive cells that migrate from the roof of the fourth ventricle and spread over the surface of the cerebellar cortex. During the first year of postnatal life this layer involutes steadily as cells migrate from it to their definitive site in the internal granular cell layer. Cases of congenital medulloblastoma in which neoplastic proliferation of the fetal granular cell layer was a prominent feature (discussed by Russell and Rubinstein 1989, pp. 251–254) would support an origin in the external granular layer, but other cell populations have been proposed. Most recently, heterotopic cell collections in the cerebellum ("dysplasias"), which are found in 85% of otherwise normal neonatal brains (Yachnis et al. 1994), have been suggested. The question of histogenesis has been comprehensively reviewed by Tomlinson et al. (1992a). Much work has been done on both cytogenetics and molecular genetics of medulloblastoma, also reviewed by Tomlinson. Culture and establishment of human medulloblastoma cell lines is difficult, and there are relatively few such lines that are well characterized. The principal animal model is a JC polyoma virus-induced tumour in hamsters (ZuRhein and Varakis 1979; Takakura et al. 1987).

Medulloepithelioma, Cerebral Neuroblastoma, Ependymoblastoma, Pineoblastoma. These are all extremely rare, highly malignant embryonal tumours that occur in very young children, generally under 5 years of age (Horten and Rubinstein 1976; Gangemi et al. 1987; Caccamo et al. 1989; Russell and Rubinstein 1989). Medulloepithelioma is distinctive in that its architecture closely resembles that of the epithelium of the neural tube; cerebral neuroblastoma is a diffuse highly cellular hemispheric tumour composed of neuroblasts, usually showing a degree of neuronal differentiation, identified either by the presence of Homer–Wright rosettes or by expression of neuronal markers such as synaptophysin on immunocytochemistry. Occasionally, neuroblastomas show focal tumour cell maturation to ganglion cells, but these do not improve the prognosis. Ependymoblastoma shows characteristic ependymal differentiation in the form of ependymal rosettes, whereas pineoblastoma may have neuroblastic rosette formation and be indistinguishable from a medulloblastoma apart from its location in the pineal gland.

Tumours Composed of Differentiated or Partially Differentiated Neuronal Cells. Although infrequent in terms of the overall incidence of CNS tumours, these occur relatively commonly in children (Russell and Rubinstein 1989). Many of the embryonal tumours discussed above may show neuronal differentiation, but the true tumours composed of neuronal cells are the gangliocytoma, ganglioglioma, central neurocytoma, olfactory neuroblastoma and the unfortunately termed dysembryoplastic neuroepithelial tumour. Unlike the embryonal tumours, which are generally highly malignant, these entities tend not to be biologically aggressive, and have a good prognosis. To confirm the diagnosis of a neuronal tumour, one must establish that any ganglion cells present are not remnants of a normal population of infiltrated cells. Neoplastic ganglion cells will be abnormally shaped and abnormally orientated and grouped: they may on occasion be binucleate or multinucleate, but further diagnostic features are abnormal distribution of Nissl substance, and a typical perikaryal surface immunoreactivity with synaptophysin (Miller et al. 1993). Another typical feature of a neuronal tumour is desmoplasia, and abundant collagen production may be seen around atypical ganglion cells, which are often arranged in lobules. As their name suggests, *gangliocytomas* are calcified slow-growing tumours composed entirely of mature ganglion cells, with no evidence of neoplastic change in the surrounding tissue. Their incidence is not well established, although they are relatively rare, forming only 0.4% in Zülch's series of 9000 tumours (1986). The so-

called "dysplastic gangliocytoma" of the cerebellum (Lhermitte–Duclos disease) is a distinct subtype that occurs in adolescents and young adults, where, in a relatively circumscribed area of cerebellum, the folia are thickened and their normal architecture distorted by intracortical accumulation of large numbers of abnormal ganglion cells. This rare lesion has several features of a malformation, but produces symptoms of a slowly expanding lesion, and for that reason tends to come to surgery. Megalencephaly may occur in association with Lhermitte–Duclos disease.

There is probably some overlap between gangliocytomas and *gangliogliomas*. Because of the neoplastic glial component, gangliogliomas grow faster than the gangliocytomas, and are more likely to produce symptoms. Recent work using specific antisera to neuronal markers in a large retrospective series has suggested that the frequency of gangliogliomas may be as high as 10.7% of paediatric CNS tumours, compared with 0.7% of adult neoplasms (Miller et al. 1993). They are characteristically seen in the temporal lobe of young patients, but intramedullary cord and brain stem gangliogliomas are also common (Epstein and Farmer 1993; Miller et al. 1993). Once again, there is very often connective tissue proliferation around islands of neuronal cells, and the glial element is generally that of a low-grade astrocytoma (Mickle 1992). However, malignant change in the astrocytoma can occur, although most authors do not find as large a proportion of malignant tumours as Miller. Long survival after surgical resection is usual after gangliogliomas, and the grade of the astrocytic elements does not appear to correlate well with prognosis (Miller et al. 1993). The desmoplastic infantile ganglioglioma is believed to be related to the desmoplastic cerebral astrocytoma, also seen in infants, and discussed above.

Central neurocytoma was recognized relatively recently, and in many cases was probably formerly diagnosed as an intraventricular oligodendroglioma or neuroblastoma, or as an "ependymoma of the foramen of Monro" (Hassoun et al. 1993). It is a well circumscribed intraventricular tumour, so far reported almost exclusively in adolescents and young adults. Cells are uniform, round and resemble oligodendroglia on routine stains. However, on electron microscopy, the tumour cells contain many dense-cored neurosecretory granules, and are now recognized to be small-cell neuronal elements rather than glial cells. Typically, they sit in a stroma that resembles neuropil and stains positively for synaptophysin. The principal differential diagnosis is oligodendroglioma or ependymoma, and the diagnosis of a neuronal tumour is confirmed by synaptophysin immunostains (Hassoun et al. 1993). It appears that the prognosis for this tumour is good in the younger patients (Figarella-Branger et al. 1992; Yuen et al. 1992).

Olfactory neuroblastoma may very rarely present as an intracranial tumour, as a result of spread through the cribriform plate, (see p. 869).

Dysembryoplastic neuroepithelial tumour is yet another distinctive lesion of young patients, surgically curable, and characteristically associated with a history of medically intractable complex partial seizures. First described by Daumas-Duport et al. (1988a), this lesion is now found to be relatively common in centres where epilepsy surgery is performed. The somewhat cumbersome title was given to indicate an association with developmental anomalies, manifest by the frequent finding of adjacent areas of dysplastic cortex. The importance of recognizing this entity is that resection, even if incomplete, appears to cure the seizures. The tumour does not recur, and more aggressive forms of treatment are unnecessary. The histology is of a multinodular intracortical tumour, which at first glance appears to be an oligoastrocytoma with admixed neurons or a ganglioglioma. The histology of this distinctive lesion is discussed in detail by Daumas-Duport (1993). Increasing use of MRI for the investigation of children with epilepsy has led to the recognition of small lesions, often impossible to classify according to existing schemes, in which the distinction between hamartoma and neoplasm is extremely difficult to make. It is important to be aware of this problem to avoid overdiagnosis, and possibly overtreatment, of such well-differentiated lesions.

Pineal Tumours. These are rare at any age, and the most common tumour at this site is a germ cell tumour (see below). The tumour that arises from true pineal cells in children is the malignant embryonal tumour, the pineoblastoma, histologically identical to the medulloblastoma, with the same propensity to seed via CSF pathways. Any tumour in the pineal region will produce hydrocephalus by obstruction to CSF flow at the level of the aqueduct.

Maldevelopmental Tumours and Tumour-like Lesions

Craniopharyngiomas occur in the region of the optic chiasm, mainly in children and young adults. In western countries they represent about 6% of paediatric intracranial tumours (Jellinger and Machacek 1982), but the incidence appears to be higher in the Far East, where they account for as many as 16.6% of tumours in children under 16 (Luo et al. 1992). A craniopharyngioma generally arises above the pituitary sella and grows upwards from the basal cisterns to involve the third ventricle. Less commonly, it extends through the sella or is entirely situated in the pituitary fossa. (See Fig. 4.81). It grows slowly and produces symptoms by compression of adjacent structures: headaches, visual disturbances, hypopituitarism and hydrocephalus are all common. The tumour may be solid, but is very commonly cystic and contains a viscous yellow-brown fluid glistening with cholesterol crystals, which is traditionally likened to motor oil. Focal calcification is common. Histologically it is an epithelial tumour, composed of bands or islands of squamous epithelium. The outer epithelial cells tend to form a pallisading basal columnar layer, while the central areas of these zones degenerate. Intercellular prickles become prominent, and the epithelial cells may appear stellate with an oedematous loose-textured background; it is this epithelium that is termed "adamantinomatous", as it resembles epithelium in the enamel organ of the tooth. Nodules of keratin may be formed. Both adamantinomatous epithelium and keratin nodules are features that are diagnostic of a craniopharyngioma, which may be helpful in a small biopsy where the main differential diagnosis is that of an epidermoid cyst. A considerable diagnostic trap for the unwary is that brain adjacent to a craniopharyngioma characteristically shows vigorous reactive gliosis, including Rosenthal fibre formation, which may be sufficiently florid to mimic a low-grade astrocytoma. In some craniopharyngiomas, examination of the gliotic surrounding brain shows small islands of apparently invasive tumour cells detached from the main tumour (Fig. 4.82). This behaviour does not indicate malignant change, but does mean that there may not be a plane of cleavage at surgery, so that total surgical excision may not be readily achieved and the tumour will recur. The origin of craniopharyngiomas and their relationship to Rathke's cleft cysts and suprasellar epidermoid cysts is uncertain: although all three lesions, in classic sites and displaying classic histological features, are entirely distinct, transitional forms between one type and another do occur, and in the absence of characteristic histological features a definitive diagnosis may not be possible. A small minority of craniopharyngiomas are papillary in type and lack adamantinomatous features. These occur in older patients: they are well circumscribed and not locally invasive; possibly for that reason they tend to have a better prognosis.

Intracranial *epidermoid cysts* are considerably less common than craniopharyngiomas in children. The cerebellopontine angle and parasellar regions are the usual sites. The epidermoid cyst wall is composed of

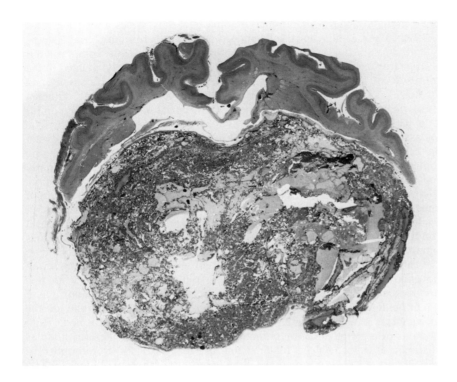

Fig. 4.81. Craniopharyngioma invading the brain, from a stillborn infant. (Courtesy of Professor E. Wildi)

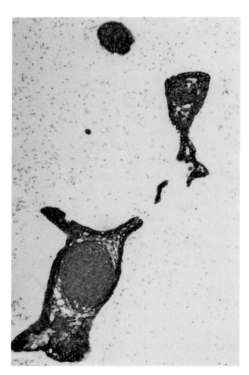

Fig. 4.82. It is common with craniopharyngiomas to find tumour infiltrating the surrounding brain, which is heavily gliotic. Here a number of tumour islands are stained by the cytokeratin marker MNF-116.

a thin outer layer of collagen, inside which lies keratinizing stratified squamous epithelium, often considerably attenuated. The lumen of the cyst is generally filled with flaky keratin, which macroscopically has a cheesy appearance and microscopically has a delicate lamellar formation, in contrast to the nodular type of keratinization that is seen in craniopharyngiomas. Craniospinal *dermoid cysts*, which are no different from dermoid cysts elsewhere in the body, are extremely rare in children.

Germ Cell Tumours

Primary intracranial germ cell tumours, which characteristically occur in children and adolescents, are rare, and the sites at which they are found are relatively inaccessible for the surgeon, so that until the advent of image-guided stereotactic biopsy published series with tissue diagnosis were small. If a tumour showed a dramatic response to a trial of radiation, biopsy was often not considered necessary (Oi and Matsumoto 1992). The germ cell tumours are usually found in the midline, principally in the pineal or suprasellar regions, and not infrequently in both sites at once (Burger et al. 1991; Sugiyama et al. 1992). The fourth ventricle and intrasellar, spinal thalamic and basal ganglia are much rarer locations (Russell and Rubinstein 1989). Germ cell neoplasms are presumed

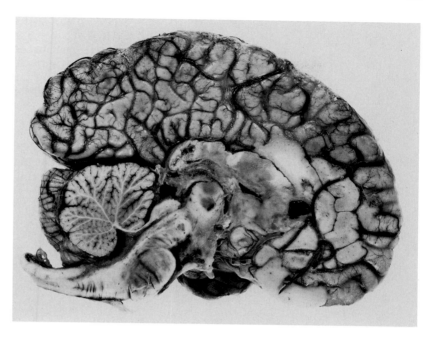

Fig. 4.83. Sagittal section through the brain of a 15-year-old boy, showing diffuse extension of a pineal germinoma through the third ventricle and into the corpus callosum. (Courtesy of Dr J.E. McLaughlin)

to originate from ectopic primordial germ cells, arrested during their migration through embryonic tissues. The tumours that occur in the brain are similar to germ cell tumours found elsewhere in the body, and the same classification system is applied, with the difference that the term germinoma is used rather than seminoma. All series of germ cell tumours show a marked male preponderance, generally about 2 : 1. For the pineal region neoplasms the proportion of males may be higher: according to Russell and Rubinstein (1989), 90% of their 45 pineal tumours occurred in males. Tumours of the pineal region present with symptoms suggestive of raised intracranial pressure, and gaze palsies. The mass compresses the aqueduct, causing hydrocephalus, and the resultant pressure on the pretectal area of the midbrain causes a conjugate upward gaze paralysis, combined with pupillary abnormalities. Germ cell tumours of the suprasellar region, on the other hand, give rise to diabetes insipidus, hypopituitarism and visual disturbances.

The largest recent series is that of Felix and Becker (1990), who performed a retrospective study of 1474 childhood brain tumours and found primary intracranial germ cell tumours in 49 patients (3.3%), 65% of which were germinomas. This is in agreement with other authors: Plantaz et al. (1992) have described 35 cases, of which 70% were germinomas, and in the series of Shen et al. (1992) germinomas comprised 78% of the 19 cases reported. Teratoma is the next most common tumour, particularly in the Far East (Oi et al. 1990; Russell and Rubinstein 1989), and in some series the most common neonatal tumour

(Buetow et al. 1990). Endodermal sinus tumours, embryonal tumours and choriocarcinomas may all be found, but are extremely rare.

Of all these tumours, the *germinoma* (Fig. 4.83) is most likely to occur in a pure form, in the absence of other germ cell elements. It is very often a well circumscribed tumour, and histologically is identical to the classic testicular seminoma (Fig. 4.84). It is composed of sheets or lobules of large round or polygonal cells with pale glycogen-rich cytoplasm and well defined cytoplasmic borders, a vesicular nucleus and prominent nucleolus. Connective tissue trabeculae intersect the lobules of cells. Characteristic of germinomas is a prominent non-neoplastic lymphocytic infiltrate, which may include variable numbers of plasma cells. For some reason suprasellar tumours appear to excite a particularly florid inflammatory response, to such an extent that this component may predominate over tumour cells. On occasion, multiple non-caseating giant cell granulomas, often containing sarcoid-like inclusions, or even reactive lymphoid follicles, may be seen. Such an inflammatory reaction may create enormous diagnostic problems in a small biopsy and, if the characteristic large tumour cells are not identified, CNS sarcoid may be considered, particularly because the favoured anatomical sites in both conditions are similar (Peeples et al. 1991), although neurosarcoid is improbable in a child. If neoplastic cells are not identified on routine stains, periodic acid–Schiff and placental alkaline phosphatase immunostains are invariably positive in germinoma tumour cells. Cytokeratin expression has

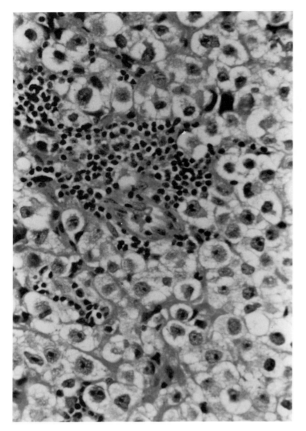

Fig. 4.84. The germinoma is identical to the testicular seminoma.

(1991), the anatomical features (demonstrated by MRI) of a pineal teratoma in a 20-year-old male suggested that the tumour must have arisen before 4 months of gestation. From comparison of an enormous series of 245 neonatal teratomas (presenting before 2 months of age) with 174 similar tumours occurring later in childhood, Wakai (1989) has concluded that there are two peaks in the age distribution of intracranial teratoma, one in the neonatal period and one at around 10 years of age. He points out that the neonatal teratomas differ from those in childhood in that they principally arise in the frontal region and lateral ventricle, whereas teratomas in older children are more likely to be situated in the pineal region. Comparison of the histological features of the two tumour groups leads Wakai to suggest that they are of different origin – that intracranial teratomas in the neonate represent fetus-in-fetu (included twins), whereas the childhood variety arises from germ cells. Histologically they may be differentiated or undifferentiated, and very often include other germ cell elements.

Nerve Sheath Tumours

For all practical purposes, these tumours are seen only in children with neurofibromatosis, when the appearances are identical to those of schwannomas and neurofibromas in adults. Malignant change in neurofibromas is a feature of NF-1.

been reported in some tumours (Russell and Rubinstein 1989; Felix and Becker 1990), and occasional large syncytiotrophoblastic cells may show positivity for human chorionic gonadotrophin, but these do not mean that the tumour is a choriocarcinoma. Alpha-fetoprotein staining is always negative. Germinomas spread readily through CSF pathways (which may lead to tumour cells being found in CSF samples), and synchronous tumours, or metastases at different intracerebral sites, are well recognized. The presence of extraembryonic differentiation into trophoblast or yolk sac elements is characteristic of *choriocarcinoma* or *endodermal sinus tumour*, and not infrequently features of different germ cell tumour types are seen in the same neoplasm. The usual site is the pineal, closely followed by the suprasellar region.

Teratomas, composed of a mixture of tissue types representative of all three germ cell layers, are more common. Fetal cases (Wakai 1989; Kuller et al. 1991) have been reported, and even prenatal diagnosis (Daita et al. 1989; Ferreira et al. 1993). In an interesting case report by Sekhon and Morgan

Meningeal Tumours

Meningiomas are rare in children. When they occur, they are found in similar sites as adult meningiomas, preferentially in the supratentorial compartment. The only difference between childhood and adult meningiomas is that the female predominance seen in older patients does not occur – if anything, meningiomas occur slightly more frequently in boys (Germano et al. 1994). The classification is the same as in adults (Kleihues et al. 1993a). Note that the "angioblastic meningioma" is now acknowledged to be a meningeal haemangiopericytoma. Some authors have suggested that a sclerosing variant exists, peculiar to children (Davidson and Hope 1989), but it seems likely that this is what is now termed the clear-cell meningioma, which is prone to undergo extensive collagenization (Scheithauer 1990). One type of meningioma which, though uncommon, may be seen in younger patients, is the papillary meningioma, characterized by foci of perivascular pseudopapillary formations in a tumour that is otherwise an ordinary meningioma. Areas of papillarity in a meningioma are indicative of aggressive behaviour, and such tumours are considered to be malignant (Scheithauer 1990).

Lymphoma and Leukaemia

Primary cerebral lymphoma is essentially a tumour of adults, and is very rarely seen in children (Hochberg and Miller 1988; Russell and Rubinstein 1989). Systemic non-Hodgkin lymphoma may secondarily involve the CNS, usually causing lymphomatous meningeal infiltration (wrongly referred to as meningitis), with tumour spreading through the subarachnoid space. The brain parenchyma is generally spared, even late in the disease. Similar infiltration of the leptomeninges by leukaemic infiltrate is a well recognized feature of relapse in acute lymphoblastic leukaemia, where cranial and spinal nerve roots as well as the brain parenchyma may also be involved.

Effects of Irradiation and Chemotherapy

The side-effects of irradiation to the neuraxis are not inconsiderable, particularly in children. They may present early, in the first few months following treatment, or be delayed. Early damage appears to involve white matter, and consists of disseminated foci of demyelination superficially resembling multiple sclerosis, often with a degree of axonal damage as well. Vessels show perivascular lymphocytic cuffing. Delayed effects may occur months to several years after treatment (Russell and Rubinstein 1989), the most serious being necrosis secondary to vascular damage, which may present clinically with symptoms of an acute mass lesion in the brain, posing the question of whether this is recurrence of the original tumour. More generalized sequelae in children who have had irradiation at an early age include cognitive defects and learning difficulties, which may be severe, and pituitary damage leading to failure of growth hormone production with resultant short stature (Kanev et al. 1991). Second CNS tumours following treatment for a tumour are increasingly recognized: in a retrospective study of 9720 children treated for acute lymphoblastic leukaemia, Neglia et al. (1991) found 43 second neoplasms, 24 of which were CNS tumours, developing after craniospinal irradiation. Chemotherapy, both systemic and intrathecal, may have a variety of adverse effects on the CNS, which are reviewed by Schochet and Nelson (1990). In particular, high-dose intrathecal methotrexate combined with radiotherapy, used in childhood leukaemia, may have profound delayed effects on cerebral white matter, producing a diffuse

necrotizing encephalomyelopathy, the pathology being maximal in the white matter (Russell and Rubinstein 1989) and consisting of multiple foci of necrosis, often confluent. Demyelination may be seen in less severely affected areas of the white matter, and the cellular reaction consists principally of microglia, lipid-laden macrophages and reactive astrocytes.

References

Adams J (1992) Head injury. In: Adams JH, Duchen LW (eds) Greenfield's neuropathology, 5th edn. Edward Arnold, London

Allen I, Brankin B (1993) Pathogenesis of multiple sclerosis – the immune diathesis and the role of viruses. J Neuropathol Exp Neurol 52: 95

Allen IV, Kirk J (1992) Demyelinating diseases. In: Adams JH, Duchen LW (eds) Greenfield's neuropathology, 5th edn. Edward Arnold, London

Altermatt HJ, Scheithauer BW (1992) Cytomorphology of subependymal giant cell astrocytoma. Acta Cytol 36: 171

Altman J (1994) Microglia emerge from the fog. Trends Neurosci 17: 47

Altman N, Naidich TP, Braffman BH (1992) Posterior fossa malformations. AJNR Am J Neuroradiol 13: 691

Armstrong DD (1993) The neuropathology of temporal lobe epilepsy. J Neuropathol Exp Neurol 52: 433

Ashwal S, Tomasi L, Schneider S, Perkin R, Thompson J (1992) Bacterial meningitis in children: pathophysiology and treatment. Neurology 42: 739

Auer RN, Hugh J, Cosgrove E, Curry B (1989) Neuropathologic findings in three cases of profound hypoglycemia. Clin Neuropathol 8: 63

Baraitser M (1990) The genetics of neurological disorders, 2nd edn. Oxford University Press, Oxford

Barkovich AJ (1990) Pediatric neuroimaging. Contemporary neuroimaging. Raven Press, New York

Barkovich AJ, Gressens P, Evrard P (1992a) Formation, maturation, and disorders of brain neocortex. AJNR Am J Neuroradiol 13: 423

Barkovich AJ, Lyon G, Evrard P (1992b) Formation, maturation, and disorders of white matter. AJNR Am J Neuroradiol 13: 447

Barkovich AJ, Good WV, Koch TK, Berg BO (1993) Mitochondrial disorders: analysis of their clinical and imaging characteristics. AJNR Am J Neuroradiol 14: 1119

Barth PG (1987) Disorders of neuronal migration. Can J Neurol Sci 14: 1

Becker LE, Yates AJ (1990) Inherited metabolic disease. In: Davis RL, Robertson DM (eds) Textbook of neuropathology, 2nd edn. Williams & Wilkins, Baltimore

Bell WE (1992) Bacterial meningitis in children. Selected aspects. Pediatr Clin North Am 39: 651

Berry CL (1992) A view of neurospinal dysraphism. Virchows Arch A Pathol Anat 420: 375

Birch JM (1990) The Li–Fraumeni cancer family syndrome. J Pathol 161: 1

Bondy ML, Lustbader ED, Buffler PA, Schull WJ, Hardy RJ, Strong LC (1991) Genetic epidemiology of childhood brain tumours. Genet Epidemiol 8: 253

Bonnin JM, Rubinstein LJ, Papasozomenos SC, Marangos PJ (1984) Subependymal giant cell astrocytoma: significance and possible cytogenetic implications of an immunohistochemical study. Acta Neuropathol 62: 185

Brett EM (1991) Paediatric neurology, 2nd end. Churchill Livingstone, Edinburgh

Brewster DR, Kwiatkowski D, White NJ (1990) Neurological sequelae of cerebral malaria in children. Lancet 336: 1039

Brody BA, Kinney HC, Kloman AS, Gilles FH (1987) Sequence of central nervous system myelination in human infancy. 1. An autopsy study of myelination. J Neuropathol Exp Neurol 46: 283

Bruni JE, del Bigio MR, Clattenburg RE (1985) Ependyma: normal and pathological. A review of the literature. Brain Res Rev 9: 1

Bruton CJ (1988) The neuropathology of temporal lobe epilepsy. Maudsley Monographs (31). Oxford University Press, Oxford

Buetow PC, Smirniotopoulos JG, Done S (1990) Congenital brain tumors: a review of 45 cases. AJR Am J Roentgenol 155: 587

Burger PC, Fuller GN (1991) Pathology – trends and pitfalls in histologic diagnosis, immunopathology, and applications of oncogene research. Neurol Clin 9: 249

Burger PC, Scheithauer BW, Vogel FS (1991) Surgical pathology of the nervous system and its coverings, 3rd edn. Churchill Livingstone, New York

Burger PC, Scheithauer BW (1994) Atlas of tumor pathology. Tumors of the central nervous system, 3rd series, fascicle 10. AFIP, Washington DC

Burns DK (1992) The neuropathology of pediatric acquired immunodeficiency syndrome. J Child Neurol 7: 332

Byard RW, Bourne AJ, Hanieh A (1991) Sudden and unexpected death due to hemorrhage from occult central nervous system lesions. Pediatr Neurosurg 92: 88

Caccamo DV, Herman MM, Rubinstein LJ (1989) An immunohistochemical study of the primitive and maturing elements of human cerebral medulloepithelioma. Acta Neuropathol 79: 248

Caplan L (1993) Stroke: A clinical approach, 2nd edn. Butterworth-Heinemann, Boston

Chiu JK, Woo SV, Ater J, Connelly J, Bruner JM, Maor MH, van Eys J, Oswald MJ, Shallenberger R (1992) Intracranial ependymoma in children: analysis of prognostic factors. J Neurooncol 13: 283

Chow CW, Klug GL, Lewis EA (1988) Subependymal giant-cell astrocytoma in children. J Neurosurg 68: 880

Copp AJ, Brook FA, Estibeiro P, Shum AS, Cockroft DL (1990) The embryonic development of mammalian neural tube defects. Prog Neurobiol 35: 363

Daita G, Yonemasu Y, Ishikawa M, Shimizu T, Yakura H (1989) Intracranial malignant teratoma diagnosed in a fetus. Neurol Med Chir 29: 1026

Dastur DK, Lalitha VS (1972) The many facets of neurotuberculosis – an epitome of neuropathology. In: Zimmerman HM (ed) Progress in neuropathology. New York, Grune and Stratton

Daumas-Duport C (1993) Dysembryoplastic neuroepithelial tumours. Brain Pathol 3: 283

Daumas-Duport C, Scheithauer BW, Chodkiewicz JP, Laws ER, Vedrenne C (1988a) Dysembryoplastic neuroepithelial tumor: a surgically curable tumor of young patients with intractable partial seizures. Neurosurgery 23: 545

Daumas-Duport C, Scheithauer BW, O'Fallon J, Kelly P (1988b) Grading of astrocytomas: a simple and reproducible method. Cancer 62: 2152

Davidson GS, Hope JK (1989) Meningeal tumors of childhood. Cancer 63: 1205

Del Bigio MR (1993) Neuropathological changes caused by hydrocephalus. Acta Neuropathol 85: 573

Di Rocco C, Iannelli A, Ceddia A (1991) Intracranial tumors of the first year of life. A cooperative survey of the 1986–1987 Education Committee of the ISPN. Childs Nerv Syst 7: 150

Duchen LW, Jacobs JM (1992) Nutritional deficiencies and metabolic disorders. In: Adams JH, Duchen LW (eds) Greenfield's neuropathology, 5th edn. Edward Arnold, London

Dulac O (1994) Epilepsy in children. Curr Opin Neurol 7: 102

Epstein FJ, Farmer JP (1993) Brain-stem glioma growth patterns. J Neurosurg 78: 408

Esiri M, Kennedy P (1992) Virus diseases. In: Adams JH, Duchen LW (eds) Greenfield's neuropathology, 5th edn. Edward Arnold, London

Evans DG, Huson SM, Donnai D, Neary W, Blair V, Newton V, Strachan T, Harris R (1992a) A genetic study of type 2 neurofibromatosis in the United Kingdom. II. Guidelines for genetic counselling. J Med Genet 29: 847

Evans DG, Huson SM, Donnai D, Neary W, Blair V, Teare D, Newton V, Strachan T, Ramsden R, Harris R (1992b) A genetic study of type 2 neurofibromatosis in the United Kingdom. I. Prevalence, mutation rate, fitness, and confirmation of maternal transmission effect on severity. J Med Genet 29: 841

Farwell JR, Dohrmann GJ, Flannery JT (1977) Central nervous system tumors in children. Cancer 40: 3123

Felix I, Becker LE (1990) Intracranial germ cell tumors in children: an immunohistochemical and electron microscopic study. Pediatr Neurosurg 16: 156

Ferreira J, Eviatar L, Schneider S, Grossman R (1993) Prenatal diagnosis of intracranial teratoma. Prolonged survival after resection of a malignant teratoma diagnosed prenatally by ultrasound: a case report and literature review. Pediatr Neurosurg 19: 84

Ferrer I, Alcantara S, Catala I, Zujar MJ (1993) Experimentally induced laminar necrosis, status verrucosus, focal cortical dysplaxia reminiscent of microgyria, and porencephaly in the rat. 94: 261

Figarella-Branger D, Pellissier JF, Daumas-Duport C, Delisle MB, Pasquier B, Parent M, Gambarelli D, Rougon G, Hassoun J (1992) Central neurocytomas. Am J Surg Pathol 16: 97

Filiano JJ, Kinney HC (1992) Arcuate nucleus hypoplasia in the sudden infant death syndrome. J Neuropathol Exp Neurol 51: 393

Fortnum HM (1992) Hearing impairment after bacterial meningitis: a review. Arch Dis Child 67: 1128

Friede RL (1989) Developmental neuropathology, 2nd edn. Springer-Verlag, Berlin

Friede RL, Mikolasek J (1978) Postencephalitic porencephaly, hydranencephaly or polymicrogyria. A review. Acta Neuropathol 43: 161

Fryer AE (1991) Tuberous sclerosis. J R Soc Med 84: 699

Fucillo DA, Sever AJ (1973) Viral teratology. Bacteriol Rev 37: 19

Gangemi M, Maiuri F, Fiorillo A, Migliorati R, Pettinati G, Del Giudice E (1987) Primary cerebral neuroblastomas. Neurochirurgia 30: 48

Germano IM, Edwards MSB, Davis RI, Schiffer D (1994) Intracranial meningiomas of the first two decades of life. J Neurosurg 80: 447

Geyer JR (1992) Infant brain tumors. Neurosurg Clin North Am 3: 781

Gilles F (1991) Perinatal neuropathology. In: Davis RL, Robertson DM (eds) Textbook of neuropathology, 2nd edn. Williams & Wilkins, Baltimore

Gilles F, Leviton A, Dooling E (1983) Development of the human brain. John Wright, Guildford, USA

Greisen G (1992) Effect of cerebral blood flow and cerebrovascular autoregulation on the distribution, type and extent of cerebral injury. Brain Pathol 2: 223

Hanefield F, Bauer HJ, Christen HJ, Kruse B, Bruhn H, Frahm J (1991) Multiple sclerosis in childhood: report of 15 cases. Brain Dev 13: 410

Hansen K, Lebech AM (1992) The clinical and epidemiological profile of lyme neuroborreliosis in Denmark 1985–1990. Brain 115: 399

Harding BN (1990) Progressive neuronal degeneration of childhood with liver disease (Alper's–Huttenlocher syndrome): a personal review. J Child Neurol 5: 273

Harding BN (1992) Malformations of the nervous system. In: Adams JH, Duchen LW (eds) Greenfield's neuropathology, 5th edn. Edward Arnold, London

Hart MN, Malamud N, Ellis WG (1972) The Dandy–Walker syndrome. Neurology 22: 771

Harwood-Nash DC (1992) Abuse to the pediatric central nervous system. AJNR Am J Neuroradiol 13: 569

Hassoun J, Soylemezoglu F, Gambarelli D, Figarella-Branger D, von Ammon K, Kleiheus P (1993) Central neurocytoma: a synopsis of clinical and histological features. Brain Pathol 3: 297

Hobbs CJ (1984) Skull fracture and the diagnosis of abuse. Arch Dis Child 59: 246

Hochberg FH, Miller DC (1988) Primary central nervous system lymphoma. J Neurosurg 68: 835

Hori A, Fischer G, Dietrich-Schott B, Ikeda K (1982) Dimyelia, diplomyelia and diastematomyelia. Clin Neuropathol 1: 23

Horten BC, Rubinstein LJ (1976) Primary cerebral neuroblastoma: a clinicopathologic study of 35 cases. Brain 99: 735

Hughes I, Jenney ME, Newton RW, Morris DJ, Klapper PE (1993) Measles encephalitis during immunosuppressive treatment for acute lymphoblastic leukaemia. Arch Dis Child 68: 775

Ilgren EB, Stiller CA (1987) Cerebellar astrocytomas. Part 1. Macroscopic and microscopic features. Clin Neuropathol 6: 185

Jacobs JM, Le Quesne PM (1992) Toxic disorders. In: Adams JH, Duchen LW (eds) Greenfield's neuropathology, 5th edn. Edward Arnold, London

Jellinger K (1987) Neuropathological aspects of infantile spasms. Brain Dev 9: 349

Jellinger K, Machacek E (1982) Rare intracranial tumours in infancy and childhood. In: Voth D, Gutjahr P, Langmaid C (eds) Tumours of the central nervous system in infancy and childhood. Springer-Verlag, Berlin

Jenkin D, Angyalfi S, Becker L, Berry M, Buncic R, Chan H, Doherty M, Drake J, Greenberg M, Hendrick B (1993) Optic glioma in children: surveillance, resection, or irradiation? Int J Radiat Oncol Biol Phys 25: 215

Johnson RT, Johnson KT (1968) Hydrocephalus following virus infection: the pathology of aqueductal stenosis developing after experimental mumps virus infection. J Neuropathol Exp Neurol 27: 591

Kanev PM, Lefebvre JF, Mauseth RS, Berger MS (1991) Growth hormone deficiency following radiation therapy of primary brain tumors in children. J Neurosurg 74: 743

Kawano N (1992) Pleomorphic xanthoastrocytoma: some new observations. Clin Neuropathol 11: 323

Kepes JJ (1993) Pleomorphic xanthoastrocytoma: the birth of a diagnosis and a concept. Brain Pathol 3: 269

Kepes JJ, Rubinstein LJ, Eng LF (1979) Pleomorphic xanthoastrocytoma: a distinctive meningocerebral glioma of young subjects with relatively favorable prognosis. Cancer 44: 1839

Kim TS, Halliday AL, Hedley-White T, Convery K (1991) Correlates of survival and the Daumas-Duport grading system for astrocytomas. J Neurosurg 74: 27

Kinney HC, Filiano JJ, Harper RM (1992) The neuropathology of the sudden infant death syndrome. A review. J Neuropathol Exp Neurol 51: 115

Kirkpatrick JB (1990) Neurologic infections due to bacteria, fungi, and parasites. In: Davis RL, Robertson DM (eds) Textbook of neuropathology, 2nd edn. Williams & Wilkins, Baltimore

Kleihues P, Burger PC, Scheithauer BW (1993a) Histological typing of tumours of the central nervous system, 2nd edn. Springer-Verlag, Berlin

Kleihues P, Burger PC, Scheithauer BW (1993b) The new WHO classification of brain tumours. Brain Pathol 3: 255

Kondziolka D, Humphreys RP, Hoffman HJ, Hendrick EB, Drake JM (1992) Arteriovenous malformations of the brain in children: a forty year experience. Can J Neurol Sci 19: 40

Koskiniemi M, Rautonen J, Lehtokoski LE, Vaheri A (1991) Epidemiology of encephalitis in children: a 20-year survey. Ann Neurol 29: 492

Koszyca B, Moore L, Byard RW (1993) Lethal manifestations of neurofibromatosis type 1 in childhood. Pediatr Pathol 13: 573

Kozlowski PB, Sher JH, Dickson DW (1990) Central nervous system in pediatric HIV infection – a multicenter study. In: Kozlowski PB, Snider DA, Vietze PM, Wisniewski HM (eds) Brain in pediatric AIDS. Karger, Basel

Kros JM, Vecht CJ, Stefanko SZ (1991) The pleomorphic xanthoastrocytoma and its differential diagnosis: a study of five cases. Hum Pathol 22: 1128

Kuller JA, Laifer SA, Martin JG, MacPherson TA, Mitre B, Hill LM (1991) Unusual presentations of fetal teratoma. J Perinatol 11: 294

Kure K, Llena JF, Lyman WD, Soeiro R, Weidenheim KM, Hirano A, Dickson DW (1991) Human immunodeficiency virus-1 infection of the nervous system: an autopsy study of 268 adult, pediatric, and fetal brains. Hum Pathol 22: 700

Lake B (1992) Lysosomal and peroxisomal disorders. In: Adams JH, Duchen LW (eds) Greenfield's neuropathology, 5th edn. Edward Arnold, London

Lallier TE (1991) Cell lineage and cell migration in the neural crest. Ann NY Acad Sci 615: 158

Larroche J-C (1962) Quelques aspects anatomiques du développement cérébral. Biol Neonat 4: 126

Larroche J-C (1991a) The central nervous system: development. In: Wigglesworth JS, Singer DB (eds) Textbook of fetal and perinatal pathology. Blackwell Scientific, Oxford

Larroche J-C (1991b) Fetal and perinatal brain damage. In: Wigglesworth JS, Singer DB (eds) Textbook of fetal and perinatal pathology. Blackwell Scientific, Oxford

Laurence KM, Martin D (1959) A technique for obtaining undistorted specimens of the central nervous system. J Clin Pathol 12: 188

Leestma JE (1988) Forensic neuropathology. New York, Raven Press

Leestma JE (1991) Viral infections of the nervous system. In: Davis RL, Robertson DM (eds) Textbook of neuropathology, 2nd edn. Williams & Wilkins, Baltimore

Levine RL, Fredericks WR, Rapoport SI (1982) Entry of bilirubin into the brain due to opening of the blood–brain barrier. Pediatrics 69: 255

Li FP, Fraumeni JF, Mulvihill JJ (1988) A cancer family syndrome in twenty-four kindreds: Cancer Res 48: 5358

Ling EA, Wong WC (1993) The origin and nature of ramified and amoeboid microglia: a historical review and current concepts. Glia 7: 9

Little WJ (1862) On the influence of abnormal parturition, difficult labour, premature birth and asphyxia neonatorum on mental and physical conditions of the child, especially in relation to deformities. Trans Obstet Soc London 3: 293

Louis DN, von Deimling A, Dickersin GR, Dooling EC, Seizinger BR (1992) Desmoplastic cerebral astrocytomas of infancy: a histopathologic, immunohistochemical, ultrastructural, and molecular genetic study. Hum Pathol 23: 1402

Ludwig CL, Smith MT, Godfrey AD, Armsbrustmacher VW (1986) A clinicopathological study of 323 patients with oligodendrogliomas. Ann Neurol 19: 15

Lund AM, Skovby F (1991) Optic gliomas in children with neurofibromatosis type 1. Eur J Pediatr 150: 835

Luo SQ, Li DZ, Dong JF (1992) Intracranial tumors in children. An analysis of 2000 cases. Chin Med J 105: 462

Manlow A, Munoz DG (1992) A non-toxic method for the demonstration gliosis. J Neuropathol Exp Neurol 51: 298

Marin-Padilla M (1991) Cephalic axial and skeletal–neutral dysraphic disorders: embryology and pathology. Can J Neurol Sci 18: 153

Marin-Padilla M, Marin-Padilla TM (1981) Morphogenesis of experimentally induced Arnold–Chiari malformation. J Neurol Sci 50: 29

Marques Dias M, Harmant-van Rijckevorsel G, Landrieu P, Lyon G (1984) Prenatal cytomegalovirus disease and cerebral microgyria: evidence for perfusion failure, not disturbance of histogenesis, as the major cause of fetal cytomegalovirus encephalopathy. Neuropediatrics 15: 18

Mastronardi L, Ferrante L, Lunardi P, Cervoni L, Fortuna A (1991) Association between neuroepithelial tumor and multiple intestinal polyposis (Turcot's syndrome): report of a case and critical analysis of the literature. Neurosurgery 28: 449–52

Matson DD, Crofton FDL (1960) Papilloma of the choroid plexus in childhood. J Neurosurg 17: 1002

McKinney RE, Katz SL, Wilfert CM (1987) Chronic enteroviral meningoencephalities in agammaglobulinemic patients. Rev Inf Dis 9: 334

Mickle JP (1992) Ganglioglioma in children. A review of 32 cases at the University of Florida. Pediatr Neurosurg 18: 310

Miller DC, Lang FF, Epstein FJ (1993) Central nervous system gangliogliomas. I: Pathology. J Neurosurg 79: 859

Misbah SA, Spickett GP, Ryba PC, Hockaday JM, Kroll JS, Sherwood C, Kurtz JB, Moxon ER, Chapel HM (1992) Chronic enteroviral meningoencephalitis in agammaglobulinemia: case report and literature review. J Clin Immunol 12: 266

Monpetit VJA, Andermann F, Carpenter S, Fawcett JS, Zborowska-Sluis D, Giberson HR (1971) Subacute necrotizing encephalomyelopathy. Brain 94: 1

Morimoto K, Mogami H (1986) Sequential CT study of subependymal giant-cell astrocytoma associated with tuberous sclerosis. J Neurosurg 65: 874

Mørk SJ, Lindegaard KF, Halvorsen TB, Lehmann EH, Solgaard T, Hatlevoli R, Harvel S, Ganz J (1985) Oligodendroglioma: incidence and biological behaviour in a defined population. J Neurosurg 63: 881

Mørk SJ, Halvorsen TB, Lindegaard KF, Eide GE (1986) Oligodendroglioma. Histologic evaluation and prognosis. J Neuropathol Exp Neurol 45: 65

Morriss-Kay CM (1981) Growth and development of pattern in the cranial neural epithelium of rat embryos during neurulation. J Embryol Exp Morphol 65 (Suppl): 225

Moser HW, Naidu S, Kumar AJ, Rosenbaum AE (1987) The adrenoleukodystrophies. Crit Rev Neurobiol 3: 29

Muller F, O'Rahilly R (1987) The development of the human brain, the closure of the caudal neuropore, and the beginning of secondary neurulation at stage 12. Anat Embryol 176: 413

Muller F, O'Rahilly R (1991) Development of anencephaly and its variants. Am J Anat 190: 193

Mustafa MM, Weitman SD, Winick NJ, Bellini WJ, Timmons CF, Siegel JD (1993) Subacute measles encephalitis in the young immunocompromised host: report of two cases diagnosed by polymerase chain reaction and treated with ribavirin, and review of the literature. Clin Infect Dis 16: 654

Naeye RL, Blanc W (1965) Pathogenesis of congenital rubella. JAMA 914: 1277

Nag S (1991) The ependyma and choroid plexus. In: Davis RL, Robertson DM (eds) Textbook of neuropathology, 2nd edn. Williams & Wilkins, Baltimore

Naidich TP, Altman NR, Braffman BH, McLone DG, Zimmerman RA (1992) Cephaloceles and related malformations. AJNR Am J Neuroradiol 13: 655

Neglia JP, Meadows AT, Robison LL, Kim TH, Newton WA, Ruymann FB, Sather HN, Hammond GD (1991) Second neoplasms after acute lymphoblastic leukemia in childhood. N Eng J Med 325: 1330

Norman MG, Ludwin SK (1991) Congenital malformations of the nervous system. In: Davis RL, Robertson DM (eds) Textbook of neuropathology, 2nd edn. Williams & Wilkins, Baltimore

O'Rahilly R, Muller F, Hutchins GM, Moore GW (1984) Computer ranking of the sequence of appearance of 100 features of the brain and related structures in staged human embryos during the first five weeks of development. Am J Anat 171: 243

Obringer AC, Meadows AT, Zackai EH (1989) The diagnosis of neurofibromatosis-1 in the child under the age of 6 years. Am J Dis Child 143: 717

Ogata H, Oka K, Mitsudome A (1992) Hydrocephalus due to acute aqueductal stenosis following mumps infection: report of a case and review of the literature. Brain Dev 14: 417

Ohama E, Ohara S, Ikuta F, Tanaka K, Nishizawa M, Miyatake T (1987) Mitochondrial angiopathy in cerebral blood vessels of mitochondrial encephalomyopathy. Acta Neuropathol 74: 226

Oi S, Matsumoto S (1992) Controversy pertaining to therapeutic modalities for tumors of the pineal region: a worldwide survey of different patient populations. Childs Nerv Syst 8: 332

Oi S, Matsumoto S, Choi JU, Kang JK, Wong T, Wang C, Chang TST (1990) Brain tumors diagnosed in first year of life in five Far-Eastern countries. Statistical analysis of 307 cases. Childs Nerv Syst 6: 79

Okazaki H, Scheithauer BW (1988) Atlas of neuropathology. Gower, New York

Parry C, Eaton J (1991) Kohl: a lead-hazardous eye makeup from the Third World to the first World. Environ Health Perspect 94: 121

Paulus W, Schlote W, Perentes E, Jacobi G, Warmuth-Metz M, Roggendorf W (1992) Desmoplastic supratentorial neuroepithelial tumours of infancy. Histopathology 21: 43

Pearl PL, Abu FH, Starke JR, Dreyer Z, Louis PT, Kirkpatrick JB (1990) Neuropathology of two fatal cases of measles in the 1988–1989 Houston epidemic. Pediatr Neurol 6: 126

Peeples DM, Stern BJ, Jiji V, Sahni KS (1991) Germ cell tumors masquerading as central nervous system sarcoidosis. Arch Neurol 48: 554

Perry VH, Andersson PB, Gordon S (1993) Macrophages and inflammation in the central nervous system. Trends Neurosci 16: 268

Philips RE, Solomon T (1990) Cerebral malaria in children. Lancet 336: 1355

Plantaz D, Kalifa C, Flamant F, Pierre-Kahn A, Habrand JL, Terrier-Lacombe MJ, Lemerle J (1992) Tumeurs germinales primitives du système nerveux chez l'enfant et l'adolescent. Etude retrospective de 35 cas de 1975 à 1989. Arch Fr Pediatr 49: 87

Powers JM (1985) Adreno-leukodystrophy (adreno-testiculo-leuko-myelo-neuropathic complex). Clin Neuropathol 4: 181

Powers JM, Liu Y, Moser AB, Moser HW (1992) The inflammatory myelinopathy of adreno-leukodystrophy: cells, effector molecules, and pathogenetic considerations. J Neuropathol Exp Neurol 51: 630

Rantala H, Uhari M (1989) Occurrence of childhood encephalitis: a population-based study. Pediatr Infect Dis J 8: 426

Raote GJ, Bhave SY (1992) Clinical profile of measles – a prospective study of 150 hospital based children. Indian Pediatr 29: 45

Rapola J (1993) Neuronal ceroid-lipofuscinoses in childhood. Perspect Pediatr Pathol 17: 7

Rawls WE, Melnick JL (1966) Rubella virus carrier cultures derived from congenitally infected infants. J Exp Med 123: 795

Riccardi VM (1987) Neurofibromatosis. Neurol Clin 5: 337

Riccardi VM, Eichner JE (1986) Neurofibromatosis. Phenotype, natural history and pathogenesis. Johns Hopkins University Press, Baltimore

Richardson EP (1990) Huntington's disease: some recent neuropathological studies. Neuropathol Appl Neurobiol 16: 451

Richardson EP (1991) Pathology of tuberous sclerosis. Neuropathologic aspects. Ann N Y Acad Sci 615: 128

Richman DP, Stewart RM, Caviness VS (1974) Cerebral microgyria in a 27-week fetus: an architectonic and topographic analysis. J Neuropathol Exp Neurol 33: 374

Roberts RO, Lynch CF, Jones MP, Hart MN (1991) Medulloblastoma: a population based study of 532 cases. J Neuropathol Exp Neurol 50: 134

Rorke LB (1983) The cerebellar medulloblastoma and its relationship to primitive neuroectodermal tumors. J Neuropathol Exp Neurol 42: 1

Rorke LB (1992a) Anatomical features of the developing brain implicated in pathogenesis of hypoxic–ischemic injury. Brain Pathol 2: 211

Rorke LB (1992b) Perinatal brain damage. In: Adams JH, Duchen LW (eds) Greenfield's neuropathology, 5th edn. Edward Arnold, London

Rorke LB (1994) A perspective: the role of disordered genetic control of neurogenesis in the pathogenesis of migration disorders. J Neuropathol Exp Neurol 53: 105

Rorke LB, Zimmerman RA (1992) Prematurity, postmaturity, and destructive lesions in utero. AJNR Am J Neuroradiol 13: 517

Rorke LB, Gilles FH, Davis RL, Becker LE (1985) Revision of the World Health Organization classification of brain tumors for childhood brain tumours. Cancer 56: 1869

Ross GW, Rubinstein LJ (1989) Lack of histopathologic correlation of malignant ependymomas with postoperative survival. J Neurosurg 70: 31

Rushing EJ, Rorke LB, Sutton L (1993) Problems in the nosology of desmoplastic tumors of childhood. Pediatr Neurosurg 19: 57

Russell DS, Rubinstein LJ (eds) (1989) Pathology of tumours of the nervous system, 5th edn. Edward Arnold, London

Rutka J (1991) The extracellular matrix: cues from the microcellular environment which can inhibit or facilitate glioma cell growth. In: Tabeuchi K (ed) Biological aspects of brain tumors. Springer-Verlag, Berlin

Scaravilli F (1992) Parasitic and fungal infections. In: Adams JH, Duchen LW (eds) Greenfield's neuropathology, 5th edn. Edward Arnold, London

Scaravilli F (ed) (1993) The neuropathology of HIV infection. Springer-Verlag, London

Schady W, Metcalfe RA, Butler P (1987) The incidence of craniocervical bony anomalies in the adult Chiari malformation. J Neurol Sci 82: 193

Schaumburg HH, Powers JM, Raine CS, Suzuki K, Richardson EP (1975) Adrenoleukodystrophy. Arch Neurol 32: 577

Scheithauer BW (1990) Tumors of the meninges: proposed modifications of the World Health Organization classification. Acta Neuropathol 80: 343

Scheithauer BW (1992) The neuropathology of tuberous sclerosis. J Dermatol 19: 897

Scherer HJ (1940) The forms of growth in gliomas and their practical significance. Brain 63: 1

Schiffer D (1993) Brain tumors. Springer-Verlag, Berlin

Schiffer D, Chio A, Giordana MT, Migheli A, Palma L, Pollo B, Soffietti R, Tribolo A (1991) Histologic prognostic factors in ependymomas. Childs Nerv Syst 7: 177

Schochet SS, Nelson J (1990) Exogenous toxic-metabolic diseases including vitamin deficiency. In: Davis RL, Robertson DM (eds)

Textbook of neuropathology, 2nd edn. Williams & Wilkins, Baltimore

Schofield DE (1992) Diagnostic histopathology, cytogenetics, and molecular markers of pediatric brain tumors. Neurosurg Clin North Am 3: 723

Schreiber D, Janisch W, Gerlch H (1982) CNS tumours in infancy, childhood and adolescence. In: Voth D, Gutjahr P, Langmaid C (eds) Tumours of the central nervous system in infancy and childhood. Springer-Verlag, Berlin

Scriver CR, Beaudet AL, Sly WS, Valle D (1989) The metabolic basis of inherited disease, vol. 2. McGraw-Hill, New York

Sekhon LH, Morgan MK (1991) Pineal teratoma and its relationship to intracerebral development. Neurosurgery 28: 594

Serville F, Benit P, Saugier P, Vibert M, Royer G, Pelet A, Chery M, Munnich A, Lyonnet S (1993) Prenatal exclusion of X-linked hydrocephalus-stenosis of the aqueduct of Sylvius sequence using closely linked DNA markers. Prenat Diagn 13: 435

Sharer LR (1992) Pathology of HIV-1 infection of the central nervous system. J Neuropathol Exp Neurol 51: 3

Sharer LR, Mintz M (1993). Neuropathology of AIDS in children. In: Scaravilli F (ed) The neuropathology of HIV infection. Springer-Verlag, London

Shaw EG, Scheithauer BW, O'Fallon JJR, Tazelaar HD, Davis HD (1992) Oligodendrogliomas: the Mayo Clinic experience. J Neurosurg 76: 428

Shen WC, Ho YJ, Lee SK, Lee KR (1992) Intracranial germ cell tumors. Chin Med J 49: 354

Shepherd CW, Scheithauer BW, Gomez MR, Altermatt HJ, Katzmann JA (1991) Subependymal giant cell astrocytoma: a clinical, pathological and flow cytometric study. Neurosurgery 28: 864

Sieb JP, Pulst SM, Buch A (1992) Familial CNS tumors. J Neurol 239: 343

Snedeker JD, Kaplan SL, Dodge PR, Holmes SJ, Feigin RD (1990) Subdural effusion and its relationship with neurologic sequelae of bacterial meningitis in infancy: a prospective study. Pediatrics 86: 163

Sørensen SA, Mulvihill JJ, Nielsen A (1986) Longterm follow up of von Recklinghausen neurofibromatosis: survival and malignant neoplasms. N Eng J Med 314: 1010

Sugiyama K, Uozumi T, Kiya K, Mukada K, Arita K, Kurisu K, Hotta T, Ogasawara H (1992) Intracranial germ-cell tumor with synchronous lesions in the pineal and suprasellar regions: report of six cases and review of the literature. Surg Neurol 38: 114

Sumi S (1970) Brain malformations in the trisomy 18 syndrome. Brain 93: 821

Sutton LN, Goldwein J, Perilongo G, Lang B, Schut L, Rorke L, Packer R (1990–91) Prognostic factors in childhood ependymomas. Pediatr Neurosurg 16: 57

Suzuki J, Kodama N (1983) Moyamoya disease – a review. Stroke 14: 104

Takakura K, Inoya H, Nagashima K, Ikeda K, Tomonaga M, Kondon K (1987) Viral neurooncogenesis. Prog Exp Tumor Res 30: 10

Takeda S, Ohama E, Ikuta F (1989) Adrenoleukodystrophy – early ultrastructural changes in the brain. Acta Neuropathol 78: 124

Taratuto AL, Monges J, Lylyk P, Leiguarda R (1984) Superficial cerebral astrocytoma attached to dura. Report of six cases in infants. Cancer 54: 2505

Tarlow IM (1937) Structure of the nerve root. I–II. Arch Neurol Psychiatr 37: 1338

Taylor TE, Molyneux ME, Wirima JJ, Fletcher A, Morris K (1988) Blood glucose levels in Malawian children before and during the administration of intravenous quinine for severe falciparum malaria. N Engl J Med 319: 1040

Tijssen CC (1986) Genetic factors and family studies in medulloblastoma. In: Zelter PM, Pochedly C (eds) Medulloblastoma in children: new concepts in tumor biology, diagnosis and treatment. Praeger Press, New York

Toffol GJ, Biller J, Adams HP (1987) Nontraumatic intracerebral haemorrhage in young adults. Arch Neurol 44: 483

Tomlinson FH, Scheithauer BW, Jenkins RB (1992a) Medulloblastoma: II. A pathobiologic overview. J Child Neurol 7: 240

Tomlinson FH, Scheithauer BW, Meyer FB, Smithson WA, Shaw EG, Miller GM, Groover RV (1992b) Medulloblastoma: I. Clinical, diagnostic, and therapeutic overview. 7: 142

Tops CM, Vasen HF, van Berge Henegouwen G, Simoons PP, van de Klift HM, van Leeuwen SJ, Breukel C, Fodde R, den Hartog Jager FC, Nagengast FM (1992) Genetic evidence that Turcot syndrome is not allelic to familial adenomatous polyposis. Am J Med Genet 43: 888

Trescher WH (1992) Ischemic stroke syndromes in childhood. Pediatr Ann 21: 374

Truwit CL, Barkovich AJ, Koch TK, Ferriero DM (1992) Cerebral palsy: MR findings in 40 patients. AJNR Am J Neuroradiol 13: 67

Van Coster R, Lombes A, De Vivo DC, Chi TL, Dodson WE, Rochman S, Orrechio EJ, Grover W, Berry GT, Schwartz JF (1991) Cytochrome C oxidase-associated Leigh syndrome: phenotypic features and pathogenetic speculations. J Neurol Sci 104: 97

VandenBerg SR (1992) Current diagnostic concepts of astrocytic tumors. J Neuropathol Exp Neurol 51: 644

VandenBerg SR (1993) Desmoplastic infantile ganglioglioma and desmoplastic cerebral astrocytoma of infancy. Brain Pathol 3: 275

VandenBerg SR, May EE, Rubinstein LJ, Herman MM, Perentes E, Vinores SA, Collins P, Park TS (1987) Desmoplastic supratentorial neuroepithelial tumors of infancy with divergent differentiation potential ("desmoplastic infantile gangliogliomas"). J Neurosurg 66: 58

Vannucci RC (1992) Cerebral carbohydrate and energy metabolism in perinatal hypoxic–ischemic brain damage. Brain Pathol 2: 229

Vieregge P, Gerhard L, Nahser HC (1987) Familial glioma: occurrence within the "familial cancer syndrome" and systemic malformations. J Neurol 234: 220

Volpe JJ (1987) Neurology of the newborn. Major problems in clinical pediatrics, 2nd edn. WB Saunders, Philadelphia.

Von Deimling A, von Ammon K, Schoenfeld D, Wiestler OD, Seizinger BR, Louis DN (1993) Subsets of glioblastoma multiforme defined by molecular genetic analysis. Brain Pathol 3: 19

Wakai S (1989) On the origin of intracranial teratomas. No To Shinkei (Brain and Nerve) 41: 947 (in Japanese)

Weller RO, Shulman K (1972) Brain damage in infantile hydrocephalus. J Neurosurg 36: 255

WHO (1992) Prevention and control of neurofibromatosis: memorandum from a joint WHO/NNFF meeting. Bull World Health Organ 70: 173

Wolf HK, Campos MG, Zentner J, Hufnagel A, Schramm J, Elger CE, Wiestler OD (1993) Surgical pathology of temporal lobe epilepsy. Experience with 216 cases. J Neuropathol Exp Neurol 52: 499

Yachnis AT, Rorke LB, Trojanowski JQ (1994) Cerebellar dysplasias in humans: development and possible relationship to glial and primitive neuroectodermal tumors of the cerebellar vermis. J Neuropathol Exp Neurol 53: 61

Younkin DP (1992) Hypoxic–ischemic brain injury of the newborn – statement of the problem and overview. Brain Pathol 2: 209

Yuen ST, Fung CF, Ng TH, Leung SY (1992) Central neurocytoma: its differentiation from intraventricular oligodendroglioma. Childs Nerv Syst 8: 383

Zülch KJ (1982) Intracranial tumours of infancy and childhood. In: Voth D, Gutjahr P, Langmaid C (eds) Tumours of the central nervous system in infancy and childhood. Springer-Verlag, Berlin

Zülch KJ (1986) Brain Tumors, 3rd edn. Springer-Verlag, Berlin

ZuRhein GM, Varakis JM (1979) Perinatal induction of medulloblastomas in syrian golden hamster by a human polyoma virus (JC). Natl Cancer Inst Monogr 51: 205

5 · Gastrointestinal System

Colin L. Berry and Jean W. Keeling

Malformations of the gastrointestinal tract are an important cause of morbidity in early life. In this field, as in cardiovascular disease, effective surgical intervention is often practicable and requires prompt diagnosis and action. Massive irreparable defects are happily rare.

A brief account of the embryology of the entire tract will first be given; some further details are included in the text where relevant.

Embryology

After the separation of the primitive endoderm from the blastodisc at about day 14, the cells of this layer form the primitive yolk sac. At around the 20th day of development, the yolk sac becomes tucked under the head fold, thus forming the *fore-gut* (Fig. 5.1). Initially, the notochord is embedded in its roof, its cranial extremity is separated from the stomatodeum by the buccopharyngeal membrane, and it is surrounded by mesoderm. More caudally situated are the pleuropericardial canals, which later become the pleural cavities. The primitive heart lies ventrally.

Formation of the tail-fold a little later defines the *hind-gut* in a comparable way. The *mid-gut* communicates directly with the extraembryonic part of the yolk sac via a broad stalk. The endoderm of all these regions gives rise to the gut epithelium and the mesoderm to the muscular, fibrous and peritoneal coats. The intraembryonic coelum on each side of the mid-gut forms the peritoneal cavity.

The endodermal part of the mouth and much of the pharynx arises from the cranial portion of the fore-gut. The branchial arches develop in the mesoderm alongside the fore-gut, and pouch-like extensions of the endoderm occur between them, ultimately giving rise to such structures as the middle ear cavity and the parathyroid and thymus glands (Figs. 5.2–5.4).

At about the 10 mm stage nasal pits are seen, and at this time the stomatodeum is bounded by the nasal folds and the mandibular and maxillary processes (Fig. 5.5). The maxillary processes then grow forward and join the medial nasal folds, forming the primitive anterior and posterior nares. The primitive palate is formed from the lower deep aspect of the frontonasal process. Masses of maxillary mesoderm grow medially as the nasal septum develops, forming the palatal processes. These processes fuse with the posterior edge of the primitive palate, and then with each other and with the lower edge of the nasal septum. The tongue projects upwards between the maxillary palatal processes for a short time and is squeezed down as these processes fuse from the front backwards (Fig. 5.6).

The ventral diverticulum that will give rise to the larynx, trachea and lungs is seen at about 3 mm. After this the caudal part of the fore-gut lengthens rapidly as the primitive oesophagus, and a longitudinal ridge develops on each side, eventually fusing and separating the respiratory diverticulum from the oesophagus. If fusion of these ridges is incomplete, abnormal communications may be formed (see p. 217). As the embryo grows and the heart descends, the oesophagus elongates rapidly. The stomach is visible as a small swelling at around 7 mm; by the 15 mm stage its form is well established, following extensive dorsal expansion, and the biliary system and pancreas are in almost adult interrelationships. The duodenum grows rapidly, its lumen becoming

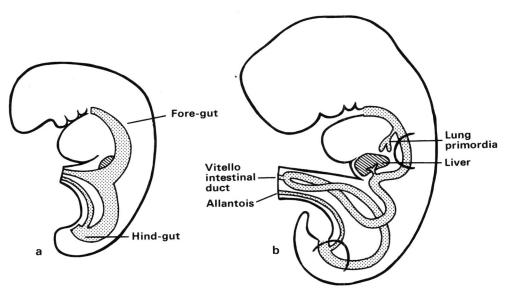

Fig. 5.1. Early development of the gastrointestinal tract showing the mid-gut loop at 3.5 mm (approx. 28 day) stage (**a**) and at the 7 mm (approx. 35 day) stage (**b**).

obliterated for a time. At about this stage the development of the liver and primitive kidney, together with elongation of the gut, results in a volume of tissue that cannot be contained within the intraembryonic coelom. The gut herniates into the extraembryonic coelom as a U-shaped loop, "based" on the superior mesenteric artery. The cranial part of the loop, from the duodenal attachment, forms the jejunum and greater part of the ileum. This limb increases markedly in size. The remaining caudal loop forms the terminal ileum, caecum and appendix,

ascending colon, and much of the transverse colon. The whole herniated loop rotates anticlockwise through 180° while herniated.

The distal part of the hind-gut is divided into the urogenital sinus and the rectum by a process analogous to that dividing oesophageal and respiratory primordia. More proximally, the left third of the transverse colon, the descending and the pelvic colon are formed from the caudal loop of the mid-gut U. At about the 10th week (42–48 mm) the region of the junction of the mid-gut loop and the hind-gut moves

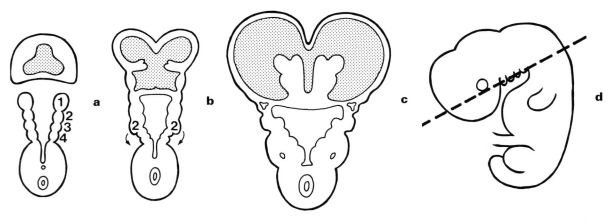

Fig. 5.2. The diagram represents an advanced embryo from below (approx. 14 mm, **c**), but the section plane is similar in each embryo illustrated (**d**: *broken line*). The branchial arches develop as shown (**a**), the second growing backwards to enclose the cervical sinus (this may persist as a pharyngeal fistula). Note that the mesodermal thickening is the branchial arch; the external cleft between these is known as the pharyngeal cleft and the interior depression as the pharyngeal pouch. These structures are transient and the first two are disappearing as the latter ones form. The structures derived from them are shown in Figs. 5.3 and 5.4.

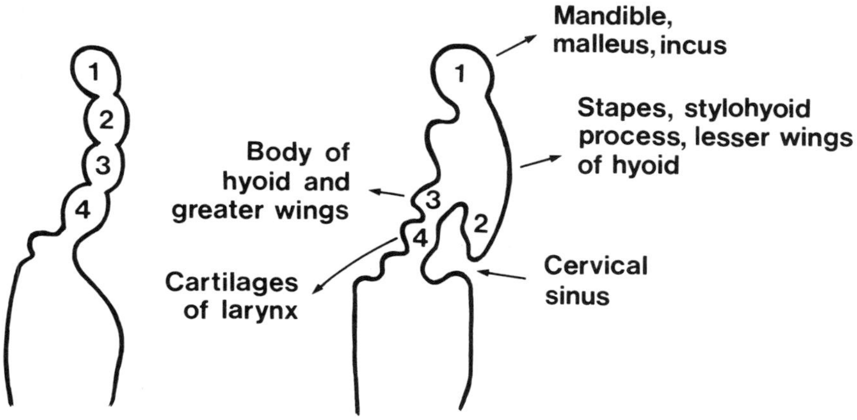

Fig. 5.3. Bony derivative of branchial arches.

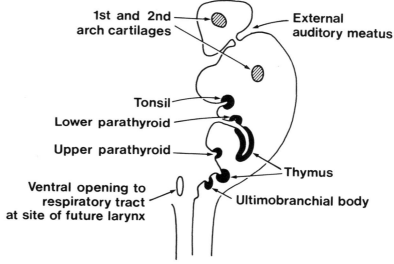

Fig. 5.4. Other derivatives of branchial arches. The only definitive structures formed from the pharyngeal pouches are the Eustachian tube and the tympanic cavity. This slice is from a later embryo.

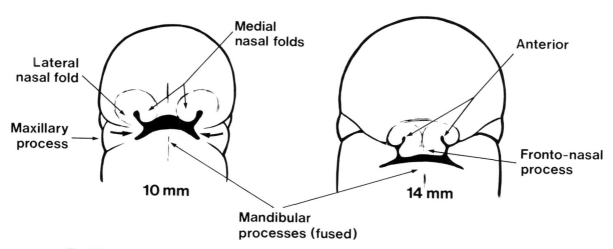

Fig. 5.5. Formation of the main components of the nose and mouth in a 10 mm (**a**) and a 14 mm embryo (**b**).

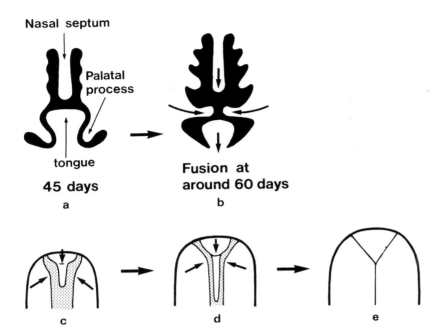

Fig. 5.6. Formation of nasal septum and palate. **a,b** The various movements that accompany this; **c–e** the ventral aspect of the palate at different stages of closure. **c** The situation at approximately 60 days (29–32 mm).

to the left and the small intestinal loops return to the abdomen, having rotated through a further 90°. The duodenal loop moves right and the caecum comes to lie in the right iliac fossa, having previously been below the right lobe of the liver after its return to the abdominal cavity. The ascending and descending mesocolons then fuse with the parietal peritoneum, and only transverse and sigmoid mesocolons remain as mesenteries into postuterine life.

Facial and Oral Abnormalities

Massive disturbance of the formation of the anterior part of the embryo is usually incompatible with life. A few anomalies of very early development (formation of the facial swellings – say 2.5 mm stage) permit further development.

The defects may be classified as follows:

1. Failure of the major facial processes
   A. Agenesis of the frontomaxillary process
      a) Cyclopia (incompatible with life)
      b) Arrhinencephaly
         i) *with medial harelip*. A true harelip, which resembles the normal condition in rabbits and which may be associated with notching of the alveolar process

and a median tooth gap. In this group the premaxilla may be absent; there is a single nasal cavity and a cleft of the hard and soft palates
         ii) *with lateral cleft lip and palate*. The maxillary process fails to move medially and there is a failure of fusion of the maxillary and palative bones, with palatal clefts in addition to lip abnormalities
   B. Abnormalities of the mandibular and maxillary swellings. A complex group including many syndromes, often discussed under the heading of branchial arch anomalies, including:
      a) *Pierre Robin syndrome*. Micrognathia with glossoptosis, hypoplasia of the mandible, usually with palatal clefts and visceral anomalies (congenital heart disease, etc.)
      b) *Treacher Collins syndrome*. Mandibulo-facial dyostosis, hypoplasia of the facial bones, malformation of the internal and external ear, and oblique palpebral fissures sloping in an antimongoloid direction (Fig. 5.7)
      c) Unilateral mandibulofacial dyostosis (Weyers)

The term "first pharygeal arch syndrome" is sometimes used to include mixed defects and the eponymous syndromes described here. Abnormalities closely resembling this group have been reproduced

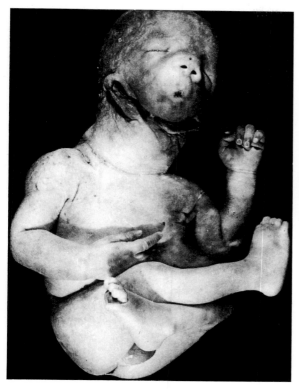

Fig. 5.7. Abnormal facial cleft in the Treacher Collins syndrome.

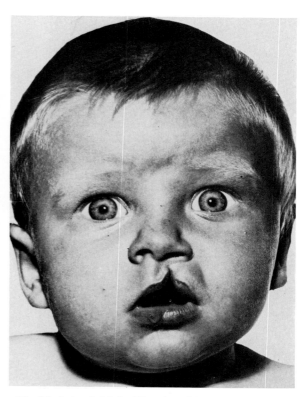

Fig. 5.8. Isolated cleft lip. Distortion of the nostril is evident.

in mice by disrupting the expression of genes for endothelin, which is presumably acting on the specific neural crest derivatives known to be defective in these cases (Kurihara et al. 1994).

2. Abnormalities of growth and fusion of the facial processes

These lesions form the commonest group, some forms occurring in approximately 1 in 1000 births.
A. Failure of fusion between the lateral nasal and maxillary swellings. An oblique fissure connecting the inner canthus with the upper lip without affecting the nose
B. Defective growth of the mandibular and maxillary swellings
C. Macrostomia. Failure of coordinated growth and fusion between the frontonasal and maxillary processes
   a) Simple cleft lip – may extend to the nostril and involve the alveolus (Fig. 5.8)
   b) Cleft lip and palate (Fig. 5.9)
   c) Isolated cleft palate (Fig. 5.10)
   Minor types are always posterior; complete types never extend beyond the incisive foramen.

These defects are not a single entity (see also p. 51). The anomalies are commoner in males (65% male, 35% female) and occur on the left more frequently than the right. The high incidence in the Japanese (1.71%) is probably related to facial shape (see the discussion on polygenically determined anomalies, p. 46). Approximately two-thirds of affected children have cleft lip and palate, one-third having cleft lip alone.

Cleft lip can exist as a unilateral or bilateral notch in the lip, or extend into the nostril and involve the bony part of the maxilla. If the cleft is bilateral the portion of the maxilla bearing the upper incisors projects upwards and outwards and gives rise to a deformity which is difficult to correct.

Cleft palate results from failure of fusion of the palatine shelves. This can affect any part of the septum and varies in severity from bifid uvula to complete absence of the palate with the nasal cavity opening into the mouth. A unilateral defect may occur with one side of the nasal cavity opening into the mouth. The soft palate alone may be cleft, but the hard palate is never cleft when the soft palate is found to be intact.

To illustrate the complexity of the interpretations of the pathogenesis of malformation in this area and

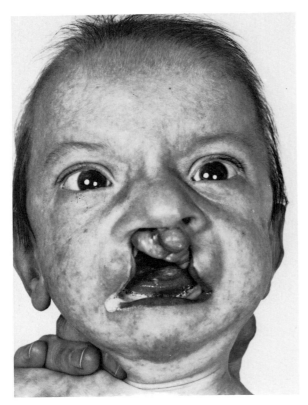

Fig. 5.9. Bilateral cleft lip and palate, with elevation and prominence of the midline structures.

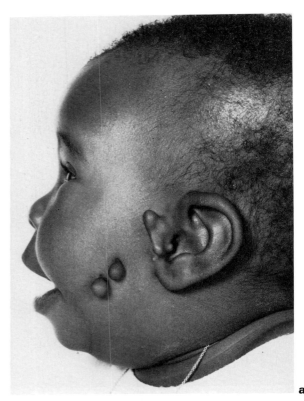

a

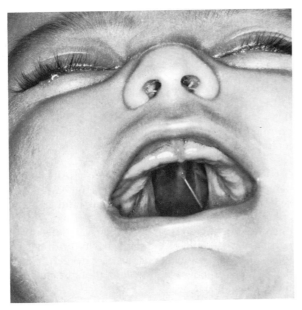

Fig. 5.10. Isolated cleft palate.

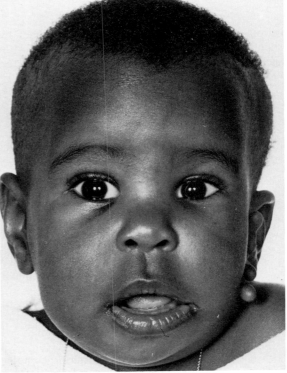

b

Fig. 5.11. Atypical development of the face.

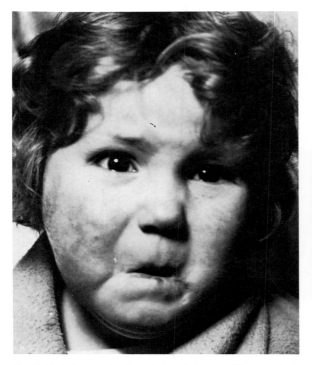

Fig. 5.12. Microstomia. Irregularity of the vermillion margin is common.

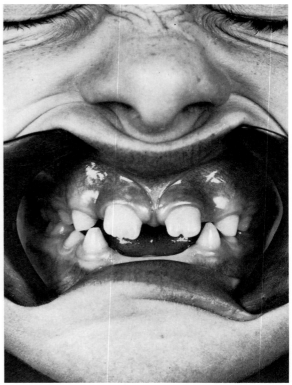

Fig. 5.13. Partial anadontia — absence of all lower and the lateral upper incisors.

to emphasize the occurrence of many atypical anomalies, Fig. 5.11 shows a child with macroglossia, unilateral accessory auricles and some facial asymmetry. Underlying bones were normal; this is not a branchial arch syndrome of the conventional type.

Microstomia

Microstomia (Fig. 5.12) has been observed in certain families and is associated with trisomy 18. The mandible is hypoplastic and association with other skeletal anomalies is documented. The mouth is often small in Down's syndrome.

Macrostomia

Massive enlargement of the mouth occurs in association with other anomalies, including absence of the tongue. The mouth may literally extend from ear to ear, and the defect is due to incomplete growth and fusion of the maxillary process with the frontonasal process.

Dentition

Apart from minor forms associated with cleft lip and palate, abnormalities of the dentition are uncommon. The two central incisors of the lower jaw may be present at birth and are then usually poorly formed.

Anodontia occurs in two forms, partial (Fig. 5.13) and complete, and is inherited as a Mendelian dominant.

Amelogenesis imperfecta also occurs in two forms, *hereditary enamel hypoplasia*, in which the teeth are abnormally shaped with sharp-pointed cusps, resulting in excessive wear, and *hereditary enamel hypocalcification*, where the soft enamel is also readily worn away. In this latter group the wear is so severe that the teeth may be eroded to gum level, and the enamel is apparently porous, being readily stained. Both deciduous and permanent dentition may be affected.

In *odontogenesis imperfecta* the teeth are also susceptible to injury; the pulp canal of their stumpy roots is obliterated by bony proliferation and they may also become discoloured (Fig. 5.14). This lesion resem-

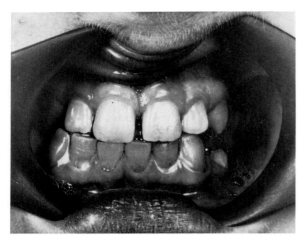

Fig. 5.14. Odontogenesis imperfecta. Discoloured lower teeth.

bles, and may form part of, the syndrome of osteogenesis imperfecta.

Discolouration of teeth also occurs after tetracycline treatment during pregnancy, usually after prolonged or regular administration. The drug is incorporated into newly growing bone and dentine and there produces fluorescence seen under ultraviolet light. Brownish-yellow tooth discolouration may occur after kernicterus.

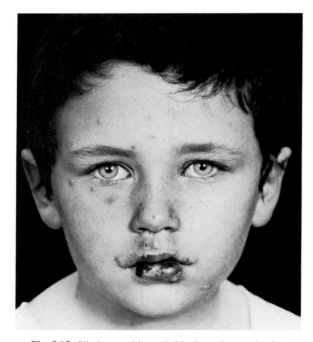

Fig. 5.15. Viral stomatitis, probably due to herpes simplex.

In Down's syndrome, growth arrest lines may be found in the teeth.

In hypophosphatasia there is early loss of deciduous teeth through bone resorption. This condition is inherited as a simple recessive characteristic.

The well defined incisor and molar abnormalities in congenital syphilis may be related to the presence of *Treponema pallidum* in the developing tooth germ (Bradlaw 1953).

Tongue

The tongue may be fixed or tied by a short frenum, but it is doubtful whether this is of clinical significance except in very gross examples. The frenum may also be congenitally absent. Macroglossia can be associated with hypothyroidism, Down's syndrome (where the mouth may also be small), glycogen storage disease and lymphangiectasia, and is part of the Beckwith–Wiederman syndrome.

Granular cell myoblastoma, neurofibroma, lingual thyroid tissue and haemangiomas may all form localized lingual swellings in infancy.

Cysts in the Mouth

Ranulae – retention cysts of the salivary gland ducts – are not uncommon. The cysts are unilocular, mucus filled, and lined with a pale secreting epithelium. They may disappear spontaneously in neonates but often require surgical removal.

Cysts lined with a respiratory type of epithelium may occur along the line of fusion of the maxillary and frontonasal process.

Infections of the Oropharynx

Vincent's angina is an acute inflammatory process affecting the mouth, from which many organisms, including anaerobic streptococci and spirochaetes, may be isolated. A necrotizing inflammatory process (noma) develops in debilitated individuals and may result in considerable perioral destruction of tissues.

Viral infections are common and have been divided by Dudgeon (1962) into infections in which:

1. The predominant lesion is oropharyngeal (Fig. 5.15)
   a) Herpes simplex stomatitis
   b) Coxsackievirus pharnygitis
   c) Adenovirus infections

2. Oropharyngeal lesions occur as part of a disseminated process:
   a) Acute exanthemas
   b) ECHOvirus infections
   c) Accidental infections (vaccinia, cowpox)

A further group of ulcerative lesions of uncertain aetiology may occur in childhood (e.g. recurrent aphthae, Stevens–Johnson syndrome, Bechet's disease.)

Most viral infections are manifest as small vesicles, often containing some leucocytes and epithelial cells, which rupture, leaving discrete ulcers with punched-out edges. In herpetic infections multinucleate cells may be seen in buccal smears.

Fungal infections are almost entirely caused by *Candida* spp., with budding yeast-like forms and pseudomycelium present in infected tissues. The oral lesions consist of flat white plaques which, when scraped, leave a flat surface with small discrete bleeding points. There is a mixed polymorph and lymphocyte infiltrate in the underlying tissues; in debilitated individuals or those with immune defects there may be very little tissue response.

Tumours of the Mouth

The term "epulis" is used to describe tumours on the gum (Fig. 5.16). These may be giant-celled fibromas or granular cell myoblastomas, the latter occasionally being present at birth. Overlying epithelial hyperplasia is seen over almost all benign gum tumours.

Malignant tumours are very rare. Kissane and Smith (1967) describe a well differentiated squamous carcinoma in a 12-year-old boy. Nasopharyngeal lymphomas may present as mouth swellings, but the commonest oral tumour in childhood is the lymphoepithelioma, an epidermal tumour with a conspicuous lymphoid infiltrate.

Iatrogenic Oral Disorders

Palatal Clefting

Midline palatal grooving and clefting are sometimes seen following long-term use of orotracheal tubes in preterm infants (Duke et al. 1976; Erenberg and Nowak 1984). Interference with contact between tongue and palate with subsequent failure of normal palatal modelling has been postulated by one group (Carrillo 1985), but it seems likely that pressure atrophy is responsible for midline clefts. Milk can accumulate in the groove and lead to inhalation pneumonitis.

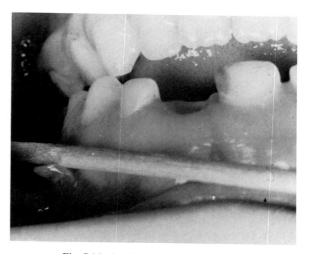

Fig. 5.16. Small fibrous tumour on gum.

Irregularity of Dentition

Enamel defects in the first dentition are described in children of low birth weight (Fearne et al. 1985) (Fig. 5.17). It is postulated that this may be the result of gingival pressure from long periods of orotracheal intubation (Moylan et al. 1980; Keeling and Bryan 1989).

Salivary Glands

Heterotopias

In an article on the histogenesis of branchial cysts, Little and Rickles (1967) have discussed the fre-

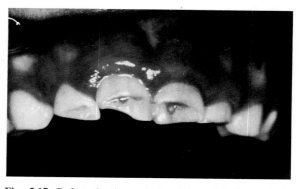

Fig. 5.17. Defects in the central and lateral incisors of the deciduous dentition in a child intubated for some weeks. (Courtesy of Dr J. Fearne)

quently observed occurrence of lymphoid tissue in salivary glands and of salivary tissue in lymph nodes. Salivary gland tissue may also occur in the middle ear (Taylor and Martin 1961).

Inflammatory Disorders

Bacterial infection is uncommon and occurs in dehydrated febrile individuals or following trauma to major salivary ducts. Mumps virus sialadenitis is accompanied by areas of focal necrosis, loss of epithelium and lymphocytic infiltration. Desquamated cells may be seen in ducts. Local lymph nodes may contain giant Warthin–Finkeldey cells during the prodromal period.

Cytomegalovirus is commonly found in salivary gland epithelium – usually ductal. Its frequency of occurrence varies widely and is apparently higher in Eastern Europe.

Tumours

In our experience the commonest neoplastic lesions occurring in salivary glands in childhood are deposits from leukaemia. Salivary neoplasms excluding haemangioma, usually of the parotid gland, are rare. An excellent review is that of Kauffmann and Stout (1963), who described pleomorphic adenomas, Warthin's tumour, mucoepidermoid carcinoma and adenoid cystic carcinoma in children. More recently Nagao et al. (1980) have described the experience of their large registry, with comparable results.

Oesophagus

Absence

Bizarre monsters may have no structure resembling an oesophagus, but otherwise this structure is always present in some form.

Double Oesophagus

The oesophagus may be doubled from pharynx to cardia. Gjørup (1934) reported a case in which a double oesophagus and partial duplication of the stomach was present; further cases of this type have since been described.

Congenital Short Oesophagus

This rare anomaly, in which part of the stomach is in the thorax, should not be confused with Barrett's oesophagus, a metaplastic epithelial change (see p. 220).

Atresia

In about 95% of cases, oesophageal *atresia* is associated with a fistula into the trachea. This defect has been classified by many authors but there is agreement that type I in Fig. 5.18 comprises around 90% of defects in all large series. Type II is the next commonest type (around 5%–8% in different studies), and all other varieties are rare. The straight-through trachea with virtual absence of the oesophagus is rarest.

The pathogenesis of the defect is generally considered to be a failure of the ventral diverticulum of the fore-gut, which will form the trachea, to separate from the oesophagus. This diverticulum appears as a longitudinal groove in the fore-gut at the 2.5 mm (4 week) stage, with caudal swellings that represent the future lung buds. The groove is then "pinched off" from the oesophagus, resulting in an over-and-under double-barrelled shotgun appearance (at around 4 mm) with progressive separation of the two barrels by a caudocephalad gradient. Partial failure of the processes of septation or separation may give rise to fistula. The rapid growth of the trachea that follows the 4–5 mm stage may cause displacement of developing oesophageal tissue and is a possible cause of atretic segments. Vascular pathogenetic actors related to the effects of obstruction due to persistence of the primitive right dorsal aorta have been considered by some to be important in the genesis of oesophageal atresia.

In the commonest form of the defect the upper oesophageal pouch ends at about the level of the second thoracic vertebra. It is often rather thick-walled, and tends to be dilated (Fig. 5.19). The fistula is often narrowed at its site of entry into the trachea, usually just above and to the left of the posterior aspect of the carina. The fistula is generally described as being lined with squamous epithelium, but in our experience of cases dying soon after birth respiratory epithelium may be found to extend well into the tract, suggesting that later appearances may be evidence of metaplasia. Rosenthal (1931) has described how squamous metaplasia may extend up to the larynx in some instances. A detailed review is that of Holder and Ashcraft (1970). Two fistulae may be present in 1%–8% of cases (Fig. 5.20) and may account for failure of an apparently successful repair (Hays et al. 1966).

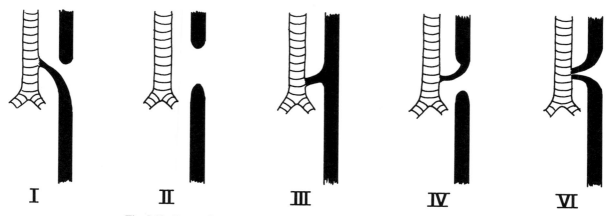

Fig. 5.18. Types of oesophageal atresia with associated tracheo-oesophageal fistula.

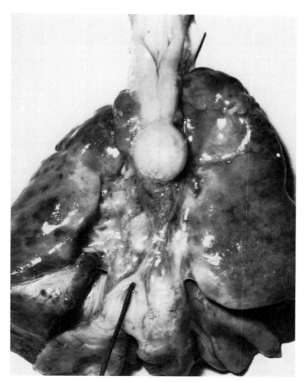

Fig. 5.19. Typical atresia with a cyst at the end of the upper pouch and area of atresia (type II).

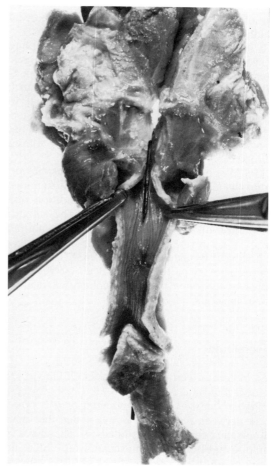

Fig. 5.20. Two fistulae into the trachea are seen, the upper containing a probe.

Associated Anomalies

Polyhydramnios is a common feature of pregnancies resulting in infants with oesophageal atresia, and occurs in about 30% of cases. Associated anomalies include Down's syndrome, and an increased incidence of congenital heart disease and anorectal anomalies is found. The prognosis is greatly affected by the presence of additional malformations.

Recent reports suggest that abnormalities of oesophageal motility are common in survivors of repair procedures (Anonymous 1978).

Stenosis

Stenosis occurs in the distal third of the viscus. It is usually due to fibrosis following peptic ulceration; ectopic gastric mucosa is not uncommon in the oesophagus. Stenosis may also follow surgery for fistula or atresia, ulceration, and fibrosis after ingestion of toxic or corrosive fluids, a common event in childhood (Fig. 5.21).

It is often difficult to establish that oesophageal stenosis is an independently occurring congenital anomaly. However, the cases described by Kumar (1963) and Paulino et al. (1963), in which cartilage rings were present outside the oesophageal wall, causing stenosis, are apparently true congenital defects. Obstruction of the lower oesophagus by membranes has also been described by Schwartz (1962).

Muscular obstruction of the oesophagus may occur in the distal third as a result of the thickening and hypertrophy of the muscularis, a condition resembling hypertrophic pyloric stenosis. The autonomic innervation of this segment is apparently normal in these cases; in rare cases the whole oesophagus can be involved (Blank and Michael 1963). The condition has been reviewed by Kreczy et al. (1990) as idiopathic hypertrophy of the oesophagus – it is commoner in adults.

Diverticula

Oesophageal diverticula are rare in childhood. They occur at three sites:

Upper oesophageal/hypopharyngeal pouches occur between the cricopharyngeus and the superior oesophageal constrictor, as in adults. They have been found to have an entire muscular wall, unlike those found in adult life, and are therefore true congenital anomalies. Frequently the lesion is confused clinically with the upper pouch of an atretic oesophagus.

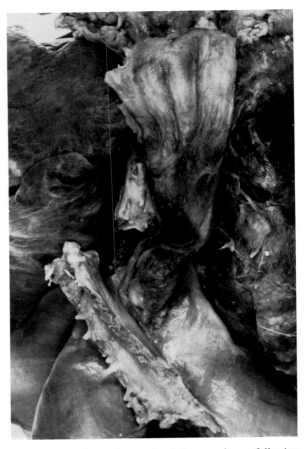

Fig. 5.21. Scarring and stenosis of the oesophagus following ingestion of strong alkali solution.

Midoesophageal pouches are thought to represent incomplete varieties of tracheo–oesophageal fistulae. They are generally small and lined with squamous epithelium.

There is an apparent connection with the so-called *oesophageal cysts*, reviewed by Cornell et al. (1950). These are found in the muscular part of the wall and bulge into the lumen. They are lined with ciliated epithelium and cartilage may be found in their walls. It seems likely that these lesions are abortive attempts to bud off accessory respiratory diverticula early in development.

Lower oesophageal diverticula are very rare, and may be lined in part with gastric epithelium and contain pancreas in their wall. They probably represent fore-gut duplication rather than true diverticula (Mendl and Evans 1962). Postinflammatory traction diverticula, formerly common and usually due to tuberculosis, are now rare.

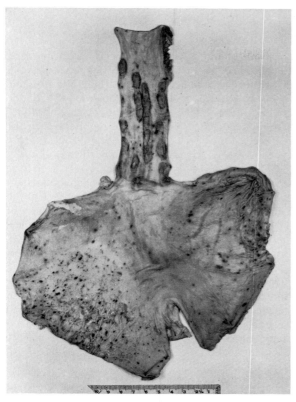

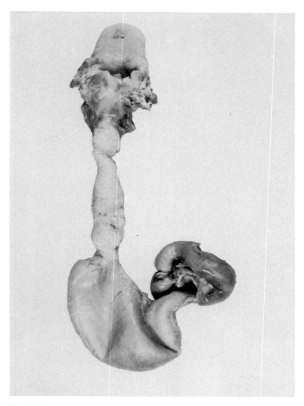

Fig. 5.22. Ulcers in the oesophagus of a leukaemic child. The stomach shows numerous petechial haemorrhages.

Fig. 5.23. Achalasia of the oesophagus in a child. The oesophagus is thick-walled and dilated.

Inflammatory Disease

Herpetic infection and moniliasis may cause oesophageal ulceration in infants, but mucosal loss in the lower third of the viscus is most commonly found after death associated with protracted vomiting, anoxia or indwelling feeding tubes. The reddened mucosa shows linear ulcers, often apparently undermined. Histologically there is often little reaction, but the picture is confused by autolytic changes (Fig. 5.22).

Achalasia

Around 5% of children with achalasia of the oesophagus are symptomatic in early life, and some cases require surgery in childhood (Swenson and Oeconomopoulos 1961). The pathology of this condition in childhood differs in no way from that in adults (Fig. 5.23).

Rupture

Rupture of the oesophagus may occur, usually posteriorly and to the left, in the lower third where the unsupported area abuts on the pleural cavity. It commonly follows episodes of repeated vomiting (Wiseman et al. 1959). Apart from this, most perforations occur as a result of surgical trauma.

Foreign Bodies

Foreign bodies in the oesophagus are usually arrested at the level of cricopharyngeus, the left main-stem bronchus, or the cardia. They are generally easily removed, but sharp objects may perforate the wall.

Oesophageal Varices

Children with portal hypertension can develop oesophageal varices. Portal vein thrombosis (Fig.

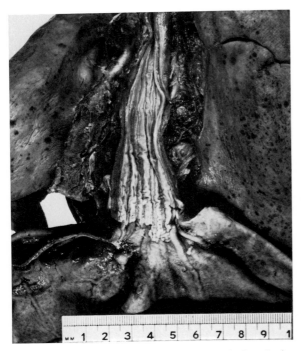

Fig. 5.24. Oesophageal varices following portal vein thrombosis in a 9-year-old child.

5.24) is the most frequent cause of portal hypertension, but it may occur in later life following hepatic changes in cystic disease. Congenitally dilated veins may also be found in the lower oesophagus (Jorup 1948).

Neoplasms

Primary oesophageal neoplasms are rare in childhood, and we have seen only leiomyomas. The oesophagus is commonly involved by spread of mediastinal neoplasms or nodal metastases. Squamous carcinoma, rhabdomyosarcoma and neurofibroma have all been reported in childhood.

Various hamartomas may be present in the oesophagus in syndromes where multiple lesions exist, for example haemangiomas in Rendu–Osler–Weber disease.

Barrett's Oesophagus

The condition known as Barrett's oesophagus has been reported in children (Dahms and Rothstein 1984), but dysplasia or neoplasia have not been seen.

Stomach

Congenital anomalies of the stomach are rare. Absence is noted in acardiac monsters, and occasionally the organ remains as a simple tube-like structure owing to failure of the later rapid growth of the greater curve. Under these circumstances the duodenum is generally found to be mobile and in the midline.

Membranous atresia of the stomach may occur at the pylorus, and it is usually diagnosed as pyloric stenosis or, if the membrane prolapses down the duodenum, as duodenal atresia. We have seen an example of gastric atresia in which the continuity of the stomach was interrupted and a fibrous cord joined the duodenum. The stomach was vastly distended. However, gastric atresias account for less than 1% of all cases of gut atresia (Parrish et al. 1968).

In the many varieties of visceral transposition the stomach may be involved (see p. 122). Isolated gastric inversion has been recorded (Lieber and Rosenbaum 1965). In cases in which a left-sided diaphragmatic defect occurs, the stomach is usually found in the thorax.

Hypertrophic Pyloric Stenosis (see also p. 52)

There is some doubt as to whether hypertrophic pyloric stenosis should really be considered a congenital defect, because it has not been reported in stillbirths and rarely presents in the first 24 h of life. However, the disease is apparently polygenically determined, with a well defined pattern of inheritance. Marked variation in racial incidence is found (see Table 5.1). There is a marked male preponderance (around 5 : 1) and a pronounced tendency for first-born children to be affected. An increase in the incidence of pyloric stenosis has been reported from several regions in the UK (Lancet Editorial 1984). Wide temporal and seasonal fluctuations have been noted in the past; continued observation will establish or refute a trend.

Table 5.1. Incidence of pyloric stenosis per 100 000 births in Hawaii

Source	Incidence
Caucasian	159
Japanese	68
Caucasian–Japanese F_1	54
Hawaiian	5
Filipino	14

Data from Morton (1970).

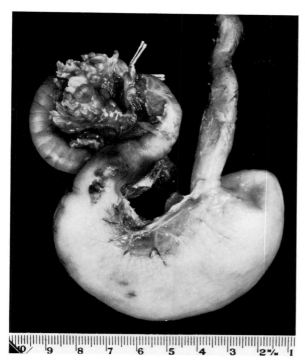

Fig. 5.25. From a case of pyloric stenosis dying at the age of 6 weeks in 1949. The stomach wall is thickened and the pylorus is seen as a discrete mass.

muscle mass is derived largely from the outer circular pyloric muscle coat, but all layers are involved. Secondary mucosal changes (oedema and ulceration) may occur in cases with a prolonged history. There have been extensive studies on the changes in autonomic innervation in the duodenum in this condition, and delayed maturation, secondary destruction and "overstimulation" of nervous tissue have all been discussed. In an extensive series of observations on serially sectioned pyloric tumours, Bodian found no evidence to support any of these hypotheses, most neuronal changes appearing to be secondary in character. It is apparent from an examination of his material that the changes in the muscle are mainly hypertrophic in character.

If the disease is not treated promptly ulceration of the mucosa of the distended stomach may occur, and hypertrophy of its muscle coats may also be found.

Diverticula

Congenital diverticula of the stomach are rare and consist of small pouches that may intussuscept and perforate. Descriptions of these lesions suggest that many are examples of reduplications (Ogur and Kolarsick 1951).

Duplications

At operation, usually at around 3 weeks of age, a fusiform mass of firm pale muscle up to 3–5 cm long is found at the pylorus (Fig. 5.25), with an abrupt return to normal gut wall distally (Fig. 5.26). The

The precise nature of enteric duplications has been obscured by a number of reports of various cystic

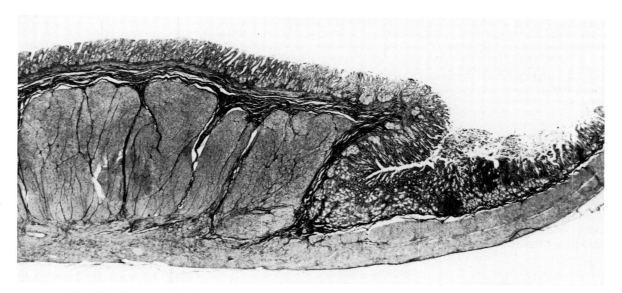

Fig. 5.26. Abrupt transition between pyloric and duodenal musculature in an untreated case of polyric stenosis.

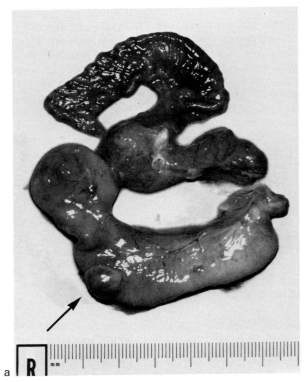

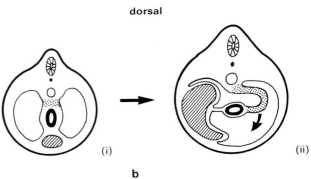

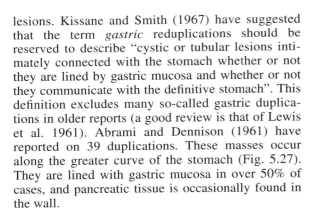

Fig. 5.27. a Nodular duplication of the stomach wall (*arrow*). Annular pancreas in also present. **b** The formation of the peritoneal reflections of the stomach from the dorsal mesogastrium (*stipple*) explains the presence of true gastric duplications only on the greater curve of the stomach. The *hatched area* is the hepatic primordium. (See also p. 227.)

lesions. Kissane and Smith (1967) have suggested that the term *gastric* reduplications should be reserved to describe "cystic or tubular lesions intimately connected with the stomach whether or not they are lined by gastric mucosa and whether or not they communicate with the definitive stomach". This definition excludes many so-called gastric duplications in older reports (a good review is that of Lewis et al. 1961). Abrami and Dennison (1961) have reported on 39 duplications. These masses occur along the greater curve of the stomach (Fig. 5.27). They are lined with gastric mucosa in over 50% of cases, and pancreatic tissue is occasionally found in the wall.

Gastric Heterotopias

Pancreatic tissue is not infrequently found in the gastric wall and has been discussed by Berant et al. (1965). We have seen a number of cases with intramural pancreatic tissue in the stomach, and are under the impression that the frequency of this anomaly varies directly with the assiduity with which it is sought. It appears to be more common in children than in adults, which may represent a sampling problem or disappearance of the tissue with age.

Gastric Perforations

Since Herbut (1943) described areas of muscular deficiency in the stomach, this finding has been considered to be a major cause of "spontaneous" gastric perforation. Some authors find frequent muscular abnormalities in cases of this type (Purcell 1962). One of us (C.L.B.) has seen such a case in a 2-year-old, presenting as sudden death following perforation. Two cases have been reported in preterm infants, both associated with defective muscularis propria (de la Fuente 1981) (Fig. 5.28). Rosser et al. (1982) described 16 cases treated during a 10-year period; half of the infants were of low birth weight.

Overdistension of the stomach with gases during resuscitation and perforation by catheters (misplaced on feeding) are the commonest cause of perforation of the stomach without previous ulceration. Dilatation due to untreated intestinal obstruction may result in necrosis and perforation due to impairment of the blood supply, which can also occur following gastric volvulus.

Foreign Bodies

Many objects may be found in the stomach of children. The well known trichobezar (Fig. 5.29) from

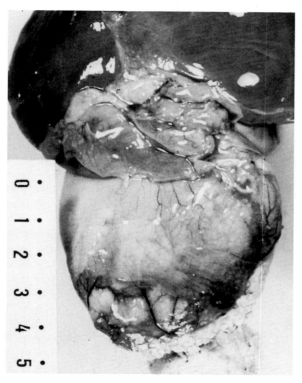

Fig. 5.28. Perforation of the stomach through an area of muscular deficiency.

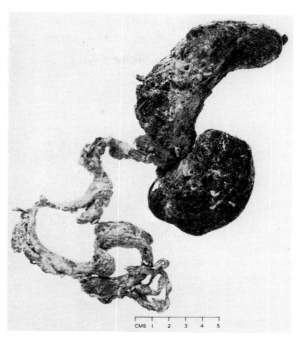

Fig. 5.29. Typical trichobezar from a 12-year-old girl with trichotillomania. Occasionally complete gastric casts are formed.

hair chewing is now less common than formerly, small wheels from plastic vehicles being more frequently found. Most objects that reach the stomach pass through it and are voided. Figure 5.30 shows an assortment of nuts, pieces of plastic, seeds, beads and leaves from the stomach of a 7-year-old boy with intestinal obstruction.

Inflammation

Accidental ingestion of medicines, which is unhappily common in children, may cause severe inflammation and ulceration of the stomach, salicylates and ferrous sulphate (Fig. 5.31) being particularly likely to cause this type of injury. Perforation and haemorrhage may occur.

Haemorrhage into the mucosa may occur in blood dyscrasias (Fig. 5.32).

Ménétrier's Disease in Children

Hypertrophic gastritis occurs in children, although it is uncommon. It is more commonly associated with cytomegalovirus infection in this age group and usually has a benign self-limiting course. Qualman and Hamoudi (1992) have reported three cases ranging in age from 22 months to 19 years.

Eosinophilic Gastritis

Eosinophilic gastritis can occur in childhood, sometimes as part of a diffuse involvement of the bowel. There is typically thickening of the pyloric or small intestinal mucosa by single or multiple foci of infiltration, by oedema and by a predominantly eosinophilic inflammatory cell mass. Blood eosinophilia is common, and malabsorption is sometimes found. Serum IgE levels may be raised. Polypoid lesions may cause intussusception. In recent years the disease has been better defined as it affects the stomach, and Goldman and Proujansky (1986) point out that the lesions are most marked in the antrum, although widespread involvement of the gut, including the oesophagus, is usual. A good review is that of Konrad and Meister (1979). From these papers it appears that there are two entities: a mucosal (allergic) form and a transmural infiltrative lesion more

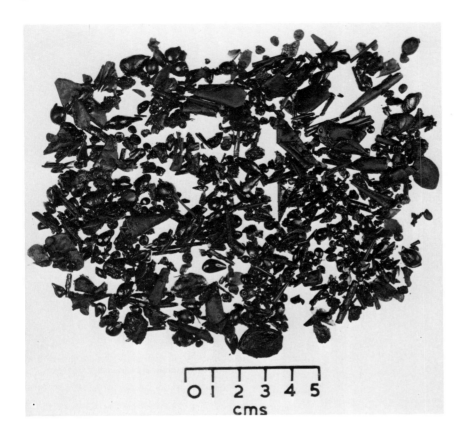

Fig. 5.30. Objects removed from the stomach at operation on a 7-year-old boy.

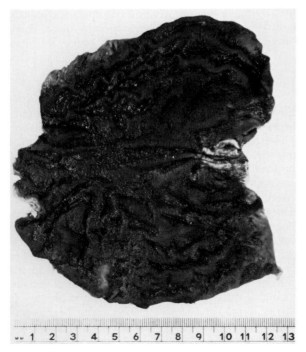

often affecting the stomach and small intestine than the whole gut. This form may perforate.

Tumours

Gastric polyps occur in the Peutz–Jeghers syndrome and are hamartomatous, as elsewhere in the gut. Achord and Proctor (1963) described a case in which death occurred from gastric carcinoma associated with the syndrome, but there is no clear evidence as to whether the tumour arose from a polyp. Williams and Knudson (1965), in reporting such a case in an adult duodenal polyp, concluded that there was very little risk of malignancy in this syndrome.

Gastric polyps may occur in some cases of familial colonic polyposis.

Neurofibromatosis may affect the stomach, and we have seen two examples of the rare gastric teratoma.

Fig. 5.31. Haemorrhagic gastritis following ingestion of ferrous sulphate in a 4-year-old boy.

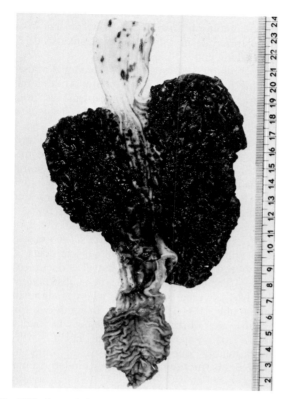

Fig. 5.32. Stomach from a case of aplastic anaemia. Haemorrhagic gastritis and some oesophageal ulceration is seen.

True hamartomas also occur (Bogomoletz and Cox 1975) (Fig. 5.33).

Leiomyomas occur in children, and leiomyosarcomas have been described (Giberson et al. 1954). However, malignant tumours are very rare, a total of about 50 cases having been reported in the world literature. Most have been carcinoma and lymphosarcoma; carcinoid tumours have been reported. J. N. Cox (personal communication) has observed a leiomyoblastoma of the stomach in a 14-year-old girl (Fig. 5.34) (see also Stout 1962).

Duodenum

Extrinsic Obstructions

In patients with malrotation of the mid-gut loop, peritoneal bands, notably those running across from the right upper quadrant of the abdomen to the caecum, which lies in the epigastrium in this syndrome, may constrict the second part of the duodenum. The con-

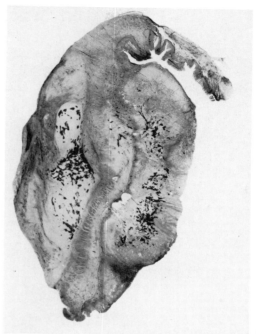

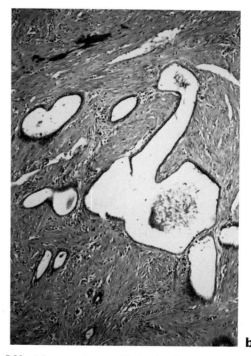

Fig. 5.33. A large cystic mass (5–6 cm) and two separate masses (2–3 cm) were found in the pyloric region. **a** A hamartoma on the mucosal and serosal aspect of the muscularis propria. **b** Cystic dilation of glands in the submucosa, surrounded by fibrous tissue and smooth muscle.

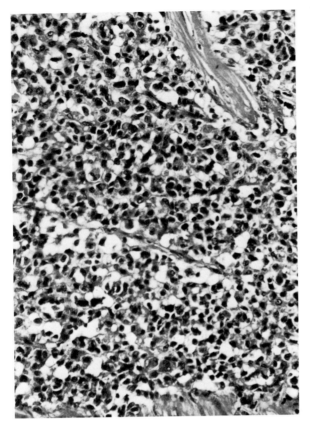

Fig. 5.34. Lipoblastoma from a 14-year-old with a left hypochondrial mass deforming the stomach on barium examination. Large regular vacuolated cells are seen. (H&E, × 240) (Reproduced by permission of Dr J.N. Cox)

dition is cured by cutting the band and completing gut rotation.

Duplications

Duplications (see p. 231) in this area are extremely rare and present as submucosal cysts bulging into the lumen, which they may ultimately obstruct.

Duodenal Atresia and Stenosis

Intestinal atresia occurs more commonly in the duodenum (1 in 5000 live births) than in the jejunum or ileum. It is commonly associated with extra-abdominal anomalies, particularly cardiac malformations and tracheo-oesophageal fistula, and anorectal anomalies are increased (Dykstra et al. 1968;

Fonkalsrud et al. 1968). Duodenal atresia occurs more commonly in trisomy 21, being present in one-third of referrals in some centres (Fonkalsrud et al. 1968; Young and Wilkinson 1968).

The commonest presentation of duodenal atresia is vomiting in the first few days of life. An abdominal radiograph characteristically demonstrates a "double bubble" as a result of gas in both the stomach and distended proximal duodenum separated by the pyloric constriction. A few cases of duodenal atresia are associated with maternal polyhydramnios in the third trimester of pregnancy and some are identified because of raised maternal serum α-fetoprotein levels in the second trimester. Both of these are the result of impaired ingestion of amniotic fluid by the fetus.

The commonest type of obstruction in the duodenum (65% of Young and Wilkinson's 1968 cases) is atresia with loss of continuity of muscle coats. The gap between the blind ends of bowel is occupied by pancreas. The next commonest type is obstruction by a mucosal covered diaphragm, whereas stenosis is found in only 10%–15% of cases. In about two-thirds of cases, the obstruction is situated beyond the ampulla of Vater (Fonkalsrud et al. 1968). Approximately one-half of cases of congenital duodenal obstruction are accompanied by annular pancreas (see below).

Peptic Ulceration

Although rare, the presence of peptic ulcers in infants and children is well documented. Up to the age of 6 years they are almost invariably acute, with haemorrhage a major presenting feature. In older children, as in adults, males are more frequently affected and duodenal lesions are commoner than gastric. A greater awareness of the presence of this type of ulcer in childhood has led to an increased frequency of obtaining typical histories of postprandial pain, and an earlier supposition that bleeding was a particularly common form of presentation in *this* age group (25%–50% in various series) is probably not justified. A family history is found in 50%–60% of the cases seen (Habbick et al. 1968; Murphy et al. 1987). More important is the presence of the Zollinger–Ellison syndrome in approximately 5% of these children (Ellison and Wilson 1964).

In infants and neonates peptic ulceration occurs acutely, often associated with severe systemic illness, and presents with haemorrhage or perforation. Fibrosis and reactive vascular changes are not seen.

Ulceration may also occur with space-occupying intracranial lesions in association with steroid therapy (Rosenlund and Koop 1970). Tolazoline therapy in preterm neonates, given to reduce pulmonary hyper-

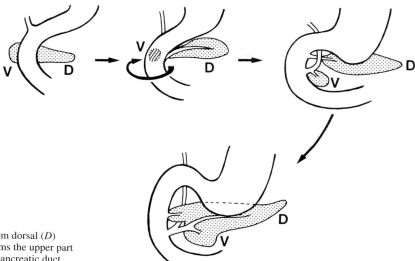

Fig. 5.35. Formation of the pancreas from dorsal (*D*) and ventral (*V*) buds. The dorsal bud forms the upper part of the head, the isthmus, body, tail, the pancreatic duct proper and the accessory duct of Santorini.

tension, may give rise to peptic ulceration, possibly due to the histamine-like structure of the drug.

Pancreas

Figure 5.35 shows how the pancreas develops from two rudiments. These appear at week 4 (3 mm), and the adult form is arrived at by week 16. Many pancreatic abnormalities are explicable in terms of failure of the normal embryological processes.

Congenital Abnormalities

If the dorsal component of the pancreas fails to develop, the gland consists of an ovoid mass in the hollow of the duodenum. In rare cases failure of fusion of the two parts of the gland may occur, in varying degrees.

Nodules of ectopic pancreas are common throughout the gastrointestinal tract and are frequently seen in trisomies 13 and 18.

Annular Pancreas

The second part of the duodenum may be completely surrounded by pancreas when the ventral part of the gland persists. The anomaly is seldom simple, and the pancreas has usually "filled the gap" left by an atretic or stenotic duodenum. The relationship of this lesion to duodenal obstruction is unclear, although it is often cited as a cause of upper-gastrointestinal obstruction in neonates. However, associated gut anomalies – mainly duodenal – may be more important (Elliott et al. 1968; Fonkalsrud et al. 1968; Young and Wilkinson 1968).

Cystic Fibrosis (Mucoviscidosis)

The generalized metabolic disease of cystic fibrosis is an autosomal recessive characteristic. The disease is caused by mutations in a single gene (at 7q22) encoding the cystic fibrosis transmembrane conductance regulator (CFTR) – a cyclic AMP-regulated chloride ion channel. The gene is on chromosome 7 and extends over approximately 250 kb of genomic DNA with 27 exons. The messenger RNA is 6.2 kb long and encodes a protein of 1480 amino acids; a specific deletion in exon 10 causes the loss of the amino acid phenylalanine at position DELTA F508 in the CFTR in the great majority of European cases. There are half a dozen other common mutations and perhaps 300 further uncommon ones. There appears to be a correlation between the type of mutation and the severity of expression of the disease; the position 508 mutation produces the severe form of the disease, and milder clinical syndromes (sinusitis, infertility as a result of congenital bilateral absence of the vas deferens) are produced by changes at other sites.

The way in which this metabolic defect accounts for the various phenotypic abnormalities of the disease relates to the fact that sweat gland, respiratory and other epithelia have decreased permeability to chloride ions. There is defective regulation of cAMP-dependent chloride channels, with failure of resorption of chloride from sweat, the production of inspissated meconium and viscid pancreatic secretions. Protein modifications may also be important, however, and abnormalities in the acidification of intracellular compartments with disturbance of Golgi functions have postulated (Barasch et al. 1991).

The tissue-specific expression of the CF gene product appears to correlate well with the pathology of the disease. High levels of expression are seen in nasal polyps and pancreas, and lower levels in lung, colon and sweat glands. Harris et al. (1991) have examined the expression of the gene in midtrimester fetuses and find high levels in the pancreas with lower levels in the gut, lungs and genital ducts. A mouse model of the disease, produced by gene targeting, has been described by Snouwaert et al. (1992). (The defective mouse gene is introduced into stem cells and can thus be used to produce a mosaic animal which can, in turn, be used to breed offspring with two copies of the mutant gene.) In this model homozygous animals (cf/cf) die within 30 days of birth with meconium ileus; changes in other systems are not marked. In the different model of Dorin et al. (1992) a milder phenotype is produced and there is heterogeneity of phenotype. (These authors used an insertional vector to introduce genetic material, which allows more variability in what is introduced.)

The incidence of cystic fibrosis is about 1 in 2500 in the UK, North America and Australia. About 15% of affected individuals present in the neonatal period with intestinal obstruction due to meconium ileus or its complication, and a similar proportion present in early childhood with malabsorption. Most of the remainder present with respiratory symptoms with or without malabsorption. The production of a viscid and abnormal mucus at many sites is characteristic. Gastrointestinal (see below), pulmonary (p. 409) and hepatobiliary lesions (p. 299) occur, and in recent years it has become evident that obstructive lesions in the duct system of the testis render males infertile. Pregnancy in affected females is difficult to manage because of pulmonary changes.

Pancreatic Changes

In infants dying in early life the pancreas may be macroscopically normal, but it is usually firm to the touch. A distinctly lobular feel is characteristic, and in those dying between 2 and 10 years of age the gland feels as if it were composed of closely interrelated hard triangles of tissue. Later fibrosis, cystic change, focal necroses and fatty infiltration blur the gross outline of the pancreas.

Histologically there is mucus plugging of distended ducts, with varying degrees of ectasia, fibrosis and calcification correlating with the severity of the disease rather than the age of the patient. Acinar destruction occurs and the islet tissue appears unduly prominent (Fig. 5.36). Stones may form in the dilated ducts. Trypsin is absent from the stools of affected individuals.

Meconium Ileus

Meconium ileus accounts for about 15% of cases of neonatal intestinal obstruction (Donnison et al. 1966) and is the mode of presentation of 13% of new cases of mucoviscidosis (McParblin et al. 1972).

Macroscopically there is a progressive dilatation of loops of small intestine by tenacious greenish meconium, which is less marked proximally and maximal in the mid-ileum, where the wall is thickened due to muscular hypertrophy. The terminal ileum is narrowed and contains hard greyish calcium-flecked pellets of meconium, while the colon is collapsed and empty (Figs. 5.37 and 5.38).

Histologically the villi are distorted by the meconium in the lumen and the mucosal glands are distended by inspissated secretions. Epithelial cells are flattened and show secondary atrophic changes.

Mortality from meconium ileus has decreased dramatically since the introduction of the Bishop–Koop anastomosis in the management of the disease. Volvulus, perforation, small intestinal atresia, meconium peritonitis and gangrene may complicate meconium ileus, and these complications are associated with a higher mortality rate. Meconium peritonitis, which can occur in utero, is manifest histologically as a serosal foreign-body reaction, often with calcification.

An association with hypertrophic pyloric stenosis is reported (McParblin et al. 1972). Peptic ulceration is more common in mucoviscidosis.

Oppenheimer and Esterley (1962) have reported meconium ileus without pancreatic disease.

Meconium Ileus Equivalent

Jensen (1962) coined the term "meconium ileus equivalent" (MIE) to describe intestinal obstruction outside the neonatal period due to sticky putty-like material in the terminal ileum. Acute obstruction is less common than episodes of constipation and colicky abdominal pain. Intussusception and volvulus may occur.

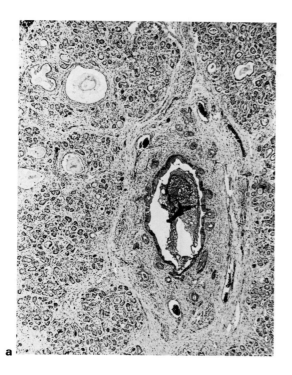

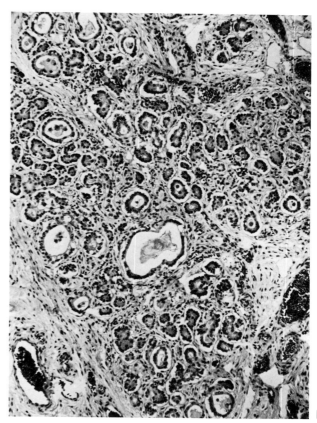

Fig. 5.36. Pancreas in cystic fibrosis. **a** Lectatic mucus-filled ducts with separation of acini by fibrous tissue. (H&E, × 40) **b** Fibrosis within lobules, with distension of smaller ducts. (H&E, × 120)

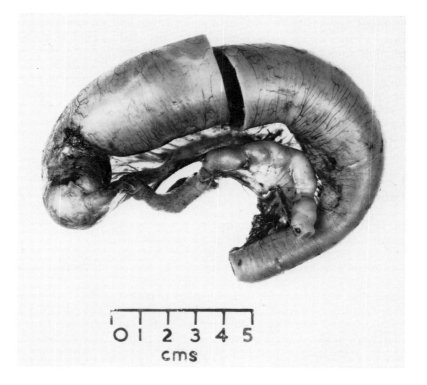

Fig. 5.37. Loop of ileum, distended by meconium, with a grossly narrowed segment distally.

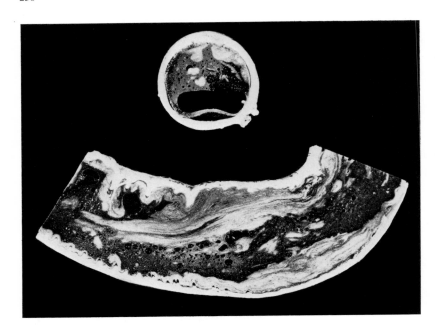

Fig. 5.38. Cut surface of fixed ileum; mucus plugging with mucosal and other debris present in the lumen.

"Cystic Fibrosis" in Preterm Infants

King et al. (1986) describe a condition of ileal obstruction by tenacious meconium and pancreatic acinar atrophy and duct dilation in six preterm infants. All had passed meconium around the time of birth and subsequently developed abdominal distension. These babies comprised 12% of neonatal necropsies during a 2-year period and there was no family history of mucoviscidosis. The authors suggest that the intestinal pancreatic changes described are pathognomonic of cystic fibrosis, but it seems likely that fluid restriction to prevent reopening of the ductus arteriosus and immaturity of intestinal function are probably responsible.

Large Bowel Strictures and High-lipase Pancreatitis

In 1993 reports began to appear of a significant problem in patients treated with capsule preparations containing high levels of lipase and other enzymes for several months. Of five cases reported by Smyth et al. (1994), four had strictures in the ascending colon, with histological findings suggestive of postischaemic ulceration repair. It is clear that other cases have occurred; the UK Committee on Safety of Medicines has knowledge of other cases. The pathogenesis of the lesion is not clear, although intralumenal distension of mucus masses has been suggested

by Smyth et al. and protease activity by Campbell et al. (1994).

Pseudocyst

In most instances pancreatic pseudocysts occur as a result of trauma. They are rare; a review in 1981 (Kagan et al.) documented only 113 cases. They are commoner in boys and associated with handlebar injuries or, in some cases, with child abuse (Bongiovi and Logosso 1969; Moossa 1975).

Presenting signs and symptoms include abdominal pain, nausea, vomiting, anorexia and weight loss. An abdominal mass may be found, and in some reports up to 80% of those affected have a raised serum amylase level at presentation (Grosfeld and Cooney 1975). Jaundice may occur.

The wall of the cyst is composed of fibrous tissue and it usually contains clear fluid; anatomically it fills the lesser sac.

Exocrine Atrophy

The combination of exocrine atrophy of the pancreas, pancytopenia and skeletal (metaphyseal) abnormalities has been reported in approximately 100 cases (Lebenthal and Shwachman 1977).

The pancreas is replaced by fat, with prominent islets persisting. The skeleton shows irregular rarefaction and condensation, notably in the femoral necks. Bone marrow abnormalities appear in the form of neutropenia, but pancytopenia has been described, as has complicating leukaemia.

Pancreatitis

Haemorrhagic pancreatitis is rare in infancy, although it may occur in leukaemia following chemotherapy or after steroid therapy. Alcoholic children are rare, although pancreatitis in an alcoholic child has been reported by Schmidt et al. (1964).

Inflammation of the pancreas occurs in mumps and in toxoplasmosis, and when the ducts are infested by roundworms. Surgical intervention to remove worms from the biliary tract is seldom useful, the duct usually being rapidly repopulated unless infestation is cleared and recurrence can be prevented. Those with experience of this problem suggest that the ducts are seldom completely obstructed by the worms present in them (D. Uys, personal communication).

Injury to the upper abdomen may also cause pancreatitis, often developing 24–36 h after injury.

Pancreatic Exocrine Tumours

Two cases of adenocarcinoma of the pancreas in childhood were reported by Benjamin and Wright (1980). Both tumours showed acinar differentiation and zymogen granules.

Small Bowel

Congenital Abnormalities

Enteric Duplications

"Enteric duplication" is the term applied to anomalies that arise early in development dorsal to the developing gut and are usually situated in a position indicating this site of origin. Thus, in parts of the gut with a persistent mesentery they are always found between its leaves. Duplications, with the exception of duodenal lesions, generally have well defined muscle coats, in which peristalsis may be seen to occur. The lining epithelium may resemble that of the adjacent gut, but gastric mucosa is often present. The lumen may or may not communicate with the gut at one or more sites. In a large review Dohn and Povlsen (1951) found that the vast majority of lesions were related to

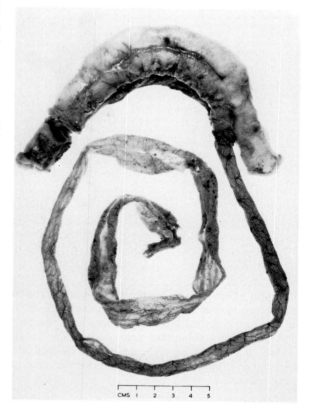

Fig. 5.39. Intestinal duplication. Part of the normal ileum is seen above an extensive, mainly thin-walled, duplication.

the small intestine, with an intrathoracic mass the next most common site (Fig. 5.39). Sites of occurrence, in descending order of frequency, are the ileum, ileocaecal region, oesophagus, jejunum and stomach.

Enteric duplications probably have their origin in the trapping of endodermal cells in the mid-dorsal area of the fore-gut, with subsequent adherence to the notochord and eventual dorsal displacement. The frequency of abnormal vertebrae is greatly elevated in children with intrathoracic reduplications, and the entire topic has been discussed by Smith (1968), who clarified the nomenclature of these lesions, and by Bentley and Smith (1960). Figure 5.40 illustrates this concept of their pathogenesis. The intrathoracic enteric diverticula are discussed in detail by Goldberg and Johnson (1963), and the "split notochord syndrome" of Bentley and Smith is a useful concept in the consideration of associated lesions, which are common. In rare instances, splitting of the notochord, with posterior gut herniation, is present at birth (Denes et al. 1967). Figure 5.41 shows a postvertebral enteric cyst removed from an adult.

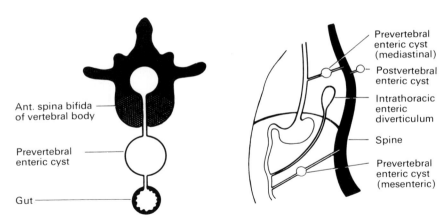

Fig. 5.40. Developmental posterior enteric remnants and spinal malformations in the split notochord syndrome. (Reproduced from Bentley and Smith 1960 by permission of the Editor of *Archives of Disease in Childhood*)

Lubolt (1958), in reviewing the literature, found that recurrent internal bleeding occurred in 20%–30% of cases of intestinal duplication. Intestinal obstruction and perforation may also occur. Sen et al. (1988), in a report of eight cases, emphasized the importance of meningitis and intraspinal sequelae in these lesions.

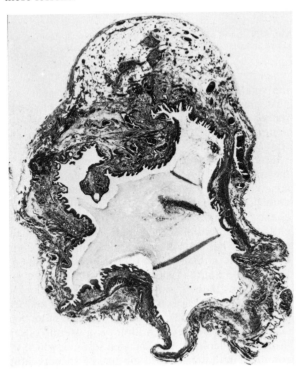

Fig. 5.41. Postvertebral enteric cyst. This lesion was removed from within the dura of a 21-year-old male with progressive paraplegia. (H&E, × 9) (Courtesy of Dr M. Squier)

Atresia and Stenosis

For many years it was assumed that during development the gut went through a stage where cell proliferation filled the lumen before recannalization established the definitive lumen. Moutsouris (1966) re-examined this hypothesis in human embryos, and found that complete obliteration of the lumen occurred only in the duodenum. This suggestion apparently afforded a less satisfactory explanation of atresia of the gut than had been thought in the past. However, experiments involving intrauterine surgery have shown that jejunal atresia accompanied by agenesis of the dorsal mesentery results from intrauterine occlusion of the superior mesenteric artery proximal to its jejunal branches. For this reason vascular changes are now propounded as a probable cause of small-bowel atresia in humans (see Louw and Barnard 1955; Abrams 1968).

Atretic and stenotic lesions of the bowel were first classified by Bland-Sutton (1889) into three types: type I, in which a "diaphragm" was formed across the gut, often involving the muscularis mucosae but not deeper layers (Figs. 5.41 and 5.42); type II, in which there was an interruption in the continuity of the gut, with a fibrous cord connecting the two "blind ends" (Figs. 5.43–5.45); and type III, in which a segment of gut and the fibrous cord were missing and in which there was, in addition, a V-shaped defect in the mesentery at the site of the atresia. Types II and III are more common than type I, but mixed types are found.

In a special form, the so-called apple-peel deformity (Fig. 5.46), a proximal jejunal or distal duodenal atresia of type III is associated with distal small intestine, which coils around the marginal artery and

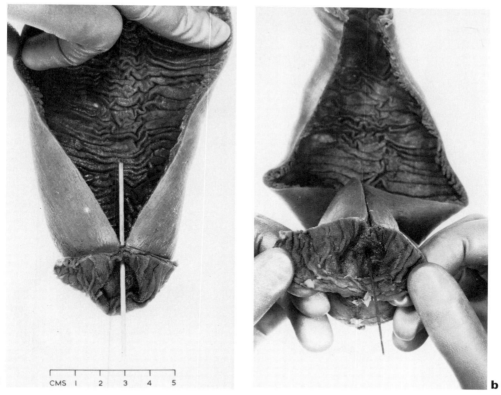

Fig. 5.42. **a** Distended jejunum with membranous atresia with a pinhole communication, resected at 10 months. In this time massive hypertrophy and dilatation of the proximal bowel had occurred. **b** The pinhole from below.

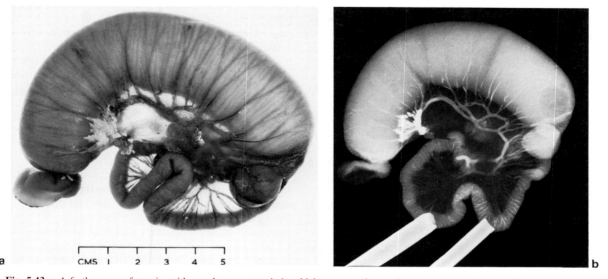

Fig. 5.43. **a** A further case of atresia, with membranous atresia in which postresection angiograms were performed. The membrane is at the site of the cystic dilatation. **b** Radiographs emphasize that vascular changes presumed to be important in the pathogenesis of complete atresias are not evident post partum in the membranous form.

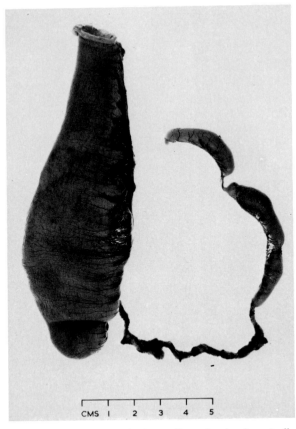

Fig. 5.44. Dilated jejunum leads to a fibrous band and eventually to two further patent segments separated by bands.

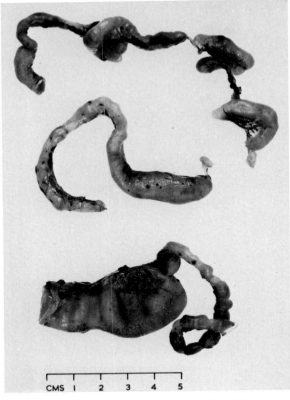

Fig. 5.45. Resections of gut from a case of multiple atresias showing blind ends and fibrous cords connecting patent bowel. A membranous atresia was present in the lowest (proximal) specimen.

receives its arterial supply distally. The mesentery is not fixed to the posterior abdominal wall.

Jejunal and ileal atresia are associated with local anomalies which predispose to volvulus and thus to local ischaemia, such as incomplete intestinal rotation, meconium ileus, vitellointestinal cord and gastroschisis (Amoury et al. 1977) or exomphalos. Extra-abdominal malformations are less commonly seen with jejunal or ileal atresia than with duodenal atresia. There is a male predominance in all types.

Stenosis of the small intestine is a well recognized late complication of necrotizing enterocolitis in preterm infants (see p. 245).

Atresia of the large bowel is very rare (Fig. 5.47). Evans (1951), in a review of 1948 reported cases of atresia, found only six of atresia in the colon. Coryllos and Simpson (1962) reviewed 20 cases and added two to the literature, and Hartman et al. (1963) reported a further 12. Benson et al. (1968) reviewed 209 instances of atresia or stenosis of the bowel and found 22 in the colon, six being of Bland-Sutton's type I, seven of type II, and eight of type III. One case of stenosis in the sigmoid was recorded. Atresia of the colon has twice been reported in association with Hirschsprung's disease (Hyde and De Lorimier 1968; Haffner and Schistad 1969). This is of some interest, as ischaemic injury has been suggested as a cause of aganglionosis.

Malrotation

Malrotation occurs in complete or incomplete forms. In the latter, the caecum lies across the stomach and duodenum and may cause high intestinal obstruction by external pressure. This abnormality is often accompanied by volvulus, and less commonly by intussusception. Where the bowel remains on a single unfixed mesentery, rotation around the superior mesenteric artery may occur with volvulus – the "maypole" or "apple-peel" bowel syndrome (Fig. 5.46). The syndrome may occur in familial clusters

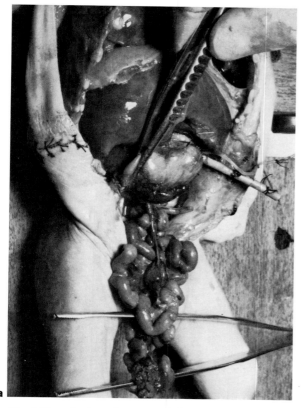

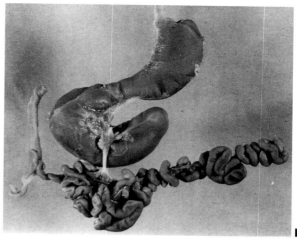

Fig. 5.46. **a** Apple-peel or maypole bowel. The intestines coil around the marginal artery, in this case the superior mesenteric. **b** Maypole bowel with stomach and duodenum.

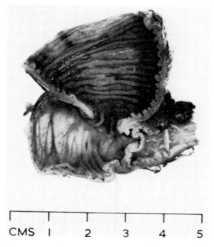

Fig. 5.47. A rare membranous atresia in the large bowel. Ileum to the *left*, caecum *below* and *right*; a membrane obstructs the proximal ascending colon.

(Blyth and Dickson 1969) and may be associated with multiple intestinal atresias (Seashore et al. 1987). Failure of intestinal rotation always accompanies abdominal wall defects such as gastrochisis, exomphalos and diaphragmatic hernia.

Meckel's Diverticulum

Meckel's diverticulum represents a partial persistence of the vitellointestinal duct and is usually found on the antimesenteric border of the ileum, about 1 m proximal to the ileocaecal valve. It represents a failure of obliteration of the duct when the mid-gut loop returns to the abdomen at 10 weeks' gestation. Other anomalies of duct obliteration are shown in Fig. 5.48; all except Meckel's diverticulum are very rare. Meckel's diverticulum is commoner in males and is a true diverticulum. The lumen is lined with

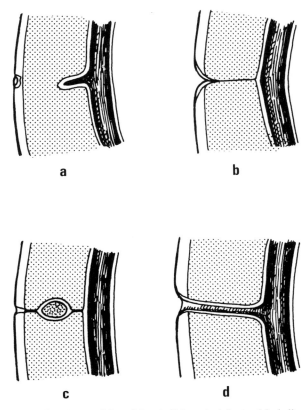

Fig. 5.48. Abnormalities of the vitellointestinal duct. **a** Meckel's diverticulum; **b** vitelline cord with umbilical sinus; **c** omphalomesenteric cyst; **d** vitelline fistula.

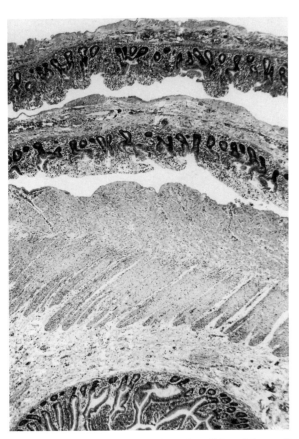

Fig. 5.49. A "Swiss roll" preparation of small bowel from a 2-year-old boy presenting with perforation. Normal bowel and areas of muscle deficiency are seen. (× 32)

epithelium similar to that of the bowel from which it arises, but areas of gastric mucosa are found in up to 50% of cases, and gastrin-producing cells may be demonstratable (Capron et al. 1977). Most diverticula are symptomless but they may form the apex of an intussusception or be the site of peptic ulceration. Seagram et al. (1968) reviewed 218 patients, 81 of whom underwent surgery for complications. Gastric mucosa was found in 64%, pancreatic tissue in 4%, and colonic mucosa in 6%. The diverticulum usually lies free, but it may be attached to the umbilicus by a fibrous cord, in which case volvulus of the small intestine around the cord is an additional hazard.

Segmental Absence of Intestinal Musculature

In segmental absence of intestinal musculature there is an abrupt change from normal bowel wall to complete absence of both muscle coats for a few centimetres. The wall is very thin and the lumen collapsed. It is an uncommon cause of intestinal obstruction in the neonate (Fig. 5.49).

We have seen similar segmental loss of muscularis propria in the intestine presenting as recurrent subacute intestinal obstruction in a young child who underwent exchange transfusion in the neonatal period and then developed necrotizing enterocolitis.

An incomplete review by Husain et al. (1992) reported three cases but confirmed that there are primary and secondary forms of this entity and that most cases occur in premature or low weight infants (see also Alvarez et al. 1982).

Short Intestine

Congenitally short intestines, usually accompanied by malrotation, have been reported (see Yutani et al. 1973). These cases have no other morphological abnormality; the gut measures 30–45 cm and the affected individuals present with vomiting, diarrhoea and failure to thrive.

The intestine may be shortened by massive resection and is reported to be short in mucoviscidosis.

Malabsorption Syndromes

Malabsorption syndromes in infants and children may be divided into two broad groups; enteropathies of the small intestine, which are disorders characterized by mucosal morphological abnormalities (Table 5.2), and those in which the intestinal mucosa is histologically normal (Table 5.3).

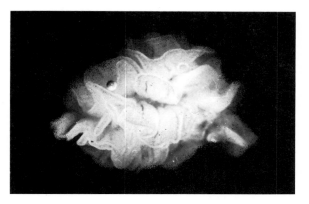

Fig. 5.50. Jejunal biopsy from an 18-month-old infant presenting with failure to thrive. Leaf-like villi and short ridges predominate but are narrow in cross-section. The epithelium was entirely normal.

Table 5.2. Causes of malabsorption with histological abnormality of the small intestine

Cause	Reference
Coeliac disease	Sakula and Shiner (1957)
Postenteritic	Rossi et al. (1980)
CMPI	Harrison et al. (1976)
Other food intolerance	Vitoria et al. (1982)
Giardiasis	Zinneman and Kaplan (1972)
Tropical sprue	
Immunological deficiencies	Ament et al. (1973)
Mucoviscidosis	Thomaidis and Arey (1963)
Histiocytosis X	Keeling and Harries (1973)
α-β Lipoproteinaemia	Lloyd (1972)
Crohn's disease	Chrispin and Tempany (1967)
Dermatitis herpetiformis	Renuala et al. (1984)
Whipple's disease	Aust and Smith (1962)
Congenital microvillus atrophy	Davidson et al. (1978)

Small intestinal enteropathy sometimes present

Malnutrition	Burman (1965)
Iron-deficiency anaemia	Naiman et al. (1964)

Table 5.3. Causes of malabsorption without intestinal mucosal abnormality

Cause	Reference
Short intestine:	
Postresection	Valman (1976)
Congenital	Yutani et al. (1973)
Enzyme defects	Holzel (1967)
Emotional deprivation	Patten and Gardner (1962)
Malrotation	Burke and Anderson (1966)
Pancreatic achylia and	
neutropenia	Shmerling et al. (1969)
Endocrine:	
Ganglioneuroma	Rosenstein and Engelman (1963)
Hypoparathyroidism	Stickler et al. (1965)

described by Chacko et al. (1960) in Indian children and subsequently in English and West Indian children residing in the UK (Burman 1965) and in white Australians (Walker-Smith 1972b). In infants, slender ridges and leaf-like villi are commonplace (Fig. 5.50). In children, a mixture of leaf-like and finger-like villi with occasional short slender ridges is found (Fig. 5.51), in contrast to the mucosal pattern in adults, where finger-like villi predominate. The immature sterological appearances are reflected in a reduced surface to volume ratio in infants (Risdon and Keeling 1974). Site-related differences in the intestinal villous pattern in infants are described (Walker-Smith 1972b), with finger-like villi being more frequent in the distal jejunum and ileum.

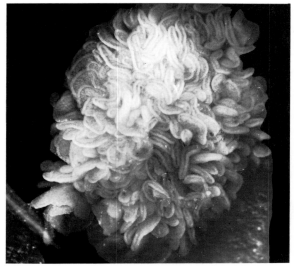

Fig. 5.51. Jejunal biopsy from a 9-year-old boy, obtained during the investigation of short stature; normal surface epihelium.

Normal Intestinal Appearances

The villous patten of the small intestine in infants and children differs from that in adults. This was first

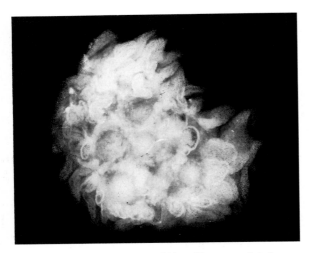

Fig. 5.52. Biopsy from a 5-year-old boy. The group of circles seen in the biopsy is produced by localized loss of villi where the mucosa is stretched over lymphoid aggregates in the submucosa.

Intestinal villi, whatever their morphological appearance, are covered by columnar epithelium with regular-sized basally arranged nuclei. The number of intraepithelial lymphocytes present lies within the adult range (Mauromichaelis et al. 1976).

The age-related variation in villous pattern in children may be responsible for some of the minor "abnormalities" described in the small intestine in conditions such as iron-deficiency anaemia and malnutrition.

Biopsy Management

Jejunal biopsies are fragile and easily distorted during processing, and will repay very careful handling. If possible they should be brought to the laboratory in the biopsy capsule and removed from it by the pathologist with a needle or ophthalmic forceps. Orientation during blocking-out is easier if the biopsy is placed mucosal surface upwards on a piece of still paper or card. It will adhere firmly in seconds. Black French art paper is particularly suitable, as it provides good contrast for both dissecting microscopic examination and photography, and its rough surface makes detachment during fixation less likely. The villous pattern is often easier to see if the biopsy is examined under fluid. Formol–saline is suitable for routine purposes and prevents autolysis of the specimen if dissecting microscopic examination is prolonged, although normal saline can be substituted if the part of the specimen is required for enzyme assay. It is not necessary to immerse the specimen and its mount in a large quantity of fluid; pipetting fluid dropwise onto

the biopsy to form a large blob can provide sufficient fluid to float out the villi.

After fixation, a large biopsy can be bisected with a scapel but still left attached to the paper during processing, as this aids orientation at the blocking-out stages. Biopsies are sectioned at right angles to the luminal surface. It is convenient to have a short ribbon of sections mounted on the same slide and stained with haematoxylin and eosin and periodic acid – Schiff (PAS) with a nuclear stain.

Common artefacts in jejunal biopsies are produced by oblique cutting (which will cause spurious shortening of villi) and stretching of the biopsy prior to fixation – which is particularly easy to do if the biopsy is superficial and does not include the muscularis mucosae for most of the length of the biopsy, as often happens when an "infant" biopsy capsule is used. When this happens the villi are usually triangular in cross-section, often with a tapering apical portion.

Siting of the biopsy is important, as duodenal villi are shorter than those of the jejunum, and minor villous shortening in a biopsy obtained without fluoroscopic monitoring should be viewed with caution.

The presence of lymphoid aggregates within the mucosa may give rise to local loss of villous pattern, the cause of which is readily apparent in the section, and may produce an abnormality on dissecting microscopic examination (Fig. 5.52). Small intestinal mucosal abnormalities are reviewed by Variend et al. (1984).

Coeliac Disease

Coeliac disease is a permanent intolerance to dietary gluten, producing a proximal small-intestinal enteropathy leading to malabsorption, with clinical and biochemical abnormalities; gluten withdrawal results in complete clinical remission and a histologically normal small-intestine mucosa (McNeish et al. 1979).

This condition was first described in children by Samuel Gee (1888), but it was not until 1950 that Dicke identified gluten, the germ protein of wheat, rye and other cereals, as the causal agent and demonstrated that its exclusion from the diet resulted in clinical remission. Subsequent investigations have shown that the most toxic component is a polypeptide with a molecular weight less than 15 000 in the α-gliadin fraction of gluten (Dissanayake et al. 1974).

Despite the precise identification of the toxic factor, the mechanism by which it produces mucosal damage is not certain. It has been suggested that a specific mucosal peptidase deficiency results in the

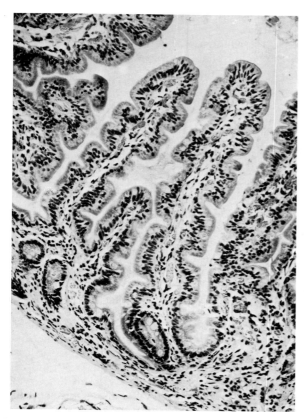

Fig. 5.53. Normal jejunal mucosa. Slender, tapering villi are covered by columnar epithelium with the nuclei of the epithelial cells arranged regularly along the basement membrane. A few round cells are seen in the lamina propria.

intracellular accumulation of a toxic peptide, leading to epithelial cell damage and mucosal abnormality. Although dipeptidase deficiency has been demonstrated in coeliac disease with return to normal after the institution of a gluten-free diet (Douglas and Peters 1970), this may be the result rather than the cause of epithelial abnormality, and a parallel may be drawn with the mucosal disaccharidase deficiency demonstrable in untreated coeliac disease.

A variety of immunological abnormalities have been demonstrated in patients with coeliac disease, including elevated levels of immunoglobulins to dietary proteins and reticulin with elevations of IgA and reduction in IgG and IgM levels (Kendrick and Walker-Smith 1970). Increased numbers of immunoglobulin-containing cells have been demonstrated in the lamina propria of the small intestine in untreated coeliac disease (Lancaster-Smith et al. 1974) and immune complexes in the basement membrane and lamina propria of the small intestine (Shiner and Ballard 1973). Doe et al. (1974) have

demonstrated immune complexes in the serum following gluten challenge in treated coeliacs, and Carswell and Logan (1973) found low levels of β_{1c} and β_{1a} globulin in untreated coeliacs. They suggest that an Arthus-type reaction occurs in the lamina propria. It is not clear whether the immunological abnormalities described are the result of the primary abnormality or whether they represent a secondary reaction to the toxic α-gliadin fraction.

Coeliac disease occurs in all areas where gluten is ingested. Its prevalence is unclear, particularly with the demonstration of symptomless cases in family studies where intestinal biopsies have been performed. Incidence estimates in the British Isles vary from 1 in 3000 births in England (Carter et al. 1957) and 1 in 300 (Myotte et al. 1973) in West Ireland. More recent studies (Littlewood et al. 1980; Stevens et al. 1987) show a substained reduction in the incidence of this disorder in different centres of the UK. Stevens et al. (1987) found a 60% reduction in incidence since 1975. Both groups of authors draw attention to the changing pattern of infant feeding, with return to breast feeding and later weaning, and to the decreased incidence of gastroenteritis in early infancy.

The familial occurrence of coeliac disease is well recognized, but the discordance of monozygotic twins for coeliac disease argues against simple Mendelian inheritance (McNeish and Nelson 1974). A positive correlation between coeliac disease and the possession of histocompatibility antigens HLA 1 and 81 has been demonstrated (McNeish et al. 1973). These findings make a polygenic basis for susceptibility to environmental factors more likely. The HLA status may explain the correlation between coeliac disease and diabetes.

The small-intestine mucosal abnormality in coeliac disease has been demonstrated at laparotomy (Paulley 1954) and confirmed by peroral biopsy (Sakula and Shiner 1957). Dissecting microscopy shows replacement of normal villi (Fig. 5.53) by a "cobblestone" appearance of the mucosa in which the mouths of crypts are seen (Fig. 5.54). Histological examination shows a "flat" biopsy (Fig. 5.55). The surface epithelium is abnormal, being low. Cuboidal epithelium with haphazard nuclear arrangement, often accompanied by infiltration of the epithelium by small, darkly staining, round cells, and patchy thickening of the basement membrane may be demonstrated by PAS staining. There is an increase in cellularity, particularly of plasma cells, in the lamina propria.

It was thought that this appearance was pathognomonic for coeliac disease, but it has since been shown that the same appearance may be produced in infants by infection (Barnes and Townley 1973), and

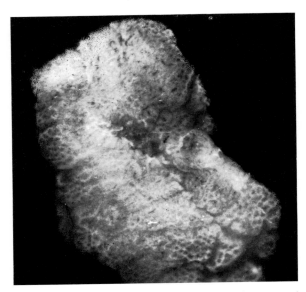

Fig. 5.54. Jejunal biopsy from a 5-year-old boy who presented with bulky offensive stools, anorexia and poor weight gain. Villi are absent and the mouths of the crypts and the cobblestone appearance of the mucosa are visible.

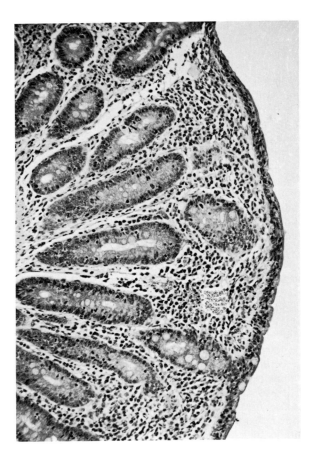

less commonly by cows' milk protein or soy protein intolerance and tropical sprue. In these conditions the changes are often patchy in distribution (Manuel et al. 1979), in contrast to coeliac disease, where the change is uniform.

The diagnosis of coeliac disease, with its implication of permanent gluten intolerance requiring life-long adherence to a gluten-free diet, must leave no room for doubt (McNeish 1980). This is particularly important following the suggestion that a gluten-free diet may reduce the risk of intestinal neoplasia, to which untreated coeliacs are susceptible (Holmes et al. 1976), and because the return to a normal diet in older children or adults may not be accompanied by clinical symptoms or signs although the small intestinal mucosa becomes abnormal. After confirming the diagnosis by intestinal biopsy and the institution of a gluten-free diet for at least 2 years, or perhaps longer in very young children, a further biopsy should be obtained while the individual is on a gluten-free diet (Fig. 5.56). Gluten should then be reintroduced (either as food or as pure powdered gluten) into the diet. A further biopsy should be obtained after 3 months, unless symptoms precipitate the need to biopsy sooner. Most children with coeliac disease will have mucosal abnormalities (Fig. 5.57) but will not necessarily yield a flat biopsy at this time, when partial rather than subtotal villous atrophy is the usual finding (Packer et al. 1978). If the biopsy is normal, a further biopsy should be considered after 2 years on a gluten-containing diet. Children who still have a normal biopsy at this time are unlikely to have coeliac disease, although occasionally a child may take longer than this to produce mucosal abnormalities (Egan-Mitchell et al. 1977).

The response to reintroduction of dietary gluten appears to be dose related. A large dose (10–20 g/day) provokes histological response in 3–6 months (Rolles and McNeish 1976; Packer et al. 1978). A small dose (2.5 g/day) results in histological abnormality in only 90% of children after 12 months (Hamilton and McNeill 1972).

Children with coeliac disease always have a flat biopsy at presentation provided that dietary manipulations have not been instituted before the biopsy is taken. The finding of less severe biopsy changes (degrees of partial villous atrophy) is so uncharacteristic in childhood that one should consider an alternative diagnosis. Very young infants who have been

Fig. 5.55. Flat small intestinal biopsy. Villi have disappeared and the surface epithelium is no longer normal. The epithelial cell height is reduced and nuclei are irregularly sited within the cell. There is an apparent increase of inflammatory cells within the lamina propria.

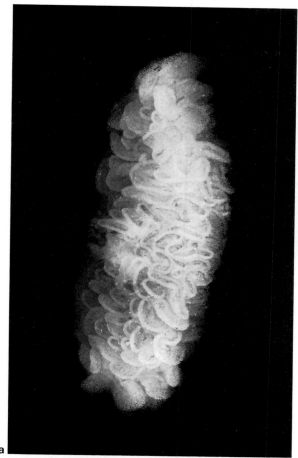

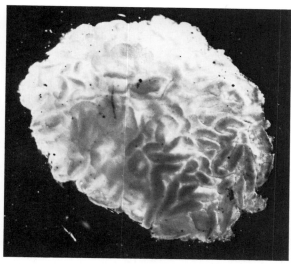

Fig. 5.57. Biopsy from an 11-year-old girl, on a gluten-free diet for 10 years, after 9 weeks on a normal diet. Thick ridges are seen throughout the biopsy; mild irregularities of surface epithelium were seen on histological examination. A biopsy taken after a further 5 weeks was completely flat.

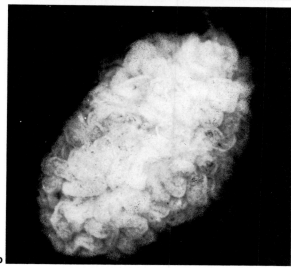

Fig. 5.56. Biopsies from a 5-year-old girl who had been on a gluten-free diet for 4 years. **a** Jejunal biopsy whilst on the diet; surface epithelium appeared normal. **b** Biopsy performed after 10 weeks on a diet containing at least 10 g natural gluten per day; the patient became anorectic and miserable. Short thick ridges predominate. The surface epithelium was irregular.

ingesting small amounts of gluten for a short period of time may be symptomatic when there is partial, not subtotal, villous atrophy (Walker-Smith et al. 1978).

Most children present before 2 years of age, and although the interval between the introduction of cereals and development of symptoms is variable most are symptomatic within 6 months. Because of the practice of very early introduction of cereals into the diet some infants present before 4 months; this group develops symptoms faster and may have an acute onset with diarrhoea and vomiting and be severely ill (Burke et al. 1965). The classic picture is of a miserable, anorectic toddler with distended abdomen, wasted buttocks and abnormal bulky stools. Older children present with short stature and iron-deficiency anaemia; they may have no gastro-intestinal symptoms.

Dermatitis herpetiformis associated with gluten enteropathy will respond to withdrawal of the allergen in children as in adults. This improvement is independent of the mucosal status; the rash may improve although the villous architecture is normal (Renuala et al. 1984).

Congenital Microvillus Atrophy

This condition, also known as microvillus inclusion disease, presents with severe intractable diarrhoea.

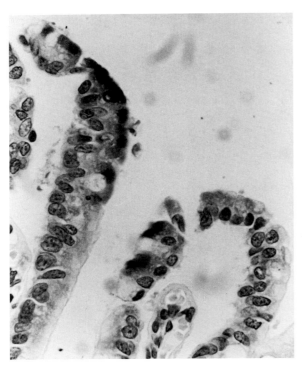

Fig. 5.58. Apical enterocytes contain packets of microvillus material at their luminal surface. (Alkaline phosphatase × 280)

Affected infants are symptomatic from birth and oral feeding exacerbates the problem. Metabolically there is impaired glucose absorption and net water and sodium excretion from the enterocyte. There is no curative treatment, and parenteral nutrition is necessary throughout life (Davidson et al. 1978; Phillips et al. 1985).

The jejunal mucosa is morphologically abnormal with partial villous atrophy, crypt hypoplasia and variable loss of the microvillus brush border over the tips of the villi. Vacuoles containing microvilli are present in the apical enterocyte cytoplasm and these and the brush border loss are demonstrable on staining for alkaline phosphatase (Phillips et al. 1985) (Fig. 5.58). On electron microscopy, microvillus-packed vacuoles, an excess of secretory granules and loss or shortening of microvilli on apical enterocytes are seen, although crypt enterocytes are relatively normal in this respect but have an excess of secretory granules. Lake (1988) has made it clear that electron microscopy is not essential for the diagnosis, but its use in rectal biopsies is advocated by Bell et al. (1991). It is clear that rectal suction biopsy is a much easier and safer procedure than jejunal biopsy in a very sick infant.

Infective Enteritis

Both bacterial and viral enteritis produce mucosal changes in the small intestine. These have been demonstrated by peroral biopsy in the acute state in a study (Barnes and Townley 1973) in which abnormalities were found in 25 of 31 infants. In five cases the biopsy was flat, and the others showed minor abnormalities and cellular infiltration of the lamina propria. The intestinal abnormalities, according to the findings of necropsy studies, are usually confined to the duodenum and jejunum, but the whole of the small intestine may be involved; there is often patchy involvement of the mucosa (Walker-Smith 1972a; Manuel et al. 1979).

Diarrhoea is often prolonged following infective enteritis in infancy because of disaccharidase deficiency induced by mucosal damage. The mucosal abnormalities may also persist for many months and may be indistinguishable from those of coeliac disease. This has probably contributed to the concept that coeliac disease can be a self-limiting condition, and make gluten challenge mandatory in the diagnosis of coeliac disease.

Allergic Enteritis

Gastrointestinal symptoms due to intolerance of cows' milk are uncommon but well recognized (Kuitunen et al. 1975). Milk-induced gastrointestinal bleeding has been reported, although the syndrome is rarely severe. The cases are rarely biopsied; changes in the small bowel are described by Maluenda et al. (1984), who found shortened villi and longer crypts. They found that only intraepithelial eosinophils were of value in discriminating allergic from non-allergic causes of mucosal change. Ament and Rubin (1972) have described an enteropathy indistinguishable from coeliac disease in soy protein intolerance. These entities may be related to allergic enteritis in general, and one group appears to affect the rectum specifically (Goldman and Proujansky 1986).

Giardiasis

Gut infestation with *Giardia lamblia* can produce a variety of symptoms, from mild diarrhoea to a frank malabsorptive picture. Poor social conditions, institutionalization, a recent holiday abroad or symptoms referable to immunological deficiency may be useful pointers in the history of such children.

Diagnosis is usually made by the demonstration of cysts in the stools or motile forms of the organism in

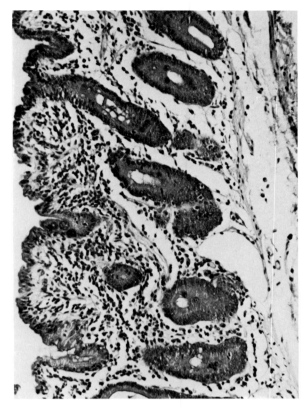

Fig. 5.59. Gardiasis. Biopsy from a 7-year-old institutionalized boy with Down's syndrome being investigated for diarrhoea. Villi are reduced in height and much thicker than normal. There is increased cellularity of the lamina propria. (H/PAS, × 240)

duodenal juice, but parasites may be demonstrable in small-intestinal biopsies.

The histological features of the biopsy are shortening of the villi (occasionally a completely flat mucosa is seen, but usually less severe degrees of villous atrophy are present (Fig. 5.59), inflammatory cell infiltration of the lamina propria, and shortening and irregularity of the surface epithelium (Fig. 5.60).

Infestation with *G. lamblia* is common in immune-deficiency states (Zinnemann and Kaplan 1972), and may be the cause of intestinal abnormalities reported as complications of immune-deficiency disorders. It has also been demonstrated in 24% of 58 coeliac patients by Carswell et al. (1973), but we have not encountered such a high rate of infestation in coeliac disease.

Immune Deficiency States

It is common in combined immunodeficiency to see complete absence of the gut lymphoid tissues (see Chapter 12). Abnormalities of the small intestinal mucosa are described in several types of immuno-deficiency (Ament et al. 1973), and lymphoid hyperplasia can occur in variable immunodeficiency syndromes. *Giardia* infestation is common.

In isolated IgA deficiency, IgA-producing cells are rarely seen in the lamina propria.

Intestinal Lymphangiectasia

A severe protein-loosing enteropathy may occur in infants with widespread abnormalities of the intestinal lymphatics, which are dilated and plexiform in affected individuals. However, less severe forms without great protein loss occur but may still be accompanied by malabsorption and evidence of immune deficiency; immunoglobulin loss may be marked. The syndrome may be caused by a number of processes that occlude the lymphatics, such as tuberculosis (Abramowski et al. 1989).

Histiocytosis X

Diarrhoea has been reported complicating histiocytosis X. Infiltration of the lamina propria and submucosa by abnormal histiocytes, including multinucleate forms, has been described. The infiltration is usually confined to the ileum, although duodenum and jejunum may be involved (Keeling and Harries 1973); in this case the normal villous pattern is lost (Fig. 5.61), although the surface epithelium remains normal. It seems likely that the diarrhoea is due to a combination of loss of absorptive area and interference with lymphatic drainage by the neoplastic proliferation.

Lymph Nodes

Mesenteric lymph nodes are often enlarged and congested in children dying from gastroenteritis. Histologically there is marked reactive change, but severe lymphoid depletion may also be seen and may not be related to the severity of the illness.

The size of the lymph nodes in the neonate is so variable that it is difficult to be certain of abnormality, but mesenteric nodes are usually clearly visible and may appear large to those performing neonatal necropsies infrequently.

Iron-deficiency Anaemia

There is considerable variation in the severity of functional and histological abnormalities of the small

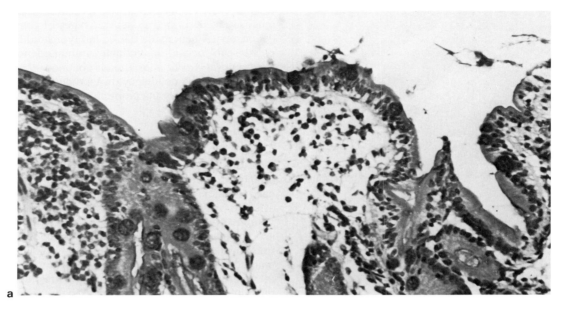

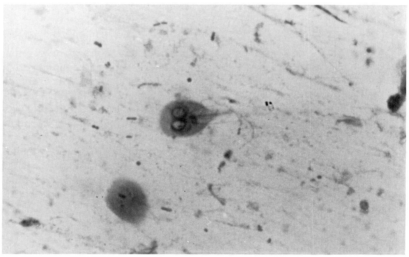

Fig. 5.60. a Same case as in Fig. 6.6. The surface epithelium is abnormal. *Giardia lamblia* are attached to the surface epithelium and lying free in the lumen. (H/PAS, × 400) **b** *G. lamblia* in duodenal aspirate. (Papanicolaou, × 1500)

intestine that are attributed to iron deficiency. Reports from the UK describe mild or equivocal histological changes (Doniach and Shiner 1957; Cameron et al. 1962). Other authors report more severe abnormalities of villous pattern (Naiman et al. 1964; Berkel et al. 1970), with normal surface epithelium. Flat biopsies have been reported in iron deficiency in Indian children (Guga et al. 1968). Intestinal parasitic infestation was excluded by three stool examinations and a concentration procedure, and although clinical improvement was recorded in response to iron therapy follow-up biopsies were not obtained. In the authors' experience of British children, those with iron-deficiency anaemia and a flat biopsy have responded to a gluten-free diet and not required iron supplements.

Malnutrition

Intestinal mucosal abnormalities, varying from minor abnormalities of the villous pattern accompanied by a normal surface epithelium to severe partial or subto-

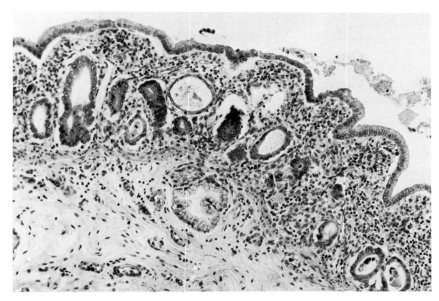

Fig. 5.61. Small intestine of an infant with skin rash, hepatosplenomegaly, lymphadenopathy and diarrhoea. She died aged 15 weeks with disseminated histiocytosis X. The small intestine shows loss of villi with infiltration of the lamina propria by abnormal histiocytes. The surface epithelium is normal.

tal villous atrophy, have been reported in kwash-iorkor (Stanfield et al. 1965). These authors report persistence of mucosal abnormalities despite a return to normal nutritional status – a finding that might cast doubt on the implied casual relationship. The frequency of infective diarrhoea in areas where severe malnutrition is most common should not be overlooked.

Resection of Small Intestine

The common causes of massive resection of small intestine in infancy are volvulus complicating malro-tation or some other congenital anomaly, and multi-ple small intestinal atresias. Successful adaptation of the remaining intestine depends on the extent and site of the resection. Hypertrophy of villi in residual ileum in animals has been described after jejunal resection, but little change occurred in the jejunum when the ileum was removed (Dowling and Booth 1967). Resection of large amounts of ileum may interrupt the enteropathic circulation of bile salts and so influence absorption. Resection of the ileocaecal valve may result in bacterial contamination of the small intestine resulting in a "blind loop" syndrome. Valman (1976) followed up children who had under-gone extensive intestinal resection in the neonatal period and found that they were shorter than their sib-lings, but of appropriate weight for their own height –

a result of prolonged postoperative malnutrition that did not persist into later life. However, Valman and Roberts (1974) demonstrated vitamin B_{12} malabsorp-tion following ileal resection in infancy, and showed that, although serum levels of the vitamin remained normal in the face of malabsorption for some years, puberty was a critical time when supplementation might be required.

Necrotizing Enterocolitis

The 1960s saw publication of a number of reports of intestinal perforation, usually colonic, complicating exchange transfusion for rhesus incompatibility or umbilical venous catheterization for other reasons (Corkery et al. 1968; Orme and Eades 1968). Since then, with the marked decrease in the number of exchange transfusions performed in neonatal nurs-eries, necrotizing enterocolitis is usually seen in the very small, sick, preterm neonate, and both small and large intestine are involved.

Caplan and MacKendrick (1993), in a review sug-gesting a major role for inflammatory mediators in the disease, cite data suggesting that almost 12% of all premature neonates weighing less than 1500 g are affected, and the disease is clearly an important cause of death in this group. The disease has been described in term neonates after cardiac catheterization and angiography during investigation for congenital heart

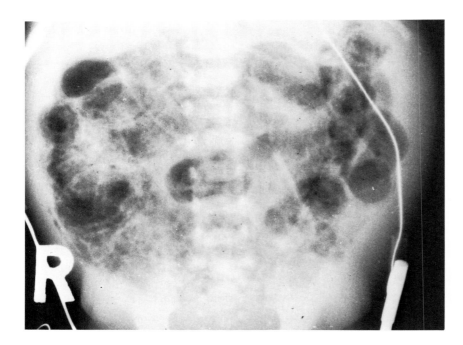

Fig. 5.62. Radiograph of a 5-day-old infant born at 36 weeks' gestation by emergency lower section caesarean section for fetal distress; asphyxiated at birth. Bloody stools and abdominal distension at 4 days. The radiograph shows abdominal distension and double contour of intestinal wall due to gas in the submucosa.

disease, and the use of hypertonic contrast medium has been implicated in its pathogenesis (Cooke et al. 1980). Epidemics of necrotizing enterocolitis in full-term neonates associated with the isolation of *Salmonella* spp. (Stein et al. 1972) and *Clostridium butyricum* (Howard et al. 1977) have been reported, but most cases are sporadic and only normal gut flora are cultured from the stools.

Three general aetiological factors have been implicated: mucosal ischaemia, a gut flora that contains organisms which invade the damaged area, and feeding that enhances bacterial growth (Book et al. 1976).

Prophylaxis with kanamycin alters bacterial flora, but does not prevent the disease (Boyle et al. 1978), which may also follow ampicillin therapy in childhood (Auritt et al. 1978). Ischaemia is of the greater significance in aetiology, and it has been suggested that the various factors that predispose to this condition (birth asphyxia, birth trauma, cyanotic heart disease, exchange transfusion, disseminated intravascular coagulation, etc.) all produce a selective ischaemia of the gut, which develops as a "protective" mechanism for the rest of the circulation, e.g. the brain or heart (Lloyd 1969).

This field has been re-explored by Sibbons et al. (1992), whose interesting studies have apparently not considered work on mediators or the effects of obstruction (Berry and Fraser 1968; Caplan and MacKendrick 1993).

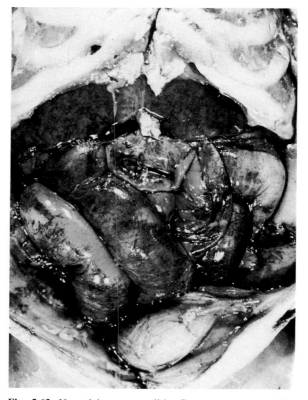

Fig. 5.63. Necrotizing enterocolitis. Gross appearance of distended loops of affected bowel.

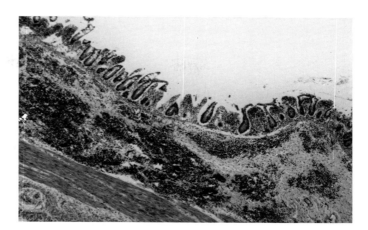

Fig. 5.64. Early stages of enterocolitis with haemorrhage and infarction of mucosa. (H&E, ×40)

The disease usually presents with ileus and abdominal distension after a period of bloody diarrhoea. Circulatory collapse is common (Fig. 5.62). The length of bowel involved is variable but the terminal ileum and ascending colon are almost always involved. The affected portion of bowel is distended and plum-coloured, with friable wall (Fig. 5.63). When it is opened, the often green-stained mucosa can be wiped off the muscularis. Perforation may occur (Kliegman and Fanaroff 1984).

The pathological findings are related to the age of the lesions. The earliest findings are irregularly shaped and sized areas of haemorrhagic infarction of the mucosa and submucosa, with variable deep extension to involve the muscularis propria and serosa

(Fig. 5.64). They are usually between 0.5 and 2 cm in diameter and frequently multiple; it is rare for them to be circumferential.

The central part of the lesion may become necrotic and grey in colour with a surrounding hyperaemic halo (Fig. 5.65). The necrotic portion of the bowel may bulge above the serosal surface and perforation may occur. Generalized peritonitis with fibrin deposition on the serosal surface of dilated loops of bowel and free pus in the peritoneal cavity may then supervene or may be localized, depending on the site of perforation.

Once necrosis of the mucosa has occurred, gas may enter the bowel wall and often spreads in the loose-textured submucosa (Fig. 5.66) but may be

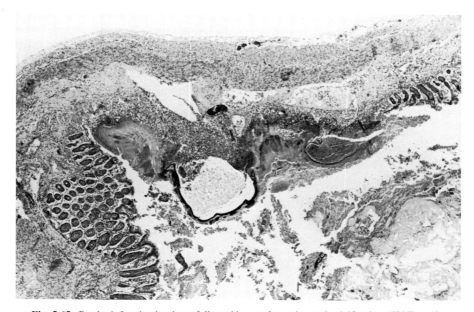

Fig. 5.65. Patchy infarction has been followed by gas formation and calcification. (H&E, ×40)

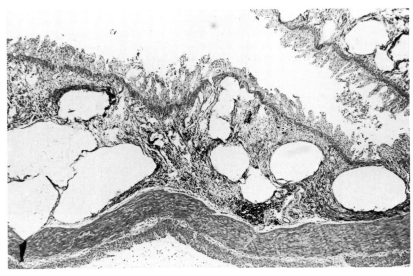

Fig. 5.66. Typical multiple gas bubbles in enterocolitis. (H&E, × 36)

present beneath the serosa. Hepatic necrosis with gas-filled cyst formation may occasionally occur. As a late sequel, stricture-producing obstruction and even atresia of the intestine may occur (see also p. 254).

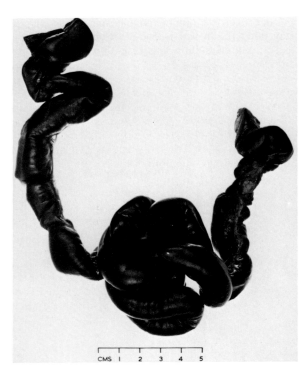

Fig. 5.67. Extensive resection of small bowel following volvulus in an infant. This was followed by malabsorption.

Massive Intestinal Infarction

Massive infarction of the intestine may occasionally follow umbilical arterial catheterization in the neonate when complicated by aortic thrombosis. This complication usually occurs in very small preterm infants whose condition necessitates prolonged catheterization, but this is not always the case.

Volvulus

Intestinal volvulus occurs more commonly in the small intestine than in the colon, and usually affects the ileum. Abnormalities of mesenteric attachment, or of gut rotation, are important predisposing causes, as are enteric duplications (Howaniety et al. 1968). Extensive resection may lead to malabsorption (Fig. 5.67). Volvulus of the small intestine due to massive loading with *Ascaris lumbricoides* has been reported (Manhani Sing 1967).

Perforation

Spontaneous perforation of the small intestine in infancy is rare, and usually complicates infarction of the bowel from any cause, or occurs in association with meconium ileus.

In recent years perforation has been associated with exchange transfusion and prolonged parenteral therapy via the umbilical veins, often appearing as part of the syndrome of enterocolitis.

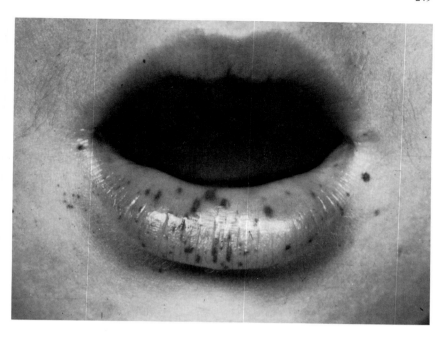

Fig. 5.68. Pigmentation around the lips in the Peutz–Jeghers syndrome.

Polypi

Solitary hamartomatous polypi are occasionally seen in the jejunum. They have a delicate branching structure with smooth muscle in the stroma and are covered by normal epithelium. They may occur as part of the Peutz–Jeghers syndrome (Figs. 5.68 and 5.69) and were found in this segment of the gut in 69% of cases in large series (Tovar et al. 1983).

Such polypi can cause haemorrhage or intussusception; they are hamartomas and not adenomatous polypi. Malignant change is apparently extremely rare and has been reported in the jejunum and stomach (Tovar et al. 1983). (See also p. 268.)

Tuberculosis

Tuberculosis of the gastrointestinal tract has become progressively less common in Europe following the introduction of effective cattle control methods and treatment of milk. It is still seen commonly in the Indian subcontinent and in Africa.

Intussusception

Intussusception is the invagination of one portion of bowel into another. Once the invagination has started, it is carried further along the bowel lumen by peristalsis. The effects of intussusception are obstruction of the intestinal lumen, vascular occlusion resulting in gangrene, perforation, peritonitis and adhesions between the two serosal surfaces, which are in apposition. Between 60% and 85% of intussusceptions occur in the first 2 years of life, with the peak incidence at around 6 months of age. In the majority of these cases no definite cause is identified. Most are ileocaecal, the ileocaecal valve having its abundant lymphoid tissue at the apex; lymphoid hypertrophy is often advanced as a causative factor. Boys outnumber girls by 2 : 1 (Bjarnason and Petterson 1968).

Porter et al. (1993) found viral inclusions with typical features of adenovirus in 19 of 35 appendices from cases of intussusception. Montgomery and Popek (1994) found lymphoid hyperplasia in half of 63 children with intussusception. They found adenovirus inclusions in five of these and in five cases with normal intestinal lymphoid tissue.

In older children a predisposing cause is usually present, a Meckel's diverticulum, a polyp, or a tumour being found at the apex of the intussusceptum. We have seen lymphosarcoma of the small intestine presenting as an irreducible intussusception; Riker and Goldstein (1968) report a similar experience.

Stevenson et al. (1967) and McGovern and Gross (1968) reported intussusception in the postoperative period as a complication of a variety of operative procedures, the majority of which were intra-abdominal.

Haemangiomas

Haemorrhage from intestinal vascular abnormalities may be a cause of severe anaemia and ill health in

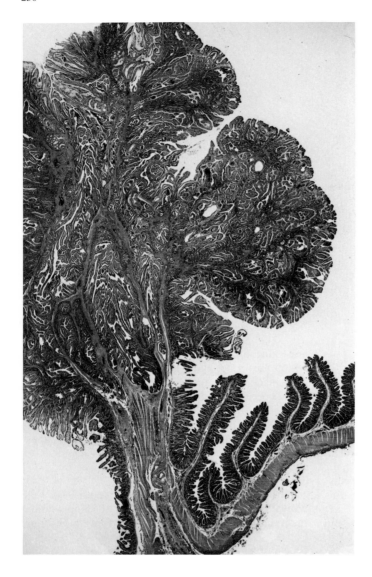

Fig. 5.69. Hamartomatous polyp in the Peutz–Jeghers syndrome. Smooth muscle is seen in the branching stroma.

childhood. Kaijser (1936) has classified these lesions into four groups:

1. Multiple phlebectasia. Varicose lesions – dilated veins in the submucosa. These are probably acquired and do not occur in childhood.
2. Cavernous haemangiomas, which may be diffuse or circumscribed.
3. Capillary haemangiomas.
4. Gastrointestinal haemangiomas associated with cutaneous lesions.

Haemangiomas of the small intestine are often multiple and may accompany angiomas in other organs. They are associated with thrombocytopenia as part of the Kippel–Trenaunay syndrome (Kuffer et al. 1968).

The angiomas are usually confined to the submucosa and present as recurrent intestinal bleeding (Nader and Margolin 1966) (Fig. 5.70), but may extend through to the peritoneal surface, causing intestinal obstruction following multiple adhesions. Useful reports are those of Rissier (1960) and Nader and Margolin (1966). A review of the investigation and management of 139 cases is given by Sparnon et al. (1984).

Lymphangiomas

Lymphangioma of the small intestine is much less common than haemangioma. A case has been reported

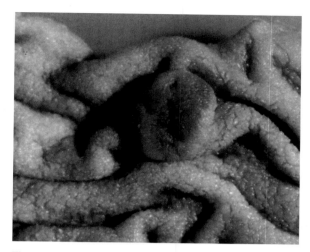

Fig. 5.70. Angioma from a child presenting with recurrent rectal bleeding.

with diarrhoea, weight loss and hypoproteinaemia (Walker-Smith et al. 1969). Localized lesions may provoke intestinal obstruction (Fig. 5.71).

Hirschsprung's Disease

Hirschsprung's disease is named after Hirschsprung, although, as with many other eponymously named diseases, there are a number of reports that antedate his report of 1887, which described two patients with megacolon. Although aganglionosis in the distal segment of the bowel was recorded only 14 years later by Tittel (1901), it was not until the work of Swenson and Bill in 1948 and Bodian et al. (1949) that the surgical and pathological findings in the disease were widely understood.

One of us (Berry 1992) has described how altered expression of homeotic genes may affect a number of developmental processes, and it seems that this type of altered gene expression may be involved in the production of the Hirschsprung phenotype. Wolgemuth et al. (1989) induced overexpression of the homeobox gene *Hox-1.4* in the mouse and produced a failure of innervation of the large bowel manifest as hypoganglionosis and megacolon, apparently due to failure either of neural crest cell migration or of gut mesenchyme to provide appropriate signals for migration (the gene is also expressed in mesenchyme). The enteric nervous system (ENS) is composed of the parasympathetic ganglia of the gut whose cells are derived from the neural crest. Colonization of the gut by neural crest cells occurs in a proximal to distal sequence, and Serbedzija et al. (1991) have shown that sacral neural crest cells contribute to the ENS as well as those of vagal (but not truncal) origin. Within the gut, colonization occurs in a dorsoventral sequence. In the spotted mouse, a further animal model of Hirschsprung's disease, excessive production of extracellular matrix components apparently restricts migration of neural crest cells into the postumbilical bowel (Payette et al. 1988). Certain of the matrix changes observed are found in the outer layer of the gut, astride the probable pathway of migration of neural crest derived cells. Payette et al provide data which suggest that there is no interference with neuronal migration directly and point out that one population of crest-derived cells, the Schwann cells, appears to migrate normally.

Two mechanisms of interference with development may thus exist, one affecting the craniocaudal positioning mechanisms of developing cell populations, resulting in a distal deficit, providing an explanation for the classic form of the disease. However, proximal dysplastic zones (see p. 256) are less readily explained. The second mechanism operates locally to interfere with cell migration selectively. Here

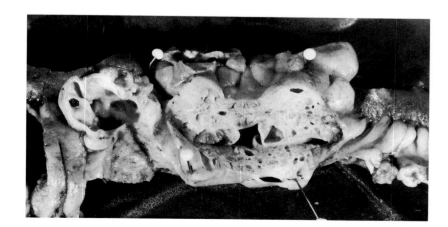

Fig. 5.71. Lymphangioma of the ileum in a boy of 15 years presenting with intestinal obstruction. Localized ectasia of lymphatics affects the whole wall and encroaches on the lumen of the intestine.

hypoplastic zones before aganglionic ones are com-
prehensible. Because the submucosal ganglia form as
a result of the migration of neurons from the original
myenteric ganglia through the circular muscle
(Gershon et al. 1980), changes in these structures
may be associated with either failure of development.

These observations illuminate the demonstration by
Angrist et al. (1993) of monogenetic inheritance in five
families with Hirschsprung's disease to a short region
situated pericentromerically on chromosome 10, in
close proximity to the locus for multiple endocrine
neoplasia type 2 (MEN2). Various associations of the
disease (with neuroblastoma, phaeochromocytoma,
Ondine's curse and Waardenburg' syndrome) seem
less surprising. Clearly, a number of related genetic
changes produce a number of phenotypes, which have
in common changes in the way in which cell populations originating in the neural crest develop; the association of the disease with deletions on chromosome
13 has also been reported. (Bottani et al. 1991).

Hirschsprung's disease occurs in around 1 in 4500
births (Spouge and Baird 1985).

Clinical and Pathological Findings

Around 3% of the cases of Hirschsprung's disease
seen at the Hospital for Sick Children, Great Ormond
Street, involve the ileum; in 1% the disease extends
proximally to the duodenum. The extensive intestinal
resection necessary in these children can prove fatal
or interfere with normal growth and nutrition.

Of 220 cases reviewed by Bodian and Carter
(1963), 82% involved the rectum and sigmoid colon
(short segment) and 18% the more proximal portion
of the bowel (long segment). Two cases of total aganglionosis of the small bowel were seen; further examples of this form have since been reported (see
Walker et al. 1966 for bibliography). It is probable
that between 3% and 8% of all cases show total
colonic involvement. In short-segment cases there is
a marked preponderance of males (8 : 1), which is
present but less marked in long-segment disease. The
proportion of affected siblings in short-segment index
cases is of the order of 1 in 20 for brothers and 1 in
100 or lower for sisters. The proportion of affected
siblings in long-segment index patients is of the order
of 1 in 10 irrespective of sex (Bodian and Carter
1963; Carter et al. 1982). There is a marked association with Down's syndrome: Graivier and Sieber
(1966) found that 3.4% of reported cases of
Hirschsprung's disease occurred in patients with
Down's syndrome, and Spouge and Baird (1985)
gave a frequency of 2.8% in a study of a large birth
cohort. Cardiovascular and skeletal and limb defects
are also increased in frequency.

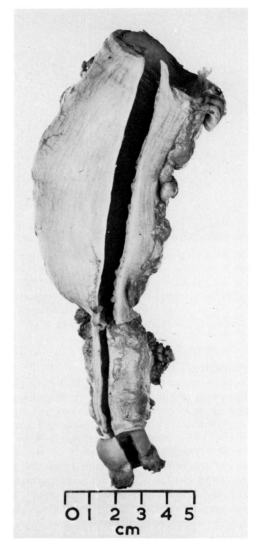

Fig. 5.72. Short-segment Hirschsprung's disease with dilated
segment, cone and narrowed zone. (Boy aged 2 years.)

The disease generally presents in the neonatal
period with intestinal obstructions, although other
presentations are seen (Ajayi et al. 1969). The mortality rate in infants with this disease has varied from
6% to 43% in various series (see Erenpries 1967),
and is related to age at diagnosis (Atwell 1968). In
neonates the extent of disease also affects prognosis;
Fraser and Wilkinson (1967) found a mortality rate
of 67% in long-segment disease, compared with 24%
in the short-segment type.

Pathological appearances vary with the length of
the segment and the duration of the disease. Typically
there is a dilated hypertrophied segment, a cone, and

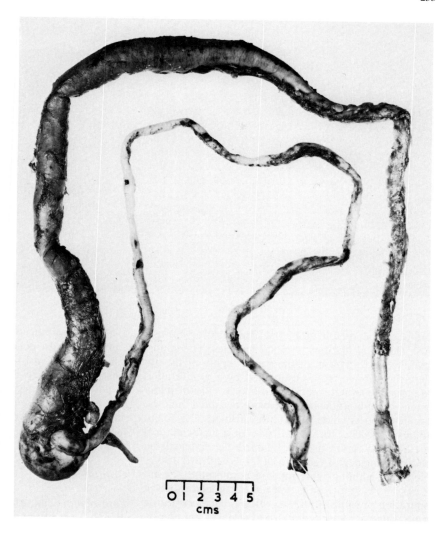

Fig. 5.73. Long-segment disease where the zonation is not marked.

a narrowed zone (Figs. 5.72 and 5.73). The basic abnormality is the complete absence of ganglion cells from the myenteric, submucosal and intramucosal plexuses in the affected segment. In the area of the myenteric and submucous plexuses large non-medullated nerves can be seen (Fig. 5.74). A short transitional zone containing scanty ganglion cells and nerve trunks is generally formed in the junctional area between collapsed and dilated and hypertrophied segments of the bowel. This zone does not correlate with the cone often seen macroscopically. There is no satisfactory explanation as to why the abnormal segment of bowel in Hirschsprung's disease is contracted. Absence of ganglion cells should leave the adrenergic system unopposed, with relaxation of the affected segment. The disease can exist in the presence of demonstrable adrenergic innervation.

Peptidergic hormones have recently been suggested as a possible cause of contraction.

"Skip" segments, i.e. patchy loss of ganglion cells, were not found in over 300 resected specimens seen at Great Ormond Street, but here are several reports of this form of the disease in the literature (Perrot and Danon 1935; Tiffin et al. 1940; Keefer and Mokrohisky 1954; Lee 1955; Chenoweth 1959; Lawrence and Van Warner 1961; Sprinz et al. 1961). In several of these cases inflammatory changes and fibrosis have been described in the area of the myenteric plexus, suggesting that they may represent an acquired disease. In some reports detailed accounts of blocking techniques are not given, and we remain sceptical about the existence of true skip lesions.

At present the diagnosis of Hirschsprung's disease is made on a combination of symptomatology, colon

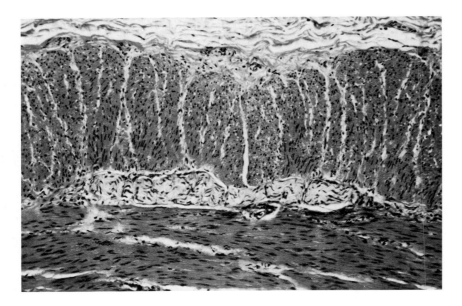

Fig. 5.74. Large nerve trunks in the myenteric plexus in Hirschsprung's disease.

radiography, rectomanometry, and histological and histochemical findings in rectal biopsies. The abnormalities of formation of the nerve supply of the gut described above are accompanied by a proliferation of parasympathetic nerves (S-2 to S-4) with many thick acetylcholinesterase-positive fibres in the lamina propria where few fibres are normally found (Fig. 5.75). This forms the basis of a histochemical method that can be used to establish the diagnosis on suction biopsies of the gut (Dobbins and Bill 1965). However, although this method is attractive, in our view it is valuable only if the result is confirmed at operation by full-thickness biopsy demonstrating aganglionosis during definitive surgery; unhappily, normal bowel has been resected on the basis of histochemical findings alone.

Histologically the diagnosis depends on the demonstration of an aganglionic segment (see Claireaux 1969). The diagnosis from full-thickness biopsy of the wall, by cryostat or processed-tissue sections, presents little difficulty when longitudinal sections are examined. Rectal submucosal biopsies require careful interpretation because of potential sources of error dependent on the normal anatomy. Hofman and Orestano (1967) and Aldridge and Campbell (1968) have described the normal innervation of the anal canal and rectum in neonates, and Smith (1968) has described its maturation. It must be remembered that a "transitional" zone, with scattered ganglion cells and nerve trunks, is seen at about the level of the internal sphincter, and that below this the gut is aganglionic. An area of up to about 1–1.5 cm above the anal valves may contain a few ganglion cells in the myenteric plexus in normal children, and

a slightly more distal extension exists in the submucous plexus. In general, a biopsy extending to the inner muscle coat will be satisfactory if taken from at least 1 cm above the anal valves. Such biopsies should be sectioned serially and examined at 10μ intervals. For suction biopsies a specimen at least 2 mm long from 3 cm above the pectinate line is necessary (Campbell and Noblett 1969).

Complications

Enterocolitis can affect both ileum and colon and is manifest as infarction and necrosis of geographical areas of mucosa (Figs. 5.76 and 5.77). During life, strips of infarcted mucosa may be shed with the stool. Resolution is incomplete and the ulcerated areas are covered with a simple cuboidal epithelium with islets of normal mucosa remaining, giving a pseudopolypoid appearance (Fig. 5.78) (see Berry 1969). This lack of resolution may be accompanied by persistent clinical symptoms and recurrent acute episodes.

Enterocolitis is the most serious single complication of Hirschsprung's disease. Its incidence is apparently related to the length of time elapsing before treatment (Fraser and Berry 1967). The pathogenesis is obscure. The disease is not related to the presence of particular pathogens in the gut, and an allergic vasculitis has been suggested as a possible cause (Berry and Fraser 1968).

Perforation is a serious complication, but modern treatment has greatly diminished its incidence. Perforation can follow stercoral ulceration or local manipulation of inspissated faeces.

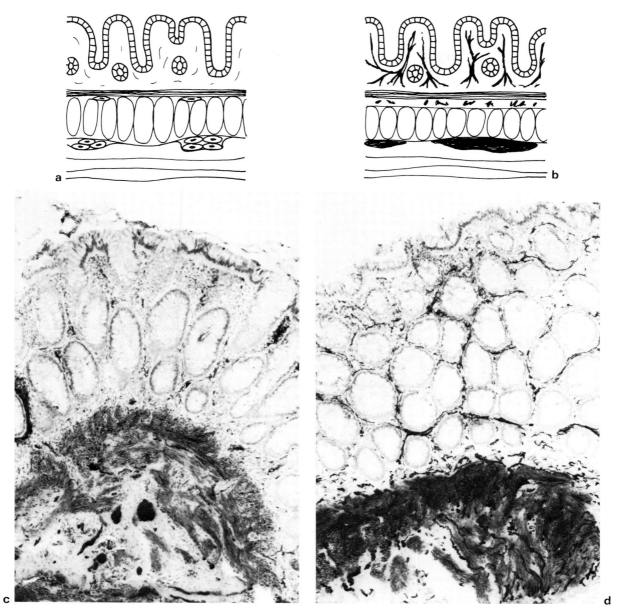

Fig. 5.75. Results of acetylcholinesterase staining in normal (**a**) and aganglionic (**b**) bowel (Hirschsprung's disease). **c** Suction rectal biopsy, normal, stained to show acetylcholinesterase activity. Note that there are few nerve fibres in the lamina propria and muscularis mucosae. Ganglion cells are clearly shown in the submucosa. (× 125) **d** Suction rectal biopsy, Hirschsprung's disease, stained to show acetylcholinesterase activity. Note the increased number of nerve fibres in the lamina propria and muscularis mucosae. (× 125)

Conditions that may be Confused with Hirschsprung's Disease

In pathological terms, diseases likely to be confused with Hirschsprung's disease are uncommon. "Ischaemic atrophy" of ganglion cells may occur, and they may be destroyed by Chagas' disease (Ehrenpreis et al. 1966). At autopsy, collapsed large bowel below a dilated, apparently obstructed, zone may be seen in the "meconium plug" syndrome (Brennan et al. 1967; Vanheeuwan et al. 1967), and "microcolon" – a collapse of the large bowel similar to that seen in long-segment disease – may occur in lower-small-bowel atresias. In all these instances

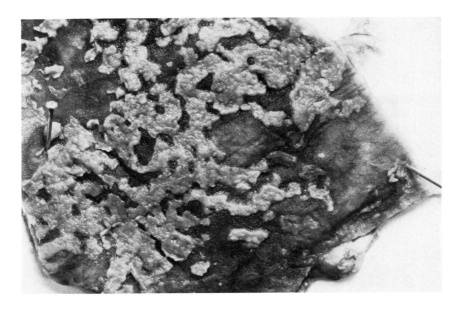

Fig. 5.76. Ilial lesions in enterocolitis associated with Hirschsprung's disease. "Geographical" surviving areas of mucosa are seen.

histopathological examination resolves the difficulty in diagnosis.

More recently, however, non-Hirschsprung causes of constipation in childhood have been considered by some to form distinct disease entities. It may be that better understanding of local developmental anatomy and a combination of good histological and histochemical studies (see Toorman et al. 1977) will confirm that there are other entities in the diagnostic gap between Hirschsprung's disease and normality, but most studies in which pathological abnormalities are suggested indicate a failure to understand normal development and anatomy rather than Hirschsprung's *forme fruste*. Decreased mobility of the colon may be found in association with gastrointestinal neurofibromatosis as part of the multiple endocrine neoplasia syndrome (Schimke et al. 1968). The so-called colonic dysplasias (Howard and Garrett 1984) are probably examples of this association. In some instances, the symptoms mimic Hirschsprung's disease, and the gross findings of megacolon with a cone in the sigmoid have been mistakenly interpreted as signs of this disease, resulting in bowel resection. It cannot be emphasized too strongly that, in our view, pathological examination by frozen section is necessary in all definitive surgical procedures.

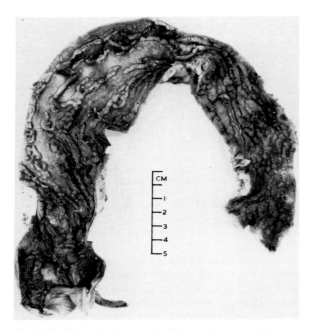

Fig. 5.77. Colonic lesion. Death 10 days after onset with some regeneration of surviving mucosa.

Intestinal Neuronal Dysplasia

Intestinal neuronal dysplasia (IND) was first used as a term to describe a clinical entity by Meier-Ruge in 1971 (Meier-Ruge 1974). He reported parasympathetic hyperganglionosis in patients with symptoms of colitis or intestinal obstruction, and in 1974 expanded the pathological concept to include hyperplasia of the submucosal and myenteric plexuses with the formation of giant ganglia, hypoplasia or aplasia of the sympathetic innervation of the myenteric plexus and the presence of isolated ganglion cells in the lamina propria and between the muscle fibres of

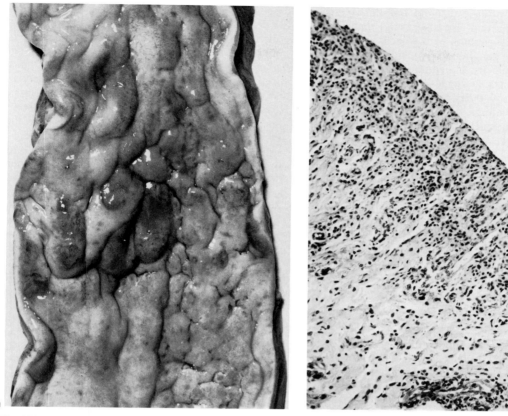

Fig. 5.78. a "Healed" enterocolitis with irregular mucosa and linear fissuring. **b** Section showing persistent ulceration and granulation tissue.

the muscularis mucosa. Other workers (Munakata et al. 1985; Briner et al. 1986) as well as the original author and his co-workers have further described this entity and suggested that it is as common as Hirschsprung's disease.

In a recent review of experience at the Children's Hospital of Pittsburg, Schofield and Yunis (1991) examined 498 consecutive rectal biopsies. They identified IND by the following criteria: slight to moderate increase in acetylcholinesterase-stained fibres within the lamina propria (and/or muscularis mucosa) and either greater than five submucosal ganglion cell clusters per high-powered field or large clusters (more than ten cells) of submucosal ganglion cells. There were 61 cases of Hirschsprung's disease and 38 biopsies satisfying the criteria adopted, which seem to be suitable for adoption as the basis of reasonable comparison between pathologists. They found no consistent clinical pattern in those affected, but were able to identify an increased frequency of twin gestation and prematurity, and of the meconium plug syndrome, and also noted five cases of gastroin-

testinal morphological abnormality. Formula/protein-sensitive enteropathy occurred in nine cases. As Schofield and Yunis point out, these findings have all been previously associated with changes satisfying their criteria for IND. On reading their clear paper, which discusses other factors associated with positive findings in the biopsies, it is difficult to disagree with the conclusion that the term IND "is at best a descriptive histopathological appearance rather than a unique clinicopathologic entity".

A further report from the Hospital for Sick Children, Great Ormond Street, identified only seven cases in 2420 patients biopsied between 1975 and 1991 (Smith 1992), compared with 54 in the much smaller series of 1115 patients reported by Scharli (1992) – a range of 0.3% to 62%.

Meier-Ruge (1992) after examining 3699 biopsies describes four types of innervation defect, aganglionosis and hypoganglionosis and two types of IND. The common type of the latter (type B) resembles that described by the criteria of the Pittsburg paper, and the author noted that in many cases of

Hirschsprung's disease (around one-third) type B IND was also present. He also found many minor anomalies in 229 patients with what is described as unclassifiable dysganglionosis, including heterotopias of neurons and plexus. If a common pathogenesis for these defects exists, as suggested by Meir-Ruge, it is difficult to see how it operates in terms of the newer experimental findings on the development of the innervation of the gut. It is tempting to ascribe differences in incidence as large as those reported to differences in criteria for diagnosis, but scrutiny of the guidelines recently established by a group of pathologists (Borchard et al. 1991) does not suggest that the differences in these series depend on this factor alone. In view of the new animal models available, the detailed prenatal and postnatal development of the hind-gut should be studied before the attribution of disease status to what may be, at least in part, changes in a normal developmental framework.

Hollow Visceral Myopathy

An uncommon cause of hypomotility of the intestine is a group of syndromes that have in common a smooth muscle myopathy (Schuffler et al. 1988). Both autosomal dominant (Schuffler and Pope 1977) and recessive (Anuras et al. 1983) forms have been described, and sporadic cases occur. Alstead et al. (1988) described an extensive family pedigree with numerous intermarriages where the disorder affected children and adolescents and appeared to behave as an autosomally recessive characteristic. Although smooth muscle myopathy is less common in childhood than in adult life, it may be symptomatic in the neonatal period (Bagwell et al. 1984).

Histological examination of the colon shows loss of definition of muscle cell margins, producing a smudged appearance. There is irregular vacuolation of muscle fibres and interstitial fibrosis, often marked in the circular coat (Alstead et al. 1988).

Malformations of the Anus and Rectum

Collectively, congenital anal and rectal defects occur with a frequency of around 1 in 5000 live births. They seem to be slightly more common in males, and Weinstein (1965) has described families in which the disease is apparently sex-linked. Cozzi and Wilkinson (1968), examining the records of 133

cases of anorectal anomalies seen at Great Ormond Street, found two instances of the disease in monozygotic twins, three affected siblings and three surviving unaffected dizygotic twins. Seven index patients had at least one sibling or other relative affected. In six of these the primary lesion was an anal stenosis, although only 16.6% of the defects were of this type. However, other studies have shown poor concordance (see Tünte 1969), and it seems likely that genetic factors are of relatively little significance.

Defects of the region have their origin in events taking place during days 50–60 of development (Fig. 5.79), and older classifications, e.g. that of Ladd and Gross (1934), were based on a mechanistic interpretation of proposed developmental failures. Thus incomplete disappearance of the anal membrane gives rise to *congenital anal stenosis* (type I); *membranous imperforate anus* (type II) results from persistence of this membrane; and more severe types in which the rectum ends blindly above an *imperforate anus* (type III) or the *bulbus analis* fails to develop (type IV), with a blind-ending rectum, were thought to be due to abnormalities of disappearance of the hind-gut or to epidermal/mesodermal induction failures, respectively. In all instances the mesodermally derived external anal sphincter was normal. More recent studies have suggested that this classification is not entirely satisfactory. The work of Bill and Johnson (1953) demonstrated that in the absence of a normal anal orifice the rectum generally communicates with the genitourinary tract or perineum (in 64 of their 70 cases of this type). The mucosal lining of such fistulae and their muscular walls suggest that "ectopic anus" would be a better descriptive term for these defects, and that they arise through a more complex process than simple failure of a major component of distal gut development: differential anterior perineal growth and altered migration of tissues are also important.

Alternative classifications to that of Ladd and Gross have been reported by Browne (1955), Partridge and Gough (1961) and Stephens and Durham Smith (1986). It is difficult to give accurate figures for the type of defect found in various series, as they are described under different titles. Of 507 anomalies described by Gross (1953), 29 were type I (congenital and stenosis), 14 of type II (membranous imperforate anus), 443 of type III, and 21 of type IV. Of the type III anomalies, 80% had associated "fistulae" to the genitourinary tract or perineum, as Bill and Johnson have noted. Partridge and Gough (1961) found 94 cases of types I and II defects, 212 of type III and five of type IV. Type III was divided broadly into cases with anorectal agenesis (114) and the so-called ectopic anus (98). Of the 114 cases of anorectal agenesis in this series, 62.3% had multiple

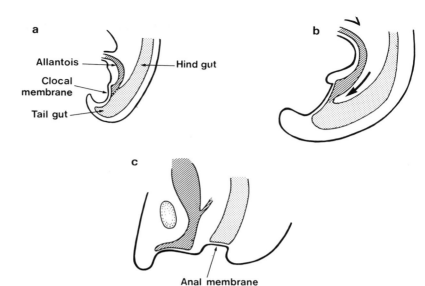

Fig. 5.79. Formation of the urogenital region during the critical stages of development. The urorectal septum fuses with the cloacal membrane at around 16 mm; the anal membrane disappears at approximately 12 weeks' gestation. **a** Week 5 of gestation, approx. 5 mm. **b** Week 7 of gestation, approx. 15 mm. *Arrow* shows growth of urorectal septum. **c** Week 8 of gestation.

congenital abnormalities, but only one of the five cases of type IV defect was accompanied by another defect. Of the 192 cases of "low" anomaly, 25% had associated malformations.

These findings are of practical importance. In the presence of "high" defects, other atresias, congenital heart disease and associated genitourinary abnormalities are likely to be found; these have been considered by Smith (1968) and Berdon et al. (1966). Vertebral abnormalities, including sacral agenesis, are also common. Figure 5.80 illustrates a high agenesis with multiple associated defects.

A detailed account of the more modern classification (see Table 5.4) may be found in the paper by Santulli et al. (1970), where the various defects are illustrated by line drawings, and a more up-to-date and extended version is seen in Stephens and Durham Smith (1986).

Rectal Prolapse

Rectal prolapse can occur in otherwise normal children during episodes of violent diarrhoea. A distinction is generally made between true prolapse – to which the short, straight, relatively unsupported rectum of children predisposes – and mucosal prolapse, a result of redundancy of the rectal mucosa.

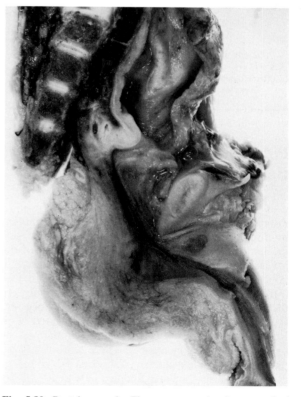

Fig. 5.80. Rectal agenesis. There was associated rectourethral fistula, oesophageal atresia with tracheo–oesophageal fistula, bilateral hydronephrosis and hydroureter, and dextrocardia with patent ductus arteriosus.

Table 5.4. Classification of anorectal anomalies

Male	Female

A. Low (translevator)
 1. *At normal anal site*
    a) Anal stenosis
    b) Covered anus, complete
	A. Low (translevator)
	 1. *At normal anal site*
	    a) Anal stenosis
	    b) Covered anus, complete

2. *At perineal site*
    a) Anocutaneous fistula (covered anus, incomplete)
    b) Anterior perineal anus
	2. *At perineal site*
	    a) Anocutaneous fistula (covered anus, incomplete)
	    b) Anterior perineal anus

	3. *At vulvar site*
	    a) Anovulvar fistula
	    b) Anovestibular fistula
	    c) Vestibular anus

B. Intermediate
 1. *Anal agenesis*
    a) Without fistula
    b) With rectobulbar fistula
	B. Intermediate
	 1. *Anal agenesis*
	    a) Without fistula
	    b) With fistula
	      i) Rectovestibula
	      ii) Rectovaginal, low

2. *Anorectal stenosis*	2. *Anorectal stenosis*

C. High (supralevator)
 1. *Anorectal agenesis*
    a) Without fistula
    b) With fistula
      i) Rectourethral
      ii) Rectovesical
	C. High (supralevator)
	 1. *Anorectal agenesis*
	    a) Without fistula
	    b) With fistula
	      i) Rectovaginal, high
	      ii) Rectocloacal
	      iii) Rectovesical

2. *Rectal atresia*	2. *Rectal atresia*

D. Miscellaneous
    Imperforate anal membrane
    Cloacal exstrophy
	D. Miscellaneous
	    Imperforate anal membrane
	    Cloacal exstrophy

Polypoid Lesions of the Large Bowel

Polypoid lesions of the large bowel are not uncommon in childhood. Louw (1968) reviewed 194 cases, the majority of which (155) were single and of the juvenile type. "Scattered multiple" polyps occurred in 25 cases, and in a further 14 instances there was diffuse involvement of the gut by many tumours. In the Louw series 13 polyps were inflammatory and four were hamartomatous, being associated with Rendu–Osler–Weber disease, neurofibromatosis or the Peutz–Jeghers syndrome. There were five lymphoid polyps. This pattern of lesions is typical of most large series (see also Shapiro 1950).

Presentation occurs most frequently between the ages of 3 and 6 years, usually with painless rectal bleeding, occasionally with passage of the polyp. When diffuse bowel involvement is excluded more than 80% of polyps are found to be in the sigmoid colon or rectum, and prolapse of the mass per rectum occurs in a significant number of cases.

The majority of childhood colonic polyps are of the *juvenile* type. These are usually single, although two or three lesions may be present. They are roughly spherical and appear reddened when compared with surrounding mucosa. They are usually about 1–2 cm in diameter, pedunculated and smooth-surfaced, and show a distinctly cystic cut surface (Fig. 5.81a, b).

Microscopically there is a single layer of epithelium overlying an abundant, often lymphocyte-infiltrated, stromal core. Glands extend into this and are often obstructed, with the formation of large mucus lakes (Fig. 5.81c). The muscularis mucosa is not included in the tumour, which may facilitate their autoamputation. Other secondary changes include ulceration of the thin epithelium with infection of the core.

The lesions may occur in a multiple form as *juvenile polyposis coli* in families in which adenomatous

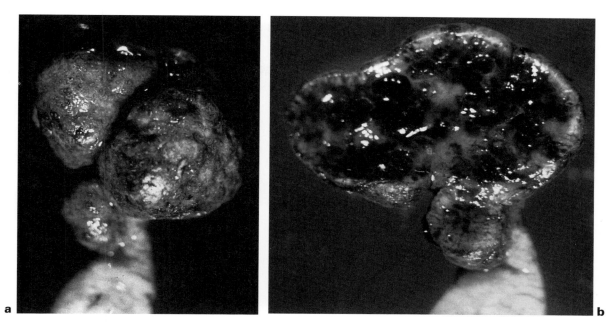

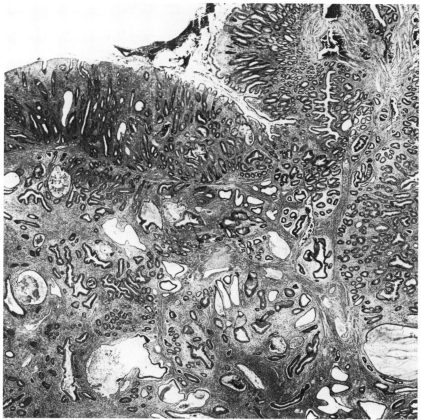

Fig. 5.81. a Juvenile polyp: it is congested, and the surface is bosselated and focally ulcerated. **b** The cut surface reveals numerous mucus-filled cysts. **c** Juvenile colonic polyp. (H&E, × 20)

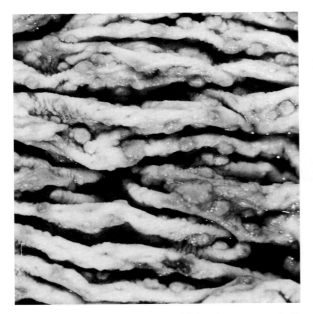

Fig. 5.82. Familial polyposis coli. Multiple polyps are seen. (× 4)

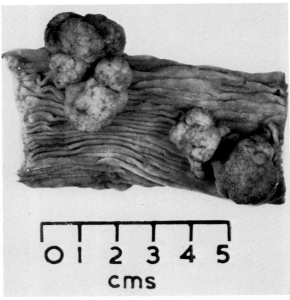

Fig. 5.83. Adenomatous polyps in segment of colon from a 7-year-old boy.

polyposis also occurs. Veale et al. (1966) have suggested that these probably hamartomatous polyps occur within the adenomatous polyposis genotype, its action being modified by a gene from a normal parent.

Adenomatous Polyps

Adenomatous lesions probably begin as areas of proliferation in the crypts of the large-bowel mucosa. The upward movement of the mass so formed pulls a number of mucosal components with it, often resulting in a poorly defined or absent stalk.

The surface is often lobulated, with intercommunicating cracks separating the lobules. The tubules of hyperplastic epithelium are closely packed; there is no increase in interstitial tissue and no tendency to cyst formation. Few goblet cells are seen, and there may be nuclear hyperchromatism in epithelial cells. The stroma may contain a few smooth muscle cells.

These lesions are rare as isolated findings in infancy, but are found in *familial polyposis coli* (Fig. 5.82). In this disease, although tumours may appear in younger individuals (Fig. 5.83), most develop after the age of 15 years, with death from associated adenocarcinoma of the large bowel occurring at around 40 years of age. However, juvenile forms are reported and adenocarcinoma of the rectum has occurred in a 12-year-old girl with this disease (Gross 1953).

From a number of studies it is apparent that the disease can be attributed to an autosomal dominant gene with high penetrance and variable expression (i.e. early- and late-onset polyposis coli, juvenile polyposis coli). Other associated connective tissue tumour may occur: osteomas, fibromas, dermoid tumours, lipomas and leiomyomas have all been described (see Gardner and Richards 1953; Gardner 1962). An association between polyposis coli and hepathoblastoma has been reported in five children who have a family history of the bowel lesion affecting the mother and maternal relatives (Kingstone et al.1983).

The polyps often present with blood loss as the major clinical problem, although other gastrointestinal complaints are common. However, the greatest danger to the individual is the premature development of adenocarcinoma of the colon, which may arise in the mucosa away from the polyps and is frequently multicentric.

The important early studies of this disease from St Mark's Hospital were reported by Dukes (1958).

Hamartomatous Polyps

Polyps associated with the Peutz–Jeghers syndrome commonly occur in the colon as well as the small bowel (p. 249). At least two children have died of adenocarcinoma apparently arising in these polyps, one gastric and one jejunal. Colonic tumours have not been reported (Tovar et al. 1983). Malignant transformation in "adenomatous" parts of the hamartomatous polyps is well documented in adults (see Perzin and Bridge 1982 for a review; Stockdale et al. 1984). Colonic tumours have occurred in young adults (Tweedie and McCann 1984).

Lymphoid Polyps

Corne (1961) reported on a series of 100 lymphoid polyps, six of which occurred in the first decade, with a further ten occurring in the second. A case of apparently familial lymphoid polyposis has also been recorded (Cosens 1958).

Appendix

Congenital Anomalies

Absence

Absence of the appendix is a rare anomaly, some 80 cases having been reported in the world literature. It is obviously compatible with a long and healthy existence: Manoil (1957) reported a case in a 90-year-old man. In the case reported by Robinson (1951) a 12 × 10 mm patch of lymphoid tissue was present in the caecal wall at the customary site of the appendiceal orifice.

Duplication

Duplication of the appendix was classified by Cave (1936) as partial duplication of the appendix alone, two separate appendices arising from a single caecum and duplication of both caecum and appendix. Watt (1959) has reviewed the many varieties of these types that have been reported.

In cases in which the caecum is duplicated there is in addition extensive duplication of the large bowel in many cases (Ravitch 1953).

Diverticula

It seems probable that reported diverticula of the appendix represent partial duplication in most instances, and not true diverticula (see Edwards 1934). However, Kissane and Smith (1967) have illustrated a true diverticulum.

Polyps

Adenomatous and juvenile polyps can occur in the appendix as in the colon.

Appendicitis

It is not proposed to discuss the aetiology of appendicitis in detail, as this has been dealt with elsewhere (see Morson 1966). There is some evidence to suggest that obstruction of the lumen is of greater practical importance in children than in adults. Hindmarsh (1954) found this to be present in 74 of 101 cases in childhood. Searches for viruses in excised appendices have not been fruitful (Jackson et al. 1966). Pinworm infestation is commonly found in childhood, and there is little evidence that such infestation is a cause of appendicitis.

Pledger and Buchan (1969) have pointed out that about 40 children a year die of acute appendicitis in England and Wales. There is an eightfold greater mortality rate in those less than 5 years old than in the 5–14 year age group – a fact of some importance because 20%–25% of all cases occur at this time of life. Fields and Cole (1967) presented 30 cases of appendicitis in children less than 3 years old, adding these to their previous experience of 38 cases at the Los Angeles County Hospital. They pointed out that perforation is often seen in the young, being found in 76% of their cases

Ulcerative Colitis

Ulcerative colitis commonly begins in childhood (around 10% of cases), and two large series of childhood cases have been reported, with 427 cases (Michener et al. 1961) and 134 cases (Langercrantz 1949). The bulk of these present at over 10 years of age, but ulcerative colitis is not rare before this; there are reports of 37 cases of the disease presenting in the first year of life. There is an excess of males, although the ratio is probably less than 2 : 1.

Of the 401 cases in Michener's series in which the course of the disease was known, 112 had died, 40 from colonic carcinoma, which had been found in 46 cases. He calculated the risk of developing carcinoma of the colon in this disease, presenting in childhood, as 556 times that in the normal population. The tendency to develop carcinoma was more pronounced with earlier onset; the mean duration of the disease

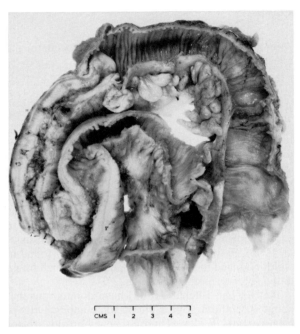

Fig. 5.84. Crohn's disease in a 9-year-old girl. The appearances are identical with those seen in adults.

the incidence of arthritis and arthralgia, erythema nososum, etc., is at least as great as that in adults. Growth retardation represents a distinctive systemic complication of this age group.

Crohn's disease of the large bowel presents in individuals less than 20 years old in one-third to one-half of reported cases (Lindner et al. 1963; Lockart-Mummary and Morson 1964). Korelitz et al. (1962, 1968) reported 25 cases in children aged 7–15 years, 16 in females and nine in males. In six cases the disease was initially confined to the colon; the rectum was spared in all. McGovern and Coulston (1968) also reported colon involvement in this disease and found sparing of the rectum in 24 cases. Sanderson and Walker-Smith (1985) have reviewed a series of Crohn's disease in British children and emphasized the relatively high frequency of the disease in those of West Indian origin.

In a study of 385 cases in childhood and adolescence Schmitz-Moormann and Schag (1990) found changes in large bowel biopsies in 84%, with a fall in the incidence of granulomas along the colon but a rise in incidence in the rectum. Granulomas were found in 42%, but chronic ulcers were less common than in adults.

before death from carcinoma occurred was 14.8 years. In 134 cases in individuals less than 15 years of age at the onset of the disease Korelitz et al. (1962) found eight carcinomas, seven of which had killed the patients. Three carcinomas were seen in the 18 cases described by Tumen et al. (1968).

The risk of carcinoma in ulcerative colitis and its prognosis when present have been discussed by Morson (1966). Onset of the disease early in life gives a greater potential time at risk of this complication and influences the management of the disease. Surgery is used more readily in therapy in childhood, owing both to this risk and to the systemic effects of the disease or therapy on growth and development (Hanley and Ray 1968).

The pathology of the disease, its complications and the extraintestinal effects found do not differ from those in cases presenting during adult life.

Crohn's Disease

Crohn's disease (Fig. 5.84) presents no distinctive pathological findings in infancy and childhood, and

Perforation of the Large Bowel

It is uncommon for perforation of the large bowel to occur in infancy and childhood, and this event generally represents a complication of ulcerative granulomatous or necrotizing colitis. Unfortunately, a number of iatrogenic causes are known. The rectum may be perforated by a thermometer. Such perforations occur in the anterior rectal wall just above the peritoneal reflection and are caused by insertion of the thermometer parallel with the floor of the cot, rather than with regard to rectal anatomy (Young 1965). Originally reported in 1957 by Segnitz, this injury has been reported several times since then (Warwich and Gilkas 1959; Miller 1962; Canby 1963). More recent reports (Greenbaum et al. 1969) have emphasized the high mortality rate. Perforation may also occur during preparation of the bowel for surgery in Hirschsprung's disease. This complication is more frequent if the gut is affected by enterocolitis (Fraser and Berry 1967). Finally, perforation may occur in the enterocolitis following exchange transfusion (see p. 245). Such cases most often involve the large bowel, although the small bowel may be affected.

Hernias

Gastroschisis

Infants with gastroschisis can be distinguished from those with omphalocele by the fact that the protruding loops of bowel are not covered by a sac of amnion (Fig. 5.85). The defect has its origin between weeks 5 and 8 of gestation and is a paraumbilical and often asymmetrical defect of the anterior abdominal wall through which loops of bowel project. In severe cases no umbilical cord is formed and any abdominal viscus (or the heart or a lung) may project from the body. Associated anomalies are common and the prognosis is poor.

Hydramnios is common in pregnancies associated with gastroschisis.

Umbilical Hernias

There are two types of umbilical hernia: hernia into the cord through the anatomical site of the return of the mid-gut loop and omphalocele. The former group is less commonly associated with serious malformation than the latter. Young (1969) found that a hernia into the cord generally contained the mid-gut loop but no other viscus, whereas an omphalocele often contained the liver (Fig. 5.86), which was itself abnormally lobulated. In major omphaloceles the bulk of the abdominal viscera are in the sac and the abdomen appears scaphoid. The umbilical cord arises from the apex of the sac. Logan et al. (1965) have described the congenital abnormalities associated with omphalocele, but imperfect rotation of the gut is common.

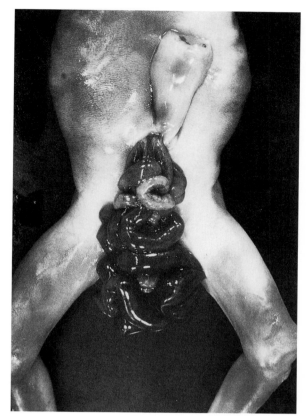

Fig. 5.85. Gastroschisis. The small intestine protrudes through a small defect to the right of the umbilical cord insertion. There is no covering sac

Diaphragmatic Hernias

This defect commonly causes pulmonary hypoplasia when the contents of the abdomen herniate into the thorax (Fig. 5.87). Midline defects thus commonly cause death from respiratory failure soon after birth, as bilateral pulmonary changes will have occurred, but recovery is possible after surgery. Nevertheless, mortality rates remain 80% in some series, leading to the development of intrauterine surgery for the condition (Harrison et al. 1990).

There are four types: anterolateral (caused by failure of development of the lateral component of the septum transversum), posterolateral (in which the pleuroperitoneal canal fails to close), pars sternalis (where the retrosternal portion of the septum transversum is deficient) and Morgagni (which is essentially a failure of adequate development of musculature around the eponymous foramen). The par sternalis anomaly is often accompanied by omphalocele.

Inguinal Hernias

Inguinal hernias occur with a frequency of 1.2 per 1000 live births (Knox 1959) and in a sex ratio of 10.3 male to 1 female. In reviewing 362 patients operated on under the age of 15 years, Gunnlaughsson et al. (1967) found that, when contralateral surgical exploration was performed at the time of operation, 60% of cases were bilateral. Although the lesion is much less common in females, Atwell (1962) was able to report 262 cases from Great Ormond Street Hospital for Sick Children. Of

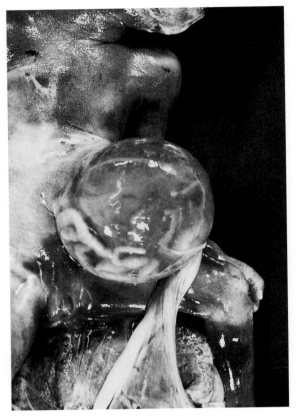

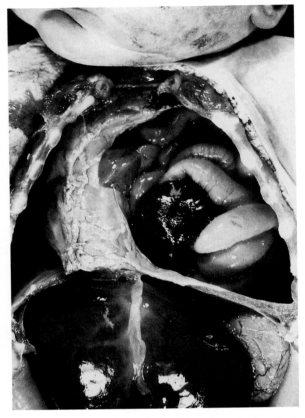

Fig. 5.86. Omphalocele. The liver and intestines protrude into a sac composed of peritoneum and amnion. The umbilical cord runs in its wall.

Fig. 5.87 Diaphragmatic hernia. Small intestine and spleen lie in the left hemithorax. The mediastinum is displaced; there was severe pulmonary hypoplasia.

these cases, 60% were right-sided, 24.4% left-sided, and only 15% bilateral. Forty-two of the hernias contained viscera at operation, and the frequency with which the ovary was present in the sac was commented on by the author.

Inguinal hernia was found in 18 of 50 cases of the Hunter–Hurler syndrome by Coran and Eraklis (1967); other conditions in which visceromegaly occurs in early life also predispose to this condition.

Pneumatosis Intestinalis

Pneumatosis intestinalis is an uncommon condition which can affect the large or small bowel of infants and children. Gas is said to be more often submucosal in infants and subserosal in adults, but in our experience either site may be involved in the young (Fig. 5.88). The gas fills cystic spaces in connective

tissue and may be found in lymphatics and blood vessels; although gas-producing organisms have been suggested as a cause of the lesions, they have seldom been isolated at autopsy. Analysis of the gas does not support a microbiological origin. Pneumatosis is a complication of other intestinal disorders, particularly proximal intestinal obstruction and necrotizing enterocolitis (Stevenson et al. 1969). It is likely that luminal gas escapes into the submucosa following loss of epithelial integrity and tracks along the course of vessels.

Malignant Tumours

Malignant gastrointestinal tumours are undoubtedly rare in childhood. As in adults, *lymphomas* are commonest, and several large series describe the frequency of ileocaecal distribution (Fig. 5.89) and male

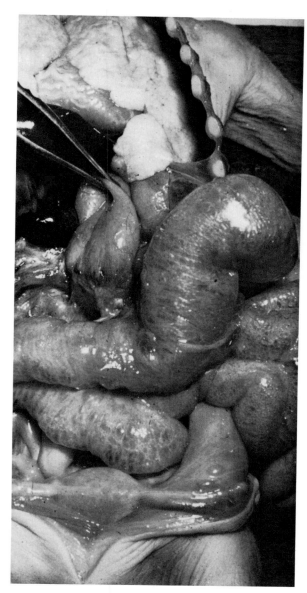

Fig. 5.88. Subserosal gas in the bowel and parietes of a female infant dying after operation for duodenal atresia. (× 280)

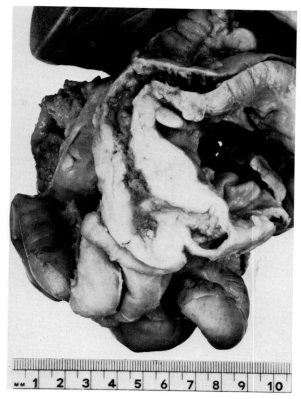

Fig. 5.89. Ileocaecal lymphosarcoma. Diffuse thickening of ileal and caecal walls with mucosal ulceration is commonly found in this condition.

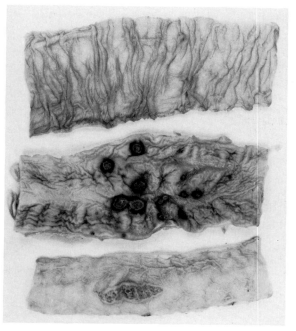

Fig. 5.90. Acute leukaemia, with deposits in ileal submucosa causing ulceration.

predominance (Berry and Keeling 1970). Carcinoid tumours are uncommon in the first two decades of life, although isolated reports exist. Although adenocarcinomas have been described, they have many unusual features and histories are sometimes atypical. Ungar (1949) reported three apparently typical tumours in an Israeli family, where the lesions resulted in death in the second decade.

Carcinoma of the jejunum has been reported in a 7-year-old boy (Büsing et al. 1977). Although the lesion was invasive but not metastatic, pulse cytophotometric investigation following DNA labelling suggested a malignant lesion. More studies of this kind might resolve the difficulties expressed about the so-called carcinomas that have been reported in association with Peutz–Jeghers syndrome.

Secondary tumours are also rare, although deposits of leukaemia may appear in the small bowel, some at the site of Peyer's patches (Fig. 5.90).

References

Abrami G, Dennison WM (1961) Duplications of the stomach. Surgery 49: 794

Abramowsky C, Hupertz V, Kilbridge P, Czinn S (1989) Intestinal lymphangiectasia in children: a study of upper gastrointestinal endoscopic biopsies. Pediatr Pathol 9 : 289

Abrams JS (1968) Intestinal atresia. Surgery 64 : 185

Achord JL, Proctor HD (1963) Malignant degeneration and metastasis in Peutz–Jeghers syndrome. Arch Intern Med 111 : 498

Ajayi OOA, Solanke TF, Seriki O, Bohrer SP (1969) Hirschsprung's disease in the neonate presenting as caecal perforation. Paediatrics 43 : 102

Aldridge RT, Campbell PE (1968) Ganglion cell distribution in the normal rectum and anal canal. J Pediatr Surg 3 : 475

Alstead EM, Murphy MN, Flanagan AM, Bishop AE, Hodgson HJF (1988) Familial autonomic visceral myopathy with degeneration of muscularis mucosae. J Clin Pathol 41 : 424

Alvarez SP, Greco MA, Genieser NB (1982) Small intestinal atresia and segmental absence of muscle coats. Hum Pathol 13 : 948

Ament ME, Rubin CE (1972) Soy protein – another cause of the flat intestinal lesion. Gastroenterology 62 : 227

Ament ME, Ochs HD, Davis SD (1973) Structure and function of the gastrointestinal tract in primary immunodeficiency syndromes: a study of 39 patients. Medicine 52 : 227

Amoury RA, Ashcraft KW, Holder TM (1977) Gastroschisis complicated by intestinal atresia. Surgery 82 : 373

Angrist M, Kauffman E, Slaugenhaupt SA, Matise TC, Puffenberger EG, Washington SS, Lipson A, Cass DT, Reyna T, Weeks DE, Sieber W, Chakravarti A (1993) A gene for Hirschsprung disease (megacolon) in the pericentromeric region of human chromosome 10. Nature Genet 4 : 351

Anonymous (1978) Oesophageal troubles after repairs in infancy. Lancet i : 700

Anuras S, Mitros FA, Nowak TV (1983) A familial visceral myopathy with external ophthalmoplegia and autosomal recessive transmission. Gastroenterology 84 : 346

Atwell JD (1962) Inguinal hernia in female infants and children. Br J Surg 1 : 294

Atwell JD (1968) The early diagnosis and surgical treatment of Hirschsprung's disease in infancy. Proc R Soc Med 61 : 339

Auritt WA, Hervada AR, Fendrick F (1978) Fatal pseudomembranous entero-colitis following oral ampicillin therapy. J Pediatr 93 : 882

Aust CS, Smith B (1962) Whipple's disease in a 3 months old infant with involvement of the bone marrow. Am J Clin Pathol 37 : 66

Bagwell CE, Filler RM, Cutz E (1984) Neonatal intestinal pseudoobstruction. J Pediatr Surg 19 : 732

Barasch J, Kiss B, Prince A, Saiman L, Gruenert D, Al-Aqwqati Q (1991) Defective acidification of intracellular organelles in cystic fibrosis. Nature 352 : 70

Barnes CL, Townley RRW (1973) Duodenal mucosal damage in thirty-one infants with gastroenteritis. Arch Dis Child 48 : 343

Bell SW, Kerner JA, Selby RK (1991) Microvillus inclusion disease. The importance of electron microscopy for diagnosis. Am J Surg Pathol 15 : 1157

Benjamin E, Wright DH (1980) Adenocarcinoma of the pancreas of childhood: a report of two cases. Histopathology 4 : 87

Benson CD, Lofti MW, Brough LAJ (1968) Congenital atresia and stenosis of the colon. J Pediatr Surg 3 : 253

Bentley JFE, Smith JR (1960) Developmental posterior enteric remnants and spinal malformations. Arch Dis Child 35 : 76

Berant M, Anead I, Jacobs J (1965) Heterotopic duodenal mucosa in the stomach. Am J Dis Child 110 : 556

Berdon WE, Hochbert B, Baker D, Grossman H, Santulli TV (1966) The association of lumbosacral spine and genitourinary anomalies with imperforate anus. AJR Am J Roentgenol 98 : 181

Berkel I, Say B, Kiran O (1970) Intestinal mucosa in children with geophagia and iron deficiency anaemia. Scand J Haematol 7 : 18

Berry CL (1969) Persistent changes in the large bowel following the enterocolitis associated with Hirschsprung's disease. J Pathol 97 : 731

Berry CL (1992) What's in a Homeobox? The development of pattern during embryonic growth. Virchows Archiv A 420 : 291

Berry CL, Fraser GC (1968) The experimental production of colitis in the rabbit; with particular reference to Hirschsprung's disease. J Pediatr Surg 3 : 36

Berry CL, Keeling JW (1970) Gastrointestinal lymphomas in childhood. J Clin Pathol 23 : 459

Bill AH Jr, Johnson RJ (1953) Failure of migration of the rectal opening as a cause for most cases of imperforate anus. Surg Gynecol Obstet 106 : 643

Bishop RF, Davidson GP, Holmes IH, Ruck BJ (1973) Virus particles in epithelial cells of duodenal mucosa from children with acute nonbacterial gastroenteritis. Lancet ii : 1281

Bjarnason G, Petterson G (1968) The treatment of intussusception: thirty years experience at Gothenburg's Children's Hospital. J Pediatr Surg 3 : 19

Bland-Sutton JD (1889) Imperforate ileum. Am J Med Sci 98 : 457

Blank E, Michael TD (1963) Muscular hypertrophy of the esophagus; report of a case with involvement of the entire esophagus. Pediatrics 32 : 595

Blyth H, Dickson JAS (1969) Apple peel syndrome (congenital intrestinal atresia). A family study of seven index patients. J Med Genet 6 : 275

Bodian M, Carter CO (1963) A family study of Hirschsprung's disease. Ann Hum Genet 26 : 261

Bodian M, Stephens FD, Ward BCH (1949) Hirschsprung's disease and idiopathic megacolon. Lancet i : 6

Bogomoletz WV, Cox JN (1975) Hamartoma of the stomach in childhood. Case report and review of the literature. Virchows Arch [Pathol Anat] 369 : 69

Bongiovi J, Logosso RD (1969) Pancreatic pseudocyst occurring in the battered child syndrome. J Pediatr Surg 4 : 220

Book LS, Herbst JJ, Jung AL (1976) Comparison of fast and slow feeding rate schedules to the development of necrotizing enteroliths. J Pediatr 89 : 463

Borchard F, Meier-Ruge W, Wiebecke B, Briner J, Munterfering H, Fodisch HF, Holschnider AM, Schmidt A, Enck P, Stolte M (1991) Innervationsstorungen des Dickdarms – Klassifikation und Diagnostic. Pathologie 12 : 171

Bottani A, Yagang X, Binkert F, Schnizel A (1991) A case of Hirschsprung disease with a chromosme 13 microdeletion, del (13) (q32.3q33.2) : potential mapping of one disease locus. Hum Genet 87 : 748

Boyle R, Nelson JS, Stonestreet BS, Peter G, Oh W (1978) Alterations in stool flora resulting from oral kanamycin prophylaxis of necrotizing enterocolitis. J Pediatr 93 : 857

Bradlaw RV (1953) The dental stigmata of prenatal syphilis. Oral Surg 6 : 147

Brennan LP, Weitzman JJ, Swenson O (1967) Pitfalls in the management of Hirschsprung's disease. J Pediatr Surg 2 : 1

Briner J, Oswald HW, Hirsig J, Lehner M (1986) Neuronal intestinal dysplasia – clinical and histochemical findings and its association with Hirschsprung's disease. Z Kinderchir 41 : 282

Browne D (1955) Congenital deformities of anus and rectum. Arch Dis Child 30 : 42

Burke V, Anderson CM (1966) Chronic volvulus as a cause of hypoproteinaemia, oedema and tetany. Aust Paediatr J 2 : 219

Burke V, Kerry KR, Anderson CM (1965) The relationship of dietary lactose to refractory diarrhoea in infancy. Aust Paediatr J 1 : 147

Burman D (1965) The jejunal mucosa in kwashiorkor. Arch Dis Child 40 : 526

Büsing CM, Haag D, Geiger H, Tschahargane C (1977) Microscopic and pulse cytophotometric investigation of a carcinoma of the jejunum in a seven year old child. Virchows Arch [Pathol Anat] 375 : 115

Cameron AH, Astley R, Hallewell M, Rawson AM, Miller CG, French JM, Hubble DV (1962) Duodeno-jejunal biopsy in the investigation of children with coeliac disease. Q J Med 31 : 125

Campbell CA, Forrest J, Musgrove C (1994) High strength pancreatic enzyme supplements and large bowel stricture in cystic fibrosis. Lancet 343 : 109 (letter)

Campbell PE, Noblett HR (1969) Experience with rectal suction biopsy in the diagnosis of Hirschsprung's disease. J Pediatr Surg 4 : 410

Canby JP (1963) Rectal perforation : a hazard of rectal temperatures. Clin Pediatr (Phila) 2 : 233

Caplan MS, MacKendrick W (1993) Necrotising enterocolitis: a review of pathogenic mechanisms and implications for prevention. Pediatr Pathol 13 : 357

Capron JP, Dupas JL, Marti R, Descombes P, Potet F (1977) Gastrin cells in Meckel's diverticulum. N Engl J Med 297 : 1126 (letter)

Carrillo P (1985) Palatal groove formation and oral endotracheal intubation. Am J Dis Child 139 : 859

Carswell F, Gibson AAM, McAlister IA (1973) Giardiasis and coeliac disease. Arch Dis Child 48 : 414

Carswell F, Logan RW (1973) Plasma B, C & B, A globulins and immunoglobulins in coeliac disease. Arch Dis Child 48: 587

Carter C, Sheldon W, Walker C (1957) The inheritance of coeliac disease. Ann Hum Genet 23 : 266

Carter CO, Evans K, Hickman V (1982) Children of those treated surgically for Hirschsprung's disease. Birth Defects 18(3b) : 87

Cave AJE (1936) Appendix vermiformis duplex. J Anat 70 : 283

Chacko CJG, Paulson KA, Mathan VI, Baker SJ (1960) The villous architecture of the small intestine in the tropics: a necropsy study. J Pathol 98 : 146

Chenoweth AI (1959) Intestinal obstruction in the neonatal period due to agenesis of the myenteric plexus. Ann Surg 149 : 799

Chrispin AR, Tempany E (1967) Crohn's disease of the jejunum in children. Arch Dis Child 42 : 631

Claireaux AE (1969) Histological techniques in the diagnosis of Hirschsprung's disease. In: Wilkinson AW (ed) Recent advances in paediatric surgery. Churchill-Livingstone, London

Cooke RWI, Meradji M, De Villeneuve VH (1980) Necrotising enterocolitis after cardiac catheterisation in infants. Arch Dis Child 55 : 66

Coran AG, Eraklis AJ (1967) Inguinal hernia in the Hurler–Hunter syndrome. Surgery 61 : 302

Corkery JJ, Dubowitz V, Lister J, Mossa A (1968) Colonic perforation after exchange transfusion. Br Med J iv : 345

Corne JS (1961) Multiple lymphomatous polyposis of the gastrointestinal tract. Cancer 14 : 249

Cornell A, Blumberg ML, Sarot IA (1950) Cysts of the esophagus: case report and review of the literature. Gastroenterology 15 : 260

Coryllos F, Simpson J (1962) Congenital atresia of the colon, review of the literature and report of two cases. Dis Colon Rectum 5 : 37

Cosens CG (1958) Gastrointestinal pseudoleukaemia: a case report. Ann Surg 148 : 129

Cozzi F, Wilkinson AW (1968) Familial incidence of congenital anorectal anomalies. Surgery 64 : 669

Dahms BB, Rothstein FC (1984) Barrett's esophagus in children. A consequence of chronic gastroesophageal reflux. Gastroenterology 86 : 318

Davidson GP, Cutz E, Hamilton JR, Gall DG (1978) Familial enteropathy: a syndrome of protracted diarrhoea from birth, failure to thrive and hypoplastic villus atrophy. Gastroenterology 75 : 783

de la Fuente AA (1981) Spontane maagperforatie bij de pasgeborene. Ned Tijdschr Geneeskd 125 : 586

Denes J, Jonh J, Leb J (1967) Dorsal herniation of the gut: a rare manifestation of the split notochord syndrome. J Pediatr Surg 2 : 359

Dissanayake AS, Jerrome DW, Offerd RE, Truelove SC, Whitehead R (1974) Identifying toxic fractions of wheat gluten and their effect on the jejunal mucosa in coeliac disease. Gut 15 : 931

Dobbins WO, Bill AH (1965) Diagnosis of Hirschsprung's disease excluded by rectal suction biopsy. N Engl J Med 272 : 990

Doe WF, Henry K, Booth CC (1974) Complement in coeliac disease. In: Hekkens W, Pena A (eds) Coeliac disease. Proceedings of the Second International Coeliac Symposium. Stenfert Kroese, Leiden, p 189

Dohn K, Povlsen O (1951) Enterocystomas: report of six cases. Acta Chir Scand 102 : 21

Doniach I, Shiner M (1957) Duodenal and jejunal biopsies. II. Histology. Gastroenterology 33 : 71

Donnison AB, Schwachman H, Gross RE (1966) A review of 164 children with meconium ileus seen at the Children's Hospital Medical Center, Boston. Pediatrics 37 : 833

Dorin JR, Dickinson P, Alton EWFW, Smith SN, et al. (1992) Cystic fibrosis in the mouth by targetted insertion of mutagenesis. Nature 359 pp 211–15

Douglas AP, Peters TJJ (1970) Peptide hydrolase activity of human intestinal mucosa in adult coeliac disease. Gut 11 : 15

Dowling RG, Booth CC (1967) Structural and functional changes following small intestinal resection in the rat. Clin Sci Mol Med 32 : 139

Dudgeon JA (1962) Oral pathology in the child: virus infections. In: Oral pathology in the child. International Academy of Oral Pathology, New York

Duke PM, Coulson JD, Santos JI, Johnson JD (1976) Cleft palate associated with prolonged orotracheal intubation in infancy. J Pediatr 89 : 990

Dukes CL (1958) Cancer control in familial polyposis of the colon. Dis Colon Rectum 1 : 413

Dykstra G, Sieber WK, Kieswelter WB (1968) Intestinal atresia. Arch Surg 97 : 175

Edwards HC (1934) Diverticula of the vermiform appendix. Br J Surg 22 : 88

Egan-Mitchell B, Fottrell PF, McNicholl B (1977) Prolonged gluten tolerance in treated coeliac disease. In: McNicholl B, McCarthy CF, Fottrell PF (eds) Perspectives in coeliac disease. MTP Press, Lancaster, p 251

Ehrenpreis J, Bentley JFR, Nixon HH (1966) Seminar on pseudo-Hirschsprung's disease and related disorders. Arch Dis Child 41 : 143

Elliott GB, Kliman MR, Elliott KA (1968) Pancreatic annulus: a sign or a cause of duodenal obstruction? Can J Surg 11 : 357

Ellison EH, Wilson SD (1964) The Zollinger–Ellison syndrome: Re-appraisal and evaluation of 260 registered cases. Ann Surg 160 : 512

Erenberg A, Nowak AJ (1984) Palatal groove formation in neonates and infants with orotracheal tubes. Am J Dis Child 138 : 974

Erenpries T (1967) Mortality in Hirschsprung's disease in infancy. J Pediatr Surg 2 : 569

Evans CH (1951) Atresias of the gastrointestinal tract. Int Abstr Surg 92 : 1

Fearne J, Bryan E, Elliman A, Elliman A (1985) Enamel defects in deciduous dentition of low birth weight infants. Presented to the Paediatric Research Societies in Europe, Munich

Fields IA, Cole NM (1967) Acute appendicitis in infants thirty-six months of age or younger. Am J Surg 113 : 269

Fonkalsrud EW, De Lorimier AA, Hays DM (1968) Congenital atresia and stenosis of the duodenum. A review compiled from the members of the Surgical Section of the American Academy of Pediatrics. Pediatrics 43 : 79

Fraser GC, Berry CL (1967) Mortality in neonatal Hirschsprung's disease with particular reference to enterocolitis. J Pediatr Surg 2 : 205

Fraser GC, Wilkinson AW (1967) Neonatal Hirschsprung's disease. Br Med J iii : 7

Gardner EJ (1962) Follow-up study of a family group exhibiting dominant inheritance for a syndrome including intestinal polyps, osteomas, fibromas, and epidermal cysts. Am J Hum Genet 14 : 376

Gardner EJ, Richards RC (1953) Multiple cutaneous and subcutaneous lesions occurring simultaneously with hereditary polyposis and osteomatosis. Am J Hum Genet 5 : 139

Gee S (1888) On the coeliac affection. St Bartholomew's Hospital Reports 24 : 17

Gershon MD, Epstein ML, Hegstrand L (1980) Colonisation of the chick gut by progenitors of enteric serotonergic neurons: distribution, differentiation and maturation within the gut. Dev Biol 77 : 41

Giberson RG, Dockerty MB, Gray HK (1954) Leiomyoma of the stomach. Surg Gynecol Obstet 98 : 186

Gjørup E (1934) Un cas d'oesophage double et estomac double. Acta Paediatr Scand 15 : 90

Goldberg HM, Johnson TP (1963) Posterior abdomino-thoracic enteric duplication. Br J Surg 50 : 445

Goldman H, Proujansky R (1986) Allergic proctitis and gastroenteritis in children. Am J Surg Pathol 10 : 75

Graivier L, Sieber WK (1966) Hirschsprung's disease and mongolism. Surgery 60 : 458

Greenbaum EI, Carson M, Kincannon WN (1969) Rectal thermometer-induced pneumoperitoneum in the newborn. Report of two cases. Pediatrics 44 : 539

Grosfeld JL, Cooney DR (1975) Pancreatic and gastrointestinal trauma in children. Pediatr Clin North Am 22 : 365

Gross RE (1953) The surgery of infancy and childhood. Saunders, Philadelphia

Guga DK, Walia BNS, Tandon BN, Deo MG, Ghai OP (1968) Small bowel changes in iron-deficiency anaemia of childhood. Arch Dis Child 43 : 239

Gunnlaughsson GH, Dawson B, Lynn HB (1967) Inguinal hernia in infants and children. Mayo Clin Proc 42 : 129

Habbick BF, Melrose AG, Grant JL (1968) Duodenal ulcer in childhood. A study of predisposing factors. Arch Dis Child 43 : 23

Haffner JF, Schistad G (1969) Atresia of the colon combined with Hirschsprung's disease. J Pediatr Surg 4 : 560

Hamilton JR, McNeill LK (1972) Childhood celiac disease: response of treated patients to a small uniform daily dose of wheat gluten. J Pediatr 81 : 885

Hanley PH, Ray JE (1968) Ulcerative colitis in children. South Med J 1231

Harris A, Chalkley G, Goodman S, Coleman L (1991) Expression of the cystic fibrosis gene in human development. Development 113 : 305

Harrison M, Kilby A, Walker-Smith JA, France NE, Wood CBS (1976) Cow's milk protein intolerance: a possible association with gastroenteritis, lactose intolerance, and IgA deficiency. Br Med J i : 1501

Harrison MR, Adzic NS, Longaker MT, Goldberg JD, Rosen MA, Filly RA, Evans MI, Golbus MS (1990) Successful repair in utero of a fetal diaphragmatic hernia after removal of herniated viscera from the left thorax. N Engl J Med 322 : 1582

Hartman SW, Kincannon WN, Greaney EM (1963) Congenital atresia of the colon. Am Surg 29 : 699

Hays DM, Wooley MM, Snyder WH (1966) Two oesophageal fistulae. J Pediatr Surg 1 : 240

Herbut PA (1943) Congenital defect in the musculature of the stomach with rupture in a newborn infant. Arch Pathol 36 : 91

Hindmarsh FD (1954) Acute appendicitis in childhood. Br Med J ii : 388

Hofman S, Orestano F (1967) Histology of myenteric plexus in relation to rectal biopsy. J Pediatr Surg 2 : 575

Holder TM, Ashcraft KW (1970) Esophageal atresia and tracheo-esophageal fistula. Ann Thorac Surg 9 : 445

Holmes GKT, Stokes PL, Sorahan TM, Prior P, Waterhouse HAH, Cooke WT (1976) Coeliac disease, gluten-free diet and malignancy. Gut 17 : 612

Holzel A (1967) Sugar malabsorption due to deficiencies of disaccharidase activity and monosaccharide transport. Arch Dis Child 42 : 341

Howaniety L, Lackmann D, Remes L (1968) Volvulus as a rare early complication of an enterogenous cyst of the newborn. Z Klin Chir 6 : 48

Howard ER, Garrett JR (1984) In: Tanner MS, Stocks RJ (eds) Neonatal gastroenterology – contemporary issues. Intercept, Newcastle Upon Tyne, p 121

Howard FM, Flynn DM, Bradley JM, Noone PE, Sjawatkowski M (1977) Outbreak of necrotising enterocolitis caused by Clostridium butyricum. Lancet ii : 1099

Husain AN, Young Hong H, Gooneratne S, Muraskas J, Black PR (1992) Segmental absence of small intestinal musculature. Pediatr Pathol 12 : 407

Hyde GA, De Lorimier AA (1968) Colon atresia and Hirschsprung's disease. Surgery 64 : 976

Jackson RH, Gardner PS, Kennedy J, McQuillin H (1966) Viruses in the etiology of acute appendicitis. Lancet ii : 711

Jensen KG (1962) Meconium ileus equivalent in a 15-year-old patient with mucoviscidosis. Acta Paediatr Scand 51 : 344

Jorup S (1948) Congenital varices of the esophagus. Acta Paediatr Scand 35 : 247

Kagan RJ, Reyes HM, Sangarapillai A (1981) Pseudocyst of the pancreas in childhood. Current advances in diagnosis. Arch Surg 116 : 1200

Kaijser R (1936) Über Hämangiome des Tractus gastrointestinalis. Arch Klin Chir 187 : 351

Kauffmann SL, Stout AP (1963) Tumors of the salivary glands in children. Cancer 16 : 1317

Keefer GP, Mokrohisky JF (1954) Congenital megacolon

(Hirschsprung's disease) Radiology 63 : 157

Keeling JW, Bryan EM (1989) Iatrogenic disease. In: Harvey D, Cooke RWI, Levitt GA (eds) The baby under 1000 g. Wright, London, p 289

Keeling JW, Harries JT (1973) Intestinal malabsorption in infants with histiocytosis X. Arch Dis Child 48 : 350

Kendrick KG, Walker-Smith JA (1970) Immunoglobulins and dietary protein antibodies in childhood coeliac disease. Gut 11 : 635

King A, Mueller RF, Heeley AF, Robertson NRC (1986) Diagnosis of cystic fibrosis in premature infants. Pediatr Res 20 : 536

Kingstone JE, Herbert A, Draper GJ, Mann JR (1983) Association between hepatoblastoma and polyposis coli. Arch Dis Child 58 : 959

Kissane JM, Smith MG (1967) Pathology of infancy and childhood. Mosby, St Louis

Kliegman RM, Fanaroff AA (1984) Necrotizing enterocolitis. N Engl J Med 310 : 1093

Knox G (1959) The incidence of inguinal hernia in Newcastle children. Arch Dis Child 34 : 482

Konrad EA, Meister P (1979) Fatal eosinophilic gastroenterocolitis in a two year old child. Virchows Arch [Pathol Anat] 382 : 347

Korelitz BI, Gribetz D, Danziger I (1962) The prognosis of ulcerative colitis with onset in childhood. I. The pre-steroid era. Ann Intern Med 57 : 582

Korelitz BI, Gribetz D, Kopel FB (1968) Granulomatous colitis in children: a study of 25 cases and comparison with ulcerative colitis. Pediatrics 42 : 446

Kreczy A, Gassner J, Mikuz G (1990) Idiopathic hypertrophy of the oesophagus in children. Virchows Archiv A 417 : 81

Kuffer FR, Starzynsk EC, Girolam A, Murphy L, Grabstald H (1968) The Klippel–Trenaunay syndrome, visceral angiomatosis and thrombocytopenia. J Pediatr Surg 3 : 65

Kuitunen P, Visakorpi JK, Savilahti E, Pelkonen P (1975) Malabsorption syndrome with cows' milk intolerance. Clinical findings and course in 54 cases. Arch Dis Child 50 : 351

Kumar R (1963) A case of congenital oesophageal stricture due to a cartilaginous ring. Br J Surg 49 : 533

Kurihara Y, Kurihara H, Suzuki H, Kodama T, Maemura K, Nagai R, Oda H, Kuwaki T, Cao W-H, Kamada N, Jishage K, Ouchi Y, Azuma S, Toyoda Y, Ishikawa T, Kumada M, Yazaki Y (1994) Elevated blood pressure and cranio-facial abnormalities in mice deficient in endothelin-1. Nature 368 : 703

Ladd WE, Gross RE (1934) Congenital malformations of anue and rectum. Am J Surg 23 : 167

Lake BD (1988) Microvillus inclusion disease: specific diagnostic features shown by alkaline phosphatase histochemistry. J Clin Pathol 41 : 880

Lancaster-Smith M, Kumar P, Clark ML (1974) Immunological phenomena following luten challenge in the jejunum of patients with adult coeliac disease and dermatitis herpetiformis. In: Hekken W, Pena A (eds) Coeliac disease. Proceedings of the Second International Coeliac Symposium. Stenfer Kroese, Leiden, p 173

Lancet Editorial (1984) Incidence of infantile hypertrophic pyloric stenosis. Lancet i : 888

Langercrantz R (1949) Ulcerative colitis in children. Nord Med 41 : 258

Lawrence AG, Van Warner DE (1961) Intussusception due to segmental againglionosis. JAMA 175 : 909

Lebenthal E, Shwachman H (1977) The pancreas: development, adaptation and malfunction in infancy and childhood. Clin Gastroenterol 6 : 397

Lee CMU Jr (1955) Megacolon with particular reference to Hirschsprung's disease. Surgery 37 : 762

Lewis PL, Holder T, Feldman M (1961) Duplication of the stomach: report of a case and review of the English literature. Arch Surg 82 : 634

Lieber A, Rosenbaum HD (1965) Situs inversus of all organs except stomach. AJR Am J Roentgenol 94 : 353

Lindner AE, Marshak RH, Wolf BS, Janowitz HD (1963) Granulomatous colitis. N Engl J Med 269 : 379

Little JW, Rickles NH (1967) The histiogenesis of the branchial cyst. Am J Pathol 50 : 533

Littlewood JM, Crollick AJ, Richards DG (1980) Childhood coeliac disease is disappearing. Lancet ii : 1359

Lloyd JK (1972) Hypolipoproteinaemia. J Clin Pathol [Suppl] 5 : 53

Lloyd JR (1969) The etiology of gastrointestinal perforations in the newborn. J Pediatr 4 : 77

Lockart-Mummary HE, Morson BC (1964) Crohn's disease of the large intestine. Gut 5 : 493

Logan WD, Crispin RH, Patterson JH, Abbot OA (1965) Ectopia cordis: report of a case and discussion of surgical management. Surgery 57 : 898

Louw JH (1968) Polypoid lesions of the large bowel in children with particular reference to benign lymphoid polyposis. J Pediatr Surg 3 : 195

Louw JH, Barnard CN (1955) Congenital intestinal atresia. Lancet ii : 1065

Lubinsky M, Severn C, Rappaport JM (1983) Fryns syndrome: a new variable multiple congenital abnormality (MCA) syndrome. Am J Med Genet 14 : 461

Lubolt W (1958) Duplication of the intestine as a cause of recurring intestinal bleeding in childhood. Paediatr Prax 7 : 449

Maluenda C, Phillips AD, Briddon A, Walker-Smith JA (1984) Quantitative analysis of small intestinal mucosa in cow's milk sensitive enteropathy. J Pediatr Gastroenterol Nutr 3 : 345

Manhani Sing A (1967) Volvulus of the small intestine due to Ascaris. Indian J Surg 29 : 328

Manoil L (1957) Congenital absence of the appendix. Am J Surg 93 : 1040

Manuel PD, Walker-Smith JA, France NE (1979) Patchy enteropathy in childhood. Arch Dis Child 20 : 211

Mauromichaelis J, Brueton MJ, McNeish AS, Anderson CM (1976) Evaluation of the intraepithelial lymphocyte count in the jejunum in childhood enteropathies. Gut 17 : 600

McGovern VJ, Coulston SJM (1968) Crohn's disease of the colon. Gut 9 : 164

McGovern JB, Gross RE (1968) Intussusception as a postoperative complication. Surgery 63 : 507

McNeish AS (1980) Coeliac disease: duration of gluten-free diet. Arch Dis Child 55 : 110

McNeish AS, Anderson CU (1974) Coeliac disease in childhood. Clin Gastroenterol 3 : 127

McNeish AS, Nelson R (1974) Coeliac disease in one of monozygotic twins. Clin Gastroenterol 3 : 143

McNeish AS, Nelson R, Macintosh P (1973) H-LA 1 and 8 in childhood coeliac disease. Lancet i : 668

McNeish AS, Harms HK, Rey J, Shmerling DH, Visakorpi JK, Walker-Smith J (1979) The diagnosis of coeliac disease. Arch Dis Child 54 : 783

McParblin JF, Dickson JAS, Swain VAJ (1972) Meconium ileus: immediate and long-term survival. Arch Dis Child 47 : 207

Meier-Ruge W (1971) Uber ein Erkrankunsbild des colons mit Hirschsprung's-symptomatik. Verh Dtsch Ges Pathol 55 : 506

Meier-Ruge W (1974) Hirschsprung's disease: its aetiology, pathogenesis and differential diagnosis. Curr Top Pathol 59 : 132

Meier-Ruge W (1992) Epidemiology of congenital innervation defects of the distal colon. Virchows Arch [A] 420: 171

Mendl K, Evans CJ (1962) Congenital and acquired epiphrenic diverticula of the oesophagus. Br J Radiol 35 : 53

Michener WM, Gage RP, Sauer WG, Stickler GB (1961) The prognosis of chronic ulcerative colitis in children. N Engl J Med 265 : 1076

Miller JA (1962) The "football sign" in neonatal perforated viscus. Am J Dis Child 104 : 311

Montgomery EA, Popek EJ (1994) Intussusception, adenovirus and children: a brief reaffirmation. Hum Pathol 25 : 165

Moossa AR (1975) Pancreatic pseodocysts in children. J R Coll Surg Edinb 19 : 148

Morson BC (1966) Cancer in ulcerative colitis. Gut 7 : 425

Morton NE (1970) Birth defects in racial crosses. In: Clarke Fraser F, McKusick VA (eds) Congenital malformations. Excerpta Medica, Amsterdam, p 264

Moutsouris C (1966) "Solid" stage and congenital intestinal atresia. J Pediatr Surg 1 : 446

Moylan FMB, Seldin EB, Shannon DC, Todres ID (1980) Defective primary dentition in survivors of neonatal mechanical ventilation. J Pediatr 96 : 106

Munakata K, Morita K, Okabe I, Sueoka H (1985) Clinical and histologic studies of neuronal intestinal dysplasia. J Pediatr Surg 20 : 231

Murphy MS, Eastham EJ, Jimenez M, Nelson R, Jackson RH (1987) Duodenal ulceration: review of 110 cases. Arch Dis Child 62 : 554

Myotte M, Egan-Mitchell B, McCarthy CF, McNicholl B (1973) Incidence of coeliac disease in the West of Ireland. Br Med J ii : 703

Nader PR, Margolin F (1966) Haemangioma causing gastrointestinal bleeding. Am J Dis Child 111 : 215

Nagao K, Matsuzaki O, Saiga H, Sugano I, Kaneko T, Katoh T, Kitamura T (1980) Histopathological studies on parotid gland tumors in Japanese children. Virchows Arch [A] 388 : 263

Naiman JL, Oski FA, Diamond LK, Vawter GF, Schwachman H (1964) The gastro-intestinal effects of iron-deficiency anaemia. Pediatrics 33 : 83

Ogur GL, Kolarsick AJ (1951) Gastric diverticula in infancy. J Pediatr 39 : 723

Oppenheimer EH, Esterley JR (1962) Observations in cystic fibrosis of the pancreas. II. Neonatal intestinal obstruction. Bull Johns Hopkins Hosp 111 : 1

Orme RL'E, Eades SM (1968) Perforation of the bowel in the newborn as a complication of exchange transfusion. Br Med J iv : 349

Packer SM, Charlton V, Keeling JW, Risdon RA, Osilure D, Rowlatt RJ, Larcher VF, Harries JT (1978) Gluten challenge in treated coeliac disease. Arch Dis Child 53 : 449

Palmiter RD (1989) Transgenic mice overexpressing the mouse homeobox-containing gene Hox-1.4 exhibit abnormal gut development. Nature 337 : 464

Parrish RA, Kanavage CB, Wells JA, Moretz WH (1968) Congenital antral membrane. Surg Gynecol Obstet 127 : 999

Partridge JP, Gough MHY (1961) Congenital abnormalities of the anus and rectum. Br J Surg 49 : 37

Patten RG, Gardner LI (1962) Influence of family environment on growth syndrome (maternal deprivation). Pediatrics 30 : 957

Paulino F, Roselli A, Aprigliano F (1963) Congenital esophageal stricture due to tracheobronchial remnants. Surgery 53 : 547

Paulley JW (1954) Observation on the aetiology of idiopathic steatorrhoea: jejunal and lymph node biopsies. Br Med J ii : 1318

Payette RF, Tennyson VM, Pomeranz HD, Pham TD, Rothman TP, Pomeranz HD, Gershon MD (1988) Accumulation of components of basal laminae: association with the failure of neural crest cells to colonise the presumptive aganglionic bowel of ls/ls mutant mice. Dev Biol 137 : 341

Perrot A, Danon L (1935) Obstruction intestinale de cause rare, chez un nourrisson. Ann Anat Pathol (Paris) 12 : 157

Perzin KH, Bridge MF (1982) Adenomatous and carcinomatous changes in hamartomatous polyps of the small intestine (Peutz–Jeghers syndrome). Cancer 49 : 971

Phillips AD, Jenkins P, Raafat F, Walker-Smith JA (1985) Congenital microvillus atrophy: specific diagnostic features. Arch Dis Child 60 : 135

Pledger HG, Buchan R (1969) Deaths in children with appendicitis. Br Med J iv : 466

Porter HJ, Padfield CJ, Peres LC, Hirschowitz L, Berry PJ (1993) Adenovirus and intranuclear inclusions in appendices in intussusception. J Clin Pathol 46 : 154

Purcell WR (1962) Perforation of the stomach in a newborn infant. Am J Dis Child 103 : 66

Qualman SJ, Hamoudi AB (1992) Pediatric hypertrophic gastropathy (Menetrier's disease). Pediatr Pathol 12 : 263

Ravitch MM (1953) Hind-gut duplication – doubling of colon and genital urinary tracts. Ann Surg 137 : 588

Renuala T, Konsnai I, Karpati S, Kuitunen P, Torek E, Savilahti E (1984) Dermatitis herpetiformis: jejunal findings and skin response to a gluten free diet. Arch Dis Child 59 : 517

Riker WL, Goldstein RI (1968) Malignant tumours of childhood masquerading as acute surgical conditions. J Pediatr Surg 3 : 580

Risdon RA, Keeling JW (1974) Quantitation of the histological changes found in small intestinal biopsy specimens from children with suspected coeliac disease. Gut 15 : 9

Rissier HL (1960) Haemangiomatosis of the intestine. Discussion, review of the literature and report of two cases. Gastroenterologia (Basel) 93 : 357

Robinson JO (1951) Congenital absence of the vermiform appendix. Br J Surg 39 : 344

Rolles CJ, McNeish AS (1976) Standardised approach to gluten challenge in diagnosing childhood coeliac disease. Br Med J i : 1309

Rosenlund ML, Koop CE (1970) Duodenal ulcer in childhood. Pediatrics 45 : 283

Rosenstein BJ, Engelman K (1963) Diarrhoea in a child with a catecholamine-secreting ganglioneuroma. J Pediatr 63 : 217

Rosenthal AH (1931) Congenital atresia of the esophagus with tracheo-esophageal fistula. Report of eight cases. Arch Pathol 12 : 756

Rosser SB, Clark CH, Elechi EN (1982) Spontaneous neonatal gastric perforation. J Pediatr Surg 17 : 390

Rossi TM, Lebenthal E, Nord KS, Fazili R (1980) Extent and duration of small intestinal mucosal injury in intractable diarrhea of infancy. Pediatrics 66 : 730

Sakula J, Shiner M (1957) Coeliac disease with atrophy of the small intestine mucosa. Lancet ii : 876

Sanderson IR, Walker-Smith JA (1985) Crohn's disease in childhood. Br J Surg 72 : S87

Santulli TV, Kiesewetter WB, Bill AH Jr (1970) Anorectal anomalies: a suggested international classification. J Pediatr Surg 5 : 281

Scharli AF (1992) Neuronal intestinal dysplasia. J Pediatr Surg Int 7 : 2

Schimke RM, Hartmann WH, Thaddeus MD, Prout TE, Rimoin DL (1968) Syndrome of bilateral pheochromocytoma, medullary thyroid carcinoma and multiple neuromas. A possible regulatory defect in the differentiation of chromaffin tissue. N Engl J Med 279 : 1

Schmidt EJ, Barros Barreto AP, Barbante PJ, Ramo OL, Concone MCMP, Queiroz AS, Carvalho AA (1964) Pancreatic lithiasis due to malnutrition and alcoholism in a child. J Pediatr 65 : 613

Schmitz-Moormann P, Schag M (1990) Histology of the lower intestinal tract in Crohn's disease of children and adolescents. Pathol Res Pract 186 : 479

Schofield DE, Yunis EJ (1991) Intestinal neuronal dysplasia. J Pediatr Gastroenterol Nutri. 12 : 182

Schuffler MD, Pope CE (1977) Studies of idiopathic pseudo-obstruction. ii. Hereditary hollow visceral myopathy: family studies. Gastroenterology 73 : 339

Schuffler MD, Pagon RA, Schwartz R, Bill AH (1988) Visceromyopathy of the gastrointestinal and genitourinary tracts in infants. Gastroenterology 94 : 892

Schwartz SI (1962) Congenital membranous obstruction of esophagus. Arch Surg 85 : 480

Seagram CGF, Louch RE, Stephens CA, Wentworth P (1968) Meckel's diverticulum: a 10-year review of 218 cases. Can J Surg 11 : 369

Seashore JH, Collins FS, Markowitz RI, Seashore MR (1987) Familial "apple peel" jejunal atresia: surgical, genetic and radiographic aspects. Pediatrics 80 : 540

Segnitz RG (1957) Accidental transanal perforation of the rectum. Am J Dis Child 93 : 255

Sen S, Bourne AJ, Morris LL, Furness ME, Ford WDA (1988) Dorsal enteric cysts. Aust N Z J Surg 58 : 51

Serbedzija GN, Burgan S, Fraser SE, Bronner-Frasser M (1991) Vital dye labelling demonstrates a sacral neural crest contribution to the enteric nervous system of chick and mouse embryos. Development 111 : 857

Shapiro S (1950) Occurrence of proctologic disorders in infancy and childhood: statistical review of 2700 cases. Gastroenterology 15 : 653

Shiner R, Ballard J (1973) Mucosal secretory IgA and secretory piece in adult coeliac disease. Gut 14 : 778

Shmerling DH, Prader A, Hitzig WH, Giedion A, Hadorn B, Kuhni M (1969) The syndrome of exocrine pancreatic insufficiency, neutropenia, metaphyseal exostosis and dwarfism. Helv Paediatr Acta 24 : 547

Sibbons PD, Spitz L, van Velzen D (1992) Necrotizing enterocolitis induced by local circulatory interruption in the ileum of neonatal piglets. Pediatr Pathol 12: 1–14

Smith ED (1968) Urinary anomalies and complications in imperforate anus and rectum. J Pediatr Surg 3 : 337

Smith J (1968) Pre- and post-natal development of the ganglion cells of the rectum and its surgical implications. J Pediatr Surg 3 : 386

Smith V (1992) Isolated intestinal neuronal dysplasia: a descriptive histological pattern or a distinct clinico-pathological entity? In: Chadzisezimovic F, Herzog B (eds) Inflammatory bowel disease – Morbus-Hirschsprung. Faulk Symposium Basel. Kluwer Academic Publishers, London, Chapter 18, pp 203–214

Smyth R, van Velzen R, Smyth AR, Lloyd DA, Heaf DP (1994) Strictures of the ascending colon in cystic fibrosis and high-strength pancreatic enzymes. Lancet 343 : 85

Snouwaert JN, Brigman KK, Latour AM, Malouf NN, Bourcher RC, Smithies O, Koller BH (1992) An animal model for cystic fibrosis made by gene targeting. Science 257 : 1083

Sparnon AL, Little KET, Morris LL (1984) Intussusception in childhood: a review of 139 cases. Aust N Z J Surg 54 : 353

Spouge D, Baird PA (1985) Hirschsprung disease in a large birth cohort. Teratology 32 : 171

Sprinz H, Cohen Z, Heaton JD (1961) Hirschsprung's disease with skip area. Ann Surg 153 : 143

Stanfield JP, Hutt MSR, Tunnicliffe R (1965) Intestinal biopsy in kwashiorkor. Lancet ii : 519

Stein H, Beck J, Solomon A, Schmaman A (1972) Gastroenteritis with necrotising enterocolitis in premature babies. Br Med J ii : 616

Stephens FD, Durham Smith E (1986) Classification, identification and assessment of surgical treatment of anorectal anomalies. Pediatr Surg Int 1 : 200

Stevens FM, Egan-Mitchell B, Cryan E, McCarthy CF, McNicholl B (1987) Decreasing incidence of coeliac disease. Arch Dis Child 62 : 465

Stevenson EO, Hays DM, Snyder WH Jr (1967) Post-operative intussusception in infants and children. Am J Surg 113 : 562

Stevenson JK, Graham CB, Oliver TK, Goldenberg VE (1969) Neonatal necrotising enterocolitis. Am J Surg 118 : 260

Stickler GB, Peyla TL, Dower JC, Sloof JP (1965) Moniliasis, steatorrhoea, diabetes mellitus, cirrhosis, gallstones and hypoparathyroidism in a 10 year old boy. Clin Pediatr 4 : 276

Stockdale AD, Ashford RFU, Leader M (1984) Gastrointestinal malignancy in association with the Peutz–Jeghers syndrome: three further cases. Clin Oncol 10 : 299

Stout AP (1962) Bizarre smooth muscle tumours of the stomach. Cancer 5 : 400

Swenson O, Bill AH Jr (1948) Resection of rectum and rectosigmoid with preservation of the sphincter for benign spastic lesions producing megacolon. Surgery 24 : 212

Swenson O, Oeconomopoulos C (1961) Achalasia of the esophagus in children. J Thorac Cardiovasc Surg 41 : 49

Taylor GD, Martin HF (1961) Salivary gland tissue in the middle ear. A rare tumour. Arch Otolaryngol 73 : 651

Thomaidis TS, Arey JB (1963) The intestinal lesions in cystic fibrosis of the pancreas. J Pediatr 63 : 444

Tiffin ME, Chandler LR, Faber HK (1940) Localized absence of the ganglion cells of the myenteric plexus in congenital megacolon. Am J Dis Child 59 : 1071

Tittel K (1901) Uber eine angeborene Missbildung des Dickdarmes. Wien Klin Wochenschr 14 : 903

Toorman J, Bots TAM, Vio PMA (1977) Acetylcholinesterase activity in rectal mucosa of children with obstipation. Virchows Arch [Pathol Anat] 376 : 159

Tovar JA, Eizaguirre I, Albert AI, Jimenez J (1983) Peutz–Jeghers syndrome in childhood: report of two cases and a review of the literautre. J Pediatr Surg 18 : 1

Tumen HJ, Valdes-Dapena A, Haddad H (1968) Indications for surgical intervention in ulcerative colitis in children. Am J Dis Child 116 : 641

Tünte W (1969) Analatresie bei Zwillingen. Z Kinderheilkd 105 : 21

Tweedie JH, McCann BG (1984) Peutz–Jeghers syndrome and metastasising colonic adenocarcinoma. Gut 25 : 1118

Ungar H (1949) Familial carcinoma of the duodenum in adolescence. Br J Cancer 3 : 321

Valman HB (1976) Diet and growth after resection of ileum in childhood. J Pediatr 88 : 41

Valman HB, Roberts PD (1974) Vitamin B_{12} absorption after resection of ileum in childhodd. Arch Dis Child 49 : 932

Vanheeuwan G, Riley WC, Glen L, Woodruff C (1967) Meconium plug syndrome with aganglionosis. Pediatrics 40 : 665

Variend S, Phillips AD, Walker-Smith JA (1984) The small intestinal mucosal biopsy in childhood. Perspect Pediatr Pathol 1 : 57

Veale AMO, McColl I, Bursey HJR, Morson BC (1966) Juvenile polyposis coli. J Med Genet 3 : 5

Vitoria JC, Camarero C, Sojo A, Ruiz A, Rodriguea-Soriano J (1982) Enteropathy related to fish, rice, and chicken. Arch Dis Child 57 : 44

Walker AW, Kempson RL, Ternberg JL (1966) Aganglionosis of the small intestine. Surgery 60 : 449

Walker-Smith JA (1972a) Uniformity of dissecting microscope appearances in proximal small intestine. Gut 13 : 17

Walker-Smith JA (1972b) Variation of small intestinal morphology with age. Arch Dis Child 47 : 80

Walker-Smith JA, Reye RDK, Soutter GB, Kenrick KG (1969) Small intestinal lymphangioma. Arch Dis Child 44 : 527

Walker-Smith JA, Kilby A, France NE (1978) Reinvestigation of children previously diagnosed as coeliac disease. In: Perspectives in coeliac disease: Proceedings of the Third International Symposium on Coeliac Disease, Galway, September 1977, p 267

Warwich WJ, Gilkas PW (1959) Neonatal transanal perforation of the rectum. Am J Dis Child 97 : 869

Watt JK (1959) Appendix duplex. Br J Surg 46 : 472

Weinstein ED (1965) Sex-linked imperforate anus. Pediatrics 35 : 715

Williams JP, Knudson A (1965) Peutz–Jeghers syndrome with metastasizing duodenal carcinoma. Gut 6 : 179

Wiseman JH, Celano ER, Hester FC (1959) Spontaneous rupture of the esophagus in a newborn infant. J Pediatr 55 : 207

Wolgemuth DJ, Behringer RR, Mostoller MP, Brinster RL, Palmiter RD (1989) Transgenic mice overexpressing the mouse homeobox containing gene Hox-1.4 exhibit abnormal gut development. Nature 337 : 464

Young DG (1965) "Spontaneous" rupture of the rectum. Proc R Soc Med 58 : 615

Young DG (1969) Anterior abdominal wall defects. In: Wilkinson AW (ed) Recent advances in paediatric surgery. Churchill-Livingstone, London, p 153

Young DG, Wilkinson AW (1968) Abnormalities associated with neonatal duodenal obstruction. Surgery 63 : 832

Yutani C, Sakurai M, Miyaji T, Okuno M (1973) Congenital short intestine: a case report and review of the literature. Arch Pathol 96 : 81

Zinnemann HH, Kaplan AP (1972) The association of giardiasis with reduced intestinal secretory immunoglobulin A. Digestive Dis 17 : 793

6 · Liver and Gallbladder

Colin L. Berry and Jean W. Keeling

Embryology

The hepatic epithelium and the extrahepatic biliary system develop from adjacent diverticula of the intestine of embryos of 0.3–0.5 mm body length (25 days). By around the 20 mm stage pseudoglandular arrangement is seen in the hepatocytes, which are mostly arranged in loose plates; haematopoiesis is established. By 30 mm, two-cell hepatic plates are well developed and ductal plates (flattened cells at the periphery of the lobules) with primitive lumens are seen in the hilum. At 150 mm portal areas, central veins, and liver plates two cells thick are clearly established, but interlobular bile ducts are confined to the hilum. However, by 200 mm ductules join the ductal plates to the interlobular ducts, the cells of the ductal plates having become larger and cuboidal.

Two inductive interactions are necessary for the formation of cells with hepatocytic morphology: prehepatic endoderm is induced by cardiac mesoderm to give rise to proliferating endodermal cells, which in turn interact with the mesoderm of the septum transversum and differentiate into hepatocytes (Houssaint 1980). The proto-oncogene *c-Jun* is essential for hepatocyte development – mouse mutants lacking the gene show apoptosis and necrosis of the hepatocytes at days 12–13 of development (Hilberg et al. 1993).

The two hypotheses of the origin of the intrahepatic bile ducts, postulate development from the main hepatic ducts or by transformation of periportal liver cells. Direct observation of the in vitro transformation of fetal liver cells into duct-like structures under the influence of mesenchyme was observed as long ago as 1934 (Doljanski and Roulet 1934), but the role of mesenchyme was uncertain until the elegant experiments of Gall and Bathal (1990). In their cultured fetal rat liver, liver explants consisting of trabeculae and endothelial cells showed evidence of maturation (including canalicular development) but little evidence of duct development unless material from the porta hepatis was included. Supplementation of the media with putative inducers of bile duct development was without effect; co-culture of stomach and pancreas or small intestine was also ineffective. Clearly there is a need for the presence of committed mesenchyme in the development of a mature system, but a hepatocytic contribution is probable.

The vascular pattern of the mature liver is established after disruption of the vitelline veins by growth of the hepatic cords in the septum transversum. Ultimately the right vitelline vein alone remains to form the hepatic vein. The umbilical veins, which enter the lateral aspect of the sinus venosus, are engulfed in the expanding liver, which provides direct venous return to the heart. The right umbilical vein and the posthepatic left vein then disappear, leaving the remnant of the left-sided vein to form the ductus venosus by fusion with a vascular pathway formed in the developing sinusoids connecting with the common hepatic vein.

The portal vein develops following selective atrophy of parts of three transverse anastomotic channels between the vitelline veins. These complex patterns of venous change have been well illustrated by Hamilton et al. (1972).

In later pregnancy, the left lobe of the liver is supplied by umbilical vein blood predominantly and the right by portal venous blood. This probably accounts for the differing relative sizes of the two lobes seen between infant and adult, and for other variations in

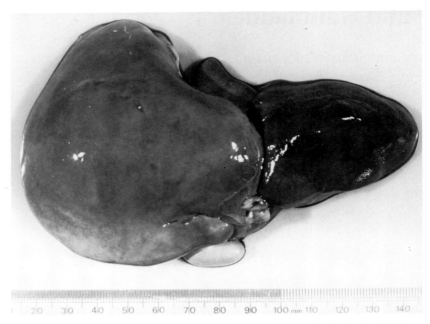

Fig. 6.1. The liver from an infant with a left-sided diaphragmatic hernia. The congested left lobe lay in the left hemithorax. The vertical groove was made by the margin of the incomplete diaphragm.

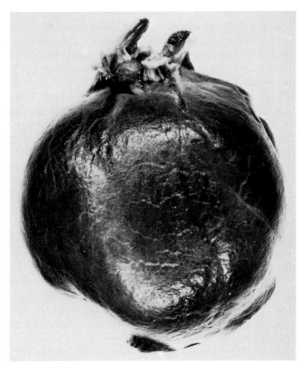

Fig. 6.2. Exomphalos. The liver is symmetrical; the whole was contained within a large exomphalos sac, which also contained the intestines. This abnormality was one of several occurring in an infant with trisomy 18.

histological appearances. Haematopoietic tissue is more prominent in the right lobe.

Anomalies of Position, Form and Size

In situs inversus totalis or situs inversus abdominis, the liver lies in the left upper quadrant and the left lobe is larger than the right. In the asplenia syndrome (see p. 122) (Ivemark 1955) the liver is symmetrical, the left lobe being increased in size and occupying the left hypochondrium.

Increase in size occurs in diaphragmatic hernia, probably because the liver is not constrained by the usual intra-abdominal pressures. If part of the liver lies in a hemithorax the shape of the liver is also abnormal, and there may be a fissure at the level of the diaphragm caused by localized pressure (Fig. 6.1). Infants with exomphalos usually have an enlarged liver for similar reasons. If part or all of the liver is contained in the exomphalos sac, the abnormal symmetry of the organ is evident (Fig. 6.2). Supernumerary lobes are not uncommon and are without functional or clinical significance, although

Reidel's lobe may be palpated on abdominal examination.

Cystic Disease

Solitary Cysts

Solitary cysts of the liver are rare and are usually an incidental finding at necropsy. Occasionally sufficient fluid may accumulate within them to give rise to an abdominal mass. They are lined by a single layer of biliary epithelium and presumably arise as a result of localized obstruction of the biliary tree. They have no effect on liver function.

Multiple Cysts

Multiple cysts of the liver in children are also uncommon. In about half the cases reported they are associated with polycystic disease of the kidneys of the adult type (Montgomery 1940; Blyth and Ockenden 1971). They rarely achieve a sufficiently large size to distort the normal contours of the liver, varying between a millimetre and several centimetres in diameter.

Infantile Polycystic Disease and Congenital Hepatic Fibrosis

The disorders of the liver characterized by proliferation, dilatation and excessive branching of the intrahepatic bile ducts without concomitant abnormality of the hepatic parenchyma have many histological similarities. On these grounds they might be considered different expressions of the basic disorder, from Von Meyenburg's complexes to infantile polycystic disease, embracing both congenital hepatic fibrosis and Caroli's disease. However, the responses of tissues to injury are not infinite and similarity of appearance cannot always be equated with common aetiology.

Kerr et al. (1961) described 13 children with "congenital hepatic fibrosis" who presented between the ages of 2.5 and 16 years (more than half before 6 years of age) with complications of portal hypertension. One of three children who died had typical infantile polycystic renal disease. They viewed 24 cases from the literature which they considered to be examples of congenital hepatic fibrosis: 15 of these had polycystic kidneys, although case 2 of Parker

(1956) seems to be an example of Meckel's syndrome. Three of the 15 cases with liver and kidney involvement were siblings. The authors stated that the presence of renal disease made the diagnosis of congenital hepatic fibrosis certain. Familial cases of congenital hepatic fibrosis have also been described by Lorimer et al. (1967), who report their findings in two sisters presenting at 30 and 34 years of age with portal hypertension. Two other siblings from this family were also thought to have the same disorder. The kidneys were of normal size but were not biopsied.

Blyth and Ockenden (1971) described a spectrum of disease in children presenting from birth to 5 years, all having cystic disease of both liver and kidneys. In their two younger groups, i.e. infants in whom the disease was obvious at birth or who presented in the first month of life, presenting signs and symptoms related to the renal abnormality, with the perinatal group dying as a result of respiratory insufficiency caused by concomitant pulmonary hypoplasia and the neonatal group from progressive renal failure. All cases had diffuse liver disease. These authors also described two further subgroups of patients, presenting at 3–6 months of age (the infantile group) and between 1 and 5 years. In the infantile group, patients presented with either chronic renal failure or increasing portal hypertension. In all cases, cystic changes were present in both liver and kidneys, but the renal disease was not as extreme as in the younger patients. Children in the juvenile group all had signs referable to portal hypertension. In this group renal tubular dilatation was minor (less than 10% of tubules involved) and portal fibrosis was more severe. Thus, although all cases had spectacular bile duct abnormalities throughout the liver, clinical signs or symptoms due to the hepatic lesion were present only in infants who survived at least several months. Time seems to be an important factor in the development of portal hypertension; whether this is the result of increasing fibrosis in the portal tracts or is merely a reflection of the time taken for the complications of portal hypertension to occur is not clear. The authors found other affected family members in several cases and suggested an autosomal recessive mode of inheritance. Their conclusion was that their cases were a spectrum of expression of the same basic disorder.

Lieberman et al. (1971) described infantile polycystic disease in 14 patients, including three from one family; five other patients had affected siblings. Seven presented before 1 month of age, the rest at up to 7 months. Five died within the first 7 months of life from respiratory or renal problems. The surviving patients were hypertensive and it was noted that kidney size decreased over a period of time. Some

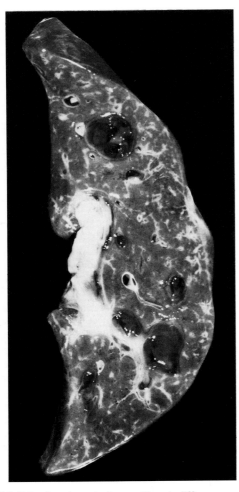

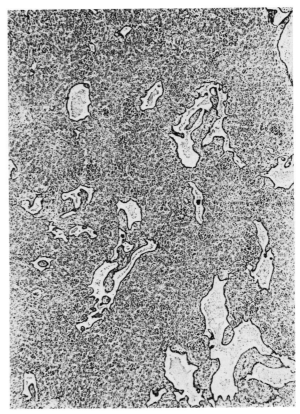

Fig. 6.4. Infantile polycystic disease in a neonate. There is irregular cystic dilatation of bile ducts in all portal areas. (H&E, × 60)

Fig. 6.3. Infantile polycystic disease. There is diffuse expansion of portal tracts of fibrous tissue. Localized dilatation of large ducts is visible.

had hepatomegaly; there was portal hypertension in two, and splenomegaly in one other case. All had the typical histology of infantile polycystic disease. The same authors described four patients with congenital hepatic fibrosis presenting between 7 weeks and 11 years 3 months, three being siblings, all with signs and symptoms of portal hypertension. The three familial cases had cystic kidneys, the cystic change being of a minor degree, as well as diffuse cystic abnormalities of the liver; in the fourth case the renal biopsy seemed to be inadequate. These authors feel that congenital hepatic fibrosis is a different disorder from infantile polycystic disease, but do not advance a very good case in support of this view.

Using quantitative methods of assessment of liver sections from patients with cystic bile duct abnormalities, Landing et al. (1980) found that the perinatal,

neonatal and infantile forms of infantile polycystic disease were distinguishable, and concluded that they represented differing presentations of the same condition. The juvenile group of polycystic disease of Blyth and Ockenden (1971) was indistinguishable from congenital hepatic fibrosis.

Following three-dimensional reconstruction of the biliary system in cystic liver disease in neonates, Jorgensen (1971, 1972) demonstrated that the abnormal biliary system was in the form of curved plates. He concluded that the basic defect was a failure of resorption of most of the fetal duct plate system of the embryo. The intrahepatic portal venous system was normal, but the amount of fibrous tissue in portal areas varied from case to case. These studies support the concept of a single basic anomaly in infantile cystic liver disease.

In infantile polycystic disease the liver is enlarged and firm with expanded portal tracts visible through the capsule. The cut surface may show cystic dilata-

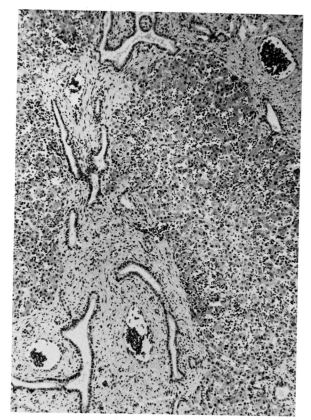

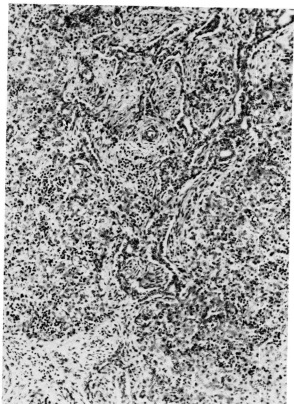

Fig. 6.5. Infantile polycystic disease. Female died aged 4 with respiratory insufficiency. The bile ducts are irregularly dilated, and there is marked portal fibrosis. The hepatic parenchyma appears normal. The kidneys in this case were typical of infantile polycystic disease. (H&E, × 108)

Fig. 6.6. Meckel's syndrome. Infant died aged 1 day with occipital encephalocele and bilateral renal enlargement with diffuse cystic change. Excessively branching undilated bile ducts are seen throughout the liver. (H&E, × 144)

tion of large bile ducts (Fig. 6.3), but this is probably present in a minority of cases. The portal areas are pale and prominent. Histologically there is spectacular dilatation and branching of the bile ducts, but there is no abnormality of the hepatic parenchyma; in particular, no intrahepatic bile retention or bile plugging is seen (Figs. 6.4 and 6.5).

In older children in whom portal hypertension is present, portal fibrosis is often more severe and the dilatation of the ducts is not as prominent as it is in neonates.

Meckel's Syndrome

Meckel's syndrome is characterized by cerebral abnormality (usually an encephalocele), cystic kidneys, cleft palate, congenital heart disease, postaxial polydactyly, and eye and other abnormalities (Opitz and Howe 1969). It is thought to be inherited

in an autosomal recessive fashion (Crawfurd et al. 1978).

Cystic change in the liver is frequently present, but the organ presents a spectrum of abnormalities ranging from hepatic enlargement with cysts visible through the capsule or readily recognizable on slicing, to a reduction in size with portal fibrosis. Histological examination may reveal diffuse cystic dilatation of bile ducts in all portal areas (Fig. 6.6) in addition to any macroscopic cysts. The absence of cysts on naked-eye inspection and failure to undertake adequate histological examination of the fetus may account for the liver's being described as normal in some cases.

Epidermoid Cysts

Epidermoid cysts are as rare in the liver in childhood as they are in adults, but they are occasionally

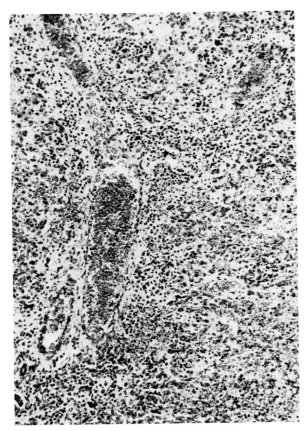

Fig. 6.7. Erythroblastosis fetalis. Within the liver of this infant with rhesus haemolytic disease, there is excessive erythropoiesis both in portal areas and within sinusoids. (H&E, × 120)

reported as cystic lesions identified on ultrasound. Their histiogenesis is unclear (Schullinger et al. 1983).

Other Disorders with Cystic Change

Diffuse dilatation of the bile ducts without parenchymal damage of biliary obstruction may occur as part of the spectrum of hepatobiliary anomalies in the trisomy 17–18 syndrome (see pp. 54, 140, 290). Hepatic abnormalities similar to cystic disease or portal fibrosis are encountered in association with other developmental abnormalities or have been described in siblings. There are several reports of an association of nephrophthisis and congenital hepatic fibrosis in siblings (Boichis et al. 1973; Witzleben and Sharp 1982).

Cystic abnormalities of the bile duct are found in Ivemark's syndrome (Ivemark et al. 1959).

Erythroblastosis Fetalis

In blood group incompatibilities between mother and fetus that cause severe haemolysis in utero (usually rhesus incompatibility) there is hepatosplenomegaly with extensive haematopoiesis in the hepatic sinusoids and within portal tracts (Fig. 6.7). An excess of iron is present in hepatocytes (Fig. 6.8). In some cases, evidence of cholestasis may be present.

Neonatal Jaundice

Unconjugated Hyperbilirubinaemia

Jaundice with unconjugated hyperbilirubinaemia occurs in 90% of full-term infants. Maximum levels occur between the 2nd and 4th days of life and seldom exceed 6 mg/100 ml (102 mmol/litre). In preterm infants higher serum levels of unconjugated bilirubin are common, and often levels of 12–14 mg/100 ml (204–238 μmol/litre) are present. Maximum levels occur later in the preterm infant, usually from the 5th to the 7th day; elevated bilirubin levels may persist until the 10th day of life.

Hyperbilirubinaemia is present in the neonate when serum levels exceed 15 mg% (225 mmol/litre) in the term baby and 12 mg% (204 mmol/litre) in the preterm infant. It is important to recognize, investigate and treat unconjugated hyperbilirubinaemia in the neonate so that kernicterus can be prevented (see Chapter 4).

Physiological hyperbilirubinaemia in the neonate is the result of a number of ill-understood factors (Lathe 1974). Increased bilirubin production occurs because of decreased erythrocyte survival, ineffective haematopoiesis and increased turnover of haem-containing enzymes. There is reduced liver cell uptake of bilirubin because of poor hepatic perfusion resulting from continuing patency of the ductus venosus and the other haemodynamic changes that occur at birth. Poor liver cell uptake of bilirubin also occurs as a result both of the relative immaturity of cell membrane transport systems and of cytoplasmic binding and glucuronidation – the major conjugation mechanism. Saturation of the excretion process may occur. Another important contributory factor is the reabsorption of unconjugated bilirubin from meconium in the gut lumen, particularly if gut emptying is slow. Poor bacterial breakdown of bilirubin in the gut is related to incomplete colonization.

Other changes may exacerbate the effects of these factors. Polycythaemia is common in infants (from late cord clamping) and will increase the load on the system; hypoxia and metabolic acidosis from any cause will further interfere with its efficiency.

There are no specific histological findings in the liver in unconjugated neonatal hyperbilirubinaemia. Liver biopsy is unlikely to be undertaken, so that the liver is seen only incidentally at necropsy. At this point, changes related to hypoxia and hypoperfusion such as fatty change and hepatocyte necrosis are present, usually in a centrilobular distribution. Severe unconjugated hyperbilirubinaemia can result in canalicular cholestasis.

Metabolic Defects Causing Unconjugated Hyperbilirubinaemia

Several defects along the degradation pathway of the haem molecule are described and are due to enzyme defects, not all of which have been specifically characterized. They give rise to jaundice in infancy and childhood. Causes of neonatal hyperbilirubinaemia are shown in Table 6.1.

Gilbert's Syndrome

Gilbert's syndrome is a benign autosomally recessive familial disorder with mild unconjugated bilirubinaemia, often without overt jaundice. It is thought that there is defective uptake of bilirubin by hepatocytes. Children are usually asymptomatic, although nausea, fatigue and upper abdominal discomfort are described in adults and are precipitated by alcohol, infection or strenuous exercise (Gilbert and Lereboullet 1901; Berk et al. 1970).

The liver is histologically normal.

Crigler–Najjar Syndrome

There are two disorders of bilirubin metabolism associated with uridine diphosphate glucuronyl transferase deficiency (Crigler–Najjar syndrome). Type I is rare and severe, with unconjugated hyperbilirubinaemia arising in the neonatal period and persisting throughout life. Severe neurological defects occur.

In type II the hyperbilirubinaemia is less severe and kernicterus does not occur.

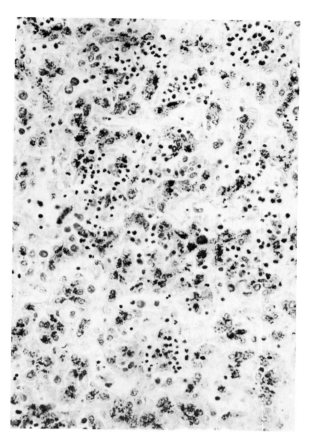

Fig. 6.8. Erythroblastosis fetalis. Much iron pigment is present within hepatocytes. Erythropoiesis is seen within sinusoids. (Pearle's reaction, × 300)

The two types appear to be genetically distinct, but both are probably inherited as autosomal recessive conditions (Crigler and Najjar 1952).

Inherited Metabolic Disease

Neonatal cholestasis is a common presentation of inherited disorders affecting a variety of metabolic pathways (see below and Chapter 14). It is important to establish or firmly refute these diagnoses because of the need to introduce an appropriate elimination diet to prevent permanent tissue injury and so that prenatal diagnosis can be undertaken in subsequent pregnancies.

Histological changes in the liver are not usually specific, although galactosaemia and fructose intolerance produce panlobular steatosis which, untreated, progresses rapidly to cirrhosis. Primary tyrosinaemia

Table 6.1. Pathogenesis of neonatal jaundice

Unconjugated hyperbilirubinaemia	Conjugated hyperbilirubinaemia
Increased bilirubin production	*Familial*
Physiological/prematurity	Cholestatic jaundice and lymphoedema
Blood group incompatibility	Cholestatic jaundice with hepatosteatosis with hyper
Internal haemorrhage	cholesterolaemia (Byler's disease)
Polycythaemia	Arteriohepatic dysplasia
Sepsis	
Haemoglobinopathies	*Metabolic*
Erythrocyte abnormalities	Galactosaemia
Drugs	Fructose intolerance
Late cord clamping	Tyrosinaemia
	α_1-Antitrypsin deficiency
Impaired transport and uptake	Cystic fibrosis
Decreased hepatic perfusion	Neimann–Pick disease
Hypoalbuminaemia	Wolman's disease
Hypoxia	Gaucher's disease
Acidosis	Zellweger syndrome
Parenteral feeding	Abnormalities of cholic acid synthesis
Physiological jaundice	
	Acquired
Inadequate conjugation	Sepsis/infection
Transient familial hyperbilirubinaemia	Drugs/parenteral feeding
Physiological jaundice	Severe haemolytic disease
High intestinal obstruction	
Hypothyroidism (cretinism)	*Idiopathic*
Drugs	Neonatal hepatitis syndrome
Crigler–Najjar syndrome	Extrahepatic biliary atresia
Breast milk jaundice	Paucity of intrahepatic bile ducts
	Choledochal cyst
Abnormal enterohepatic circulation	
Low intestinal obstruction	*Other*
(anatomical or mechanical)	Chromosomal abnormalities (trisomy 13, 18, 21, 45 XO)
Cystic fibrosis	Hepatic tumours
Altered bacterial flora in gut	

After Rushton (1987).

and disorders leading to secondary tyrosinaemia give rise to widespread giant cell transformation and cholestasis.

Wilson's Disease

Hepatolenticular degeneration is a rare inherited (autosomal recessive) disorder of copper metabolism in which copper is deposited in the liver, brain, cornea and kidneys. When the disease presents in childhood, the symptoms are usually manifestations of liver damage – subacute or chronic hepatitis or cirrhosis. Jaundice and portal hypertension with oesophageal varices and hypersplenism may occur. Biochemical abnormalities of liver function may be demonstrated, and depend on the degree of liver damage. Serum copper and caeruloplasmin levels are low and urinary copper increased. There is sometimes copper deposition in the cornea in older children. Treatment with oral penicillamine effectively removes copper from the body and produces clinical improvement when started early in the disease.

Histological abnormalities produced in the liver in Wilson's disease are cirrhosis, an increase in fibrous tissue, and striking vacuolation of hepatocyte nuclei caused by glycogen accumulation (Walshe 1962).

Galactosaemia

Galactosaemia is an inherited disorder of carbohydrate metabolism resulting from deficiency of the enzyme galactose-1-phosphate uridyl transferase. It is inherited in an autosomal recessive fashion and occurs at a rate of 1 per 4000 births in the UK. There is defective conversion of galactose to glucose, with accumulation of galactose-1-phosphate and galactosuria. High levels of galactose in the blood induce liver injury by trapping uracil nucleotides in toxic intermediary metabolites (UDP-glucosamine).

The infants are well at birth, although in utero damage may have occurred from maternal galactose ingestion (Allen et al. 1980). There is usually vomiting, failure to thrive, jaundice and hepatomegaly. If the disorder is not recognized and galactose ingestion continues, cirrhosis develops, with liver failure and signs of portal hypertension. A few infants are asymptomatic in the neonatal period, and the disease is recognized only when cirrhosis is established.

Cataracts usually form, and affected infants are susceptible to infection. Treatment is by lifelong restriction of galactose (Anonymous 1982); most untreated infants die in infancy.

The earliest histological abnormality is steatosis and ductular transformation or periportal hepatocytes. This is followed by portal fibrosis, widespread hepatocyte degeneration and irregular collapse of lobular architecture, macronodular cirrhosis and extensive ductular transformation of hepatocytes (Fig. 6.9).

α_1-Antitrypsin Deficiency

α_1-Antitrypsin is a polymorphic glycoprotein (mol. wt. 45 000) synthesized in the liver. It migrates as an α^2-globulin on paper electrophoresis. It has protease-inhibitor activity (trypsin, collagenase, elastase, thrombin and plasmin are all inhibited).

The production of this glycoprotein is governed by a pair of completely penetrant co-dominant autosomal alleles with about 50 variant alleles on the long arm of chromosome 14 (Cox et al. 1982) known as the Pi (protease inhibitor) system. The subtypes are designated by letter according to their electrophoretic mobility: PiF (fast), PiM (medium), PiS (slow), and PiZ (ultraslow). Most people are of the genotype PiMM, and PiZZ corresponds to the clinical homozygous deficiency state. The frequency of the PiZZ phenotype is said to be 1 in 3460 in England and Wales so that about 230 α_1-antitrypsin-deficient infants are born each year (Cook 1974). Between 10% and 20% of these infants develop liver disease. α_1-Antitrypsin deficiency was described in association with infantile cirrhosis (Sharp et al. 1968), and shortly afterwards in four infants with neonatal hepatitis, which in two children progressed to cirrhosis (Johnson and Alper 1970). Subsequently, a relationship between α_1-antitrypsin deficiency and some cases of adult liver disease was also demonstrated (Berg and Eriksson 1972). An association between pulmonary emphysema in young adults and low serum α_1-antitrypsin levels was noted by Laurell and Eriksson (1963). It was thought that individuals with low α_1-antitrypsin levels might be healthy or might develop liver or lung disease, but not both. This view has subsequently been shown to be erroneous in both children (Glasgow et al. 1971) (Fig. 6.11) and adults (Cohen et al. 1973).

The relationship between Pi phenotype and the development of liver disease is complex, but

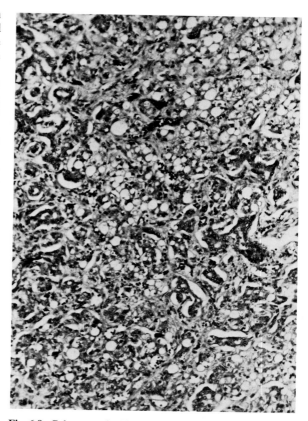

Fig. 6.9. Galactosaemia. There is portal fibrosis with some apparent bile duct reduplication and ductular change in degenerating hepatocytes. Marked fatty degeneration of hepatocytes is present.

10%–20% of PiZZ individuals present with conjugated hyperbilirubinaemia in the neonatal period and have been shown to have intrahepatic cholestasis with giant cell transformation of hepatocytes on liver biopsy. Neonatal presentation with a bleeding diathesis is also described (Hope et al. 1982). A characteristic appearance of the liver in these infants is the presence of PAS-positive diastase-resistant globules in the cytoplasm of hepatocytes, particularly those adjacent to portal areas (Fig. 6.10). These globules seem to be a precursor of α_1-antitrypsin not excreted by the hepatocytes. Peptide mapping has shown that this molecule differs from that of PiMM individuals in that a glutamic acid molecule in the normal is replaced by lysine in the PiZZ individual. That this material is antigenically similar to α_1-antitrypsin can be demonstrated by immunohistochemical methods based on fluorescein- or peroxidase-labelled antihuman α_1-antitrypsin: the globules were said not to be present in infants under 12 weeks of age (Talbot and Mowat 1975), but have subsequently been demonstrated in the liver of a fetus with PiZZ phenotype at

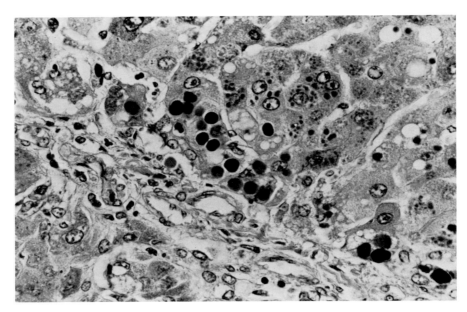

Fig. 6.10. a_1-Antitrypsin deficiency. Diastase-resistant PAS-positive globules are seen in the cytoplasm of periportal hepatocytes. (PAS, $\times 576$)

20 weeks' gestation (Roberts 1985). Cottrall et al. (1974) found α_1-antitrypsin deficiency to be as common as extrahepatic biliary atresia in conjugated hyperbilirubinaemia in infancy in a study in southeast England. A similar histological abnormality has been described in an infant with PiZnull (Z–) phenotype (Burn et al. 1982). Psacharopoulos et al. (1983) have followed families of infants with severe liver disease and found that 28% died within 4 years, a similar proportion were alive with established cirrhosis and a further 21% had persistent liver disease. Of PiZZ siblings, 78% developed chronic liver disease in infancy.

Intrahepatic cholestasis of infancy in α_1-antitrypsin deficiency can progress to cirrhosis (Fig. 6.11). The deficiency may be found in individuals with cirrhosis with no history of jaundice in the neonatal period (Cottrall et al. 1974), although anicteric liver damage beginning in early life cannot be ruled out. Aagenaes et al. (1974) suggest that in α_1-antitrypsin deficiency liver disease may be present in utero, and that the low birth weight in infants with neonatal hepatitis and α_1-antitrypsin deficiency compared with apparently normal infants with low serum α_1-antitrypsin levels is evidence for prenatal damage. They also describe a slow but definite deterioration towards cirrhosis in all their patients, despite initial improvement in liver function tests and apparent well-being. Cottrall et al. (1974) found that the prognosis in neonatal intrahepatic cholestasis was worse in patients with α_1-antitrypsin deficiency than in the rest of the group.

A review covering the biochemical and clinical aspects of α_1-antitrypsin deficiency is given by Morse (1978a, b).

Glycogen Storage Disease

Hepatomegaly and histological abnormality occur in several of the glycogen storage diseases (GSDs) (see Chapter 16, p. 853). In type 1 GSD (usually glucose-6-phosphatase deficiency) there is marked hepatomegaly with steatosis. These children develop multiple hepatic adenomas, and hepatocellular carcinoma may occur (Howell et al. 1976).

Both types 2A and 3 exhibit hepatomegaly with increased glycogen content of hepatocytes, but fibrosis and fatty change are usually absent. Progression to cirrhosis in adult life has been reported in a few individuals in type 3 GSD (Fellows et al. 1983). In type 6B, similar changes with mild to moderate steatosis are found. Type 4 GSD is rare. It has the most severe liver involvement, with bile stasis, excess glycogen and cirrhosis usually leading to death from liver failure during the first 2 years of life (Andersen 1956).

Disorders of Fat Oxidation

In conditions in which inadequate glycogen is present in the liver as the metabolic source of energy production, long-chain fatty acids are mobilized from

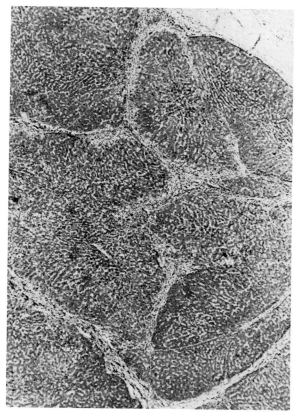

Fig. 6.11. Cirrhosis in a_1-antitrypsin deficiency. Female aged 12 years. Giant cell hepatitis in infancy. Portal fibrosis by 16 months. Cirrhosis by 3 years of age. Death from respiratory insufficiency due to emphysema. (H&E, × 36)

adipose tissue and are oxidized in mitochondria. The first step in this metabolic path is a dehydrogenation, and three distinct dehydrogenases deal with long-, medium- and short-chain acyl CoA esters. Genetically determined abnormalities in all three dehydrogenases have now been described, with medium-chain acyl CoA deficiency (MCAD) the commonest (Stanley et al. 1983; Anonymous 1986).

This disease commonly presents with episodic encephalopathy and hepatomegaly, and the illness is often wrongly diagnosed as Reye's syndrome. Sudden infant death (SID) may occur, but some affected individuals have never been acutely ill.

Defective degradation of very long chain fatty acids has been demonstrated in the cerebrohepato-renal syndrome of Zellweger (Moser et al. 1984). The liver abnormalities in this condition are portal fibrosis with irregularity of the margin of portal tracts and a mild increase of iron within hepatocytes. Similar hepatic changes are seen in the glutaricacidaemias; steatosis is sometimes present (Goodman et al. 1982).

Disorders of Carnitine Metabolism

Long-chain fatty acids enter the mitochondria via a carnitine-dependent step, and if this substrate is deficient disorders of fat metabolism may occur. Carnitine deficiency and carnitine palmitoyl transferase deficiency may present with an encephalopathy resembling Reye's syndrome. Sudden death may occur in these conditions.

Urea Cycle Enzyme Deficiencies

An important group of inherited metabolic diseases is the urea cycle enzyme deficiencies, as the presentation is frequently sudden death in a family with a history of previous sudden death. Hepatomegaly and hyperammonaemia may suggest Reye's syndrome, but the hepatic architecture is undisturbed. The biochemical types include ornithine carbamoyl transferase deficiency, carbamoyl-phosphate synthetase 1 deficiency, ornithinaemia, citrullinaemia and argininosuccinicaciduria (Syderman 1981).

Neonatal Haemochromatosis

Excess iron deposition in the liver and other organs accompanied by hepatitis fibrosis, liver cell necrosis and spectacular giant cell transformation of surviving hepatocytes was first described in the English literature by Fienberg (1960). He described the necropsy findings in two unrelated sib pairs who all died in the first 3 days of life. By 1986, Blisard and Barlow found 56 more published cases, including several sib pairs, and added two further cases. The amount of iron present is greatly in excess of that seen in hereditary tyrosinaemia and Zellweger syndrome. The extent of fibrosis is comparable with that of congenital syphilis. The basic defect has not been identified, but its occurrence in sibships and distinctive histological features suggest that this is a distinct disorder.

Dubin–Johnson Syndrome

In the Dubin–Johnson syndrome there is defective excretion of conjugated bilirubin from the hepatocytes into the bile canaliculi. There is mild fluctuating jaundice in childhood, which may become more severe in later life. Nausea, malaise, anorexia and hepatomegaly occur, but infrequently. The disease is inherited as an autosomal recessive condition. The prognosis is good.

The liver is greenish black on naked-eye examination, and hepatocytes contain lipochrome pigment within lysosomes. The pigment is apparently a melanin. The liver architecture is normal (Dubin and Johnson 1954).

Rotor's Syndrome

Clinically and biochemically Rotor's syndrome resembles the Dubin–Johnson syndrome, but without the accumulation of pigment in hepatocytes (Rotor et al. 1948).

Giant Cell Transformation and Intrahepatic Cholestasis

"Giant cell hepatitis" is a term that has fallen into disrepute, particularly with clinicians. However, one can find fault with the synonyms "neonatal hepatitis" and "neonatal hepatitis syndrome" for the same reasons; all these terms appear to insist on an infective aetiology when in practice none is found in most cases. The commonest predisposing factor in one large series was an inherited defect of transport inhibitor enzyme (Mowat et al. 1976). "Obstructive cholangiopathy of infancy" is etymologically correct and all-embracing, but rather clumsy.

Giant cell hepatitis and extrahepatic biliary atresia were for many years regarded as distinct entities and, although it has long been recognized that giant cell transformation in the neonatal liver can have many aetiologies, not all of them infectious, biliary atresia was regarded as a congenital anomaly. It is now recognized that in biliary atresia the bile ducts develop normally and atresia is a secondary phenomenon, usually developing during intrauterine life, although in some cases the damage occurs postnatally. Some workers think that the same aetiological factors may be responsible for both extrahepatic biliary atresia and neonatal hepatitis, the type of damage produced being determined by the timing and severity of the insult, and the type of response the fetus is able to mount (Landing 1974; Mowat et al. 1976). This view is not universally accepted; Danks et al. (1977), while accepting that the majority of cases of neonatal hepatitis are attributable to unidentified intrauterine infective agents, think that the agents responsible for extrahepatic biliary atresia are different, although similarly operative in utero. Although it seems that giant cell hepatitis and biliary atresia may be two ends of the same spectrum, it is still important for the clinician to be able to distinguish between these disorders. With new surgical techniques, increasing numbers of infants with biliary atresia can be treated (Kasai et al. 1972), although subsequent reports on the outcome have not been so optimistic (Howard and Mowat 1977). Routine tests of biliary function are poor discriminants in this situation, but Manolaki et al. (1983) have found the combination of percutaneous needle liver biopsy and the rose bengal secretion test to be completely reliable. It has been suggested that laparotomy should be avoided in infants with giant cell hepatitis, as this predisposes to cirrhosis (Boggs and Lawson 1974). However, such a causal relationship is by no means established, as five of the 14 cases in this report were familial, which would, of itself, give an unfavourable prognosis (Danks et al. 1977).

The causes of conjugated hyperbilirubinaemia in the neonate are given in Table 6.1. The frequency of aetiological factors in the hepatitis syndrome of infancy found in two large published series of cases, together with the cases of extrahepatic and intrahepatic biliary atresia seen over the same periods, are given in Table 6.2.

The main histological feature is giant cell transformation of hepatocytes, which can involve only part of a lobule or be very extensive, with few mononuclear forms remaining (Fig. 6.12). Similarly, hepatocyte necrosis may be minimal, and seen clearly only on sections stained for reticulin, or may be widespread with fibrous replacement of liver cells. There is inflammatory cell infiltration of both hepatic lobule and portal tracts, and in many cases, particularly those with an infective aetiology, haematopoiesis persists. Intracellular bile retention and bile plugging may be present. In only a small proportion of cases is it possible to visualize the aetiological agent, e.g. cytomegalovirus (CMV), herpes virus, varicella zoster virus, or perhaps *Toxoplasma gondii* or *Treponema pallidum*. Virus cultures, serological techniques and observation of extrahepatic disease may enable a definite diagnosis to be made in other cases. Some infants with neonatal hepatitis make a full recovery, about a third develop cirrhosis (Fig. 6.13) and succumb to its various complications, and in 10%–20% of cases the disease runs a fulminant course in the neonatal period. When so little is known about the underlying abnormality, in many cases an accurate assessment of the prognosis is difficult. Danks et al. (1977) found that the prognosis was poor among infants with persistent jaundice and acholic stools. The presence of a second disease (Table 6.3) had serious implications. Deutsch et al. (1985) followed up patients with neonatal cholestasis without

Table 6.2. Frequency of aetiological factors in neonatal conjugated hyperbilirubinaemia

	Mowat et al. (1976)		Danks et al. (1977)
Extrahepatic biliary atresia		32	55
Intrahepatic biliary atresia		1	11
Choledochal cyst		2	
Neonatal hepatitis		102	105
Idiopathic	70		69
α_1-Antitrypsin deficiency	24		8
Galactosaemia	1		6
Tyrosinaemia	1		—
Cytomegalovirus	1		13
Hepatitis B virus	2		1
Rubella virus	2		2
Toxoplasmosis	2		2
Coxsackie B_2 virus	—		1
Coxsackie B_4 virus	—		1
Parainfluenza 3 virus	—		1
Syphilis	—		1
Total		137	171

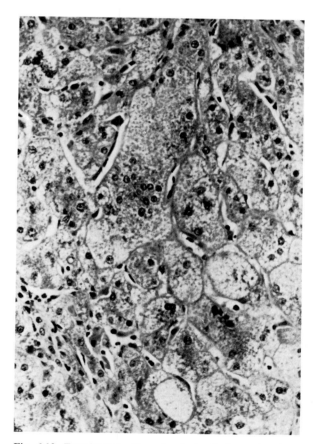

Fig. 6.12. Tyrosinaemia. There is giant cell change involving hepatocytes throughout the lobule. (H&E, × 360)

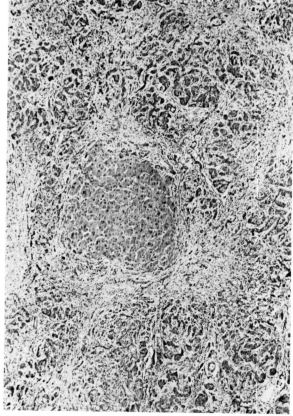

Fig. 6.13. Cirrhosis following giant cell hepatitis in infancy. Male aged 5 years, hepatitis in infancy, chronic liver damage apparent from 16 months of age. Giant cell transformation is present in the central regenerative nodule. (H&E, × 57)

Table 6.3. Other diseases seen in infants with idiopathic neonatal intrahepatic cholestasis

	Mowat et al. (1976)	Danks et al. (1977)
Total no. with idiopathic neonatal hepatitis	70	59
No. with other disease	9	24
Rhesus incompatibility	—	6
Down's syndrome	4	4
Chondrodysplasia punctata	—	3
Sepsis	3	—
Cystic fibrosis	2	2
Fibromatosis	—	2
Cystenosis	—	1
Niemann–Pick disease	—	1
Hepatic haemangioendothelioma	—	1
Polycystic kidneys	—	1
Hydrocephalus	—	1
Congenital heart disease		1
Multiple congenital abnormalities	—	1

atresia. Of babies with non-familial idiopathic disease, 22% died within 12 months, half of these deaths being due to liver failure; a further 8% died later. Nearly half of familial idiopathic cases were dead within 1 year of presentation. The best outcome was observed in infants whose hepatitis had an infectious aetiology, although infants with CMV infection had sequelae in other systems.

Obstructive Jaundice

Paucity of Intrahepatic Bile Ducts

Atresia of the intrahepatic bile ducts is an uncommon cause of obstructive jaundice in childhood, being

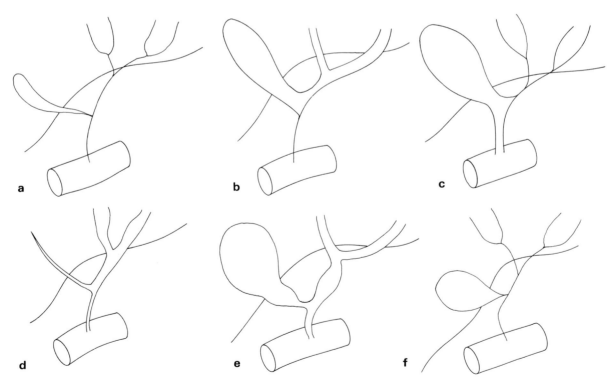

Fig. 6.14. Biliary atresia. Various degrees of extrahepatic obstruction: **a** complete atresia of the extrahepatic biliary tree with hypoplasia of the gallbladder; **b, c** localized atresia; **d** hypoplasia of the extrahepatic biliary system; **e** localized narrowing at the distal end of the common bile duct. **f** A gallbladder of normal size may be found in the presence of atresia of the whole of the extrahepatic biliary system.

found in only one of 137 cases prospectively studied by Mowat et al. (1976). In the cases described by Sass-Kortsak et al. (1956) and Rosenthal et al. (1961), bile ducts were uniformly absent from portal areas throughout the liver, and bile plugging of peri-portal bile canaliculi was present. Inflammatory cell infiltration of portal areas was absent, as was hepatic parenchymal necrosis. The extrahepatic biliary system was normal.

Some infants without intrahepatic bile ducts have many cutaneous xanthomas, which may appear before 1 year of age and are always associated with prolonged elevation of serum cholesterol levels (Rosenthal et al. 1961). Danks et al. (1977) found intrahepatic biliary atresia in 11 of 171 babies with neonatal jaundice in a comprehensive study in Victoria over an 11 year period. All the affected infants had odd facies. Eight had pulmonary valve stenosis or atresia. Two of the infants were brother and sister. Alagille et al. (1975) have reported similar cases with mid-facial hypoplasia and cardiovascular anomalies. Danks et al. (1977) suggest that the intra-hepatic bile ducts in these cases are susceptible to injury, perhaps by a variety of agents, atresia being the end result. Paucity of intrahepatic bile ducts is found without facial or cardiovascular dysmorphism. A biochemical defect in bile elimination may be the primary disorder and ductular atrophy a secondary phenomenon (Harris and Anderson 1960). The progress of hepatic dysfunction in this group of children is variable; in many it follows a benign course.

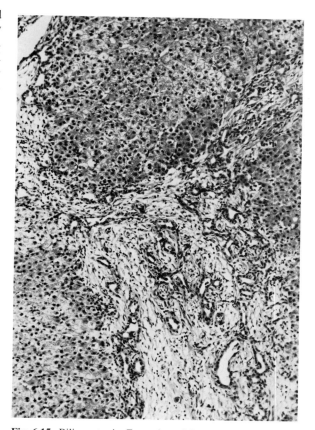

Fig. 6.15. Biliary atresia. Expansion of the portal area by fibrous tissue within which many small bile ducts are present. (H&E, × 57)

Extrahepatic Biliary Obstruction

Extrahepatic biliary obstruction usually presents with conjugated hyperbilirubinaemia and acholic stools from birth, although in a small number of cases the infant is initially normal and obstructive jaundice starts in early postnatal life. The commonest cause of extrahepatic biliary obstruction is extrahepatic biliary atresia, affecting all or part of the extrahepatic biliary system (Fig. 6.14). In a few cases, obstruction of the extrahepatic bile ducts is caused by a choledochal cyst (see p. 308), a situation that can be remedied sur-gically and should be sought actively in every case. Where biliary obstruction is localized, it may be pos-sible to effect satisfactory bile drainage by anasto-mosing part of the duct system or the gallbladder to the small intestine. Where there is widespread extra-hepatic biliary atresia, clearance of the fibrosed ducts and fibrous tissue from the porta hepatis to the intes-tine by way of a Roux-en-Y procedure may relieve the obstruction (Kasai et al. 1972), although ascending cholangitis is a problem in some cases.

Of the cases reported by Alagille (1984), 37% are alive at least 5 years after surgery, although most had abnormal liver biopsies; cirrhosis and absent or reduced bile ducts were present in most cases. Occasionally extrahepatic biliary obstruction is pro-duced by inspissated mucus in the biliary tree in mucoviscidosis or by bile plugs or sludging in the extrahepatic ducts.

Histologically there is expansion of the portal areas by fibrous tissue and proliferation of interlobular bile ducts and small ductules at the periphery of portal areas (Fig. 6.15). These ducts often contain bile, and the bile duct plugging within the hepatic lobule is fre-quently seen. There may be inflammatory cell infiltration in the portal areas: this is not a florid change and the inflammatory cells are not usually seen in the parenchyma. Giant cell transformation of hepatocytes may be present, being usually focal in distribution and rarely conspicuous (Fig. 6.16).

If the obstruction is not relieved, portal fibrosis progresses to biliary cirrhosis and death results from hepatic failure or intercurrent infection. In the late

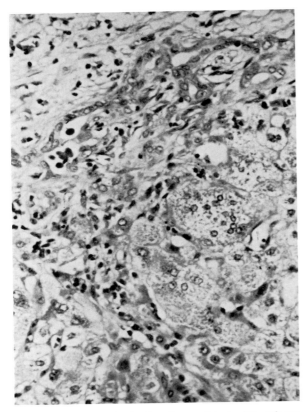

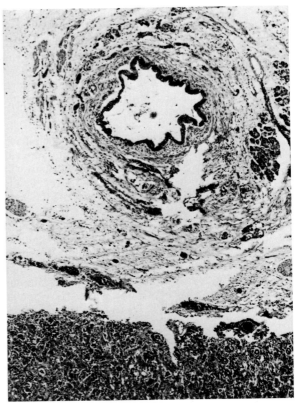

Fig. 6.16. Biliary atresia. A minor degree of giant cell transformation of hepatocytes may be present. Note absence of inflammation within the lobule. (H&E, × 360)

Fig. 6.17. Trisomy 18. Female died 1 day. Multiple congenital abnormalities. The common bile duct is hypoplastic. (H&E, × 60)

stages of the disease bile duct proliferation is not as florid as at the outset.

A liver biopsy exhibiting the changes caused by extrahepatic biliary obstruction does not usually present any diagnostic problem; any giant cell transformation of hepatocytes is usually minor in degree, and inflammatory infiltration is confined to the portal areas, being absent in the lobule, whereas bile duct proliferation is marked and uniform throughout the biopsy. When errors are made, the problem seems to be that of over-interpreting the patchy and usually minor ductular proliferation in hepatitis as due to extrahepatic obstruction (Brough and Bernstein 1974). Ductular proliferation may be widespread in α_1-antitrypsin deficiency, but the absence of interlobular duct proliferation and the presence of diastase-resistant PAS-positive globules in the cytoplasm of periportal hepatocytes indicate the correct diagnosis. Brough and Bernstein (1974) counsel against assessment of possible bile duct proliferation on sections stained by trichrome methods as this tends to accen-

tuate small bile radicles. In their hands it has contributed to over-interpretation of minor degrees of ductular proliferation.

Other Causes

A spectrum of liver abnormalities may occur in the trisomy 17–18 syndrome. Weichsel and Luggatti (1965) described extrahepatic biliary atresia in an infant with 17–18 trisomy. In the cases described by Alpert et al. (1969), three of ten infants with cytogenetically proven 17–18 trisomy had hepatitis with giant cell transformation, bile stasis and hepatocellular necrosis. They also described hepatitis in four of nine phenotypic cases and biliary atresia in two others (Fig. 6.17 and 6.18). Cystic dilatation of intrahepatic bile ducts with no inflammation, giant cell transformation of hepatocytes, and bile plugging is occasionally present (Fig. 6.19).

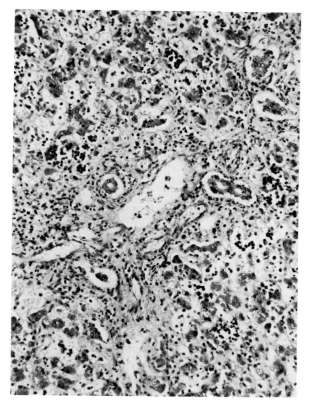

Fig. 6.18. The same case as in Fig. 7.19. Portal areas are expanded. There is some proliferation of bile ducts and loss of hepatocytes with fibrous replacement within the lobule. (H&E, × 156)

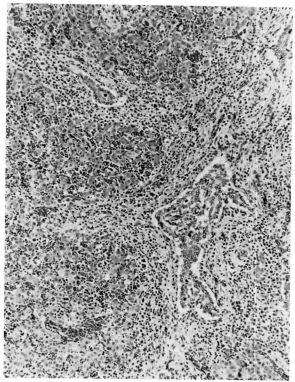

Fig. 6.19. Trisomy 18. Expansion of portal areas. The bile ducts are excessively branching and somewhat dilated, and some contain bile plugs. The extrahepatic biliary tree was patent. (H&E, × 108)

Sclerosing cholangitis, characterized by radiographic evidence of stenosis and local dilatation of intrahepatic bile ducts, is described in a group of infants with neonatal cholestasis which progressed to cirrhosis with partial hypertension (Amedee–Manesme et al. 1987). Initially, liver biopsy showed absence of interlobular bile ducts.

Intravenous Alimentation

Intravenous administration of fat (e.g. Intralipid) as part of a total parenteral nutritional regimen results in its uptake by reticuloendothelial cells throughout the body. The material can be demonstrated by fat stains in spleen, lymph nodes and thymus, and in the Kupffer cells. On routine staining the Kupffer cells are distended and easily seen within the sinusoids (Fig. 6.20). The cytoplasm has a foamy appearance

because of the accumulation of fat globules (Fig. 6.21).

Jaundice complicating parenteral nutrition with amino acid mixtures with and without lipid emulsions was first recognized by Peden et al. (1971), and there have been many subsequent reports. Bernstein et al. (1977) included liver biopsy in the investigation of their cases. Hepatic immaturity seems to be an important factor and, although all the cases reported by Bernstein et al. (1977) had necrotizing enterocolitis, this had occurred as a complication of prematurity rather than an aetiological factor in disturbing liver function. Cholestatic jaundice develops after several weeks of intravenous alimentation, and maximum serum bilirubin levels are seen 7–15 weeks from the onset of treatment. Recovery occurs after cessation of intravenous feeding.

The histological appearance of the liver is that of cholestasis with bile plugging and intracellular bile retention (see Fig. 6.20). Some of the intracellular brown pigment is lipofuscin (Fig. 6.22). Giant cell transformation of hepatocytes is often present and

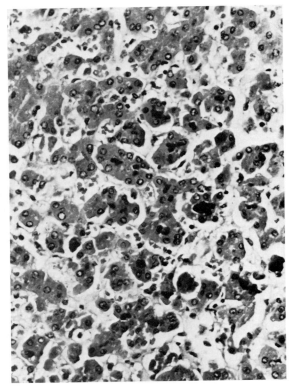

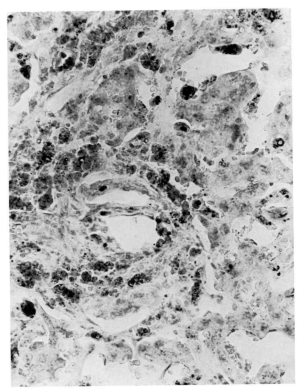

Fig. 6.20. Intravenous alimentation. The sinusoids are distended and Kupffer cells are prominent; their cytoplasm is foamy. Bile plugs are prominent. (H&E, × 360)

Fig. 6.21. Intravenous alimentation. Fat droplets are seen within Kupffer cells. (Oil Red O, × 144)

may be widespread. Patchy liver cell necrosis is present in some cases. There is no accompanying inflammatory cell infiltration, but haematopoiesis is seen in portal areas and is an indication of the immaturity of the patient.

Electron microscopic examination of the liver reveals matrix-rich giant mitochondria, mitochondrial heterogeneity, and damage to microsomal membranes. These findings are non-specific indicators of hepatocellular injury.

Infections

Listeriosis

The liver is usually involved in perinatal infection with *Listeria monocytogenes*. The infection is acquired from the maternal genital tract in the few weeks before delivery. Miliary creamy-white necrotic granulomas are visible through the liver capsule.

Gram-positive bacilli can be demonstrated within the necrotic foci in histological sections.

Syphilis

Intr auterine syphilitic infection of the fetus produces hepatomegaly, and examination of the neonatal liver reveals extensive replacement of hepatic parenchyma by fibrous tissue, which begins as an expansion of portal areas (Fig. 6.23) and extends to produce cirrhosis. Giant cell transformation of hepatocytes occurs, and in severe cases isolated multinucleate cells surrounded by fibrous tissue are seen (Fig. 6.24). (See page 733.)

Viral Hepatitis

Type A

Viral hepatitis A is of worldwide distribution and is endemic in many areas. Transmission is usually

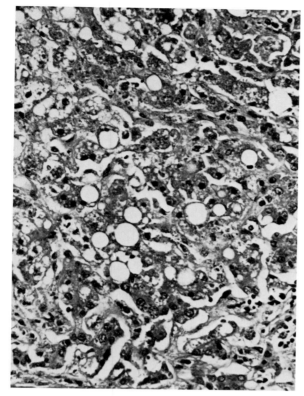

Fig. 6.22. Intravenous alimentation. Pigment retention and fatty change are seen within hepatocytes. (H&E, × 144)

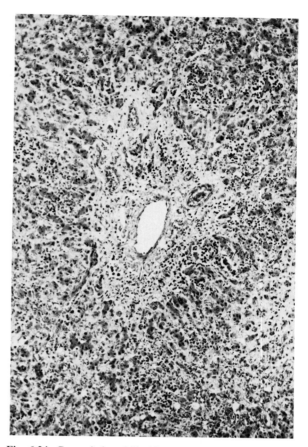

Fig. 6.24. Congenital syphilis (the same case as in Fig. 6.23). Giant cell transformation of hepatocytes and extensive fibrosis. (H&E, × 120)

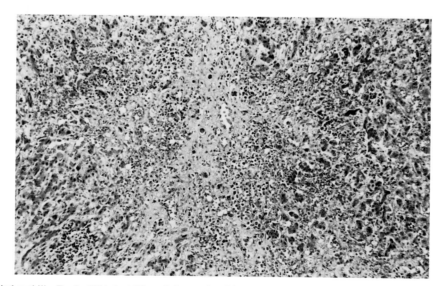

Fig. 6.23. Congenital syphilis. Fresh stillbirth at 34 weeks' gestation. Maternal WR-positive. Treated 2 weeks before delivery. There is marked fibrosis of portal tracts which extends into the lobule. Extensive hepatocyte necrosis. (H&E, × 120)

by the faecal/oral route, so that crowded conditions and poor standards of hygiene facilitate spread. In these conditions infection in childhood is likely.

In children the disease is frequently mild, and jaundice does not necessarily occur, particularly in infants. In rare cases the infection is fulminant, with rapidly deepening jaundice. If death occurs at this stage the histological picture is that of extensive hepatic necrosis, as in adults. Although most patients seem to recover completely, postnecrotic cirrhosis develops in some cases.

Type B

Viral hepatitis B is not a common problem in paediatric practice in Britain. There are, however, particular circumstances in which this type of hepatitis may occur.

Infection may occur in the perinatal period, and the infant's limited immune competence at this time may be a contributory factor. Most of the infants who have developed hepatitis B in the perinatal period have been born to mothers with clinical hepatitis in the last trimester of pregnancy, and it is probable that infection occurs intrapartum by contamination with maternal blood or ingestion of bloody liquor (Cossart 1974). Neonatal infection with type B hepatitis may progress to cirrhosis (Wright et al. 1970).

A small proportion of infants born to mothers who are carriers of hepatitis B surface antigen also become HBsAg-positive. The susceptibility to vertical transmission of hepatitis B surface antigen may be genetically determined; a survey in London seems to indicate an increased susceptibility among the offspring of Chinese mothers (Woo et al. 1979). None of these infants developed signs of biochemical abnormalities suggestive of liver disease.

Perinatal hepatitis B infection may follow the transfusion of blood that is HBA positive (Dupuy et al. 1975). This can readily be prevented by using only screened donor blood or blood products, but chronic, often subclinical, liver disease remains a problem in some countries with a high incidence of hepatitis among children requiring repeated blood transfusion, e.g. those with thalassaemia (Masera et al. 1980). Children with malignant disease and who may be receiving immunosuppressive therapy and at the same time require many transfusions with blood or blood products are particularly vulnerable.

Institutionalized children form another group at risk for hepatitis B infection, particularly the mentally handicapped, among whom adequate standards of hygiene may be difficult to maintain. Children with Down's syndrome, who are particularly susceptible to infections, constitute a very vulnerable group.

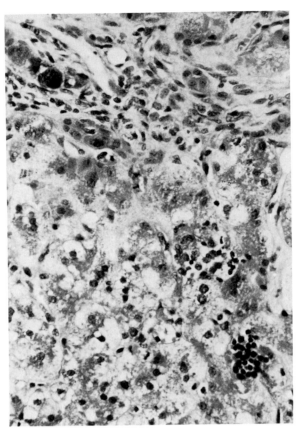

Fig. 6.25. Cytomegalovirus infection producing giant cell hepatitis. There is giant cell transformation of hepatocytes. Haematopoiesis persists within the lobule. An intranuclear viral inclusion is seen in biliary epithelium within the portal tract (*top right*). (H&E, × 576)

Cytomegalovirus Infection

Cytomegalovirus (CMV) infection of the liver in the neonate may be part of a generalized infection acquired in utero and manifested at birth, or may be acquired just before or during delivery. Infection may also result from blood transfusion in utero or in the neonatal period, and may be subsequently transmitted to the non-immune mother by her infant (Tobin et al. 1975). It occurs in older children who are treated with immunosuppressive drugs and who require frequent blood transfusion.

In the neonate, CMV infection is often histologically manifested as a neonatal hepatitis syndrome; giant cell transformation of hepatocytes and inflammatory cell infiltration of the parenchyma occur, and an occasional typical intranuclear viral inclusion may be seen in bile duct epithelium or in a periportal hepatocyte (Fig. 6.25).

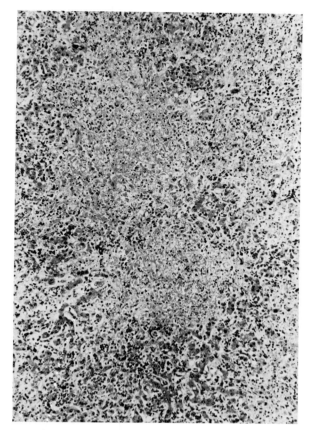

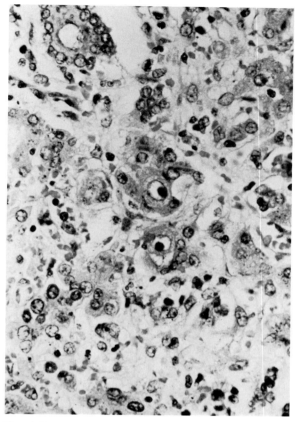

Fig. 6.26. Cytomegalovirus hepatitis. An infant born at 26 weeks' gestation, who died aged 63 days with disseminated infection. Focal necrosis is visible within the liver. (H&E, × 144)

Fig. 6.27. Cytomegalovirus infection (the same case as in Fig. 6.25). Intranuclear viral inclusions are present in hepatocytes at the periphery of a necrotic focus. There is marked inflammatory cell infiltration within the lobule. (H&E, × 576)

Cytomegalovirus infection may, however, produce severe acute hepatic disease as part of a generalized infection, the hepatitis resembling that produced by herpes simplex (CMVs are members of the same group). Areas of necrosis may be seen throughout the liver and intranuclear viral inclusions are readily apparent, usually at the perimeter of the necrotic focus (Figs. 6.26 and 6.27).

Herpes Simplex

The neonate is usually protected from herpes simplex infection by maternal antibody, so infection rarely occurs. Severe generalized infection can occur in the infant of a non-immune mother (Leading article 1969). The disease has a high mortality rate, and hepatitis is usually present.

The characteristic features are focal necrosis; intranuclear viral inclusions are seen in the cells at the margins of these areas.

Enteroviral Infections

Infants and children are susceptible to infection. Serotypes commonly encountered are Coxsackie B_{1-5} and echovirus 11, although types 9, 6, 14, 19 and 31 may cause fatal neonatal infection. Liver involvement in the form of acute necrosis is usual in the syndrome characterized by hypotension and haemorrhagic infarction (Nagington et al. 1978). Echovirus 11 is the responsible organism in most cases (Berry and Nagington 1982). Neonatal meningitis and renal haemorrhage with small vessel thrombosis of kidneys and adrenals were found in an outbreak in a special care baby unit (Nagington et al. 1978). Hepatitis may

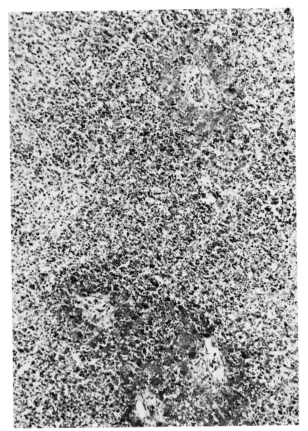

Fig. 6.28. Echo II hepatitis. Term male infant. Sudden deterioration on day 6 with pallor, hypothermia and hepatomegaly. Generalized bleeding tendency, jaundice and convulsions at age 8 days. Extensive parenchymal necrosis is present. Hepatocytes survive only in periportal areas. (H&E, × 144)

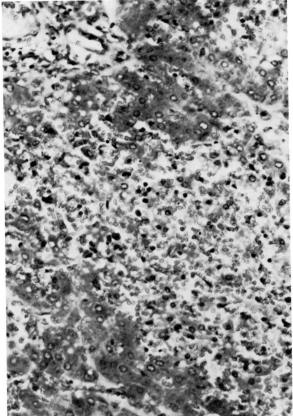

Fig. 6.29. Echo II hepatitis. Focal necrosis with diffuse inflammatory cell infiltration. (H&E, × 360)

occur, with sudden collapse, jaundice and haemorrhage. There is widespread necrosis of the hepatic parenchyma, which is largely centrilobular in distribution with mixed inflammatory cell infiltration (Figs. 6.28 and 6.29).

Adenovirus Infection

Jaffe et al. (1987) have reported a distinctive histopathological appearance in the liver of children who have had liver transplantation and develop adenovirus hepatitis (four of 20 patients from whom adenovirus was cultured). Adenovirus type 5 was involved in all four cases. Circumscribed lesions were scattered throughout the liver (Fig. 6.30a). In these there were polymorphs and macrophages, but few lymphocytes. At the margin of the lesions infected liver cells could be identified (Fig. 6.30b).

Reye's Syndrome

The association of acute encephalopathy and fatty degeneration of the viscera was described by Reye et al. in 1963, and must be considered in the differential diagnosis of convulsions or altered consciousness, particularly if accompanied by severe vomiting proceeding rapidly to coma, in a child who has been previously well. There may be evidence of a mild infective illness. Papilloedema is commonly found, but there are no localizing central nervous system signs. There may be mild to moderate hepatomegaly and hypoglycaemia is usual, as are reduced prothrombin activity and a markedly raised aspartate aminotransferase level. The blood ammonia level may also be elevated. A liver biopsy demonstrating severe panlobular fatty change confirms the diagnosis but is rarely done, either because the clinician does

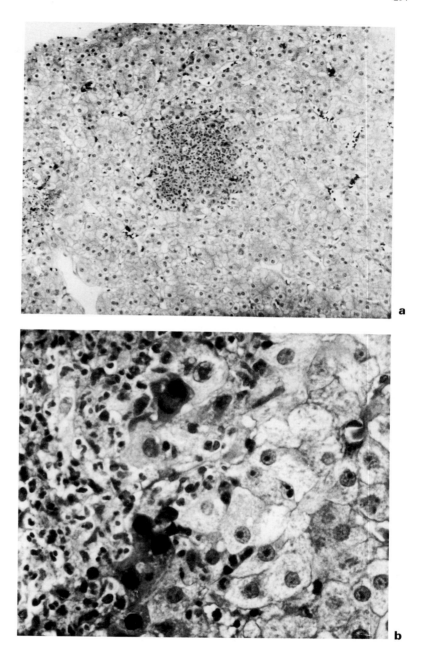

Fig. 6.30. a Focal area of necrosis in the liver. (H&E, × 149) **b** Margin of lesion showing altered hepatocytes. (H&E, × 240) (Biopsy by courtesy of Dr R. Jaffe)

not consider the diagnosis of Reye's syndrome or because of reluctance to undertake such a procedure in the face of reduced prothrombin activity. The clinical diagnosis appears to be made more often than is justified by the pathological findings, and diagnostic criteria such as those of Lichtenstein et al. (1983) should be used.

The necropsy findings are those of severe cerebral oedema in the absence of any inflammatory cell infiltration of brain or meninges, hepatomegaly with severe panlobular fatty degeneration and accumulation of lipid in renal tubules.

The principal epidemiological features of Reye's syndrome in the USA appear to be an equal sex distribution, a median age of 8–9 years and an association with recent influenza B and also, to a lesser extent, with influenza A. Varicella is an important associated infection. The case fatality ratio is around 20%. In the UK, however, the median age is around 14 months, the mortality rate is higher at 50%, and a

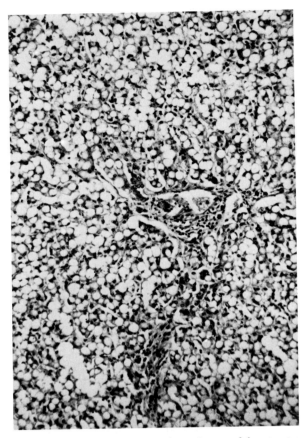

Fig. 6.31. Kwashiorkor. Severe fatty change of hepatocytes throughout the lobule. There is periportal round-cell infiltration. Liver architecture is normal. (H&E, × 150)

wider range of viruses seem to be involved as prodromal events, suggesting that different diagnostic criteria may be used in the two countries.

The relationship of the syndrome to the ingestion of aspirin was first quantified in a US Public Health Services study. A pilot scheme showed that 93% of children with Reye's syndrome had a history of aspirin ingestion compared with 46% of controls; however, there were serious flaws in the study, where it was possible that a preferential diagnosis of Reye's syndrome might have been made if a history of aspirin ingestion was available. Nevertheless, the information was used as the basis for a campaign in which parents were warned against giving aspirin to children, especially those with influenza or varicella. Fewer children received aspirin and reports of the syndrome declined substantially (Hurwitz et al. 1985; Remmington et al. 1986).

Further evidence of a possible role for aspirin in the syndrome is seen in an increased risk of its

manifestation in children with connective tissue disorders treated with long-term salicylate therapy (Rennebohm et al. 1985).

Kwashiorkor

Severe fatty degeneration of the liver is almost universal in kwashiorkor, when up to 50% of the wet weight of liver may be fat (Waterlow 1948). This is probably a reflection of abnormal triglyceride transport secondary to reduced plasma lipoprotein levels.

Histological appearances are those of panlobular accumulation of fat in small vacuoles distending the hepatocytes (Fig. 6.31). Hepatic architecture is not disturbed, but periportal round-cell infiltration may be present. Focal hepatocellular necrosis is occasionally present. The liver returns to normal following resumption of normal nutritional status (Cook and Hutt 1967).

Cirrhosis

Cirrhosis of the liver in childhood is uncommon. In comparison with adults, a much greater proportion of cases complicate a recognized liver disease or metabolic abnormality involving the liver. The majority of cases follow the hepatitis syndrome of infancy (see Fig. 6.9), particularly when this is a manifestation of α_1-antitrypsin deficiency (see Fig. 6.14) and biliary atresia (see Fig. 6.15). Cirrhosis is a rare complication of viral hepatitis, but is common in galactosaemia and may occur in Wilson's disease and the mucopolysaccharidoses. It is a late complication of thalassaemia major (see below).

Cirrhosis in mucoviscidosis is uncommon. Its special features are described below.

Indian childhood cirrhosis is an almost universally fatal condition affecting children in the first 5 years of life in the subcontinent (Bhave et al. 1982). There are 10 clinicopathological criteria for diagnosis (Bhagwat et al. 1983). These are:

1. Age (10–24 months at presentation)
2. Firm smooth hepatomegaly extending 3 cm or more below the costal margin
3. Sharp leafy edge to the liver
4. Splenomegaly
5. Serum glutamine oxaloacetic transaminase (GOT) level greater than 260 IU

6. Periportal to panlobular coarse hepatocytic orcein-positive deposits
7. Mallory's hyaline with satellitosis
8. Excess copper by qualitative or quantitative methodology with normal serum ceruloplasmin
9. Dissecting fibrosis of liver lobules
10. Macrovesicular and microvesicular fat in the absence of recent steroid therapy or significant hypoalbuminaemia

Using a scoring system with one point for each criterion, the diagnosis requires eight points.

The disease is commoner in rural areas and is thought to be due to excess storage in the liver of copper derived from cooking utensils and containers. It has been reported in the UK (Klass et al. 1980).

The histological picture varies from massive hepatic necrosis in the acute stage to portal cirrhosis. The presence of cytoplasmic hyaline degeneration indistinguishable from Mallory's alcoholic hyaline degeneration by histological stains and histochemical methods (Nayak et al. 1969) is unique among the childhood cirrhoses and has been interpreted as an index of toxic injury to the hepatocyte.

Hepatocellular carcinoma is a rare but well recognized sequel of cirrhosis in childhood. As in adults, its occurrence is probably related to the length of survival and not to any specific underlying abnormality (Keeling 1971).

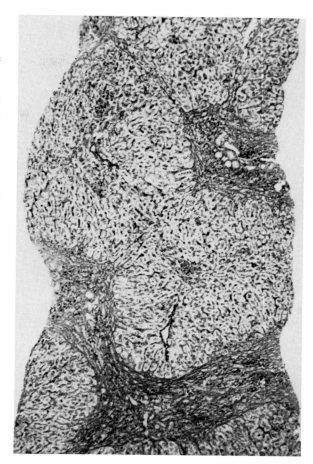

Fig. 6.32. Thalassaemia. Cirrhosis present in a needle liver biopsy.

Thalassaemia

In thalassaemia major, as a result of transfusion overload, there is progressive iron deposition within the liver with increasing age. Iron accumulates within hepatocytes and also within macrophages in portal areas. There is a gradual increase in portal fibrous tissue (Fig. 6.32) with progression to cirrhosis in individuals who survive into their second or third decade. Risdon et al. (1975) found a linear relationship between the extent of fibrosis and the age of the patients, and an exponential relationship between both the rate and extent of hepatic fibrosis and the amount of iron deposited in the liver. They concluded that the reduction in liver iron concentration produced by chelation therapy produced a considerable reduction in the rate of fibrosis within the liver.

Reports from Italy (De Virgiliis et al. 1980; Masera et al. 1980) suggest that chronic active or chronic persistent hepatitis following hepatitis B infection may contribute to deterioration in liver function in patients with thalassaemia. Acute infection was largely subclinical, but the incidence of subsequent chronic liver disease was higher among patients with thalassaemia than among non-thalassaemic individuals. It has been suggested that interaction between low-dose infection and iron overload might play a part in perpetuating chronic liver disease in thalassaemic subjects (De Virgiliis et al. 1980).

Mucoviscidosis

There is some liver involvement in most children with cystic fibrosis, although the majority are asymptomatic. The pathogenetic mechanism of the liver disease is similar to that producing pathological changes in other organs, namely the production of viscid secretions by mucus-producing cells in the biliary tract, which obstruct bile flow and give rise to

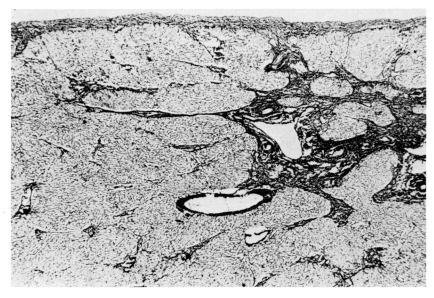

Fig. 6.33. Mucoviscidosis in a male who died, aged 12 years, with bronchiectasis and bronchopneumonia. Patch portal fibrosis is visible beneath the liver capsule. (Gordon and Sweet's reticulin stain, × 36)

a localized cholangitis and portal fibrosis. On the whole, the severity of liver involvement in cystic fibrosis is related to length of survival, but one may find minimal liver damage in adolescents who have very extensive lung damage and complete fatty replacement of the pancreas.

Focal Portal Fibrosis

Focal portal fibrosis of local biliary cirrhosis is the commonest hepatic lesion in mucoviscidosis, and is usually discovered as an incidental finding at laparotomy or necropsy.

Fibrosis often occurs just beneath the capsule of the liver (Fig. 6.33). Portal tracts are irregularly expanded by fibrous tissue, and fibrous bands run between adjacent portal areas. The involved portal tracts contain elevated numbers of bile ducts. Mucus is sometimes seen within the ducts or duct epithelial cells, but concretions are rare.

Biliary Cirrhosis

Some children with cystic fibrosis develop biliary cirrhosis during childhood. Jaundice is uncommon and biochemical tests of liver function usually yield normal results, the signs and complications of portal hypertension being the presenting features (di Sant'Agnese and Blanc 1956).

The liver has an irregular nodularity; the fibrous scars may produce fissuring resembling the hepar lobatum of congenital syphilis (Craig et al. 1957).

There is marked portal fibrosis, and within the fibrous tissue there are very many dilated bile ducts filled with inspissated material (Fig. 6.34), an appearance pathognomic of cystic fibrosis. There is bile plugging within the lobules in many cases; regenerative nodules are not conspicuous. Fatty change of the parenchyma is variable and probably reflects the general nutritional status of the patient.

Neonatal Jaundice

In a small number of patients with cystic fibrosis, obstructive jaundice in the neonatal period is the mode of presentation, but it is more commonly seen at this age in infants presenting with meconium ileus or ileal atresia (Oppenheimer and Esterly 1975). The jaundice may be persistent (Valman et al. 1971).

The histological appearance of the liver at this time is typical of extrahepatic biliary obstruction, with proliferation of small bile radicles in portal areas, bile plugging, and perhaps a minor degree of giant cell transformation of hepatocytes in the presence of a demonstrably patent extrahepatic biliary tree. Mucus in the bile ducts around the porta hepatis may produce marked localized dilatation of the ducts, which is usually transient (Oppenheimer and Esterly 1975).

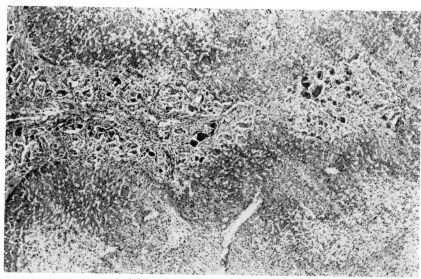

Fig. 6.34. Mucoviscidosis. There is marked bile duct proliferation and dilatation within portal areas. Many ducts are filled with inspissated material. (H&E, × 36)

Nodular Regenerative Hyperplasia

This change is an unusual alteration in liver architecture, with proliferative nodules separated by atrophic parenchyma, often associated with Felty's syndrome, rheumatoid arthritis and haematological disorders. It may rarely occur in the fetus (Galdeano and Drut 1991).

Budd–Chiari Syndrome

The clinical course and appearances of the liver are similar in childhood to those seen in the adult. Occasional causes of Budd–Chiari syndrome in children are congenital anomalies, such as stenosis of a hepatic vein and anomalous valves and sphincters. More commonly it complicates other diseases, such as tumours or leukaemia, sickle cell disease, polycythaemia and allergic vasculitis.

Trauma

The liver of infants and children is more susceptible to trauma than that of the adult because of its relatively large size and the poor protection offered by the developing rib cage.

The liver may be damaged during delivery, and subcapsular haematomas with or without haemoperitoneum are not uncommon, particularly in preterm infants presenting by the breech. Liver damage may follow vigorous external cardiac massage in the neonate, when a linear haematoma along the costal margin or extensive haemorrhage beneath the capsule of the right lobe is produced (Fig. 6.35). Metabolism of a subcapsular haematoma may produce jaundice.

In older children, laceration of the liver may be the result of non-penetrating injuries to the abdomen, usually as a result of road traffic accidents, but falls and non-accidental injury can also produce liver damage.

The mortality rate from laceration of the liver is high, often because of failure of diagnosis, although prompt surgical intervention may be successful (Sparkman 1954).

Aflatoxicosis

In 1991 an outbreak of aflatoxin poisoning occurred in Malaysia associated with contamination of a form of noodle during the Nine Emperor Gods Chinese festival. There were 13 deaths (one in an adult), and massive hepatic necrosis and bile duct proliferation were seen in the children who died, closely resembling the changes seen in animals poisoned with this mycotoxin (Chao et al. 1991).

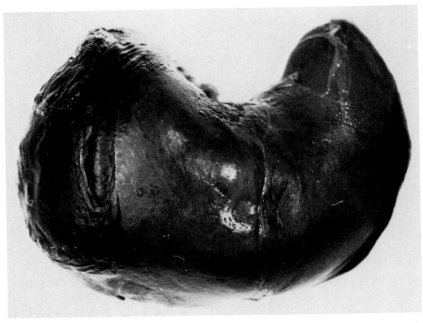

Fig. 6.35. Large subcapsular haematoma of the right lobe of the liver in a male born at 28 weeks, who died aged 2 days.

Tumours

Hepatoblastoma

See p. 892.

Hamartoma

Hamartomas of the liver are of two basic types: angiomas, which form the larger group, with mesenchymal, composed of liver and fibrous tissue. They occur in around 6% of livers of those dying in early life (Berry 1987).

Angiomas are tumours of infancy (Dehner and Ishak 1971). They are often large at the time of birth (Fig. 6.36) and may rupture during delivery, causing death by exsanguination (Claireaux 1960). Some are the cause of cardiac failure in the neonatal period because of shunting (Figs. 6.37–6.39) (Bamford et al. 1980) with a high cardiac output (Linderkamp et al. 1976), and others are palpated as an abdominal mass which is often rapidly enlarging. Resection of a single large tumour and the surrounding liver may be necessary to control heart failure, but ligation of its supply vessels may be possible. The lesions may be accompanied by a consumptive coagulopathy due to clotting within the angioma or an isolated thrombocy-

topenia occurring as a result of increased mechanical destruction of platelets in the abnormal vessels. There may be jaundice, which in some cases is obstructive in type. Angiomas are frequently single, but may be multiple (Balazs et al. 1978). They may be capillary, cavernous or mixed.

Regression following steroid therapy has been documented (Goldberg and Fonkalsrud 1969), and flattening of endothelial cells, with loss of capillary buds and increased stromal fibrosis, followed steroids and radiotherapy in the case described by Balazs et al. (1978).

The mesenchymal hamartoma, which presents as an abdominal mass, is the next most common type (Yandza and Valuyer 1986). It may enlarge rapidly as cystically dilated duct elements fill with fluid. These lesions are more commonly solid in appearance, with a myxoid stroma containing epithelial-lined duct-like structures and thin-walled vessels (Fig. 6.40). Haematopoiesis may be present and cause some diagnostic confusion.

Other malformations reported as accompanying hepatic hamartomas include tracheo-oesophageal fistula and annular pancreas (Keeling 1971), atrial septal defect, patent ductus arteriosus, meningomyelocele, renal agenesis, hypoplastic mandible and cutaneous angiomas (cited by Linkerkamp et al. 1976). All are commonly occurring malformations and there seems to be no specific association.

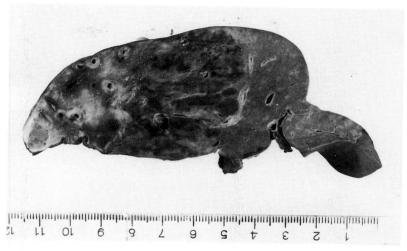

Fig. 6.36. Massive vascular hamartoma in the liver of a neonate.

Hepatocellular Carcinoma

Hepatocellular carcinoma occurs in the older child, usually presenting after the age of 6 years. The symptoms are vomiting, abdominal pain, loss of weight and abdominal distension; jaundice occurs late in the disease. The liver is usually palpably enlarged, and a liver scan may demonstrate the site of the tumour. Liver function tests are usually normal although the serum α_1-fetoprotein level may be raised.

Hepatocellular carcinomas can arise in a previously normal liver or in one with pre-existing disease. Cirrhosis, itself the sequel to extrahepatic biliary atresia or hepatitis in infancy, may predispose to the development of carcinoma in some cases. Hepatocellular carcinoma has been found in children with a variety of metabolic disorders, including glycogen storage disease, Niemann–Pick disease and hereditary tubular dysplasia (Fanconi's disease) (Keeling 1971).

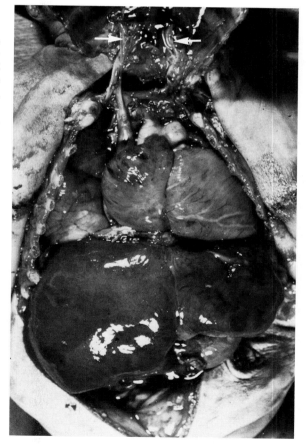

Fig. 6.37. Female born at 36 weeks. Hepatomegaly with prominent left lobe at 2 h. Cardiomegaly. A left ventricular angiocardiogram showed enormously dilated internal mammary arteries supplying an arteriovenous malformation of the left lobe of the liver. Died aged 3 days with disseminated intravascular coagulation despite ligation of feeding vessels. There is marked hepatomegaly with irregular contour to the left lobe and cardiomegaly. Both internal mammary arteries (*arrows*) are dilated and tortous.

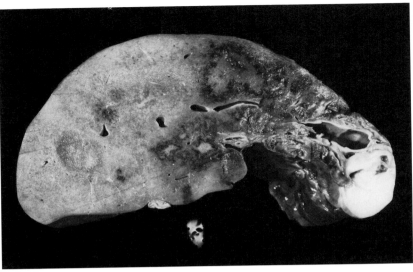

Fig. 6.38. Arteriovenous malformation. Slice of liver showing the left lobe replaced by irregular vascular channels. Areas of infarction are present in the right lobe.

Within the liver there may be a solitary tumour mass (Fig. 6.41) or multiple tumour nodules throughout the organ. These are lobulated, yellow–tan in colour and appear to be encapsulated. Histologically and at the ultrastructural level the liver cell carcinoma

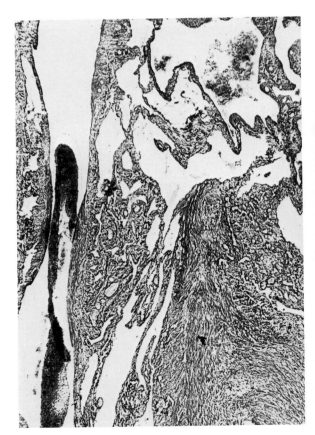

Fig. 6.39. Histological section showing irregular vascular channels. (Gordon and Sweet's reticulin method, × 81)

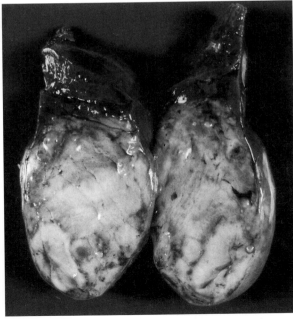

Fig. 6.40. Mesenchymal hamartoma filling most of the right lobe of the liver (the usual site). (Courtesy of Professor J.N. Cox)

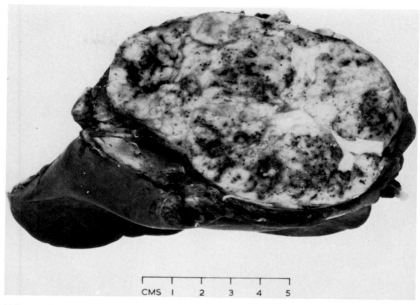

Fig. 6.41. Hepatocellular carcinoma. Lobulated tumour with multiple small haemorrhages scattered throughout. (Reproduced from Keeling 1971, by permission of the Editor of the *Journal of Pathology*)

of older children is identical with that found in the adult (Fig. 6.42), and quite distinct from hepatoblastoma of the infant liver, which may differentiate along a largely hepatocellular line (Misugi et al. 1967; Ito and Johnson 1969). At present, treatment of these tumours is disappointing, irrespective of the presence or absence of pre-existing liver disease. Tumours with fibrolamellar histology have a better prognosis.

Rhabdomyosarcoma

Rhabdomyosarcoma also occurs in the liver of the older child. It is thought to arise from the muscle in the wall of the intrahepatic bile ducts. Symptoms include jaundice, which may be severe, anorexia, abdominal pain and swelling.

A single mass, often in the vicinity of a large bile duct, may be present, or there may be multiple widely separated tumour nodules throughout the liver (Fig. 6.43). The tumour is cream in colour and firm; translucent polypoid nodules may protrude into the lumen of an adjacent bile duct (Fig. 6.44). In some tumours, cystic degeneration is a prominent feature.

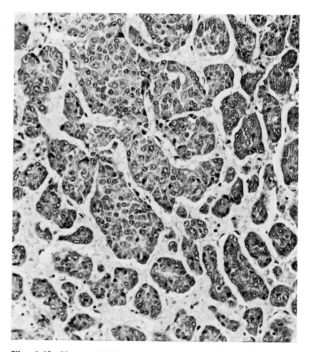

Fig. 6.42. Hepatocellular carcinoma. Large cells with abundant cytoplasm having a trabecular configuration. (H&E, × 100)

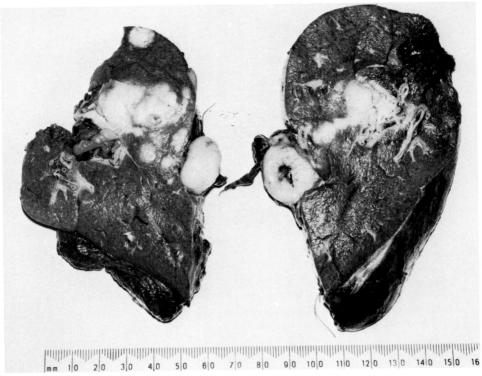

Fig. 6.43. Rhabdomyosarcoma from 6-year-old boy who presented with obstructive jaundice and hepatomegaly. The cut surface of the liver shows multiple tumour nodules.

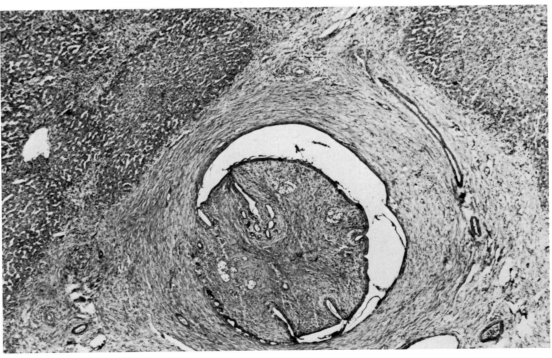

Fig. 6.44. Rhabdomyosarcoma. An epithelial covered tumour nodule protrudes into a dilated bile duct. (H&E, × 48)

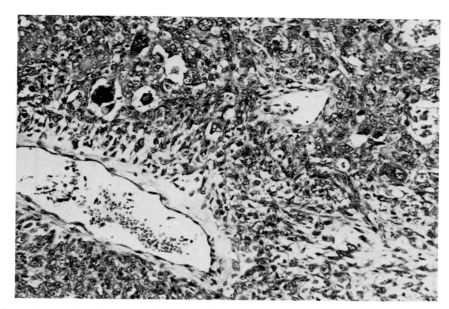

Fig. 6.45. Rhabdomyosarcoma. There is marked cellular and nuclear pleomorphism. Cytoplasmic degeneration is seen at the lower right. (H&E, × 100) (Reproduced from Keeling 1971, by permission of the Editor of the *Journal of Pathology*)

Histologically, the tumour is composed of large mesenchymal cells with large pale-staining nuclei exhibiting considerable pleomorphism (Fig. 6.45). The cytoplasm of the cells may be densely eosinophilic or foamy. "Tadpole" or elongated "strap" cells are often present, but cytoplasmic striations are not seen in these tumours as commonly as in rhabdomyosarcomas arising in the urogenital tract.

These tumours metastasize to lymph nodes in the porta hepatis. Haematogenous spread to the lungs may occur early in the disease.

Malignant Mesenchymal Tumour

Malignant mesenchymal tumours also occur in older children, presenting as an abdominal mass, often with fever and pain (Stanley et al. 1973). Arteriography reveals poor perfusion, and on resection the tumours are seen as large, partly cystic, mucoid masses. Histologically they are poorly differentiated. Bizarre giant cells are seen in a myxoid stroma, with many spindle cells forming a background of varying density (Fig. 6.46).

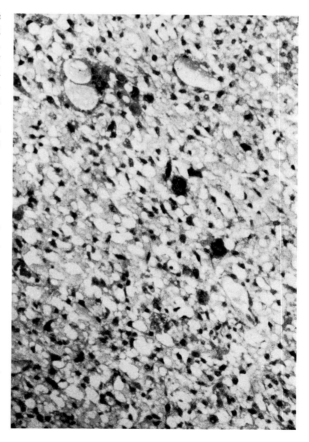

Fig. 6.46. Malignant mesenchymal tumour from a 12-year-old girl presenting with shoulder-tip pain. Death occurred 6 months later after two resections. Myxoid tissue with bizarre large cells. (H&E, × 240)

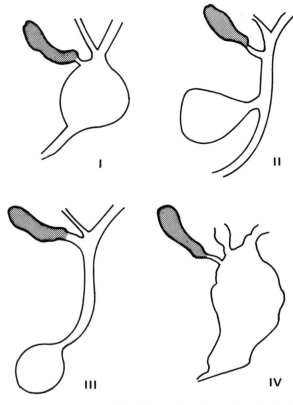

Fig. 6.47. Forms of choledochal cyst. Type I: saccular or fusiform dilatation below the level of the confluence of the main hepatic ducts. Type II: diverticulum from the side of the common bile duct. Type III: dilatation at the lower end of the common duct. Type IV: dilatation of the intrahepatic and extrahepatic biliary tree (Caroli's disease). (After Powell et al. 1981)

Teratoma

True teratomas of the liver are very rare, and must be distinguished from hepatoblastoma with squamous metaplasia and osteoid formation. Both benign (Yarborough and Evashnick 1956) and malignant tumours (Misugi and Reinger 1965) have been described.

Gallbladder

Congenital Anomalies

Congenital abnormalities of the gallbladder are very rare and take the form of septation and duplication. Complete duplication of the gallbladder may occur,

each having its own spiral valve and cystic duct, which may empty into the common bile duct or directly into the duodenum. It is usually of no consequence in infancy but may give rise to problems in the presence of acquired disease.

An externally normal gallbladder may be divided internally by an intraluminal septum composed of muscle and covered by biliary epithelium. A diverticulum may arise from the gallbladder or from the cystic duct. It is distinguished from Rokitansk-Aschoff sinus by the presence of a muscular wall.

Choledochal Cysts

A choledochal cyst is a focal dilatation of the common bile duct, which may take the form of a fusiform or eccentric saccular dilatation or may be pedunculated. There is enormous variation in size, from those having a volume of only a few millilitres to enormous cysts containing several litres of bile-stained fluid. Large cysts may be palpable per abdomen or visualized by ultrasound or radiological techniques. The cysts probably arise as a result of the formation of an abnormal pancreaticobiliary junction allowing reflux of pancreatic secretions into the biliary tree. The common form of the junction is acutely angled with a long common channel extending for 2–3 cm before entry into the duodenum. Reflux occurs and cyst fluid often has high amylase levels (Kato et al. 1980). The various forms of choledochal cyst are shown in Fig. 6.47. Twenty-five per cent of patients present in the first year of life and 60% before the age of 10 years (Lee et al. 1969; Spitz 1978). Presenting symptoms include obstructive jaundice, particularly in the neonate, upper abdominal pain, and a mass in the right hypochondrium. Complications include cholangitis, biliary cirrhosis and calculi. Rupture may occur. The incidence of carcinoma in the cysts or biliary tract is high.

The diagnosis is usually confirmed by ultrasound, but radiological examination may aid preoperative diagnosis, and the cyst may displace the right kidney downwards or the duodenum anteriorly and medially.

The cysts are lined with biliary epithelium but this is frequently disrupted by inflammation. The wall consists of smooth muscle and fibrous tissue.

Cholecystitis

Cholecystitis is extremely rare in infancy and childhood and resembles acute inflammation of this viscus in the adult.

Cholelithiasis

Cholelithiasis in children usually occurs as a complication of haemolytic anaemia or sickle cell disease. It is described in preterm neonates treated with diuretics and by intravenous alimentation (Whitington and Black 1980).

Spontaneous perforation of the common bile duct is an occasional neonatal surgical emergency (Howard et al. 1976).

References

Aagenaes O, Fagerhol M, Elgjo K, Munthe E, Hovig T (1974) Pathology and pathogenesis of liver disease in α_1-antitrypsin deficient individuals. Postgrad Med J 50: 365

Alagille D (1984) Extrahepatic biliary atresia. Hepatology 4: 7S

Alagille D, Odievre M, Gautier M, Dommergnes JP (1975) Hepatic ductular hypoplasia associated with characteristic facies, vertebral malformations, retarded physical, mental and sexual development, and cardiac murmur. J Pediatr 86: 63

Allen JT, Gillett M, Holton JB, King GS, Pettit BR (1980) Evidence of galactosaemia in utero. Lancet i: 603

Alpert LI, Strauss L, Hirschhorn K (1969) Neonatal hepatitis and biliary atresia associated with trisomy 17–18 syndrome. N Engl J Med 280: 16

Amedee-Manesme O, Bernard O, Brunelle F, Hadchouel M, Polonovski C, Baudon JJ, Beguet P, Alagille D (1987) Sclerosing cholangitis with neonatal onset. J Pediatr 111: 225

Andersen DH (1956) Familial cirrhosis of the liver with storage of abnormal glycogen. Lab Invest 5: 11

Anonymous (1982) Clouds over galactosaemia. Lancet ii: 1379

Anonymous (1986) Sudden infant death and inherited disorders of fat oxidation. Lancet ii: 1073

Balazs Marta, Denes J, Lukacs VF (1978) Fine structure of multiple neonatal haemangioendothelioma of the liver. Virchows Arch [A] 379: 157

Bamford MFM, de Bono D, Pickering D, Keeling JW (1980) An arteriovenous malformation of the liver giving rise to persistent transitional (fetal) circulation. Arch Dis Child 55: 244

Berg NO, Eriksson S (1972) Liver disease in adults with α_1-antitrypsin deficiency. N Engl J Med 287: 1264

Berk PD, Bloomer JR, Howe RB, Berlin NI (1970) Constitutional hepatic dysfunction (Gilbert's syndrome). A new definition based on kinetic studies with unconjugated radiobilirubin. Am J Med 49: 296

Bernstein J, Chang CH, Brough AJ, Heidelberger KP (1977) Conjugated hyperbilirubinaemia in infancy associated with parenteral alimentation. J Pediatr 90: 361

Berry CL (1987) Liver lesions in an autopsy population. Hum Toxicol 6: 209

Berry PJ, Nagington J (1982) Fatal infection with Echovirus 11. Arch Dis Child 57: 22

Bhagwat AG, Walisa BNS, Koshy A, Banerjee K (1983) Will the real Indian childhood cirrhosis please stand up? Cleve Clin 50: 323

Bhave SA, Pandit AN, Pradhan AM et al. (1982) Liver disease in India. Arch Dis Child 57: 922

Blisard KS, Barlow SA (1986) Neonatal hemochromatosis. Hum Pathol 17: 376

Blyth H, Ockenden BG (1971) Polycystic disease of kidneys and liver presenting in childhood. J Med Genet 8: 257

Boggs JD, Lawson EE (1974) Long-term follow up of neonatal hepatitis: safety and value of surgical exploration. Paediatrics 53: 650

Boichis H, Passwell J, David R et al. (1973) Congenital hepatic fibrosis and nephronophthisis. Q J Med 62: 221

Brough AJ, Bernstein J (1974) Conjugated hyperbilirubinemia in early infancy. A reassessment of liver biopsy. Hum Pathol 5: 507

Burn J, Dunger D, Lake B (1982) Liver damage in a neonate with α_1-antitrypsin deficiency due to phenotype PiZ null (Z-). Arch Dis Child 57: 311

Chao T-C, Maxwell SM, Wong S-Y (1991). An outbreak of aflatoxicosis and boric acid poisoning in Malaysia: a clinico-pathological study. J Pathol 164: 225

Claireaux AE (1960) Neonatal hyper-bilirubinaemia. Br Med J i: 1528

Cohen KL, Rubin PE, Echevarria RA, Sharp HL, Teague PO (1973) α_1-antitrypsin deficiency, emphysema and cirrhosis in an adult. Ann Intern Med 78: 227

Cook GC, Hutt MSR (1967) The liver after kwashiorkor. Br Med J iii(i): 454

Cook PJL (1974) Genetic aspects of the Pi system. Postgrad Med J 50: 362

Cossart YE (1974) Acquisition of hepatitis B antigen in the newborn period. Postgrad Med J 50: 334

Cottrall K, Cook PJL, Mowat AP (1974) Neonatal hepatitis syndrome and α_1-antitrypsin deficiency: an epidemiological study in south-east England. Postgrad Med J 50: 376

Cox DW, Markovic VD, Teshima IE (1982) Genes for immunoglobulin heavy chains and for α_1-antitrypsin are localised to specific regions of chromosome 14q. Nature 297: 428

Craig JM, Haddad H, Shwachman H (1957) The pathological changes in the liver in cystic fibrosis of the pancreas. Am J Dis Child 93: 357

Crawfurd M d'A, Jackson P, Kohler HG (1978) Case report: Meckel's syndrome (dysencephalia splanchnocystica) in two Pakistani sibs. J Med Genet 15: 242

Crigler JF, Najjar VA (1952) Congenital familial non-haemolytic jaundice with kernicterus. Paediatrics 10: 169

Danks DM, Campbell PE, Jack I, Rogers J, Smith AL (1977) Studies of the aetiology of neonatal hepatitis and biliary atresia. Arch Dis Child 52: 360

Dehner LP, Ishak KG (1971) Vascular tumours of the liver in infants and children. Arch Pathol 92: 101

Deutsch J, Smith AL, Danks DM, Campbel PE (1985) Long term prognosis for babies with neonatal liver disease. Arch Dis Child 60: 447

De Virgiliis S, Fiorelli G, Gargion S, Gornacchia G, Sanna G, Cossu P, Murgia V, Cao A (1980) Chronic liver disease in transfusion-dependent thalassaemia: hepatitis B virus marker studies. J Clin Pathol 33: 949

di Sant' Agnese PA, Blanc WA (1956) Distinctive type of biliary cirrhosis of the liver associated with cystic fibrosis of the pancreas. Recognition through signs of portal hypertension. Pediatrics 15: 387

Doljanski L, Roulet FR (1934) Uber die gestaltende Wechselwirkung zwischen dem Epithel und dem Mesenchyme, Zugleich ein Beitrag zur Histogenese der sogenannten "Gallengang swucherungen". Virchows Arch A Pathol Anat Histopathol 292: 256

Dubin IN, Johnson FB (1954) Chronic idiopathic jaundice with unidentified pigment in liver cells. Medicine 33: 155

Dupuy JM, Frommmel D, Alagille D (1975) Severe viral hepatitis type B in infancy. Lancet i: 191

Fellows IW, Lowe JS, Ogilvie AL, Stevens A, Toghill PJ,

Atkinson M (1983) Type III glycogenosis presenting as liver disease in adults with atypical histological features. J Clin Pathol 36: 431

Fienberg R (1960) Perinatal idiopathic hemochromatosis: giant cell hepatitis interpreted as an inborn error of metabolism. Am J Clin Pathol 33: 480

Galdeano S, Drut R (1991) Nodular regenerative hyperplasia of fetal liver: a report of two cases. Pediatr Pathol 11: 479

Gall JAM, Bathal PS (1990) Development of intrahepatic bile ducts in rat foetal liver explants in vitro. J Exp Pathol 71: 41

Gilbert A, Lereboullet P (1901) La cholémie simple familiale. Sein Med (Paris) 21: 241

Glasgow JFT, Hercz A, Levison H, Lynch MJ, Sass-Kortsak A (1971) α_1-Antitrypsin (AT) deficiency with both cirrhosis and chronic obstructive lung disease in two sibs. Pediatr Res 5: 427

Goldberg SJ, Fonkalsrud E (1969) Successful treatment of hepatic hemangioma with corticosteroids. JAMA 208: 2473

Goodman SI, Stene DO, McCabe ERB, Norenberg MD, Shikes RH, Stumpf DA, Blackburn GK (1982) Glutaric acidemia type II: clinical, biochemical and morphologic considerations. J Pediatr 100: 946

Hamilton WJ, Boyd JD, Mossman HW (1972) Human embryology. Heffer, Cambridge, p 342

Harries JT (ed) (1977) Essentials of paediatric gastroenterology. Churchill Livingstone, Edinburgh, p 327

Harris RC, Anderson DH (1960) Intrahepatic bile duct atresia. Paper presented at the Annual Meeting of the American Pediatric Society, 5 May 1960

Hilberg F, Aguzzi A, Howells N, Wagner EF (1993) c-Jun is essential for normal mouse development and hepatogenesis. Nature 365; 179

Hope PL, Hall MA, Millward-Sadler GH, Normand ICS (1982) α_1-antitrypsin deficiency presenting as a bleeding diathesis in the newborn. Arch Dis Child 57: 68

Houssaint E (1980) Differentiation of the mouse hepatic primordium. 1. An analysis of tissue interactions in hepatocyte differentiation. Cell Differ 9; 269

Howard ER, Mowat AP (1977) Extrahepatic biliary atresia: recent developments in management. Arch Dis Child 52: 825

Howard ER, Johnston DI, Mowat AP (1976) Spontaneous perforation of common bile duct in infants. Arch Dis Child 51: 883

Howell RR, Stevenson RE, Philiky RL, Berry DH (1976) Hepatic adenomata in patients with type I glycogen storage disease (Von Gierke's). J Am Med Assoc 236: 1481

Hurwitz ES, Barrett MJ, Bregman D, Gunn WJ, Schonberger CB, Fairweather WR, Drage JS, La Montaigne JR, Kaslow RA, Burlington DB, Winnan GV, Parker RA, Phillips K, Pinsky P, Dayton D, Dowle WR (1985) Public Health Service study on Reye's syndrome and medications: report of the pilot phase. N Engl J Med 313: 849

Ito J, Johnson WW (1969) Hepatoblastoma and hepatoma in infancy and childhood. Light and electron microscopic studies. Arch Pathol Lab Med 87: 259

Ivemark BI (1955) Implications of the agenesis of the spleen on pathogenesis of cono-truncal anomalies in childhood. Acta Paediatr Scand 44 [Suppl 104]: 1

Ivemark B, Oldfelt V, Zetterstrom R (1959) Familial dysplasia of kidneys, liver, and pancreas: a probably genetically determined syndrome. Acta Paediatr 48: 1

Jaffe R, Konery B, Kunz R, Esquivel CO, Starzl TE (1987) The pathology of adenovirus hepatitis in paediatric liver transplantation. Society for Paediatric Pathology abstract. Lab Invest 56: 3P

Johnson AM, Alper CA (1970) Deficiency in childhood liver disease. Pediatrics 46: 921

Jorgensen M (1971) A case of abnormal intrahepatic bile duct arrangement submitted to three-dimensional reconstruction. Acta Pathol Microbiol Scand [A] 79: 303

Jorgensen M (1972) Three-dimensional reconstruction of intrahepatic bile ducts in a case of polycystic disease of the liver in an infant. Acta Pathol Microbiol Scand [A] 80: 201

Kasai M, Watanabe J, Ohi R (1972) Follow-up studies of long-term survivors after hepatic portoenterostomy for "non-correctable", biliary atresia. J Pediatr Surg 10: 173

Kato T, Hebiguchi T, Kassai M (1980) Etiology of congenital choledochal cyst. Tohoku J Exp Med 141: 135

Keeling JW (1971) Liver tumours in infancy and childhood. J Pathol 103: 69

Kerr DNS, Harrison CV, Sherlock S, Milnes Walker R (1961) Congenital hepatic fibrosis. Quart J Med 30: 91

Klass HJ, Kelly JK, Warnes TW (1980) Indian childhood cirrhosis in the United Kingdom. Gut 21: 344

Landing BH (1974) Considerations of the pathogenesis of neonatal hepatitis, biliary atresia and choledochal cysts: the conception of infantile obstructive cholangiopathy. Prog Paediatr Surg 6: 113

Landing BH, Wells TR, Claireaux AE (1980) Morphometric analysis of liver lesions in cystic disease of childhood. Hum Pathol 2: Suppl 549

Lathe GH (1974) Newborn jaundice: bile pigment metabolism in the fetus and newborn infant. In: Davis GA, Dobbing J (eds) Scientific foundation of paediatrics. Heinemann, London, p 105

Laurell CB, Eriksson S (1963) The electrophoretic α_1-globulin pattern of serum in α_1-antitrypsin deficiency. Scand J Clin Lab Invest 15: 132

Leading article (1969) Br Med J ii: 204

Lee SS, Min PC, Kim GS, Hong PW (1969) Choledochal cyst. A report of nine cases and review of the literature. Arch Surg 99: 19

Lichtenstein PK, Heubi DE, Daugherty CC, Farrell MK, Sokol RJ, Rothbaum R, Suchy FJ, Balistreri WF (1983) Grade I Reye's syndrome. A frequent cause of vomiting and liver dysfuntion after varicella and upper respiratory tract infection. N Engl J Med 309: 133

Lieberman E, Salinas-Madrigal L, Gwinn JL, Brennan LP, Fine RN, Landing BH (1971) Infantile polycystic disease of the kidneys and liver. Medicine 50: 277

Linderkamp O, Hopner F, Klose H, Riegel KC, Hecker W (1976) Solitary hepatic hemangioma in a newborn infant complicated by cardiac failure, consumption coagulopathy, microangiopathic hemolytic anemia, and obstructive jaundice. Eur J Pediatr 124: 23

Lorimer AR, McGee J, McAlpine SG (1967) Congenital hepatic fibrosis. Postgrad Med J 43: 770

Manolaki AG, Larcher VF, Mowat AP, Barrett JJ, Portmann B, Howard ER (1983) The prelaparotomy diagnosis of extrahepatic biliary atresia. Arch Dis Child 58: 591

Masera G, Jean G, Conter V, Terzoli S, Mauri RA, Cazzaniga M (1980) Sequential study of liver biopsy in thalassaemia. Arch Dis Child 55: 800

Misugi K, Reinger CB (1965) A malignant true teratoma of liver in childhood. Arch Pathol 80: 409

Misugi K, Okajima H, Misugi N, Newton WA Jr (1967) Classification of primary malignant tumours of liver in infancy and childhood. Cancer 20: 1760

Montgomery AH (1940) Solitary nonparasitic cysts of the liver in children. Arch Surg 41: 422

Morse JO (1978a) α_1-Antitrypsin deficiency. I. N Engl J Med 299: 1045

Morse JO (1978b) α_1-Antitrypsin deficiency. II. N Engl J Med 299: 1099

Moser AE, Singh I, Brown FR et al. (1984) The cerebrohepatorenal (Zellweger) syndrome. Increased levels and impaired degradation of very-long-chain fatty acids and their use in prenatal diagnosis. N Eng J Med 310: 1141

Mowat AP, Psacharopoulos HT, Williams R (1976) Extrahepatic

biliary atresia versus neonatal hepatitis. Review of 137 prospectively investigated infants. Arch Dis Child 51: 763

Naginton J, Wreghitt TG, Gandy G, Robertson NCR, Berry PJ (1978) Fatal echovirus II infections in outbreak in a special care baby unit. Lancet ii: 725

Nayak NC, Sagreiya K, Ramalingaswami V (1969) Indian childhood cirrhosis. Arch Pathol 88: 631

Opitz JM, Howe JJ (1969) The Meckel syndrome (dysencephalia splanchnocystica, the Gruber Syndrome). Birth Defects 5: 167

Oppenheimer EH, Esterly JR (1975) Hepatic changes in young infants with cystic fibrosis: possible relation to focal biliary cirrhosis. J Pediatr 5: 683

Parker RGF (1956) Fibrosis of the liver as congenital anomaly. J Pathol 71: 359

Peden VH, Witgleben CL, Skelton MA (1971) Total parenteral nutrition. J Pediatr 78: 180

Powell CS, Sawyers JL, Reynolds VH (1981) Management of adult choledochal cysts. Ann Surg 193: 666

Psacharopoulos HT, Mowat AP, Cook PJL, Carlile PA, Portman B, Rodeck CH (1983) Outcome of liver disease associated with α_1-antitrypsin deficiency (PiZ). Implications for genetic counselling and antenatal diagnosis. Arch Dis Child 58: 882

Remmington PL, Rowley D, McGee H, Hall NN, Monto AS (1986) Decreasing trends in Reye's syndrome and aspirin use in Michigan 1979 to 1984. Pediatrics 77: 93

Rennebohm RM, Heubi JE, Dougherty CC, Daniels SR (1985) Reye's syndrome in children receiving salicylate therapy for connective tissue disease. J Pediatr 107: 877

Reye RDK, Morgan G, Baral J (1963) Encephalopathy and fatty degeneration of the viscera: a disease entity in children. Lancet ii: 749

Risdon RA, Barry M, Flynn DM (1975) Transfusional iron overload: the relationship between tissue iron concentration and hepatic fibrosis in thalassaemia. J Pathol 116: 83

Roberts PL (1985) PiZZ α-antitrypsin deficiency in a 20 week fetus. Hum Pathol 16: 188

Rosenthal IM, Spellberg MA, McGrew EA, Rozenfeld IH (1961) Absence of interlobular bile ducts. Report of a case of probable intrahepatic bile duct agenesis with severe hypercholesterolemia, xanthomatosis, and glomerular lipid deposition. Am J Dis Child 101: 228

Rotor AB, Manahan L, Florentin A (1948) Familial non-hemolytic jaundice with direct van der Bergh reaction. Acta Med Philippina 5: 37

Rushton DI (1987) Liver and gallbladder. In: Keeling JW (ed) Fetal and neonatal pathology. Springer, Berlin, p 340

Sass-Kortsak A, Bowden DH, Brown RJK (1956) Congenital intrahepatic biliary atresia. Pediatrics 17: 383

Schullinger JN, Wigger HJ, Price JB, Benson M, Harris RC (1983) Epidermoid cysts of the liver. J Pediatr Surg 18: 240

Sharp H, Freier E, Bridges R (1968) α_1-globulin deficiency in a familial infant liver disease. Pediatr Res 2: 298

Sparkman RS (1954) Hepatic rupture: report of 8 cases with survival. Am Surg 139: 690

Spitz L (1978) Choledochal cyst. Surg Gynecol Obstet 144: 444

Stanley CA, Hale DE, Coates PM (1983) Medium chain acyl CoA dehydrogenase deficiency in children with non-ketotic hypoglycemia and low carnitine levels. Pediatr Res 17: 877

Stanley RJ, Dehner LP, Hesker AE (1973) Primary malignant mesenchymal tumours (mesenchymoma) of the liver in childhood. Cancer 32: 973

Stocker TJ, Ishak KG (1981) Focal nodular hyperplasia of the liver: a study of 21 pediatric cases. Cancer 48: 336

Syderman SE (1981) Clinical aspects of disorders of the urea cycle. Pediatrics 68: 284

Talbot IC, Mowat AP (1975) Liver disease in infancy: histological features and relationship to α_1-antitrypsin phenotype. J Clin Pathol 28: 559

Tobin JO'H, Macdonald H, Brachey M, Macauley D (1975) Cytomegalovirus infection and exchange transfusion. Br Med J iv: 404

Valman HB, France NE, Wallis PG (1971) Prolonged neonatal jaundice in cystic fibrosis. Arch Dis Child 46: 805

Walshe JM (1962) Wilson's disease: the presenting symptoms. Arch Dis Child 37: 253

Waterlow JC (1948) Fatty liver disease in infants in the British West Indies. HMSO, London (Medical Research Council special report series, no. 263)

Weichsel ME, Luggatti L (1965) Trisomy 17–18 syndrome with congenital extrahepatic biliary and congenital amputation of the left foot. J Pediatr 67: 324

Whitington PF, Black DD (1980) Cholelithiasis in premature infants treated with parenteral nutrition and furosemide. J Pediatr 97: 647

Witzleben CL, Sharp AR (1982) "Nephronophthisis–congenital hepatic fibrosis": an additional hepatorenal disorder. Hum Pathol 13: 728

Woo D, Cummins M, Davies PA, Harvey DR, Hurley R, Waterson AP (1979) Vertical transmission of hepatitis B surface antigen in carrier mothers in two west London hospitals. Arch Dis Child 54: 670

Wright R, Perkins JR, Bower BD, Jerrome DW (1970) Cirrhosis associated with the Australia antigen in an infant who acquired hepatitis from her mother. Br Med J iv: 719

Yandza T, Valuyer J (1986) Benign tumours of the liver in children: analysis of a series of 20 cases. J Pediatr Surg 21: 419

Yarborough SM, Evashnick G (1956) Case of teratoma of the liver with 14 years post-operative survival. Cancer 9: 848

7 · Respiratory System

Jerry N. Cox

Development and Structure

Our knowledge of the development of the respiratory system has unfolded rapidly in recent years following the application of modern techniques in molecular biology and genetics. Some of these, together with highly specific immunocytochemistry, are now readily applied to material obtained for diagnostic purposes, with great practical medical benefit.

The respiratory system comprises the nose, nasopharynx, larynx, trachea, bronchi and lungs. In considering the pathology, it can be divided into two parts: the upper respiratory system, comprising the nose, nasopharynx, larynx and trachea; and the lower respiratory system, comprising the bronchi and lungs.

Face and Nasopharynx

The development of the face and nasopharynx is dealt with on pp. 210–214.

Larynx

Between the 3rd and 4th weeks of gestation (about 3 mm) the respiratory primordia, including the tracheobronchial groove, make their appearance caudal to the hypobronchial eminence. At the end of the 4th week the epithelial component of the larynx develops rapidly with the appearance of the hypopharyngeal eminences on either side, indicating the site of the right and left arytenoid swellings, forming the primitive laryngeal aditus.

Towards the end of the 5th week and during the 6th week, the *epiglottis* makes its appearance as a midventral prominence at the base of the third and fourth arches, cephalic to the glottis. The arytenoid swellings continue to grow towards the base of the tongue, enfolding the epiglottis during the process. At this stage of development, actively proliferating epithelium temporarily obliterates the entrance to the larynx. In the ensuing weeks, the growth of the larynx proceeds rapidly, and the lumen is re-established. However, the entrance becomes ovoid, and there is a persistent interarytenoid notch in the sagittal plane. By the 10th week, the essential elements of the larynx are established, and the vocal cords appear on either side of the laryngeal lumen.

The larynx now grows much more slowly, and it is not until the last trimester of intrauterine life that it attains its definitive form, but it remains high in the neck. The laryngeal cartilages make their appearance at about the 10th week from the 4th and 6th pairs of the brancheal arches.

Trachea

The tracheobronchial groove appears early during the 4th week of gestation. At this stage, it has a blunted caudal end but an extensive communication with the ventrocaudal part of the pharynx. The future trachea, represented by the distal portion of the groove, lies ventral to and parallel with the oesophagus from which it is separated by the tracheo-oesophageal septum. The blunted end forms the *primary bronchial (lung) buds*. Tracheo-oesophageal separation occurs during the 4th and 5th weeks.

The endodermal outgrowth from the pharynx gives rise to the epithelial lining and glands of the trachea; the cartilage, muscle and connective tissue investing the organ are derived from the surrounding mesenchyme.

Cartilage rings are identifiable during the 10th week. The epithelial glands are not apparent until about the 4th month, and during subsequent weeks they assume their final characteristics. By the 5th month, the main anatomical features of the trachea are established.

Lungs

The *pulmonary primordia* or *lung buds* appear towards the end of the 3rd and beginning of the 4th week of gestation at the caudal end of the tracheo-bronchial groove. They are generally asymmetrical, inclining to the right, and made up of two lobes, a large right and a smaller left lobe, separated by a shallow sulcus. During the following weeks and up to the 7th week, by a series of monopidial and irregular dichotomous branchings, the principal bronchi appear, establishing the basic organization of the mature lung into lobar and segmental units. At this stage there are ten principal branches on the right and eight on the left. Between the 10th and 14th weeks, there is active division and ramification of the bronchi, producing about 70% of the bronchial generations. By the 16th week, the bronchial tree is fully developed and the lung has a glandular appearance. Capillaries rapidly penetrate the epithelium, and the glandular appearance becomes canalicular. The number of bronchial generations is now complete and is actually in excess of the final number found in adults; by a process of alveolarization some of the non-respiratory bronchioles are transformed into respiratory bronchioles, finally leaving some 27 generations.

In experimental animals many growth factors and cytokines have been shown to play an essential role in growth, differentiation and maturation of various organs, including the lower respiratory system. In the human fetus, as in various animal species, *epidermal growth factor*, a growth-promoting polypeptide, seems to be among the principal polypeptides in stimulating epithelial proliferation, differentiation and/or chloride and fluid exchange of the developing airway which finally leads to maturation. Its action is through the activation of *epidermal growth factor receptors*, which are already present on the epithelium of the conducting airways during the first trimester (12–13 weeks) of gestation. Activation of these receptors catalyses phosphorylation of many intracellar substances, chief among them *lipocortin–1*, which has many actions (such as binding of calcium, acidic phospholipids and actin filaments), but inhibits phospholipase A2 activity, which may affect local prostaglandin synthesis. *Transforming growth factor* α, which also appears early during the first trimester of gestation, may function as the predominant ligand for epidermal growth factor receptor during early fetal lung development. *Insulin-like growth factors I and II*, regulatory peptides which are present early in the fetal lung during development, also play an important role in the control of cell proliferation, differentiation and exchange between the cell surface and extracellular fluids. Through the specific *insulin growth factor binding proteins*, by various complex mechanisms, they are involved in the regulation of cell growth, as well as the control of response to substances or factors that may alter lung growth, differentiation and proliferation. These various elements, controlled by specific genes, may have a paracrine/autocrine effect on the normal developing lung. The cell adhesive glycoprotein, *fibronectin*, a promotor of cell migration and differentiation during early lung development, may also be under the control of these growth factors. The entire process from the beginning is constantly under the genetic control of a programmed sequence of events during lung development. Certain gene(s) regulate the positional identity of the organ in early embryogenesis, while others control the various phases of proliferation and differentiation (pseudoglandular, canalicular and saccular) by way of the epithelial–mesenchymal interactions and cell–cell contacts through specific cellular receptors.

The bronchial tree is now represented by the two main bronchi; these are subdivided into lobar bronchi, segmental bronchi, lobular bronchi and alveolar ducts. The first 19 of these form the conducting airway, whose main role is to convey air to and from the lungs, and which do not take part in gas exchange. The first seven divisions are cartilaginous in type; the remaining twelve are membranous non-respiratory bronchioles and terminal bronchioles. The following four (generations 20–23) are respiratory bronchioles and, like the remaining four (generations 24–27), which form the alveolar ducts, participate in gas exchange.

At birth, the respiratory unit is the primitive alveolus or "saccule", of which there are about 25 million; further development continues, increasing in rate at about 2 months after birth, resulting in the maximum number of alveoli (about 300 million) at the age of 8 years (see pp. 14–18 for illustrations). The results of recent studies suggest that alveolar formation begins in utero by the 30th week of gestation; however, alveolar formation remains principally a postnatal event. Thus, from these data, five stages of intrauterine lung development have been proposed:

1. *Embryonic*, 26th day to 6th week
2. *Pseudoglandular*, 6th to 16th week
3. *Canalicular*, 17th to 28th week

4. *Saccular*, 28th to 36th week
5. *Alveolar*, after the 36th week

The postnatal period can be divided into two phases: birth to the 18th month, during which there are major shifts in the volumetric proportions of the parenchymal compartments, more intense during the first 6 months of life; and from 18 months to adulthood, when there is proportionate growth of all components in a linear fashion. Epithelial keratin expression in the developing lung may be of value in better defining the various stages of lung development and maturity.

As the pulmonary primordia appear, and subsequently divide and proliferate, the bronchi invade the mass of mesenchymal tissue along the midline and thus create the future mediastinum. Growth continues into the developing pleural cavities, and eventually the surface becomes covered by mesothelial cells which are continuous with those of the pleura.

The mesenchymal tissues encircling the bronchi give rise to the cartilaginous elements, smooth muscle layers, and the supporting connective tissue. This connective tissue becomes very scanty as one approaches the periphery of the bronchial tree. The cartilaginous elements make their appearance about the 7th week, and are fully established by the 25th week. Discountinuous elastin microfibrils first appear around primitive bronchioles at about week 10 of gestation and at about week 20 they can also be observed at the primordium of secondary crests as amorphous material. By week 28 they make their appearance in the saccular walls as thin bundles and are more prominent around the terminal bronchioles. At term, they are present in the primitive alveolar septae.

Mucus-secreting structures are recognizable by the 13th week of intrauterine life, when goblet cells are observed in the epithelium of the trachea and the proximal and intrasegmental bronchi. They seem to grow most rapidly between weeks 14 and 28; at birth they are not found distal to the bronchi. Recently, it has been shown that human bronchi express, like other mucus-secreting organs, a single or two closely related mucin genes, which may be useful in the regulation of mucin gene expression in certain disease states.

The blood supply to the respiratory primordium appears at about week 5 (5 mm) as a capillary network arising from the sixth arch. These vessels take up position next to the branches of the bronchial system, and remain interrelated throughout development. These are the pulmonary artery branches, which are referred to as conventional branches. Besides these arteries, there are additional vessels – supernumerary or accessory arteries – which appear

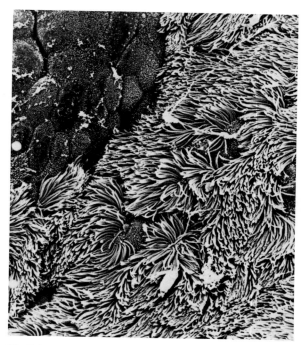

Fig. 7.1. Scanning electron micrograph showing cilia of bronchiolar epithelial surface. Clara cell surface, upper left-hand corner. (× 2500) (Courtesy of Dr Y. Kapanci)

about the 12th week and arise from the hilus. Both systems are complete by the 16th week. Vascular growth and proliferation are under a variety of external factors which may stimulate the growth of vascular endothelial cells. Signals mediated by polypeptide growth factors and physical interactions may take their origin from the endothelial cells themselves in conjunction with specific cell surface molecules.

The blood supply to the developing lungs drains into a venous plexus, forming a single pulmonary vein that empties into the heart. This vein finally becomes incorporated into the future left atrium, and its main branches on each side form the superior and inferior pulmonary veins.

The pseudostratified columnar epithelium of the large airways is made up of various types of cell. The most common is the ciliated cell, which continues into the respiratory bronchioles, where it is somewhat flatter or cuboidal. These cells are covered by cilia (Fig. 7.1), which are partly anchored by dynein arms and contractile elements to the apical portion of the cell (Fig. 7.2). Contractile elements are also present within cilia. Ciliary movements play an important role in the defence mechanism of the respiratory system, and its absence is associated with certain disease entities.

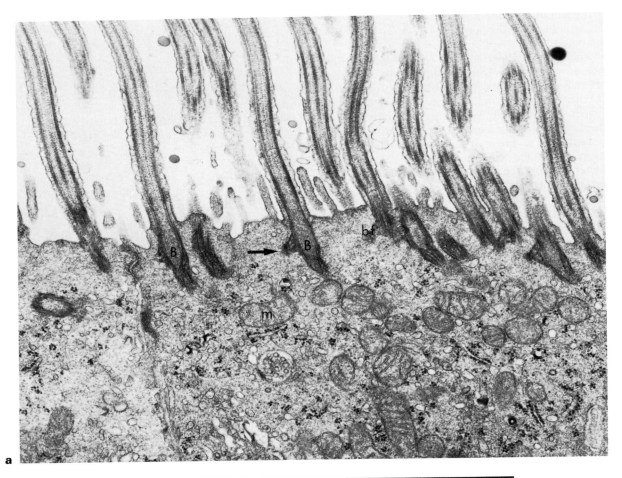

a

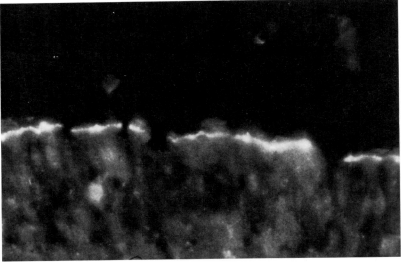

b

Fig. 7.2. a Electron micrograph showing basal bodies (*B*) and basal feet (*bf*) of cilia. Microfilaments and microtubules (*arrow*) can be seen radiating from the basal feet. Mitochondria (*m*) are also present. **b** Immunofluorescent staining of human bronchial epithelium with AAA serum showing a subciliary fluorescent band of actin. (× 400) (Courtesy of Dr Y. Kapanci)

Between isolated or small groups of ciliated cells are the goblet cells, which empty their secretion on the epithelial surface. Against the basal membrane and between the basal portions of the two previous cell types mentioned are the basal cells, which are reserve cells capable of replacing either the ciliated or the goblet cells as necessary.

Three other cell types are also encountered within the respiratory epithelium throughout the tracheobronchial tree. The first is the *Kulchitsky-like* (argyrophil) *cell*, which may occur singly or in groups of two or three. These cells are more prevalent in fetuses and newborns than in the adult, are more commonly referred to as *neuroendocrine cells*, and form part of the dispersed neuroendocrine (APUD) system.

Cell clusters of similar cells are better known as *neuroendocrine bodies*, and together they form the pulmonary neuroendocrine system exerting local paracrine influence by way of synaptic (neurocrine) controls with possible complex responses to nervous influences (Fig. 7.3). They first appear between the 8th and 10th weeks of gestation and attain their maximum density just before term. They contain secretory granules containing monoamines and/or serotonin as well as bombesin, calcitonin and leuenkephalin, the latter mainly within the neuroendocrine cells. They have a sensory innervation with both afferent and efferent terminals. Although their role is not clearly understood, they seem to react as chemoreceptors in response to hypoxia, hyperoxia and hypercapnia therefore regulating ventilation–perfusion ratios in the lung by action on the bronchiolar or bronchial smooth muscle. These cells are considered to be precursors of bronchial carcinoids and have been associated with oat-cell carcinomas.

Clara cells are the second type and are found in greater numbers in the bronchioles. They are non-ciliated dome-shaped cells containing granules (Fig. 7.4). Recent studies have shown that these cells synthesize, stock and secrete proteinaceous substances identical to those of type II epithelial cells and thus may contribute to the surfactant layer. They also act as stem cells in the process of bronchiolar repair.

The third type is the *brush cell* (type III cell), characterized by its pronounced microvillous covering. This cell type, though rare, has been described at all levels of the airway including the acinus. Its precise function is unknown.

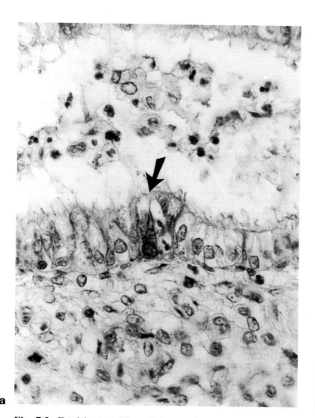
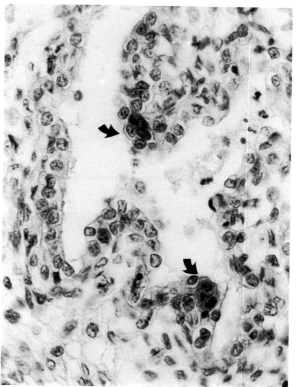

Fig. 7.3. Fetal lung at 32 weeks' gestation. **a** Neuroendocrine cell (*arrow*). (Grimelius, × 600) **b** Neuroepithelial body stained for bombesin (*arrow continued overleaf*).

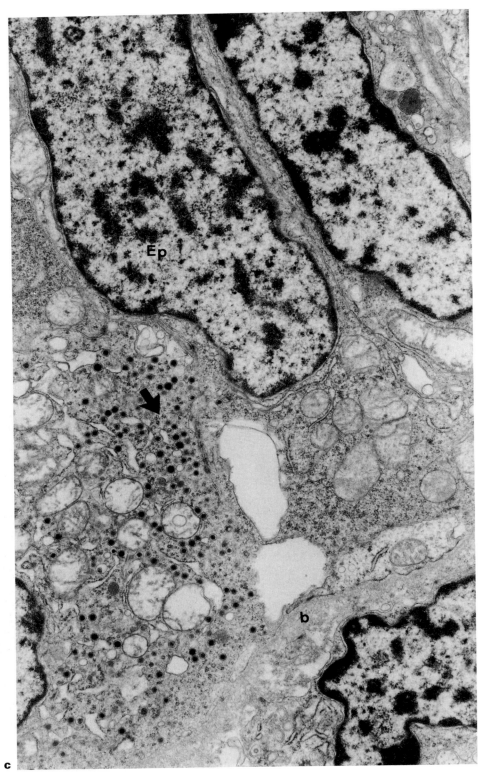

Fig. 7.3. (continued). **c** Electron micrograph (× 600) of a neuroendocrine cell (*bottom left*) showing numerous spherical granules (*arrow*) of variable densities. *Ep*, epithelial cell; *b*, basement membrane. (TEM, × 21 716)

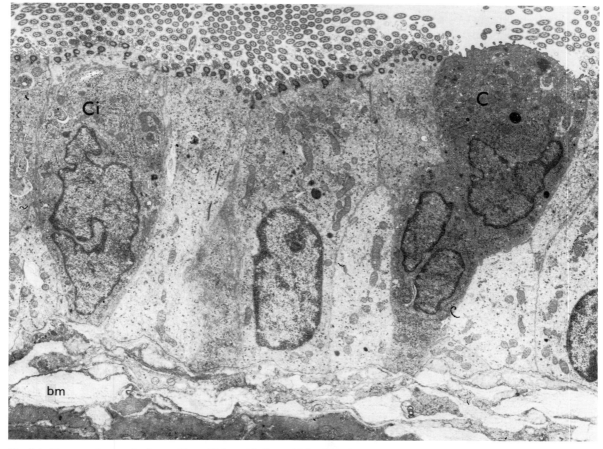

Fig. 7.4. Electron micrograph of normal bronchiolar epithelium with its ciliated cells (*Ci*) and a Clara cell (*C*) on the right. Note the basal membrane (*bm*). (× 6300) (Courtesy of Dr Y. Kapanci)

At this point, it is necessary to describe briefly the terminal respiratory unit and the interalveolar septum. The terminal respiratory unit consists of the structures that are distal to the terminal bronchiole. Each terminal bronchiole gives off two to five orders of respiratory bronchiole. The last respiratory bronchiole leads into the first alveolar ducts, which vary in number between two and five. Each alveolar duct opens into as many as 10–16 alveoli. The aveoli are separated by an interalveolar septum made up of three parts: the alveolar epithelium, capillary and interstitial tissue.

Alveolar epithelium is made up of two cell types. Type I cells or squamous pneumocytes have a broad thin cytoplasmic sheet and nuclei that often protrude above the epithelial surface. These cells cover about 90% of the alveolar surface. Type II cells, or granular pneumocytes, are more numerous than type I cells, but because of their configuration – round or cuboidal – they occupy only about 5% of the alveolar surface.

They are characterized by surface microvilli and the presence of cytoplasmic osmiophilic lamellar bodies, suggesting a secretory function. These bodies, which appear in the cells at about the 25th week of gestation, are associated with the production of surface-active material (surfactant), a substance that plays an important role in lung expression. Type II pneumocytes are also considered to play an important role in epithelial regeneration. Both cell types are attached to a continuous basement membrane.

The alveolar septa are provided with a single capillary network. The capillary has a basement membrane, which is covered by a single layer of endothelial cells; pericytes are present in the capillary wall (Fig. 7.5).

The interstitial tissue contains some collagen and elastic fibres, among which are found contractile interstitial cells or myofibroblasts. There are also some macrophages in varying numbers within the interstitium (see General References).

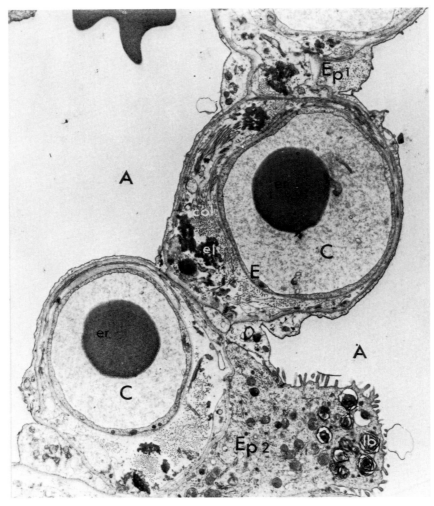

Fig. 7.5. Electron micrograph of human alveolar septum. The alveolar spaces (*A*) are lined with type I (*Ep 1*) and type II (*Ep 2*) epithelial cells, the latter containing lamellated bodies (*lb*). Capillaries (*C*) contain erythrocytes (*er*) and are lined with endothelial cells (*E*). Collagen fibres (*col*) and elastic fibres (*el*) are conspicuous. (× 5700) (Courtesy of Dr Y. Kapanci)

Nose and Nasopharynx

Congenital Abnormalities of the Nose

Illustrations of various malformations of the nose have been documented by Patten (1968) and Potter (1962) (Fig. 7.6). *Congenital absence* of the nose and anterior nasopharynx is a rare condition. Gifford et al. (1972) described two cases and reviewed the literature on the subject. In *cyclopia*, another rare condition, in which there is fusion of the eyes, there is a proboscis-like cylindrical fleshy mass hanging from the nasal region or the forehead in place of the nose. Sometimes this bears a single central orifice repre-

senting a nostril, but in other instances there is no external opening. In most cases there is no communication with the nasopharynx (Landing 1957; Potter 1962). Rontal and Duritz (1977) described a case in which a lateral proboscis replaced one of the nostrils. Cyclops have also been described in association with chromosomal abnormalities, and principally with trisomies (Arakaki and Waxman 1969). In a somewhat milder form of cyclopia, *cebocephaly*, there is hypoplasia of the maxillary bones and nose associated with a lissencephalic brain with fusion of the cerebral hemispheres and internal hydrocephaly. *Frontonasal dysplasia*, another relatively rare condition, may or may not be associated with cleft lip and cleft palate. The condition appears to be a developmental defect not necessarily related to chromosomal

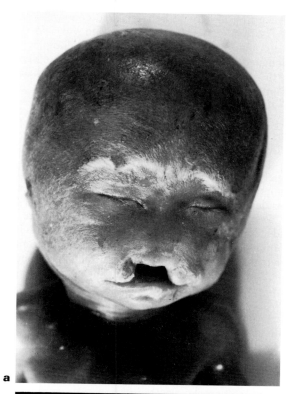

a

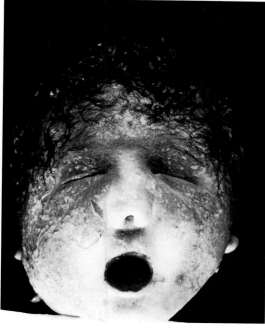

b

Fig. 7.6. a Absence of the nose of a polymalformed female fetus of 22 weeks' gestation with trisomy 13. **b** Male fetus of 36 weeks' gestation with malformed nose and a central dimple but no nasal openings.

abnormalities (Sedano et al. 1970). *Aplasia* (hypoplasia) of the alae nasi is rare and often associated with other abnormalities, including deafness and abnormal endocrine function (Johanson and Blizzard 1971) and cardiac anomalies with situs inversus and severe hypoproteinaemia (Helin and Jodal 1981). *Craniofrontonasal dysplasia* (craniosynostosis, ocular hypertelorism, broad nasal root, with a bifid nasal tip or median nasal groove) is another rare syndrome which does not seem to follow a Mendelian mode of inheritance (Sax and Flannery 1986). Cleft lip and palate are discussed on pp. 51).

Choanal atresia can be divided into two main types. Anterior atresias are found when the epithelial plugs between the developing medial and lateral nasal placodes are not absorbed in the embryo. Posterior (choanal) atresia, by far the most common form although still a rare anomaly, is usually situated at the level of the sphenoid, vertical vomer and palatine bones adjacent to the nasopharynx. Choanal atresia is often found in association with certain syndromes or chromosomal abnormalities such as the CHARGE association or the trichorhinophalangeal syndrome type 1 (Langer–Giedion syndrome) (Marchau et al. 1993; Morgan et al. 1993). It is an important cause of neonatal asphyxia; it can be relieved by a simple surgical procedure or by prompt medical management (Winther 1978; Stahl and Jurkiewicz 1985; Ferguson and Neel 1989).

The anomaly occurs as a result of bony overgrowth, an excess of hyperplastic cartilage, or membranous proliferations, or results from combinations of these factors. It is most commonly unilateral, with a right-sided predominance, but may be bilateral, complete or incomplete. It has been known to be inherited as a dominant trait in certain families. Choanal atresia has a female predominance (estimated at 2 : 1), and is often associated with other congenital anomalies, mainly of the cardiovascular system, face and, in rare instances, the kidney (Qazi et al. 1982; Stahl and Jurkiewicz 1985; Ferguson and Neel 1989).

Dermoid cysts of the nose are rare. They may be the cause of a widened nasal septum, septal deviation or duplication (Taylor and Erich 1967; Hoshaw and Walike 1971; Szalay and Bledsoe 1972), and are classified according to location into: *superficial*, found mainly in the perpendicular plate of the ethmoid bone or the quadrangular cartilage; and *deep* or *septal*, found within the columella and the vomer. They may also be observed in Jacobson's organ or the nasopalatine region of the floor of the nose (Pratt 1965; Sing and Pahor 1977). Some communicate with the dermis by a fistulous tract opening in the midline of the nasal bridge or by a small dimple in the skin (MacGregor and Geddes 1993; Cauchois et al. 1994). Macroscopically, they are round or oval,

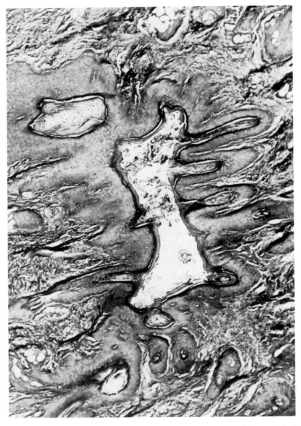

Fig. 7.7. Fistulous tract of nasal dermoid cyst lined with stratified squamous epithelium in an 8-year-old boy. (H&E, × 35)

firm or rubbery masses which, on histological examination, show a cavity lined with stratified squamous epithelium (Fig. 7.7).

Acquired Disease

Nasal deformities in the neonatal period are generally associated with mechanical ventilation and are the direct complications of nasal endotracheal tubes (Gowdar et al. 1980). In infants and children, the majority of acquired pathological conditions are associated with infections or trauma. Chemical irritants or obstructions of the nares by foreign bodies are also important in this age group. In infections, bacterial or virological studies of secretions or scrapings will often indicate the pathogenic agent responsible, but many pathogens (bacterial or viral) can now be detected by the indirect immunofluorescence and/or the enzyme-linked immunosorbent assay (ELISA) technique (Popow-Kraupp et al. 1986). Both tuberculosis and congenital syphilis of the nose have become

rare entities, at least in industrialized countries. The nasal lesions formerly encountered in yaws in the developing countries have been almost completely eliminated; however, leprosy still remains a problem, and the diagnosis can often be established from nasal scrapings (Barton and Davey 1976; Olson et al. 1979).

Hypertrophic or "Hyperplastic" Rhinitis

Hypertrophic or "hyperplastic" rhinitis is a relatively common condition among adolescents, and has been considered to be associated with chronic infection of the nose or the paranasal sinuses. However, there is evidence that it might be related to a hypersensitivity reaction and that hormonal factors may be important. New radiological techniques and especially computed tomography are valuable in arriving at a correct diagnosis (Williams and Williams 1969; Nguyen et al. 1993).

Excised mucosa shows squamous metaplasia of the epithelium together with glandular atrophy. There is marked submucosal oedema with some fibrosis and a varying degree of chronic inflammation.

Rhinoscleroma

Rhinoscleroma is a slowly progressive chronic granulomatous disease often beginning as a bilateral lesion in the nose with nasopharyngeal extension. The larynx and trachea are also often involved. Though endemic in Eastern Europe, Central and South America, Africa and the Far East, it can be encountered in any part of the globe and can affect either sex of any race at any age. There is a slight female preponderance. The condition is encountered most frequently among those living in poor socioeconomic conditions or with impaired immune function. The disease affects the mucous membranes, causing hyperplasia and hypertrophy of the surface epithelium. As it progresses, an atrophic rhinitis develops, with the formation of nodular granulation tissue, which, in most cases, obstructs and destroys the nares.

Histologically, the lesions are divided into three stages, which depend on the clinical phase of the disease. The first is the catarrhal–atrophic stage, in which there is squamous epithelial metaplasia accompanied by a mixed subepithelial inflammatory reaction including polymorphonuclears and some granulation tissue. Second is the granulomatous stage, characterized by a pseudoepitheliomatous hyperplasia and a mixed chronic inflammatory reaction associated with numerous large histiocytes or

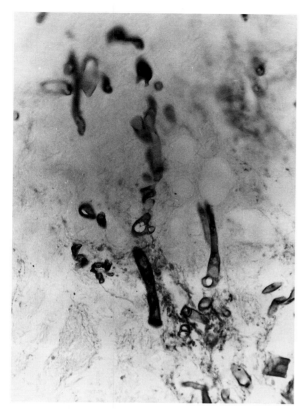

Fig. 7.8. Mucomycosis. The fungus may go unnoticed unless special stains (PAS, Grocott) are employed. (Grocott, × 310) (Courtesy of Dr J. Briner).

foam cells (Mikulicz cells) with a central nucleus and a clear vacuolated cytoplasm. Some of these histiocytes contain several gram-negative encapsulated bacilli (*Klebsiella rhinoscleromatis*), which are considered to be the cause of the disease. The bacilli, although apparent in gram-stained tissue, are distinct in sections stained by silver impregnation techniques or by the periodic acid–Schiff (PAS) stain. Specific immunohistological techniques are useful, and the organisms are readily observed on electron microscopy. Thirdly, there is sclerotic stage, resembling the granulomatous stage, leading to nasal deformity or destruction may ensue with extension into the adjacent structures, including the bony skeleton, and eventually leading to severe disabilities or stenosis in the late fibrotic stages (Andraca et al. 1993).

Mucomycosis by its presentation (a purulent brownish nasal discharge, sometimes with bleeding) may resemble clinically the first stage of rhinoscleroma. However, special stains (PAS, Grocott) will illustrate the fungus (Fig. 7.8). It may be the cause of nasal obstruction, septal nasal perforation or cerebral involvement.

Sinus Histiocytosis with Massive Lymphadenopathy

Sinus histiocytosis with massive lymphadenopathy or Rosai–Dorfman disease is a benign condition that sometimes involves the nasal cavities and paranasal sinuses with extension into the maxillary sinus, retro-orbital space and even the brain. It is usually accompanied by massive lymphadenopathy, principally in the cervical region. The condition has a worldwide distribution, but appears to be more common in developing countries or in patients with an immunodeficiency state or condition and in autoimmune disorders. Although all ages may be affected, there is a predilection for infants and children. Both sexes are about equally involved. Histologically, the tissue crossed by fibrous bands is infiltrated by large histiocytes mixed with lymphocytes and occasional lymphoid aggregates without germinal centres. The histiocytes, isolated, in groups or sheets, have a clear cytoplasm containing a large indented nuclei with a prominent nucleoli (Fig. 7.9). The cytoplasm is PAS positive and stained with S100 protein and occasionally with CDI. Emperipolesis is a common feature, with lymphocytes and plasma cells present in the cytoplasm. These lymphocytes are CD4 and CD8 positive, indicating their T-cell nature. An occasional atypical histiocyte resembling the Reed–Sternberg cell has been described. The aetiology of the condition is unknown, but some authors have incriminated the Epstein–Barr virus, while others favour the association of a dysimmunity state with an inflammatory state (Foucar et al. 1990; Paulli et al. 1992). Involvement of the subglottis and trachea have also been documented in a 17-year-old boy (Leighton and Gallimore 1994).

Lethal Midline Granuloma or Non-healing Midline Granuloma

A mixed group of conditions (inflammatory, neoplastic and vasculitic) have been described under this non-specific title, but using detailed immunohistochemical studies it has been shown that in the majority of cases non-Hodgkin's lymphomas (B- or T-cell types) or malignant histiocytosis is the most frequent underlying pathological condition (Fu and Perzin 1979; Aozasa and Inoue 1982; Ishii et al. 1982; Weis et al. 1986). Fu and Perzin have emphasized the need to take many sections from outside the necrotic area to arrive at a correct diagnosis. However, it is necessary in all cases to exclude the possibility of *Wegener's granuloma*, which often presents clin-

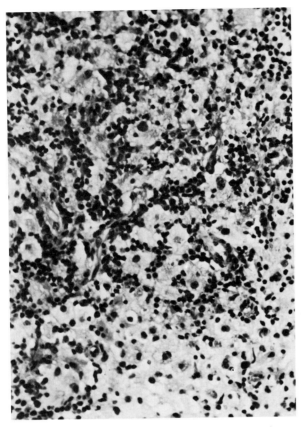

Fig. 7.9. Sinus histiocytosis in a 9-year-old boy, presenting as polypoid nasal masses with extensive involvement of the surrounding tissues and destruction of the adjacent bony structures. (H&E, × 160)

ically in this way. Baliga et al. (1978) collected eight childhood cases of Wegener's granuloma from the literature, and three of these were of the generalized type. Moorthy et al. (1977) were able to collect seven cases of the generalized type and added two of their own. Recently, Nespoli et al. (1979) described another case in a 27-month-old girl, the youngest on record. Histologically, the condition is characterized by angiocentric angiodestructive aseptic necrosis, which likewise involves the kidneys and in many instances the lungs (Crissman et al. 1982).

Tumours

Neoplasms of the nose and nasopharynx in infancy and childhood are rare; however, tumours of the surrounding tissue (brain, meninges, bony skeleton) may protrude into the nasal cavity or nasopharynx, producing symptoms, mainly obstructive.

Nasal Polyps

Nasal polyps are not true neoplasms but are associated with chronic nasal inflammation or repeated allergic reactions within the nasal cavity. They may also be associated with vascular disturbances in the mucosa or be the result of mechanical obstruction. They are frequently encountered in certain systemic diseases, the principal of which is fibrocystic disease of the pancreas (mucoviscidosis) (Berman and Colman 1977). These last authors, among others, have suggested that one should always look for cystic fibrosis in children presenting with nasal polyps. Although their aetiology in this condition is not fully understood, it has been stated to be associated with iodide therapy; however, this has not been supported in all series (Finn et al. 1981; David 1986). Tos et al. (1977) could not find differences between nasal polyps from cases of cystic fibrosis and those of other origins; however, Oppenheimer and Rosenstein (1979) have shown histochemical differences between polyps in cystic fibrosis and those of atopic patients.

Polyposis forms an integral part of *Kartagener's syndrome* (Siewert–Kartagener), a hereditary condition with autosomal recessive inheritance involving different genetic determinants and affecting equally both sexes without racial predisposition. Patients present with situs inversus, chronic bronchitis with bronchiectasis (bilateral), rhinosinusitis, nasal polyposis and chronic recurrent otitis media, with absence or underdevelopment of the frontal sinuses and a high percentage of infertility in males due to spermatozoal immotility. In this syndrome, there is partial or complete lack of ciliary motility of the epithelial cells lining the upper and lower respiratory system and the middle ear as well as the tails of spermatozoa. Ciliary dysfunction is considered to be the cause of the disease, and is due to the absence of, or abnormalities in, the ciliary dynein arms (outer, inner or both) normally rich in ATPase (Fig. 7.10), the radial spokes and an abnormal internal structural arrangement of the microtubular doublets within the cilia. This condition has also been reported in dogs (Afzelius et al. 1984; Pysher and Neustein 1984; Sturgess and Turner 1984; Popper et al. 1985; Eavey et al. 1986; Sturgess et al. 1986). Kartagener's syndrome is now considered to be part of the more general "immotile cilia syndrome", also referred to as the "dyskinetic cilia syndrome" or "ciliary dyskinesis", comprising a heterogeneous group of disorders exhibiting a spectrum of ciliary structural anomalies associated with a range of abnormalities in ciliary motility and defects in the granulocyte locomotory system. There is absence of, or diminished, cilial motility; various structural abnormalities of cilia associated with chronic infec-

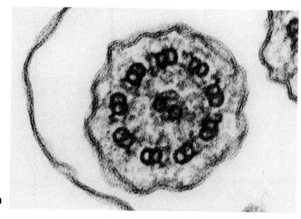

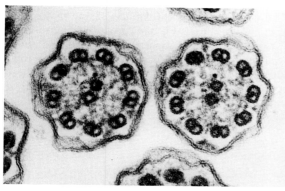

Fig. 7.10. a Normal cilium showing 9 + 2 doublets and presence of all the dynein arms. **b** Case of Kartagener's syndrome showing total absence of all the dynein arms, both inner and outer. (× 82 800)

tion of the upper and lower respiratory system with bronchiectasis; and male infertility, irrespective of situs inversus, associated with headache and some sensory disturbances. Genetic factors may play a role in some of the various ultrastructural variations observed (Eavey et al. 1986; Sturgess et al. 1986; Torikata et al. 1991; Verra et al. 1993; Rayner et al. 1995).

Most nasal polyps arise from the mucosa of the ethmoidal cells at the level of the middle meatus or in the paranasal sinuses. They may be single or multiple, unilateral or bilateral, and either sessile or pedunculated. They are often the source of nasal bleeding or obstruction, and may cause displacement and even destruction of the bones limiting the nasal cavity (Winestock et al. 1978). On gross inspection, they present as smooth round or oval myxomatous masses, yellowish in colour. Histologically there is hypertrophy of the mucous membrane covered by columnar ciliated epithelium, sometimes with squamous metaplasia. The stroma is very loose, fibrillar and oedematous. There is stromal atypia in some cases, which may be falsely interpreted as sarcoma (Compagno et al. 1976). The vessels are dilated, and there are scattered aggregates of lymphocytes and plasma cells with eosinophils (Fig. 7.11). The submucosal glands are generally hyperplastic, but may be atrophic in some areas.

Choanal polyps are a different clinical entity. They generally arise from the mucosa of the maxillary sinuses and project towards the posterior choanae. Their histology is very similar to that of other nasal polyps.

In tropical and subtropical countries, many mycotic infections of the nose in children can present as nasal polyps (Engzell and Jones 1973). Histological examination often reveals granulation tissue, sometimes with granulomas and/or foci of necrosis. Special staining techniques (silver impregnation or PAS) are often necessary for identifying the particular fungus (Fig. 7.11c). Cultures may be necessary in establishing the diagnosis (see Chapter 14, pp. 729).

Epithelial Tumours

Epithelial tumours of the nasal cavity are rare in the paediatric age group. *Papillomas* are occasionally observed in childhood with a marked preponderance for male subjects. The lesions have been known by many synonyms, but currently they are commonly referred to as *inverted papillomas*. In most of the older literature, this term was applied to lesions presenting an inverted growth pattern and situated principally on the lateral walls of the nasal cavity, while those having a fungating exophytic growth pattern and located on the septum were referred to as septal papillomas. The pathological features, clinical presentations and behaviour, apart from their growth pattern, are similar and therefore do not warrant different names. The tumour is usually unilateral, can be localized or diffused, papillary or lobulated, or occasionally pedunculated. Histologically, there is marked proliferation of basal cells, which may partially or completely replace the ciliated cells by a stratified squamous epithelium. This hyperplastic epithelium produces invaginations within the fibrous stroma, and intercellular "microcysts" are not an uncommon feature (Fig. 7.12). Mitotic figures are relatively few and nuclei atypia rare. There are sometimes varying degrees of dyskeratosis and some hyperkeratotic areas. Many of these tumours appear to be histologically benign but are locally aggressive. Clinically they behave as malignant tumours, and aggressive surgery is indicated because inadequate removal is followed by local recurrences and squamous cell carcinoma is known to develop from these lesions. There is increasing evidence that these types of

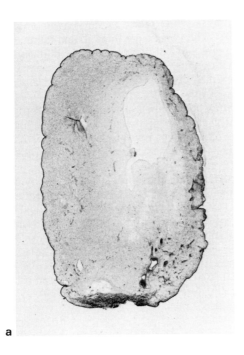

a

lesions may be associated with one or more specific types of human papillomaviruses (Kelly et al. 1980; Perzin et al. 1981; Eavey 1985; de Villiers et al. 1986; Kahn et al. 1986).

Squamous cell carcinoma of the nasal cavity is very rare in childhood. We have observed a case in a 9-year-old boy who presented with a large polypoid necrotic mass obstructing the right nostril and causing extensive destruction of the corresponding maxilla (Fig. 7.13). Carcinoma of the nasopharynx, however, is more prevalent, even though Jaffé (1973a) recorded only three cases in his review of 178 tumours of the head and neck in children.

In childhood *carcinomas of the nasopharynx* are more common in the Far and Middle East, and especially in Africa, where they may represent about 15% of all nasopharyngeal carcinomas. These tumours do occur in other areas but are rare. They cause nasal obstruction, deafness, cranial nerve palsy, and protosis. There is a male predominance and a high incidence of distant metastases. Patients with these tumours have high antibody titres to Epstein–Barr

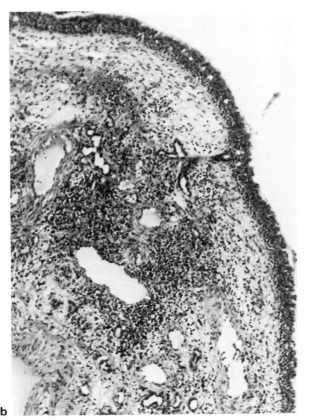

b

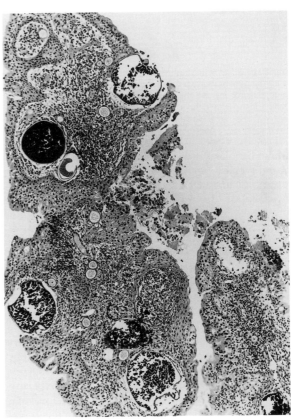

c

Fig. 7.11. a Nasal polyp from a 12-year-old boy with cystic fibrosis. **b** Nasal polyp in a child with chronic sinusitis. **c** Rhinosporidosis in a male patient from Sri Lanka (HCE, × 50) (Courtesy of Dr J. Briner)

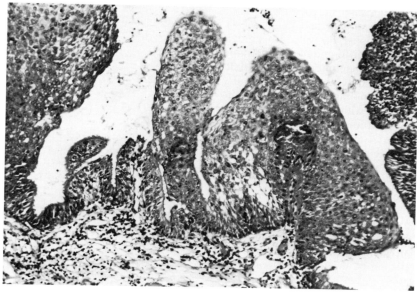

Fig. 7.12. Nasal papilloma in a 14 year-old girl with papillomatosis of the laryngotracheal tree discovered at age 3. Note the numerous "microcysts". (H&E, × 160)

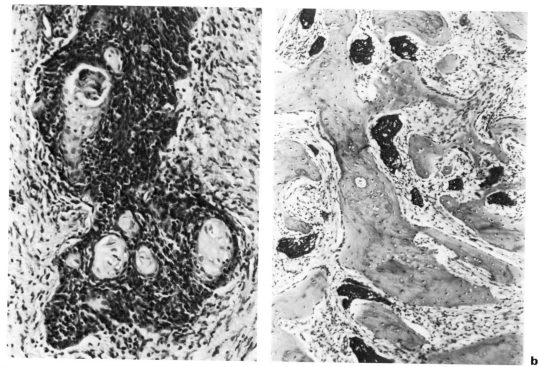

Fig. 7.13. a Squamous-cell carcinoma of the nasal cavity in an 11-year-old boy. (H&E, × 225); **b** Infiltration and destruction of the adjacent bones. (H&E, × 60)

virus, and the virus can also be identified in the tumour and other cells (Niedobitek and Young 1994).

Carcinomas of the nasopharynx vary in histological appearance. The well differentiated epidermoid carcinoma is more often encountered in the adult, whereas in childhood the tumours are generally poorly differentiated, resembling transitional cell carcinoma. The cells are large with an almost inconspicuous cytoplasm, and sometimes they have a syncytial appearance. Their nuclei are quite large, round or oval with prominent nucleoli. Some cases may have the appearance of a lymphoepithelial carcinoma of the *Schmincke–Regaud* type; others may be anaplastic in character (Pick et al. 1974). By the use of antibodies (keratin antibodies, leucocyte common antigen, desmin, myoglobin, etc.), it is now possible to arrive at a precise diagnosis of this often undifferentiated carcinoma (Miettinen et al. 1982; Shi et al. 1984; Ziegels-Weissman et al. 1984; Frierson et al. 1986; Micheau 1986).

Intranasal mixed tumours (*pleomorphic adenomas*) have also been reported in children. The histology is similar to that of pleomorphic tumours of the major salivary glands, but they have a relatively lower rate of recurrence (Compagno and Wong 1977).

The majority of nasopharyngeal tumours (benign or malignant) in childhood are derived from the supporting tissues and from neighbouring structures – for example, the nasopharyngeal papillary adenocarcinoma (Wenig et al. 1988).

Vascular Tumours

Haemangiomas of the nose and nasopharynx are occasionally encountered in infancy and childhood. They can arise anywhere in the nasal cavity but have a predilection for the anterior nasal septum, and are a frequent cause of bleeding. They may present as extremely vascular sessile or pedunculated polyps causing obstruction and are sometimes associated with cutaneous haemangiomas (Strauss et al. 1981) *Benign haemangioendothelioma* has also been described in children. In these highly cellular tumours the capillaries are lined with prominent but uniform endothelial cells (Fu and Perzin 1974a).

Juvenile nasopharyngeal angiofibroma is a rare haemangiomatous tumour occurring principally in adolescent males and is more common in fair-skinned and red-headed individuals. Although benign, it is often locally aggressive and may displace and distort adjacent structures and even erode bone. It occasionally appears before puberty, but grows rapidly during this period and may regress in later years, undergoing hyalinization, fibrosis and or myxomatous changes. These clinical features have suggested hormonal

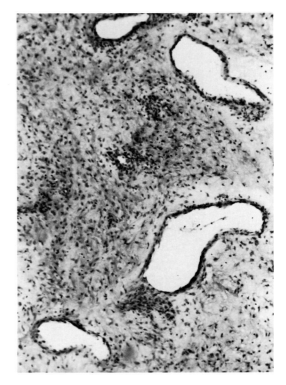

Fig. 7.14. Juvenile nasopharyngeal angiofibroma in a 13-year-old boy. Note the fibrocytic stroma with the stellate cells and the scattered vessels devoid of muscular layers. (H&E, × 160)

dependence, even though the tumour has been reported in adults and in females. Bilateral carotid angiography is one of the most useful diagnostic aids (Conley et al. 1968; Hicks and Nelson 1973; Fu and Perzin 1974a; Sessions et al. 1981).

The pathology of this lesion has been described in detail (Taxy 1977; Arnold and Huth 1978). It generally develops as a solitary, sessile, somewhat lobulated mass in the region of the sphenoethmoidal recess or the choana, from where it may protrude into the nasal cavity, producing obstruction. It can extend into neighbouring structures. Histologically, the angiofibroma is covered by normal nasopharyngeal epithelium and is composed of numerous distended vessels lined with a flattened endothelium in a relatively dense fibrous stroma. The vessel walls are devoid of elastic fibres, and their muscular coats are irregular, incomplete or even absent in smaller vessels, as demonstrated by specific immunohistochemistry. The stroma is fibrocytic in appearance, with a varying amount of collagen fibres but little or no elastic fibres and numerous S100 positive nerve fibres. The stromal cells are myofibroblasts staining positive with Vimentin and smooth muscle actin (Beham et al. 1993) (Fig. 7.14). Taxy (1977) and

Arnold and Huth (1978) have recently described the ultrastructure of these tumours. Angiofibromas create many therapeutic problems due to bleeding, local extension and a high rate of local recurrence (Sessions et al. 1981; Chandler et al. 1984; Jones et al. 1986). Androgen receptors have been demonstrated in these tumours (Lee et al. 1980), suggesting that they may be androgen dependent. Recently, Kumagami (1991) has demonstrated oestradiol in the stromal cells and Schiff et al. (1992) have localized an angiogenic growth factor in the endothelial cells by immunohistochemical techniques. This benign lesion may undergo sarcomatous transformation into a malignant fibrous histiocytoma after irradiation or combined therapy (Spagnolo et al. 1984). Nasopharyngeal angiofibroma must be distinguished from fibromatosis of the region usually encountered in younger children and more so in infancy. The lesion may mimic haemangioma, which must be considered in the differential diagnosis.

Angiofollicular lymph node hyperplasia (Castleman's disease) of the nasopharynx is rare and could easily be mistaken for juvenile nasopharyngeal angiofibroma clinically. The tumour, however, is composed of lymphoid tissue covered by respiratory epithelium. Within this tissue are numerous variably sized germinal centres with hyalinized central zones (Fig. 7.15). The germinal centres are surrounded by concentric rings of lymphocytes (B-cells), and the interfollicular zones are made up mainly of T-lymphocytes. Among these are groups of plasmacytoid monocytes. The tissue is richly vascularized and some of these vessels may have hyalinized walls (Chen and Kuo 1993).

Lymphangioma of the nasal cavity is extremely rare but may sometimes be seen in adolescents and has been reported in infancy (Beneck et al. 1985). It presents as a polypoid mass covered by normal respiratory epithelium; in a fibrous stroma there are numerous dilated lymphatic vessels lined with flattened endothelial cells (Fig. 7.16).

Haemangiopericytoma has also ben recorded in the nasal cavity (Fu and Perzin 1974a). Benveniste and Harris (1973) reviewed the literature and found ten cases, one of which was in a 4-year-old girl. They added one case of their own, which occurred in a newborn. Compagno (1978) has reviewed the subject of haemangiopericytomas of the nasal cavity, and found that although they do occur in childhood they are more common among adults.

Fibrous Tumours

Fibrous tumours are exceedingly rare in children. Fu and Perzin (1976b) did not find any cases of *fibroma*

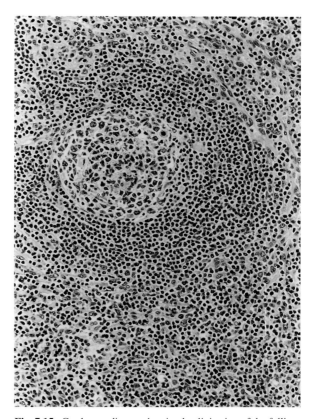

Fig. 7.15. Castleman disease showing hyalinization of the follicular zone surrounded by rows of mononuclear cells in an "onion skin" fashion. (H&E, × 50)(Courtesy of Dr J. Briner)

in the paediatric age group in their material, but observed three cases of *fibromatosis*. Townsend et al. (1973) described a case of what they referred to as a histocytoma in a 3-year-old boy and Rice et al. (1974) recorded a case in a 13-year-old girl. Jaffé (1973a) has reported a case of *malignant histiocytoma* of the nose in an infant. The histological picture usually shows fibroblast-like cells with a histiocytic component presenting a wide range of morphologic changes (Perzin and Fu 1980).

Fibrosarcoma is also very rare. Fu and Perzin (1976b) found only one case below 15 years of age among their 13 patients, and made reference to two others in children (Fig. 7.17).

Muscular Tumours

Smooth-muscle tumours (*leiomyoma* and *leiomyosarcoma*) of the nasal cavity are rare. There were no cases in children in the series of Fu and Perzin (1975). Striated-muscle tumours are more common. Fu and Perzin (1976a) described one case of *rhabdomyoma* and found another in the literature; Canalis

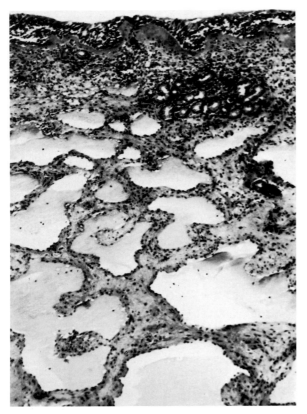

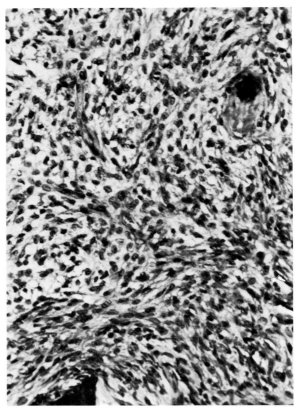

Fig. 7.16. Lymphangioma in a 15-year-old. (H&E, × 60)

Fig. 7.17. Slow-growing fibrosarcoma of the nasal cavity in a 13-year-old boy. (H&E, × 225)

et al. (1978) have reviewed the literature on *rhabdomyosarcoma* in this region and found 96 recorded cases, 56 of which were well documented, and added four of their own. Rhabdomyosarcomas can occur in the nose or nasopharynx, and often present as polypoid masses (Jaffé 1973a; Fu and Perzin 1976a; Kuruvilla et al. 1990), often with a history of repeated local resection. The predominant histological pattern encountered is of the embryonal type and could easily be mistaken for a chronic inflammatory reaction. Immunohistochemistry could be a valuable asset in arriving at the correct diagnosis, and the use of suitable markers (myoglobin, desmin, skeletal muscle actin, and fetal, slow and fast myosins) for one or more of the striated myofibrilar proteins would indicate the degree of differentiation of the neoplastic rhabdomyoblastic cells. Ultrastructural studies will also help to confirm the diagnosis. The tumours infiltrate the surrounding structures extensively, making resection difficult, if not impossible, in most cases (Donaldson et al. 1973; Liebner 1976; Bale et al. 1983; Eusebi et al. 1986; Bussolati et al. 1987).

Tumours of Cartilaginous and Osseous Nature

Tumours of cartilaginous and osseous nature are uncommon in the nasal cavity in children. *Chondromas* have been mentioned in the literature (Fu and Perzin 1974c) and are usually found in the nasal septum as a polypoid mass. Histologically, it is difficult to determine whether these lesions are neoplasms or merely hypertrophic areas of the cartilaginous septum or heterotopic islets of cartilage. *Chondrosarcoma* was observed in four children by Fu and Perzin (1974c), who collected 25 documented cases from the literature, including some children. *Chordomas* are uncommon in the nasopharynx, and even more so in childhood. Although the histology is characteristic in most cases (Fig. 7.18), it can present difficulty, especially when mixed with other tissue components, mainly cartilaginous foci (Heffelfinger et al. 1973).

Both *fibrous dysplasia* and *ossifying fibroma* are extremely rare. Fu and Perzin (1974b) reported eight cases of these two conditions presenting in the first

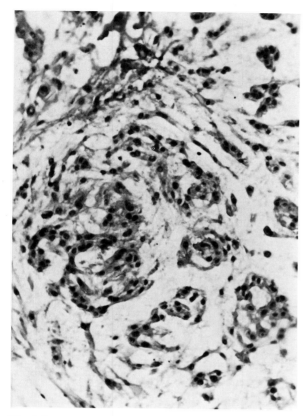

Fig. 7.18. Chordoma of the paranasal sinuses (Courtesy of Dr C. Bozic) (H&E, × 225)

two decades. Ossifying fibroma, although a benign tumour, provokes extensive local bone destruction. The tumour is made up of bony trabeculae separated by abundant fibrous tissue (Dehner 1973). This tissue is quite cellular, containing numerous spindle-shaped fibroblasts, sometimes arranged in whorls.

There are occasional rare mitotic figures. Other types of benign osseous tumours, and *osteosarcomas* and *myxomas*, have been encountered in childhood (Fu and Perzin 1974b, 1977).

Other Tumours

Heterotopic nervous tissue or so-called "nasal glioma", can be found in the nasopharyngeal region. It is a rare congenital abnormality of mature neural tissue and can be found intranasally or extranasally or both and may be multiple. Heterotopic nervous tissue can also be observed in other regions of the head and neck, and when located in the nasopharynx are often associated with malformations of the head and face. Histologically, the tissue is composed of

various components including glial tissue, neuronal cells, ependyma, choroid plexus (Fig. 7.19a), retinal-like elements, oligodendroglia and even calcification (Fig. 7.19b). These tumours are usually polypoid, pale, soft or rubbery and are often received in fragments. In older patients they may be firm and somewhat fibrous. Most cases are observed in children with a high percentage of cases arising in and around the nasal cavity.

Heterotopic nervous tissue must be distinguished from encephalocele. However, although the malformation may be distinguished from the heterotopia by the presence of meninges or tissue organization, there remain intermediate forms where the decision remains a problem (Patterson et al. 1986; Yeoh et al. 1989).

Primary meningiomata of the nasal cavities and sinuses are rare. Ho (1980) found seven cases described in children and Taxy (1990) found two other cases. Although glomus tumour of the region is very rare it must be taken into consideration among the differential diagnoses of these various lesions (Hayes et al. 1993).

Olfactory neuroblastoma or aesthesioneuroblastoma, has also been described in children. Bailey and Barton (1975) presented a case in a 6-year-old boy and reviewed the literature. They found 25 cases occurring before the age of 20 years, three in the first decade and 22 in the second. These tumours appear to arise from the basal layer of the olfactory sensory epithelium in the upper nasal cavity above the middle turbinate and are of neural crest origin. Even though they may be related to the childhood neuroblastoma of other regions, they are quite distinct biologically, although arginine vasopressin has recently been recovered from such a tumour (Chaudhry et al. 1979; Elkon et al. 1979; Singh et al. 1980). Histologically the tumour consists of groups or nests of neuroblasts, which have a lymphocytoid appearance. The cells have a round or oval nucleus with coarse or thin chromatin; the cytoplasm is scanty, the stroma is fibrillary, and there may be pseudo-rosettes around some fibrillar elements (Fig. 7.20). Immunohistochemistry and electron microscopic studies are now mandatory to differentiate this entity from undifferentiated carcinomas, lymphomas, embryonal rhabdomyosarcomas and other small-cell tumours of the region. These tumours may extend into the adjacent paranasal sinuses but rarely metastasize (Levine et al, 1986; Taxy et al. 1986; Lloreta et al. 1992; Kleinclaus et al. 1993). Siwersson and Kindblom (1984) have recently described an *oncocytic carcinoid* of the nasal cavity, another rare tumour, associated with a bronchial carcinoid in a 13-year-old girl.

Teratomas of the nasopharynx are rare and can be the cause of neonatal asphyxia and hygroma coli;

332

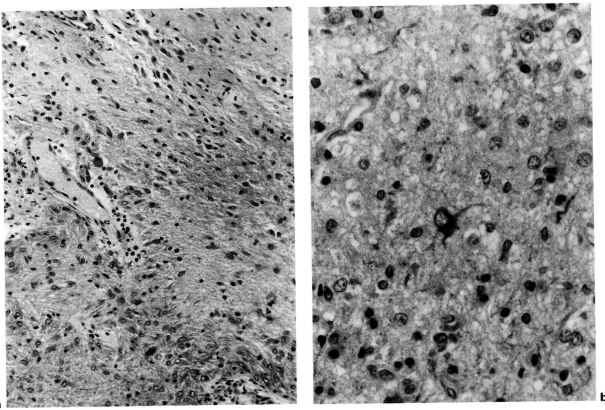

Fig. 7.19. a So-called nasal glioma of the nasal cavity of a 14-week-old male infant. There are many calcified areas. (H&E, × 50)
b Ganglion cell with neurofilaments. (S-100 protein, × 78)

they may go unnoticed and present symptoms only during childhood. These tumours are generally of the adult or mature type, but other types have also been described (Zerella and Finberg 1990; Tharrington and Bossen 1992; Jaarsma et al. 1994; Rothschild et al. 1994).

Malignant lymphomas (non-Hodgkin's) are not uncommon in childhood and occasionally affect the nasopharynx, presenting in either a nodular or a diffuse form (Wollner et al. 1976). The introduction of monoclonal antibodies has helped in identifying the B- and T-cell variants and in separating this group of tumours from plasma cell granuloma (a benign condition) and the undifferentiated carcinomas (Fellbaum et al. 1989; Ratech et al. 1989; Seider et al. 1991; Arber et al. 1993; Niedobitek and Young 1994).

In Africa, however, lymphoblastic lymphoma (*Burkitt's lymphoma*) is prevalent in the paediatric age group, and may first present as a simple isolated mass or multiple tumours in the jaw, maxilla, nasal cavity or nasopharynx, with distortion and destruc-

tion of the bones (Burkitt 1970). The histological, cytological and ultrastructural features of this fascinating tumour, together with the environmental factor(s) that may play a role in its aetiology, have all been fully documented (Epstein and Achong 1970; Wright 1970). The histology is characteristic, with sheets of immature lymphoblasts among which are scattered large histiocytes, giving the tumour the characteristic "starry sky" appearance. The histocytes have an abundant clear vesicular cytoplasm containing phagocytosed cellular elements (Fig. 7.21).

Larynx and Trachea

Congenital Malformations

Congenital Laryngeal Atresia

Congenital laryngeal atresia is an extremely rare condition; few cases have been recorded in the literature,

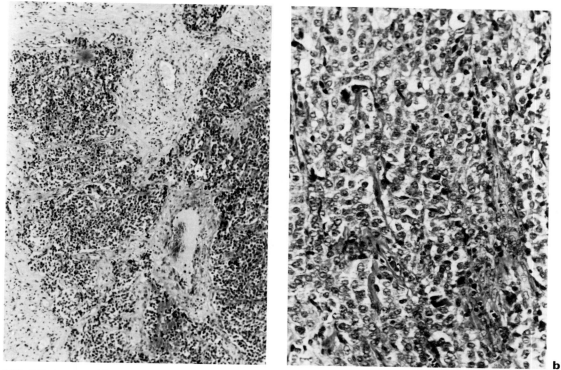

Fig. 7.20. Olfactory neuroblastoma (aesthesioneuroblastoma) in an 11-year-old boy. (H&E, **a** × 40, **b** × 120) (Courtesy of Dr C. Bozic)

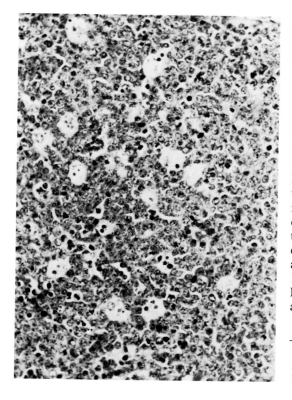

and these have often presented in association with other congenital anomalies (Fox and Cocker 1964; Morimitsu et al. 1981; Schlesinger and Tucker 1986). The atretic zone can be localized in the glottic, supraglottic or subglottic region, or it can affect the entire larynx. The cricoid cartilage may form a diaphragm across the stenosed larynx. We have seen a case in which this diaphragm was pierced by a small hole. The condition results from the failure of resorption of epithelium during the 7th and beginning of the 8th week of intrauterine life. Partial resorption of the lamina may lead to *stenosis*, which usually occurs in the subglottic region with narrowing of the inferior margin of the cricoid cartilage. Two main histological variants can be observed: cartilaginous and soft-tissue anomalies. This abnormality is more frequently encountered than atresia. Both conditions are often associated with other anomalies (Landing and Dixon 1979; Walton et al. 1985; Wigglesworth et al. 1987). Malformation of the epiglottis (bifid, anomalous accessory cartilages) may be associated with these

Fig. 7.21. Burkitt's lymphoma, with its "starry-sky" appearance, in a 9-year-old African boy. (H&E, × 120)

and other anomalies (Healy et al. 1976; Templer et al. 1981).

Laryngomalacia (flabby larynx) is one of the main causes of stridor in the perinatal period. It is associated with three well defined anatomical abnormalities characterized by: a flaccid epiglottis, which may be hypoplastic, long and with cartilage deficiency; poorly supported arytenoids; and short aryepiglottic folds. All of these are responsible for narrowing of the larynx during inspiration. Two distinct groups have been recognized: a congenital form in neonates with symptoms shortly after birth and another observed in older infants and children. The condition is associated with other respiratory disorders and certain syndromes (Landing and Dixon 1979; Nussbaum and Maggi 1990). Hypercellularity with staining abnormalities of the cartilaginous matrix have been noted in a familial case of laryngomalacia.

Laryngeal Webs

Laryngeal webs are much more common than atresias, but may be considered to be lesser degrees of the same lesion. They, like atresia and stenosis, are causes of cyanosis, stridor or other signs of respiratory distress in the newborn. Webs are usually thin bands situated at the anterior portion of the vocal cords, partially obstructing the laryngeal orifice. They result from failure of normal separation of the two vocal cords. Occasionally they are observed on the posterior portion. They have been reported in families and in association with various congenital anomalies (Gay et al. 1981) Histologically these webs are made up of dense connective tissue, sometimes containing skeletal muscle and numerous capillaries. The proximal surface is covered with squamous epithelium, and the distal surface with respiratory epithelium.

There have been occasional case reports or reviews of the relatively rare condition of *cleft larynx*, but the abnormality may be more prevalent than the literature suggests. The length of the cleft varies widely. In some cases it presents as a slit in the posterior midline of the cricoid cartilage, resulting in a communication between the larynx and the superior portion of the (often atretic) oesophagus. In other cases, it extends to the level of the trachea as far as the carina, resulting in an oesophagotrachea. This abnormality is known to run in families; it affects mostly girls and has been reported in siblings and occasionally associated with hamartoma, tracheo-oesophageal fistula, congenital heart anomalies or part of a clinical syndrome. The clinical symptoms (stridor, feeding difficulties, recurrent aspiration) generally appear shortly after birth, but can go unnoticed until childhood. In severe cases, prompt treatment is needed. Surgical repairs have been attempted with some success (Novak 1981; Holinger et al. 1985; Tyler 1985; Corbally 1993).

Laryngeal Cysts and Laryngoceles

Laryngeal cysts (mucocele), like laryngoceles (aerocele), are generally located at the level of the laryngeal ventricle, and there is often some confusion between the two conditions. Cysts are closed cavities and do not have an outlet into the laryngeal lumen, in contrast to laryngoceles. These abnormalities can protrude into the lumen or be situated within the wall of the larynx. Less commonly they are found at any level in the neck; they attain a considerable size, displacing adjacent organs, Stell and Maran (1975) reviewed the literature on laryngocele and found some 139 cases described in both children and adults. Cysts may increase in diameter as their mucus content increases, and laryngoceles can also vary in size, depending on the quantity of air trapped inside them. Most cysts are supraglottic, whereas subglottic (retention) cysts have been documented principally among premature infants as a complication of prolonged intubation with subglottic stenosis (Miller et al. 1989; Smith et al. 1990a; Civantos and Holinger 1992; Chu et al. 1994). Histologically both cysts and laryngoceles are lined with respiratory epithelium.

Tracheal Agenesis

Total or partial absence of the trachea is a rare abnormality with just over 60 cases reported in the literature. Tracheal atresia can be divided into three anatomical types based on the chronology of the development and separation of the trachea from the oesophagus during intrauterine life. In type I the upper trachea is atretic but the normal lower trachea, with the bronchi and lungs, connects to the oesophagus; in type II, the whole trachea is absent and the bronchi join in the midline forming a unique trunk which opens into the oesophagus (the majority of cases fall into this category); in type III, the trachea is absent and the bronchi arise separately from the oesophagus. Tracheal agenesis may occur in association with a number of malformations, including laryngeal anomalies or atresia, ventricular septal defects or other congenital cardiac malformations, aberrant lung lobation, abnormalities of the upper gastrointestinal tract and pancreas, and central nervous system malformations, and especially in association with the Pallister–Hall, VATER and VACTERL syndromes. Tracheal hypoplasia has also been described in patients with chromosomal abnormalities (Holinger et al. 1987; Downing 1992; Wells et al. 1992; Davis et al. 1992; Aboussouan et al. 1993).

Tracheal Stenosis

Tracheal stenosis occurs in several forms and is often associated with abnormalities of the main stem bronchi or other major or minor congenital malformations (Smith et al. 1984; Chambran et al. 1988; Hoffer et al. 1994). The condition may present as one or several continuous complete or solid tracheal rings at any level of the tracheal tree, with narrowing of the segment involved. In rare instances the trachea is completely cartilaginous, and the lungs have been found to be abnormal in some cases (Fig. 7.22). Associated anomalies are not uncommon and the condition can be observed in association with many syndromes. Tracheal stenosis may also be the result of compression by an abnormal adjacent vessel (displaced aorta, vascular rings and anomalous left pulmonary artery).

Tracheomalcia and Bronchomalacia

Tracheomalacia and bronchomalacia are conditions in which the tracheobronchial tree shows abnormal flaccidity and softness of the cartilaginous framework (defective calcium deposits), with a tendency to collapse during respiration. Tracheomalacia may be divided into two main groups: *primary* (affecting normal infants, premature babies and the dyschondroplasias) and *secondary* (associated with tracheo-oesophageal fistula, arterial compression or vascular rings or other compression) (Grundfast et al. 1981; Cogbill et al. 1983; Benjamin 1984; Denneny 1985; Sotomayor et al. 1986). When the anomaly affects the larynx it is known as *laryngomalacia*. Hypercellularity with staining abnormalities of the cartilage matrix have been noted in a familial case of laryngomalacia. *Congenital tracheal diverticulum*, although rare, must be considered among the differential diagnoses. The lesion is composed of smooth muscle and cartilage, and may occur alone or in association with other congenital anomalies of the tracheobronchial tree.

Tracheo-oesophageal Fistula

Tracheo-oesophageal fistula is a relatively common congenital malformation, with various anatomical presentations that may or may not be associated with

oesophageal atresia. Tracheal abnormalities are not uncommon and include cartilage deficiency with an increase in the extent of the muscle in the membranous part of the tracheal ring. The condition has been reported in twins (Holden and Wooler 1970; Sundar et al. 1975; La Salle et al. 1979; Wailoo and Emery 1979; Sankaran et al. 1983; Whalen et al. 1987). Emery and Haddadin (1971) and Maeta et al. (1977) have shown that there is extensive squamous metaplasia of the tracheal epithelium, especially in cases with associated oesophageal atresia (see also p. 217). This condition is often associated with other malformations involving various systems, thus giving rise to complex patterns.

Acquired Lesions

Traumatic

Various *foreign bodies* can lodge in the larynx or trachea in children and provoke symptoms of obstruction.

Lesions induced by *endotracheal intubation* (Fig. 7.23) are common in infants treated in intensive care units for the respiratory distress syndrome or for other neonatal respiratory difficulty. The lesions may be localized in the larynx at the level of the vocal cords, but are more often observed in the subglottic region or in the trachea. Less severe lesions consist of erosion of the mucosa; in the more severe forms the submucosa is ulcerated and infiltrated by inflammatory cells. The cartilage may be severely eroded in areas, and perforation can occur. These lesions are becoming less frequent because of better techniques and modifications of the materials used in tube manufacture; however, healed lesions may cause severe scarring and subglottic or tracheal stenosis and/or deformation. Histologically, there are various degrees of destruction of the cartilage plates with extensive scar tissue covered by a hyperplastic squamous epithelium. These lesions are more common and appear to be more severe in premature babies, especially when ventilated over long periods (Hwang et al. 1988; Wiswell et al. 1989; Weber et al. 1991).

High-frequency jet ventilation may also cause severe damage to the trachea and main stem bronchi with extensive necrosis leading to tracheobronchi obstruction by a mixed basophilic membrane (Fig. 7.23c) made up of mucus, fibrin, damaged necrotic tissue and blood. The distal airways show extensive squamous cell metaplasia (Delafosse et al. 1988; Wiswell et al. 1988; Polak et al. 1989; Davis et al. 1990; Keszler et al. 1991).

Corrosive agents (acids and alkalis) ingested accidentally and vomited may subsequently be aspirated,

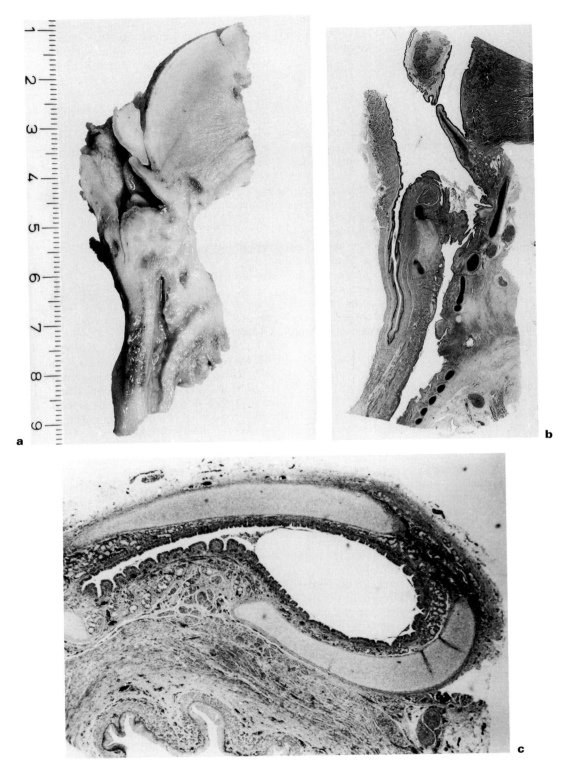

Fig. 7.22. a Gross specimen showing marked stenosis of the upper deformed portion of the trachea. **b** Histological section showing the abnormal cartilage rings, absent in places. (**a, b** Courtesy of Professor C.L. Berry) **c** Stenosis and malformation of the trachea in a case of VATER complex.

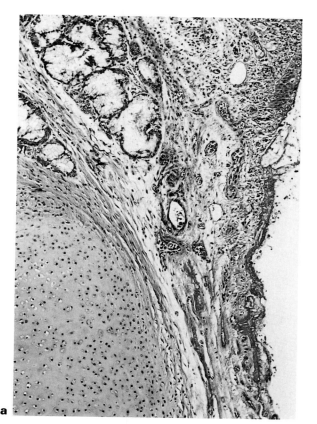

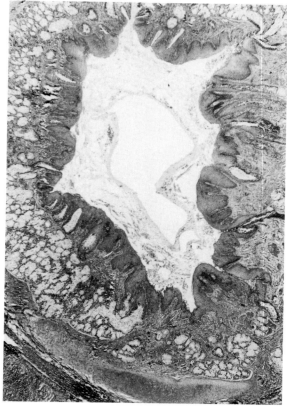

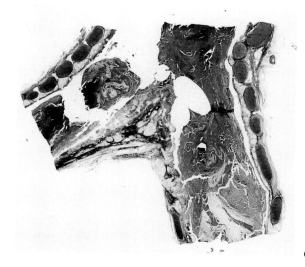

Fig 7.23. a Severe ulceration of the tracheal mucosa covered by fibrin and infiltrated by chronic inflammatory cells. Ten days' endotracheal intubation. (H&E, × 60) **b** Twenty-seven days' intubation leading to tracheal stenosis and severe and extensive squamous metaplasia of the epithelium. (H&E, × 25) **c** Extensive destruction of the tracheal and bronchial walls in a case of high jet ventilation.

causing oedema and necrosis of the laryngeal and tracheal mucosa. Lysol and kerosene cause similar lesions, the latter especially in developing countries. In rare instances, toxic gases may be the cause of irritation of the mucosa with oedema, congestion and a secondary inflammatory reaction (Greene and Stark 1978). Various foreign bodies when aspirated can cause severe damage to the treachea, larynx and main bronchi, sometimes resulting in perforation, but more often in secondary aspiration pneumonia (Van Asperen et al. 1986; Esclamado and Richardson 1987).

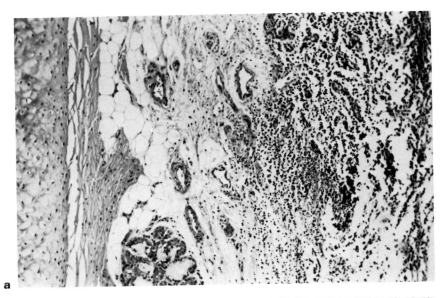

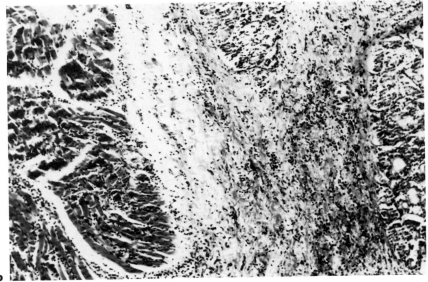

Fig. 7.24. Acute epiglottis in an 8-month-old boy. (H&E, × 90) **a** Acute inflammation with ulceration and oedema of the epiglottic mucosa. **b** Inflammation of the subglottic region with extension into the deep muscle layers.

Infections

Acute infections of the larynx and trachea, including the epiglottis (*laryngotracheo-bronchitis*), may be life-threatening and require prompt medical or surgical attention (Bass et al. 1974; Scheidemandel and Page 1975; Cantrell et al. 1978; Cohen and Chai 1978; Liston et al. 1983; Diaz 1985). Various microorganisms have been recovered, the most common being *Haemophilus influenzae*, α-haemolytic streptococci, β-haemolytic streptococci group A, *Staphylococcus aureus*, pneumococci and Neisseria. Vaccine against *Haemophilus influenzae* type b,

among others, has considerably diminished the frequency of these agents as potential pathogens. In many developing countries, *Corynebacterium diphtheriae* still plays an important role in infections of this region.

Anatomically, changes in the epiglottis are the most striking; however, both the larynx and the trachea are also usually involved. The epiglottis is markedly swollen, oedematous and congested. Its edges are rounded, and there is partial stenosis of the laryngeal orifice as a result. The larynx is also oedematous, and the vocal cords may touch in the middle. Histologically there is marked oedema of the submucosal tissues of the epiglottis and larynx, extending into the trachea. A diffuse polymorphonuclear infiltration extending into the deeper layers may be seen, usually sparing the cartilaginous structures. The lesions are non-specific (Fig. 7.24). With *C. diphtheriae* infection there is necrosis of the mucosa, and a pseudomembrane, composed of a fibrin network in which there are leucocytes and numerous bacteria is present.

Virus infections usually affect the subglottic region and are characterized by oedema with marked congestion and some round-cell infiltration; associated bacterial infection is common.

The larynx and trachea may be the site of non-specific granulomas in cases of acute and chronic infections. In the developing world tuberculosis of the region may be encountered, and the lesions usually present as mucosal ulcerations with the characteristic appearance. Cohen et al. (1978c) have described a case of Wegener's granulomatosis of the larynx in a 12-year-old girl with the diffuse systemic form of the disease. Mycotic lesions of the larynx and trachea may present as ulcerations (Vitale et al. 1993) or pseudocarcinomatous hyperplasia of the mucosa especially in patients with AIDS or those with some other immunodeficiency state. Viral infections, mainly herpes and cytomegalovirus, may also be observed in such patients.

Tumours

Tumours of the larynx and trachea are quite uncommon among infants and children.

Epidermoid cysts of the vocal cords are occasionally observed in children, and may cause dysphonia. They may be unilateral or bilateral, and are often associated with glottic sulcus and/or mucosal bridges. Although there is still debate concerning their origin, some consider them congenital anomalies. Histologically, they resemble epidermoid cysts elsewhere (Monday et al. 1983; Bouchayer et al. 1985).

Epithelial Tumours. Papilloma is by far the most common tumour of this area and is more appropriately referred to as *juvenile laryngotracheal papillomatosis*, because multiple lesions are the rule. These tumours occur more frequently among children whose mothers present with condyloma acuminata during pregnancy and in recent years evidence has accumulated that one or more types of papillomaviruses (HPV6, HPV7, HPV16, HPV18, HPV30, HPV33) may be associated with these lesions. The viruses can often be demonstrated in the apparently normal adjacent epithelium, explaining the possible repeated recurrences. Papillomatosis often begins as a single wart on the vocal cords and spreads along the mucosa of the larynx to reach the trachea and even the main stem bronchi. The warts may disappear spontaneously at puberty, but are frequently recurrent despite repeated excisions. Squamous cell carcinomas are known to develop from these lesions, especially after irradiation. In such instances it is not always easy to identify the area of carcinomatous transformation, in spite of widespread metastases (Crissman et al. 1988; Chaput et al. 1989; Basheda et al. 1991; Dickens et al. 1991; Simon et al. 1994).

Histologically there is marked hyperplasia of the squamous epithelium with some degree of keratosis and parakeratosis associated with koilocytosis but no hyperkeratosis. The hyperplastic epithelium is thrown into folds about a thin stalk of connective tissue containing few capillaries and a few chronic inflammatory cells. Focal dysplastic areas can be observed in cases followed over several years (Fig. 7.25).

Squamous cell carcinoma of the larynx in children is extremely rare. Large national surveys of tumours in children have failed to find this tumour; however, there are some cases in the literature (Orton 1947; Jones and Gabriel 1969; Jaffé 1973b; Askin 1975). In a review of the recorded cases, Gindhart et al. (1980) collected 54 cases and added one of their own. The origin is often in the vocal cords and there is a male predominance (3 : 2), usually with advanced disease at diagnosis (Shvero et al. 1987; Ohlms et al. 1994). X-ray irradiation for juvenile papillomas may be a predisposing factor. There have also been reports indicating that carcinomas in the supraglottic area in adults have developed in laryngoceles (Micheau et al. 1975). The histological appearance of this tumour is similar to that of other squamous cell carcinomas. Weber and Grillo (1978) treated a case of squamous cell carcinoma of the trachea in a 13-year-old girl, and Olmedo et al. (1982) an adenoid cystic carcinoma in a 16-year-old girl.

Briselli et al. (1978), in a review of the literature on tracheal *carcinoids*, found one reported case in a 13-year-old adolescent girl.

Vascular Tumours. Haemangiomas of the larynx and trachea, although uncommon, are important lesions because of the diagnostic problems they present and the high mortality rate among infants with these lesions. They may be observed at birth or shortly thereafter, grow progressively with age, and usually present some months after birth. They are occasionally associated with haemangiomas in other sites including the skin, head and neck. They are most often localized in the subglottis, but may also involve the supraglottic region. The lesion may be confined to the submucosa, or appear as sessile, flat, pinkish or bluish masses in the mucosa, and may be the cause of

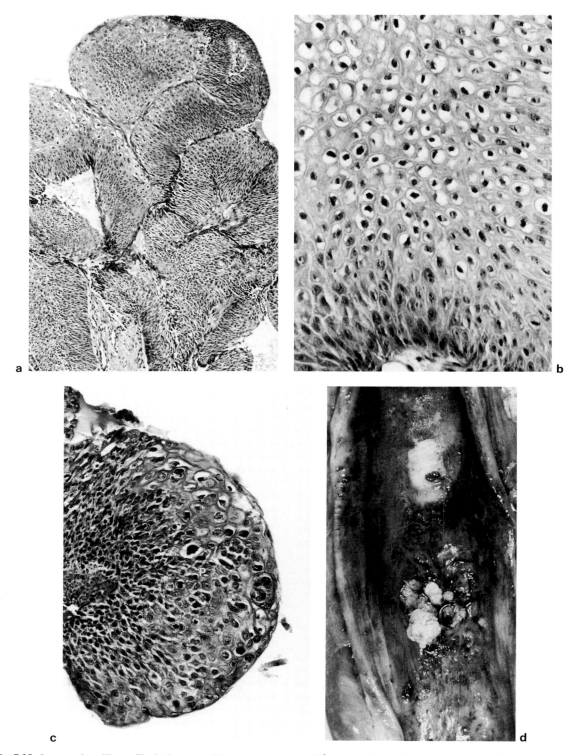

Fig. 7.25. Laryngeal papilloma. The lesions were discovered at the age of $2\frac{1}{2}$ years and led to the patient's death at 25 years from extensive metastatic squamous cell carcinoma. **a** Papillomas extending from the larynx into the main stem bronchi at age 12 years. (H&E, × 35) **b** Note severe koilocytosis in biopsy at age 16 years. (H&E, × 225) **c** Severe dysplastic changes with intraepithelial neoplasia. (H&E, × 225) **d** Bouquet of multiple tracheal papillomas at the time of death, with marked scarring above and below the lesions as a result of repeated biopsies.

airway obstruction. In tracheal lesions there may be extension into the perichondrium and/or beyond the tracheal rings. Spontaneous or partial regressions have been observed between the ages of 1 and 8 years, with slow resolution in others by 12–15 years of age. There is a marked female predominance. Biopsy is not recommended because of the haemorrhage that may result. Recently, various new treatements have been introduced in the management of these lesions. The histology is that of haemongiomas elsewhere (Ezekowitz et al. 1992; Ohlms et al. 1994; Sie et al. 1994).

Lymphangiomas of the larynx in infancy and childhood are rare and are usually associated with cystic hygroma or cavernous lymphangioma of the head and neck region. They can occasionally be found as isolated tumours, or present as a laryngocele or a saccular cyst (Jaffé 1973b; Moore and Cobo 1985; Cohen and Thompson 1986; Donegan et al. 1986). Jaffé (1973b) had also observed a *haemangiopericytoma* in a 3-month-old boy.

Tumours of Nervous Origin. Neurofibromas of the larynx may occur and are sometimes associated with neurofibromatosis (von Recklinghausen's disease). In recent reviews of this subject (Jafek and Stern 1973; Maisel and Ogura 1974) there were four recorded cases in the paediatric age group, one of which occurred in a 3-month-old boy, and Stanley et al. (1987) added two more cases from their series. Neurilemmoma is also extremely rare in this age group: Horovitz et al. (1983) in a review of the literature could only find one recorded case in a 6-year-old girl, and Stanley et al. (1987) reported three more occurring in the second decade of life.

Tumours of Muscular Origin. Granular cell myoblastoma of the larynx has been reported in children by Booth and Osborn (1970), Nasser et al. (1970) and Thawley and Osborn (1974). The tumour has also been documented in the trachea in children. These tumours appear to have a familial occurrence, and all races seem to be affected. Several tissues or organs may be simultaneously involved. Immunohistochemistry has shown that these tumours are probably of Schwann cell origin rather than muscular (Thaller et al. 1985; Muthuswamy et al. 1986; Nathrath and Remberger 1986; Rifkin et al. 1986, Stanley et al. 1987)

Leiomyoma of the trachea is extremely rare (Bouros et al. 1987) and Kitamura et al. (1969) could find only nine published cases, one of which was in a 15-year-old patient presented by Unger (1952). *Rhabdomyosarcoma*, although an uncommon tumour, is perhaps more prevalent than most other soft-tissue

tumours of these parts. There have been reports of this tumour occurring in the larynx of children (Wayoff and Labaeye 1973; Frugoni and Ferlito 1976; Fu and Perzin 1976a; Canalis et al. 1978), as well as in the trachea (Ho and Rassekh 1980).

Cartilaginous Tumours. Chondroma and chondrosarcoma tumours of the larynx and trachea have been recorded in adults but are exceptional in childhood (Simpson et al. 1979).

Chemodectomas. Non-chromaffin paraganglia of possible Kultschitzky cell origin sometimes occur in the larynx. Hohbach and Mootz (1978) found 23 recorded cases in the literature, one of which occurred in a 14-year-old boy, and added one of their own.

Other Tumours. In their review of tracheal tumours Gilbert et al. (1953) found nine cases of *fibroma* among children. Cohen et al. (1978a) described a case of *fibrous histiocytoma* in the trachea of a $2\frac{1}{2}$ year old girl, and Sandstrom et al. (1978), in their review, found one case in a 15-year-old girl. Rosenberg et al. (1981) described two cases of *fibromatosis* of the larynx in neonates and retrieved six from the literature, some of which had been previously reported as either fibroma or fibrosarcoma. The difficulty in the histological diagnosis, especially when some lesions show evidence of local invasion or malignant changes, indicates the importance of immunohistochemistry and electron microscopy in the study of these lesions (Pollak et al. 1985; Tan-Liu et al. 1989). Witwer and Tampas (1973) described a case of tracheal *fibroxanthoma* in a 5-year-old boy, and discovered a second case in the literature. *Pleomorphic adenoma*, a benign mixed tumour, has been described in both the larynx and the trachea in children (Som et al. 1979; Heifetz et al. 1992). Sarcomas, including rhabdomyosarcomas of the larynx and trachea have been documented in this age group (Gorenstein et al. 1980a; Olmedo et al. 1982; Abramowsky and Witt 1983; Dodd-O et al. 1987), and one cannot over-emphasize the importance of immunohistochemistry and ultrastructural examinations as aids to a correct diagnosis. *Liposarcoma*, an extremely rare tumour of the region, has not been described in children (Esclamado et al. 1994).

Cohen et al. (1978d) described a case of a primary *lymphosarcoma* of the larynx in a girl aged 4 years 7 months, and also reported on a *solitary plasmacytoma* affecting the larynx and upper trachea in a 15-year-old girl treated for systemic lupus erythematosus (Cohen et al. 1978b).

Lungs

Congenital Abnormalities

Congenital abnormalities of the lungs are varied and often complex. They may be isolated to the lungs but it is not uncommon to find such abnormalities associated with other organ or system malformation.

There is no general agreement on the classification of pulmonary agenesis. Schneider (1912) first attempted to divide the abnormality into three groups:

1. Agenesis, in which there is complete absence of bronchi, alveolar tissue and their blood supply
2. A group in which a rudimentary bronchus arose from the trachea with no pulmonary tissue investing its tips
3. A group with a poorly developed main bronchus invested by a fleshy mass of ill-developed pulmonary tissue

This classification was subsequently modified by Boyden (1955), who recommended a system based on the degree of developmental arrest. There were also three categories:

1. Complete absence of one or both lungs (agenesis)
2. Suppression of all but a rudimentary bronchus (aplasia)
3. Abortive growth (hypoplasia)

Spencer (1977a, b) proposed yet another classification, based on the categories of anomalies:

1. Bilateral complete agenesis
2. Unilateral agenesis, which is further subdivided into three groups, which are identical with Schneider's three groups
3. Lobar agenesis and other lesser forms of congenital abnormality

We shall follow this last general classification.

Bilateral or *complete pulmonary agenesis* is a very rare condition, and there are few recorded cases. The laryngotracheal tree may terminate blindly at the level of the larynx or trachea, or even at the main stem bronchi. The pulmonary artery normally takes its origin from the right ventricle, but terminates in the thoracic aorta by way of the ductus arteriosus. The bronchial arteries and pulmonary veins are usually absent, and there are other associated abnormalities affecting the cardiovascular system, upper gastrointestinal system, anus, urogenital system, musculoskeletal system and spleen. It may also be observed in association with some syndromes

(VACTERL), and polyhydramnios has been documented in two cases, one of which presented with hydrops fetalis (Engellenner et al. 1989). There are now 12 cases on record and they all seem to be part of the same developmental field defect (Toriello and Bauserman 1985; Toriello et al. 1985).

Unilateral pulmonary agenesis is much more common than complete agenesis, and is not compatible with normal life. This condition has been referred to by several names in the numerous case reports or reviews on the subject. According to Spencer's (1977a, b) classification there are three subgroups, each of which corresponds to one of Schneider's (1912) three groups, described above. There may be other associated abnormalities involving the cardiovascular system, gastrointestinal tract, ipsilateral facial bones, vertebral column and upper limbs and their associated muscles, and urogenital system, as well as diaphragmatic agenesis or hernia. Over 260 cases of this condition are described in the literature (Say et al. 1980; Mardini and Nyhan 1985; Toriello et al. 1985). Agenesis of one lobe with abnormality of the bronchial tree has also been described (Maesen et al. 1993). The life expectancy of these patients depends on the severity of the associated malformations and the problem of infections in the existing lung. Ryland and Reid (1971) and Hislop et al. (1979) have further shown that in existing lung tissue there is bronchial reduction with an increase in alveolar density. The pulmonary artery in their case also showed a reduction in both the conventional and the supernumerary branches, which was more marked for the former group of vessels.

Minor Abnormalities

Abnormal lobulation is not an uncommon finding in post-mortem material, and is often the result of lobar fusions or accessory fissures. It is generally associated with other congenital malformations, usually cardiovascular, e.g. Ivemark's syndrome, Fallot's tetralogy, polysplenia and situs inversus (Landing and Wells 1973). The bronchial tree of these abnormal lungs also shows variations from the normal bronchial pattern, and it must be emphasized that many accessory lobes (azygos, cardiac, left middle) are variations of normal lobulation.

There is an uncommon condition in which the lungs are fused in the midline behind the apex of the heart, giving them a *horseshoe* appearance. The condition (25 cases) is described in association with dextrocardia and other cardiac anomalies, as well as bronchial, parenchymal and pleural anomalies and the VATER association (Hawass et al. 1990; Hassberg et al. 1992; Ersoz et al. 1992; Figa et al.

1993). The condition is also often associated with the *Scimitar syndrome* (anomalous drainage of the right pulmonary vein to the inferior vena cava, often subdiaphragmatic, right lung hypoplasia and other cardiac and vascular anomalies), another rare condition which may present with symptoms in early infancy or childhood or may be completely asymptomatic. It has been described in families (Cabrera et al. 1989; Redington et al. 1990; Yamaguchi et al. 1990; Dupuis et al. 1993; Trinca et al. 1993).

Accessory supernumerary bronchus (bronchus cardiacus superior dexter or *sinister)* is a rare anomaly in which the accessory bronchus takes its origin directly across from the orifice of the right (left) upper lobe bronchus. The condition must be distinguished from the much commoner *displaced bronchi* in which the bronchi take off from unusual sites (Maesen et al. 1983). Congenital bronchial atresia is not altogether uncommon, but is most often discovered in adults. The atretic bronchus often appears as a series of cystic dilatations reminiscent of bronchiectasis (Jederling et al. 1986).

Pulmonary Hypoplasia

A decrease in lung volume and weight is generally referred to as pulmonary hypoplasia due to a developmental abnormality resulting in a reduction in numbers and/or size of the acini. Both lungs may be involved (oligohydramnios), or the lesion may be unilateral (diaphragmatic hernia) in which case the lesion is usually apparent, whereas, in the former, the lungs may appear normal on gross inspection although there is a marked reduction in volume and weight when compared with those of other fetuses of comparable gestational age. There are many ways of assessing pulmonary hypoplasia. Lung weight is still the simplest, but this is subject to variations depending on the pathological lesions. Wet lung weight to body weight ratio is widely accepted as a simple method, available to all in spite of the variations that may occur in cases with lung pathology or in hydrops fetalis. The normal values range between 0.018 and 0.025 with wide variations.

Other methods include alveolar radial count or its modified versions which are easily reproducible, lung tissue maturity (quantitative biochemical assays of desaturated phosphatidylcholine, ultrastructural studies of acinar cellular lining), morphometric evaluation of the acini, DNA estimation of cell number and elastic tissue distribution. A significant number of cases, unilateral, or bilateral, are associated with malformations forming a heterogeneous group of abnormalities including cases associated with syndromes, with or without chromosomal anomalies.

Hypoplasia with oligohydramnios from prolonged leaks of amnotic fluids, renal agenesis, renal polycystic disease, renal dysplasia or congenital urinary tract abnormalities with obstruction is perhaps the best documented form. Hypoplasia in oligohydramnios is associated with markedly diminished lung volume, and small acinar size and surface area for gestational age. The lungs are structurally and biochemically immature with a lag in the appearance of several elements making up the developing pulmonary parenchyma. As in other cases of pulmonary hypoplasia, there is extension of the muscular arteries into the intra-acinar level together with an increase of medial arterial thickness.

Reduction in the intrathoracic space may be the consequence of congenital diaphragmatic hernia (unilateral), polycystic kidney and liver disease, immune and non-immune hyrops with polyhydramnios, pleural effusions, the chondrodysplasias, neonatal hypophosphatasia, intrathoracic tumours and abdominal wall defects. In this group, hypoplasia in diaphragmatic hernia (Fig. 7.26) is the best documented. There is delay in pulmonary maturity with a diminished number of airways, blood vessels and acinar numbers in the ipsilateral lung, although the contralateral may be within normal limits with an increase in alveolar numbers (Fig. 7.27).

The condition is also observed with anencephaly and other neuromuscular conditions, in which cases there is pulmonary immaturity and acinar developmental delay. However, there are cases in which no apparent cause is evident. In Down's syndrome, pulmonary hypoplasia is associated with a reduction in number and size of the acini, which is responsible for the postnatal development of subpleural emphysema or cysts. Recent studies suggest that loss of lung fluid and decrease in fetal breathing movements are important factors in the genesis of pulmonary hypoplasia, but other factors (genetic programme disturbances, hormonal cell-mesenchymal interactions) may be important contributing factors (Cooney and Thurlbeck 1982; Page and Stocker 1982; Cooney and Thurlbeck 1985; George et al. 1987; Wigglesworth et al. 1987; Silver et al. 1988; Argyle 1989; Nicolini et al. 1989; Nakamura et al. 1990; Haidar et al. 1991; Rosenak et al. 1991; Wigglesworth et al. 1991; Barth and Rüschoff 1992; Husain and Hessel 1993; Foster et al. 1994; Di Fiore and Wilson 1995).

Accessory Lungs and Pulmonary Sequestration

Müller (1918) defined *accessory lung* as an organlike mass of pulmonary tissue with its own pleura, separated from the rest of the lung. The accessory

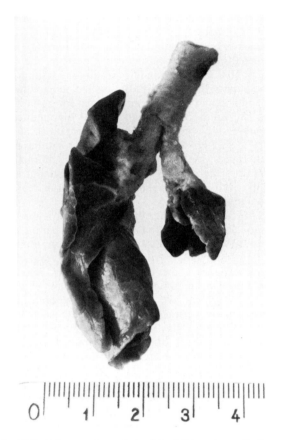

Fig. 7.26. Pulmonary hypoplasia of the left lung in a patient presenting with a large left diaphragmatic hernia. (Courtesy of Dr C. Bozic)

lung may connect with either the tracheobronchial tree or the fore-gut. *Pulmonary sequestration*, on the other hand, describes a piece of lung which, although lying within the same pleura as the normal lung, is not connected to its bronchial system or derivatives. The sequestrated tissue receives its blood supply from a systemic artery. This condition must be distinguished from *ectopic* or *herniation lung tissue*, which has been described in the neck and thoracic regions in association with iniencephaly and certain syndromes (Landing and Dixon 1979; Bridger et al. 1992). Sequestered lung may be located within the main lung (*intralobar sequestration*) or separate from it (*extralobar sequestration*). It is possible, from these broad definitions, to separate four main pathological entities without considering minor variations or combined abnormalities. These are:

1. Accessory lung with connections to the tracheobronchial tree

2. Accessory lung with bronchi arising from fore-gut derivatives
3. Extralobar pulmonary sequestration
4. Intralobar pulmonary sequestration

These various lesions used to be considered rare abnormalities, and were usually accidental findings at autopsy. They were sometimes discovered during treatment of a repeated pulmonary infection or during the course of certain radiographic procedures. As radiographic procedures and techniques improve, the lesions are discovered more frequently, and have been reported at all ages. Pulmonary sequestration is sometimes associated with funnel-chest deformity and other anomalies (Gerle et al. 1968; Accard et al. 1970; Felson 1972; Dutau et al. 1973; Jaubert de Beaujeu et al. 1973; Iwa and Watanabe 1979; Savic et al. 1979).

Accessory Lung with Connections to the Tracheobronchial Tree

The accessory bronchus takes its origin from the normal tracheobronchial tree and terminates in a mass of poorly defined pulmonary tissue. The latter may be cystic or may resemble a hamartoma. Examples of this type of abnormality have been described by Cotton et al. (1956) and Herxheimer (1901).

Accessory Lung with Bronchi Arising from Fore-gut Derivatives

The accessory bronchus originates from fore-gut derivatives, usually the lower (occasionally the upper) portion of the oesophagus or the stomach. The tissue lies outside and separate from the lung proper. Histologically it is made up of tubular structures lined by ciliated respiratory-type epithelium. The bronchus leading to the accessory lung may be lined by squamous epithelium similar to that of the oesophagus or by gastric-type mucosa, depending on its origin. The artery supplying the accessory lung generally arises from the aorta (Grans and Potts 1951; Boyden et al. 1962; Gerle et al, 1968; Pai et al. 1971; Kobler and Ammann 1977; Stocker et al. 1978).

Extralobar Pulmonary Sequestration

These masses consist of bronchial and alveolar structures, often lying behind the lung. They may be located at any level from the neck to the diaphragm.

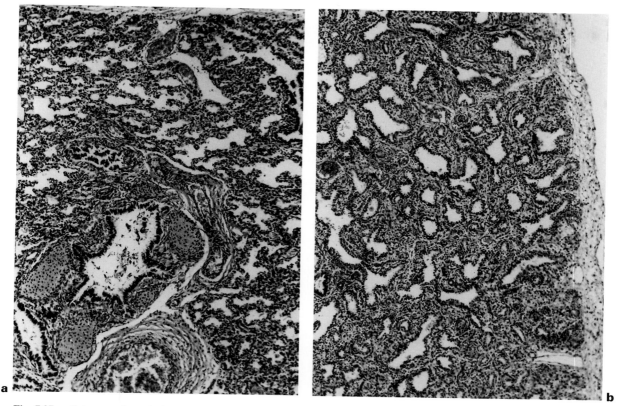

Fig. 7.27. a Pulmonary hypoplasia (diaphragmatic hernia) showing abnormal peripherial bronchial cartilage plates with grouping of reduced bronchial and bronchiolar branches. (H&E, × 20) **b** Pulmonary hypoplasia (Down's syndrome, 20 weeks' gestation) showing marked reduction in number and size of acini together with delay in maturation. (H&E, × 20)

The majority have been found on the left, and they are frequently associated with diaphragmatic hernia or some other congenital malformation. The arterial supply to the sequestrated tissue is usually by a number of small branches from the thoracic or abdominal aorta, but occasionally from the subclavian or intercostal arteries. The venous drainage is by way of the azygos system (Accard et al. 1970; Jaubert de Beaujeu et al. 1970; Merlier et al. 1970; Bliek and Mulholland 1971; Stocker and Kagan-Hallet 1979).

Intralobar Pulmonary Sequestration

This is a relatively common abnormality. The sequestrated pulmonary tissue does not communicate with the tracheobronchial tree and is contained within the pleura of the normal lung. It is usually situated in the lower lobes and mostly on the left, although other lobes may contain the lesions. The posterior basal segment is most frequently involved. This abnormality is rarely associated with other malformations.

The sequestrated tissue frequently consists of a single cystic cavity or a group of interconnecting cysts. Less commonly, a solid mass of tissue is found, which is not separable from the surrounding normal lung. This mass contains dilated bronchus-like spaces lined with respiratory-type epithelium whose walls sometimes contain cartilage plates. Alveolus-like structures are also observed.

The artery supplying the sequestrated tissue is usually prominent, taking its origin from the thoracic or abdominal aorta, or occasionally from the intercostal arteries. The supplying artery is generally short, of large diameter, and has an elastic structure similar to that of the pulmonary artery. The venous drainage is by way of the pulmonary venous system (Pryce 1946; Pryce et al. 1947; Buchanan 1959; Zelefsky et al. 1971; Dutau et al. 1973).

The embryogenesis and pathogenesis of these abnormalities are still a matter of debate, and there are many theories on their formation. With the advent of routine ultrasound examinations during pregnancy, the diagnosis of this condition is now often made during intrauterine life (Pryce et al. 1947; Delarue et al. 1959; Gebauer and Mason 1959; Kyllonen 1964; Gerle et al. 1968; Lebrun et al. 1985; Mendoza et al. 1986b).

Cysts

Lung cysts remain a controversial subject with no satisfactory classification available, although several have been proposed. They can be divided into two main groups, congenital and acquired, the latter being by far the most common. There is still some difficulty in deciding whether a cyst is congenital or acquired, especially when it is discovered after the neonatal period. One can only be sure that a cyst is congenital if it is discovered in a fetus or newborn, as acquired cysts can occur in the first months of life after pulmonary infection, particularly staphylococcal or viral infections, pulmonary infarctions, or maldevelopment of the distal airways, especially in association with cardiovascular malformations in Down's syndrome. In older children the distinction between the two becomes almost impossible. They can affect only a portion of the lung or of a lobe, and can be single or multiple. Either sex may be affected (Bâle 1979; Stocker 1987; Gonzalez et al. 1991).

Spencer (1977b) has presented a temporary classification based on pathology. His groups are:

A. Congenital, further subdivided into four types:
   1. Central and peripheral
   2. Lymphangiomatous
   3. Cystic change in an intralobular sequestrated or accessory lung, and enterogenous cysts
   4. Congenital cystic adenomatoid malformation

B. Acquired cysts.

There are also four large subgroups of this class, which will not be discussed further here.

Central cysts are often referred to as bronchogenic. They are usually observed in the mediastinum near the hilus or a main bronchus, and appear to have been derived from a large bronchus. Less commonly they occur in the wall of the oesophagus or in the subcutaneous tissue of the chest wall or neck. They are most often single cysts, variable in size, and do not necessarily communicate with the tracheobronchial tree but may simply be attached by a fibrous band. Histologically the cysts are lined by a pseudostratified columnar epithelium, the wall consisting of smooth muscle bundles, cartilage plates and abundant

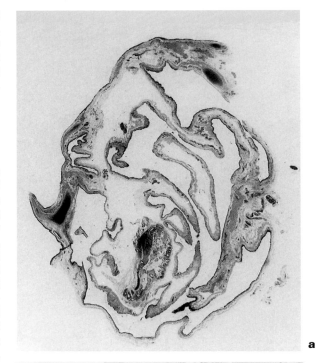

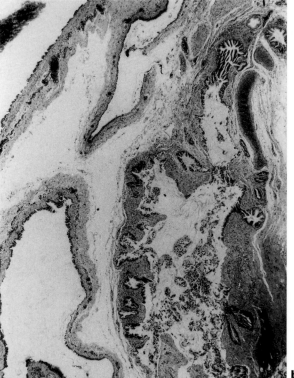

Fig. 7.28. a Central bronchogenic cyst from a newborn presenting with symptoms of respiratory distress. (H&E, × 4) **b** The cysts resemble normal bronchial wall in places. Note the cartilage plates and normal appearing bronchial mucosa. (H&E, × 20)

elastic fibres. There are also numerous subepithelial glands, which explain the presence of mucus in the lumen (Fig. 7.28). The changes caused by infection may be superadded.

Peripheral cysts probably develop as a result of disturbance in the growth of the bronchial tree at a late stage of intrauterine life or even after birth. They are usually multiple, and may affect both lungs, a lobe or part of a lobe, or even an entire lung (Fig. 7.29a). Microscopically they may communicate with a parent bronchus, and they are a form of honeycomb lung of infancy. Histologically, they are lined with ciliated or cuboidal respiratory epithelium. Their wall consists of connective tissue in which there are many elastic fibres and a few small cartilage plates but practically no smooth muscle fibres. Subepithelial mucus glands are usually absent (Fig. 7.29b).

Cystic Adenomatoid Malformation

Cystic adenomatoid malformation is a relatively rare condition, and has often been included with congenital cystic disease of the lung or pulmonary sequestration. It is now considered a hamartoma and in some instances may be associated with dysplastic or neoplastic tissues and other congenital malformations such as extralobar sequestration, renal agenesis, malformation of the urogenital tract and cardiac anomalies. The diagnosis is now made in utero by ultrasound as the condition is known to be associated with anasarca and maternal polyhydramnios. The abnormality is usually unilateral, affecting one or more lobes, usually the lower lobe (Stocker et al.

1987; Carles et al. 1992a; Heydanus et al. 1993; Zangwill and Stocker 1993; Thorpe-Beeston and Nicolaides 1994), but more than one lobe may be involved. The lesions may be bilateral and occupy variable proportions of the lobes, as in a case we have seen recently. The condition has also been described in adults (Pulpeiro et al. 1987). Tumours are known to develop in or in association with this malformation (Stephanopoulos and Catsaras 1963; Ueda et al. 1977).

Kwittken and Reiner (1962) were among the first to attempt to define the condition histologically, and included an increase of terminal respiratory structures with intercommunicating cysts of various sizes lined with respiratory-type or cuboidal epithelium, polypoid formation of the mucosa and an increased

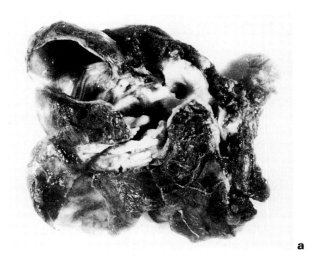

a

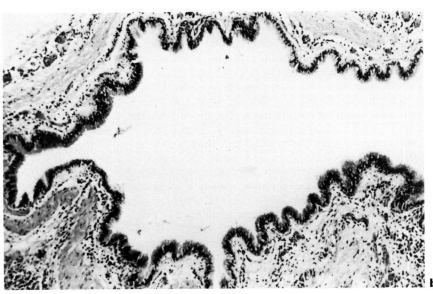

Fig. 7.29. a Peripheral bronchial cysts in a 3-month-old child. **b** Wall of peripheral bronchogenic cyst from a 4-year-old boy. (H&E, × 35) (Courtesy of Dr.C. Bozic)

b

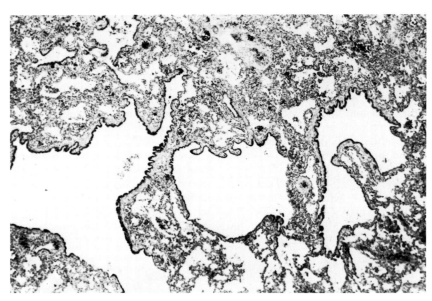

Fig. 7.30. Congenital cystic adenomatoid malformation, corresponding to type II lesions of Stocker et al. (1977), from a 3-day-old baby girl. (H&E, × 25) (Courtesy of Dr C. Bozic)

amount of elastic fibres in the wall beneath the epithelium. There was usually absence of cartilage and there were no inflammatory cells.

In 1973, Van Dijk and Wagenvoort described three cases of this condition and proposed a new classification into cystic, intermediate and solid types. Stocker et al. (1977) reviewed 38 cases and proposed a different classification. These authors also grouped their cases into three distinct categories, based on clinical, gross and histological criteria. *Type I* lesions presented only a few large thick-walled cysts containing air or fluid. These cysts were lined with ciliated pseudostratified columnar epithelium with numerous polypoid projections in the lumen. The wall contained smooth-muscle fibres and elastic tissue, but very few cartilage plates. There were smaller cysts adjacent to the larger ones, and large alveolus-like structures were observed between the cysts. Sometimes these alveolus-like structures communicated with the smaller cysts. The blood vessels were normal. *Type II* lesions presented as numerous evenly spaced cysts, generally less than 1 cm in diameter. They communicated with the normal bronchial tree. The cysts were lined with cuboidal or tall columnar ciliated epithelium, with rare areas of pseudostratification (Fig. 7.30). The wall consisted of a thin layer of loose fibromuscular tissue, and in this there were dense concentrations of elastic tissue beneath the epithelium. The cysts appeared to communicate with structures resembling respiratory bronchioles and alveolar ducts. Cartilage was not observed as a part of the lesion but rather as a normal

component of the bronchi. There is a subgroup of the type II lesion containing bands of striated muscle fibres throughout the lesion, lying close to the bronchiole-like cysts and blood vessels from which may develop the rhabdomyosarcomas described in association with this lesion. *Type III* lesions were less numerous and presented as bulky and firm masses of pulmonary tissue occupying almost the entire lobe or lobes and containing very small visible cysts (less than 0.5 cm). The cysts were similar to bronchioles in size and distribution, and were lined in areas with ciliated cuboidal epithelium or, in most places, with non-ciliated cuboidal epithelium (Fig. 7.31). Electron microscopic studies of these cells (Olson and Mendelsohn 1978) have shown that they are composed primarily of granular pneumocytes (type II) and few type I pneumocytes. They resembled the glandular structure of the developing lung and were separated by a loose connective-tissue stroma with a few elastic fibres and occasional smooth-muscle fibres. Cartilage was absent.

In their series, Stocker et al. (1977) found that type I and type II lesions were by far the most frequently observed. They also noted that type I lesions were larger, involving almost the entire lobe or lobes with no adjacent normal pulmonary tissue. Furthermore, type I lesions were more commonly associated with other congenital malformations.

Two additional types (0 and IV) have been added to the present classification (Stocker 1994). Type 0 affects the proximal tracheobronchial tree. The cysts are lined by a ciliated pseudostratified columnar epithe-

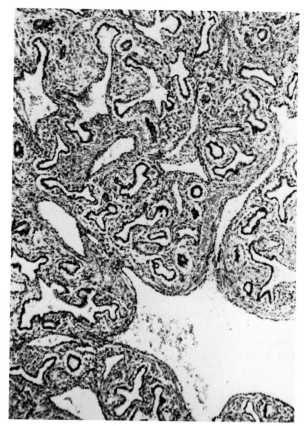

Fig. 7.31. Type III lesion of congenital cystic adenomatoid malformation (classification of Stocker et al. 1977) from a premature baby boy. (H&E, × 60)

lial lining with goblet cells. Mucus cells and cartilage are always present but there is absence of striated muscle. Type IV cysts are peripheric, lined by flattened type I pneumocytes and low cuboidal epithelial cells. The walls are variable in thickness with many vessels whose walls also vary in thickness.

Pulmonary Lymphangiectasis

Pulmonary lymphangiectasis is not uncommon. Clinically it presents as respiratory distress in the neonate. Infants with this anomaly rarely survive beyond 24 h; however, cases have been recorded of survival for some weeks or even years. There is a net male predominance. The abnormality has been described in association with other congenital malformations (asplenia, cystic renal disease, anomalous pulmonary drainage) or restricted to the lung. This has led some authors to separate the condition into three categories: a generalized form, a form associated with obstructive cardiovascular anomalies with abnormal pulmonary venous connections, and an idiopathic form isolated to the lung. When unique and localized it is referred to as *lymphangioma* and, when diffuse, occupying one or more lobes, as *lymphangiectasis*.

The aetiology is obscure, and various theories are proposed as to its pathogenesis, including obstruction of the pulmonary venous flow, obstruction of the pulmonary lymphatics, and anomalous pulmonary development with failure or regression of the developing lymphatic network. It has been described in association with pulmonary hypertension in the neonate, pleural effusions or chylothorax, and it has been reported in siblings. The condition may be widespread involving bone, soft tissue and/or viscera and is then referred to as *lymphangiomatosis* (Stocker et al. 1978; Karmazin et al. 1989; Kelso et al. 1991; Stark and Mark 1992; Ramani and Shah 1993; Verlaat et al. 1994).

Macroscopically both lungs are generally involved, although there are a few reported cases in which only one lung has been involved. The lungs are large and firm, with a grossly lobulated or nodular surface. Between the lobules, one can observe the lymphatic network, with multiple round or ovoid cystic cavities lying beneath the pleura and containing fluid. The cut surface may appear relatively normal or show a honeycomb appearance with thickening of the intralobular septa, which may contain numerous cysts, resembling interstitial emphysema. Histologically the septa are thickened throughout the lung, and they contain a lace-like network of distended lymphatic vessels of variable sizes extending into the intrapleural space (Fig. 7.32). The lymphatics are thin-walled, lined with a single layer of endothelial cells, and do not have valves. Muscle fibres are absent from the thickened septa, and there is no lymphoid tissue present.

Heterotopic Tissue in the Lungs

There are few recorded cases of ectopic tissue within the pulmonary parenchyma. Heterotopic brain tissue has been observed in the lungs in anencephaly and in other cerebral malformations. Heterotopic glial tissue may be multifocal, unilateral or bilateral (Okeda 1978; Kanbour et al. 1979; Gonzalez-Crussi et al. 1980). Striated muscle in the lung has been documented both in adults and in childhood. Of the 20 cases so far described, eight have been in the paediatric age group (Chi and Shong 1982). Congenital adrenal tissue in the lung has been reported, and two of the cases presented with adrenal cytomegaly in both the adrenals and the heterotopic tissue (Armin and Castelli 1984). Heterotopic liver in the lung is also rare (Mendoza et al. 1986a), as is heterotopic thyroid tissue (Bando et al. 1993).

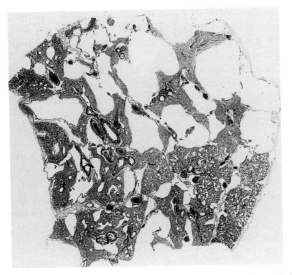

Fig. 7.32. Lymphangiectasis. There is diffuse dilatation of the lymphatics occupying the entire lobe, forming dilated cysts in many areas. (H&E, × 3)

Lobar Emphysema

Lobar emphysema is also referred to in the literature as regional infantile emphysema or congenital obstructive emphysema, and the condition is due to air-trapping by a check-valve. The lesion can involve one or several segments, one or multiple lobes, or even an entire lung; the upper lobes are most often affected, with a slight predominance on the left. In rare cases both lungs have been involved. The condition is observed principally in neonates and infants. Clinically it manifests itself as a rapidly progressive respiratory distress syndrome, with dyspnoea and cyanosis leading to cardiorespiratory failure. On radiographs the affected area is hyperlucent, and there is compression atelectasis of the adjacent pulmonary parenchyma with displacement of the mediastinum toward the opposite side. A relatively high incidence of associated malformations, including cystic adenomatoid malformation, is recorded in these patients (Lincoln et al. 1971; Strunge 1972; Sulayman et al. 1975; Young et al. 1978; Moyland and Shannon 1979).

Although the underlying mechanism causing this condition is not always clear, obstruction of the bronchus leading to the involved segment, lobe or lung is an important cause. Extrinsic factors that can obstruct the bronchus include anomalous mediastinal blood vessels, enlarged lymph nodes, bronchogenic mediastinal cysts, and enteric duplications (Gerami et al. 1969; Schapiro and Evans 1972; Desvignes et al. 1974; Powell and Elliott 1977). Intrinsic causes include mucus plugs or redundant bronchial mucosal folds. More common, however, are structural defects in the bronchial wall, which may be overlooked unless careful histological studies of the main bronchus leading to the involved emphysematous zone are performed. The bronchus may be atretic or stenosed, or it may have abnormal cartilages, with cartilage present as hypoplastic or fragmented cartilage plates affecting either a localized area or several bronchi. The hypoplasia may be partial or total. Bronchomalacia may be included among the defects causing lobar emphysema as well as obstruction caused by secondary vascular disease. Emphysema in this age group has been recorded with Down's syndrome, in siblings and in a mother and daughter. Within recent years attempts at clearly defining the condition have been made in order to understand its physiopathology better. (Berlinger et al. 1987; Toran et al. 1989; Gonzalez et al. 1991).

By quantitative analyses of lungs with congenital lobar emphysema or "apparent" emphysema, Hislop and Reid (1970, 1971) and Henderson et al. (1971) were able to illustrate other causes. These various authors were able to separate combinations of anatomical lesions that may be associated with congenital lobar emphysema. They described the *"polyalveolar"* lobe (*acinus giantism*), in which there was an increase in alveolar number, and further showed that unilateral congenital emphysema can be present in a hypoplastic lung with contralateral compensatory emphysema. Silver et al. (1988) have described what they referred to as *perinatal pulmonary hyperplasia* associated with laryngeal atresia. Lung development was far advanced for the gestational age.

Neonatal Pathological Conditions

It is impossible to over-emphasize the importance of radiographic examination of the body or the thorax before autopsy to enable the pathologist to exclude certain abnormalities within the thoracic cavity. The need to test the pleural spaces for pneumothorax is evident in view of the widespread use of assisted ventilation and, because useful information can be gained from bacteriological and virological studies, material from the trachea, bronchi and lungs and blood from the heart may be cultured. These examinations often supply valuable information and are often helpful in cases where the gross pathology is uninformative.

Amniotic Fluid and Meconium Aspiration

It is well established that the fetal lung secretes a liquid that occupies the terminal air spaces and airways and whose composition and viscosity are different from those of the plasma and amniotic fluid (Adams 1966; Adamson et al. 1969a). There has been considerable controversy as to whether there are spontaneous fetal respiratory movements in utero, with mixing of the amniotic fluid with that of the fetal lung. Recent studies using various methods (mainly ultrasonic monitoring) have shown that fetal breathing movements in utero occur both in experiemental animals and in humans. These movements, which are associated with contractions of both the diaphragmatic and the intercostal muscles, have been detected early in gestation and they become more regular with advancing gestational age. Because of the high viscosity of lung fluid and the short duration of inspiration, normal breathing is insufficient to clear the tracheal dead space, and therefore the tidal volume is very small. It is mainly during gasping under various adverse conditions that relatively large volumes of anmiotic fluid may be inspired by the fetus (Benacerraf and Frigoletto 1986; Mortola 1987; Natale et al. 1988; Wiswell and Bent 1993). The amniotic fluid may sometimes be stained with meconium, suggesting fetal distress or acidosis. However, Miller et al. (1975) and Seppälä and Aho (1975) have suggested that the passage of meconium is not always a result of hypoxia or fetal distress, but may be a spontaneous or even a physiological phenomenon. Whatever the determining factors may be, the amount of meconium released and the quantity of meconium-stained amniotic fluid aspirated by the fetus depend largely on the duration and intensity of the stimulating factor.

Aspiration of amniotic fluid or meconium-stained fluid occurs mainly in mature or postmature infants, but can also be observed in the premature. It is generally associated with fetal anoxia, which may in turn be related to cerebral haemorrhage, vagal reflex, intrauterine pneumonia, congenital heart disease or other malformation, or drugs administered to the mother during pregnancy or at delivery. Aspiration may result in intrauterine death or the meconium aspiration syndrome of the newborn, which could be due to the inhibition of surfactant function by the aspirated meconium resulting in a decrease in lung–thorax compliance (Clark et al. 1987; Sun et al. 1993). The meconium aspiration syndrome is not infrequently associated with persistent pulmonary hypertension (persistent fetal circulation) (Reid 1986; Perlman et al. 1989; Swaminathan et al. 1989). The lung may show little on gross examination; however,

the presence of meconium on the perianal region, within the external ear, or on other parts of the body and the placenta is an indication that intrauterine fetal distress or anoxia has occurred. The external ear should always be examined for meconium in a neonate; if the body has been washed postnatally, as often happens, traces can be discovered with a swab. The histological lesions are variable and include aspiration of amniotic fluid into the terminal airways, which are distended and contain fluid, a few squamous epithelial cells, and some cellular debris, and show congestion of surrounding capillaries. When meconium is aspirated, the distal airways are distended, containing masses of meconium with some squamous epithelial cells; the trachea and large bronchi may contain large meconium plugs; the bronchioles and terminal airways are also distended and are partly or completely filled with squamous epithelial cells and a little meconium (Fig. 7.33). In both instances there is congestion of the capillaries. Muscularization of the intra-acinar pulmonary arteries when present is consistent with persistant pulmonary hypertension.

When squames are observed in the distal airways of infants several weeks after birth, it is, of course, possible that there might have been a period of intrauterine fetal distress with aspiration of amniotic fluid.

Perinatal Pneumonia

Pneumonia in still born and newborn infants is a relatively common finding at autopsy. It is responsible for the deaths of 5%–20% of infants dying within the first 24–48 h of extrauterine life, and may be found in as many as 30% of stillbirths. Most authors refer to pneumonia occurring in those dying within 48 h of birth as intrauterine or congenital pneumonia, and associate it with aspiration of infected amniotic fluid in utero, maternal sepsis, or infection acquired during passage through the birth canal (intrapartal infection). The term *neonatal pneumonia* is reserved for pneumonia occurring during the first days or weeks after birth, but not after the first month of age. It is generally associated with infections acquired from the environment (delivery room and nursery).

In most infants dying in the immediate neonatal period, between 24 and 48 h of age, it is impossible to distinguish between the two groups.

Most intrauterine pneumonia is the result of infection ascending from the birth canal into the amniotic sac. It is associated with premature rupture of the membranes and prolonged labour, conditions that favour chorioamnionitis, the incidence of which

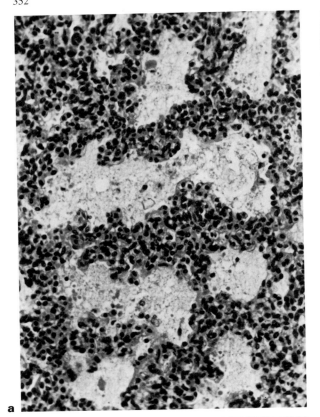

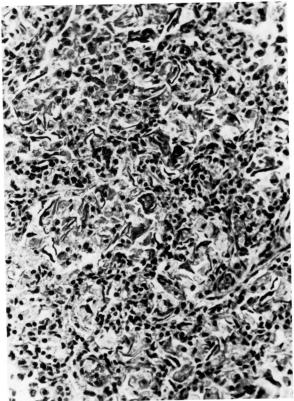

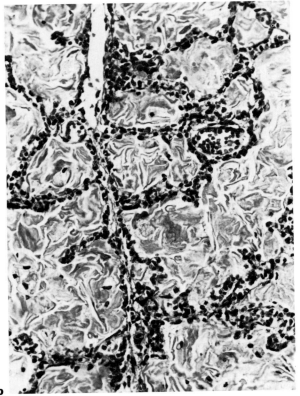

Fig. 7.33. Lungs in neonatal asphyxia. (H&E, × 225) **a** Progressive respiratory distress in a full-term infant. Alveolar saccules are filled with amniotic fluid but contain little debris. **b** Severe respiratory distress with marked extension of alveolar saccules filled with squamous epithelial cells. **c** Prolonged respiratory distress. There is a giant cell reaction associated with secondary inflammation.

increases significantly after 24 h. Congenital pneumonia has also been observed in prolonged labour with intact membranes or where there have been obstetric manoeuvres during labour. In the remaining cases, infection is transplacental and is often associated with clinical symptoms in the mother, e.g. pyelonephritis.

Premature infants appear to be more susceptible to intrauterine pneumonia.

The commonest causative organisms are *Escherichia coli*, β-haemolytic streptococci group B, *Streptococcus faecalis*, *Staphylococcus aureus*, *Klebsiella–aerobacter*, *Pseudomonas aeruginosa* and, less frequently, *Haemophilus influenzae* and pneumococci. Numerous other pathogens have been isolated occasionally, including viruses, fungi, chlamydia and mycoplasmas (Alt et al. 1984; Campognone and Singer 1986; Tomashefski et al. 1989; Itoh et al. 1990; Webber et al. 1990; Bang et al.

1993; Eschenbach 1993; Primhak et al. 1993; Sanchez 1993; Wright and Butt 1994).

Gross inspection of the lungs reveals nothing apart from occasional localized pleurisy. Histologically, the distal airways are filled with a polymorphonuclear-rich inflammatory reaction, which may or may not contain squames. The most striking feature characterizing this type of pneumonia is the absence of fibrin, which has created doubt as to whether the histological picture is a true inflammatory response to infection or caused by aspiration of amniotic elements containing polymorphonuclear (maternal) leucocytes. Recent studies have now established that the inflammatory cells within the airspaces, as well in the interstitium, are of fetal origin and could be the fetal response to infection, toxins and/or chemotactic mediators or combinations, including meconium toxicity, inducing a pulmonary inflammatory reaction characteristic of intrauterine pneumonia. Peribronchial lymphoid hyperplasia may be an associated phenomenon, as well as an increase in the number of polymorphonuclear cells in the liver (Arnon et al. 1993; Grigg et al. 1993; Bohin and Field 1994; Scott et al. 1994; Stallmach and Karolyi 1994). The alevolar septa, bronchioles and bronchi are not involved. Bacteria are not usually observed in sections and, if present, are few (Fig. 7.34). In neonatal pneumonia the exudate contains fibrin, and interstitial inflammatory changes with monocytic cell infiltration can be seen. The bronchi and bronchioles may be surrounded by or infiltrated with mononuclear cells. Necrosis is common but may occur with the formation of microabscesses and/or pneumothorax, notably in staphylococcal infections

Pulmonary Haemorrhage

The real incidence of massive pulmonary haemorrhage in the newborn is not known; there are wide variations in the individual series studied. It is sometimes found in stillborn infants, but is most common among those dying in the first 48 h of life. Premature infants and those small for gestational age are the most often affected. Symptoms may appear immediately after or within a few hours of birth and resemble a severe respiratory distress syndrome.

Although fluid escaping from the nose and mouth may resemble blood, chemical analyses have shown it to be a mixture of plasma filtrate and a small quantity of blood, comparable with haemorrhagic oedema fluid (Adamson et al. 1969b; Fedrick and Butler 1971b; Cole et al. 1973).

Several aetiologies have been proposed for this condition. It has been described in association with prenatal and perinatal asphyxia or anoxia, bacterial or viral infection, cerebral oedema and/or intraventricular haemorrhage, hypothermia, cardiac anomalies (patent ductus arteriosus or ventricular septal defect), haemorrhagic disease of the newborn, hyaline membrane disease and hyperammonaemia (Esterly and Oppenheimer 1966; Adamson et al. 1969b; Chessels and Wigglesworth 1971; Fedrick and Butler 1971b; Cole et al. 1973; Sheffield et al. 1976). The recent studies of Cole et al. (1973) and those of Trompeter et al. (1975) suggest that massive pulmonary haemorrhage in the neonate covers a spectrum of conditions that may rapidly lead to acute left ventricular failure owing to asphyxia. This is followed by an increase in pulmonary capillary pressure and pulmonary haemorrhage. It would appear that infants treated with synthetic surfactant therapy for idiopathic respiratory distress syndrome (IRDS) are more prone to develop pulmonary haemorrhage (Coffin et al. 1993; Pinar et al. 1993).

On gross examination the lungs are heavy, fleshy and of normal size. They may have one or several dark haemorrhagic areas; in most instances an entire lobe or several lobes may be involved. The trachea and large bronchi often contain blood-stained fluid. Histologically, the distended distal airways, bronchioles and some bronchi are filled with erythrocytes. The alveolar septa are markedly congested and show zones of interstitial haemorrhage (Fig. 7.35). Hyaline membranes, squames and mild inflammatory reactions have all been observed in association with this condition.

Idiopathic Respiratory Distress Syndrome (IRDS)/Hyaline Membrane Disease

Idiopathic respiratory distress syndrome, with its well defined clinical presentation, was once the most frequent cause of death among neonates, especially the premature. The principal anatomic finding in these cases was hyaline membrane disease in the lung. Better understanding of some of the possible mechanisms of the condition and the enormous progress in perinatal intensive care units have reduced the death rate due to this disorder considerably, and in well equipped centres there are relatively few infants dying with hyaline membrane disease alone. Such deaths show a male preponderance, probably due to a slower lung maturation in male fetuses; in addition the second-born of twins appears to be at greater risk, as well as postmature infants. A familial predisposition has also been documented.

Prenatal identification of infants at risk, the better understanding of lung development and maturation have now made it possible to design new approaches in the treatment of this disorder, resulting in more favourable outcomes. The cases that now come to autopsy usually present with associated pathological conditions and/or complications (Farrell and Avery

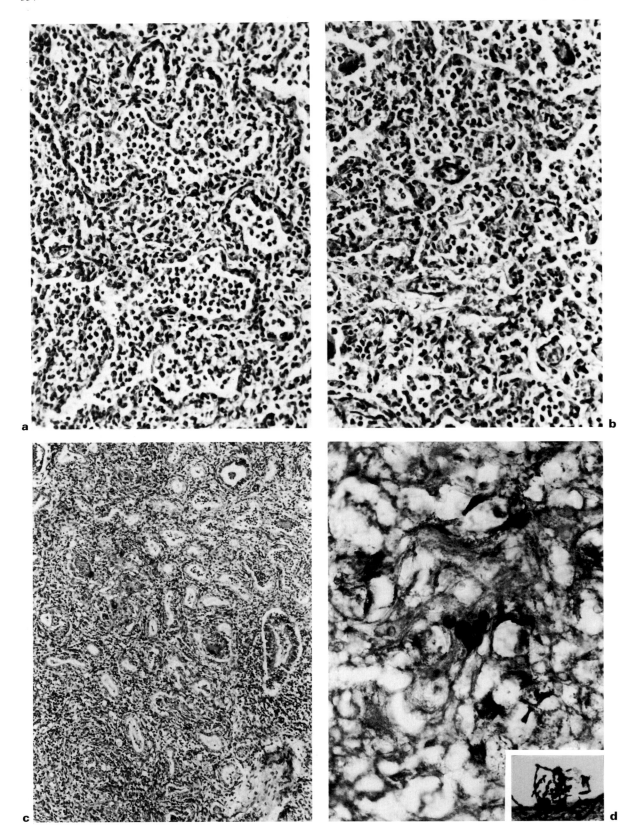

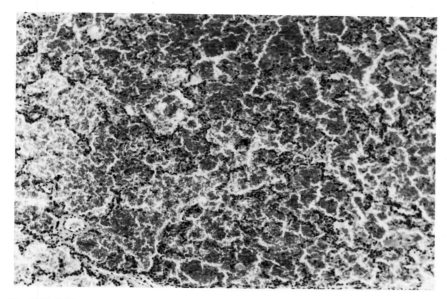

Fig. 7.35. Diffuse intra-alveolar haemorrhage of unknown origin in a newborn infant. (H&E, × 90)

1975; Bonikos et al. 1976; Northway et al. 1990; Seo et al. 1990; Van Lierde et al. 1991; Dobashi et al. 1993).

It is generally accepted that there are three main predisposing factors among infants who present with the respiratory distress syndrome:

1. *Prematurity* or *immaturity*. Infants of low birth weight (800–1500 g) appear to be more susceptible to this disorder than infants born at or near term. It should be noted that the condition has seldom been recorded in fetuses below 800 g and has not been seen in stillborn infants.
2. *Caesarean section*. There is still much controversy as to whether caesarean section per se predisposes to hyaline membrane disease; the evidence suggests that it does, and that this is more apparent following certain indications for section (fetal distress, maternal bleeding and placenta praevia). Catecholamines and other hormones that play an essential role in the

preparation of the fetus for adaptation to extrauterine life are low or lacking and seem to be responsible, at least in part, for the incidence of the condition in this group.
3. *Maternal diabetes*. Here again, hyaline membrane disease may simply be the reflection of the high rate of premature delivery and caesarean section among this group. However, it is well established that these infants are both hyperglycaemic and hyperinsulinaemic due to the disturbance in glucose metabolism. Furthermore, there is growing evidence to suggest that insulin affects type II pneumocytes, causing a delay in their maturation and a diminution in desaturated phosphatidylcholine, phosphatidylglycerol and surfactant apoproteins (Farrell and Avery 1975; Rosan 1975; deMello et al. 1987; Nakamura et al. 1988; van Golde et al. 1988; Margraf et al. 1990).

Histopathology. Hyaline membranes apparently do not appear in stillborns, although some authors have interpreted necrotic cellular debris in such cases as the first changes leading to hyaline membrane disease. An infant must breathe for a short period before the clinical manifestations of the syndrome begins or hyaline membranes develop. Some authors have described their presence as early as 8 and 30 min (McAdams et al. 1973; de la Monte et al. 1986).

On gross inspection, the lungs are airless, reddish grey in colour, resembling liver and rubbery in consistency, but there is little or no change in weight and

---

Fig. 7.34. a Intrauterine pneumonia in a stillborn fetus. The alveolar saccules are distended and filled with polymorphonuclear leucocytes. Conspicuous absence of fibrin. **b** Intrauterine pneumonia with giant cells, probably of viral origin, in a 2-day-old infant whose mother presented with a temperature of unknown origin. No bacteria present. (H&E, × 225) **c** Intrauterine penumonia with granulomatous appearance and numerous giant cells. (H&E, × 160) **d** Grocott stain showing mycotic elements within the giant cells (× 650.) *Inset*, placental infection.

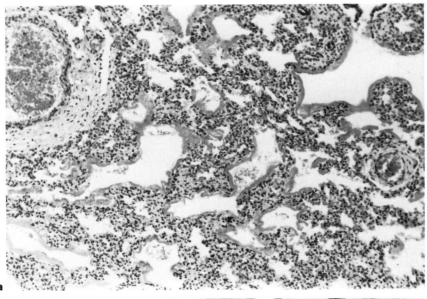

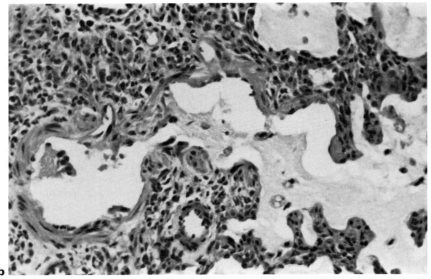

Fig. 7.36. Lungs in respiratory distress syndrome. **a** Some alveolar saccules are lined with hyaline membranes; other are collapsed. (H&E, × 90) **b** Organization of hyaline membranes invested by fibroblasts. (H&E, × 120)

size. Infants who succumb within the first 2 h after birth present diffuse bilateral atelectasis. The terminal airways are occasionally recognizable, distended and present necrosis of the respiratory epithelium and/or destruction and desquamation of their epithelial cells, taking on a basophilic appearance. Hyaline membranes may not be conspicuous at the early stages. Oedema fluid may be seen in some airspaces as well as in the interstitial tissues. The capillaries are usually dilated and there are often foci of haemorrhages. The lymphatics are generally dilated. One must be cautious, however, at this stage, to exclude an eventual intrauterine or perinatal infection (usually by group B streptococcus), which may present similar histological features, in which case a Gram stain could be useful. The airways may contain numerous polymorphonuclears.

After about 12 h the lesions are more extensive; dilated distal bronchioles and terminal airways are more conspicuous and alternate in an irregular fashion with atelectatic zones. The membranes are now quite conspicuous, extensive and confluent, and may be observed in atelectatic areas. They appear as homogeneous eosinophilic bands on the denuded thickened basal membrane, or epithelial cells of the distal bronchioles and terminal air spaces are seen below, containing epithelial cellular debris and pyknotic nuclei (Fig. 7.36).

Interstitial and intraluminal haemorrhages are common findings. Arterioles appear contracted and the veins are congested. Lymphatics are usually dilated. In infants dying after 12 h the lesions are even more widespread, and the hyaline membranes are extensive, thicker and well defined.

Beyond 36 h of life the first signs of repair appear. Type II pneumocytes begin to regenerate at the margins of denuded areas and beneath the hyaline membranes; by day 3 these changes are well defined. The membranes become fragmented and resorption is in process (phagocytosis by macrophages). There is active interstitial fibroblastic proliferation, and this, with type II pneumocyte cell regeneration, seems to incorporate the membranes into the alveolar wall, leading to fibrosis of varying degree. Meanwhile, the oedema has diminished considerably. Tubular myelin and surfactant apoproteins are now prominent in the proliferating hyperplastic type II pneumocytes (Lauweryns 1969; Lauweryns et al. 1971; Finlay-Jones et al. 1973; Nilsson et al. 1978; Robertson 1987; deMello et al. 1987; Nakamura et al. 1988; Margraf et al. 1990).

The chemical composition of hyaline membranes has been extensively documented. They are weakly PAS-positive and rich in fibrin deposits, being most readily identified by fluorescent or electron microscopy. Conventional stains for fibrin (Mallory phosphotungstic acid haematoxylin) are often disappointing. Hyaline membranes have also been shown to contain high quantities of tyrosine, α_1-antitrypsin and C_3 fractions of complement (Gitlin and Craig 1956; Berezin 1969; Lauweryns 1970; Demarquez et al. 1976; Singer et al. 1976).

In hyperbilirubinaemic premature infants with the respiratory distress syndrome, the hyaline membranes lining the distal airways may appear yellowish; hence the name *yellow pulmonary hyaline disease*. The condition is most often encountered among premature babies with a moderate bilirubinaemia who have been ventilated and received relatively high levels of oxygen for long periods. The membranes attain this colour as a result of increased permeability of the air–blood barrier in the lung to a serum protein–bilirubin complex. Yellow hyaline membranes stain positively for bile (Morgenstern et al. 1981; Turkel and Mapp 1983).

The pathogenesis of hyaline membrane disease is probably variable. Hyaline membranes have been described in association with or complicated by the aspiration of amniotic fluid, premature rupture of the membranes, neonatal asphyxia with acute anoxia and acidosis, hypothermia, intrauterine infection, congenital heart disease leading to rapid heart failure, pul-

monary hypoperfusion, birth injury, erythroblastosis fetalis and deficient lung fibrinolytic activity (plasminogen activator). Immunological factors and neuroendocrine disorders have also been incriminated (Lieberman 1969; Fedrick and Butler 1970a; Ambrus et al. 1974; Farrell and Avery 1975; Kenny et al. 1976; Berkowitz et al. 1978).

However, the most important single contributory factor in the pathogenesis of the respiratory distress syndrome is the absence or low level of *surfactant (surface-active materials)*. The role of surfactant in the normal lung is well established. The terminal air spaces in the normal newborn infant, like the alveoli in adults, are lined with a surfactant (Fig. 7.37), which maintains their stability by lowering surface tension at the air–liquid interface, thus preventing alveolar collapse during pulmonary expansion. It has been noted that the lungs of newborn infants dying with hyaline membrane disease are consistently lacking or deficient in surfactant and surfactant apoproteins, which are normally secreted by the granular pneumocytes and Clara cells. Between 20 and 24 weeks' gestation, these cells make their appearance in the terminal spaces of the developing lung. Soon afterwards there is a marked decrease in the glycogen content of the type II cells, and osmiophilic lamellar inclusion bodies appear within the cytoplasm, representing the first morphological expression of the secretory activity of these cells. About the same period, surface-active materials, mainly phospholipids and surfactant apoproteins, can be recovered from the pulmonary fluid of the fetus or from the amniotic fluid in small quantities. They can also be identified in the fetal lung by immunohistochemistry. From then on the number of granular pneumocytes, and to a lesser degree Clara cells, increases rapidly, and by 30 weeks they are normally producing large quantities of surfactant, which attain their maximum levels at about the 35th week of gestation (Fig. 7.38).

Apocrine epithelial antigen (AEA) can be detected in type II cell membranes early in fetal lung before the occurrence of detectable surfactant. Anti-AEA also stains reactive material in hyaline membranes. Furthermore, the type II cells contain few intermediate keratin filaments; these vary in quality and quantity, depending on the development and maturation of the cells. The most active component of surfactant is dipalmitoyl phosphatidylcholine (saturated lecithin). This substance can already be detected in very small quantities between 18 and 20 weeks' gestation, and increases in amount with advancing gestational age. As a result, the determination of this phospholipid in amniotic fluid is now widely used to evaluate fetal lung maturity and predict which infants are at risk. Its value is expressed as a ratio of lecithin to sphingomyelin (L/S) (Rosenthal et al. 1974; Hallman et al.

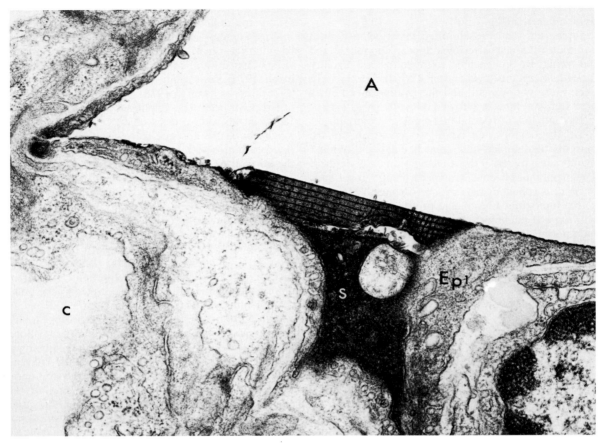

Fig. 7.37. Electron micrograph of surfactant (*S*) lining the alveolar surface. *A*, alveolus; *C*, capillary; *EP*₁, epithelial cell type 1. (× 41 000) (Courtesy of Dr Y. Kapanci)

1989; Bowie et al. 1991; Bender et al. 1994; Miyamura et al. 1994).

The regulation of lung phospholipid biosynthesis depends on certain enzymes, principally phosphatidic acid phosphohydrolase, within the granular pneumocytes. This enzyme can also be detected in the lung and amniotic fluids; its level increases with gestational age. Its concentration in amniotic fluid can also be used as an indicator of lung maturity as it rises in parallel with the L/S ratio. Phosphatidylglycerol is another good marker, as are amniotic fluid prolactin, surfactant apoproteins and lamellar body concentrations (Hallman et al. 1989; Dubin 1990; Bowie et al. 1991; van Kreel 1991; Fakhoury et al. 1994; Bender et al. 1994).

Surfactant contains variable amounts of phosphatidylethanolamines, phosphatidylglycerol and sphingomyelins (70%–80%) as well as neutral lipids (mainly cholesterol). Besides the active phospholipid component (dipalmitoyl phosphatidylcholine), surfactant also contains small amounts of carbohydrates

and many proteins in varying quantities. It is now evident that the protein, which makes up about 10% of purified surfactant, is composed of two equal fractions, one of serum albumin, secretory IgA and IgG and the other of a species of associated apoproteins, four of which have so far been identified. These surfactant proteins (SP), designated SP-A, B, C and D, play an important role in the morphological structure and function of surfactant.

SP-A, a hydrophilic highly immunogenic family of glycoproteins, is cloned on chromosome 10(10q). It is synthesized and secreted by type II pneumocytes and bronchiolar Clara cells. The collagen-like sequences on its amino-terminal end make it structurally homologous to CIq and can thus enhance FcR and CRI mediating phagocytosis. Its non-collagenous terminal domain is responsible for its inhibitory effect on lipid secretion and binding to type II pneumocytes. Although it can be identified in fetal lung by 12 weeks' gestation, it is detected in substantial quantities only during the last trimester at about 34

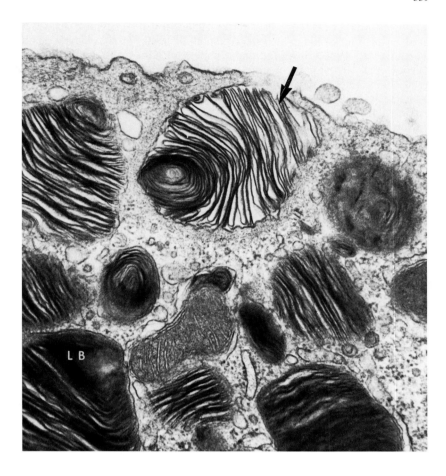

Fig. 7.38. Electron micrograph of granular pneumocyte (type II cell), showing numerous lamellated bodies (*LB*), one of which (*arrow*) is undergoing exocytosis. (× 68 000) (Courtesy of Dr Y. Kapanci)

weeks. It is regulated by a number of hormones and growth factors (glycocorticoids, cAMP, insulin, interferon γ, EGF and TGF β). It cooperatively enhances the activities of the hydrophobic apoproteins (SP-B and SP-C), but acts specifically as a regulator of function in surfactant metabolism and participates in the formation of tubular myelin and in the local defence mechanisms of the host. The type II pneumocytes express high-affinity receptors for SP-A in the surfactant recycling process.

SP-B, a highly immunogenic hydrophobic surfactant apoprotein, is associated with surfactant phospholipids. The genes for it are located on chromosome 2 and its mRNA is detectable early during the second trimester of gestation, well before its appearance as morphologically recognizable lamellar bodies and earlier than mRNA for SP-A, and is synthesized by both type II pneumocytes and bronchiolar Clara cells; its production is enhanced by glucocorticoids. Its biologically active form is derived from a much larger precursor protein and has the function of facilitating a reduction in surface tension. When associated with SP-A, it plays a major role in the transfor-

mation of the multilayered membranes of lamellar bodies into tubular myelin.

SP-C is a hydrophobic surfactant apoprotein synthesized by type II pneumocytes; genes for it are located on chromosome 8. mRNA is detectable early during the second trimester of gestation. It is markedly enhanced by glucocorticoids and is effective in facilitating phospholipid absorption.

SP-D, a hydrophilic collagenous glycoprotein, is encoded in chromosome 10 at the locus that also includes SP-A. It is secreted by both type II pneumocytes and Clara cells and is expressed during the canalicular phase of lung development. It is under the regulation of hormonal and growth factors and its mRNA can be upregulated by glycocorticoids. As a member of the C-type lectin family, which recognizes pathogens with carbohydrate-containing surfaces, it may have a prominent role in pulmonary defences against gram-negative bacteria and certain viruses. Furthermore, it interacts with macrophages through its carbohydrate binding domain and may have a significant clinical role in the respiratory distress syndrome both in the neonatal period and in adults. (Kuroki et al. 1988; Possmayer 1988; Strunk et al. 1988; Van Golde et al. 1988; Ryan et al. 1989; Tenner et al. 1989; Hawgood and Clements 1990; Oomen et al. 1990; Otto-Verberne et al. 1990; Kuroki et al. 1991; Phelps and Floros 1991; Weaver 1991; Venkatesh et al. 1993; Deterding et al. 1994; Kuan et al. 1994; Crapo and Wright 1995).

Surfactant metabolism is complex and at present many aspects remain speculative. The intracellular phase takes place in the type II pneumocytes, where endoplasmic reticulum and the Golgi apparatus play an important role in the production of structured lamellar bodies. Intra-alveolar secretion of surfactant is under the stimulus of several agents, including adrenergic agonists, cholinergic agents, mechanical factors, and prostaglandins. Once in the alveolar space intra-alveolar metabolism takes place and the secreted lamellar bodies are transformed into tubular myelin structures in the presence of calcium. The events at this stage, although not clearly understood, suggest that there is clearance of some of the material, degradation and incorporation by alveolar macrophages of a portion, and recycling and reprocessing of the remainder by type II pneumocytes, Clara cells and perhaps other parenchymal cells. Thus surfactant composition is both morphologically and functionally heterogeneous, and there are differences in form and activity which correlate with apoprotein content. It has three main functions: as a tenso-active material, as an anti-oedema barrier, and as an active and important agent in pulmonary defence. In addition, there are several secondary roles, in control of transepithelial transport of water and ions, in metabolism of xenobiotics, in defence against oxidative agents, in synthesis of components of the extracellular matrix, in reparation of cellular damage and in the defensive functions associated with alveolar macrophages, among others (Wright and Clement 1987; van Golde et al. 1988; Joyce-Brady and Brody 1990; Kobayashi et al. 1990; Voorhout et al. 1991; Kuroki et al. 1992; Wirtz and Schmidt 1992; Hawgood et al. 1993; Kondepudi and Johnson 1993; Murata et al. 1993; Neagos et al. 1993; Scott et al. 1993; Risco et al. 1994).

Glucocorticoids are known to accelerate lung maturation in the fetus by activating the synthesis and secretion of pulmonary surfactant, and administration of glucocorticoids (cortisol, dexamethasone) to mothers of premature infants at risk or to very premature babies has lowered significantly the incidence of respiratory distress syndrome in these groups. The effect appears to be a result of interaction between pulmonary interstitial fibroblasts, which are in direct contact with the type II pneumocytes and produce the *fibroblast pneumocyte factor*, which stimulates the type II cells. This activity, mediated by several

enzymes, accelerates the maturation of the granular pneumocytes, using the glycogen stored within the cells and resulting in a marked increase of lamellar inclusion bodies and maturation of the air–blood barrier. Thyroid hormones also accelerate fetal lung maturation, with early disappearance of glycogen from type II pneumocytes. Their administration results in a decrease in the incidence of respiratory distress syndrome, but the mechanism is unknown. It is possible that there is an interaction between the two hormones acting in synergy at different chemical sites or through the interstitial fibroblasts, which have surface receptors for both endogenous and exogenous corticosteroids whereas thyroid hormones have nuclear binding sites. Sex hormones also appear to play a role in lung maturation. Oestrogen accelerates lung maturation apparently by direct action on the lung or in cooperation with interstitial lung fibroblasts, which are partly responsible for sex difference in surfactant synthesis by type II pneumocytes. It has been shown that fibroblasts from female fetuses produce more fibroblast pneumocyte factor than those from males. Insulin receptors are also present on type II pneumocytes and are known to play an important role in the presence of high levels of insulin. Fetuses of diabetic mothers are both hyperglycaemic and hyperinsulinaemic, and this results in a diminished production of surfactant in this category, thus leading to respiratory distress syndrome (Van Golde et al. 1988; Shimizu et al. 1991; Kari et al. 1994).

It is generally accepted that pulmonary surfactant is deficient in infants presenting with hyaline membrane disease; however, it is not certain what factor(s) may be responsible for its absence from the lungs. Absence may be the result of inadequate production and secretion or of delayed synthesis in the immature lung. These speculations about the cause of the condition have led to the introduction of various therapeutic approaches to the mother as a prenatal preventive measure or to the newborn.

It is now apparent that respiratory distress syndrome in premature babies has clinical and physiopathological features similar to those encountered in the adult respiratory distress syndrome. The mechanisms by which the lung respond to various injuries (primary or secondary) are similar in infants, children and adults, although the response may be variable depending on the many factors involved in the process (Royall and Levin 1988; Donnelly and Haslett 1992; Davis et al. 1993).

Various lesions are found in association with hyaline membrane disease. *Pulmonary infection* is common in infants dying with this condition. The pulmonary infiltration may be mild or may involve large areas of several lobes or the entire lung.

Squamous debris may be observed in the terminal air spaces, suggesting the aspiration of amniotic fluid. *Pulmonary haemorrhage*, although less common, can also be associated with hyaline membrane disease. The haemorrhage can be focal, but occasionally presents as massive lesions. Pulmonary infection and haemorrhage can coexist with hyaline membranes (Fedrick and Butler 1970a).

Intraventricular haemorrhage is commonly associated with hyaline membrane disease. It is observed mainly among premature infants, especially among those weighing less than 1500 g. When associated with hyaline membrane disease, intraventricular haemorrhage is often the cause of death among infants dying early in the course of the illness, usually within the first 24 h of life (Fedrick and Butler 1970b; Machin 1975; Anderson et al. 1976; Wigglesworth et al. 1976; Leviton et al. 1977). *Tentorial tears* occur with elevated frequency in infants with hyaline membrane disease, mostly among infants of advanced gestational age, at or near term. Many of these cases have presented obstetric difficulties at the time of delivery (Barson 1978).

Complications Associated with Therapy. Bronchopulmonary dysplasia remains the most significant complication in premature babies of low birth weight (below 1500 g) receiving oxygen at high concentrations and artificial ventilation at high pressures for long periods (3–4 weeks). The morphological changes are variable and depend on a number of elements, including gestational age, duration and mode of treatment, and possible associated infections. Macroscopically the general appearance depends on the many factors described above, but the cut surface reveals collapsed areas alternating with emphysematous zones. Both the clinical and pathological features have been divided into phases or stages, but with much overlapping.

Histologically, in the early stages of the disease there is necrosis of the epithelial cells lining the distal bronchi, bronchioles and terminal airways, associated with an interstitial oedema involving the vessel walls. There is widespread capillary damage with intraluminal and interstitial haemorrhages. At later stages the interstitial oedema has regressed, but it leaves marked thickening following fibroblastic and myofibroblastic proliferation (Fig. 7.39) associated with a predominantly mononuclear inflammatory reaction. Regenerative changes of the bronchial and bronchiolar epithelium take place with some degree of hyperplasia and squamous metaplasia. In severe cases there is obliterative bronchitis and bronchiolitis, often associated with marked squamous metaplasia of the epithelium. The muscular layers of the bronchi and bronchioles are thickened and there is fibrosis of

the adventitia. There is fibrous thickening of the alveolar septae (often infiltrated by inflammatory cells), and the alveoli may contain macrophages and inflammatory cells. The lung parenchyma presents areas of hyperexpansion and/or emphysematous zones. Hyperplasia and hypertrophy of the pulmonary arteries and arterioles are not uncommon findings. The lymphatics may appear normal or somewhat distended and surrounded by inflammation. There is muscularization of the intra-acinar arterioles, indicative of pulmonary hypertension. In infants with bronchopulmonary dysplasia who have survived for long periods, fibrosis is usually very extensive and hyperexpansion is more widespread. There is marked reduction in the peripheral arterial density.

Pneumothorax, pneumomediastinum with pneumopericardium and sometimes gas embolism are complications generally related to positive pressure ventilation especially among very low birth weight babies. They may be responsible for the high morbidity and mortality rates in this age group; retrolental fibroplasia is related to oxygen toxicity.

Although the heart may be normal in size, there is often hypertrophy of either the right or the left ventricle or both, sometimes associated with transient systemic hypertension. There may also be areas of scarring, predominantly in the papillary muscles. The ductus arteriosus, especially in the very premature, may remain patent and present abnormalities of its wall (necrosis, abnormal elastic lamina) resulting in additional complications (left to right shunting) with unfavourable outcomes. For these reasons many centres insist on closing the ductus either by surgery or by medication. The neuroendocrine cells, and especially the neuroendocrine bodies of the lung, are usually increased in number (Rosan 1975; Bonikos et al. 1976; Anderson and Engel 1983; Stocker 1986; Westgren et al. 1986; Erickson et al. 1987; Northway 1990; Northway et al. 1990; Gorenflo et al. 1991; Van Lierde et al. 1991; Crapo and Wright 1995).

Interstitial pulmonary emphysema is often associated with barotrauma due to positive pressure ventilation in the very premature baby, resulting in air leaks and dissection of the lung parenchyma mainly along the bronchovascular bundles. The condition may be acute, occurring within the first week, or persistent over longer periods. In the acute phase, the air cysts may be located in one or more lobes or involve both lungs; they are usually peripheral in the form of numerous bullae of variable sizes scattered below the distended pleura. Histologically they are located in the region of the interlobular septa and peribronchial spaces, resulting in compression of the neighbouring structures (Fig. 7.40a). In persistent interstitial emphysema the bullae are numerous, of variable size, often widespread and larger than those seen in baro-

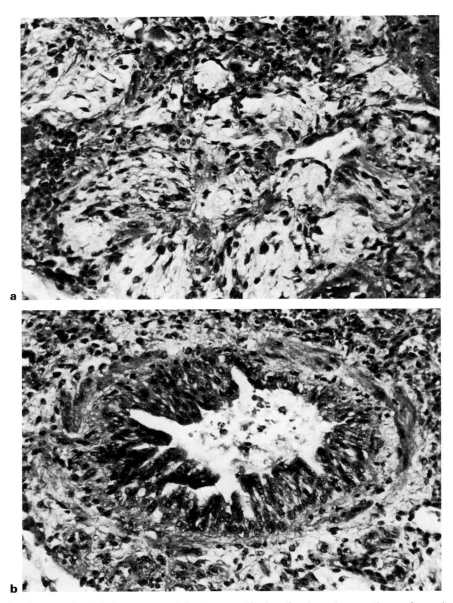

Fig. 7.39. Bronchopulmonary dysplasia in a premature infant as a complication of prolonged oxygen therapy for respiratory distress syndrome. **a** Alveolar saccules obliterated by proliferating fibroblastic tissue. **b** Metaplasia of the bronchial epithelium. (H&E, × 225)
Continued on next page

trauma, and involve most of the lung, often associated with bronchopulmonary dysplasia. On section, the cut surface may present a Swiss cheese appearance. Histologically, the bullae are bordered by a fibrous wall of variable thickness lined by foreign body giant cells, alone or in strings (Fig. 7.40b). The adjacent parenchyma is generally compressed (Stocker and Madewell 1977; Stocker 1986; Morisot et al. 1990).

Three elements appear to have major roles in the pathogenesis of the lesions: the developmental immaturity of the lung parenchyma, barotrauma due to high ventilation pressures, and oxygen toxicity. Recent studies suggest that high ventilation pressures on the epithelial structures of the distal airways (which are undergoing continuous differentiation and maturation) cause epithelial disruption at the time when the various components of surfactant are

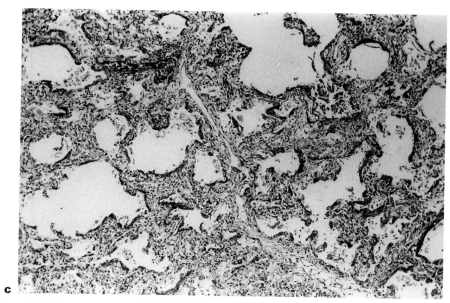

Fig. 7.39. (*continued*) **c** Marked alveolar thickening associated with thick scarred areas and organizing hyaline membranes in the lung of a 628-g premature infant after 5½ weeks' survival. (Masson's trichrome, × 20)

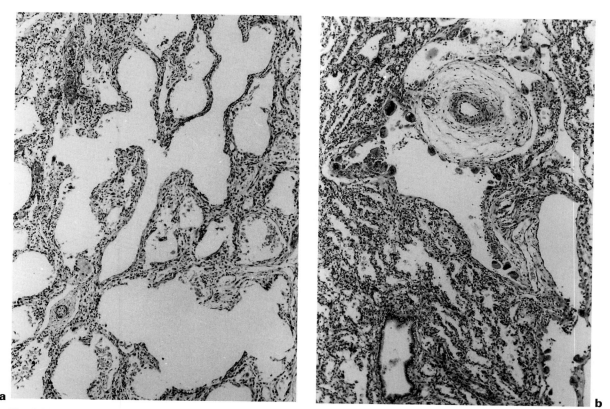

Fig. 7.40. a Acute interstitial pulmonary emphysema showing radial cystic dilatations bordered in places by compressed airspaces. (H&E, × 20) **b** Persistent interstitial pulmonary emphysema. The irregular cystic walls are lined by giant cells, alone or in strings. (H&E, × 50)

incompletely organized. The high levels of oxygen delivered create toxic radicals whose action at the immature cell junctions causes disruption of cellular contacts at sites where the concentration of protective antioxidant enzymes and factors promoting lung differentiation and regeneration are low, leading to lung tissue damage. This encourages an inflammatory reaction with the accumulation of neutrophils and macrophages in the lumen of the airways. The proteolytic enzymes liberated by the neutrophils may cause further damage to the lung parenchyma, and the cytokines and growth factors secreted by the macrophages may result in an excess production of fibronectin and provoke pulmonary fibrosis.

Specific immunohistochemistry on fetal lung tissue has shown that the superoxide dismutases are closely related to lung maturation and that copper–zinc superoxide dismutase is low in intensity and area distribution in both hyaline membrane disease and bronchopulmonary dysplasia, whereas manganese superoxide dismutase is unaltered in hyaline membrane disease but increased in bronchopulmonary dysplasia. These results have produced a change of attitudes in the prevention and treatment of these conditions (Walti et al. 1989; Margraf et al. 1990; Northway 1990; Papadopoulos et al. 1990; Dobashi et al. 1993; Jacobson et al. 1993; Groneck et al. 1994). Several authors have now turned their attention to the nutritional states of premature babies prone to develop bronchopulmonary dysplasia; others have concentrated on antioxidant protection. Vitamins A, C and E together with some metallic ions have been introduced as preventive and therapeutic measures to enhance the premature lung's defence mechanisms and favour a more appropriate repair (Frank and Sosenko 1988; Kurzner et al. 1988; Fariss 1990; Northway 1990; Shenai and Chytil 1990).

Late sequelae of bronchopulmonary dysplasia are as follows. Alveolar septal fibrosis may be variable in quantity and distribution, and is usually more severe in infants of very low birth weight. There are important residual or active lesions of the tracheobronchial tree, often with squamous metaplasia of the mucosa associated with a chronic mononuclear inflammatory reaction. Ulceration of the mucosa is an occasional finding. Hyperplasia of the bronchial and bronchiolar muscle layers is constant, sometimes with scarring of the submucosal tissue. Bronchial gland hyperplasia is prominent. Alveolar septal fibrosis may be minimal, moderate or severe, and in some cases diffuse with scarred areas. The alveoli often contain macrophages, some of which contain iron pigment, as well as inflammatory cells. Some cases present with emphysematous or cystic lesions consistent with persistent pulmonary emphysema,

and this has led some authors to postulate that these features in longstanding cases are the pathological correlates of the radiological images classically described in the Wilson–Mikity syndrome. Others have shown, however, that this syndrome is associated with a high incidence of intrauterine infection. The important point is that the alveolar population is reduced, large and simplified, and that there is a severe and persistent reduction in alveolar multiplication with little evidence of compensatory alveolar development, resulting in decreased lung volume and size. There is also an abnormal distribution of elastic fibres. The arteries and arterioles show thickening of their muscular layers and muscularization of the intra-acinar arterioles, whose lumen may be significantly reduced. Perivascular fibrosis is prominent, together with that of the interlobular septa, which often extend to the thickened pleura. Secondary infection, bacterial and/or viral, may provoke further lung injury and be detrimental to these patients (Stocker 1986; Erickson et al. 1987; Fujimura et al. 1989; Nakamura et al. 1990; Margraf et al. 1991; Gillan and Cutz 1993).

Although most survivors of bronchopulmonary dysplasia have apparently normal development, others suffer from various symptoms. These children may have weights below those of age-matched controls, and their head circumference is also somewhat smaller. Some patients are more susceptible to frequent and repeated lung infections; others present with exercise-induced bronchospasm with air trapping. Neurological sequelae are a major problem and may be non-progressive or progressive. In the former, there are deficiencies in coordination, a greater need for academic support, and hearing abnormalities (among others); in the latter, there is a progressive encephalopathy with seizures, movement disorders with progressive neurologic deterioration and even death (Perlman and Volpe 1989; Northway et al. 1990; Blayney et al. 1991; Vohr et al. 1991; Giffin et al. 1994; Crapo and Wright 1995).

Within recent years *extracorporeal membrane oxygenation* has become an established mode of therapy for neonatal respiratory failure (meconium aspiration, congenital diaphragmatic hernia, persistent pulmonary hypertension, shock, respiratory distress syndrome) in neonates unresponsive to conventional treatment. There are several complications which may result from the use of this treatment, of which the most common are central nervous system haemorrhages, infarcts and haemorrhages in various organs. In the lung, interstitial and intra-alveolar haemorrhages associated with hyaline membrane formation appeared within the first 2 days, and reactive epithelial hyperplasia of the distal airways, squamous metaplasia and smooth muscle hyperplasia occurred between the second and third days, followed by interstitial fibrosis after a week. Various other lesions have been described after longer applications of this treatment (Chou et al. 1993; Beca and Butt 1994; Kanto 1994; Walsh-Sukys et al. 1994).

Surfactant replacement therapy is now widely used for the treatment of respiratory distress syndrome and also as a preventive measure for neonates of very low birth weight susceptible to develop the syndrome. Since its introduction there has been a significant decline in morbidity and mortality rate among premature newborns. There are numerous compositions of surfactants, many of which carry special brand names, and several collaborative group studies are in progress. Several reports have indicated a slight increase of pulmonary haemorrhage among infants receiving surfactant therapy. Haemorrhage appears to be more prevalent in the intra-alveolar spaces, but some authors have not observed any difference between intra-alveolar and septal spaces. Globular deposits of hyaline material were observed in the alveolar spaces by some authors but no hyaline membranes, whereas others, like ourselves, have noticed typical hyaline membranes in some infants as well as haemorrhages (Pinar et al. 1993; Pramanik et al. 1993; Raju and Langenberg 1993; Pappin et al. 1994; Berry et al. 1994; Gortner et al. 1994; Thornton et al. 1994). Prenatal glucocorticoid administered to mothers at risk, in combination with exogenous surfactant therapy to the newborn, has recently been introduced and gives favourable results. (Jobe et al. 1993; Leviton et al. 1993; Kari et al. 1994; Schwartz et al. 1994).

Persistent pulmonary hypertension (persistent fetal *circulation*) may be the cause of respiratory failure in the newborn. It is often described in association with meconium aspiration syndrome, perinatal asphyxia, intrapartum infection, congenital diaphragmatic hernia and elective repeat caesarean delivery. It is most often encountered in those born at term or in post-term infants who present with shunting across the foramen ovale and/or ductus arteriosus accompanied by severe hypoxaemia. Morphologically the right ventricle is usually hypertrophic, and the characteristic histological finding is muscularization of intra-acinar pulmonary arteries, which are normally non-muscularized or only partially muscularized (Fig. 7.41a). Treatment in a number of centres consists of administration of *nitric oxide*, which is known rapidly and selectively to relieve pulmonary vasoconstriction; Other centres have used extracorporeal membrane oxygenation. The lungs in infants receiving nitric oxide in this setting may show hyperplasia of the bronchial and bronchiolar mucosa with a depletion of goblet cells together with a marked hyperplasia of type II pneumocytes (Fig. 7.41b).

These changes may be apparent as early as 2 days after establishment of treatment (Heritage and Cunningham 1985; Haworth 1987, 1993; Pison et al. 1993; Roberts and Shaul 1993; Zopal et al. 1994).

Pulmonary hypertension may also be observed in infants and children with cardiac malformations of various types, bronchopulmonary dysplasia, SIDS, sickle cell disease, intravenous drug addiction and congenital myotonic dystrophy among others (Williams et al. 1979; Dupuis et al. 1993; Haworth 1993; Rais-Bahrami et al. 1994).

Common Infections

Bacterial

The antibiotic era has dramatically modified the morphological appearances of inflammation of the pulmonary parenchyma. This is especially true in the industrialized nations, where both mortality and morbidity rates have been significantly reduced. In many developing nations, however, these modifications are less spectacular and classic pathological lesions can still be encountered among infants and children and the aged, principally because of inadequate medical services and poor handling of antibiotics. Inflammation of the lung in infants and children is by far the most common pathological lesion observed at autopsy, and may be the primary cause of death or a terminal episode accompanying other pathological conditions.

In lobar *pneumonia*, a lobe, an entire lung or both lungs may be involved at any one time. The lesions usually begin in the terminal air spaces or alveoli and spread to adjacent tissue. The involved lobes show lesions at the same stage of evolution. In the case of *bronchopneumonia*, the primary inflammatory reaction begins in the distal respiratory tract, extending into the surrounding parenchyma; lesions are generally at various stages of evolution. It is not necessary to describe the typical pathological features of pneumonia, with its characteristic four stages, but certain specific features should be considered.

Streptococcus. Streptococcal infections are an important cause of pulmonary infections among infants and children. *Streptococcus pneumoniae* is the principal cause of lobar pneumonia in this age group, especially after the first year of life, when over 90% of cases of pneumonia are related to this organism. Bacteria can be demonstrated in the lung in large numbers in the early stages of the disease. The various products and toxins produced by organisms are responsible for their virulence, independently or in combinations. Pneumococcal pneumonia may be

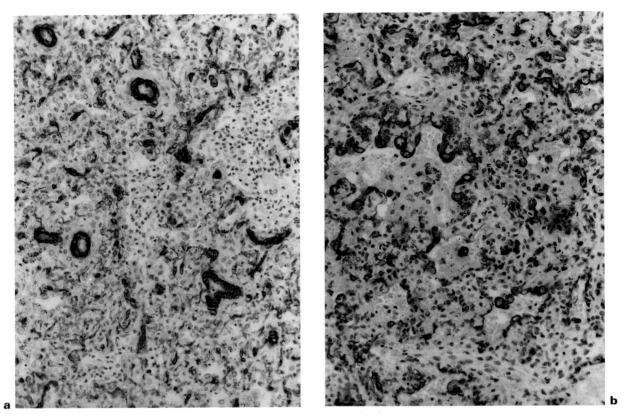

Fig. 7.41. a Persistent pulmonary hypertension: thickened muscularized intra-acinar arteries with stenosis of their lumini. (Smooth muscle α-actin, × 160) **b** Hyperplasia of type II pneumocytes after 36 hours of NO treatment, keratin CAM-5.4, × 160.

found to be associated with viral or other infectious agents when infants are carefully investigated. Lung abscesses and empyema are significant complications and septicaemia may occur in rare instances, especially in the neonatal period. (Naylor and Wagner 1985; Tomashefski et al. 1989; Webber et al. 1990; Johnston 1991; Boulnois 1992).

Other types of streptococcal infection (β-haemolytic) can occasionally cause lobar pneumonia, but are more often the cause of bronchopneumonia. The involved lung is oedematous but the inflammatory response is moderate, with only scattered aggregates of polymorphonuclear leucocytes. Interstitial haemorrhages are common, and typical and atypical hyaline membranes may form. Gram-positive cocci are identifiable (Cayeux 1972; Franciosi et al. 1973; Ablow et al. 1976; Slack and Mayon-White 1978).

Staphylococcus. Staphylococcal infections usually produce bronchopneumonia. The great majority of cases occur within the first year of life, and may occur in small epidemics, especially among children in hospital. Staphylococcal infection is commonly

associated with cystic fibrosis or other underlying conditions (Bryan and Reynolds 1984).

The affected lung is consolidated and shows focal haemorrhagic areas. The pleura may be covered by a fibrinous exudate, and empyema is not rare. The alveoli are usually filled with erythrocytes, oedema fluid and a few polymorphonuclear leucocytes. Sometimes macrophages are abundant, containing numerous microorganisms. Necrosis, often leading to abscess formation, is common. Interstitial emphysema and pneumatoceles are frequent complications of staphylococcal infections, and may cause pneumothorax (Oliver et al. 1959; Klein 1969; Boisset 1972; Gooch and Britt 1978; Asher et al. 1982).

Haemophilus. *Haemophilus influenzae* infection of the lung is increasing in frequency in the paediatric age group. It may be a cause of the respiratory distress syndrome in the neonate (Speer et al. 1978). The bacillus is a common inhabitant of the nasopharynx, and often causes acute laryngotracheobronchitis and bronchopneumonia. All lobes of the lungs can be involved, but the lower lobes are most often affected.

Well defined nodules around bronchi and bronchioles filled with pus are seen, with destruction of the bronchiolar epithelium and a mucopurulent exudate in the lumen. The bronchial and bronchiolar walls are infiltrated by mononuclear cells, chiefly lymphocytes, and some polymorphonuclear leucocytes. The inflammatory reaction extends into the surrounding alveoli, where oedema and interstitial haemorrhage may be found. Thrombosis of small vessels occurs in the acute phase of infection, and longstanding infections may produce obstruction of the bronchioles (Nicholls et al. 1975; Asmar et al. 1978b; Bale and Watkins 1978; Lilien et al. 1978). The recent introduction of a *H. influenzae* type B polysaccharide vaccine for children, which appears to give effective coverage except in those who present with some form of immune deficiency or other genetic factors, may have some effect on the frequency of this condition in the near future. Recent studies suggest that *H. influenzae* infection is principally a secondary infection to other bacterial and viral infections (Granoff et al. 1986; Korppi et al. 1992; Sawyer et al. 1994).

Escherichia. *Escherichia coli* is an important cause of gastrointestinal infections and septicaemia in the newborn period, and such infections are usually accompanied by neonatal (intrauterine) pneumonia. Histologically, the alveoli are filled with polymorphonuclears and macrophages, and are rich in fibrin. *E. coli* pneumonia is common after the 4th week of life. It can occasionally cause a pneumatocele (Klein 1969; Kuhn and Lee 1973).

Klebsiella. *Klebsiella pneumoniae* (Friedländer's bacillus) occasionally causes bronchopneumonia in infants and children. It is often associated with other bacterial or viral infections and is important in children with immunodeficiency states or in those receiving cytotoxic drugs for the treatment of malignancy. The lung in these cases shows many consolidated nodules of variable sizes disseminated in one or more lobes of both lungs. In the acute phase there is marked oedema extending into the interlobar spaces, alveolar destruction and a polymorphonuclear leucocyte infiltration. *Klebsiella* bacilli are numerous in gram-stained sections. These lesions often lead to abcess formation, and pneumatoceles may be encountered (Papageorgiou et al. 1973; Barter and Hudson 1974).

Pseudomonas. *Pseudomonas aeruginosa (Bacillus pyocyaneus)* affects premature infants and may be the cause of epidemics in nurseries. It is often found in children treated with broad-spectrum antibiotics, steroids or cytotoxic drugs. The lungs show firm irregular nodules, greenish-yellow in colour, scattered throughout the parenchyma, which is oedematous. The pleural cavities may contain a haemorrhagic pleural effusion. Histologically, the nodules often show a central necrotic zone and a polymorphonuclear leucocytic infiltrate surrounded by haemorrhagic areas. The distal arteries contain fibrinous thrombi, and organisms are frequently observed in the vessel walls.

Moraxella catarrhalis (Branchamella). Commonly known as *Neisseria catarrhalis*, this commensal microorganism of the upper respiratory tract may also be the cause of pulmonary infections, often in association with viral infection in childhood (Korppi et al. 1992).

Listeria. *Listeria monocytogenes* is a gram-positive motile bacillus, which has been associated with epidemics of abortion and encephalitis in animals. The exact distribution of the disease is not known, and its prevalence seems to be much higher in continental Europe than in the UK, the USA and Canada. Human infection is supposedly contracted by contact with infected animals, although proof of this means of transmission has not often been established (see also p. 736).

The disease can affect both infants and adults, and presents in various clinical forms. Epidemics have been described mostly in relation with contaminated food or food products, and in most instances, of the many known serotypes, type 4b is the most frequently incriminated. The condition is also described in debilitated patients, the immunocompromised and those with acquired immune deficiency syndrome (AIDS). In paediatrics, it is most common in the perinatal period, presenting either in a generalized form (*granulomatosis infantiseptica*) or as meningitis. Infection usually occurs during the second half of pregnancy and may be the cause of premature delivery, stillbirth or repeated abortions. Intrauterine infection can be acquired transplacentally, resulting in widespread lesions of various organs, or via the membranes, when the lung and gastrointestinal tract are mainly involved, probably as a result of aspiration and ingestion of infected amniotic fluid. Infection may also be acquired during delivery as the infant passes through the birth canal. Such infants usually present with meningitis in the first 10 days of life (Khong et al. 1986; Klatt et al. 1986a; Schlech 1986; McLauchlin 1990a, b; Svare et al. 1991).

In listerial infection, the lung may be normal in appearance or it may be heavy and firm with numerous minute whitish nodules on both the pleural and the cut surfaces. Haemorrhagic areas may also be observed. Similar lesions may be seen on the skin,

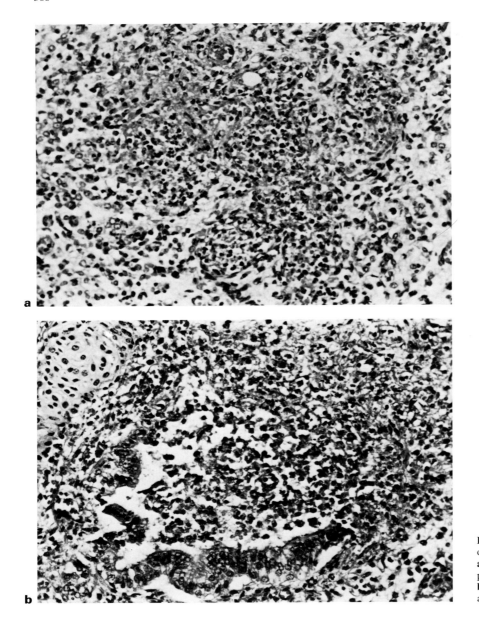

Fig. 7.42 Listeriosis in a 3-day-old baby girl. (H&E, × 120)
a Confluent microabscesses in the pulmonary parenchyma.
b Necrosis of the bronchial wall and adjacent tissue.

where they present as a purpuric rash, and in other organs and the placenta.

Microscopically, the nodules are focal areas of necrosis or small granulomas, occasionally surrounded by congested vessels or haemorrhagic zones. The bronchi may be ulcerated or involved in the granulomatous process (Fig. 7.42). The necrotic tissue contains cellular debris and pyknotic nuclei and some mononuclear leucocytes. Gram staining reveals numerous gram-positive bacilli; some of the rods may appear gram-negative, and some take the shape of a comma. The vessel wall may be involved in the necrotic process, resulting in focal haemorrhages.

Legionnaires' Disease. Since the discovery of pneumonia called by the Legionnaires' disease bacterium, *Legionella pneumophila,* several other species have been identified (*L. micdadei, L. longbeachae, L. wadsworthii,* etc.) and there are some 28 known species, but in humans. *L. pneumophila* is by far the most prevalent cause of infection at all ages. It is known to occur in epidemics or sporadically, and, although it is not an uncommon cause of pneumonia, the exact mode of transmission is still not clearly defined. The disease is often associated with contamination of water distribution systems, cooling towers and air conditioners. Pulmonary damage is due apparently to tissue-destructive protease liberated by the organism, leading to the various histological pictures observed in this condition. The aetiological agent is a gram-negative bacterium, which has special staining qualities in tissues and requires special media for its culture. The lungs show areas of consolidation and resemble lungs affected by confluent bronchopneumonia or lobar pneumonia, often with a fibrinous pleuritis. Pleural effusion is common. The alveoli contain an exudate that is rich in polynuclear leucocytes, macrophages and fibrin. Extensive lysis of the exudate, in areas, is a common feature, and abscess formation is not altogether uncommon. The oedematous and congested alveolar septa show areas of necrosis and an inflammatory reaction. Hyaline membranes may be associated with the lesions. Bronchial necrosis is common in affected areas. Legionnaires' disease bacterium can be demonstrated in the cells of the inflammatory exudate and cytoplasmic debris by the Dieterle silver stain (Fig. 7.43) or by immunohistochemical techniques. The majority of fatal cases have so far been diagnosed in adults, but children have also been affected. It is observed in patients after organ transplants, those receiving corticotherapy or cytotoxic drugs and in AIDS (Muldoon et al. 1981; Baskerville et al. 1986; Muder et al. 1986; Korvick and Yu 1987; Williams et al. 1987; Ezaki et al. 1990; Halablab et al. 1990).

Chlamydiaceae. This family of obligate intracellular bacterial parasites depends on the host cell for ATP metabolites. It is made up of three distinct species of *Chlamydia*:

1. *C. trachomatis*, responsible primarily for urogenital and conjunctival diseases in humans, may also be the cause of upper and/or lower respiratory disease especially in infancy and those with immunodeficiency states
2. *C. psittaci* (*ornithosis*), aetiologic organism of infection in birds and transmissible to humans
3. *C. pneumoniae* (TWAR strains), known to cause upper and lower respiratory infections, including pneumonia in humans, especially in the young, the immunocompromised and the aged

The organisms present in two forms: an infectious metabolically inactive form, the *elementary body*, and a non-infectious metabolically active intracellular form, the *reticulate body*. They have a worldwide distribution, but appear to be more prevalent among peoples of lower socioeconomic status.

C. trachomatis is known to colonize the lower genitourinary tract in humans. In pregnancy the organisms may attain the uterine mucosa, resulting in chorioamnionitis and eventually intrauterine infection

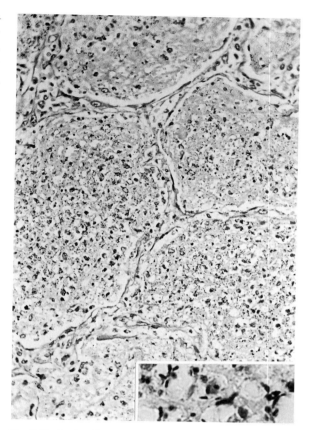

Fig. 7.43. *Legionella pneumophila* pneumonia. The alveoli are filled with inflammatory cells and necrotic tissue containing large quantities of bacteria stained by the Dieterle technique. (× 363; *inset* × 513)

of the fetus, with possible premature delivery and low birth weight of the fetus. However, most infections appear to occur during the passage of the fetus in the birth canal at normal delivery. Symptoms may therefore occur between the first and third weeks after delivery and they are non-specific. In infancy *C. trachomatis* may be associated with other pulmonary infections (viral, mycoplasmal, bacterial), conjunctivitis, diarrhoea and sepsis. The pulmonary lesions are non-specific. Diagnosis is usually made by serological examination (IgG, IgM) or on tissue sections by Giemsa or iodine stains. Immunohistochemistry and ultrastructural studies are useful in confirming the diagnosis.

C. psittaci is not altogether uncommon among bird fanciers (psittacosis, parrot fever), who may present with a febrile illness, high fever, episodes of persistent cough and frequent headaches accompanied by bronchopneumonia. The pulmonary lesions are non-specific, and the diagnosis is usually made on serological examination or immunohistochemistry.

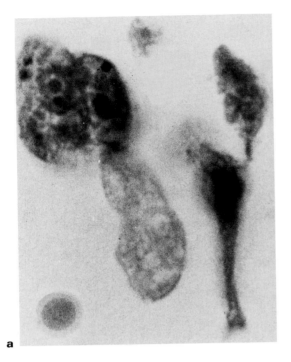

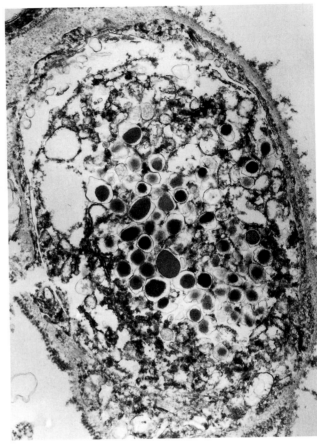

Fig. 7.44. a *C. pneumoniae* in intra-alveolar macrophages. (Giemsa × 330) **b** Ultrastructure showing oval forms surrounded by a wide halo suggestive of *C. pneumoniae*. (Electron micrograph, × 6560, reduced)

C. pneumoniae (TWAR) is associated with infections of the upper respiratory tract (sinusitis, pharyngitis) and the lungs, where it is responsible for bronchitis and pneumonia especially among young adults, the aged and the immunocompromised (AIDS, transplant patients). The infection is often associated with other pulmonary infections, primarily viral, in which case it may present as ARDS, multinodular bronchopneumonia or necrotizing pneumonia. Pneumothorax and mediastinal emphysema may be associated complications, and the condition may be the cause of chronic obstructive pulmonary disease. The disease can be both endemic and epidemic, and has a growing list of extrapulmonary manifestations. Its role in coronary artery disease is under investigation. Diagnosis is usually made by specialized serological tests and isolation from culture systems. Special stains, immunohistochemistry, molecular biology techniques and ultrastructural studies are additional methods applied on BAL fluids or lung biopsies (Fig. 7.44) as important aids in arriving at a correct diagnosis (Chi et al. 1987; Madan et al. 1988; Grayston et al. 1990; Klingebiel et al. 1989; Lundemose et al. 1989; Griffin et al. 1990; Kazanjians and Mark 1990; Shurbaji et al. 1990; Donders et al. 1991; Matsumato et al. 1991; Straumann Kunz et al. 1991; Marrie 1993; Blasi et al. 1994; Herrmann et al. 1994).

Viral

Viral infections of the respiratory system are very common among infants and children. The viruses involved are varied, and new strains are isolated and identified each year. They usually affect the entire respiratory system and can cause severe damage to the lung parenchyma. The lesions produced by many viruses are histologically similar, and as a result one cannot rely solely on histological changes to establish a diagnosis with certainty. Furthermore, viral infections of the lung are not infrequently associated with one or more bacterial infections.

Where a viral infection is suspected, tissue should be taken for culture and for immunological and ultrastructural studies if adequate facilities exist. Serum should also be preserved for appropriate examination. It is only by the isolation or identification of the virus that a definitive diagnosis can be established.

Cytomegalovirus Infection. Cytomegalovirus (DNA virus) is a member of the herpesvirus group, of which there are at least seven members (herpes simplex virus type I and II, varicella zoster virus, cytomegalovirus, Epstein–Barr virus and human herpesvirus 6 (HHP-6 and HHV-7)). It has a worldwide distribution and appears to be more prevalent among the lower socioeconomic group. Infection by the virus in childhood may be acquired in utero (congenital), perinatally or postnatally (see also p. 739):

1. *Congenital (intrauterine) infection* may occur in as many as 1%–2% of all newborns. Severe intrauterine infection, especially in the early part of the first half of pregnancy, may be the cause of death of the fetus in utero owing to disseminated disease. It has now become evident that maternal acquired immunity before pregnancy provides protection for the fetus. At birth these newborns are often asymptomatic of infection and the sequelae are limited and much less severe, although some may have viraemia and/or secrete the virus in their saliva for months or even years after birth. Infants whose mothers present with a primary infection during pregnancy are more likely to present symptoms at birth, with severe sensorineural hearing loss and severe handicap as a result of various neurological symptoms due to brain damage of varying degrees. These observations have further stimulated questions about vaccination campaigns against this virus. The disease has also been reported in siblings from consecutive pregnancies.

2. *Perinatal infection* is believed to be acquired during delivery, probably from the cervix, as the infant passes through the birth canal, and it is assumed that infants infected in this way are usually asymptomatic. Accumulating evidence now points to the fact that infection is not limited to the mucosa of the birth canal, but that uterine mucosa and endothelial cells may serve as reservoirs for the virus, and that environmental factors, virus reactivation during pregnancy and maternal antibody may all have important roles in the timing of primary infections. Furthermore, like many authors, we have been able to demonstrate by immunohistochemistry widespread placental involvement where at birth the infant was clinically normal. The reasons for the type of clinical presentation (symptomatic/asymptomatic) is still uncertain. Maeda et al. (1994), found that immedi-

ate early antigens (proteins) were seldom demonstrated in intrauterine cytomegalovirus infection; this may result from the dynamics of viral replication. These depend on the duration of the infection and the immaturity of the immune response.

3. *Postnatal infection* is considered to be common, and is generally asymptomatic. The mode of transmission is varied and infants in daytime maternal homes as well as adolescents with a high frequency of promiscuity are usually exposed to a high rate of infection. Among the most frequently incriminated is blood transfusion, in which case the patient may present with a syndrome referred to as *cytomegalovirus mononucleosis*. This has clinical and haematological features resembling those of infectious mononucleosis, but there is a negative Paul–Bunnell reaction. Infection by the virus is also prevalent among infants receiving chemotherapy for malignant disease in immunodeficiency states, in those with monoclonal macroglobulinaemia, and in those with renal allografts treated with immunosuppressive agents. Many of these patients present with interstitial pneumonitis.

Cytomegalovirus infection of the lung has also been observed with other pulmonary conditions, such as hyaline membrane disease, congenital syphilis, bacterial or viral pneumonias, and *Pneumocystis carinii* infection. It is one of the most common infections encountered after transplantation of organs, as well as among patients with AIDS, and is responsible for high morbidity and mortality rates among these patients, often in association with other viral (including HHV-6), mycotic and/or bacterial infections. Its transmission through blood transfusions is of great hazard, especially to recipients of organ transplants (Gorelkin et al. 1986; Griffiths and Grundy 1987; Paradis et al. 1988; Porter et al. 1990; Demmler 1991; Fowler et al. 1992; Yow and Demmler 1992; Huang et al. 1993; Bauman et al. 1994; Furukawa et al. 1994).

On gross examination the lungs may show little change unless affected by some other condition. Histologically the diagnosis may go unnoticed if one is not attentive. The presence of the characteristic viral inclusion with its clear halo (owl's eye) in some other organ (kidney, liver, pancreas, salivary gland, etc.) may draw the pathologist's attention to possible pulmonary involvement. Careful examination will reveal an occasional grossly hyperplastic alveolar cell with its intranuclear inclusion. In severe disseminated pulmonary disease the virus is observed in the nuclei or cytoplasm of the enlarged alveolar lining cells and is sometimes seen free in the alveoli (Fig. 7.45). In the early stages, the intranuclear inclusions are aci-

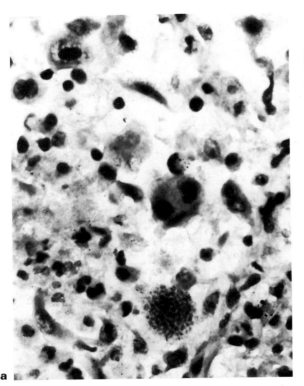
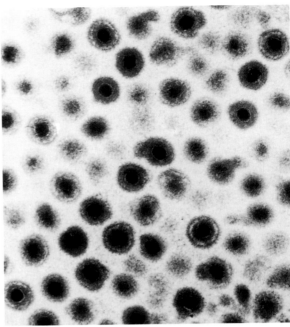

Fig. 7.45. a Cytomegalovirus inclusion disease in a 6-day-old premature girl. (In situ hybridization, × 430) **b** Electron micrograph showing the virus elements. (Courtesy of Dr J. Briner)

dophilic, but they become basophilic with time. The acidophilic intranuclear inclusion body stains purple with Masson's trichrome, and the intracytoplasmic inclusions stain intensely with PAS stain or Giemsa. Gomori's methenamine silver and Masson–Goldner stains are also helpful in identifying the virus. More specific staining with the immunoperoxidase antibody technique, in situ hybridization (alone or in combination), molecular biology and ultrastructural examination can help to identify the many strains of this structurally diverse collection of viruses. The cytoplasm of the infected cell is basophilic and granular. There is no inflammatory reaction unless secondary infection occurs. Bronchial and bronchiolar epithelial cells may be infected in addition to the epithelial cells of the peribronchial glands. Viral inclusions can often be demonstrated in endothelial cells of blood vessels.

Human Herpesvirus 6 (HHV-6). This recently identified herpesvirus is ubiquitous in the human population, with over 90% seroconversion by 3 years. There are two types (A and B), which are highly prevalent and last for a lifetime. The virus is known to be the causative agent of exanthem subitum (roseola) in infancy, often associated with a febrile illness and sometimes with seizures and encephalopathy. It may, on occasion, present with a mononucleosis-like syndrome or, more likely, a varied spectrum of ill-defined clinical manifestations which could, in some instances, lead to a fatal outcome. Fever, otitis and upper and lower respiratory tract symptoms are the most characteristic presentations, often associated with gastroenteritis, hepatitis and even viraemia. Pneumonitis is often documented in association with the virus, especially in the immunocomprised host and transplant patients, principally after bone marrow transplantation. Although HHV-6 is genetically similar to cytomegalovirus, with which it shares many characteristics, it is distinct biologically, immunologically and by molecular analysis from other herpesviruses. The virus can be demonstrated in peripherial mononuclear cells and saliva in older children and adults, and its genome and DNA in salivary and bronchial glands, which may explain latent infections. It has also been localized in macrophages in lymph nodes (Hodgkin's disease, Kikuchi lymphadenitis). Very recently lymphotropic herpesvirus (human herpes virus-7, HHV-7) has been identified, making the future very bright for surprises as to the role of these viruses in the pathology of the respiratory system (Pruksananoda et al. 1992; Agut 1993; Akashi et al. 1993; Cone et al. 1993; Dewhurst et al. 1993; Drobyski et al. 1994; Asano et al. 1994; Ward and Gray 1994; Asano et al. 1995).

Measles (Rubeola) Pneumonia (see also p. 771). Measles is caused by an RNA virus of the myxovirus group. The disease is still common in countries with low socioeconomic status and those with little or no immunization programmes, and it occurs in epidemics. In these countries, pulmonary complications are common and the mortality rate is high, especially among children suffering from various types of malnutrition. Secondary bacterial infection is common and is responsible for the high mortality rate in many series. Fatal cases have been described in apparently healthy children and in adults or patients with immunological disorders, including those receiving cytotoxic or immunosuppressive treatments for malignancies. The majority of these patients do not present the exanthema characteristic of the disease and have not necessarily had previous contact with patients suffering from the disease.

Atypical pulmonary lesions are known to occur and persist in individuals receiving killed measles vaccine, and fatal cases of measles pneumonia have been recorded after the administration of live measles vaccine to infants with immunodeficiency disorders (Mihatsch et al. 1972). In recent years the condition has made its reappearance among young army recruits and adolescents in countries where vaccination programmes were not properly carried out.

The main feature of the pulmonary lesion is the multinucleated syncytial giant cell, which should be distinguished from the pathognomonic giant (Warthin–Finkeldey) cell observed in the lymphoid tissues during the prodromal stage of the disease or in the very early phase of the rash. Hecht's giant-cell pneumonia was formerly considered to be a separate entity; however, recent studies have shown that the virus responsible for this condition is identical with that observed in cases of measles pneumonia, and therefore it is now generally admitted that the two conditions are the same. Immunohistological staining with specific measles antibody can now be used to identify the viral inclusions not only in the lung but in the gastrointestinal epithelium and other organs (Gustafson et al. 1987; Drut and Drut 1988; Radoycich et al. 1992; Rupp et al. 1993; Frenkel et al. 1994).

Macroscopically the lungs are heavier than normal. They show homogeneous firm greyish-white consolidated areas, variable in size, sometimes occupying an entire lobe or lung. The lesions are generally bilateral.

Microscopically there is interstitial pneumonia with oedema of the interstitium and alveolar wall. The inflammatory infiltrate consists mainly of mononuclear cells. The numerous multinucleated syncytial giant cells have a crescent shape and are found lining the alveolar wall, the alveolar ducts and the distal bronchioles. These giant cells may contain 10–50 or even 100 nuclei. Intranuclear and intracytoplasmic eosinophilic bodies are conspicuous, and stain with the phloxine–tartrazine stain. The alveolar spaces are rich in oedema fluid mixed with fibrin, and hyaline membranes may be present (Fig. 7.46), giving the characteristic features of diffuse alveolar damage. The bronchial and bronchiolar epithelia show degenerative changes in places, and in other areas there is marked epithelial hyperplasia with loss of ciliated epithelium. Squamous metaplasia may be prominent. There is a peribronchial mononuclear infiltration with hyperplasia of the lymphoid tissue. It is not unusual to observe endothelial hyperplasia of the small vessels with some degree of stenosis. The lesions may, however, present a spectrum of histological features different from those observed normally: areas of organizing diffuse alveolar damage and/or zones of interstitial pneumonia with a moderate number of giant cells in which viral inclusions cannot be demonstrated. Serology and ultrastructural examinations are necessary to make the correct diagnosis.

Influenza Pneumonia. Influenza can occur sporadically, but often occurs in epidemics. During these outbreaks fatal cases may occur in children, in particular in the immunosuppressed. Several types of virus are known to be responsible for infection of the respiratory system, and new strains and subgroups are isolated each year. Mutational modifications take place in the polypeptide surface antigens, giving rise to antigenic variations requiring constant adaptation of new vaccines (CDC 1994). The virus provokes an interstitial pneumonitis, which can progress to haemorrhagic pneumonia and death. Pneumonia due to superimposed bacterial infection is the main cause of death (Hers and Mulder 1961; Aherne et al. 1970; Lindsay et al. 1970; Zinserling 1972; Joshi et al. 1973; Laraya-Cuasay et al. 1974; Sabin 1977; Foy et al. 1979).

Macroscopic examination of the lungs may reveal nothing in the early phase of the disease; in the full-blown disease they are heavy, reddish and markedly haemorrhagic, with abundant oedema. The bronchi and bronchioles are congested, and the epithelium of the main bronchi may be ulcerated. Their lumen may be filled with a thick yellow blood-stained exudate. Histologically, congestion of the capillaries is a prominent feature. The capillaries are extremely dilated; the septa are oedematous and thickened and

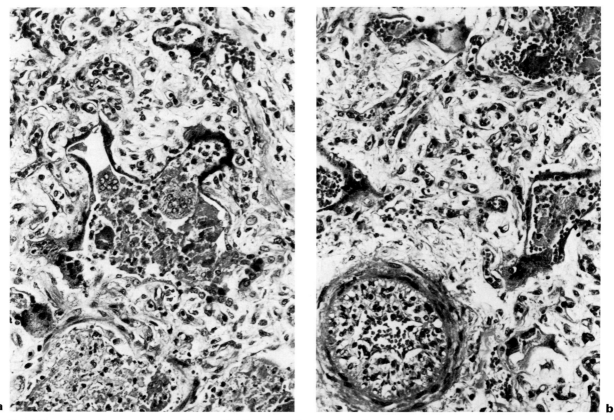

Fig. 7.46. a Giant-cell penumonia in a 12-year-old African girl. The syncytial cells contain intranuclear and intracytoplasmic inclusion bodies consistent with those of measles. **b** Arteritis and endothelial proliferation associated with giant-cell pneumonia. (H&E, × 225)

contain mononuclear inflammatory cells. There are areas of focal necrosis with interstitial haemorrhage. Hyperplasia of the alveolar lining cells is conspicuous, and there is some desquamation into the alveolar spaces, where fibrin, erythrocytes, macrophages and mononuclear cells may be seen. Hyaline membranes are also present. In some areas the alveolar epithelium regenerates. The bronchi and bronchioles show marked congestion, with areas of mucosal necrosis, oedema of their wall, and a diffuse mononuclear infiltrate. Squamous metaplasia of the bronchial epithelium is an indication of regeneration; simultaneously there is epithelial hyperplasia of the bronchioles and alveolar ducts. Healing of the lesions may lead to alveolar fibrosis. Delage et al. (1979) described a giant cell pneumonia due to parainfluenza type 3 virus in infants with immunodeficiency diseases, which histologically resembled measles pneumonia.

Rhinoviruses. These viruses are often the cause of an influenza-like infection of the upper respiratory tract in infants and children. Neonates and premature babies are particularly subject to infection. The disease often runs a benign course, but fatal cases can occur. The viruses may cause an interstitial pneumonia or bronchopneumonia affecting one or more lobes or an entire lung, and the involvement is often bilateral (Fig. 7.47). Rhinoviruses have been associated with the sudden infant death syndrome.

Adenovirus. Adenovirus infection of the respiratory system is relatively common among infants and children and in young adults. The disease is hardly ever fatal, although it may cause severe chronic lung damage, including chronic bronchitis, bronchiolitis and bronchiolitis obliterans, sometimes associated with pulmonary fibrosis. The upper respiratory tract is often the site of infection by the virus. The disease appears to be more common in countries of low socioeconomic status, and especially among children suffering from severe malnutrition or other debilitating conditions. It may be the cause of fatal pneumonia in the newborn and has been documented in

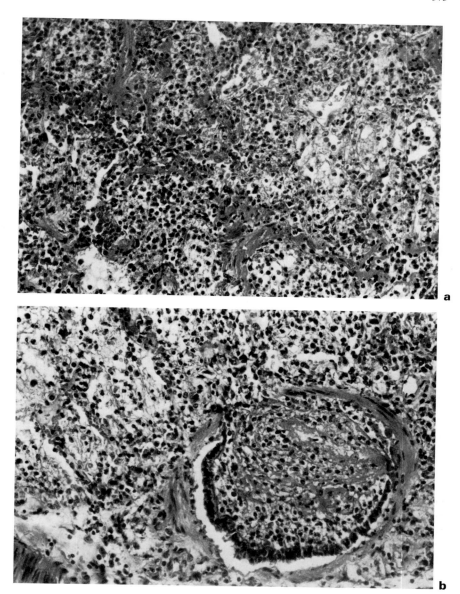

Fig. 7.47. Rhinovirus pneumonia in a 4-year-old African girl. (H&E, × 120) **a** Extensive necrosis of the alveolar wall with distension of the alveolar spaces filled mainly with mononuclear cells. **b** Necrosis of the bronchial wall with bronchiolitis obliterans.

sudden infant death syndrome (SIDS) as well as the immunocompromised host and transplant recipients. It has also been described in association with other viruses, including measles, and/or bacteria. Numerous strains of adenovirus have been isolated with some 41 serotypes identified, and although several types are known to cause respiratory disease in humans only a few have been recorded as being responsible for fatal diseases in children (Sun and Duara 1985; Landry et al. 1987; Green and Williams 1989; Hoggs et al. 1989; Shikes and Ryder 1989; Van Lierde et al. 1989; Mistchenko et al. 1992; An et al. 1993).

Macroscopically the lungs are heavy and firm, with bilateral grey consolidated zones mainly occupying the posterior lower lobes. The parenchyma is markedly oedematous, and the trachea and large bronchi are hyperaemic and ulcerated in places. Their lumen is often filled with thick mucoid material that is rich in fibrin. Histologically there is extensive denudation of the epithelium lining the bronchi and bronchioles, with occasional vesicles in the residual mucosa. In other areas, there is widespread eosinophilic necrosis of the mucosa, which may form a pseudomembranous layer in places. The inflammatory reaction in the wall may be mild or moderate,

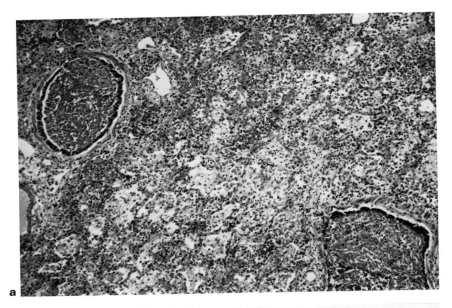

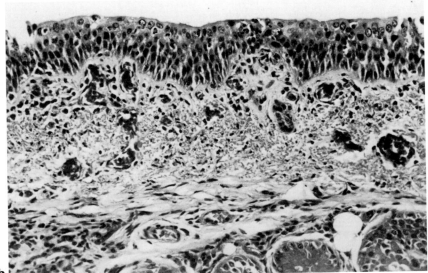

Fig. 7.48. Respiratory syncytial virus pneumonia in a 22-month-old boy with Reye's syndrome. **a** Bronchitis and bronchiolitis obliterans with pneumonitis. (H&E, × 35) **b** Squamous-cell metaplasia of the tracheal epithelium. (H&E, × 225) (Courtesy of Dr J.W. Keeling)

and consists of lymphocytes, plasma cells and some histiocytes. In some instances polymorphonuclear leucocytes may be conspicuous. The alveolar ducts and alveoli are filled with eosinophilic material containing oedema fluid mixed with fibrin and dense hyaline membranes. Parenchymal necrosis may be focal or widespread, with little or no inflammatory reaction. The alveoli and bronchioles contain desquamated necrotic granular pneumocytes, macrophages and damaged epithelial cells, whose nuclei may show nuclear inclusion bodies. These inclusion bodies are of two types: eosinophilic inclusions, well defined and surrounded by a clear halo rim (Feulgen-nega-

tive), and basophilic, amorphous inclusions (smudge nuclei) without a halo (Feulgen-positive). The bodies may be observed in the nuclei of the cellular debris, but principally in the nuclei of the desquamated bronchial and bronchiolar epithelial cells and in the regenerating hyperplastic epithelium. Immunohistochemical labelling, in situ hybridization and electron microscopic studies are valuable aids in diagnosis.

Respiratory Syncytial Virus. This virus is known to have a worldwide distribution and is one of the most important causes of acute respiratory disease among infants and children, especially the premature and those less than 6 months of age. Although it is not often fatal it can cause a diffuse interstitial-type bronchopneumonia or pneumonia. Very often infection is asymptomatic; it has been described in association with SIDS, Reye's syndrome and bronchopulmonary dysplasia. It is the most common cause of severe pulmonary lesions among premature infants and the immunocompromised host. Most fatal cases have been documented in the neonatal period or in infancy. (Groothuis et al. 1988; Nielson and Yunis 1990; An et al. 1993; Jamjoon et al. 1993; Midulla et al. 1993; Moler et al. 1993; Murguia de Sierra et al. 1993; Sigurs et al. 1995).

Macroscopically the lungs show focal areas of consolidation indistinguishable from those seen in most other conditions. Histologically, there is hyperplasia of the epithelium lining the medium-sized bronchi and bronchioles, with desquamation, cellular debris and/or a dense granular eosinophilic material filling the lumen (Fig. 7.48). The wall is sometimes infiltrated by mononuclear cells, with some polymorphonuclear leucocytes. There is also marked shedding of the epithelial cells lining the alveoli, into a lumen sometimes filled with a dense oedematous fluid. Cytoplasmic inclusion bodies may be observed at the periphery of the bronchial, bronchiolar and alveolar pneumocytes, the peribronchial glandular epithelium and the syncytial giant cells protruding into the bronchial lumen or lining the alveoli or bronchiolar walls. There are no nuclear inclusion bodies as in adenovirus infections. Areas of necrosis may be prominent, and these are infiltrated by lymphocytes, plasma cells and macrophages, which play an essential role in the host defence. Very large multinucleated giant cells may border the bronchial and alveolar lesions, mimicking measles pneumonia. Specific immunohistologic staining, in situ hybridization and ultrastructural studies may be necessary to differentiate the two conditions.

Varicella (Chickenpox) Pneumonia. Varicella is a common childhood infection, which is seldom fatal. Specific serological examinations aided by immunohistochemistry and electron microscopic studies are very useful complements to arrive at the correct diagnosis. It is estimated that the mortality rate among infants and children is 1%, whereas it is probably between 10% and 50% among adults. Varicella pneumonia, which may manifest itself a few days after the rash, is considered to be the most serious complication among adults and pregnant women, and it can be accompanied by secondary bacterial infection. In both children and adults the disease may run a fatal course in patients who are receiving steroids or cytotoxic drug therapy for malignancies.

Virus can be transmitted to the fetus in utero and can result in congenital varicella (fatalities occur as a result of pneumonia). Newborns who develop the rash 5 days or more after birth have a higher mortality rate than those who develop the rash within the first 4 days. Varicella infection has become one of the most serious infectious problems among transplant recipients, and in such patients the infection may appear alone or in association with other viral and/or bacterial infections. It is also often reported in patients with AIDS (Charles et al. 1986; Preblud 1986; Alkalay et al. 1987; Saito et al. 1989; Martin et al. 1991; Enders et al. 1994; Puchhammer-Stöckl et al. 1994).

Macroscopically, the lungs are often oedematous, enlarged and rose-coloured, with firm dark-red areas. The bronchi contain abundant blood-stained mucus. Histologically the thickened oedematous alveolar septa show areas of necrosis in places, while in others the alveolar spaces are filled by a dense eosinophilic serous fluid mixed with fibrin and numerous desquamated hyperplastic alveolar epithelial cells with occasional multinucleated giant cells (Fig. 7.49). The bronchi, bronchioles and blood vessels in the involved areas are often necrotic. Intranuclear acidophilic inclusion bodies can be seen in the hypertrophied alveolar cells and in the tracheal and bronchial epithelium as well as endothelial cells of capillaries and other blood vessels. Specific immunohistochemistry and electron microscopy are very useful aids towards correct diagnosis. The inflammatory reaction is moderate and is composed chiefly of mononuclear cells. Healing of the necrotic areas may leave granulomatous lesions, but more often calcified nodules disseminated within the pulmonary parenchyma.

Herpes Simplex Virus (see also pp. 177, 678). There are two antigenically different types of herpes simplex virus known to affect humans (type 1 and type 2). Herpes type 2 virus appears to be venereally transmitted, and as a result is responsible for most congenital herpes virus infection. Fetuses and neonates infected by the virus in utero may present with a fatal disseminated form of the disease involving the brain, liver, adrenals, gastrointestinal tract, lungs and myocardium. It may be the cause of hydrops and is also responsible for cystic degeneration of the brain. Herpes simplex virus infection of the fetus or newborn may be acquired during passage through an infected birth canal, or in utero as a result of premature rupture of the membranes with ascending transplacental transmission. Subclinical latent intrauterine endometrial infection may also infect the conceptus. Transplacental transmission may not be uncommon, as most cases are asymptomatic at birth and the search for the virus may not be undertaken in

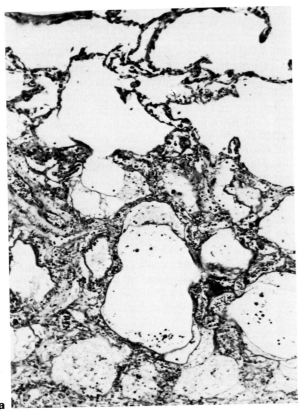 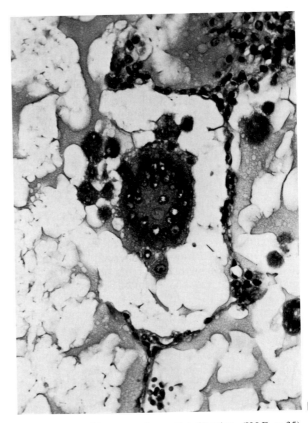

a

b

Fig. 7.49. Varicella pneumonia. **a** Extensive necrosis of the alveolar walls with mild mononuclear cell infiltration. (H&E, × 35) **b** Interstitial giant-cell pneumonitis with intranuclear inclusion bodies. (H&E, × 225)

macerated fetuses, their placentae, membranes or umbilical cords. The period during which infection is transmitted seems to play an important role in the outcome in the fetus or newborn. Small intranuclear calcifications in necrotic areas in a macerated fetus, without an inflammatory reaction, may be the only sign indicating the possibility of herpes viral infection (Benjamin 1989; Kimura et al. 1991; Malm et al. 1991; Martin et al. 1991; Gibbs and Mead 1992; Kulhanjian et al. 1992; Hyde and Giacoia 1993; Nicoll et al. 1994; Malm et al. 1995).

Macroscopically the lungs may appear normal; however, areas suggestive of bronchopneumonia are sometimes conspicuous, and in some cases the cut surface shows some miliary whitish nodules. Microscopically there are multiple round or oval foci of necrosis. Inflammatory cells may be absent or occasionally found at the periphery of the involved zone. The exudate is made up principally of mononuclear inflammatory cells. Bronchioles in the area may undergo necrosis, while in other areas of the lung the bronchial and bronchiolar epithelium is hyperplastic. Focal areas of squamous metaplasia can also be seen. Eosinophilic intranuclear bodies are sometimes seen

in the hyperplastic epithelial cells or in the necrotic cells at the periphery of the lesions (Fig. 7.50). In patients who survive, calcification of the necrotic area may occur. Immunohistochemistry, in situ hybridization and molecular biological techniques are vital aids, not only in making the diagnosis, but also in extending our knowledge to improve our understanding of this infection.

Echovirus (see also p. 781). Echovirus infection may have many clinical presentations, including upper respiratory tract infection with or without pneumonia, and may be the cause of perinatal death.

Histologically, tracheobronchitis, bronchiolitis and an interstitial-type pneumonia are the main findings, in association with lung oedema and congestion. Echovirus II is one of the most frequent offenders and may be associated with SIDS (Jones et al. 1980; Berry and Nagington 1982; Wreghitt et al. 1984).

Parvovirus. Human parvovirus B19 is now known to be related to several clinical conditions in the adult as well as in children (aplastic anaemia, erythema infectiosum), and can be the cause of transplacental infection of the fetus leading to cardiac failure, hydrops

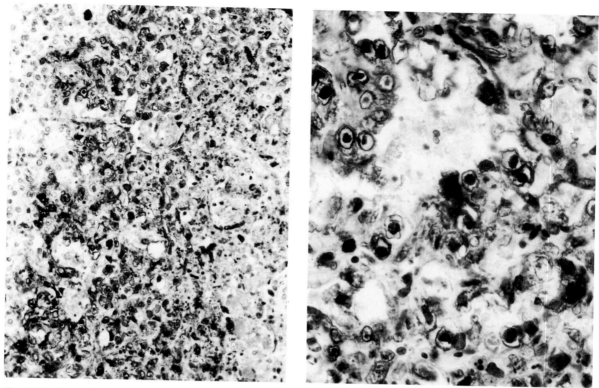

Fig. 7.50. Congenital herpetic infection in a 12-day-old infant. **a** There are extensive multifocal necrotic areas within the lung parenchyma. On the external borders of these zones, the cells are heavily infected. (Immunoperoxidase, × 115) **b** Note the nuclear inclusions. (× 290)

fetalis (non-immunological or other common known causes), intrauterine death and termination in abortion, and is associated with a raised maternal serum α-feto-protein level. It is common in patients with sickle cell anaemia. As the virus (DNA) has a strong affinity for the rapidly dividing erythroblasts, it can be found within the nuclei of these cells in the bone marrow, liver and spleen, as well as in the circulating erythro-blasts in the microcirculation of every organ including the lung (Fig. 7.51a). The nuclei are markedly swollen, containing intranuclear viral inclusions, which may stain blue, lilac or red with haematoxylin with eosin, depending on their size, and bright red with phlox-ine–tartrazine even on macerated material. They may also be identified on electron microscopy (Fig. 7.51b) and by specific DNA probes, which have shown that there is a wide diversity of B19 viruses in the infected fetus. Haemosiderosis of the liver and spleen – evidence of haemolysis – is also observed (Hassam et al. 1990; Berry et al. 1992; Mark et al. 1993; Rogers et al. 1993; Umene and Nunoue 1993).

Hantavirus. This recently recognized group of viral zoonosis may cause severe pulmonary lesions which could lead to death in children (Khan et al. 1995).

Mycoplasmal

Mycoplasmas are members of the class Mollicutes, family *Mycoplasmataceae*, sharing common proper-ties with both bacteria and viruses. There are many strains.

Mycoplasma pneumoniae infection is endemic; it occurs in epidemics and has a worldwide distribution. It affects mainly the respiratory system, especially in children and young adults, but can cause many non-respiratory infections. Pulmonary infection can be mild or severe, causing bronchopneumonia or pneu-monia (primary atypical pneumonia). Atelectasis, bullous emphysema, pulmonary abcesses and pleuri-tis with pleural effusion are associated complications. Meningoencephalitis is a common complication of mycoplasma infection. Myocarditis with pericarditis and pancreatitis have also been described, as well as severe anaemia, thrombocytopenia, disseminated intravascular coagulation and glomerulitis; the latter often in AIDS by *M. Fermentans.* Fatal cases have been documented, many of them in patients with immunodeficiency states or sickle cell anaemia. Transplacental infection has been reported. The diag-nosis, in disease of the respiratory system, is usually

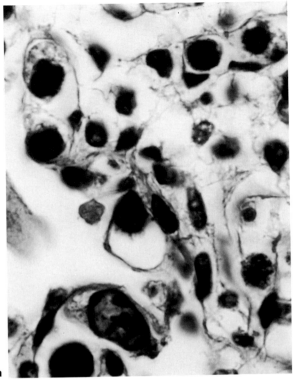
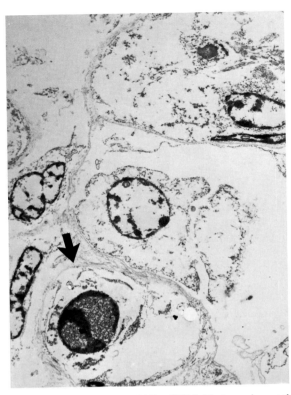

a   b

Fig. 7.51. **a** Parvovirus infection showing the infected circulating normoblasts in the lung tissue. (H&E, × 980) **b** Electron micrograph showing the virus particles within the nucleus of the normoblast. (Courtesy of Dr P. Burton)

made by isolation of the organisms from material taken from the upper respiratory tract or bronchial secretions and by specific immunological and serological tests. These examinations have indicated that the condition is far more prevalent than was once estimated, with a non-negligible morbidity and mortality rate. The organism can now be identified by appropriate immunohistochemistry and by ultrastructural studies (Lutsky et al. 1986; Brasfield et al. 1987; Bauer et al. 1991; Foy 1993).

Macroscopically, the lungs are markedly oedematous, reddish and heavy. Focal zones of intrapulmonary haemorrhage can be seen, sometimes associated with areas of bronchopneumonia. The bronchi and bronchioles are congested, and the distal branches can be partially obliterated by a thick oedematous fluid rich in mucus and mucopus.

Microscopically, the lesions are often indistinguishable from those of viral pneumonias, hence the term "atypical viral pneumonia". The alveolar septa are markedly thickened by a dense oedematous fluid and are infiltrated by lymphocytes, plasma cells and macrophages. The alveolar spaces contain numerous hyperplastic desquamated alveolar cells mixed with erythroctyes, macrophages and fibrin. Lysis of the desquamated alveolar cells is prominent in places, and hyaline membranes are observed in some areas. Single or grouped organisms may be recognized in the nuclei of the modified alveolar epithelial cells or those of the bronchial mucosa. Bronchiolitis is prominent and widespread. There is marked congestion of the vessels, some of which may contain fibrinous thrombi or show necrosis of their walls.

There is now growing interest in *Ureaplasma urealyticum* and pulmonary infection and sepsis in the newborn, principally those of low birth weight (below 1250 g). The organism is known to colonize the lower genital tract in most women and especially among those of low socioeconomic status. Transmission to the fetus may be: in utero secondary to an ascending infection via the transplacental route; during normal delivery and passage through a birth canal heavily infected; or postnatally by nosocomial transmission (horizontal). Infection of the fetus in utero is often associated with chorioamnionitis, and on occasion with a febrile illness of the mother. *U. urealyticum* infection of the newborn, especially in premature infants, is often associated with respiratory distress syndrome, sepsis and meningitis. It may be responsible for diffuse pneumonitis and/or interstitial fibrosis, sometimes with pulmonary haemorrhage. Together with *Mycoplasma hominis*, it has been associated with development of persistent pulmonary hypertension and bronchopulmonary dysplasia in the newborn (Waites et al. 1989; Brus et al. 1991; Walsh et al 1991; Eschenbach 1993; Ollikainen et al. 1993; Sànchez 1993; Waites et al. 1993; Wang et al. 1993a).

Fungal

Mycotic infection of the lung in childhood are uncommon, and the majority of such infections encountered are secondary or opportunist infections. However, a few cases of congenital infection have been described with some species of fungus. In most instances the particular mycotic infection is observed in association with children receiving antibiotic or steroid treatment or in those suffering from some form of chronic debilitating disease. In recent years there has been an increasing number of reports among children treated with immunosuppressive drugs or cytotoxic agents for malignancies. These infections are more common in tropical and subtropical zones, where certain species of fungus are prevalent. Special stains (Gram, PAS, Grocott's silver methenamine) may be necessary to identify the organisms in sections; culture and immunological studies are essential in determining the exact species involved.

Moniliasis (Candida). Several species of *Candida* can affect humans, but *C. albicans* is usually responsible for pulmonary lesions in the paediatric age group. Both congenital and neonatal pulmonary moniliasis have been described. In childhood the lesions may be localized in the tracheobronchial tree, where the fungus may produce ulceration of the mucosa, or in the pulmonary parenchyma, with the formation of microabcesses. In severe cases, there is diffuse pulmonary and sometimes vascular involvement. Associated bacterial infection is common, and in these cases an inflammatory infiltrate is often pronounced. In the neonatal period moniliasis may be associated with prolonged umbilical vein catheterization, which is also seen in older children who have had other intravenous catheters in place for long periods (Smith and Congdon 1985; Knox et al. 1987). The condition is a particular hazard to immunocompromised patients (those with AIDS, those subject to immunosuppression therapy and transplant recipients).

Pulmonary Aspergillosis. This condition is also uncommon in children, and it has been observed mainly as an opportunistic infection. It can be a complication of tuberculosis, pneumatocele and/or an infected bronchogenic cyst. Eosinophilia is a common feature of the condition.

As in adults, the disease may present in several forms: allergic bronchopneumonia, which is extremely rare; aspergilloma, a more common entity; and disseminated or septicaemic pulmonary aspergillosis. The morphological features are identical to those observed in adult cases. In recent years there has been a marked increase of the condition among children treated for malignancies, those with AIDS and transplant recipients, as well as those with cystic fibrosis and chronic granulophthisis (Neijens et al. 1989; Denning and Stevens 1990; Kurup and Kumar 1991; Loire et al. 1993; Cowie et al. 1994; Miller et al. 1994; Simmonds et al. 1994).

Pulmonary thrombi containing fungal hyphae, sometimes associated with infarction, are the most striking features (Fig. 7.52). There is sometimes necrosis of the vessel wall with secondary infection of the surrounding tissue in disseminated infection.

Histoplasmosis. Two forms of histoplasmosis are thought to exist: *H. capsulatum* (North American form) and *H. duboisii* (African form).

The North American form of *H. capsulatum* has a worldwide distribution and is known to be endemic in certain regions. The clinical and radiological features are non-specific and can resemble those of a viral lung infection or, in some instances, tuberculosis. The disease is common in children and can cause death in endemic areas. It may present as:

1. An acute influenza-like illness with a variable outcome (usually the infection is benign)
2. A chronic pulmonary infection with one or more pulmonary cavities, resembling tuberculosis, in which secondary calcification is frequently observed; it may even present as a non-caseating granulomatous lesion resembling sarcoidosis
3. Disseminated histoplasmosis, with widespread dissemination by the bloodstream, generally affecting younger children, and often rapidly fatal

The disease is also described in association with AIDS. The organism can now be identified by an immunoperoxidase histoplasma antibody stain (Body et al. 1988; Loyd et al. 1988; Wheat et al. 1989).

African histoplasmosis, *H. duboisii*, is more restricted to the tropical and subtropical belt of Africa. The organisms occasionally produces pulmonary lesions, which are mainly granulomatous; in rare instances cavities develop (Oddo et al. 1990).

Pulmonary Pneumocystic Carinii (Interstitial Plasma Cell Pneumonia). Pneumocystic carinii has recently

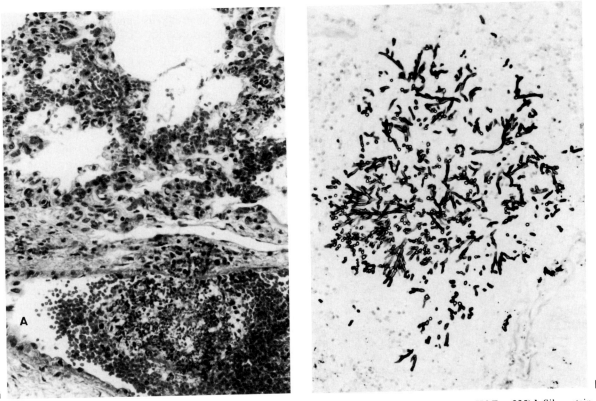

Fig. 7.52. Pulmonary aspergillosis in an 8-month-old boy. **a** Thrombosis with infiltration of vessel wall (*A*). (H&E, × 225) **b** Silver stain to show fungi. (Grocott, × 360)

been shown to be a diverse group of exotic fungi, which may include several species. It has a worldwide distribution and appears to be a saprophyte in the lungs of several domestic animals as well as humans. Its mode of transmission still remains unclear; however, it is generally accepted that the organisms may reach the lungs by inhalation. Whatever the route may be, in humans, exposure occurs early and most children by the age of 3 present serum antibodies to the organism. The disease is known to be endemic in some areas, and it is not uncommon among the inmates of institutions. Epidemics have been described, principally in Central Europe. The lung is the organ most often affected, but the organisms have been observed in the regional lymph nodes and, in severe disseminated cases, the bone marrow, liver, spleen, adrenals and kidneys. Multiple organ failure may ensue.

The condition has been described among premature babies and debilitated infants, especially those with congenital immunological abnormalities, recurrent infections or severe malnutrition. The disease has been severe and rapidly progressive, with a high mortality rate in most cases reported. *P. carinii* has been reported in siblings, and transplacental transmission has been documented. Effective therapy has now greatly modified the course of the disease.

At present, *P. carinii* is most commonly encountered as an opportunistic infection in immunodeficient subjects, especially those with AIDS and organ transplant recipients, and after prolonged antibiotic and chemotherapies. It has also been described in association with congenital heart disease, severe aplastic anaemia, systemic lupus erythematosus and acute disseminated Langerhans' cell histiocytosis, and in association with various bacterial infections, cytomegalovirus infection, and infection by *Candida albicans*.

The clinical and radiological features are nonspecific and may be accompanied by lung cavities, pneumatoceles, pneumothorax and/or pleural effusion. The organisms may be recovered from the latter. Serological and immunological studies are often necessary for establishing the diagnosis, and BAL fluids and lung biopsy can be additional assets (Millard and Heryet 1988; Limper et al. 1989; Davey and Masur

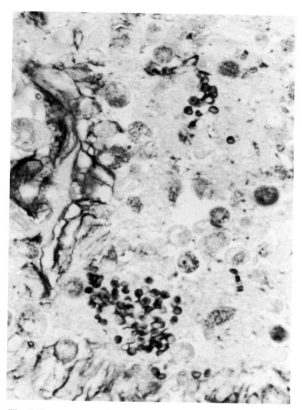
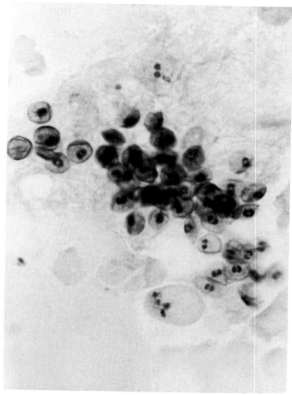

a

b

Fig. 7.53. *Pneumocystis carinii* pneumonia in a case of treated leukaemia. **a** The alveoli are filled with a granular material, foam cells and cellular debris. (H&E, × 650) **b** Abundant *P. carinii* of various forms in intra-alveolar exudate. (Grocott)

1990; Telzak et al. 1990; Chave et al. 1991; Leong et al. 1991; Walzer 1991a, b; Hidalgo et al. 1992; Murray and Schmidt 1992; Martin 1993; Smyth et al. 1994; Stringer 1993).

Macroscopically, the lungs are heavier than normal, firm, oedematous and may show focal reddish or brownish-grey areas of consolidation. In severe cases the lesions may be diffused, involving one or more lobes or the entire lung, but there are numerous variations between the two extremes. Emphysematous areas may be conspicuous, associated sometimes with pneumothorax and/or mediastinal emphysema. The hilar lymph nodes are often swollen.

Histologically, there is some degree of hyperplasia of the alveolar lining cells, with desquamation into the alveolar spaces mixed with macrophages in the early stages or in mild infection. The organisms can be observed within the macrophages or alveolar cells when stained with the appropriate stains (PAS, Grocott and specific monoclonal antibody). The interstitial inflammatory reaction is usually mild and composed chiefly of lymphocytes, plasma cells and macrophages. In the severe form, the alveoli are distended and filled with an exudate of foamy material mixed with desquamated cells and macrophages. The organisms are seen in large numbers within the cells, but are present mainly in the amorphous debris (Fig. 7.53). The alveolar wall is thickened, cellular, even fibrosed in places, and diffusely infiltrated by mononuclear cells and macrophages. Cysts and trophozoites may be identified, not only within the cells, but also in the scarred areas. Giant cells and non-caseating granulomas have been observed, and calcification has been recorded in these lesions and the hilar lymph nodes, where organisms can be seen. Survivors may show pulmonary fibrosis of varying degrees, sometimes with organisms.

Other Mycoses. Blastomycosis, mucormycosis, paracoccidioidomycosis, nocardiosis, etc, may be responsible for pulmonary lesions in infants and children, especially in humid tropical countries; however, they are unusual (Powell and Schuit 1979; Ramos et al. 1981).

Parasitic

The lung is commonly affected by parasitic disease, and in many tropical countries parasites or their eggs can be observed in the lung parenchyma. The extent of pulmonary involvement is variable.

Toxoplasmosis of the Lung. Toxoplasma gondii is a protozoon, a member of the sporozoa group. The parasite has a worldwide distribution and infects many animal species. In humans it has a wide spectrum of manifestations, varying from subclinical or mild infection to severe generalized disease. Although the mode of transmission is not fully understood, the organisms may be acquired in utero or during childhood, and various surveys have shown that over 90% of some populations, notably those living in hot humid climates, have antibodies to the parasite.

Infection of the mother during pregnancy may result in intrauterine death, stillbirth or neonatal death in about 10% of cases. Should the parasite be acquired during the first 6 months of gestation transplacental transmission is infrequent, but the lesions are severe in the fetuses and infants who do acquire the disease. After the 6th month there is a much higher rate of transplacental transmission, and the infection is more often benign or asymptomatic in the offspring. A few reports have suggested that persistent maternal infection results in repeated abortion in successive pregnancies, but this has not been substantiated. Congenital toxoplasmosis may cause perinatal death, serious abnormalities of the central nervous system and the eyes (chorioretinitis) or latent disease. Because of the significant morbidity and mortality rates in the perinatal period, various routine immunological tests have been devised to detect the disease during pregnancy or in the neonatal period. Over 60% of infants born to mothers who have the disease during pregnancy show no evidence of infection. Infants may acquire the disease during passage through the birth canal or in childhood. In many countries emphasis is now placed on the routine screening of pregnant women and those of childbearing age. Toxoplasma infection is not uncommon among patients with malignant disease or other conditions requiring corticosteroid drugs and/or cytotoxic or immunosuppressive agents. In these patients the disease often runs a fatal course if not treated adequately. (Pinon et al. 1987; Berger et al. 1992; Thulliez et al. 1992).

Macroscopically, the lungs can appear normal or show reddish firm, sometimes confluent, nodules. Areas of consolidation have been observed in the diffused neonatal form of the disease. Microscopically, the alveolar spaces are filled with desquamated epithelial lining cells and macrophages. The alveolar wall is thickened, containing numerous macrophages with many plasma cells and lymphocytes, and few eosinophils and polymorphonuclear leucocytes. Toxoplasma pseudocysts may be seen free in the alveolar spaces, but occur principally in the cytoplasm of the desquamated alveolar cells and macrophages. Sometimes they can be seen in the cytoplasm of the swollen endothelial cell.

Amoebic Lung Abscesses. The protozoon *Entamoeba histolytica* (class Rhizopoda) is endemic in tropical and subtropical countries. It is also known to exist in certain temperate countries, and in recent times has been encountered more frequently than before, as a result of rapid air travel and the shifting of populations.

The parasite attacks principally the colon (see p. 793), but can spread to the liver by way of the portal system, and can eventually reach the lung and brain. The disease has been observed at all ages, but there are no figures for its true incidence. Intestinal infection in children is not altogether uncommon, but secondary spread to the liver with formation of liver abscesses is rare, and pulmonary involvement is even less common. The lung is infected from an amoebic liver abscess. The liver capsule overlying the abscess may adhere to the diaphragm, and eventually the abscess ruptures into the thoracic cavity, extending into the pulmonary parenchyma. A bronchopulmonary fistula has been observed in certain instances. There is little or no secondary inflammatory reaction (Abioye and Edington 1972; Jessee et al. 1975; Strauss and Bove 1975; Woodruff 1975; Shabot and Patterson 1978).

Other Parasites

Several other parasites can be observed in the lungs during childhood. The lung may be involved in the life-cycle of some of these parasites, or it may be infected secondarily by the eggs, larvae or adult parasites.

Hydatid cystic disease (*Echinococcus granulosus*) is one of the most important of these. This parasite has a worldwide distribution, and there is a high morbidity in areas where the disease is endemic. *E. multilocularis*, another species, is limited to certain parts of Europe, including Switzerland. The larval form of *E. granulosus* is responsible for the classic hydatid cyst, whereas *E. multilocularis* is associated with the alveolar (multilocular) hydatid cyst (Poole and Marcial-Rojas 1971).

Four types of schistosomes are known to affect humans: *Schistosoma mansoni* and *S. haematobium*, *S. japonicum* and *S. intercalatum*.

Eggs of *S. mansoni* and *S. haematobium*, and to a lesser extent of *S. japonicum*, have been described in the lungs of patients harbouring the parasites in endemic zones. In some cases the eggs lodge in the alveolar wall of the interstitial tissue with little or no reaction; in others they may produce a granulomatous reaction with marked septal fibrosis. Embolism of the eggs in the pulmonary circulation is one cause of pulmonary hypertension. The adult worms can occasionally be observed in the lumen of the pulmonary vessels, with little or no reaction of the endothelial cells (Berthoud 1972; Cowper 1973; Pettersson et al. 1974).

The larvae of *Strongyloides stercoralis* have been reported in the lungs of infants and children in association with hyperinfection, especially among those suffering from severe malnutrition or receiving treatment with cytotoxic or immunosuppressive agents (Boyd et al. 1978; Burke 1978; Scowden et al. 1978).

Larvae of *Ascaris lumbricoides* can be observed in the lungs in children infested with this parasite. The larvae reach the lung by way of the blood vessels and can be seen in the capillaries or free in the alveolar wall, where there is sometimes an inflammatory reaction with numerous eosinophils. The larvae of *A. lumbricoides* must be distinguished histologically from those of *S. stercoralis* (Arean and Crandall 1971).

In endemic zones where *filariasis* is a major problem, microfilariae can be identified in the lung. The organisms are often free in the alveolar wall or in the capillaries. Occasionally there is a secondary inflammatory reaction around the microfilariae. Filiarasis of the lung is often associated with pulmonary eosinophilia (Webb et al. 1960; Meyers et al. 1977).

There are several types of *pentastomiasis*, and the causative parasites are known to inhabit the nasopharynx of birds and mammals in various parts of the world. Humans may become infected secondarily, and the second-stage larva may be found in several organs, including the lung (Fig. 7.54) (Self 1969).

Recently a case of *capillariasis* (*Capillaria acrophila*) was described in a child in Iran by Aftandelians et al. (1977). Pulmonary paragonimiasis may be encountered in children coming from the Far East (Mayer 1979).

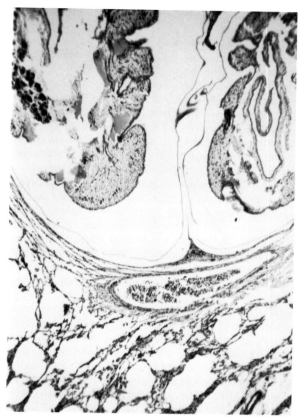

Fig. 7.54. Pulmonary pentastomiasis in a 6-year-old African girl with fatal disseminated infestation. (H&E, × 25)

increasingly in respiratory distress syndrome and bronchopulmonary dysplasia. It may be helpful in the diagnosis of Langerhans' cell histiocytosis (histiocytosis X), in which the cells stain for OKT6, CD1a and S-100 protein, but it is in no way specific. The technique has the advantage of permitting rapid diagnosis of various kinds of infection, with the possibility of promoting therapeutic intervention. In addition, study of the cellular population in the fluid obtained makes data available on immune status and the evolution of some specific conditions. These, together with the study of the other components making up the fluid, have become important tools in both normal and pathological conditions.

Bronchoalveolar Lavage

In children, bronchoalveolar lavage (BAL) is widely used in sarcoidosis, AIDS, asthma, extrinsic allergic alveolitis (hypersensitivity pneumonitis), transplant patients (renal, bone marrow, cardiac) and now

Acquired Immune Deficiency Syndrome

In the paediatric age group with AIDS, the pulmonary lesions have been the best documented, and these appear to be somewhat different from those observed in adults. The thymus, lymph node, gastrointestinal tract, brain and spinal cord are also severely affected (see also p. 821).

The pulmonary lesions may take one of several forms. Opportunistic infections are not uncommon and may be the only pathological findings, with *Pneumocystis carinii* often heading the list, or in association with some viral infections, principally cytomegalovirus infection, or mycotic infections (*Candida, Aspergillus*), *Toxoplasma*, and/or bacterial infections (*Haemophilus influenzae, Mycobacterium avium intracellulare*). By far the most common lesion, however, is *pulmonary lymphoid hyperplasia* (PLH), which consists of nodular peribronchial lymphoid hyperplasia with or without germinal centres scattered about the lung fields. The alveolar septa are infiltrated by mild to moderate amounts of mononuclear cells. The next most common finding is the *lymphoid interstitial pneumonitis* (LIP) characterized by a diffuse mononuclear infiltrate of the alveolar wall and peribronchiolar spaces. The infiltrate is composed of lymphocytes, immunoblasts and plasma cells often containing Russell bodies. Some alveolar spaces may be filled with macrophages and desquamated alveolar cells, and the alveolar wall may be lined by metaplastic cuboidal cells and infiltrated by varying quantities of mononuclear cells, thus taking on the appearance of *desquamative interstitial pneumonitis* (DIP). The alveolar infiltration may be accompanied by scattered nodular aggregates of lymphoid tissue, sometimes centred on germinal centres. In general there may be great overlapping of these various histological appearances within the same lung or even within a given lobe. Lesions consistent with pulmonary hypertension may be present, especially among intravenous drug users; the lesions may be widespread. Malakoplakia has also been described with this syndrome.

Some areas may take on the appearance of secondary alveolar proteinosis (partial staining for surfactant apoprotein), especially when this is associated with *Pneumocystis carinii* or *Mycobacterium tuberculosis*.

It has been shown recently that a monoclonal antibody (anti-P18) labels cytoplasmic and membranal viral proteins in lymphoid tissue associated with AIDS or AIDS-related complex (ARC), and this could be a valuable aid in diagnosing the condition in infants with a negative serology. Several new tests have been added to those already existing (Anderson and Lee 1988; Beers et al. 1990; Mills and Masur 1990; Murray and Mills 1990; Schwartz et al. 1990; Travis et al. 1990; Garcia et al. 1991; Klapholz et al. 1991; Kovacs et al. 1991; Russler et al. 1991; Speich et al. 1991; Polos et al. 1992; Sepkowitz et al. 1992; Travis et al. 1992; Karlinsky and Mark 1993; Yousem 1993).

The Lung in Transplantations

Lung transplantation and heart–lung transplantation have become relatively common procedures worldwide, as well as transplantations of other organs isolated or in combinations. Although the control of rejection is one of the principal element, determining management, secondary infections in these immunocompromised patients often cause significant morbidity and mortality. Major problems may arise in the interpretation of lung biopsies, and it is not always easy to differentiate rejection from opportunistic infections. Bacterial, fungal, viral and parasitic infections must be taken into consideration when evaluating a lung biopsy for rejection. Immunohistochemistry, in situ hybridization, molecular biology and ultrastructural techniques on biopsy material or BAL are often necessary to arrive at a diagnosis. In cases coming to autopsy, other pathological conditions must also be taken into consideration, principally *bronchiolitis obliterans*, its consequences and complications, as well as associated bronchial and vascular lesions (Tazelaar and Yousem 1988; Clelland et al. 1990; Fend et al. 1990; Weiss et al. 1990; Abernathy et al. 1991; Groussard 1993).

Pulmonary Lesions after Bone Marrow Transplantation

Pulmonary complications are responsible for a considerable proportion of the morbidity and mortality among bone marrow transplant patients. These complications are more prevalent among those receiving allogenic marrow transplantation than those receiving syngenic autologous transplantation.

Many predisposing factors have been incriminated, including pretreatment radiotherapy. Total body irradiation in a single dose would appear to predispose to a higher frequency of pulmonary complications than fractionated irradiation. Chemotherapy due to drug toxicity on the lung parenchyma may also be a contributing factor.

The symptoms are generally non-specific, with fever, cough, dyspnoea and tachypnoea. Chest radiography may be unrevealing, but more often shows bilateral nodular infiltrates. BAL is of great value in arriving at a rapid diagnosis.

The pulmonary lesions are variable and consist of:

1. *Opportunistic Infection.* One or more pathogens may be involved, including bacteria (atypical mycobacteria, *Legionella*, etc.), fungi (*Candida, Aspergillus* spp., *P. carinii*), viruses (cytomegalovirus,

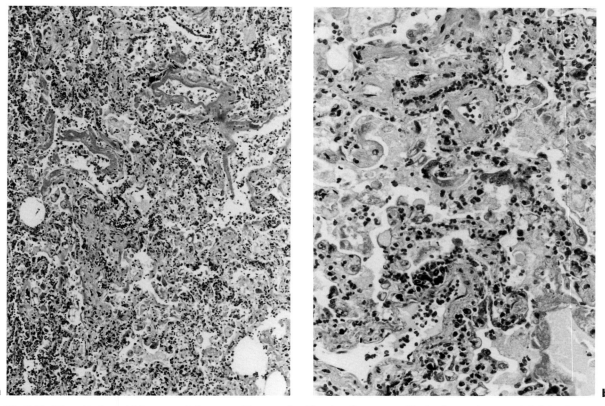

Fig. 7.55. Idiopathic interstitial pneumonia in a case of bone graft. **a** The alveoli are covered by hyalin membranes and their lumina are filled with desquamated alveolar cells and macrophages. Mononuclear cells are observed in the alveolar wall in small groups. (H&E, × 60). **b** The hyperplastic alveolar cells are evident, some taking on a giant cell appearance.

herpes simplex, Epstein–Barr, parvovirus 19, respiratory syncytial virus, HHV-6 and HHV-7).

2. *Interstitial Pneumonitis (Idiopathic)*. No infectious agent can be identified by the various means at our disposal. The lung tissue presents thickening of the alveolar wall, infiltrated by mononuclear cells or aggregates of lymphocytes. There is marked hyperplasia of the alveolar lining cells, some having a giant cell appearance (Fig. 7.55). No viral inclusions can be identified even by *in situ hybridization* or by ultrastructural means. The alveoli often contain a granular oedematous fluid with numerous desquamated alveolar cells accompanied by several macrophages. Here and there one observes a moderate peribronchial and/or peribronchiolar mononuclear infiltrate. The condition may present in one of two forms: with severe clinical symptoms with diffuse radiological involvement and a rapid fatal course, or with discrete or mild clinical symptoms, evolving chronically, and not leading to death. In this case the lung usually presents diffuse fibrous thickening of the alveolar wall.

3. *Bronchiolitis Obliterans*. The terminal bronchi and bronchioles are obliterated by proliferating fibrous tissue with focal or complete necrosis of the wall or complete scarring. This lesion is usually associated with late acute or chronic graft-versus-host disease. (Roy et al. 1989; Holland et al. 1990; Jochelson et al. 1990; Benz–Lemoine et al. 1991; Burgart et al. 1991; Gucalp et al. 1991; Rosenfeld and Young 1991; Corrin 1992; Garaventa et al. 1992; Harrington et al. 1992; Ezri et al. 1994).

Bronchus-associated Lymphoid Tissue (BALT)

Bronchus-associated lymphoid tissue, also referred to as idiopathic follicular bronchitis or follicular bronchiectasis, may be encountered in fetuses, premature babies and even abortuses, and in the majority of cases it is associated with intrauterine infection and chorioamnionitis. It is a relatively frequent finding in SIDS and may also be observed in infants, children and adults with immunodeficiency states, autoimmune conditions or hypersensitivity states.

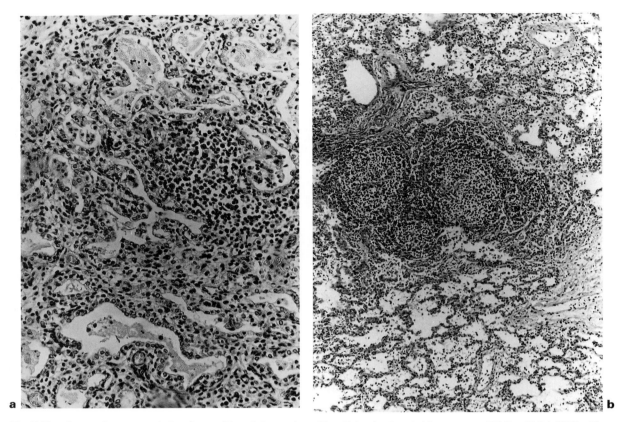

Fig. 7.56. a Intrauterine pneumonia in a fetus at 27 weeks' gestation with well develop lymphoid aggregates. (H&E, × 125) **b** SIDS with well developed peripheral lymphoid follicules in the lung, age 15 months. (H&E, × 50)

The condition is thought to be induced by infection in some cases and by antigenic stimulus in others, and therefore may represent a host defence mechanism of the lung. Histologically there is lymphoid tissue or lymphoid follicles in close proximity to the bronchial and/or bronchiolar epithelium, most often in the region of their bifurcation or along their channel (Fig. 7.56). A mild or moderate bronchitis and or bronchiolitis may be associated (Emery and Dinsdale 1974; Yousem et al. 1985; Pabst 1992; Gould and Isaacson 1993; Holt 1993; Kinane et al. 1993).

Diffuse Interstitial Pneumonia (Desquamative Interstitial Pneumonia)

Diffuse interstitial pneumonia in infancy and childhood is a rare condition in this age group, and many of the histological patterns are similar, in many respects, to those observed in adults; in the latter, it has a worldwide distribution and carries many synonyms (Hamman–Rich syndrome, diffuse fibrosing alveolitis, fibrotic lung disease, interstitial pulmonary fibrosis, cryptogenic alveolar fibrosis, idiopathic pulmonary fibrosis). Diffuse interstitial pneumonia has been described in association with pathological changes in other organs in some cases, especially among patients suffering from Sjögren's syndrome, chronic active hepatitis, Hashimoto's thyroiditis, ulcerative colitis. It has also been described in families, and in most of these cases it seems to have an autosomal dominant mode of inheritance. Histological patterns are often indistinguishable from those produced by drug allergic reactions and certain viral pneumonias (Katzenstein 1985; Burkhardt 1989; Burkhardt and Cottier 1989; Dunnill 1990; Smith et al. 1990; Cherniack et al. 1991; Thompson et al. 1992). The condition may present in an acute form (desquamative interstitial pneumonia), which is distinct from the chronic interstitial pneumonias but may represent a spectrum of the same disease process. Lung biopsies and BAL have become valuable aids in confirming diagnosis (Robinson et al. 1988; Hällgren et al. 1989; Katzenstein et al. 1995).

The disease has been documented in both infancy and childhood, sometimes with repeated relapses; it

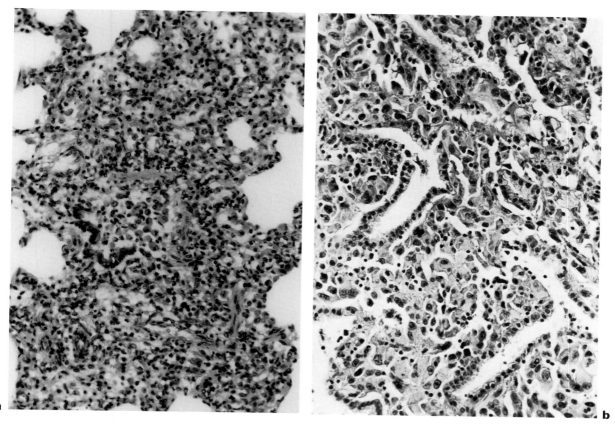

Fig. 7.57. a Acute desquamative interstitial pneumonia in a 5-week-old infant. Note the partial obstruction of the bronchiole containing macrophages and the few inflammatory cells extending into the thickened alveoli. (H&E, × 55) **b** Desquamative interstitial pneumonia in a 7-month-old boy, which progressed to diffuse pulmonary fibrosis by the 20th month. (H&E, × 225)

has also been described in association with segmental glomerulosclerosis (Hewitt et al. 1977; Steinkamp et al. 1990; Sheth et al. 1992; Usui et al. 1992). Recently, Schroeder et al. 1992 have described a cellular interstitial pneumonitis in infants which they consider a different entity from those described above.

Hewitt et al. (1977) reviewed the literature on cases of fibrosing alveolitis occurring in childhood. All pertinent features of the disease in the paediatric age group were evaluated, and a comparison of fibrosing alveolitis in children and adults was made.

Macroscopically the lungs are heavier than normal, firm, non-crepitant and airless. They are greyish in colour and in the late stages present a honeycomb appearance. Macroscopically, in the early phase, the air spaces are distended, filled with desquamated, PAS-positive, granular pneumocytes (type II cells) and some macrophages (CD68+) which may contain haemosiderin pigment. The alveoli are lined with hyperplastic alveolar cells, some of which show cuboidal metaplasia. The alveolar wall is thickened

and infiltrated by a mononuclear exudate but there are no polymorphonuclear leucocytes (Fig. 7.57). There is no necrosis, and hyaline membranes are not found. Lymphoid aggregates may be conspicuous, and follicles with prominent germinal centres are frequently observed, especially in the crytogenic phase.

During the late stages, the alveolar wall shows varying degrees of thickness and fibrosis. The extent of these changes depends on the evolution and duration of the disease. Reticulin and collagen fibres are increased; elastic fibres are numerous and thickened. There is an active proliferation of smooth-muscle cells. Some alveoli may become obliterated by the process, while others become cyst-like, leading to the typical honeycomb appearance. The bronchiolar epithelium may show metaplasia, and the bronchial wall is usually thickened as a result of muscular hyperplasia. The bronchi and bronchioles are often surrounded by lymphoid follicles.

Platelet aggregates have been observed in capillaries in the early phase. In general, vessel walls are thickened due to muscular hyperplasia with moderate

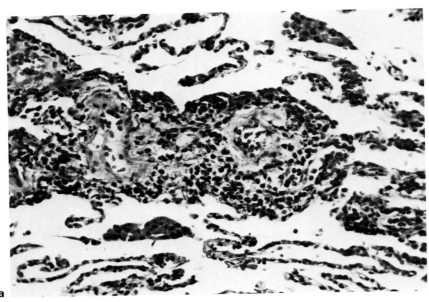

a

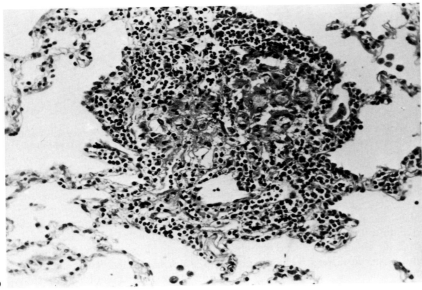

b

Fig. 7.58. a Hypersensitivity pneumonitis associated with animal furs, principally horsehair, in an 11-year-old girl. (H&E, × 180) **b** Hypersensitivity pneumonitis associated with pigeon proteins (pigeon fancier's lung) in a 13-year-old girl. (H&E, × 180)

to severe fibrosis. In the late stages, the large and medium-sized vessels are thickened and fibrosed.

Extrinsic Allergic Alveolitis (Hypersensitivity Pneumonia)

Extrinsic allergic alveolitis is an inflammatory reaction of the distal airways to various inhaled antigenic materials. A variety of agents, including proteins of animal and avian origin, fungi and thermophilic organisms, have been incriminated as responsible for the lesions, and new aetiological agents continue to

be identified. Extrinsic allergic alveolitis is often an occupational hazard; however, social and environmental factors are also contributory elements. Although the majority of cases have been reported in adults, infants and children are also affected. The condition is not infrequently encountered among adolescent drug abusers who inhale various narcotics, often contaminated with other substances, or among "sniffers". It has also become more prevalent among those exposed to an excessive quantity of hairspray.

Extrinsic allergic alveolitis is mainly associated with type III immune reaction, and the pathogenesis is believed to involve both immune-complex disease and cellular hypersensitivity (cell-mediated) reactions in the terminal air spaces in association with complement (C_3). Genetic and environmental factors seem to play an important role and may determine the host's response to the particular antigenic insult. HLA antigens and antibodies to the P_1-erythrocyte antigen also appear to be of some importance, at least in some cases, in determining the response of the host. Antigen, immunoglobulins (mainly IgG with smaller quantities of IgA and IgM) and complement (C_3) can be detected in the lungs of patients suffering from the disease. Their identification depends partly on the sensitivity of the tests, and in particular on the evolution of the disease process. They are more frequently found in the early stage of the disease, before extensive phagocytic infiltration or fibrosis has occurred. The condition is thought to be the result of a complex series of immunological events in which the alveolar macrophages, T-lymphocytes, neutrophils and their secretions have a role under well defined genetic factors.

Pathologically it is not possible to distinguish between immune-complex disease and cellular hypersensitivity lesions in the lung. Furthermore, in the late stages of the disorder, it is not possible to differentiate between extrinsic allergic alveolitis and fibrosing alveolitis.

Diagnosis is made on the basis of the clinical and immunological findings in susceptible individuals. The radiological findings are non-specific. The presence of specific antigens in the serum is of prime importance; the analysis of cells and proteins from BAL may be helpful and more so their T-cell components. Predominantly CD8+ T-lymphocytes in BAL is highly suggestive of an acute phase of hypersensitivity pneumonitis, whereas an increased number of CD4+ T-lymphocytes would favour a fibrotic process which on histology would be indistinguishable from idiopathic pulmonary fibrosis. Microbiological and specific immunohistological studies may be of help in arriving at an aetiological diagnosis, and this can be strengthened by specific skin tests (Lipscomb et al. 1986; Salvaggio and de Shazo 1986; Coleman and Colby 1988; Semenzato et al. 1988; Selman et al. 1990; Murayama et al. 1993).

Macroscopically, the lungs present features similar to those of fibrosing alveolitis. However, in most cases, lung tissue is obtained by biopsy for histological and immunological studies during the course of the disease. Microscopically, there is a wide variability in the lesions, depending on the state of the disease. In the early stages there is oedema of the alveolar wall, which is thickened and infiltrated by aggregates of lymphocytes, some plasma cells, and many histiocytes with a foamy cytoplasm. The alveolar spaces and bronchiolar lumen may contain few desquamated epithelial cells with some histiocytes (Fig. 7.58). At a later stage the inflammatory reaction is more prominent, histiocytes are more numerous, and there are well developed lymph follicles, sometimes with well defined germinal centres. Epithelioid-cell granulomas with foreign body-type giant cells are now conspicuous and may contain cholesterol clefts. Some giant cells may also be seen in the alveolar spaces among the few histiocytes and desquamated epithelial cells. Schauman bodies may occasionally be present. The small bronchi and bronchioles are also involved in the inflammatory disease process, with features characteristic of organizing pneumonia. Their walls are thickened and infiltrated by mononuclear cells and histiocytes, and bronchiolitis obliterans may occur as the disease progresses. Small vessels may also participate in the reaction, and arteritis with eventual thickening and fibrosis of the vessel wall is sometimes observed.

In the late stages, there is moderate to severe thickening of the alveolar wall, which is rich in collagen and reticulin fibres. The inflammatory reaction is now patchy or almost absent, and granulomas are no longer present. Remodelling of the parenchyma and formation of cystic spaces gives rise to the honeycomb appearance, which is indistinguishable from that seen in fibrosing alveolitis.

Eosinophilic Pneumonias

Eosinophilic pneumonias are a group of allergic inflammatory reactions in the lungs, characterized by a marked eosinophilic exudate in the lung parenchyma, which must be distinguished from the hypereosinophilic syndrome; they can occur with or without blood eosinophilia. The clinical manifestations may be variable and are often non-specific; however, two modes of presentation, acute and chronic, have been documented. The classic fluffy peripheral radiological features and/or peripheral computed tomographic images are often diagnostic of the condition, and BAL fluids often contain a high percentage of eosinophils. The disease generally responds to corticosteroids. Löffler's syndrome describes a particular clinical presentation.

The eosinophilic pneumonias occur in childhood. They are generally associated with certain drug reactions, fungi or parasitic diseases, but there are other instances where the aetiology remains unknown or uncertain. Various drugs, including penicillin, sulphonamides and p-aminosalicylic acid, have been described in association with this entity, and among the fungi Aspergillus fumigatus appears to be the most important offender. Numerous parasites known to cause blood eosinophilia (tropical eosinophilia) are associated with the condition; among the most common are microfilariae and the larvae of *Ascaris lumbricoides, Strongyloides stercoralis, Ascaris duodenale, Toxocara canis* and *Toxocara cati.*

The pulmonary lesions may be caused by a local immunological type I or type III reaction. There is diffuse inflammation in the pulmonary parenchyma. Eosinophils usually predominate, and histiocytes are also present. Focal areas of necrosis can be observed, and granulomas are not uncommon. The most striking feature in many cases is fibrinoid necrosis of the peripheral arteries and arterioles in and about the lesions. In parasitic infections, sections of microfilariae or larvae can sometimes be identified within the granulomas (Alfaham et al. 1987; Jederlinic et al. 1988; Allen et al. 1989; Naughton et al. 1993; Winn et al. 1994).

Wegener's Granulomatosis

A relatively uncommon condition of unknown aetiology, Wegener's granulomatosis has been described in children. The disease is generally characterized by a pathological triad of necrotizing granulomas of the upper and lower respiratory tracts, systemic vasculitis and glomerulonephritis. The disease can be limited to the lungs, which may have nodules of variable sizes presenting with central necrosis resembling infarcts but with little haemorrhage. There is necrotizing granulomatous bronchitis and bronchiolitis, and angiitis of both arteries and veins of medium and small size often containing fibrin and/or thrombi within their lumen. Capillaritis is a common associated finding. Deposits of IgG and C_3 can be demonstrated in both the alveolar and the vessel walls. In the disseminated or generalized form, the disease shows widespread necrotizing and granulomatous vasculitis of arteries and veins of the upper and lower respiratory tracts, as well as most other organs or systems, including the joints, and central and peripheral nervous systems. In the lung, the necrotic areas of variable size can be isolated or confluent, or involvement could be diffuse affecting an entire lobe. These lesions may present haemorrhagic areas, sometimes massive or confluent and of different ages. These areas usually contain aggregates of chronic inflammatory cells of variable quantities, sometimes mixed with few polymorphonuclear cells but numerous monocytes. Giant cells of foreign body type are often seen on the periphery of the lesions. Stains for fungi and acid-fast bacilli are always negative. The vascular lesions may vary from fibrinoid necrosis of the vessel wall with an inflammatory cell infiltrate, a granulomatous vasculitis, to a scarred obliterative vasculitis, or

combinations of these, and may be associated with diffuse pulmonary haemorrhage. The association of Wegener's granulomatosis with the antineutrophil cytoplasmic antibodies directed to the neutrophil cytoplasmic enzyme, proteinase 3, makes it possible to differentiate this condition from some of the entities presenting with diffuse pulmonary haemorrhage. The limited form of this condition must be distinguished from *lymphatoid granulomatosis*, which has also been reported in childhood. Lymphatoid granulomatosis is characterized by an infiltrative process of the lung by small lymphocytes, plasma cells, histiocytes and atypical lymphoreticular cells associated with necrotizing angiocentric and angiodestructive lesions. Extrapulmonary involvement, especially of the skin and brain, is not uncommon. The sensitivity and specificity of the *antineutrophil cytoplasmic antibodies* in the diagnosis of this disease is now well established (Travis et al. 1987; Mark et al. 1988; Hoffman et al. 1992; Yoshimura et al. 1992; Dreisen 1993; Rottem et al. 1993).

Asthma

Bronchial asthma, a complex syndrome, is characterized by paroxysms of dyspnoea, wheezing and cough due to airway hyper responsiveness resulting in variable airway obstruction, usually over short periods and reversible. Bronchial hyperresponsiveness may also be present with this condition. It appears to be on the increase.

Asthma is now divided into two categories: extrinsic or IgE mediated (atopic or allergic), and intrinsic (non-atopic). The condition can be induced or triggered by a large variety of stimuli, including allergens (indoor or outdoor pollutions, foods, aerosols), medicaments (β-agonists, methotrexate, aspirin), chemical irritants (various gases, e.g. ozone), physical stimuli (exercise, cold air), infections (viruses, fungi, bacteria), psychologic status and many others.

There is accumulated evidence that the inflammatory mechanisms in asthma depend largely on various inflammatory cell types, principally the eosinophil and its secretion products (major basic proteins, eosinophil cationic protein, eosinophil peroxidase, eosinophil-derived neurotoxin), which serve as important proinflammatory mediators. Other cell types (mast cells, neutrophils, macrophages, platelets, lymphocytes) also play essential roles in the pathophysiology of the condition. Significant mucociliary clearance impairment and circulation adhesion molecules are also important factors in the exacerbations of the disease. The presence of Creola bodies (non-ciliated fragments of bronchial epithelium), Curshmann's spiral (condensed mucus bands),

Charcot–Leyden crystals and eosinophils in the sputum and/or BAL fluids are of clinical importance in the clinical diagnosis. Bronchial biopsy has now become an important tool in the diagnosis of the condition (Jeffery et al. 1989; Djukanovic et al. 1990; Jeffery 1991; Laitinen and Laitinen 1991; Messina et al. 1991; Aikawa et al. 1992; Kuwano et al. 1993; Gaillard et al. 1994; Janson et al. 1994; McBride et al. 1994; Montefort et al. 1994; Suissa et al. 1994; Sigurs et al. 1995).

Macroscopically, the lungs are very large, distended, filling the thoracic cavity, but they are not heavy unless superadded infection has occurred. Microscopically, the lesions are non-specific and largely confined to the medium-sized and small bronchi. The distal airways are distended, partially or totally obliterated by a thick, tenacious mucus (mucoid impaction) plug containing macrophages, desquamated epithelial cells, eosinophils (granulated and non-granulated), lymphocytes and sometimes neutrophils. In cases of sudden death the bronchial lumen may be free. There is a marked increase in goblet cells of the distal bronchial and bronchiolar epithelium, with hypersecretion of mucus. Mast cells, eosinophils and lymphocytes can be seen in the epithelium. The basement membrane appears to be thickened, but is supported by a hyaline-like collagen (collagens III and V and fibronectin, but no laminin) deposit containing reticulin but no elastic fibres. Submucosal glands are markedly enlarged showing hypersecretion. The smooth muscle of the bronchial wall shows varying degrees of hypertrophy, and aggregates of chronic inflammatory cells accompanied by eosinophils and mast cells stream across the bundles (Fig. 7.59). The blood vessels are congested and their walls are sometimes oedematous; there is an increase of nerve fibres containing substance P, but an absence of fibres containing VIP. The bronchioles and alveoli in the immediate vicinity of the bronchial lesions may be thickened and infiltrated by lymphocytes, plasma cells and some eosinophils; they may be distended. The large bronchi also show goblet-cell hyperplasia, and there can be some degree of squamous metaplasia. The peribronchial glands are also hyperplastic.

Idiopathic Pulmonary Haemosiderosis (Ceelen's Disease)

Idiopathic pulmonary haemosiderosis is an uncommon disorder of unknown aetiology. It has been reported mainly in infants and children and among young adults. The disease is characterized by repeated widespread intrapulmonary haemorrhages leading to respiratory distress, haemoptysis and severe iron-deficiency anaemia.

In children the majority of cases occur before the age of 10 years, and the incidence is about equal in both sexes; among adults there is a male predominance. The clinical symptoms are variable but the severity may increase, leading to marked disability and eventually to a fatal outcome. Some cases are asymptomatic. The radiological appearance is not diagnostic for the condition. The prognosis is unpredictable, and in the chronic stages pulmonary fibrosis may result. The condition has been described in association with myocarditis, and some cases have presented with diabetes. Chromosomal abnormalities and familial cases have been reported.

The diagnosis is usually made by elimination, as other conditions (mitral stenosis, pulmonary hypertension, veno-occlusive disease, etc.) can be accompanied by pulmonary haemosiderosis. The pathogenesis is unknown; however, some authors have proposed an immunological mechanism at the level of the basal membrane of the alveolar capillaries. This would suggest a mechanism similar to that occurring in Goodpasture's syndrome; however, immunoglobulins and complement have not been demonstrated on the basal membranes in idiopathic pulmonary haemosiderosis. Other authors have envisaged a connective tissue abnormality limited to the elastic tissue in the lung, and principally at the level of the small vessels. Cows' milk proteins acting as allergens on the capillary wall have been suggested as causative agents, but there is no conclusive evidence to support this theory; some reports have described the condition in association with coeliac disease. Within recent years the association with systemic lupus erythematosus in older children has been documented, and one report has shown acute alveolar capillaritis and focal alveolar necrosis in such cases. Ultrastructural studies in one case have shown mineral deposits (iron and calcium) on an altered basement membrane (Kjellman et al. 1984; Miller et al. 1986; Myers and Katzenstein 1986; Cutz 1987; Travis et al. 1987; Bonsib and Walker 1989; Travis et al. 1990; Harrity et al. 1991).

Macroscopically, the lungs are firm, somewhat nodular and reddish-brown in colour. The hilar lymph nodes are enlarged and brown. Microscopically, the changes depend on the stage of the disease. Initially the distended alveolar spaces are filled with numerous macrophages laden with haemosiderin. Macrophages are accompanied by erythrocytes, indicating recent haemorrhages, which are also observed in the bronchiolar wall. Intra-alveolar fibrin deposits can be demonstrated by means of special stains or immunofluorescence. The alveolar wall is oedematous and somewhat thickened, and contains iron-filled histiocytes. This thickening is accentuated by the hyperplasia of the alveolar epithe-

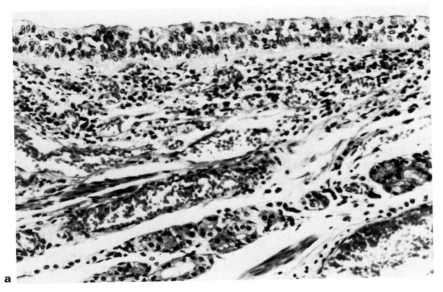

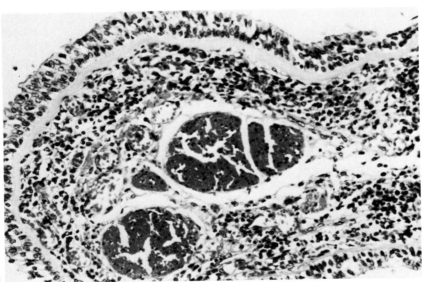

Fig. 7.59. A 17-year-old female patient, hospitalized for asthma on many occasions since the age of 3. (H&E, × 225) **a** Hyperplasia of goblet cells and marked thickening of the basement membrane. **b** Similar changes in the main stem bronchus. Note the marked muscular hypertrophy.

lial cells (mainly type II cells), which appear cuboidal. The capillary basement membrane shows some degree of thickening. There is no tissue necrosis or vasculitis. During the later stages, the thickening of the alveolar wall is more apparent, and fibrosis may be marked. There is an increase in collagen and reticulin fibres, accompanied by thick fragmented elastic fibres. Intra-alveolar and interalveolar haemorrhages may be widespread. Haemosiderin pigment deposits are abundant at this point, diffuse, and also observed in the interlobular spaces. Fibrotic nodules, some of which are siderotic, can be identified, and elastic tissue fragments are also impregnated by the pigment. Foreign-body giant cells containing elastic

fragments are seen in the alveolar spaces and elsewhere in the parenchyma. There are few inflammatory cells, and they are observed in the alveolar wall or the peribronchial and perivascular spaces, often associated with histiocytes containing haemosiderin pigment. Mastcells and eosinophils are sometimes prevalent.

Goodpasture's Syndrome

Goodpasture's syndrome is a rare condition characterized by pulmonary haemorrhages and acute glomerulonephritis. The disease has a predilection for young adults, and males are predominantly affected. The condition has also been recorded in infants and children.

The clinical symptoms closely resemble those of idiopathic pulmonary haemosiderosis but, in addition, the patients present with proteinuria and haematuria, indicating renal involvement. They may present with pulmonary disease only, especially when the condition is in its acute phase. In such patients antiglomerular basement membrane antibody is helpful in diagnosis. An influenza-like infection often precedes the symptoms, but the aetiological factors are many and varied. The course of the disease is variable and depends on the stage, but it often has a rapidly fatal outcome. The disease has been described in children with sickle cell disease (Albelda et al. 1985; Travis et al. 1987; Bonsib and Walker 1989; Travis et al. 1990; Harrity et al. 1991; Rosenblum and Colvin 1993).

Macroscopically, the lungs are heavy and there are subpleural haemorrhages in the acute stages, but later reddish-brown firm areas are found. The cut surface shows numerous old and recent haemorrhages scattered throughout the lung. Microscopically, the alveolar spaces are distended, filled with erythrocytes and macrophages laden with haemosiderin pigment. Fibrin strands can be identified by special stains or immunofluorescence. The alveolar wall is oedematous, generally thickened, and may be infiltrated in some cases by few inflammatory cells, mainly lymphocytes with few plasma cells and histiocytes. Polymorphonuclear leucocytes are rare. The alveolar epithelial cells are hyperplastic, cuboidal or even multilayered. Scattered foci of alveolar wall necrosis are occasionally observed and vasculitis has been reported. The histology is variable and by no means specific. Arteritis, when present, may be suggestive of periarteritis nodosa or some form of hypersensitivity reaction, and thus make diagnosis difficult. Immunofluorescent staining for immunoglobulins reveals the presence of extensive fluorescence for IgG and β_1c on the alveolar basement membrane and capillary basement membrane as a linear almost continuous pattern. Similar patterns are also observed on the glomerular basement membrane and portions of Bowmans capsule (see p. 473).

Aspiration Pneumonia

Although considered a rare condition, aspiration pneumonia may be more prevalent than is readily admitted. The condition may often go unrecognized and be incorrectly diagnosed as some other disease. The pulmonary lesions depend largely on the material

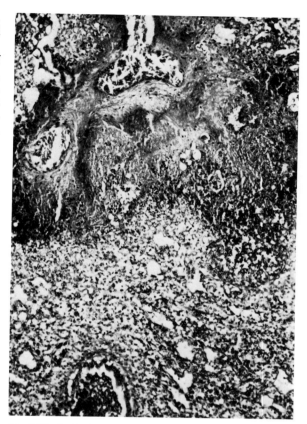

Fig. 7.60. Aspiration pneumonia due to aspiration of gastric juice, causing necrosis of the pulmonary parenchyma (*left*). (H&E, × 60)

inhaled, the quantity and the time elapsing between the episode(s) and medical examination.

Gastric secretions or contents may be inhaled into the lungs and may be the cause of severe respiratory insufficiency, occasionally resulting in death of the patient. Inhalation of gastric contents in infants and children is more likely to occur among those who suffer with dysphagia, diaphragmatic hernias, gastro-oesophageal reflux, or pyloric or oesophageal stenosis; in mentally retarded, wasted and debilitated children; in certain comatose states and during or after general anaesthesia; and in any condition associated with repeated vomiting.

When pure gastric secretion, with its high hydrochloric acid content, is inhaled into the lung, oedema results immediately with stasis, followed by widespread haemorrhage. Destruction of the tracheobronchial mucosa ensues, and within hours a diffuse inflammatory reaction occurs in the pulmonary parenchyma. The lesions contain few or no bacteria and are caused by the action of the hydrochloric acid on the lung tissue (Fig. 7.60).

In mild cases there is usually consolidation, which finally resolves, leaving mild pulmonary fibrosis; in severe cases there may be abscess formation. The lungs may eventually become fibrosed, with significant changes in pulmonary function.

In instances in which the gastric secretions are mixed with foreign material (partially digested food), the pulmonary lesions depend largely on the quantity of foreign material aspirated and on whether the process is acute or chronic. In the acute stage the lesions are non-specific, and the only indication of the pathogenesis is the presence of food particles (vegetables, meat, etc.) identifiable in histological sections. In chronic aspiration, there is often a foreign body giant cell reaction, some cells containing particles of foreign material.

Numerous microorganisms (including saprophytic anaerobes) are commonly associated with aspiration of foreign material. Abscesses are quite common in the lungs of these patients. The right lung is most often involved, and principally the lower segment of the right upper lobe and superior segment of the right lower lobe. The presence of saprophytic organisms can cause putrefaction of the lung tissue, giving it a characteristic foul odour (Awe et al. 1966; Cameron et al. 1967; Sladen et al. 1971; Bartlett et al. 1974a; Kaplan et al. 1978; Nelson 1984).

Exogenous Lipid (Lipoid) Pneumonia. This occurs when oily substances of different chemical natures are inhaled or aspirated into the lower respiratory system. The oily substance may be of vegetable, animal or mineral origin, and the tissue reaction produced will vary according to the lipids involved. Vegetable oils generally produce little or no pulmonary reaction; animal oils, which are rapidly hydrolysed to give fatty acids, produce necrosis of the tissue with a severe inflammatory reaction. Mineral oils, which are not hydrolysed but emulsified, produce little or no necrosis but do lead to extensive fibrosis.

Lipoid pneumonia is more common among infants and old people but may be observed at all ages. In childhood the disease is usually associated with the intake of cod liver oil, oily nasal sprays or drops, and mineral oils used as laxatives. It is also the result of repeated inhalation by infants of milk or milk products, resulting in severe respiratory distress, and can lead to severe bronchopneumonia. The condition is more common in debilitated or mentally retarded infants, especially those affecting swallowing, palatal or cough mechanisms, and also in cases of anorexia nervosa. It has also been reported in fire eaters and in patients employing excessive quantities of lip gloss. The condition has been documented in many patients in countries where there is practice of ethnic customs or habits particular to their societies. Deposits of fat droplets have also been described in pulmonary arteries, capillaries, macrophages, lymphatics and regional lymph nodes, especially in infants or children who have received intravenous fat emulsions (Levene et al. 1980; Shulman et al. 1987; Brown et al. 1994; Spickard and Hirschmann 1994).

The pulmonary lesions are described as diffused (infantile) and localized (adult type). The lesions are generally located in the lower segment of the upper and middle right lobes and/or the apical segments of the lower right and/or left lobes. However, both lungs may be involved to varying degrees.

The clinical manifestations are often misleading, and the radiological patterns are non-diagnostic. Lipophages or free lipids may be recovered from the sputum, and macrophages laden with lipid droplets may be seen in material from bronchial washings. Macroscopically, the area involved is fairly well delimited, heavy and firm. It is often grey or yellowish in colour, with a thickened pleural or significant pleural adhesion, and enlarged hilar lymph nodes may also be yellow. Microscopically, the lesions are variable, depending on the oily substance involved. The alveoli may be distended and filled with macrophages with a clear cytoplasm (foam cells) and occasionally free fat globules. The macrophages may be slightly positive with PAS or negative, light blue with Sudan black B, and orange with oil red O stains. The alveolar wall can be thickened, somewhat congested, and oedematous. The inflammatory reaction is also variable. When there is secondary bacterial infection, both the alveolar spaces and alveolar wall contain polymorphonuclear leucocytes and lymphocytes, with few plasma cells. When the pneumonitis is due to animal or mineral oils, the inflammatory reaction is more intense and there is active remodelling of the alveolar walls, which show varying degrees of thickening. In the chronic stages there is diffuse fibrosis with emphysematous blebs and/or bronchiectasis, the latter due largely to elastic tissue degeneration of the walls of the bronchi and bronchioles. The lesions usually progress to the mural stage of fibrosing alveolitis. Foreign-body giant cells can be observed in the chronic stages.

Endogenous Lipid (Lipoid) Pneumonia. This is the result of the accumulation of lipid substances, principally cholesterol and its esters, in the alveolar spaces, as a result of their liberation from damaged alveolar cells and bronchiolar epithelium. The condition is usually observed in cases of bronchial obstruction, most often by a malignant or chronic inflammatory process with lung tissue damage. It has also been described with secondary pulmonary hypertension, certain drugs (amiodarone), fat emboli, lipid storage disorders and immune deficiency states. Macroscopically, the lesion is golden yellow, and histologically cholesterol crystals are numerous within macrophages and giant cells, and there are few among the cellular debris, hence the name *golden* or *cholesterol* pneumonia.

The lesion can be distinguished from exogenous lipoid pneumonia by special histochemical techniques. The macrophages in the alveolar spaces, rich in fine fat droplets, are strongly PAS-positive after amylase digestion; they stain intensely with oil red O, black with Sudan black, and are birefringent under polarized light.

Because of its various clinical presentations, macroscopic appearance and histological and ultra-structural features, endogenous lipoid pneumonia is now considered by some authors as one of the phases making up the spectrum of *alveolar proteinosis*. They may have a common pathophysiological basis – alteration of pulmonary surfactant metabolism in which repeated gastro-oesophageal reflux plays an important role (Verbeken et al. 1989; Fisher et al. 1992; Spickard and Hirschmann 1994).

Pulmonary Alveolar Proteinosis (Idiopathic Alveolar Phospholipoproteinosis).   The rare condition of pulmonary alveolar proteinosis (PAP) is characterized by the accumulation in the alveolar spaces and bronchioles of large amounts of an amorphous material rich in lipids and proteins, leading to severe respiratory insufficiency. There is a male predominance.

The symptoms of PAP are non-specific and variable. They may regress spontaneously or proceed to progressive pulmonary insufficiency, and sometimes death if not adequately treated. The radiological pattern is not diagnostic for the condition, and pulmonary function tests are suggestive of a restrictive type of disease.

Although the aetiology of PAP is unknown, it has been considered as a form of lung response to a variety of agents, but two types are now recognized: a primary form of unknown aetiology, and a secondary form reported in association with tuberculosis and neoplasms often with bronchial obstruction in the lung as well as a number of mycotic, viral or parasitic agents. *Nocardiosis* is by far the most prevalent among these infections. *Aspergillosis, cryptococcosis, mucormycosis, candidosis, cytomegalic inclusion pneumonitis* and *pneumocytis* have also been reported, but less frequently. In childhood the condition is very often associated with some form of immune abnormality or haematological disorder, and has also been reported in siblings, suggesting a genetic disorder of autosomal recessive inheritance, for example lysinuric protein intolerance. It has also been documented in patients with AIDS.

Primary PAP is now considered a familial congenital condition most often in full-term infants who present with the respiratory distress syndrome at birth or shortly thereafter. These infants are resistant to all forms of intensive-care treatment, and death ensues within days or weeks later. The condition may be observed in siblings and both sexes may be affected. It has been shown recently that in the majority of cases there is an abnormal expression of SP-B gene product with little or no staining for SP-B, while SP-A, SP-C and SP-D show increased staining. In one case, however, the pattern was different suggesting that although the disease is related to a dysfunction of surfactant apoproteins, it may be heterogeneous and more than one gene, and/or other mechanisms, may be involved (deMello et al. 1994; de la Fuente 1994).

Extensive research on the amorphous material in the alveolar spaces has shown that it is quite heterogeneous and complex, composed of insoluble lipids, proteins and carbohydrates with large quantities of cellular debris, macrophages and granular pneumocytes (type II). The lipid concentration is several times that observed in normal lungs or in other pathological conditions and is composed principally of phospholipids. The proteins are largely surfactant apoproteins (A, B, C, D) associated with immunoproteins from the serum. The other constituents are disintegrating granular pneumocytes and macrophages with various types of inclusion body, including lamellar bodies tubular myelin and several other structures such as membraneous vesicles, electron-dense bodies and amorphous material (Gilmore et al. 1988; Rubinstein et al. 1988; Verbeken et al. 1989; Fisher et al. 1992; Parto et al. 1993).

The excessive production of surfactant, or its accumulation as a result of impaired removal or combination of both abnormalities, may be implicated in the pathogenesis of the condition or an alveolar macrophage catabolic defect. A defect in the processes during the formation of tubular myelin must also be considered (Ruben and Talamo 1986; Zijlstra et al. 1987; Gilmore et al. 1988).

Macroscopically, the lungs are enlarged and firm with consolidated areas. The cut surface is moist, revealing yellowish-grey zones alternating with dark red areas. Microscopically the alveolar spaces and bronchioles are distended with an abundant quantity of amorphous eosinophilic granular material in which cellular debris is associated with varying numbers of granular pneumocytes at different stages of disintegration and numerous macrophages (Fig. 7.61). The alveolar wall is not altered and shows no inflammatory reaction. It is mainly lined by cuboidal or flattened type II pneumocytes.

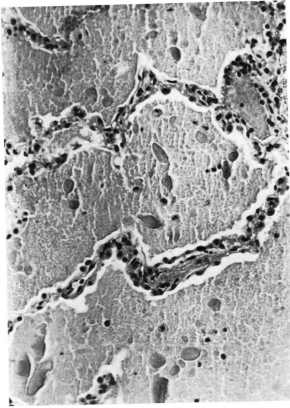

Fig. 7.61. Alveolar lipoproteinosis with distended alveoli full of an eosinophilic proteineous material. Absence of inflammatory reaction. (Courtesy of Dr Bozic) (H&E, × 225)

resistant and also positive with Von Kossa and Prussian blue stain (Fig. 7.62).

Kerosene Pneumonia. Kerosene is a by-product of petroleum and is the cause of a significant form of pneumonitis in childhood. Kerosene is widely used for fuel and lighting in many developing countries or areas not supplied with gas or electricity. Infants and children may inadvertently swallow the substance, which causes severe irritation of the stomach followed by severe vomiting and regurgitation. Under these circumstances the substance can be inhaled and reach the distal airways, producing a diffuse necrotizing pneumonitis. Death may follow due to pulmonary, gastrointestinal or central nervous system effects.

In the respiratory system, there is an immediate, marked, diffuse oedema with congestion of the lungs. This is followed by widespread necrosis of the pulmonary parenchyma, with a severe inflammatory response. The exudate is rich in fibrin and polymorphonuclear leucocytes, and fibrin may line the alveolar ducts and bronchioles. The lesions are generally bilateral, but are more frequently located in the right lung than in the left. There is extensive necrosis of the bronchial and bronchiolar epithelium, accompanied by infiltration of the walls by mononuclear cells and polymorphs. Necrosis of the peripheral vessels with haemorrhages is common, and in the healing stages the vessel walls are usually markedly thickened and sclerosed. Patients who survive show extensive pulmonary fibrosis (Press et al. 1962; Nouri and Al-Rahim 1970).

The intra-alveolar granular material, like that observed in endogenous lipid pneumonia, is strongly PAS-positive even after amylase digestion, and is metachromatic when stained with toluidine blue, and stains black with Sudan black B. Under polarized light, there are numerous doubly refractile crystals, mainly cholesterol. The macrophages also contain large quantities of this lipoprotein material in their cytoplasm, as shown by special stains and ultrastructural studies. Surfactant apoprotein labelling both in lung tissue sections and BAL fluid is of considerable importance in differentiating primary (uniform, diffuse labelling) from secondary (focal, patchy labelling) in this condition. In chronic stages of the disease pulmonary fibrosis ensues.

Malakoplakia, a rare granulomatous inflammatory disease of unknown aetiology, may occasionally involve the lung (Byard et al. 1990) and must be distinguished from these lesions. It is characterized by the presence of large foamy histiocytes containing the characteristic intracytoplasmic Michaelis–Gutmann inclusions which are strongly PAS-positive, diastase

Powder Aspiration. Occasionally, the aspiration of powder can cause respiratory distress in infants under 2 years of age; a relatively high mortality rate is associated with this condition. The accidental aspiration of talcum powder (rich in zinc oxide) causes bronchial obstruction, and after a relatively long latent period produces massive bronchitis with bronchiolitis. Oedema and congestion of the lungs may precede the inflammatory reaction. When there is complete obstruction of the bronchial lumen atelectasis ensues, and if death does not occur compensatory emphysema follows (Pfenninger and D'Apuzzo 1977; Motomatsu et al. 1979).

Pulmonary talc granulomatosis is not an uncommon finding in chronic adolescent drug addicts who administer narcotics mixed with talc or mixtures containing talc by intravenous injection. Pulmonary thromboembolism may be another complication which can lead to severe pulmonary hypertension. Electron-probe radiography may be of help in identifying the elements involved, as may X-ray

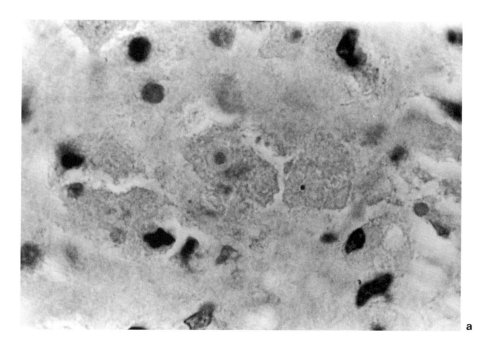

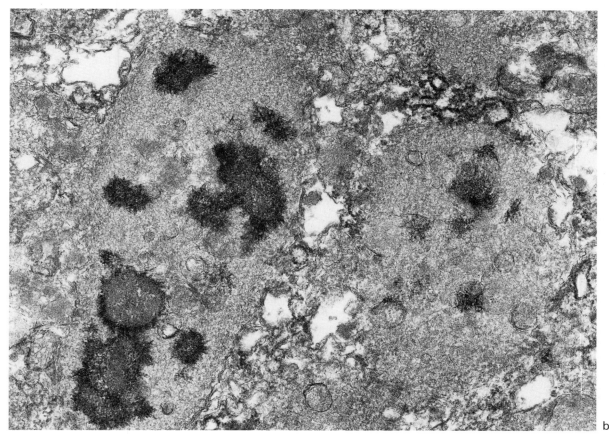

Fig. 7.62. a Malakoplakia showing alveolar macrophages containing classical cytoplasmic Michaelis–Gutmann inclusions. (PAS, × 340)
b Ultrastructure of Michaelis–Gutmann inclusions of variable form and size. (Electron micrograph, × 39 000)

diffractometry and scanning electron microscopy (Berner et al. 1981; Ghadially et al. 1984).

Starch in the Lungs. Dain et al. (1970) have described the presence of starch granules in the lungs of newborns treated with positive pressure ventilation for respiratory distress syndrome, chiefly hyaline membrane disease. They suggested that the source of the starch was the sterile gloves used in handling the endotracheal catheter. The substance was not usually recognizable with routine haematoxylin and eosin stains, but exhibited the characteristic maltese crosses when observed under polarized light. The starch granules may be free in the alveolar spaces or intermingled with the bronchial and alveolar exudate in the early stages. After a few days they are found in macrophages or in foreign-body giant cells within the alveoli.

Paraquat Lung

Paraquat (1,1-dimethyl-4,4-dipyridilum dichloride) is a herbicide. When ingested, it causes a rapid onset of diffuse pulmonary fibrosis, with severe respiratory failure and death within weeks of intake. The substance may be swallowed accidentally by children, and it can be taken up through the skin.

Paraquat causes ulceration of the mouth and upper gastrointestinal tract, with vomiting and diarrhoea. These symptoms are accompanied by acute renal failure, jaundice and increasingly severe dyspnoea with cyanosis, leading to marked pulmonary insufficiency within days. Cerebral symptoms may also be present. Paraquat is poorly absorbed by the intestine, and is excreted in the urine. The substance is metabolized in the liver and reaches the lungs from the circulation. It causes hepatic necrosis and damage to the adrenals, myocardium and renal tubules. It accumulates in the lungs and muscles.

The pulmonary lesions and the prognosis in general seem to depend on the serum concentration of the active substance ingested. In general, pulmonary fibrosis occurs over a variable period, preceded by pulmonary oedema and haemorrhage. Surfactant is lacking, following destruction of the type II cells or granular pneumocytes, which seems to follow that of the type I cells (Bus and Gibson 1984; Skillrud and Martin 1984; Fukuda et al. 1985; Hirai et al. 1985; Martin and Howard 1986; Matters and Scandalios 1986; Bismuth et al. 1987; Vale et al. 1987) mainly due to the toxic effect of superoxide species.

Macroscopically, the appearance depends on the time lapse after the intake of the substance, because little if any of the substance reaches the lungs by way of the bronchial tree. Within the first 4 days the lungs are heavy congested and oedematous. Later they show areas of consolidation, or appear solid with a somewhat rubbery consistency, and within weeks they take on a honeycomb appearance.

Microscopically, in the first few days, there is congestion with marked oedema of the alveolar wall. Interalveolar and intra-alveolar haemorrhages are conspicuous. The alveolar spaces are filled with a fibrinous exudate containing desquamated alveolar lining cells (some of which are undergoing degeneration) and numerous macrophages and erythrocytes. Polymorphonuclear leucocytes and aggregates of lymphocytes and plasma cells may be seen. Hyaline membranes are prominent, lining both the alveolar spaces and the distal airways. There is destruction of the epithelial lining of the distal bronchi and bronchioles. Some of these lesions may be due to oxygen therapy. In later stages of the disease there is a very active, but variable, organization of the intra-alveolar exudate. The alveolar spaces are invaded by an active fibroblastic proliferation resembling the pattern of growth seen in a tissue culture. These cells have been referred to as "profibroblasts" and are probably myofibroblasts. Finally the alveolar space is obliterated by a fibrous process with collagen, reticulin fibres and a few elastic fibres. There is also a rich capillary network, and a few foci of chronic inflammatory cells are present. Simultaneously a similar process takes place in the alveolar wall, and eventually it is impossible to distinguish the alveolar wall from the alveolar space. As the lesion progresses there is continuous remodelling of the alveolar structure leading to diffuse pulmonary fibrosis, with an increase in collagen and reticulin fibres; and, although the lesions have a heterogenous distribution, they may resemble honeycomb (Takahashi et al. 1994).

The bronchial and bronchiolar walls are also affected by the fibrotic process, and can be obliterated. Bronchiectasis may occur, and other bronchi and bronchioles may show epithelial proliferation and hyperplasia. Small pulmonary arteries show thickening and fibrosis of their walls. Arterioles show distinct muscular hyperplasia.

Lung Abscesses

There are many possible causes of lung abscesses in childhood, including bronchial obstruction by an inhaled foreign body, by an inspissated mucus plug, or by infected material associated with some surgical procedure in the mouth or oropharynx. The majority of abscesses are located in the lower segments of the

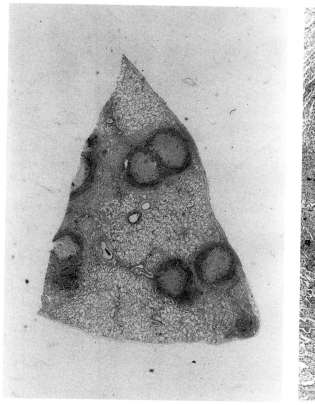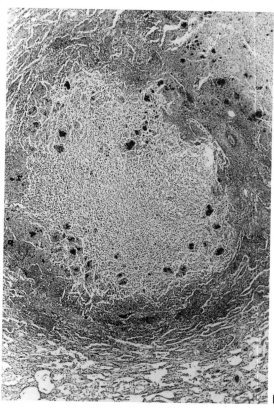

Fig. 7.63. a Multiple microabscesses, confluent in places, and formation of a pseudocapsule of compressed parenchyma. (H&E, ×4) **b** Abscess showing a necrotic central zone filled with neutrophils. Bacterial colonies are located in the necrotic areas, peripheral zones and lung parenchyma. (H&E, ×50)

upper lobes or the upper segments of the lower lobes, and they are more often found on the right side. Whatever the source, the material is generally accompanied by a mixture of both anaerobic and aerobic microorganisms. Necrosis of the bronchial wall takes place at the site of obstruction, with active bacterial proliferation and a marked inflammatory exudate. The related distal airways collapse and become necrotic, and a purulent inflammatory reaction develops. The centre of the lesion undergoes liquefaction, and partial drainage may take place by way of the eroded bronchus (Fig. 7.63).

In chronic cases the wall of the abscess is surrounded by a dense fibrous layer bordered by granulation tissue. The cavity may be lined with a squamous epithelial lining in continuity with the epithelial lining of the bronchus.

Lung abscesses may also be associated with bacterial pneumonia or bronchopneumonia. *Staphylococcus aureus*, which is known to cause extensive tissue destruction, is by far the most common offender. Other microorganisms commonly responsible for

such lesions are *Klebsiella pneumoniae*, *Pneumococcus* and *Pseudomonas*.

Septic emboli may affect the lung in septicaemia, and in childhood an important cause is thrombophlebitis around an indwelling catheter. *Staphylococcus aureus* is most often associated with these abscesses (Pryce 1948; Mark and Turner 1968; Bartlett et al. 1974b; Brook and Finegold 1979; Asher et al. 1982).

Granulomatous Lesions

Numerous agents are known to produce granulomatous lesions in the lung (Ulbright and Katzenstein 1980). In certain instances special staining techniques make it possible to identify the agent responsible for the lesions within the granulomas, and infectious causes including *Mycobacterium tuberculosis*, coccidioidomycosis, aspergillosis, blastomycosis and histoplasmosis are discussed elsewhere.

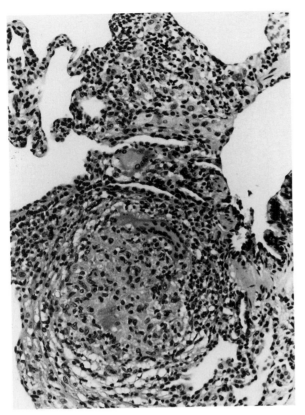

Fig. 7.64. Non-caseating granulomatous lesions in a male patient. The adjoining lung tissue is involved in the process. (H&E, × 125) (Courtesy of Dr J. Briner).

Sarcoidosis (Boeck's Sarcoid, Besnier–Boeck–Schaumann Disease)

Sarcoidosis has a worldwide distribution, the incidence varying from one area to another, and even within the same region. The clinical and radiological features of the condition have been extensively documented. The disease usually presents as a slowly progressive chronic inflammatory reaction affecting the skin (erythema nodosum), lungs, lymph nodes and uveal tract. Spontaneous healing may occur after a long period. Less frequently, the disease also affects many other organs or systems (heart, kidney, skeletal muscles, central nervous system, bone and joints – arthralgia). The symptoms are often variable and may go unnoticed; in many instances the disease is an accidental finding on routine chest radiographs or at autopsy.

A female predominance has been indicated by some authors, but others claim that there is an equal male-to-female ratio. The disease has been reported in families, and there are strong indications that it is more common among negroes. Sarcoidosis is not common in childhood; it is prevalent among children in their teens and rare in infants below 5 years of age.

Descriptions of the disease in childhood show no features distinguishing it from the condition seen in adults. Severe obstructive vascular lesions in the lung may lead to pulmonary hypertension. Elevated serum angiotensin-converting enzyme activity is a common finding in active disease, and immunohistological staining for this enzyme will reveal positive staining of epithelioid and giant cells within the granulomata. BAL fluid as well as lung and skin biopsies show an increased ratio of helper/suppressor (cytotoxic) T cells, suggesting an increased activity of cell-mediated immunity; alveolar macrophages show a reduced capacity to produce arachidonic acid metabolites. Ultrastructural studies have revealed tadpole-shaped structures in granulomatous lung disease, consistent with sarcoidosis (Smith et al. 1983; Dewar et al. 1984; Allen et al. 1986; Pattishall et al. 1986; Van Maarsseven et al. 1986; Viale et al. 1986; Bachwich et al. 1987).

Chronic Granulomatous Disease

Chronic granulomatous disease is characterized by severe, chronic and recurrent infections, usually involving the skin, lung, liver, bone and lymph nodes, but any organ can be involved. The first clinical symptoms generally appear during the first year of life, and the disease may run a fatal course before the age of 10 if inadequately treated.

The condition occurs in a number of forms, with variable modes of inheritance, but a recessive mode of transmission is most commonly found (see p. 635).

In the lung, pneumonia or bronchopneumonia with abscess formation may be present. There may also be numerous non-caseating granulomas with foreign-body giant cells, together with many histiocytes containing lipid pigments (Fig. 7.64). On the periphery of the lesions are lymphocytes, and occasionally central necrosis can be identified containing few polymorphonuclear leucocytes. Fungal infection is not an uncommon complication (Landing and Shirkey 1957; Holmes et al. 1966; Thompson and Soothill 1970; Schlegel 1975; Dilworth and Mandell 1977; Moskaluk et al. 1994).

BCG Granulomas

Generalized BCG infection is a rare complication of BCG vaccination in childhood. It has been reported to have a fatal outcome in some instances, mainly among infants with some form of immune abnormality. Inadequate preparation of the vaccine may be responsible for the condition. The lung, the intestine and bones, as well as other organs, are the site of numerous granulomas, which may show caseation. Groups of acid-fast bacilli can be observed in the epithelioid cells and/or in the necrotic areas (Passwell et al. 1976; Genin et al. 1977; Torriani et al. 1979; Hanimann et al. 1987).

Rheumatic Pneumonitis

There is still no unanimity as to whether the pulmonary lesions observed during the course of acute rheumatic fever are specific for the condition, although they are generally referred to as rheumatic pneumonitis.

The radiological images of diffuse pulmonary consolidation are in no way specific, and the morphological features may resemble those seen in a number of other conditions. Associations with the clinical aspects of the disease are the only guiding factors. The lesions are generally observed in cases presenting with severe valvular involvement or fulminant pancarditis (Massumi and Legier 1966; Grunow and Esterly 1972).

Macroscopically, the lungs are oedematous, large and heavy. They are often reddish in colour and rubbery in consistency. Microscopically, the lesions are widespread. The alveolar spaces are filled with a thick fibrinous exudate, which is haemorrhagic in some areas. There are fibrin strands and a few desquamated alveolar cells with some macrophages containing pigment granules. Scattered groups of inflammatory cells, chiefly mononuclear cells, are often present. Some of the alveolar spaces and alveolar ducts are lined with thick bands of hyaline membranes. The alveolar walls are thickened, oedematous and congested. Intraseptal and intra-alveolar haemorrhages are constant findings. Alveolar wall necrosis has been observed in a number of cases, and in many of these fibrinoid necrosis of the wall of the distal branches of the pulmonary artery is present (Fig. 7.65). In advanced stages there are signs of organization of the intra-alveolar exudate, characterized by the penetration of fibroblasts. The epithelium of the distal bronchi and bronchioles may show evidence of necrosis, and their walls may be infiltrated by a few mononuclear cells or surrounded by peribronchial lymphoid tissue. During regeneration there is metaplasia of the bronchial epithelium.

These lesions are in no way specific, and there is still some doubt as to whether they are primary lesions. Aschoff nodules are not identified with this pneumonitis.

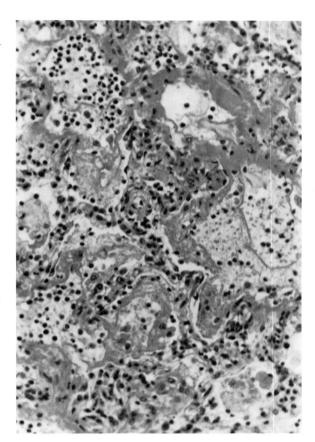

Fig. 7.65. Rheumatic pneumonitis in a 12-year-old boy with extensive pancarditis and severe valvular lesions. (H&E, × 120)

Pulmonary Alveolar Microlithiasis

Pulmonary alveolar microlithiasis is a relatively rare pulmonary condition of unknown aetiology. The disease has a worldwide distribution and has been described in all races. All ages are affected, and it has been documented at birth. It was formerly thought that adults were principally affected, but the disease seems to be more prevalent among children in Japan. it has an equal distribution between the sexes or perhaps a slight male predominance. There is a familial tendency, suggesting that some genetically determined disturbance of metabolism may be present, although there are no abnormalities of the metabolism of calcium and phosphorus in these patients. The disease is often asymptomatic, and may be discovered at routine chest radiography or when dyspnoea of unknown origin is investigated. Surveys in families may reveal new cases. There is generally a significant discrepancy between the severe radiographic changes and the absent or mild clinical symptoms. Pulmonary function tests give variable

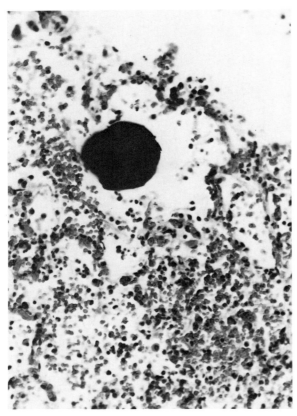

Fig. 7.66. Pulmonary microlithiasis in a girl of 2 years 5 months. (Courtesy of Dr C. Bozic) (H&E, × 180)

results, depending largely on the stage of the disease, its distribution and the extent of the lesions. Evolution is also quite varied, extending over a period of a few months or years or even several decades as the pulmonary function deteriorates. There is no satisfactory treatment (Sears et al. 1971; Onadeka et al. 1977).

Macroscopically, the lungs are much heavier than normal, very hard in consistency, and reddish in colour. The lesions may predominate in the lower lobes, but all lobes can be affected. Microscopically the lesions vary with the stage of evolution. In the early stages the alveolar spaces are filled with psammoma-like bodies, which are darker in their centres. These bodies are strongly PAS-positive, and stain intensely for calcium with the von Kossa stain. They are known as calcospherites, and are different from the *corpora amylacea* associated with chronic congestive heart failure or pulmonary fibrosis. The alveolar wall shows little or no histological modification at this stage (Fig. 7.66). Later the calcospherites not only appear as laminated bodies with radial striations, but also show extensive calcification, with ossification

occurring at the periphery. The alveolar walls are thickened, fibrosed, disrupted in places, and infiltrated by mononuclear cells (chiefly monocytes and lymphocytes). Giant cells may be observed in some instances, and calcospherites may be incorporated within the thickened alveolar wall or situated in the proximity of small vessels.

The condition can now be diagnosed by BAL and/or transbronchial biopsy. Ultrastructural studies have shown that the psammoma-like bodies are composed partially of hydroxyapatite crystals; chemical analyses have shown that calcospherites are composed mainly of calcium phosphates with small quantities of iron and fat. Surfactant apoprotein has been demonstrated immunohistochemically as a component of these structures (Cale et al. 1983; Mascie-Taylor et al. 1985; Akino et al. 1990; Ucan et al. 1993).

Pulmonary calcification can also be observed in children undergoing long-term haemodialysis and/or peritoneal dialysis. The diagnosis is not readily made on chest radiographs, but can be confirmed by radionuclide pulmonary scintigrams (Drachman et al. 1986).

Pulmonary Alveolar Septal Calcinosis

Pulmonary alveolar septal calcinosis, an uncommon metastatic pulmonary calcification, may be observed in the paediatric age group and often goes undiagnosed clinically. The condition is observed as a complication in many clinical settings such as primary or secondary hyperparathyroidism, chronic renal insufficiency, vitamin D intoxication, milk alkali syndrome, and primary or secondary conditions of the haematopoietic and lymphatic systems (Northcutt et al. 1985; Sinniah et al. 1986). Histologically, there is focal or diffuse calcification of the alveolar septa as well as the vessels and bronchial walls (Fig. 7.67). Emphysema may be prominent in areas, and metastatic calcifications are often seen in other organs such as the heart, kidney, liver and gastrointestinal tract.

Pulmonary Arterial Calcification

Calcification of the pulmonary arterial trunk and/or its branches has been documented in cases of idiopathic arterial calcification in newborns and infants. The lesions may be multifocal and are more prominent in the main and secondary branches (Fig. 7.68). Thromboses, sometimes calcified, are frequent findings, often associated with pulmonary infarcts (Carles et al. 1992b; Beguin 1994). Recently, in utero pulmonary arterial calcification in monochorionic twins has been described (Popek et al. 1993).

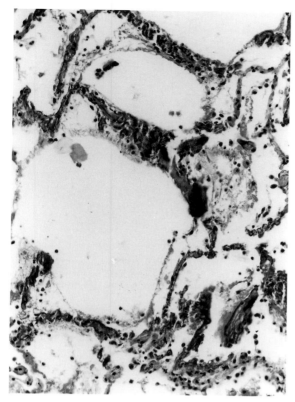

Fig. 7.67. Alveolar septal calcinosis involving also pulmonary arteries in a case of severe chronic renal failure. (H&E, ×50) (courtesy of Dr J. Briner)

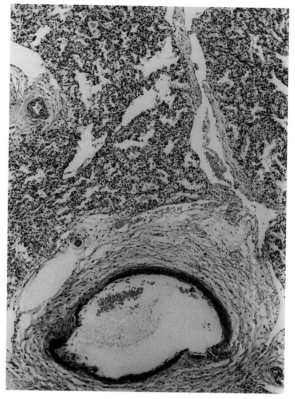

Fig. 7.68. Pulmonary arterial calcification at 32 weeks' gestation in a male fetus with diffuse arterial calcification and calcified thrombus resulting in extensive infarction in several organs, including the lungs. (H&E, × 20)

Bronchial Lesions

Intrauterine (Congenital) Bronchiolitis Obliterans

Bronchiolitis obliterans is not uncommon. It has been described in numerous conditions and is associated mainly with various inflammatory reactions of the respiratory tract. Bacterial and viral infections are chiefly responsible for the lesions, and all age groups can be affected.

Intrauterine bronchiolitis obliterans is rare, and only a few reports are recorded. The aetiology is not known; however, it is generally accepted that intrauterine infection may be responsible for the lesions (Sir 1962; Nezelof et al. 1970; Sueishi et al. 1974; Rosen and Gaton 1975).

Macroscopically, the lesions are observed in premature infants or in the immediate neonatal period. The lungs are diffusely consolidated and heavy, and appear dark red with some haemorrhagic areas. Microscopically, there are areas of intrauterine pneumonia. Some of the alveoli are filled with squames accompanied by polymorphonuclear leucocytes. Occasional giant cells with vacuolated cytoplasm may be present. The distal bronchi and bronchioles are obliterated by polypoid masses consisting of granulation tissue projecting into the lumen from an area of damaged wall. Some of the lesions show various degrees of organization, with fibroblasts, collagen fibres and hyalinization being present. Vascular penetration from the base of insertion of the polyp may be apparent (Fig. 7.69).

The bronchial epithelium shows signs of regeneration, sometimes with squamous metaplasia; in other areas there is evidence of hypersecretion. The bronchial wall and surrounding tissues are infiltrated with polymorphonuclear leucocytes and some lymphocytes. The lesions of bronchiolitis obliterans in children are similar to those observed in adults (Hardy et al. 1988; Marinopoulos et al. 1991).

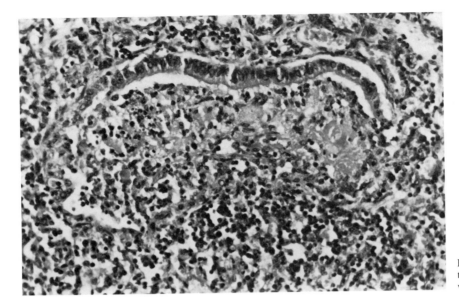

Fig. 7.69. Intrauterine bronchiolitis obliterans in a newborn infant who lived for 12 h. (H&E, × 180)

Bronchitis and Bronchiolitis

Inflammation of the lower respiratory tract is extremely common in infants and children, and all levels of the bronchial tree are liable to injury by the agent or agents responsible. Bacterial infections have been considered to be responsible for most of the lesions; however, it is now well established that viral infections are the major cause of bronchitis and bronchiolitis in childhood and the principal cause in infancy. Secondary bacterial infections may be associated with viral infection.

The development of better tissue culture techniques and specific serological tests have resulted in the isolation and identification of the various viruses responsible for the lesions. Direct and indirect immunofluorescence antibody techniques and in situ hybridization have proved useful in the diagnosis of viral infections.

Respiratory syncytial virus infection is the commonest in infants during the first 2 years of life. Other viruses known to cause these illnesses include *adenovirus, parainfluenza viruses, influenza A and B viruses* and *measles virus*. Other organisms, e.g. *Bordetella pertussis* and *Mycoplasma pneumoniae*, can produce severe infections. Physical, chemical or gaseous injury to the distal airway may be responsible for similar lesions.

The clinical symptoms are in no way specific for any one virus. There is generally an upper respiratory tract infection with a catarrhal reaction, raised temperature, cough, dyspnoea and wheezing. Diffuse interstitial pneumonia is sometimes present, and hyperventilation may be observed. The radiological patterns are non-specific.

Although the mortality rate is relatively low for many of these infections, morbidity can be high and repeated infections may be responsible for significant abnormalities of lung function. The physiopathological features of the condition have been well documented and it has been shown that the respiratory difficulties are related principally to the obstruction of the distal bronchi and bronchioles. The severity of the lesions in infancy depends largely on the anatomical structure of the lung at that age. Other factors, including immunological ones, may also be important (Aherne et al. 1970; Becroft 1971; Gardner et al. 1973; Simpson et al. 1974; Kaul et al. 1978; Wohl and Chernick 1978).

Microscopically, the bronchial and bronchiolar mucosa show patchy or widespread ulceration with necrosis of the epithelium. Signs of regeneration are characterized by the proliferation of epithelial cells, which become cuboidal. The walls of the distal airways are congested, oedematous and infiltrated by mononuclear cells. The lumen may be partially or completely obliterated by an exudate composed of cellular debris, fibrin, some mucus and a large number of inflammatory, principally mononuclear, cells. Patchy atelectatic foci may be present when obstruction is complete. There is also peribronchial and peribronchiolar inflammatory infiltration extending from the walls of the affected airways into the surrounding pulmonary parenchyma, resulting in localized zones of pneumonia (Fig. 7.70).

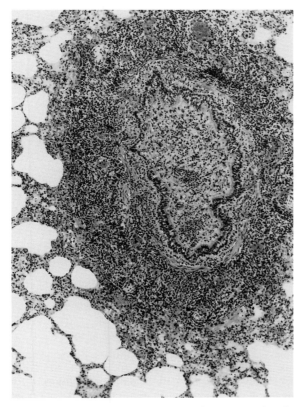

Fig. 7.70. Acute bronchitis with diffuse inflammatory infiltration of the entire bronchial wall and the surrounding lung parenchyma. The bronchial lumen is filled with numerous neutrophils in the mucus plug. (H&E, × 20)

These lesions are common to the majority of viruses involved; however some viruses (adenovirus, influenza A virus) may produce severe residual lung damage with extensive destruction of the distal bronchi and bronchioles and obliteration of the lumen. In chronic disease there is organization of the intraluminal material, resulting in bronchiolitis obliterans. In this case there is vascular granulation tissue initially, which progresses to fibrous scarring with partial or complete obliteration of the affected distal bronchi and bronchioles.

Bronchiectasis

Bronchiectasis is not uncommon in infants and children, and it is often associated with chronic and frequently repeated lung infections. There is much controversy and debate on the aetiology and pathogenesis. Some authors maintain that there are two forms of the disease: *congenital*, related to malformations in the bronchial wall as a result of absent or deficient cartilage plates, and *acquired*, associated with acute respiratory infection resulting in severe pulmonary damage with sequelae. Most authors consider the lesions to be acquired in most cases, with only a very small percentage attributable to congenitally determined defects. In support of this hypothesis, it is true to say that bronchiectasis has never been observed at birth or in the neonatal period. In almost all cases, including most of those described as congenital, the condition has developed after a period of acute bronchitis or pneumonia during infancy (generally within the first 2 years of life). Obstruction (extrinsic or intrinsic) of a bronchus or of bronchi may also be associated with the development of bronchiectasis.

The disease begins in infancy, often during the first or second year of life, after an attack of what is generally referred to as bronchitis or pneumonia. In well documented cases, the association of the development of bronchiectasis with syncytial virus, adenovirus, influenza virus, measles, pertussis or *Mycoplasma pneumoniae* infections has been established. Sequelae of tuberculosis infection with parenchymal destruction and fibrosis could be responsible for the disease, as well as aspergillus and other fungal infections.

Bronchiectasis may affect only a small percentage of infants or children after viral epidemics, and is not apparent immediately after infection. Host as well as immunological factors probably play an important role in the development of the lesions. The stage of lung development may be an additional factor.

The disease may be progressive, with a high incidence of chronic and frequent recurrent infections of the respiratory tract. Cough is often associated with wheezing. Haemoptysis is a variable finding. In the chronic stages of the disease, dyspnoea occurs on exercise, and finger clubbing may be seen. Radiography, and principally bronchography, is important in establishing the diagnosis, and repeated examinations may be necessary to follow its evolution.

Bronchiectasis has been observed in association with certain syndromes, notably the unilateral hyperlucent lung (Swyer–James syndrome or McLeod's syndrome), a clinical and radiological entity that was once thought to be congenital but is now recognized as being a sequela of various insults to the lung, including viral infections, tuberculosis, *Mycoplasma pneumoniae*, foreign-body aspiration, ingestion of hydrocarbons, and radiotherapy. It is also an integral part of Kartagener's syndrome, a condition with familial tendency, in which bronchiectasis is associated with situs inversus, chronic paranasal sinusitis and ciliary dysfunction. The Williams–Campbell and Stevens–Johnson syndromes may also be associated with bronchiectasis, and to a lesser extent the

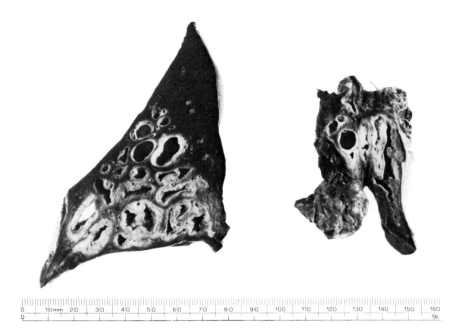

Fig. 7.71. Significant bronchiectasis in an 18-month-old infant. (Courtesy of Dr C. Bozic)

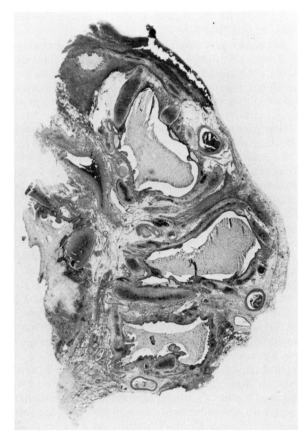

Fig. 7.72. Bronchiectasis with fibrosis and chronic inflammation of the wall containing lymphoid follicles. (H&E, × 25)

Ehlers–Danlos and Marfan syndromes. Bronchiectasis has also been described with certain immuno-deficiency states, as well as pulmonary injury after ingestion or inhalation of certain toxic substances or drugs. It has recently been described in an infant after intoxication by inhalation of acrolein (Barker and Bardana 1988; Mahut et al. 1993; Nikolaizik and Warner 1994).

Bronchiectasis is associated with small-airway disease, with obstruction of the involved airways and bronchiolitis obliterans. Atelectasis of the parenchyma distal to the obstruction is often encountered. There is hypersecretion of mucus distal to the occlusion, with subsequent infection leading to abscess formation and foci of pneumonia. Destruction and weakening of the bronchial walls occur proximal to the lesions, with profound remodelling of the surrounding tissue as a result of chronic inflammation. Subsequently there is dilatation of these bronchi, due in part to the negative intrathoracic pressure and the traction exerted by the surrounding fibrous tissue. The basic physiopathological problem in bronchiectasis is one of perfusion/ventilation associated with airtrapping.

Macroscopically, dilated bronchi may be cylindrical in form or show saccular dilation, or both. The changes are often severe and widespread. They may be unilateral or bilateral, and may affect one or more lobes or segments. The left lower lobes, the lingula, the right middle lobe and the posterior basal segments are most frequently involved (Fig. 7.71). Microscopically there is marked dilation of the bronchi, and mucus with an inflammatory exudate may occupy the lumen. The bronchial epithelium is variable from one area to another, being generally hyperplastic and lined with tall columnar cells whose cytoplasm contains large amounts of mucus. In other areas squamous metaplasia may be conspicuous. The wall is infiltrated by a dense mononuclear infiltrate, which is more prominent in the submucosa. In some instances the inflammatory reaction is overwhelming and consists of lymphocytes extending into the surrounding parenchyma. Well developed lymphoid follicles with prominent germinal centres can be seen in this infiltration (Fig. 7.72). The submucosal glands are usually atrophic but some glands may be dilated, containing large quantities of mucus englobing inflammatory cells. The bronchial muscular layer is hypertrophied in some places and atrophied in others. Fibrous bands may encircle, dissect or completely replace the muscle bundles. The peribronchial elastic fibres are fragmented and disorganized. In some instances, especially in areas where the dilatation is saccular, the bronchial wall is completely destroyed and the regenerated epithelium, which may show squamous metaplasia, covers a layer of granulation tissue with no other supporting structures.

The bronchial arteries show extensive hypertrophy of their walls; the pulmonary arteries in the neighbourhood may have been destroyed in the inflammatory process or may show severe endarteritis. As a result there is shunting of blood by bronchopulmonary anastomoses, leading to pulmonary hypertension.

In cases of congenital bronchiectasis there is hypoplasia of the involved lung. The inflammatory reaction is scanty and the cartilage plates are poorly developed. The most striking feature is marked hypertrophy of the bronchial muscle, which appears disorganized. Lymphangiectasis may be an associated abnormality.

Cystic Fibrosis of the Pancreas (Mucoviscidosis)

Cystic fibrosis (CF) may be manifest at birth as intestinal obstruction resulting from meconium ileus, but pulmonary involvement is by far the most serious complication of the disease, and is responsible for the high morbidity and mortality rate. Pulmonary manifestations may be recognized during early infancy but may go unnoticed until adolescence or adult life.

The patients usually present with repeated chronic pulmonary infections, which become progressively more severe. Areas of bronchopneumonia may never resolve as other areas are affected. These pulmonary infections are often accompanied by severe pansinusitis, with or without nasal polyp formation. *Staphylococcus aureus* has been considered to be responsible for most infections, but recently it has been appreciated that other organisms are more important as the patients grow older, and that viruses may participate in promoting and/or maintaining secondary bacterial infections. *Pseudomonas aeruginosa* is the organism most often incriminated in these cases, and *Haemophilus influenzae* is also known to play an important role. Although the non-mucoid strains of *P. aeruginosa* seem to colonize the airways in the first instance, the mucoid strains predominate later during the course of the infection. They are associated with the active inflammatory and obliterature process in the lung, leading to bronchiolitis obliterans and alveolitis. The antigen produced from antigen–antibody complexes, which can be localized in many tissues in these patients, including the lung, and it is considered that some of the pulmonary damage may result from these complexes. *P. aeruginosa* also produces a number of enzymes (esterase, protease), which are capable of acting locally on the pulmonary parenchyma as well as the host defence mechanisms. *P. cepacia* also creates important problems among these patients, and mycoplasmal and other infections may be aggravating or complicating factors in most of these infections. Gastrooesophageal dysfunction in the form of gastrooesophageal reflux is now known to contribute significantly in the severity of the pulmonary lesions as well as hypersensitivity to *Aspergillus fumigatus*, which may be responsible for an allergic bronchopulmonary reaction in these patients.

The frequent, repeated and chronic pulmonary infections are the result of obstruction of the bronchial tree, in particular the distal airways, by a thick, viscoid mucus or mucopurulent secretion maintained largely by *P. aeruginosa*. Subsequently bronchopneumonia, bronchiectasis and bronchiolectasis, loss of lung elasticity and diffuse emphysema (more important in the upper lobe), with modifications in pulmonary function tests, develop. Immune complexes seem to play a minor role in the pathogenesis of the lesions. Pulmonary hypertension follows, leading to right ventricular hypertrophy associated with biventricular scarring. In most cases hypertrophy of the carotid body is found. Pneumothorax may be a troublesome complication. The ultrastructure of cilia in both nasal and bronchial epithelium in patients with cystic fibrosis may show various nonspecific anomalies, including compound cilia, excessive cytoplasmic matrix, abnormal number and arrangement of microtubular doublets and rippled ciliary contours, abnormalities which have also been described in chronic inflammation of the respiratory tract (Sturgess and Turner 1984; Baltimore et al. 1989; Elborn and Shale 1990; Hoiby and Koch 1990;

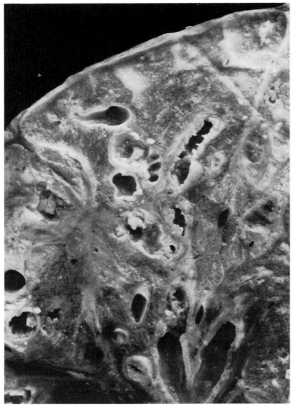

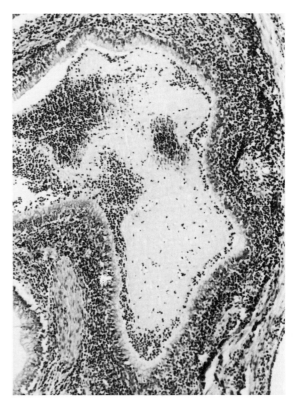

Fig. 7.73. Bronchiectasis and pulmonary consolidation in a 14-year-old boy with cystic fibrosis.

Fig. 7.74. Bronchiectasis in cystic fibrosis. Increased number of goblet cells and mucopus obliterating the lumen. The inflammatory exudate contains numerous polymorphonuclear leucocytes. (H&E, × 35)

Gustafsson et al. 1991; Betancourt and Beckerman 1992; Fuller et al. 1992; Tizzano and Buchwald 1992; Tomashefski et al. 1992; Tizzano 1993; Mrouch and Spock 1994).

Macroscopically, the entire lung is involved. It is large, reddish and emphysematous, especially at the anterior margin, while the posteriorly sited lobes may show areas of atelectasis. There are areas of consolidation, and the bronchi and bronchioles are dilated, containing abundant viscous mucus (Fig. 7.73). Abscesses are sometimes present. Microscopically, the most striking feature is diffuse bronchial and bronchiolar dilatation, with the lumen completely obliterated by adherent mucus plugs. The inspissated mucus secretions contain numerous inflammatory cells, chiefly polymorphonuclear leucocytes, but including eosinophils, lymphocytes and some plasma cells. Bacteria can be identified by gram staining.

The lesions involve the distal bronchi and bronchioles initially. These become obliterated, causing atelectasis of some of the pulmonary parenchyma distal to the obstruction. The larger bronchi are then affected, and as a result of repeated episodes of chronic inflammation there is partial destruction of the bronchial wall with cylindrical dilatation of the involved segments. These changes may involve one or more lobes, or the entire lung (Fig. 7.74).

The bronchial mucosa is covered by hypertrophic and hyperplastic mucus-secreting cells whose cytoplasm is filled with a strongly PAS- and Alcian blue-positive mucus. Squamous metaplasia of the mucosa may be observed in places. The bronchial wall is generally fibrous and thinned, but isolated areas show signs of muscular hypertrophy. Chronic inflammatory cells are abundant.

Areas of bronchopneumonia are found, and resolution of these zones leaves alveolar wall scarring. Abscesses are sometimes observed in the vicinity of affected airways or within the parenchyma. Most of the lung outside these areas is markedly emphysematous. Pulmonary arteries show the changes associated with moderate pulmonary hypertension.

Lung Involvement in Metabolic Diseases (see also p. 837–866)

The lung is known to be involved in Gaucher's disease, an inherited deficiency of the enzyme gluco-cerebrosidase whose gene is located on chromsome I. The many mutations observed in this disease are responsible for the various clinical presentations and manifestations that exist in this condition. The lungs may be involved in all forms. In the more severe cases there may be large areas of consolidation, and an entire lobe or lung may be involved; in others the lesions are limited. Histologically, there is a diffuse infiltration of the alveolar spaces by Gaucher cells and numerous histiocytes (Fig. 7.75). Alveolar walls may also be infiltrated by histiocytes and some Gaucher cells. Some of the distal bronchi and bronchioles may also contain these cells (Beutler 1992).

In other forms of sphingolipidosis (Niemann–Pick), pulmonary involvement is more common, however, and it has also been seen in Fabry's disease (Bartimmo et al. 1972; Martin et al. 1972). The pulmonary parenchyma shows consolidated areas in which the alveoli are filled with foam cells. Lung involvement has also been recorded in cases of gangliosidosis (Volk et al. 1975) and mucopolysaccharidosis (de Montis et al. 1972). Recently, pulmonary vascular obstruction has been described in association with cholesteryl ester storage disease in a 15-year-old girl (Michels et al. 1979).

Tumours

Although primary lung tumours are uncommon in infancy and childhood, both benign and malignant tumours have been described in this age group. Metastatic tumours are more prevalent.

Benign

Vascular

Haemangiomas of the lung are extremely rare. Most of the lesions described as haemangiomas or angiomas of the lungs in infants and children are congenital developmental defects of the pulmonary vasculature, which are referred to under several synonyms: pulmonary arteriovenous fistulae or aneurysms, congenital arteriovenous varix and pulmonary haemangiomatosis.

A significant proportion of patients with these lesions present with coexisting vascular anomalies in other organs (mucous membranes, skin, brain), forming part of a more generalized syndrome of hereditary telangiectasia of the Rendu–Osler–Weber type. Familial occurrence has been recorded.

Vascular anomalies are generally located in the periphery of the lung or in the subpleural zones, and may involve extrapulmonary structures (mediastinum, pericardium, thymus and spleen). They are more common in the lower lobes, may present as localized structures, single or multiple, and are often bilateral with the appearance of either a low-grade neoplasm or a hamartomatous lesion. They may be the cause of primary pulmonary hypertension. An elevated incidence of cerebral abscesses has been reported among patients with these lesions (White et al. 1989; Galliani et al. 1992).

Microscopically, the lesions may resemble capillary or cavernous angiomas, the latter becoming distended as a result of large arteriovenous anastomoses (Fig. 7.76). These abnormal vessels are lined with flattened endothelial cells, and the structure of their walls varies, being arterial and venous in different areas.

Congenital alveolar capillary dysplasia, also referred to as *congenital alveolar dysplasia*, is a developmental anomaly of the alveolar capillaries of the lung affecting full-term infants, and is among the causes of the syndrome of persistent fetal circulation (persistent pulmonary hypertension) in the newborn. The lungs, especially the lobes, are usually abnormal, accompanied by congenital pulmonary vascular abnormalities – mainly abnormal or malpositioned pulmonary veins and their branches. The lesion is characterized by a marked reduction in the number of alveolar capillaries and an increase in the thickness of the septa. The few capillaries are rarely in contact with the normal alveolar epithelium. The intra-acinar arterioles are thickened, muscularized and accompanied by large, abnormal, dilated veins. (Khorsand et al. 1985; Carter et al. 1989; Langston 1991). *Pulmonary acinar dysplasia*, another maldevelopmental process, in which there is an abortive development or arrest in the differentiation of the alveolar acini, has been reported (Rutledge and Jensen 1986).

Sclerosing haemangioma of the lung (Liebow and Hubbell 1956) is a circumscribed pulmonary lesion described in the literature under several synonyms (histiocytoma, fibroxanthoma, alveolar angioblastoma, mast-cell granuloma), depending on the histological patterns exhibited.

These lesions have been reported in children. They are often described in the lower lobes, but can be located in any lobe and occur mainly in the periphery of the lung. Most patients are asymptomatic and the

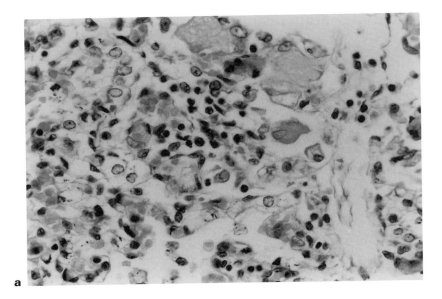

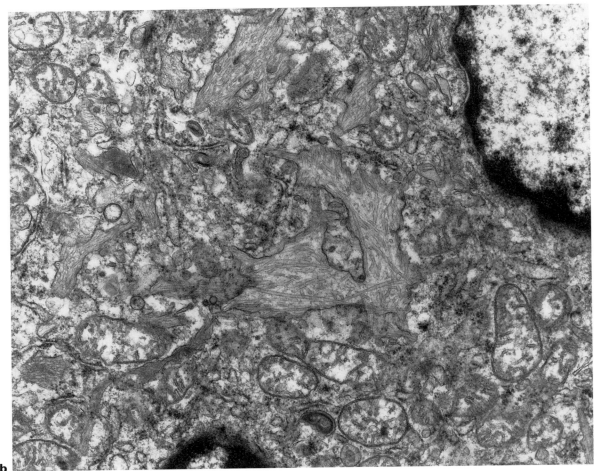

Fig. 7.75. a Gaucher cells and other macrophages in the alveolar lumen associated with few mononuclear cells. (H&E, × 300) **b** The lung in Gaucher's disease, showing the characteristic elements. (Electron micrograph, × 31 000)

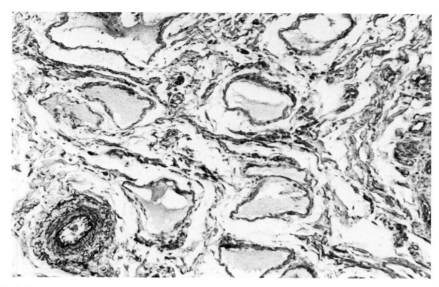

Fig. 7.76. Pulmonary arteriovenous shunt (pulmonary varix) in a newborn with cardiac malformation. (V6–Élastin, × 120)

tumours are discovered on routine chest radiography. Haemoptyses have been recorded as the most common clinical symptom.

The pathogenesis of the lesions is unknown and their aetiology remains obscure. Some authors still regard them as pseudoinflammatory reactions; others consider them to be vascular lesions in various stages of sclerosis with secondary epithelial proliferation, or as a proliferation of undifferentiated pulmonary epithelial and mesenchymal tissues with secondary changes, and yet others regard them as of mesothelial origin. These various morphological variations point to the great heterogeneity of the lesions: the different components may be variable in quantity in any given lesion. Recent ultrastructural studies have shown lamellar bodies within the lining cells similar to those observed in type II pneumocytes, and microvilli on the luminal surfaces of others. Immunohistochemical studies have confirmed that many of the lining cells are analogous to those of bronchiolar epithelial cells and type II pneumocytes and that they also contain surfactant apoproteins. Clara cells have also been identified among the type II pneumocytes. These recent findings have led some authors to consider these lesions as hamartomas, distinct from pulmonary histiocytomas. Although Haas et al. (1972) concluded from their observations that the lesions were primarily angiomatous in nature, Hill and Eggleston (1972) considered the primary lesions to be of epithelial origin with the other changes a secondary phenomenon. Recent immunohistochemical and ultrastructural findings would support the latter view; thus, some authors consider these lesions as hamartomas, distinct

from pulmonary histiocytomas, and others have suggested "benign sclerosing pneumocytoma" or "type II pneumocytoma" as being more appropriate terms (Noguchi et al. 1986; Nagata et al. 1987; Yousem et al. 1988; Alvarez-Fernandez et al. 1989; Satoh et al. 1989).

Macroscopically, sclerosing haemangiomas are solitary, circumscribed, round or oval masses, firm or rubbery in consistency, yellow in colour, with tan or haemorrhagic areas. Multiple lesions, sometimes presenting as a principal mass with satellite nodules have been described, as well as bilateral tumours. Calcification and even ossification have been observed in some cases.

Microscopically, there may be papillary structures lined with alveolus-like mesenchymal cells, cuboidal and/or columnar in appearance, mainly at the periphery of the lesions. The supporting stroma is fibroblastic with some histiocytes, and contains many irregular dilated capillaries with an angiomatous appearance. In other areas the stroma is composed of numerous spindle cells separated by large bands of collagen. Hyalinization may occur in other regions, where the vessels may be seen as slit-like openings. Mitotic figures are few, and there is no cellular atypia. Evidence of both recent and old haemorrhage is seen. Plasma cells, lymphocytes and mast cells have been observed scattered throughout lesions of this type.

Plasma-cell granuloma, although a relatively uncommon tumour, is perhaps the most common benign tumour of the lung in childhood. The lesion, in which plasma cells predominate, must be distinguished from its malignant counterpart, the pulmonary plasmacytoma. Plasma-cell granuloma has been considered to be a postinflammatory pseudotumour, and some authors use the term "plasma-cell pseudotumour" when referring to the lesion. It has also been mistakenly called a fibroxanthoma, because of the presence of numerous fat-laden histiocytes, and has further been confused with sclerosing haemangioma and other fibrohistiocytic lesions.

The majority of plasma-cell granulomas have been reported in children, with apparently no predominance between the sexes. The youngest patient thus far was 13 months old, and there appears to be an increase in frequency with age. Although the aetiology is unknown, the condition is thought to be infectious in nature and it has been described in association with Q-fever pneumonia and *Mycoplasma pneumoniae* and *Coxiella burnetti* infections. Immunoperoxidase staining has shown the polyclonal nature of the plasma cells, indicating an inflammatory reactive process rather than one of a neoplastic nature. Clinically the condition is asymptomatic unless it produces obstruction of bronchi, causing dyspnoea. It is often discovered during routine chest radiography, and presents as a solitary circumscribed parenchymal mass or coin lesion. The prognosis is generally good, and surgery is the treatment of choice (Lebecque et al. 1987; Warter et al. 1987; Dardick et al. 1989; Anthony 1993; Haver and Mark 1994).

Macroscopically, the lesions are firm or rubbery in consistency, round or oval, and yellowish-white or grey in colour. They may appear brownish owing to haemorrhages, and occasionally show central necrotic zones. They may also contain fine granular calcification. The lesions are usually peripheral and intraparenchymatous, but may sometimes involve bronchi, causing obstruction.

Microscopically, the tumour is made up of mature plasma cells with some lymphocytes and mononuclear cells. Russell bodies may be conspicuous, but the plasma cells, immunohistochemically, are polyclonal. Polymorphonuclear leucocytes are occasionally observed. Histiocytes may be prominent, grouped together and located among fibroblasts arranged in whorls and supported by dense collagen bundles. Many of the histiocytes are laden with fat globules, giving the lesion a xanthomatous pattern. Mast cells are scattered throughout the tumour and some eosinophils may be present. Lymphoid follicles with germinal centres are sometimes visible. Iron pigment-laden macrophages may be prominent as a result of haemorrhages. The lesions may bulge into the adjacent alveolar spaces and may sometimes attain the bronchial and vascular walls, mainly venous, with intraluminal protrusions.

Lymphangioleiomyomatosis (lymphangiomyomatosis) is a rare clinicopathological entity with a worldwide distribution. The disease has been described almost exclusively in females of childbearing age, and rarely in males. Cases have been described before the age of 20 and the clinical symptoms often begin during childhood. The lesions are not confined to the lung, but may involve extrapulmonary structures, mainly the lymph nodes and lymphatics, but the uterus, ovaries and liver have also been documented. The condition has been reported in association with renal angiomyolipomas as well as with multiple soft tissue tumours and endocrine tumours, and this has led some authors to suggest the possibility that it may form part of the tuberous sclerosis complex; however, there are no proofs that the conditions are interrelated. Oestrogen and progesterone receptors have been documented on smooth muscle cells, which form part of the lesion, but their expression is variable from one case to another and depends somewhat on the techniques employed. In spite of these variations, hormonal therapy, among others, still remains the treatment of choice (Vincent et al. 1987; Colley et al. 1989; Berger et al. 1990; Cagnano et al. 1991; Ohori et al. 1991).

The clinical symptoms may go unrecognized for some time. The patients present with breathlessness, recurrent pneumothorax, and sometimes haemoptyses. Chylothorax is not an uncommon finding in this condition, and may be associated with chylous ascites. Pulmonary haemorrhages have also been recorded. The disease follows a relentlessly progressive course, with death from respiratory failure. The period over which this occurs is variable. Most patients affected die within 10 years of discovery; however, some have survived for more than 20 years.

Extensive hypertrophy and proliferation of smooth muscle in the wall of lymphatic vessels are the principal histological characteristics of the abnormality, but some authors have suggested that the proliferating cells in the lung may be derived from immature pluripotent myoid stromal cells or myofibroblasts. However, the cellular heterogeneity of the lesions would suggest one of two possibilities as proposed by some authors: either there are different degrees of differentiation from the same phenotypic cell line or there is coexistence of different cell types. Immunohistochemistry and molecular biology could be very instructive (Sherrier et al. 1989; Fukuda et al. 1990; Bonetti et al. 1991; Cagnano et al. 1991; Ohori et al. 1991; Bonetti et al. 1993; Matthews et al. 1993).

Macroscopically, the most characteristic picture is one of honeycombing of the entire lung, with enlarged hilar lymph nodes. Morphometric studies have shown abnormalities similar to those of centriacinar emphysema (Sobonya et al. 1985). The pleura is thickened and the lymphatics are prominent and well defined. Microscopically the alveolar septa and other involved areas are diffusely thickened by proliferation and hyperplasia of smooth-muscle-like cells, some of which may form nodules about myoid stromal cells. The tumour cells stain variably with desmin, actin and vimentin, or in combinations. Some cells having epithelioid-like features have been shown to express melanoma-related antigens, which appear ultrastructurally as electron-dense membrane-bound granules. A tumour may therefore present various histological and immunohistochemical variations in different regions. The lesions may surround the lymphatics in the interlobular spaces (Fig. 7.77), the bronchial wall or the pulmonary vessels. When the veins are involved, venous obstruction may result. Intra-alveolar haemorrhages may follow, and numerous haemosiderin-laden macrophages may be observed in the alveolar spaces.

Muscular

Smooth- or striated-muscle tumours of the lung are exceedingly rare. *Leiomyoma*, the smooth muscle variant, may originate from the tracheobronchial tree or the lung parenchyma. In the tracheobronchial tree it may grow within the wall or protrude within the lumen forming a polypoid mass resulting in bronchial obstruction with distal bronchiectasis and secondary infection associated with haemoptysis, dyspnoea, fever and clubbing of the fingers. There is a female predominance. The tumours appear to originate from the smooth muscles of the bronchi or bronchioles or ultimately from the wall of the pulmonary vessels, and may be associated with cyst formation. Histologically, the lesions are characteristic of smooth-muscle tumours elsewhere; however, immunohistochemistry may be necessary to exclude carcinoids (Vera-Román et al. 1983; Uyama et al. 1988; Gotti et al. 1993; Kim et al. 1993).

Another group of smooth-muscle tumours is seen in young women of childbearing age and young men. There is much controversy over the many synonyms by which these lesions are known: "low-grade" leiomyosarcoma with malignant potential, the so-called benign metastasizing leiomyoma, fibroleiomyomatosis hamartoma, and more recently a specific entity composed of extrauterine smooth-muscle neoplasms with multifocal origin. Oestrogen and progesterone receptors have been demonstrated in the cells of some of these tumours, and they are known to be responsive to hormonal influences, such as pregnancy, oophorectomy and hormonal manipulations. The lesions are sometimes single but often multiple, diffuse and bilateral. The nodules may be variable in

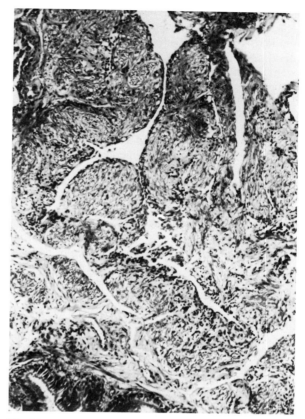

Fig. 7.77. Lymphangioleiomyomatosis from a female patient presenting with symptoms from the age of 11 years, with chylus effusion. (H&E, × 225)

size and therefore may go unrecognized, or be discovered on routine chest radiographs. Histologically, they resemble leiomyomas or fibroleiomyomas, but a classic leiomyosarcoma (cellular atypia, mitotic counts, epithelioid nests, necrosis, haemorrhage) must be excluded. Immunohistochemistry is mandatory to arrive at a correct diagnosis and especially to exclude other tumours. Ultrastructural studies may be helpful (Cho et al. 1989; Gal et al. 1989).

Congenital multiple fibromatosis (*infantile myofibromatosis*) has also been described in association with multiple congenital mesenchymal tumours or fibromatosis. The lesions are present at birth or within the first weeks after birth. New lesions may occur in the perinatal period or a few months later, but spontaneous resolutions have been documented as well as death in some cases. There is a strong male predominance, and the condition has been described as having both an autosomal and a recessive mode of inheritance with some sporadic cases. The nodules are multiple, firm, yellowish or greyish-white, of variable size and distributed throughout the lung.

Similar lesions are also seen in various organs, including the skin, muscle, bone and viscera. The tumours are located adjacent to bronchioles and blood vessels, and may show central necrosis and even calcification. They may be responsible for severe respiratory distress in the neonatal period (Chung and Enzinger 1981; Jennings et al. 1984; Goldberg et al. 1988).

Congenital peribronchial myofibroblastic tumour is a term coined recently by McGinnis et al. (1993) as representative of a distinct clinicopathological entity in the neonatal period. Their gross appearance together with their immunohistological and ultrastructural features of the cells making up the lesions point to their myofibroblastic origin. These authors have grouped all the tumours commonly referred to as *bronchopulmonary fibrosarcoma, congenital fibroleiomyosarcoma, hamartoma of lung* or *massive congenital mesenchymal malformation* under this umbrella, separating them from true leiomyosarcomas seen in older children.

Granular cell myoblastoma is a very rare benign tumour of the respiratory tract, may be single or multicentric, and is sometimes associated with lesions involving the tongue, skin and other soft tissues. The tumour has been reported in childhood; the histology and histogenesis is similar to that described for other sites (Redjaee et al. 1990; Guillou et al. 1991; Deavers et al. 1995).

Pulmonary tumours of *nervous* origin are very rare, even though those arising in the mediastinum are common in childhood. Isolated cases of intrapulmonary tumours of nervous origin have been recorded in infancy and childhood. They include neurofibromas (often associated with generalized neurofibromatosis), neurilemmoma and benign schwannoma. Immunohistochemistry is valuable in arriving at a correct diagnosis (Gay and Bonmati 1954; Neilson 1958; Bartley and Arean 1965; Massaro et al. 1965).

Others

Fibromas of the lung are very rare. When present, they may be located peripherally in the pulmonary parenchyma or the bronchial wall. The tumour has been reported in children. It is composed mainly of fibrocytes supported by collagen fibres, with some myxomatous areas (Roenspies et al. 1978).

Chondromas are benign well differentiated hyaline cartilage outgrowths arising from the cartilaginous plates of bronchi, and are often lined with bronchial epithelium. They have been observed in childhood and present as polypoid or lobulated masses, projecting into the bronchial lumen and causing stenosis or bronchial obstruction.

Chondromas must be distinguished from chondromatous hamartomas, benign lesions made up largely of cartilage. They are considered to be hamartomas, although they continue to grow after body growth ceases. Their histogenesis is still unsettled. The lesions are relatively common and are most frequently described in adults, with a peak incidence between the fourth and sixth decades; nevertheless, they do sometimes present in childhood.

Chondromatous hamartoma has been described by several synonyms (chondromas, fibroadenoma, lipochondroadenoma, adenochondroma), depending on the predominant tissue in the lesion. They are most commonly located in the lung parenchyma towards the periphery (intrapulmonary), and less frequently in the bronchial wall (endobronchial). The lesions are usually single and either lung may be affected. There is a male preponderance. Multiple tumours have also been described, but they are less common, often bilateral, and are observed almost exclusively in females. It is necessary to exclude Carney's triad (pulmonary chondroma, gastric leiomyosarcoma and extra-adrenal paraganglioma) in young females with pulmonary chondroma (Raafat et al. 1986).

The clinical features are non-specific and depend largely on the size and localization of the tumour. Although radiography may be of little help, computed tomography may better delineate the lesion (King et al. 1982; Austin et al. 1994).

Macroscopically, the tumour is variable in size and is generally made up of a round or oval mass with a smooth surface, often lobulated. It is whitish in colour, somewhat translucent, firm in consistency, well circumscribed, and separated from the surrounding parenchyma by a pseudocapsule. Microscopically, the greater portion is composed of lobules of well differentiated hyaline cartilage interrupted by cleft-like spaces lined by cuboidal or columnar epithelium resembling that of the respiratory tract. The remainder of the tumour is made up of an admixture of various amounts of fibrous tissue, fat tissue, muscle bundles (striated and smooth), and occasionally metaplastic bone and aggregates of lymphocytes. Calcification may occur occasionally.

Recent ultrastructural studies by Stone and Churg (1977) have shown that the epithelial component of the chondromatous hamartoma is made up of cells resembling those lining the distal bronchioles and alveoli of adult lung.

Intrapulmonary teratomas are rare. Day and Taylor (1975) found only 19 recorded cases of intrapulmonary teratoma in the literature, and added one of their own. In their review they reported one malignant terotama in an infant: the ages in the other cases ranged from 16 to 66 years. The left upper lobe was most commonly involved, and of the 16 cases for whom adequate histological descriptions are provided nine tumours were benign and seven malignant.

Teratomas in the lung are usually large masses of greyish-white fleshy tissue, sometimes surrounding cystic cavities of variable diameter. Tissue derivatives of the three embryonic germ layers may be identified histologically. In a case described by Day and Taylor (1975) the tumour seems to have developed in ectopic thymic tissue within the lung. Besides the two additional cases described by Holt et al. (1978) and Präuer et al. (1983), there have been some cases described in the Chinese and Japanese literature and more recently by Kayser et al. (1993) in an adult.

Malignant

Primary

Haemangiopericytoma of the lung is exceedingly rare and most of the cases published have been described in adults with occasional cases in children. The sex distribution is about equal. The tumours may attain considerable size before symptoms appear, sometimes associated with paraneoplastic symptoms. The histological diagnosis can be difficult, but immunohistochemistry and ultrastructural studies are of considerable help. The course of the disease is unpredictable and its prognosis variable, but total excision remains the treatment of choice, with radiotherapy and chemotherapy when there are metastases (Yousem and Hochholzer 1987; Rusch et al. 1989).

Primary fibrosarcoma of the lung is uncommon in childhood and may involve the bronchial tree (endobronchial or transbronchial) or intraparenchymal. The endobronchial lesions may cause obstruction resulting in pulmonary atelectasis with distal secondary infection or endogenous lipoid pneumonia as complications. The intraparenchymal masses are often well circumscribed lobulated masses (Pettinato et al. 1989; Cohen and Kaschula 1992). Macroscopically, the lesions are firm, greyish-white to yellowish, with occasional haemorrhagic areas. Histologically the lesions are cellular, composed principally by fusiform or oval spindle cells with little cytoplasm. Immunohistochemistry is mandatory for arriving at a correct diagnosis. There is a strong cytoplasmic positivity for Vimentin, indicating their fibroblastic nature, but are negative with the other intermediate filaments.

Malignant fibrous histiocytoma, a common soft tissue sarcoma, may originate in the lung; some 40 cases have been described in this organ, two of which

were in teenagers. Either lung may be affected, and the tumour may present as a single mass or occupy an entire lobe. Histologically the storiform–pleomorphic type predominates, but the lesion may be made up of the various components with dominant features of one or more of the four components (Yousem and Hochholzer 1987; McDonnell et al. 1988). The tumour is aggressive, often infiltrating the chest wall and mediastinum, with frequent vascular invasions. It must be differentiated from spindle cell sarcoma or carcinosarcoma, and immunohistochemistry can be helpful. The prognosis is generally poor.

Primary leiomyosarcoma of the lung is also very rare in childhood. The lesion may originate in the bronchial or vascular wall as well as the pulmonary parenchyma, principally in the peribronchial mesenchyma. Certain authors prefer to refer to these tumours in the perinatal period as *congenital peribronchial myofibroblastic tumour*, indicating their myofibroblastic nature. The tumour may be the cause of bronchial obstruction in the newborn and could be associated with polyhydramnios and non-immune hydrops fetalis (Jimenez et al. 1986; Gal et al. 1989; Pettinato et al. 1989; Khong and Keeling 1990; McGinnis et al. 1993; Klaveren et al. 1994).

Histologically, it is important to differentiate this tumour from fibrosarcoma and certain tumours of neurogenic origin. Special stains, especially immunohistochemical staining for vimentin, desmin and antibodies to muscle-specific actin are necessary for arriving at a correct diagnosis. Ultrastructural studies, tissue cultures and flow cytometry are all useful aids in confirming the diagnosis. Leiomyosarcoma tends to metastasize by way of the blood stream; involvement of the lymphatic system appears to be infrequent.

Primary rhabdomyosarcoma in childhood is rare. The tumour may be endobronchial, parenchymatous or both. It is often described in association with cystic lesions of the lung – principally bronchogenic cysts, congenital cystic adematoid malformation and mesenchymal cystic hamartoma – but is probably more often encountered with solid lesions like pulmonary mesenchymomas, pleuropulmonary blastoma (in childhood) and pulmonary blastoma (adult type) (Hartman and Schochat 1983; Allan et al. 1987; Pettinato et al. 1989; Domizio et al. 1990). Immunohistochemistry (myoglobin, desmin, actin and vimentin) and ultrastructural studies are most helpful in arriving at a correct diagnosis, especially in infancy and early childhood.

Rhabdomyomatosis dysplasia, the presence of nontumoral striated muscle fibres in the lungs, has been described in association with congenital cystic adenomatoid malformations, hypoplastic lungs with anomalous vascular anomalies and major cardiopul-

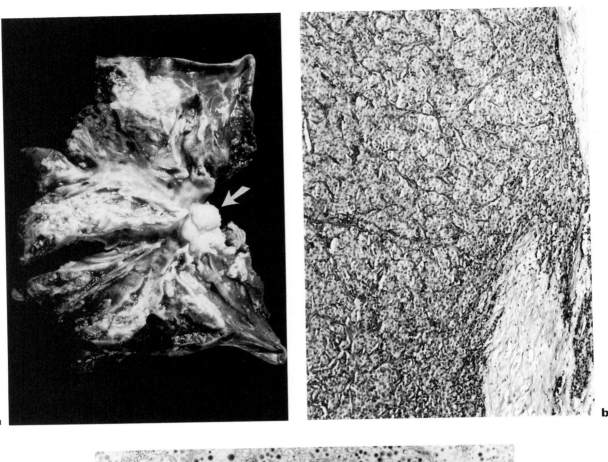

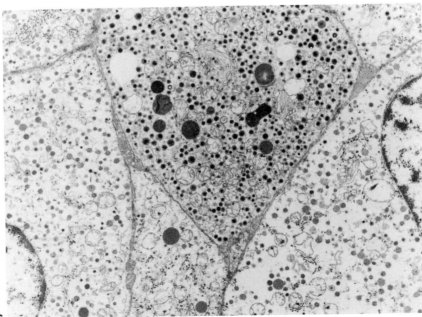

Fig. 7.78. **a** Carcinoid tumour in a 9-year-old girl; it is obliterating the bronchi, resulting in bronchiectasis and severe peripheral infection with abscess formation. **b** Tumour showing the classic picture of nests of tumour cells separated by thin fibrous bands. (H&E, × 120) **c** Electron micrograph showing the tumour cells laden with dense granules of variable sizes and densities. (× 48 404)

monary malformations. Either lung may be affected and the lesions may be bilateral. The striated muscle fibres or bundles may be patchy, and may affect one lobe or an entire lung. It has also been documented with abnormalities involving the diaphragm and with intralobular and extralobular sequestration (Chellam 1988; Drut et al. 1988; Chen et al. 1991; Meacham et al. 1991).

A primary pulmonary embryonal liposarcoma has been described in a 9-year-old girl who presented with the adrenogenital syndrome (Wu et al. 1974), and this tumour has also been reported in the pediatric age group by Lagrange et al. (1988) and Ruiz-Palomo et al. (1990).

Chondrosarcoma of the lung is rare and the cases reviewed by Daniels et al. (1967) included one in a 17-year-old girl.

The term *bronchial adenoma* is now generally used to include five distinct neoplasms arising in the bronchus. Each of these lesions forms a well defined entity. A total of 58 cases has been reported in childhood (Wellons et al. 1976).

The five tumour types are:

1. Mucous gland adenoma
2. Bronchial carcinoid
3. Cylindroma or adenoid cystic carcinoma
4. Mucoepidermoid tumour
5. Papillary adenoma

A possible sixth type, alveolar adenoma or bronchioloalveolar cell adenoma, has been recently described (Yousem and Hochholzer 1986; Miller 1990; Hancock et al. 1993).

Mucous gland adenoma is the only truly benign lesion of the group, and is also the rarest. Courtin et al. (1987) collected 34 cases from the literature and added one of their own. These tumours, rare in childhood, take their origin in the submucosal glands of the large bronchus, and involve both the glands and their ducts. They may cause obstruction of the bronchial lumen or stenosis by compression.

Carcinoid tumours are most common among this group, representing 80%–85% of all bronchial adenomas. They take their origin from the Kulchitsky cells (APUD) in the bronchial mucosa and have been reported at all ages. Lawson et al. (1976) subdivided this tumour into three histological subgroups, while others (Valli et al. 1994) suggest four based on the cellular morphology. Carcinoids are known to be of low-grade malignancy, and may metastasize to neighbouring lymph nodes or other sites after a long period (Fig. 7.78). The carcinoid syndrome has been reported in some cases (Ricci et al. 1973), and acromegaly has been associated with this tumour. Most go unnoticed as they infiltrate the bronchial

wall and adjacent tissue or proliferate into the lumen until large enough to cause obstruction with atelectasis, infection and bronchiectasis (Wang et al. 1993b). Some undergo calcification or ossification. Haemoptysis is the most frequent clinical symptom and is associated with intraluminal growth.

Cylindroma is rare, accounting for about 12%–15% of all bronchial adenomas. They are derived from the mucus-secreting cells of the mucosa of the larynx and tracheobronchial tree, but mainly the large bronchi, and histologically they resemble tumours of the major salivary glands, having that characteristic histological pattern. The tumour, although of low-grade malignancy, may slowly infiltrate the surrounding tissues with metastases to the lymph nodes and other organs. It is considered that cylindrinoma, especially the solid pattern, is the most aggressive of the three malignant types, followed by the carcinoid (Schmitt et al. 1989; Ishida et al. 1990).

Mucoepidermoid carcinoma, with its origin in the larger airways, is the least common of these tumours (less than 5%) and has been documented in children (Yousem and Hochholzer 1987; Heitmiller et al. 1989; Corrao and Mark 1990).

Papillary adenoma may present as a single or as multiple well defined nodules in one or both lungs. Histologically, the lesions have a papillary appearance with fibrovascular buddings lined by cuboidal and columnar epithelial cells. These have been shown, by immunohistochemistry and electron microscopic studies, to be composed of both Clara cells and type II pneumocytes (Dempo et al. 1987; Fukuda et al. 1992; Hegg et al. 1992; Kurotaki et al. 1993).

Primary carcinoma of the lung is rare in childhood. Niitu et al. (1974) reviewed the literature, which included 39 cases, including their own in a boy of 15 years 7 months. The youngest patient in the Japanese series was 2 years 3 months old; the youngest reported case is in an infant of 5 months.

The condition is usually discovered during chest radiography for ill-defined clinical symptoms, and is often misinterpreted for long periods before the correct diagnosis is made with growth of the tumour. There is an equal distribution between the sexes. Undifferentiated carcinoma is the commonest histological type in western countries, whereas in Japan adenocarcinoma has been prevalent; however, it must be mentioned that in many western reports the tumour was unclassified. Squamous-cell carcinoma was rare. Metastases to one or both lungs or to distant organs have been reported. It is important to emphasize that some of the cases described as adenocarcinomas might prove to be carcinoids if reviewed critically. Long periods of survival have been

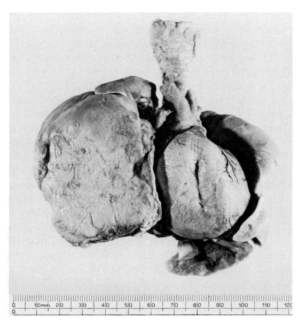

Fig. 7.79. Pulmonary blastoma occupying the inferior and middle lobes of the right lung in a 6-month-old boy. (Courtesy of Dr C. Bozic)

reported after surgery for localized tumours. Spencer et al. (1980), in a review of 21 cases of non-invasive bronchial epithelial tumours, found one case in a boy of 7. These tumours are usually undifferentiated neoplasms, and in the case of the boy described the peripheral tumour appeared to be composed of a complex papillary process covered by cuboidal non-ciliated columnar epithelial cells bearing a striking resemblance to Clara cells, with local invasion.

Malignant small-cell tumour of the thoracic wall (Askin's tumour), a highly aggressive tumour with origin in the chest wall and/or lung parenchyma, is rare. The tumour has a female predominance and appears to take its origin from the nerve sheath without involvement of the ribs. The tumour is usually bulky and lobulated; histologically, it may resemble one of many of the small round-cell tumours (Ewing's sarcoma, lymphoma, metastatic neuroblastoma, embryonal rhabdomyosarcoma). Recent studies have shown that this tumour, like Ewing's sarcoma, shares microscopic neuroectodermal tumour and they may form a single group of the same tumours (Tsokos 1992; Dehner 1993; Ramani et al. 1993; Perlman et al. 1994).

Pulmonary blastoma is a rare primary lung tumour and has been described in infants and children. Barnard (1952) coined the term "embryoma" because of its histological resemblance to fetal lung, but Spencer (1961) suggested the term "blastoma",

assuming that the tumour arose from mesodermal blastoma similar to that of nephroblastoma. There is still much debate as to whether it is derived from the endoderm or a pluripotent pulmonary blastoma.

The tumours are usually bulky, nodular, intrapulmonary masses, which occasionally involve the bronchus. They are often solitary, sometimes multiple, located either at the periphery, centrally or both. They are generally variable in colour, well defined but unencapsulated, and may present haemorrhagic areas or cystic-like zones.

Histologically, they present two distinct components, which may be variable in composition. In the biphasic form, glandular or tubular structures lined by columnar cells with a brush border but no cilia are evident. The cells are rich in glycogen. The glands and stroma may take on an endometrioid appearance in areas. The stromal component may be made up of either a spindle cell-like sarcomatous tissue or a primitive embryonic mesenchyme embedded in an abundant myxoid matrix. Mesenchymal structures (cartilage, bone, striated muscle cells, fat) undergoing differentiation or neoplastic changes may be apparent.

In some cases the tumour may be composed mainly of epithelial elements forming glands or connecting tubules supported by a thin mature connective tissue structure, giving it the aspect of a well differentiated fetal adenocarcinoma; this was formally considered to be a separate entity, but is now accepted as a variant of pulmonary blastoma. These lesions may be single but are generally multiple and often bilateral. Neuroendocrine cells and morulas have been identified in both types and have shown immunoreactivity for regulatory peptides.

The clinical course is generally impredictable and, although the prognosis is poor, the outcome depends somewhat on the grading of the tumour (Heckman et al. 1988; Chejfec et al. 1990; Yousem et al. 1990; Koss et al. 1991).

Pulmonary blastoma of the adult type is rarely encountered in the paediatric age group, but they are seen in older children. Manivel et al. (1988) drew attention to the fact that the tumours referred to as blastomas in childhood were different from those normally observed in adults, especially among those below the age of 12 years. These tumours originate principally in the pleura and mediastinum or both, but rarely in the lung parenchyma, hence the name "pleuropulmonary blastoma". These tumours are solid, bulky, well circumscribed, lobulated and surrounded by a fibrous capsule, often the visceral pleura occupying an entire lobe or lung. They are firm or rubbery in consistency, greyish-white, and sometimes present large areas of necrosis and zones of old and recent haemorrhages (Fig. 7.79). They are usually in the

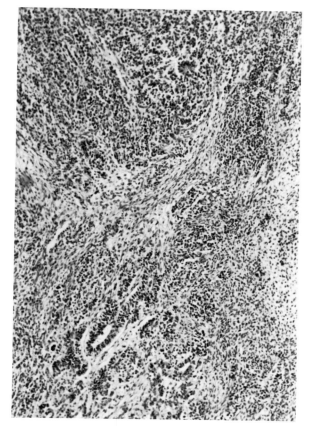

Fig. 7.80. Pleuropulmonary blastoma with entrapped epithelial nests in a diffuse proliferative, undifferentiated, mixed blastomal and abundant loose mesenchymal stroma. (H&E, × 60)

IgM. This was corrected after surgical resection of the tumour. Microscopically the tumour is made up of plasma cells at various stages of maturation. Lymphocytes may be present, occasionally forming well defined lymphoid follicles.

Veliath et al. (1977) described a *primary lymphosarcoma* of the lung in a 5-year-old girl in whom a diagnosis was made on tissue obtained by percutaneous needle biopsy of a right pulmonary mass. The child was well 1 year later, following radiotherapy and chemotherapy.

The 8½-year-old girl described by Liebow et al. (1972) with *lymphomatoid granulomatosis* of the lung was found, 2 years later, to have an eosinophilic granuloma of the skull. Furthermore, DeRemee et al. (1978) consider lymphomatoid granulomatosis to be identical pathologically with polymorphic reticulosis. It appears that one should be extremely cautious before making this diagnosis, which should be suggested only in the absence of other histological entities.

Intrapulmonary thymoma, although a very rare tumour, has been reported in children. It is often an incidental finding on chest radiography, presenting as a solitary mass. Immunohistochemical studies are important in differentiating this tumour from lymphomas and germ cell tumours (Kung et al. 1985).

Lipomas of the lung are rare. Lagrange et al. (1988) have described a lipoblastic liposarcoma in a 20-year-old woman, while Guinee et al. (1995) have documented various forms of lipomatous lesions of the lung in adults.

vicinity of or within cystic structures, with invasion of neighbouring tissues or adjacent structures.

Histologically, the tumour is characterized by a diffuse proliferation of undifferentiated blastemal cells with a storiform or alveolar pattern and areas of mesenchymal neoplastic differentiation (rhabdomyosarcomatous, chondrosarcomatous, leiomyosarcomatous, mesenchymomatous, liposarcomatous or combinations). The glandular and/or epithelial structures within the tumour are non-neoplastic but entrapped bronchial and bronchiolar elements of the lung (Fig. 7.80). The tumours are frequently described in association with cystic lung disease, principally with congenital cystic adenomatoid malformation type I, bronchogenic cysts or simple or multicystic lesions (Bove 1989; Domizio et al. 1990; Cohen et al. 1991; Delahunt et al. 1993; Hachitanda et al. 1993; Seballos and Klein 1994).

Solitary pulmonary plasmacytoma is extremely rare. Baroni et al. (1977) reported a case in a 14-year-old boy, associated with an abnormal secretion of

Metastases

The metastases of many childhood tumours are blood-borne, and they generally produce massive secondaries in the lung. These may be limited in number, or occasionally there is a diffuse dissemination of small lesions scattered throughout the parenchyma. Metastases to the lung are common in *Wilms' tumour, hepatoblastoma, osteosarcoma, Ewing's sarcoma* and *sarcomas of soft tissues*. *Neuroblastoma* spreads to the lung less readily, but is a common tumour, so pulmonary deposits are frequently found (Vassilopoulou-Sellin et al. 1993; Cohen 1994; Fassina et al. 1994; Heij et al. 1994; Massimino et al. 1995).

In childhood *leukaemia* the vessels of the lung contain leukaemic cells, and these cells may be seen infiltrating the alveolar wall. Perivascular aggregates can be observed in severe cases. *Non-Hodgkin's lymphomas* may also be localized in the lung, either as a primary lesion or, more often, as a secondary infiltration. *Hodgkin's disease* in childhood may involve the lung and infiltrate the parenchyma, forming nodules, or produce peribronchial or bronchial infiltrations with bronchial stenosis. The differential diagnoses of these various entities and their subgroups can be made with precision only by the use of detail and careful immunohistochemical labelling of the various cell types (Weiss et al. 1985; Weis et al. 1986).

Histiocytosis X and Similar Conditions

Langerhans' cell histiocytosis (histiocytosis X), formally referred to as histiocytosis X, frequently involves the lung. In acute disseminated Langerhans' cell histiocytosis, the pulmonary lesions are diffuse and bilateral; they often appear in successive crops and can be associated with pneumothorax. There may be numerous areas of necrosis with abscess formation. Microscopically there are numerous Langerhans' cells with large giant cells, containing a yellowish granular pigment in their cytoplasm. The inflammatory infiltrate may be minimal away from areas of necrosis, but scattered polymorphonuclear eosinophils sometimes accompany the lesion.

Multifocal Langerhans' cell histiocytosis invariably involves the lung. The lesions are bilateral and diffuse, with formation of granulation tissue containing numerous Langerhans' cells, sometimes associated with active fibrosis and a chronic inflammatory infiltrate. Accompanying macrophages often have a xanthomatous appearance. Lung involvement is always accompanied by lesions of other organs or systems.

Unifocal Langerhans' cell histiocytosis (eosinophilic granuloma) is generally described in bones. It has long been recognized that it can occur as an isolated lesion in the lung. The majority of cases have been reported in adults, with a male preponderance. Radiography of the chest reveals disseminated nodules in both lung fields, which are more prominent in the hilar region. High-resolution computed tomography and isotope ventilation/perfusion scanning are extremely helpful in diagnosing the condition at an earlier stage. Sometimes cavities of variable sizes are apparent, and emphysema is not infrequent. During the late stages of the disease fibrosis with honeycombing may be conspicuous. Pneumothorax and pleural effusion have been recorded in a number of cases.

Macroscopically the lungs show numerous small cavities throughout the parenchyma. There is also nodular fibrosis with a classic honeycomb appearance in some cases. Microscopically, in the early stages of the condition there is focal or nodular infiltration mainly around bronchioles and small vessels in the periphery, with some involvement of the pleura. More often there is a spectrum of lesions with vari-

able amount of Langerhans' and mononuclear cells. Neutrophils are sometimes present. The Langerhans' cells are numerous in the cellular phase and may be few or totally absent in the late fibrotic stage, thus making diagnosis difficult. Some Langerhans' cells may have a foamy granular cytoplasm with pigment granules. The nuclei are large and folded; nucleoli are prominent. There is a moderate infiltration of lymphocytes and plasmocytes, accompanied by varying quantities of eosinophils scattered throughout the granulation tissue. Fibroplastic proliferation is also evident. Distal bronchi and bronchioles and the vessels in adjacent areas are involved in the granulomatous process and may be partially or completely obliterated. Similar lesions are sometimes observed in the pleura.

Recent studies have suggested that there may be a neutrophilic chemotactic defect in these patients due to some intrinsic impairment associated probably with an increased frequency of HLA antigens Bw61 and Cw7. Langerhans' cells are antigen-presenting (accessory) cells of the dendritic cell/Langerhans' cell lineage, which partially degrade protein antigens and express the peptides on their surface in association with HLA molecules. It is now well established that in all cases the diagnosis is based on the identification of Langerhans' cells in the lesions. These large cells are lobulated with grooved nuclei and with well defined granules (Fig. 7.81a). They stain with S-100 protein and OKT6 and strongly express the CD1a surface antigen, and ultrastructurally they contain the characteristic X-bodies or Birbeck granules (Fig. 7.81b). Giant cells may be conspicuous and the inflammatory reaction variable, containing neutrophils, eosinophils in variable quantities and some mononuclear cells. Although BAL fluid examination has been proposed by some authors, its usefulness is limited because several other pathological conditions may be accompanied by the presence of Langerhans' cells in the fluid. Lung biopsy (transbronchial or preferably open) produce more specific results (Rancy and D'Angio 1989; Foucar and Foucar 1990; McLelland et al. 1990; Ha et al. 1992; Soler et al. 1992; Goerdt et al. 1993; Travis et al. 1993; Emile et al. 1995).

Recently, William et al. (1994) have detected clonal histiocytes in all forms of Langerhans' cell histiocytosis, indicating that this condition is probably a clonal neoplastic disorder with highly variable biological behaviour.

Pleural Tumours

Mesothelioma of the pleura is very rare in childhood. In a retrospective study, Grundy and Miller (1972)

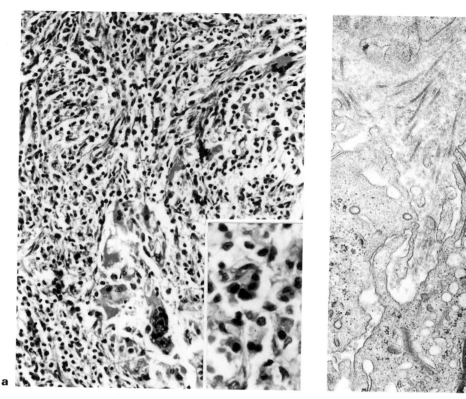

Fig. 7.81. a Histiocytosis X in a $7\frac{1}{2}$ year-old boy. **a** Note the granulomatous-like infiltration with numerous histiocytes and some giant cells. *Inset*, giant cell and typical histiocyte. (H&E, × 225) **b** Histiocyte with the classic Bw granule or X-bodies, confirming the diagnosis. (× 31 960)

were able to collect 13 well documented cases of malignant mesothelioma in the USA. Eight of the patients were 16 years of age or less and the remaining five were 17 years old. The youngest patient was 4. There are now over 30 cases recorded in the literature, with a significant male predominance. Histologically the majority of tumours showed a fibrous pattern, which is often described in the literature in the paediatric age group, but mixed types have also been documented (Dische et al. 1988; Lin-Chu et al. 1989). One must exclude an eventual secondary infiltration of the pleural cavities by a peritoneal mesothelioma in these patients (Nishioka et al. 1988; Geary et al. 1991).

The tumour often progresses without clinical symptoms until late in the course of the disease, when the patient presents with thoracic pain, sometimes dyspnoea, and pleural effusion. Death usually takes place within 12 months of the initial symptoms. Although malignant mesothelioma in adults is often related to environmental factors, principally exposure to asbestos (Whitewall et al. 1977), no such relationship was found in the cases studied by Grundy and Miller (1972). Li (1977), in a review of second

malignant tumours after treatment of malignancy in childhood, recorded mesothelioma arising 16 years after radiotherapy and, similar to the case described by Anderson et al. (1985), 13 years after both chemotherapy and radiotherapy for Wilms' tumour. Mesotheliomas have been reported in a family, in siblings and in a pair of twins, suggesting that in some instances there may be hereditary predisposition (Martensson et al. 1984).

The microscopic pattern is often mixed, as can be elegantly demonstrated by histochemical and immunohistochemical techniques. This finding is confirmed by ultrastructural studies showing that these tumours are derived from both epithelial and fibroblastic components of the mesothelial layer and thus exclude a pulmonary adenocarcinoma (Brown et al. 1993; Moch et al. 1993a, b).

Malignant mesenchymoma of the pleura has been described by Darling et al. (1967; cited in Holdsworth Mayer et al. 1974) in a 3-month-old girl. This tumour showed the histological patterns encountered in similar tumours at other sites.

Fibroma or *benign localized mesothelioma* of the pleura, although rare, has been recorded in childhood.

The tumours can occur singly but are sometimes multiple and bilateral, and are known to evolve over very long periods, and may recur after excision. Fibromas of the pleura are variable in size and usually nodular, firm and yellowish-white. They take their origin from the subendothelial areolar tissues, and have been observed both on the visceral and parietal layers as well as within the pulmonary parenchyma (Scattini and Orsi 1973; Yousem and Flynn 1988). Spontaneous regression has been recorded in some cases. Microscopically they are composed of proliferating fibroblasts supported by thick collagen bundles and reticulin fibres, sometimes set in a myxoid ground substance. Mitotic figures may be prominent but metastases do not occur and the prognosis is favourable, supporting the benign nature of these lesions.

Mesenchymal hamartoma of the chest wall takes its origin from one or more ribs and may be the cause of chest wall deformity in the neonatal period. Cohen et al. (1992) in a review of the literature found 33 cases described in infancy and added three of their own. The lesion may be diagnosed during intrauterine life by echography and can be the cause of pulmonary hypoplasia and also respiratory distress in the newborn. It is generally lobulated, circumscribed, single or multiple, with a benign behaviour (D'Ercole et al. 1994; Dounies et al. 1994). Histologically, the lesion is composed of chondroid tissue with foci of hyaline cartilage, areas undergoing ossification associated with an important vascular component.

General References: Development and Structure

Adamson IYR, King GM (1986) Epithelial–interstitial cell interactions in fetal rat lung development accelerated by steroids. Lab Invest 55: 145

Adriaensen D, Scheuermann DW (1993) Neuroendocrine cells and nerves of the lung. Anat Rec 236: 70

Bourbon JR, Farrel PM (1985) Fetal lung development in the diabetic pregnancy. Pediatr Res 19: 253

Boyden EA (1969) The pattern of the terminal air spaces in a premature infant of 30–32 weeks that lived nineteen and a quarter hours. Am J Anat 126: 31

Burri PH (1985) Morphology and respiratory function of the alveolar unit. Int Arch Allerg Appl Immunol 76 (Suppl. 1): 2

Caniggia I, Liu J, Han R, Buch S, Funa K, Tanswell K, Post M (1993) Fetal lung epithelial cells express receptors for platelet-derived growth factor. Am J Respir Cell Mol Biol 9: 54

Cooney TP, Thurlbeck WM (1982a) The radial alveolara count method of Emery and Mihtal: a reappraisal. 1. Postnatal lung growth. Thorax 37: 572

Cooney TP, Thurlbeck WM (1982b) The radial alveolar count method of Emery and Mithal: a reappraisal. 2. Intrauterine and early postnatal lung growth. Thorax 37: 580

D'Amore PA (1992) Mechanisms of endothelial growth control. Am J Respir Cell Mol Biol 6: 1

Desai R, Wigglesworth JS, Aber V (1988) Assessment of elastic maturation by radioimmunoassay of desmosine in the developing human lung. Early Hum Dev 16: 61

Dilly SA (1984) Scanning electron microscope study of the development of the human respiratory acinus. Thorax 39: 733

Dormans JAWA (1985) The alveolar type III cell. Lung 163: 327

Dunnill MS (1982) The problem of lung growth. Thorax 37: 561

Haidar A, Wigglesworth JS, Krausz T (1990) Type IV collagen in developing human lung: a comparison between normal and hypoplastic fetal lungs. Early Hum Dev 21: 175

Heath D (1974) The Clara cell. Thorax 29: 147

Hislop AA, Wigglesworth JS, DeSaia R (1986) Alveolar development in the human fetus and infant. Early Hum Dev 13: 1

Jany BH, Gallup MW, Yan PS, Gum JR, Kim YS, Basbaum CB (1991) Human bronchus and intestine express the same mucin gene. J Clin Invest 87: 77

Johnson MD, Gray ME, Carpenter G, Pepinsky RB, Stahlman MT (1990) Ontogeny of epidermal growth factor receptor and lipocortin-1 fetal and neonatal human lungs. Hum Pathol 21: 182

Langston C, Kida K, Reed Maud, Thurlbeck WM (1984) Human lung growth in late gestation and in the neonate. Am Rev Respir Dis 129: 607

Lauwerns JM, Van Ranst L, Verhofstad AAJ (1986) Ultrastructural localization of serotonin in the intrapulmonary neuroepithelial bodies of neonatal rabbits by use of immunoelectron microscopy. Cell Tissue Res 243: 455

Minoo P, King RJ (1994) Epithelial–mesenchymal interactions in lung development. Annu Rev Physiol 56: 13

Murray JF (1976) The normal lung: the basis for diagnosis and treatment of pulmonary disease. Saunders, Philadelphia, p 1

Nakatani Y (1991) Pulmonary endocrine cells in infancy and childhood. Pediatr Pathol 11: 31

Nexo E, Kryger-Baggesen N (1989) The receptor for epidermal growth factor is present in human fetal kidney, liver and lung. Regul Pept 26: 1

Price WA, Moats–Staats BM, D'Ercole AJ, Stiles AD (1993) Insulin-like growth factor binding protein production and regulation in fetal rat lung cells. Am J Respir Cell Mol Biol 8: 425

Roman J, McDonald JA (1992) Expression of fibronectin, the integrin $\alpha 5$, and α-smooth muscle actin in heart and lung development. Am J Respir Cell Mol Biol 6: 472

Stahlman MT, Gray ME (1993) Colocalization of peptide hormones in neuroendocrine cells of human fetal and newborn lungs: an electron microscopic study. Anat Rec 236: 206

Stahlman MT, Orth DN, Gray ME (1989) Immunocytochemical localization of epidermal growth factor in the developing human respiratory system and in acute and chronic lung disease in the neonate. Lab Invest 60: 539

Stiles AD, Smith BT, Post M (1986) Reciprocal autocrine and paracrine regulation of growth of mesenchymal and alveolar epithelial cells from fetal lung. Exp Lung Res 11: 165

Thurlbeck WM (1982) Postnatal human lung growth. Thorax 37: 564

Warburton D, Lee M, Berberich MA, Bernfield M (1993) Molecular and embryology and the study of lung development. Am J Respir Cell Mol Biol 9: 5

Woodcock-Mitchell J, Mitchell JJ, Reynolds SE, Leslie KO, Low RB (1990) Alveolar epithelial cell keratin expression during lung development. Am J Respir Cell Mol Biol 2: 503

Zeltner TB, Burri PH (1987) The postnatal development and growth of the human lung. II. Morphology. Respir Physiol 67: 269

Zeltner TB, Caduff JH, Gehr P, Pfenninger J, Burri PH (1987) The postnatal development and growth of the human lung. I. Morphometry. Respir Physiol 67: 247

References

Abernathy EC, Hruban RH, Baumgartner WA, Reitz BA Hutchins GM (1991) The two forms of bronchiolitis obliterans in heart–lung transplant recipients. Hum Pathol 22: 1102

Abioye AA, Edington GM (1972) Prevalence of amoebiasis at autopsy in Ibadan. Trans R Soc Trop Med Hyg 66: 754

Abiow RC, Driscoll SG, Effmann EL, Gross I, Jolles CJ, Vaux R, Warshaw JB (1976) A comparison of early-onset group B streptococcal neonatal infection and the respiratory distress syndrome of the newborn. N Engl J Med 294: 65

Aboussouan LS, O'Donovan PB, Moodie DS, Gragg LA, Stoller JK (1993) Hypoplastic trachea in Down's syndrome. Am Rev Respir Dis 147: 72

Abramowsky CR, Witt WJ (1983) Sarcoma of the larynx in a newborn. Cancer 51: 1726

Accard JL, Toty L, Personne C, Hertzog P (1970) Etude d'une série de 35 séquestrations avec référence aux formes particulières. Ann Chir Thorac Cardiovasc 9: 501

Adams FH (1966) Functional development of the fetal lung. J Pediatr 68: 794

Adamson TM, Boyd RDH, Platt HS, Strang LB (1969a) Composition of alveolar liquid in the foetal lamb. J Physiol 204: 159

Adamson TM, Boyd RDH, Normand ICS, Reynolds EOR, Shaw JL (1969b) Haemorrhagic pulmonary oedema ("massive pulmonary haemorrhage") in the newborn. Lancet i: 494

Aftandelians R, Roafat F, Taffazoli M, Beaver PC, (1977) Pulmonary capillariasis in a child in Iran. Am J Trop Med Hyg 26: 64

Afzelius BA, Carlsten J, Karlsson S (1984) Clinical, pathologic, and ultrastructural features of situs inversus and immotilecilia syndrome in a dog. J Am Vet Med Assoc 184: 560

Agut H (1993) Puzzles concerning the pathogenicity of human herpesvirus 6. N Eng J Med 329: 203

Aherne W, Bird T, Court SDM, Gardner PS, McQuillin J (1970) Pathological changes in virus infections of the lower respiratory tract in children. J Clin Pathol 25: 7

Aikawa T, Shimura S, Sasaki H, Ebina M, Takishima T (1992) Marked goblet cell hyperplasia with mucus accumulation in the airways of patients who died of severe acute asthma attack. Chest 101: 916

Akashi K, Eizuru Y, Sumiyoshi Y, Minematsu T, Hara S, Harada M et al. (1993) Brief report: severe infectious mononucleosislike syndrome and primary human herpesvirus 6 infection in an adult. N Engl J Med 329: 168

Akino T, Mizumoto M, Simuzu Y et al. (1990) Pulmonary corpora amylacea contain surfactant apoprotein. Path Res Pract 186: 687

Albelda SM, Gefter WB, Epstein DM, Miller WT, (1985) Diffuse pulmonary hemorrhage: a review and classification. Radiology 154: 289

Alfaham MA, Ferguson SD, Sihra B, Davies J (1987) The idiopathic hypereosinophilic syndrome. Arch Dis Child 62: 601

Alkalay AL, Pomerance JJ, Rimoin DL (1987) Fetal varicella syndrome. J Pediatr 111: 320

Allan BT, Day DL, Dehner LP (1987) Primary pulmonary rhabdomyosaracoma of the lung in children. Report of two cases presenting with spontaneous pneumothorax. Cancer 59: 1005

Allen JN, Pacht ER, Gadek JE, Davis WB (1989) Acute eosinophilic pneumonia as a reversible cause of noninfectious respiratory failure. N Engl J Med 321: 569

Allen RKA, Chai SY, Dunbar MS, Mendelsohn FAO (1986) In vitro autoradiographaiac localization of angiotensin-converting enzyme in saracoid lymph nodes. Chest 90: 315

Alt R, Eryny P, Messer J, Willard D (1984) Infections bactériennes néo-natales. Etude cinétique de la C, réactive protéine et de l'orosomucoide. Presse Med 13: 1373

Alvarez-Fernandez E, Carretero-Albinana L, Menarguez-Palanca J (1989) Sclerosing hemangioma of the lung: an immunohistochemical study of intermediate filaments and endothelial markers. Arch Pathol Lab Med 113: 121

Ambrus CM, Weintraub DH, Choi TS, Eisenberg B, Staub HP, Courey NG, Foote RJ, Goplerud D, Moesch RV, Ray M, Bross IDJ, Jung OS, Mink IB, Ambrus JL (1974) Plasminogen in the prevention of hyalaine membrane disease. Am J Dis Child 127: 189

An SF, Gould S, Keeling JW, Fleming KA (1993) Role of respiratory viral infection in SIDS: detection of viral nucleic acid by in situ hybridization. J Pathol 171: 271

Anderson VM, Lee H (1988) Case 1 lymphocytic interstitial pneumonitis in pediatric AIDS Pediatr Pathol 8: 417

Anderson WR, Engel RR (1983) Cardiopulmonary sequelae of reparative stages of bronchopulmonary dysplasia. Arch Pathol Lab Med 107: 603

Anderson JM, Bain AD, Brown JK, Cockburn F, Forfar JO, Machin GA, Turner TL (1976) Hyaline-membrane disease, alkaline buffer treatment and cerebral intraventricular haemorrhage. Lancet i: 117

Anderson KA, Hurley WC, Hurley BT, Ohrt DW (1985) Malignant plueral mesothelioma following radiotherapy in a 16-year-old boy. Cancer 56: 273

Andraca R, Edson RS, Kern EB (1993) Rhinoscleroma: a growing concern in the United States? Mayo Clinic Experience. Mayo Clin Proc 68: 1151

Anthony PP (1993) Inflammatory pseudotumour (plasma cell granuloma) of lung, liver and other organs. Histopathology 23: 501

Aozasa K, Inoue A (1982) Malignant histiocytosis presenting as lethal midline granuloma: immunohistological study. J Pathol 138: 241

Arakaki DT, Waxman SH (1969) Trisomy D in a cyclops. J Pediatr 74: 620

Arber DA, Weiss LM, Albujar PF, Chen YY, Jaffe ES (1993) Nasal lymphomas in Peru. High incidence of T-cell immunophenotype and Epstein–Barr virus infection. Am J Surg Pathol 17: 392

Arean VM, Crandall CA (1971) Ascariasis. In: Marcial-Rojas PA (ed) Pathology of protozoa and helminthic disease with clinical correlation. Williams & Wilkins, Baltimore, p 769

Argyle JC (1989) Pulmonary hypoplasia infants with giant abdominal wall defects. Pediatr Pathol 9: 43

Armin A, Castelli M (1984) Congenital adrenal tissue in the lung with adrenal cytomegaly. Case report and review of the literature. Am J Clin Pathol 82: 225

Arnold W, Huth F (1978) Electron microscope findings in four cases of nasophryngeal fibroma. Virchows Arch [Pathol Anat] 379: 285

Arnon S, Grigg J, Silverman M (1993) Pulmonary inflammatory cells in ventilated preterm infants: effect of surfactant treatment. Arch Dis Child 69: 44

Asano Y, Suga S, Yoshikawa T, Yazaki T, Uchikawa T (1995) Clinical features and viral excretion in an infant with primary human herpesvirus 7 infection. Pediatrics 95: 187

Asano Y, Yoshikawa T, Suga S, Kobayashi I, Nakashima T, Yazaki T, et al. (1994) Clinical features of infants with primary human herpesvirus 6 infection (exanthem subitum, roseola infantum). Pediatrics 93: 104

Asher MI, Spier S, Beland M, Coates AL, Beaudry PH (1982) Primary lung abscess in childhood. A long-term outcome of conservative management. Am J Dis Child 136: 491

Askin FB (1975) Nose, nasopharynx, larynx and trachea. In: Kissane JM (ed) Pathology of infancy and childhood. Mosby, St Louis, p 464

Asmar BI, Slovis TL, Reed JO, Dajani AS (1978b) Haemophilus infuenzae type B pneumonia in 43 children. J Pediatr 93: 389

Assimes IK, Rosales JK (1980) Congenital tracheal diverticulum. A case report. Ann Otol Rhinol Laryngol 89: 406

Aterman K, Patel S (1970) Striated muscle in the lung. Am J Anat 128: 341

Austin JR, deTar M, Rice DH (1994) Pulmonary chondroid hamartoma presenting as an inflatable neck mass. Case report and clinicopathologic analysis. Arch Otolaryngol Head Neck Surg 120: 440

Awe WC, Fletcher WS, Jacob SW (1966) The pathophysiology of aspiration pneumonitis. Surgery 60: 232

Bachwich PR, Lynch JP Kunkel SL (1987) Arachidonic acid metabolism is altered in sarcoid alveolar macrophages. Clin Immunol Immunopathol 42: 27

Bailey BJ, Barton S (1975) Olfactory neuroblastoma management and prognosis. Arch Otolaryngol 101: 1

Bale JF Jr, Watkins M (1978) Fulminant neonatal *Haemophilus influenzae* pneumonia and sepsis. J Pediatr 92: 233

Bâle PM (1979) Congenital cystic malformation of the lung: a form of congenital bronchiolar ("adenomatoid") malformation. Am J Clin Pathol 71: 411

Bale PM, Parsons RE, Stevens MM (1983) Diagnosis and behaviour of juvenile rhabdomyosarcoma. Hum Pathol 14: 596

Baliga R, Chang CH, Bidani AK, Perrin EV, Fleischmann LE (1978) A case of generalized Wegner's granulomatosis in childhood: successful therapy with cyclophosphamide. Pediatrics 61: 286

Baltimore, RS, Christie CDC, Walker Smith, GJ (1989) Immunohistopatholigic localization of *Pseudomonas aeruginosa* in lungs from patients with cystic fibrosis. Implications for the pathogenesis of progressive lung deterioration. Am Rev Respir Dis 140: 1650

Bando T, Genka K, Ishikawa K, Kuniyoshi M, Kuda T (1993) Ectopic intrapulmonary thyroid. Chest 103: 1278

Bang AT, Bang RA, Morankar VP, Sontakke PG, Solanki JM (1993) Pneumonia in neonates: can it be managed in the community? Arch Dis Child 68: 550

Barker AF, Bardana EJJr (1988) Bronchiectasis: update of an orphan disease 1,2. Am Rev Respir Dis 137: 969

Barnard WG (1952) Embryoma of lung. Thorax 7: 299

Baroni CD, Mineo TC, Ricci C, Guarino S, Mandelli F (1977) Solitary secretary plasmacytoma of the lung in a 14-year-old boy. Cancer 40: 2329

Barson AJ (1978) Tentorial tears as a problem for the paediatrician. Paper presented at the twenty-eighth meeting of the Paediatric Pathology Society, Bristol

Barter RA, Hudson JA (1974) Bacteriological findings in perinatal pneumonia. Pathology 6: 223

Barth PJ, Rüschoff J (1992) Morphometric study on pulmonary arterial thickness in pulmonary hypoplasia. Pediatr Pathol 12: 653

Bartimmo EE Jr, Guisan M, Moser KM (1972) Pulmonary involvement in Fabry's disease: a reappraisal. Follow-up of a San Diego kindred and review of the literature. Am J Med 53: 755

Bartlett JG, Gorbach SL, Finegold SM (1974a) The bacteriology of aspiration pneumonia. Am J Med 56: 202

Bartlett JG Gorbach SL, Tally FP, Finegold SM (1974b) Bacteriology and treatment of primary lung abscess. Am Rev Respir Dis 109: 510

Bartley TD, Arean VM (1965) Intrapulmonary neurogenic tumours. J Thorac Cardiovasc Surg 50: 114

Barton RPE, Davey TF (1976) Early leprosy of the nose and throat. J Laryngol 90: 953

Barton Rogers B, Mark Y, Oyer CE (1993) Diagnosis and incidence of fetal parvovirus infection in an autopsy series: I Histology. Pediatr Pathol 13: 371

Basheda SG, Mehta AC, De Boer G, Orlowski JP (1991) Endobronchial and parenchymal juvenile laryngotracheo-bronchial papillomatosis. Effect of photodynamic therapy. Chest 100: 1458

Baskerville A, Conlan JW, Ashworth LAE, Dowsett AB (1986) Pulmonary damage caused by a protease from *Legionella pneumophila*. Br J Exp Pathol 67: 527

Bass JW, Steele RW, Wiebe RA (1974) Acute epiglottitis. A surgical emergency. JAMA 229: 671

Bauer FA, Wear DJ, Angritt P, Lo S-C (1991) *Mycoplasma fermentans* (Incognitus strain) infection in the kidneys of patients with acquired immunodeficiency syndrome and associated nephropathy: a light microscopic, immunohistochemical, and ultrastructural study. Hum Pathol 22: 63

Bauman NM, Kirby–Keyser LJ, Dolan KD, Wexler D, Gantz BJ, McCabe B F et al. (1994) Mondini dysplasia and congenital cytomegalovirus infection. J Pediatr 124: 71

Beca J Butt W (1994) Extracorporeal membrane oxygenation for refractory septic shock in children. Pediatrics 93: 726

Becroft DM (1971) Bronchiolitis obliterans, bronchietasis and other sequelae of adenovirus type 21 infection in young children. J Clin Pathol 24: 72

Beers MF, Sohn M, Swartz, M (1990) Recurrent pneumothorax in AIDS patients with pneumocystis pneumonia. A clinicopathologic report of three cases and review of the literataure. Chest 98: 266

Beguin G (1994) Calcification arterielle idiopathique infantile. Nouvelles donne es morphologiques, hypothese étiologique et revue de la littérature. Thesis – Geneva 1–88

Beham A, Fletcher CDM, Kainz J, Schmid C, Humer U (1993) Nasopharyngeal angiofibroma: an immunohistochemical study of 32 cases. Virchows Archiv A [Pathol Anat] 423: 281

Benacerraf BR, Frigoletto FD (1986) Fetal respiraotry movements: only part of the biophysical profile. Obstet Gynecol 67: 556

Benatre A, Laugier J, Grangeponte MC (1978) La maladie de membranes hyalines. Rôle du complément. Rev Fr Mal Respir 6: 67

Bender TM, Stone LR, Amenta JS (1994) Diagnostic power of lecithin/sphingomyelin ratio and fluorescence polarization assays for respiratory distress syndrome compared by relative operating characteristic curves. Clin Chem 40: 541

Beneck D, Abati AD, Greco MA (1985) Lymphangioma presenting as a nasal polyp in an infant. Arch Pathol Lab Med 109: 773

Benikos et al. 1976

Benjamin B (1984) Tracheomalacia in infants and children. Ann Otol Rhinol Laryngol 93: 438

Benjamin DR (1989) Case 4 herpes simplex tracheobronchitis and pneumonitis. Pediatr Pathol 9: 773

Benveniste RJ, Harris HE (1973) Nasal hemangiopericytoma. Arch Otolaryngol 98: 358

Benz-Lemoine E, Delwail V, Castel O, Guilhot F, Robert R, Grollier G et al. (1991) Nosocomial Legionnaires disease in a bone marrow transplant unit. Bone Marrow Transplant 7: 61

Berezin A (1969) Histochemical study of the hyaline membrane of newborn infants and of that produced in guinea pigs. Biol Neonate 14: 90

Berger R, Störchler D, Rudin C (1992) Cord blood screening for congenital toxoplasmosis: detection and treatment of asymptomatic newborns in Basel, Switzerland. Scand J Infect Dis 84: 46

Berger U, Khaghani A, Pomerance A, Yacoub MH, Coombes RC (1990) Pulmonary lymphangioleiomyomatosis and steroid receptors. An immunocytochemical study. Am J Clin Pathol 93: 609

Bergman B, Hender T (1978) Antepartum administration of terbutaline and the incidence of hyaline membrane disease in preterm infants. Acta Obstet Gynecol 57: 217

Berkowitz RL, Kantor RD, Beck GJ, Warshaw JB (1978) The relationship between premature rupture of the membranes and the respiratory distress syndrome. An update and plan of management. Am J Obstet Gynecol 131: 503

Berlinger NT, Proto DP, Thompson TR (1987) Infantile lobar emphysema. Ann Otol Rhinol Laryngol 96: 106

Berman JM, Colman BH (1977) Nasal aspects of cystic fibrosis in children. J Laryngol Otol 91: 133

Berner A, Gylseth B, Levy F (1981) Talc dust pneumoconiosis. A case report. Acta Pathol microbiol Immunol Scand[A]89: 17

Berry PJ, Nagington J (1982) Fatal infection with echovirus II. Arch Dis Child 57: 22

Berry DD, Pramanik AK, Philips JB III, Buchter DS, Kanarek KS, Easa D et al. (1994) Comparison of the effect of three doses of a synthetic surfactant on the alveolar–arterial oxygen gradient in infants weighing 1250 grams with respiratory distress syndrome. J Pediatr 124: 295

Berry JP, Gray ES, Porter HJ, Burton PA (1992) Parvovirus infection of the human fetus and newborn. Semin Diagn Pathol 9: 4

Berthoud S (1972) Les multiples aspects de la bilharziose. A propos de quelques cas observés à Genéve. Praxis 61: 809

Betancourt D, Beckerman RC (1992) Immunologic features of the lungs in cystic fibrosis. Immunology and Allergy Clinics of North America 12: 249

Beutler E (1992) Gaucher disease: new molecular approaches to diagnosis and treatment. Science 256: 794

Biggs JSG, Hemming J, McGeary H, Gaffney TJ (1974) Human amniotic and fetal neonatal pharyngeal fluids. J Obstet Gynaecol Br Cwlth 81: 70

Bismuth C, Scherrmann JM, Garnier R, Baud FJ, Pontal PG (1987) Elimination of paraquat. Hum Toxicol 6: 63

Blasi F, Boschini A, Cosentini R, Legnani D, Smacchia C, Ghira C et al. (1994) Outbreak of *Chlamydia pneumoniae* infection in former injection-drug users. Chest 105: 812

Blayney M, Kerem E, Whyte H, O'Brodovich H (1991) Bronchopulmonary dysplasia: improvement in lung function between 7 and 10 years of age. J Pediatr 118: 201

Bliek AJ, Mulholland DJ (1971) Extralobal lung sequestration associated with fetal neonatal respiratory distress. Thorax 26: 125

Body BA, Spicer A, Burgwyn CM (1988) Immunoidentification of *Histoplasma capsulatum* and *Blastomyces dermatitidis* with commercial exoantigen reagents. Arch Pathol Lab Med 112: 519

Bohin S, Field DJ (1994) The epidemiology of neonatal respiratory disease. Early Hum Develop 37: 73

Boisset G (1972) Subpleural emphysema complicating staphylococcal and other pneumonias. J Pediatr 81: 259

Bonetti F, Chiodera PK, Pea M, Martignoni G, Bosi F, Zamboni G et al. (1993) Transbronchial biopsy in lymphangiomyomatosis of the lung. HMB45 for diagnosis. Am J Surg Pathol 17: 1092

Bonetti F, Pea M, Martignoni G, Zamboni G, Iuzzolino P (1991) Cellular heterogeneity in lymphangiomyomatosis of the lung (Letter). Hum Pathol 22: 727

Bonikos DS, Bensch KG, Northway WH Jr. Edwards DK (1976) Bronchopulmonary dysplasia: the pulmonary pathologic sequel of necrotizing bronchiolitis and pulmonary fibrosis. Hum Pathol 7: 643

Bonsib SM, Walker WP (1989) Pulmonary–renal syndrome: clinical similarity amidst etiologic diversity. Mod Pathol 2: 129

Booth JB, Osborn DA (1970) Granular cell myoblastoma of the larynx. Acta Otolaryngol 70: 279

Bouchayer M, Cornut G, Witzig E, Loire R, Roch JB, Bastian RW (1985) Epidermoid cysts, sulci, and mucosal bridges of the true vocal cord: a report of 157 cases. Laryngoscope 95: 1087

Boulnois GJ (1992) Pneumococcal proteins and the pathogenesis of disease caused by *Streptococcus pneumoniae*. J Gen Microbiol 138: 249

Bouros D, Gazis A, Blatsios V, Melissinos C (1987) Leiomyoma of the trachea. Eur J Respir Dis 71: 206

Bove KE (1989) Case 6. Sarcoma arising in pulmonary mesenchymal cystic hamartoma. Pediatr Pathol 9: 785

Bowie LJ, Shammo J, Dohnal JC, Farrel E Vye MV (1991) Lamellar body number density and the prediction of respiratory distress. Am J Clin Pathol 95: 781

Boyd WP Jr. Campbell FW, Trudeau WL (1978) *Strongyloides stercoralis* hyperinfection. Am J Trop Med Hyg 27: 39

Boyden EA (1955) Developmental anatomy, physiology and pathology. Development anomalies of the lung. Am J Surg 80: 79

Boyden EA, Bill AH Jr, Creighton SA (1962) Presumptive origin of a left lower accessory lung from an esophageal diverticulum. Surgery 52: 323

Brasfield DM, Stagno S, Whitley RJ, Cloud G, Cassell G, Tiller RE (1987) Infant pneumonitis associated with cytomegalovirus, *Chlamydia, Pneumocytis, and Ureaplasma*: follow-up. Pediatrics 79: 76

Bridger JE, Kreczy A, Wigglesworth JS (1992) Transthoracic Herniation of the fetal lung. Bagpipe lung. Pediatr Pathol 12: 417

Briselli M, Mark GJ, Grillo HC (1978) Tracheal carcinoids. Cancer 42: 2870

Brook I, Finegold SM (1979) Bacteriology and therapy of lung abscess in children. J Pediatr 94: 10

Brown RW, Clark GM, Tandon AK, Allred DC (1993) Multiple-marker immunohistochemical phenotypes distinguishing malignant pleural mesothelioma from pulmonary adenocarcinoma. Hum Pathol 24: 347

Brown AC, Slocum PC, Putthoff SL, Wallace WE, Foresman BH (1994) Exogenous lipoid pneumonia due to nasal application of petroleum jelly. Chest 105: 968

Brus F, van Waarde WM, Schoots C, Oetomo SB (1991) Fatal ureaplasmal pneumonia and sepsis in a newborn infant. Eur J Pediatr 150: 782

Bryan CS, Reynolds KL, (1984) Bacteremic nosocomial pneumonia: analysis of 172 episodes from a single metropolitan area. Annu Rev Respir Dis 129: 668

Buchanan MC (1959) Sequestration of the lung. Arch Dis Child 34: 137

Burgart LJ, Heller MJ, Reznicek M, Greiner TC, Teneyck CJ, Robinson RA (1991) Cytomegalovirus detection in bone marrow transplant patients with idiopathic pneumonitis. A clinocopathologic study of the clinical utility of the polymerase chain reaction on open lung biopsy specimen tissue. Am J Clin Pathol 96: 572

Burke JA (1978) Strongyloidiasis in childhood. Am J Dis Child 132: 1130

Burkhardt A (1989) Alveolitis and collapse in the pathogenesis of pulmonary fibrosis. Am Rev Respir Dis 140: 513

Burkhardt A, Cottier H (1989) Cellular events in alveolitis and the evolution of pulmonary fibrosis. Virchows Archiv B Cell Pathol 58: 1

Burkitt DP (1970) General features and facial tumours. In: Burkitt DP, Wright D (eds) Burkitt's lymphoma. Livingstone, Edinburgh, p 6

Bus JS, Gibson JE, (1984) Paraquat: model for oxidant-initiated toxicity. Environ Health Perspect 55: 37

Bussolati G, Papatti M, Forschini MP, Eusebi V (1987) The interest of actin immunocytochemistry in diagnostic histopathology. Basic Appl Histochem 14: 596

Byard RW, Thorner PS, Edwards V Greenberg M (1990) Pulmonary malacoplakia in a child. Pediatr Pathol 10: 417

Cabrera A, Sarrionandia JJ, Idigoras G et al. (1989) Scimitar syndrome in the newborn child and infant. Rev Esp Cardiol 42: 322

Cagnano M, Benharroch D, Geffen DB (1991) Pulmonary lymphangioleiomyomatosis. Report of a case with associated multiple soft-tissue tumors. Arch Pathol Lab Med 115: 1257

Cale WF, Petsonk EL, Boyd CB (1983) Transbronchial biopsy of pulmonary alveolar microlithiasis. Arch Intern Med 143: 358

Cameron JL, Anderson RP, Zuidema GD (1967) Aspiration pneumonia. A clinical and experimental review. J Surg Res 7: 44

Campognone P, Singer DB (1986) Neonatal sepsis due to nontypable *Haemophilus influenzae.* Am J Dis Child 140: 117

Canalis RF, Jenkins HA, Hemenway WG, Lincoln C (1978) Nasopharyngeal rhabdomyosarcoma. A clinical perspective. Arch Otolaryngol 104: 122

Cantrell RW, Bell RA, Moricka WT (1978) Acute epiglottis-intubation versus tracheostomy. Laryngoscope 88: 994

Carles D, Dallay D, Serville F et al. (1992a) Malformation adenomatoïde kystique du poumon, agénésie rénale bilatérale et hypoplasie du coeur gauche. Ann Pathol 12: 367

Carles, D, Servile F, Dubecq JP, Alberti EM, Horovitz J, Weichhold W (1992b) Idiopathic arterial calcification in a stillborn complicated by pleural hemorrhage and hydrops fetalis. Arch Pathol Lab Med 116: 293

Carter G, Thibeault DW, Beatty EC Jr, Kilbride HW, Huntrakoon M (1989) Misalignment of lung vessels and alveolar capillary dysplasia: a cause of persistent pulmonary hypertension. J Pediatr 114: 293–300

Cauchois R, Laccourreye O, Bremond D, Testud R, Küffer R, Monteil JP (1994) Nasal dermoid sinus cyst. Ann Otol Rhinol Laryngol 103: 615

Cayeux P (1972) Infections néonatales à streptocoques du groupe B constatations étiologiques. A propos de 77 observations. Arch Fr Pediatr 29: 391

CDC (1994) Update: influenza activity – United States and world-wide, 1993–94 season, and composition of the 1994–95 influenza vaccine. JAMA 271: 1070

Chambran P, Binet JP, Narcy P et al. (1988) Sténose trachéale congénitale par anneaux circulaires complets. Trachéoplastie à l'aide de péricarde autologue. Presse Med 17: 1810

Chandler JR, Goulding R, Moskowitz L, Quencer RM (1984) Nasopharyngeal angiofibromas: staging and management. Ann Otol Rhinol Laryngol 93: 322

Chaput M, Ninane J, Gosseye S et al. (1989) Juvenile laryngeal papillomatosis and epidermoid carcinoma. J Pediatr 114: 269

Charles RE, Katz RL, Ordonez NG, Mackay B (1986) Varicella–Zoster infection with pleural involvement. A cytologic and ultrastructural study of a case. Am J Clin Pathol 85: 522

Chaudhry AP, Haar JG, Koul A, Nickerson PA (1979) Olfactory neuroblastoma (esthesioneuroblastoma). A light and ultrastructral study of two cases. Cancer 44: 564

Chave J-P, David S, Wauters J-P, Van Melle G, Francioli P (1991) Transmission of *Pneumocystis carinii* from AIDS patients to other immunosuppressed patients: a cluster of *Pneumocystis carinii* pneumonia in renal transplant recipients. AIDS 5: 927

Chejfec G, Cosnow I, Gould NS, Husain AN, Gould VE (1990) Pulmonary blastoma with neuroendocrine differentiation in cell morules resembling neuroepithelial bodies. Histopathology. 17: 353

Chellam VG (1988) Rhabdomyomatous dysplasia of the lung. A case report with review of the literature. Pediatr Pathol 8: 391

Chen TC Kuo T (1993) Castleman's disease presenting as a pedunculated nasopharyngeal tumor simulating angiofibroma. Histopathology 23: 485

Chen MF, Onerheim R, Wang NS, Hütner I (1991) Rhabdomyomatosis of newborn lung. A case report with immunohistochemical and electronmicroscopic characterization of striated muscle cells in the lung. Pediatr Pathol 11: 123

Cherniack RM, Colby TV, Flint A, Thurlbeck WM, Waldron J, Ackerson L et al. (1991) Quantitative assessment of lung pathology in idiopathic pulmonary fibrosis. Am Rev Respir Dis 144: 892

Chessels MJ, Wigglesworth JS (1971) Haemostatic failure in babies with rhesus isoimmunisation. Arch Dis Child 46: 38

Chi JG, Shong YK (1982) Diffuse striated muscle heteroplasia of the lung. An autopsy case. Arch Pathol Lab Med 106: 641

Chi EY, Kuo C-C, Grayston JT (1987) Unique ultrastructure in the elementary body of Chlamydia sp. strain. TWAR J Bacteriol 169: 375

Cho KR, Woodruff JD, Epstein JI (1989) Leiomyoma of the uterus with multiple extrauterine smooth muscle tumors: a case report suggesting multifocal origin. Hum Pathol 20: 80

Chou P, Blei ED, Shen-Schwarz S, Gonzalez-Crssi F, Reynolds M (1993) Pulmonary changes following extracorporeal membrane oxygenation: autopsy study of 23 cases. Hum Pathol 24: 405

Chu L, Gussack GS, Orr JB, Hood D (1994) Neonatal Laryngoceles. A cause for airway obstruction. Arch Otolaryngol Head Neck Surg 120: 454

Chung EB, Enzinger FM (1981) Infantile myofibromatosis. Cancer 48: 1807

Civantos FJ, Holinger LD (1992) Laryngoceles and saccular cysts in infants and children. Arch Otolaryngol Head Neck Surg 118: 296

Clark DA, Nieman GF, Thompson JE, Paskanik AM, Rokhar JE, Bredenberg CE (1987) Surfactant displacement by meconium free fatty acids: an alternative explanation for atelectasis in meconium aspiration syndrome. J Pediatr 110: 765

Clelland CA, Higenbottam TW, Stewarat S, Scott JP, Wallwork J (1990) The histological changes in transbronchial biopsy after treatment of acute lung rejection in heart–lung transplants. J Pathol 161: 105

Coffin CM, Schechtman K, Cole FS, Dehner LP (1993) Neonatal and infantile pulmonary hemorrhage: an autopsy study with clinical correlation. Pediatr Pathol 13: 583

Cogbill TH, Moore FA, Accurso FJ, Lilly JR (1983) Primary tracheomalacia. Ann Thorac Surg 35: 538

Cohen SR, Chai J (1978) Epiglottis: twenty-year study with tracheotomy. Ann Otol 87: 461

Cohen SR, Thompson JW (1986) Lymphangiomas of the larynx in infants and children. A survey of pediatric lymphangioma. Ann Otol Rhinol Laryngol 95: 1

Cohen SR, Landing BH, Isaacs H (1978a) Fibrous histiocytoma of the trachea. Ann Otol Rhinol 87: 2

Cohen SR, Landing BH, Isaacs H, King KK, Hanson V (1978b) Solitary plasmacytoma of the larynx and upper trachea associated with systemic lupus erythematosus. Ann Otol Rhinol Laryngol 87: 11

Cohen SR, Landing BH, King KK, Isaacs H (1978c) Wegener's granulomatosis causing laryngeal and tracheobronchial obstruction in an adolescent girl. Ann Otol Rhinol Laryngol 87: 15

Cohen SR, Landing BH, Byrne WJ, Feig S, Isaacs H (1978d) Primary lymphosarcoma of the larynx in a child. Ann Otol Rhinol Laryngol 87: 20

Cohen M, Emms M, Kaschula RO (1991) Childhood pulmonary blastoma: a pleuropulmonary variant of the adult-type pulmonary blastoma. Pediatr Pathol 11: 737

Cohen MC, Drut R, Garcia C, Kaschula ROC (1992) Mesenchymal hamartoma of the chest wall: a cooperative study with review of the literature. Pediatr Pathol 12: 525

Cohen MC, Kaschula ROC (1992) Primary pulmonary tumors in childhood: a review of 31 years' experience and the literature. Pediatr Pulmonol 140: 222

Cohen MD (1994) Current controversy: is computed tomography scan of the chest needed in patients with Wilm's tumor? Amer J Pediatr Hemato-Oncol 16: 191

Cole VA, Normand ICS, Reynolds EOR, Rivers RPA (1973) Pathogenesis of hemorrhagic pulmonary edema and massive pulmonary haemorrhage in the newborn. Pediatrics 51: 175

Coleman A, Colby TV (1988) Histologic diagnosis of extrinsic allergic alveolitis. Am J Surg Pathol 12: 514

Colley MH, Geppert E, Frankin W A (1989) Immunohistochemical detection of steroid receptors in a case of pulmonary lymphangioleiomyomatosis. Am J Surg Pathol 13: 803

Compagno J (1978) Hemangio pericytoma – like tumors of the nasal cavity: a comparison with hemangiopericytoma of soft tissues. Laryngoscope 88: 460

Compagno J, Wong RT (1977) Intranasala mixed tumors (pleomorphic adenomas). A clinicopathologic study of 40 cases. Am J Clin Pathol 68: 213

Compagno J, Hyams VJ, Lepore ML (1976) Nasal polyposis with stromal atypia: review and follow-up study of 14 cases. Arch Pathol Lab Med 100: 244

Cone RW, Hackman RC, Huang M-L, Bowden RA, Meyers JD, Metcalf M et al. (1993) Human herpesvirus 6 in lung tissue from patients with pneumonitis after bone marrow transplantation. N Engl J Med 329: 156

Conley J, Healey WV, Blaugrund SM, Perzin KH (1968) Nasopharyngeal angiofibroma in the juvenile. Surg Gynecol Obstet 126: 825

Cooney TP, Thurlbeck WM (1982) The radial alveolar count of Emery and Mithal: a reappraisal. II Intrauterine and early postnatal lung growth. Thorax 37: 580

Cooney TP, Thurlbeck WM (1985) Lung growth and development in anencephaly and hydranencephaly. Am Rev Respir Dis 132: 596

Corbally MT (1993) Laryngo-tracheo-eosophageal cleft. Arch Dis Child 68: 550

Corrao WM, Mark EJ (1990) Case records of the Massachusetts General Hospital (Case 21-1990). N Engl Med 322: 1512

Corrin B (1992) Bronchiolitis obliterans organizing pneumonia. A British view. Chest 102: 7S

Cotton BH, Spaulding K, Penido JRF (1956) An accessory lung: report of a case. J Thorac Surg 23: 508

Courtin P, Janin A, Sault MC, Pruvot FR, Degreef JM, Gosselin B (1987) Adénome bronchique pur. Etude anatomoclinique et ultrastructurale d'un cas. Ann Pathol 7: 315

Cowie F, Meller ST, Cushing P, Pinkerton R (1994) Chemoprophylaxis for pulmonary aspergillosis during intensive chemotherapy. Arch Dis Child 70: 136

Cowper SG (1973) Bilharziasis (schistosomiasis) in Nigeria. Trop Georgr Med 25: 105

Crapo JD (1986) Morphologic changes in pulmonary oxygen toxicity. Annu Rev Physiol 48: 721

Crapo JD and Wright JR (1995) SP-A deficiency. A cause or consequence of inflammation in bronchopulmonary dysplasia? Am J Respir Crit Med 151: 595

Crissman JD, Weiss MA, Gluckman J (1982) Midline granuloma syndrome. A clinicopathologic study of 13 patients. Am J Surg Pathol 6: 335

Crissman JD, Kessis T, Shah KV et al. (1988) Squamous papillary neoplasia of the adult upper aerodigestive tract. Hum Pathol 19: 1387

Cutz E (1987) Idiopathic pulmonary hemosiderosis and related disorders in infancy and childhood. Perspect Pediatr Pathol 11: 47

de la Fuente AA (1994) Full term SIBS with neonatal RDS. Abstract – 40th Annual Meeting Pediat Path Soc

Deavers M, Guinee D, Koss MN, Travis WD (1995) Granular cell tumors of the lung. Clinicopathologic study of 20 cases. Am J Surg Pathol 19: 627

deMello DE, Nogee LM, Heyman S, Krous HF, Hussain M, Merritt TA et al. (1994) Molecular and phenotypic variability in the congenital alveolar proteinosis syndrome associated with inherited surfactant protein B deficiency. J Pediatr 125: 43

D'Ercole C, Boubli L, Potier A, Borrione C-L, Leclaire M, Blanc B (1994) Pathologie tumorale thoracique foetale. A propos d'un cas d'hamartome thoracique. Medecine Foetale et Echographie en Gynecologie 19: 17

Dain DW, Randall JL, Smith JW (1970) Starch in the lungs of newborns following positive-pressure ventilation. Am J Dis Child 119: 218

Daniels AC, Conner GH, Straus FH (1967) Primary chondrosarcoma of the tracheobronchial tree. Report of a unique case and brief review. Arch Pathol 84: 615

Dardick I, Guindi M, Barr JR, Hickey NM, Sachs HJ (1989) An unusual tumor of the lung. Ultrastruct Pathol 13: 325

Davey RT Jr, Masur H (1990) Recent advances in the diagnosis, treatment, and prevention of *Pneumocystis carinii* pneumonia. Antimicrob Agents Chemother 34: 499

David TJ (1986) Nasal polyposis, opaque paranasal sinuses and usually normal hearing: the otorhinolaryngological features of cystic fibrosis. JR Soc Med 79 (suppl 12): 23

Davis JM, Metlay LA, Dickerson B, Penney DP, Notter RH (1990) Early pulmonary changes associated with high-frequency jet ventilation in newborn piglets. Pediat Res 27: 460

Davis S, Bove KE, Wells TR, Hartsell B, Weinberg A, Gilbert E (1992) Tracheal cartilaginous sleeve. Pediatr Pathol 12: 349

Davis SL, Furman DP, Costarino AT Jr (1993) Adult respiratory distress syndrome in children: associated disease, clinical course, and predictors of death. J Pediatr 123: 35

Day DW, Taylor SA (1975) An intrapulmonary teratoma associated with thymic tissue. Thorax 30: 582

de la Monte SM, Hutchins GM, Moore GW (1986) Respiratory epithelial cell necrosis is the earliest lesion of hyaline membrane disease of the newborn. Am J Pathol 123: 155

de Montis G, Garnier P, Thomassin N, Job JC, Rossier A (1972) La mucolipidose type II (maladie des cellules à inclusion). Etude d'un cas et revue de la littérature. Ann Pediatr 19: 369

De Remee RA, Weiland LH, McDonald TJ (1978) Polymorphic reticulosis, lymphomatoid granulomatosis. Two diseases or one? Mayo Clin Proc 53: 634

de Villiers EM, Neumann C, Le J-Y, Weidauer H, Zur Hausen H (1986) Infection of the oral mucosa with defined types of human papillomaviruses. Med Microbiol Immunol 174: 287

Dehner LP (1973) Tumors of the mandible and maxilla in children. I. Clinicopathologic study of 46 benign lesions. Cancer 31: 364

Dehner LP (1993) Primitive neuroectodermal tumor and Ewing's Sarcoma. Am J Surg Pathol 17: 1

Delafosse C, Chevrolet J-C, Suter P, Cox JW (1988) Necrotising tracheobronchitis: a complication of high frequency jet ventilation. Vichows Arch [A] 413: 257

Delage G, Brochu P, Pelletier M, Jasmin G, Lapointe N (1979) Giant-cell pneumonia caused by parainfluenza virus. J Pediatr 94: 426

Delahunt B, Thomson KJ, Ferguson AF, Neale TJ, Meffan PJ, Nacey JN (1993) Familial cystic nephroma and pleuropulmonary blastoma. Cancer 71: 1338

Delarue J, Paillas J, Abelanet R, Chomette G (1959) Les bronchopneumopathies congénitales. Bronches 9: 114

Demarquez JL, Arsene–Henry–Fizet D, Babin JP, Allain D, Bentegeat J, Moulinier J, Martin C (1976) Alpha-1 antitrypsine et détresse respiratoire idiopathique du nouveau-né. Etude dans le sérum et dans le poumons. Arch Fr Pediatr 33: 359

deMello DE, Chi EY, Doo E, Lagunoff D (1987) Absence of tubular myelin in lungs of infants dying with hyaline membrane disease. Am J Pathol 127: 131

Demmler GJ (1991) Summary of a workshop on surveillance for congenital cytomegalovirus disease. Rev Infect Dis 13: 315

Dempo K, Satoh M, Tsuji S, Mori M, Kuroki Y, Akino T (1987) Immunohistochemical studies on the expression of pulmonary surfactant apoproteins in human lung carcinomas using monoclonal antibodies. Pathol Res Pract 182: 669

Denneny JC (1985) Bronchomalacia in the neonate. Ann Otol Rhinol Laryngol 94: 466

Denning DW, Stevens DA (1990) Antifungal and surgical treatment of invasive aspergillosis: review of 2121 published cases. Rev Infect Dis 12: 1147

Desvignes C, Hummel J, Jamet G, Levasseur P, Rojas-Miranda A, Verley J, Merlier M (1974) Emphysème pulmonaire et atrésie

430

bronchique. A propos de quatre observations. Ann Chir Thorac Cardiovasc 13: 135

Deterding RR, Shimizu H, Fisher JH, Shannon JM (1994) Regulation of surfactant protein D expression by glucocorticoids in vitro and in vivo. Am J Respir Cell Mol Biol 10: 30

Dewar A, Corrin B, Turner-Warwick M (1984) Tadpole shaped structures in a further patient with granulomatous lung disease. Thorax 39: 466

Dewhurst S, McIntyre K, Schnabel K, Hall CB (1993) Human herpesvirus 6 (HHV-6) variant B accounts for the majority of symptomatic primary HHV-6 infections in a population of US infants. J Clin Microbiol 31: 416

Diaz JH (1985) Croup and epiglottitis in children: an anesthesiologist as diagnostician. Anesth Analg 64: 621

Dickens P, Srivastava, G, Loke SL, Larkin S (1991) Human papillomavirus 6, 11, and 16 in laryngeal papillomas. J Pathol 165: 243

DiFiore JW, Wilson JM (1995) Lung liquid, fetal lung growth, and the congenital diaphragmatic hernia. Pediatr Surg Int 10: 2

Dilworth JA, Mandell GL (1977) Adults with chronic granulomatous disease of "childhood". Am J Med 63: 233

Dische MR, Guttenberg ME, Gordon R (1988) Case 4 malignant pleural mesothelioma in a child. Pediatr Pathol 8: 437

Djukanovic R, Roche WR, Wilson JW, Beasley CRW, Twentyman OP, Howarth PH et al. (1990) Mucosal inflammation in asthma. Am Rev Respir Dis 142: 434

Dobashi K, Asayama K, Hayashibe H, Munim A, Kawaoi A, Morikawa M et al. (1993) Immunohistochemical study of copper-zinc and manganese superoxide dismutases in the lungs of human fetuses and newborn infants: developmental profile and alterations in hyaline membrane disease and bronchopulmonary dysplasia. Virchows Archiv A [Pathol Anat] 423: 177

Dodd-O JM, Wieneke KF, Rosman PM (1987) Laryngeal rhabdomyosarcoma. Case report and literature review. Cancer 59: 1012

Domizio P, Liesner RJ, Dicks-Mireaux C, Risdon RA (1990) Malignant mesenchymoma associated with a congenital lung cyst on a child: case report and review of the literature. Pediatr Pathol 10: 785

Donaldson SS, Castro JR, Wilbur JR, Jesse RH Jr (1973) Rhabdomyosarcoma of head and neck in children. Combination treatment by surgery, irradiation and chemotherapy. Cancer 31: 26

Donders GGG, Moerman P, de Wet GH, Hooft P, Goubau P (1991) The association between Chlamydia cervicitis, chorioamnionitis and neonatal complications. Arch Gynecol Obstet 249: 79

Donegan JO, Strife JL, Seid AB, Cotton RT, Dunbar JS (1986) Internal laryngocele and saccular cysts in children. Ann Otol Rhinol Laryngol 89: 409

Donnelly SC, Haslett C (1992) Cellular mechanisms of acute lung injury: implications for future treatment in the adult respiratory distress syndrome. Thorax 47: 260

Dounies R, Chwals WJ, Lally KP et al. (1994) Hamartomas of the chest wall in infants. Ann Thorac Surg 57: 868

Downing GJ (1992) Tracheal agenesis with diaphragmatic hernia. Am J Med Genet 42: 85

Drachman R, Baillet G, Gangadoux M-F, de Vernejoul PaulBroyer M (1986) Pulmonary calcifications in children on dialysis. Nephron 44: 46

Dreisen RB (1993) New perspectives in Wegener's granulomatosis. Thorax 48: 97

Drobyski WR, Knox K-K, Majewski D, Carrigan DR (1994) Brief report: fatal encephalitis due to variant B human herpesvirus-6 infection in a bone marrow-transplant recipient. N Engl J Med 330: 1356

Drut R, Drut RM (1988) Measles pneumonia in a newborn. Pediatr Pathol 8: 553

Drut RM, Quijano G, Drut R, Las Heras J (1988) Rhabdomyomatous dysplasia of the lung. Pediatr Pathol 8: 385

Dubin SB (1990) Assessment of fetal lung maturity; in search of the Holy Grail. Clin Chem 36: 1867

Dunnill MS (1960) The pathology of asthma with special references to changes in the bronchial mucosa. J Clin Pathol 13: 27

Dunnill MS (1990) Pulmonary fibrosis. Histopathology 16: 321

Dupuis C, Charaf LA, Breviere GM, Abou P (1993) "Infantile" form of the scimitar syndrome with pulmonary hypertension. Am J Cardiol 71: 1326

Dutau G, Rochiccioli P Petel B, Fanic H, Fabre J, Dalous A (1973) Séquestration pulmonaire de l'enfant. A propos d'une observation avec étude bronchologique, angiographique et anatomique. Ann Pediatr 20: 373

Eavey RD (1985) Inverted papilloma of the nose and paranasal sinuses in childhood adolescence. Larynsoscope 95: 17

Eavey RD, Nadol JB, Holmes LB, Laird NM, Lapey A, Joseph MP, Strome M (1986) Kartagener's syndrome. A blinded, controlled study of cilia ultrastructure. Arch Otolaryngol Head neck Surg 112

Edman JC, Kovacs, Masur H, Santi DV, Elwood HJ, Sogin ML (1988) Ribosomal RNA sequence shows Pneumocystis carinii to be a member of the fungi. Nature 334: 519

Elborn JS, Shale DJ (1990) Lung injury in cystic fibrosis. Thorax 45: 970

Elkon D, Hightower SI, Lim ML, Cantrell RW, Constable WC (1979) Esthesioneuroblastoma. Cancer 44: 1087

Elrad H, Beydoun SN, Hagen JH, Cabalum MT, Aubry RH, Smith C (1978) Fetal pulmonary maturity as determined by fluorescent polarization of amniotic flud. Am J Obstet Gyencol 132: 681

Emery JL, Dinsdale F (1974) Increased incidence of lymphoreticular aggregates in lungs of children found unexpectedly dead. Arch Dis Child 49: 107

Emery JL, Haddadin AJ (1971) Squamous epithelium in respiratory tract of children with tracheo-oesophageal fistula. Arch Dis Child 46: 236

Emile J-F, Wechsler J, Brousse N, Boulland ML, Cologon R, Fraitag S et al. (1995) Langerhans' cell histiocytosis. Definitive diagnosis with the use of monoclonal antibody 010 on routinely paraffin-embedded samples. Am J Surg Pathol 19: 636

Enders G, Miller E, Cradock-Watson J, Bolley I, Ridehalgh M (1994) Consequences of varicella and herpes zoster in pregnancy: prospective study of 1739 cases. Lancet 343: 1548

Engellenner W, Kaplan C, van de Vegte GL (1989) Pulmonary agenesis association with nonimmune hydrops. Pediatr Pathol 9: 725

Engzell VCG, Jones AW (1973) Rhinosporidiosis in Uganda. J Laryngol Otol 87: 795

Epstein MA, Achong BG (1970) The fine structure of cultured Burkitt lymphoblasts of established in vitro stains. In: Burkitt DP, Wright D (eds) Burkitt's lymphoma. Livingstone, Edinburgh, p 118

Erickson AM, de la Monte SM, Moore GW Hutchins GM (1987) The progression of morphologic changes in bronchopulmonary dysplasia. Am J Pathol 127: 474

Erosoz A, Soncul H, Gokgoz L, Kalaycioglu S, Tunaoglu S, Kaptanoglu M et al. (1992) Horseshoe lung with left lung hypoplasia. Thorax 47: 205

Eschenbach DA (1993) Ureaplasma urealyticum respiratory disease in newborns. Ureaplasma urealyticum and premature birth. Clin Infect Dis 17: S100

Esclamado RM, Richardson MA (1987) Laryngotracheal foreign bodies in children. A comparison with bronchial foreign bodies. Am J Dis Child 141: 259

Esclamado RM, Disher MJ, Ditto JL, Rontal E, MacClatchey KD (1994) Laryngeal liposarcoma. Arch Otolaryngol Head Neck Surg 120: 422

Esterly JR Oppenheimer EA (1966) Massive pulmonary haemorrhage in the newborn. I. Pathologic considerations. J Pediatr 69: 3

Eusebi V, Rilke F, Ceccarelli C, Fedeli F, Schiaffino S, Bussolati G (1986) Fetal heavy chain skeletal myosin. An oncofetal antigen expressed by rhabdomyosarcoma. Am J Surg Pathol 10: 680

Ezaki T, Hashimoto Y, Yamamoto H, Lucida ML, Liu SL, Kusunoki S et al. (1990) Evaluation of the microplate hybridization method for rapid identification of Legionella species. Eur J Clin Microbiol Infect Dis 9: 213

Ezekowitz RAB, Mulliken JB, Folkman J (1992) Interferon α therapy for life-threatening hemangiomas of infancy. N Engl Med 326: 1456

Ezri T, Kunichezky S, Eliraz A, Soroker D, Halperin D, Schattner A (1994) Q J Med 87: 1

Fadel HE, Saad SA, Nelson GH, Davis HC (1986) Effect of maternal–fetal disorders on lung maturation. I. Diabetes melitus. Am J Obstet Gynecol 155: 544

Fakhoury G, Daikoku NH, Benser J, Dubin NH (1994) Lamellar body concentrations and the prediction of fetal pulmonary maturity. Am J Obstet Gynecol 170: 72

Fariss MW (1990) Oxygen toxicity: unique cytoprotective properties of vitamin E succinate in hepatocytes. Free Radical Biology and Medicine 9: 333

Farrell PM, Avery ME (1975) Hyaline membrane disease. Am Rev Respir Dis 111: 657

Fassina AS, Rupolo M, Pelizzo MR, Casara D (1994) Thyroid cancer in children and adolescents. Tumori 80: 257

Fedrick J, Butler NR (1970a) Certain causes of neonatal death. I. Hyaline membranes. Biol Neonate 15: 229

Fedrick J, Butler NR (1970b) Certain causes of neonatal death. II Intraventricular haemorrhage. Biol Neonate 15: 257

Fedrick J, Butler NR (1971b) Certain causes of neonatal death. IV. Massive pulmonary haemorrhage. Biol Neonate 18: 243

Fellbaum Hansmann ML, Lennert K (1989) Malignant lymphomas of the nasal cavity and paranasal sinuses. Virchows Archiv A [Patho Anat Histopathol] 414: 399

Felson B (1972) The many faces of pulmonary sequestration. Semin Roentgenol 7: 3

Fend F, Prior C, Margreiter R, Mikuz G (1990) Cytomegalovirus pneumonitis in heart–lung transplant recipients: histopathology and clinicopathologic considerations. Hum Pathol 21: 918

Ferguson JL, Neel HB, III (1989) Choanal atresia; treatment trends in 47 patients over 33 years. Ann Otol Rhinol Laryngol 98: 110

Figa FH, Yoo SJ, Burrows PE, Turner-Gomes S, Freedom RM (1993) Horseshoe lung – a case report with unusual bronchial and pleural anomalies and a proposed new classification. Pediatr Radiol 23: 44

Finlay-Jones JM, Papadimitriou JM, Barter RA (1973) Pulmonary hyaline membrane: light and electron microscopic study of the early stage. J Pathol 112: 117

Finn DG, Hudson WR, Balylin G (1981) Unilateral polyposis and mucoceles in children. Laryngoscope 91: 1444

Fisher M, Roggli V, Merten D, Mulvihill D, Spock A (1992) Coexisting endogenous lipoid pneumonia, cholesterol granulomas and pulmonary alvelar proteinosis in a pediatric population. Pediatr Pathol 12: 365

Fishman AP (1978) UIP, DIP and all that. N Engl J Med 298: 843

Forrest JB, Rossman CM, Newhouse MT, Ruffin R (1979) Activation of nasal cilia in immotile cilia syndrome. Am Rev Resp Dis 120: 511

Foster MJ, Caldwell AP, Staheli J, Smith DH, Gardner JS, Seegmiller RE (1994) Pulmonary hypoplasia associated with reduced thoracic space in mice with disproportionate micromelia (DMM). Anat Rec 228: 454

Foucar E, Rosai J, Dorfman R (1990) Sinus histiocytosis with massive lymphadenopathy (Rosai–Dorfman disease): review of the entity. Semin Diagn Pathol 7: 19

Foucar K, Foucar E (1990) The mononuclear phagocyte and immunoregulatory effector (M-PIRE) system concepts. Semin Diagn Pathol 7: 4

Fowler KB, Stagno S, Pass R-F, Britt WJ, Boll TJ, Alford CA (1992) The outcome of congenital cytomegalovirus infection in relation to maternal antibody status. N Engl J Med 326: 663

Fox H, Cocker J (1964) Laryngeal atresia. Arch Dis Child 39: 641

Foy HM (1993) Infections caused by Mycoplasma pneumoniae and possible carrier state in different populations of patients. Clin Infect Dis 17: S37

Foy HM, Cooney MK, Allan I, Kenny GE (1979) Rates of pneumonia during influenza epidemics in Seattle, 1964 to 1975. JAMA 241: 253

Franciosi RA, Knostman JD, Zimmerman RA (1973) Group B streptococcal neonatal and infant infections. J Pediatr 82: 707

Frank L, Sosenko IRS (1988) Undernutrition as a major contributing factor in the pathogenesis of bronchopulmonary dysplasia. Am Rev Respir Dis 138: 725

Frenkel LM, Nielsen K, Garakian A, Cherry JD (1994) A search for peristent measles, mumps, and rubella vaccine virus in children with human immunodeficiency virus type I infection. Arch Pediatr Adolesc Med 148: 57

Frierson HF, Mills SE, Fechner RE, Taxy JB, Levine PA (1986) Sinonasal undifferentiated carcinoma. An aggressive neoplasm derived from Schneiderian epithelium and distinct from olfactory neuroblastoma. Am J Surg Pathol 10: 771

Frugoni P, Ferlito A (1976) Pleomorphic rhabdomyosarcoma of the larynx. A case report and review of the literature. J Laryngol 90: 687

Fu YS, Perzin KH (1974a) Non-epithelial tumors of the nasal cavity, paranasal sinuses and nasophrynx: a clinicopathologic study. I. General features and vascular tumors. Cancer 33: 1275

Fu YS, Perzin KH (1974b) Non-epithelial tumors of the nasal cavity, paranasal sinuses and nasopharynx: a clinicopathologic study. II. Osseous and fibro-osseous lesions, including osteoma, giant cell tumor and osteoblastoma. Cancer 33: 1289

Fu YS, Perzin KH (1974c) Non-epithelial tumors of the nasal cavity, paranasal sinuses and nasopharynx: a clinicopathologic study. III. Cartilaginous tumors (chondroma, chondrosarcoma). Cancer 34: 453

Fu YS, Perzin KH (1975) Non-epithelial tumors of the nasal cavity, paranasal sinuses and nasopharynx: a clinocopathologic study. IV. Smooth muscle tumors (leiomyoma, leiomyosarcoma). Cancer 35: 1300

Fu YS, Perzin KH (1976a) Non-epithelial tumors of the nasal cavity, paranasal sinuses and nasopharynx: a clinocopathologic study. V. Skeletal muscle tumors (thabdomyoma and rhabdomyosarcoma). Cancer 37: 364

Fu YS, Perzin KH (1976b) Non-epithelial tumors of the nasal cavity, paranasal sinuses and nasopharynx: a clinicopathologic study. VI. Fibrous tissue tumors (fibroma, fibromatosis, fibrosarcoma). Cancer 37: 2912

Fu YS, Perzin KH (1977) Non-epithelial tumors of the nasal cavity, paranasal sinuses and nasopharynx: a clinocopathologic study. VII. Myxomas. Cancer 39: 195

Fu YS, Perzin KH (1979) Non-epithelial tumors of the nasal cavity, paranasal sinuses and nasopharynx: a clinicopathologic study. X. Malignant lymphomas. Cancer 43: 611

Fujimura M, Takeuchi T, Kitajima H, Nakayama M (1989) Chorioamnionitis and serum IgM in Wilson–Mikity syndrome. Arch Dis Child 64: 1379

Fukuda Y, Ferrans VJ, Schoenberger CI, Rennard SI, Crystal RG (1985) Patterns of pulmonary structural remodelling after experimental paraquat toxicity. The morphogenesis of intraalveolar fibrosis. Am J Pathol 118: 452

Fukuda Y, Kawamoto M, Yamamoto A, Ishizaki M, Basset F, Masugi Y (1990) Role of elastic fiber degradation in emphysema-like lesions of pulmonary lymphangiomyomatosis. Hum Pathol 21: 1252

Fukuda T, Ohnishi Y, Kanai I, Watanabe T, Kitazawa M, Okamura A, et al. (1992) Papillary adenoma of the lung. Histological and ultrastructural findings in two cases. Acta Pathol Jpn 42: 56

Fuller CM, Howard MB, Bedwell DM, Frizzell RA, Benos DJ (1992) Antibodies against the cystic fibrosis transmembrane regulator. Am J Physiol 262: C396

Furukawa T, Jisaki F, Sakamuro D, Takegami T, Murayama T (1994) Detection of human cytomegalovirus genomein uterus tissue. Arch Virol 135: 265

Gal AA, Brooks SJ, Pietra GG (1989) Leiomyomatous neoplasms of the lung: a clinical, histologic, and immunohistochemical study. Mod Pathol 2: 209

Gaillard D, Ruocco S, Lallemand A, Dalemans W, Hinnrasky J, Puchelle E (1994) Immunohistochemical localization of cystic fibrosis transmembrane conductance regulator in human fetal airway and digestive mucosa. Pediatr Res 36: 137

Galliani CA, Beatty JF, Grosfeld JL (1992) Cavernous hemangioma of the lung in an infant. Pediatr Pathol 12: 105

Gandy G, Jacobson W, Gairdner D (1970) Hyaline membrane disease. I. Arch Dis Child 45: 241

Garaventa A, Porta F, Rondelli R, Dini G, Meloni G, Bonetti F, et al. (1992) Early deaths in children after BMT Bone Marrow Transplant 10: 419

Garcia LW, Hemphil RB, Marasco WA, Ciano PS (1991) Acquired immunodeficiency syndrome with disseminated toxoplasmosis presenting as an acute pulmonary and gastrointestinal illness. Arch Pathol Lab Med 115: 459

Gardner PS, Court SDM, Brocklebank JT, Downham MAPS, Weightman D (1973) Virus gross-infection in paediatric wards. Br Med J ii: 571

Gay BB Jr, Bonmati J (1954) Primary neurogenic tumors of the lung and interlobar fissures: a review of clinical and radiologic findings in reported cases with addition of two new cases. Radiology 63: 43

Gay I, Feinmesser R, Cohen T (1981) Laryngeal web, congenital heart disease and low stature. Arch Otolaryngol 107: 510

Geary WA, Mills SE, Frierson HF Jr, Pope TL (1991) Malignant peritoneal mesothelioma in childhood with long-term survival. Am J Clin Pathol 95: 493

Gebauer PW, Mason CB (1959) Intralobar pulmonary sequestration associated with anomalous pulmonary vessels: a non entity. Dis Chest 35: 282

Genin C, Touraine JL, Berger F, Bryon PA, Valancogne A, Philippe N, Monnet P (1977) BCGite généralisée dans un déficit immunitaire mixte et grave: évolution défavorable malgré une tentative de greffe de moelle osseuse. Arch Fr Pediatr 34: 639

George DK, Cooney TP, Chiu BK, Thurlbeck WM (1987) Hypoplasia and immaturity of the terminal lung unit (acinus) in congenital diaphragmatic hernia 1–3. Am Rev Respir Dis 138: 947

Gerami S, Richardson R, Harrington B, Pate JW (1969) Obstructive emphysema due to bronchogenic cysts in infancy. J Thrac Cardiovasc Surg 58: 432

Gerle RD, Jaretzki A III, Ashley A, Berne A S (1968) Congenital broncho-pulmonary foregut malformation. N Engl J Med 278: 1413

Gervaix A, Suter S (1991) Epidemiology of invasive Haemophilus influenza type b infections in Geneva, Switzerland, 1976–1989. Pediatr Infect Dis J 10: 370

Ghadially FN, Murphy F, Lalonde JMA (1984) Diagnosis of pulmonary talcosis by electron-probe X-ray analysis. J Submicrosc Cytol 16: 773

Gibbs RS, Mead PB (1992) Preventing neonatal herpes – current strategies. N Engl J Med 326: 946

Giffin F, Greenough A, Yuksel B (1994) Prediction of respiratory morbidity in the third year of life in children born prematurely. Acta Paediatr 83: 157

Gifford GH Jr, Swanson L, MacCollum DW (1972) Congenital absence of the nose and anterior nasopharynx. Report of two cases. Plast Reconstr Surg 50: 5

Gilbert JG, Mazzarella LA, Feit LJ (1953) Primary tracheal tumors in the infant and adult. Arch Otolaryngol 58: 1

Gillan JE, Cutz E (1993) Abnormal pulmonary bombesin immunoreactive cells in Wilson–Mikity syndrome (pulmonary dysmaturity) and bronchopulmonary dysplasia. Pediatr Pathol 13: 165

Gilmore LB, Talley FA, Hook GER (1988) Classification and morphometric quantitation of insoluble materials from the lungs of patients with alveolar proteinosis. Am J Pathol 133: 252

Gindhart TD, Johnston WH, Chism SE, Dedo HH (1980) Carcinoma of the larynx in childhood. Cancer 46: 1683

Gitlin D, Craig JM (1956) The nature of the hyaline membrane in asphyxia of the newborn. Pediatrics 17: 64

Goerdt S, Kolde G, Bonsmann G, Hamann K, Czarnetzki B, Andreseen R, et al. (1993) Immunohistochemical comparison of cutaneous histiocytoses and related skin disorders: diagnostic and histogenetic relevance of MS-1 high molecular weight protein expression. J Pathol 170: 421

Goldberg NS, Bauer BS, Kraus H, Crussi FG, Esterly NB (1988) Infantile myofibromatosis: a review of clinicopathology with perspective on new treatment choices. Pediatr Dermatol 5: 37

Gonzalez OR, Gonzalez-Gomez I, Recalde AL, Landing BL (1991) Postnatal development of the cystic lung lesion of Down's syndrome: suggestion that the cause is reduced formation of peripheral air spaces. Pediatr Pathol 11: 623

Gonzalez-Crussi F, Boggs JD, Raffensperger JG (1980) Brain heterotopia in the lungs. A rare cause of respiratory distress in the newborn. Am J Clin Pathol 73: 281

Gooch JJ, Britt EM (1978) Staphylococcus aureus colonization and infection in newborn nursery patients. Am J Dis Child 132: 893

Gorelick MH, Baker MD (1994) Epiglottitis in children, 1979 through 1992. Effects of Haemophilus influenzae type b immunization. Arch Pediatr Adolesc Med 148: 47

Gorelkin L, Chandler FW Ewing EP (1986) Staining qualities of cytomegalovirus inclusions in the lungs of patients with the acquired immunodeficiency syndrome: a potential source of diagnostic misinterpretation. Hum Pathol 17: 926

Gorenflo M, Vogel M, Obladen M (1991) Pulmonary vascular changes in bronchopulmonary dysplasia a clinicopathologic correlation in short- and long-term survivors. Pediatr Pathol 11: 851

Gorenstein A, Neel HB, Weiland LH, Devine KD (1980a) Sarcomas of the larynx. Arch Otolaryngol 106: 8

Gortner L, Pohlandt F, Bartmann P, Bernsau U, Proz F, Hellwege H-H et al. (1994) High-dose versus low-dose bovine surfactant treatment in very premature infants. Acta Paediatr 83: 135

Gotti G, Haid MM, Paladini P, Di Bisceglie M, Volterrani L, Sforza V (1993) Pedunculated pulmonary leiomyoma with large cyst formation. Ann Thorac Surg 56: 1178

Gould SJ, Isaacson PG (1993) Bronchus-associated lymphoid tissue (BALT) in human fetal and infant lung. J Pathol 169: 229

Gowdar K, Bull MJ, Schreiner RL, Lemons JA, Gresham EL (1980) Nasal deformities in neonates. Their occurrence in those treated with nasal continuous positive airway pressure and nasal endotracheal tubes. Am J Dis Child 14: 954

Granoff DM, Shackelford PG, Suarez BK, Nahm MH, Cates KL, Murphy TV, Karasic R, Osterholm MT, Pandey JP, Daum RS and the Collaborataive Group (1986) Hemophilus influenzae type B disease in children vaccinated with type B polysaccharide vaccine. N Engl J Med 315: 1584

Grans SL, Potts WJ (1951) Anomalous lobe of lung arising from the esophagus. J Thorac Surg 21: 313

Grayston JT, Campbell LA, Kuo C-C, Mordhorst CH, Saikku P, Thom DH et al. (1990) A new respiratory tract pathogen: *Chlamydia pneumoniae* strain TWAR J Infect Dis 161: 618

Green WR, Williams AW (1989) Neonatal adenovirus pneumonia. Arch Pathol Lab Med 113: 190

Greene R, Stark P (1978) Trauma of the larynx and trachea. Radiol Clin North Am 16: 309

Griffin M, Pushpanathan C, Andrews W (1990) *Chlamydia trachomatis* pneumonitis: a study and literature review. Pediatr Pathol 10: 843

Griffiths PD, Grundy JE (1987) Molecular biology and immunology of cytomegalovirus. Biochem J 241: 313

Grigg J, Arnon S Chase A, Silverman M (1993) Inflammatory cells in the lungs of premature infants on the first day of life: perinatal risk factors and origin of cells. Arch Dis Child 69: 40

Groneck P, Götze-Speer B, Oppermann M, Eiffert H, Speer CP (1994) Association of pulmonary inflammation and increased microvascular permeability during the development of bronchopulmonary dysplasia: a sequential analysis of inflammatory mediators in respiratory fluids of high-risk preterm neonates. Pediatrics 93: 712

Groothuis JR, Gutierrez KM, Lauer BA (1988) Respiratory syncytial virus infection in children with bronchopulmonary dysplasia. Pediatrics 82: 199

Groothuis JR, Simoes EAF, Hemming VG and the Respiratory Syncytial Virus Immune Globulin Study Group (1995) Respiratory syncytial virus (RSV) infection in preterm infants and the protective effects of RSV immune globulin (RSVIG). Pediatrics 95: 463

Groussard O (1993) Le rejet pulmonaire au cours des transplantations pulmonaires et cardiopulmonaires. Ann Pathol 13: 8

Grundfast KM, Mumtaz A, Kanter R, Pollack M (1981) Tracheomalacia in an infant with multiplex congenital (Larsen's) syndrome. Ann Otol Rhinol Laryngol 90: 303

Grundy GW, Miller RW (1972) Malignant mesothelioma in childhood. Report of 13 cases. Cancer 30: 1216

Grunow WA, Esterly JR (1972) Rheumatic pneumonitis. Chest 61: 298

Gucalp R, Ciobanu N, Sparano J, Motyl M, Carlisle P, Wiernik PH (1991) Disseminated aspergillosis after fungemia in a patient with extragonadal germ cell tumor undergoing autologous bone marrow transplantation. Cancer 68: 1842

Guillou L, Gloor E, Anani PA, Kaelin R (1991) Bronchial Granular-cell tumor. Report of a case with preoperative cytologic diagnosis on bronchial brushings and immunohistochemical studies. Acta Cytol 35: 375

Guinee Jr DG, Thornberry DS, Azumi N, Przygodzki RM, Koss MN, Travis WD (1995) Unique pulmonary presentation of an angiomyolipoma. Analysis of clinical, radiographic, and histopathologic features. Am J Surg Pathol 19: 476

Gustafson TL, Lievens AW, Brunell PA, Moellenberg RG, Buttery CMG, Schulster LM (1987) Measles outbreak in a fully immunized secondary-school population. N Engl J Med 316: 771

Gustafsson PM, Fransson SG, Kjellman N-IM, Tibbling L (1991) Gastro-oesophageal reflux and severity of pulmonary disease in cystic fibrosis. Scand J Gastroenterol 26: 449

Ha SY, Helms P, Fletcher M, Broadbent V, Pritchard J (1992) Lung involvement in Langerhans' cell histiocytosis: prevalence, clinical features, and outcome. Pediatrics 89: 466

Haas JE, Yunis EJ, Totten RS (1972) Ultrastructure of a sclerosing hemangioma of the lung. Cancer 30: 512

Hachitanda Y, Aoyoma C, Sato JK, Shimaa H (1993) Pleuropulmonary blastoma in childhood. A tumor of divergent differentiation. Am J Surg Pathol 17: 382

Hagwood S, Latham D, Borchelt J et al. (1993) Cell-specific posttranslational processing of the surfactant-associated protein SP-B. Am J Physiol 264: L290

Haidar A, Ryder TA, Wigglesworth JS (1991) Epithelial cell morphology and airspace size in hypoplastic human fetal lungs associated with oligohydramnios. Pediatr Pathol 11: 839

Halablab MA, Richards L, Bazin MJ (1990) Phagocytosis of *Legionella pneumophila*. J Med Microbiol 33: 75

Hällgren R, Bjermer L, Lundgren R, Venge P (1989) The eosinophil component of the alveolitis in idiopathic pulmonary fibrosis. Am Rev Respir Dis 139: 373

Hallman M, Ajorma P, Hoppu K, Teramo K, Akino T (1989) Surfactant proteins in the diagnosis of fetal lung maturity. II. The 35 kd protein and phospholipids in complicated pregnancy. Am J Obstet Gynecol 161: 965

Hancock BJ, Di-Lorenzo M, Youssef S, Yazbeck S, Marcotte JE, Collin PP (1993) Childhood primary pulmonary neoplasms. J Pediatr Surg 28: 1133

Hanimann B, Morger R, Baerlocher K, Brunner CH, Giver T, Schopfer K (1987) BCG – Osteitis in der Schweiz. Schweiz Med Wochenschr 117: 193

Hardy KA, Schidlow DV, Zaieri N (1988) Obliterative bronchiolitis in children. Chest 93: 460

Harrington RD, Hooton TM, Hackman RC, Storch GA, Osborne B, Gleaves CA et al. (1992) An outbreak of respiratory syncytial virus in a bone marrow transplant center. J Infect Dis 165: 987

Harrity P, Gibert-Barness E, Cabalka A, Hong R, Zimmerman J (1991) Isolated pulmonary Goodpasture sydrome. Pediatr Pathol 11: 635

Hartman GE, Shochat SJ (1983) Primary pulmonary neoplasma of childhood: a review. Ann Thorac Surg 36: 108

Hassam S, Briner J, Tratschin JD, Siegel G, Heitz PU (1990) In situ hybridization for the detection of human parvovirus B19 nucleic acid sequences in paraffin-embedded specimens. Virchows Archiv B [Cell Pathol] 59: 257

Hassberg D, Steil E, Sieverding L, Rosendahl W (1992) Combination of scimitar syndrome and horseshoe lung. A rare but typical finding. Case report and review of the literature. Klin Pädiatr 204: 434

Hawass ND, Badawi MG, al-Muzrakchi AM, al-Sammarai AI, Jawad AJ, Abdullah MA et al. (1990) Horseshoe lung: differential diagnosis. Pediatr Radiol 20: 580

Haver KE, Mark EJ (1994) Inflammatory pseudotumour. Case records of the Massachusetts General Hospital. N Engl Med 330: 1439

Hawgood S, Clements JA (1990) Pulmonary surfactant and its apoproteins. J Clin Invest 86: 1

Hawgood S, Latham D, Borchelt J, Damm D, White T, Benson B, Wright JR (1993) Cell-specific posttranslational processing of the surfactant-associated protein SP-B. Amer J Physiol 264: L290

Haworth SG (1987) Understanding pulmonary vascular disease in young children. Int J Cardiol 15: 101

Haworth SG (1993) Pulmonary hypertension in childhood. Eur Respir J 6: 1037

Hayes MMM, van der Westhuizen N, Holden GP (1993) Aggressive glomus tumor of the nasal region. Report of a case with multiple local recurrences. Arch Pathol Lab Med 117: 649

Hüllgren R, Bjermer L, Lundgren R, Venge P (1989) The eosinophil component of the alveolitis in idiopathic pulmonary fibrosis. Am Rev Respir Dis 139: 373

Healy GB, Holtand GP, Tucker JA (1976) Bifid epiglottis: a rare laryngeal anomaly. Laryngoscope 86: 1459

Heckman CJ, Truong LD, Cagle PT, Font RL (1988) Pulmonary blastoma with rhabdomyosarcomatous differentiation: an electron microscopic and immunohistochemical study. Am J Surg Pathol 12: 35

Heffelfinger MJ, Dahlin DC, MacCarty CS, Beabout JW (1973) Chordomas and cartilaginous tumors at the skull base. Cancer 32: 410

Hegg CA, Flint A, Singh G (1992) Papillary adenoma of the lung. Am J Clin Pathol 97: 383

Heifetz SA, Collins B, Matt BH (1992) Pleomorphic adenoma (benign mixed tumor) of the trachea. Pediatr Pathol 12: 563

Heij HA, Vos A, de Kraker J, Voute PA (1994) Pronostic factors in surgery for pulmonary metastases in children. Surgery 115: 687

Heitmiller RF, Mathisen DJ, Ferry JA, Mark EJ, Grillo HC (1989) Mucoepidermoid lung tumors. Ann Thorac Surg 47: 394

Helin I, Jodal U (1981) A syndrome of congenital hypoplasia of the alae nasi, situs inversus, and severe hypoproteinemia in two siblings. J Pediatr 99: 932

Henderson R, Hislop A, Reid L (1971) New pathological findings in emphysema of childhood. III. Unilateral congenital emphysema with hypoplasia and compensatory emphysema of contralateral lung. Thorax 26: 195

Heritage CK, Cunningham MD (1985) Association of elective repeat cesarean delivery and persistent pulmonary hypertension of the newborn. Am J Obstet Gynecol 152: 627

Herrmann B, Salih MAM, Yousif BE, Abdelwahab O, Mardh P-A (1994) Chlamydial etiology of acute lower respiratory tract infections in children in the Sudan. Acta Paediatr 83: 169

Hers JFP, Mulder J (1961) Broad aspects of the pathology and pathogenesis of human influenza. Am Rev Respir Dis 83: 84

Herxheimer G (1901) Ueber einen Fall von echter Nebenlunge. Zentralbl Allg Pathol 12: 529

Hewitt CJ, Hull D, Keeling JW (1977) Fibrosing alveolitis in infants and childhood. Arch Dis Child 52: 22

Heydanus R, Stewart PA, Wladimiroff JW, Los F (1993) Prenatal diagnosis of congenital cystic adenomatoid lung malformation: a report of seven cases. Prenat Diagn 13: 65

Hicks JL, Nelson JF (1973) Juvenile nasopharyngeal angiofibroma. Oral Surg 35: 807

Hidalgo HA, Helmke RJ, German VF, Mangos JA (1992) Pneumocystis carinii induces an oxidative burst in alveolar macrophages. Infect Immun 60: 1

Hill GS, Eggleston JC (1972) Electron microscopic study of so-called pulmonary sclerosing hemangioma. Cancer 30: 1092

Hirai KI, Witschi H, Coté MG (1985) Mitochondrial injury of pulmonary alveolar epithelial cells in acute paraquat intoxication. Exp Mol Pathol 43: 242

Hislop A, Reid L (1970) New pathological findings in emphysema of childhood. I. Polyalveolar lobe with emphysema. Thorax 25: 682

Hislop A, Reid L (1971) New pathological findings in emphysema of childhood. II. Overinflation of a normal lobe. Thorax 26: 190

Hislop A, Hey E, Reid L (1979) The lungs in congenital bilateral renal agenesis and dysplasia. Arch Dis Child 54: 32

Ho KL (1980) Primary meningioma of the nasal cavity and paranasal sinuses. Cancer 46: 1442

Ho K-L, Rassekh ZS (1980) Rhabdomyosarcoma of the trachea: first reported case. Hum Pathol 11: 572

Hoffer ME, Tom LWC, Wetmore RF, Handler SD, Potsic EP (1994) Congenital tracheal stenosis. The otolaryngologist's persepctive. Arch Otolaryngol Head Neck Surg 120: 449

Hoffman GS, Kerr GS, Leavitt RS, Hallahan CW, Lebovics RS, Travis WD et al. (1992) Wegener granulomatosis: an analysis of 158 patients. Ann Intern Med 116: 488

Hoggs JC, Irving WL, Porter H, Evans M, Dunnill MS, Fleming K (1989) In situ hybridization studies of adenoviral infections of the lung and their relationship to follicular bronchiectasis. Am Rev Respir Dis 139: 1531

Hohbach C, Mootz W (1978) Chemodectoma of the larynx. A clinicopathological study. Virchows Arch [Pathol Anat] 378: 161

Hoiby N, Koch C (1990) *Pseudomonoas aeruginos* infection in cystic fibrosis and its management. Thorax 45: 881

Holden MP Wooler GH (1970) Tracheo–oesophageal fistula and oesophageal atresia; results of 30 years' experience. Thorax 25: 406

Holdsworth Mayer CM, Favara BE, Holton CP, Rainer WG (1974) Malignant mesenchymoma in infants. Am J Dis Child 128: 847

Holinger LD, Tansek KM, Tucker GF (1985) Cleft laryx with airway obstruction. Ann Otol Rhinol Laryngol 94: 622

Holland HK, Wingard JR, Saral R (1990) Herpesvirus and enteric viral infections in bone marrow transplantation. Clinical presentations, pathogenesis, and therapeutic strategies. Cancer Invest 8: 509

Holmes B, Que PG, Windhurst DB, Good RA (1966) Fatal granulomatous disease of childhood – an inborn abnormality of phagocytic function. Lancet i: 1225

Holt PG (1993) Development of bronchus associated lymphoid tissue (BALT) in human lung disease: a normal host defence mechanism awaiting therapeutic exploitation? Thorax 48: 1097

Holt S, Deverall PB, Boddy JE (1978) A teratoma of the lung containing thymic tissue. J Pathol 126: 85

Horovitz AG, Khalail KG, Verani RR, Guthrie AM, Cowan DF (1983) Primary intratracheal neurilemoma. J Thorac Cardiovasc Surg 85: 313

Hoshaw JW, Walike TC (1971) Dermoid cysts of the nose. Arch Otolaryngol 93: 487

Huang L-M, Lee C-Y, Chang M-H, Wang J-D, Hsu C-Y (1993) Primary infection of Epstein–Barr virus, cytomegalovirus, and human herpesvirus-6. Arch Dis Child 68: 408

Husain AN, Hessel G (1993) Neonatal pulmonary hypoplasia: an autopsy study of 25 cases. Pediatr Pathol 13: 475

Hwang WS, Trevenen CL, McMillan DD, Garvey P (1988) The histopathology of the upper airway in the neonate following mechanical ventilation. J Pathol 156: 189

Hyde SR, Giacoia GP (1993) Congenital herpes infection: placental and umbilical cord findings. Obstet Gynecol 81: 852

Ishida T, Yano T, Sugimachi K (1990) Clinical applications of the pathological properties of small cell carcinoma, large cell carcinoma and adenoid cystic carcinoma of the lung. Semin Surg Oncol 6: 53

Ishii Y, Yamanaka N, Ogawa K, Yoshida Y, Takami T, Matsuura A, Isago H, Kataura A, Kikuchi K (1982) Nasal T-cell lymphoma as a type of so-called "lethal midline granuloma". Cancer 50: 2336

Itoh K, Aihara H, Takada S, Nishino M, Lee Y, Negishi H et al. (1990) Clinicopathological differences between early-onset and late-onset sepsis and pneumonia in very low birth weight infants. Pediatr Pathol 10: 757

Iwa T, Watanabe Y (1979) Unusual combination of pulmonary sequestration and funnel chest. Chest 76: 314

Jaarsma AS, Tamminga RYJ, de Langen ZJ, van der Laan T, Nikkels PGJ, Kimpen JLL (1994) Neonatal teratoma presenting as hygroma colli. Eur J Pediatr 153: 276

Jacobson JD, Troug WE, Benjamin DR (1993) Increased expression of human leukocyte antigen-DR on pulmonary macrophages in bronchopulmonary dysplasia. Pediatr Res 34: 341

Jafek BW, Stern FA (1973) Neurofibroma of the larynx occurring with venereal disease: report of a case. Arch Otolaryngol 98: 77

Jaffé BF (1973a) Pediatric head and neck tumors: a study of 178 cases. Laryngoscope 83: 1644

Jaffé BF (1973b) Unusual laryngeal problems in children. Ann Otol 82: 637

Jamjoom GA, al-Semrani AM, Board A, al-Frayh AR, Artz F, al-Mobaireek KF (1993) Respiratory syncytial virus infection in young children hospitalized with respiratory illness in Riyadh. J Trop Pediatr 39: 346

Janson C, Björnsson E, Hetta J, Boman G (1994) Anxiety and depression in relation to respiratory symptoms and asthma. Am J Respir Crit Care Med 149: 930

Jaubert de Beaujeu M, Mollard P, Campo-Paysan A (1970) Aspects particuliers des séquestrations pulmonaires. Chir Thorac Cardiovasc 9: 515

Jaubert de Beaujeum M, Chavrier Y, Korkmaz G (1973) Séquestrations pulmonaires chez l'enfant. Réflexions à propos de 10 observations. Ann Chir Infant 14: 341

Jederlinic PJ, Sicilian L, Gaensler EA (1988) Chronic eosinophilic pneumonia. A report of 19 cases and a review of the literature. Medecine 67: 154

Jederling PJ Sicilian LS, Baigelman W, Gaensler EA (1986) Congenital bronchial atresia. A report of 4 cases and a review of the literature. Medicine 65: 73

Jeffery PK (1991) Morphology of the airway wall in asthma and in chronic obstructive pulmonary disease. Am Rev Respir Dis 140: 1745

Jeffrey PK, Wardlaw AJ, Nelson FC , Collins JV, Kay AB (1989) Bronchial biopsies in asthma. An ultrastructural, quantitative study and correlation with hyperreactivity. Am Rev Respir Dis 140: 1745

Jennings TA, Sabetta J, Duray PH, Enzinger FM, Collins S (1984) Infantile myofibromatosis. Evidence for an autosomal-dominant disorder. Am J Surg Pathol 8: 529

Jessee WF, Ryan JM, Fitzgerald JF, Grosfeld JL (1975) Amebic abscess in childhood. Clin Pediatr 14: 134

Jimenez JF, Uthman EO, Townsend JW, Gloster ES, Seibert JJ (1986) Primary bronchopulmonary leiomyosarcoma in childhood. Arch Pathol Lab Med 110: 348

Jobe AH, Mitchell BR, Gunkel JH (1993) Beneficial effects of the combined use of prenatal corticosteroids and postnatal surfactant on preterm infants. Am J Obstet Gynecol 168: 508

Jochelson M, Tarbell NJ, Freedman AS, Rabinowe SN, Takvorian T, Soiffer R et al. (1990) Acute and chronic pulmonary complications following autologous bone marrow transplantation in non-Hodgkin's lymphoma. Bone Marrow Transplant 6: 329

Johanson A, Blizzard R (1971) A syndrome of congenital aplasia of the alae nasi, deafness, hypothyroidism, dwarfism, absent permanent teeth and malabsorption. J Pediatr 79: 982

Johnston RB Jr (1991) Pathogenesis of pneumococcal pneumonia. Rev Infect Dis 13: S509

Jones DG, Gabriel CE (1969) The incidence of carcinoma of the larynx in persons under twenty years of age. Laryngoscope 70: 251

Jones MJ, Kolb M, Votava H, Johnson RL, Smith TF (1980) Intrauterine echovirus type II infection. Mayo Clin Proc 55: 509

Jones GC, De Santo LW, Bremer JW, Neel HB (1986) Juvenile angiofibromas. Behavior and treatment of extensive and residual tumors. Arch Otolaryngol 112: 1191

Joshi VV, Escobar MR, Stewart L, Bates RD (1973) Fatal influenza A2 viral pneumonia in a newborn infant. Am J Dis Child 126: 839

Joyce-Brady MF, Brody JS (1990) Ontogeny of pulmonary alveolar epithelial markers of differentiation. Dev Biol 137: 331

Kahn T, Schwarz E, Zur Hausen H (1986) Moleclar cloning and chacterization of the DNA of a new human papillomavirus (HPV 30) from a laryngeal carcinoma. Int J Cancer 37: 61

Kanbour AI, Barmada MA, Klionsky B, Moossy J (1979) Anencephaly and heterotopic central nervous tissue in lungs. Arch Pathol Lab Med 103: 116

Kanto WP Jr (1994) A decade of experience with neonatal extracoporeal membrane oxygenation. J Pediatr 124: 335

Kaplan SL, Gnepp DR, Katzenstein ALA, Feigin RD (1978) Miliary pulmonary nodules due to aspirated vegetable particles. J Pediatr 92: 448

Kari MA, Hallman M, Eronen M, Teramo K, Virtanen M, Koivisto M et al. (1994) Prenatal dexamethasone treatment in conjunction with rescue therapy of human surfactant: a randomized placebo-controlled multicenter study. Pediatrics 93: 730

Karlinsky JB, Mark EJ (1993) Casse records of the Massachusetts General Hospital. Case 23-1993. N Engl J Med 328: 1696

Karmazin N, Panitch HB, Balsara RK, Faerber EN, de Chadarevian J-P (1989) De novo circumscribed pulmonary lobar cystic lymphatic anomaly in a young boy. A possible sequel of bronchopulmonary dysplasia. Chest 95: 1162

Katzenstein A-LA (1985) Pathogenesis of "fibrosis" in interstitial pneumonia: an electron microscopic study. Hum Pathol 1015: 1024

Katzenstein A-LA, Gordon LP, Oliphant M, Swender PT (1995) Chronic pneumonitis of infancy. A unique form of interstitial lung disease occurring in early childhood. Am J Surg Pathol 19: 439

Kaul A, Scott R, Gallagher M, Scott M, Clement J, Ogra PL (1978) Respiratory syncytial virus infection – rapid diagnosis in children by use of indirect immunofluorescence. Am J Dis Child 132: 1088

Kayser K, Gabius HJ, Hagemeyer O (1993) Malignant teratoma of the lung with lymph node metastasis of the ectoderm compartment: a case report. Anal Cell Pathol 5: 31

Kazanjians PH, Mark EJ (1990) Case records of the Massachusetts General Hospital. Case 48-1990. N Engl J Med 323: 1546

Kelly JH, Joseph M, Carrol E, Goodman ML, Pilch BZ, Levinson RM, Strome M (1980) Inverted papilloma of the nasal septum. Arch Otolaryngol 106: 767

Kelso JM, Kerr DJ, Lie JT, Sachs MI, O'Connell EJ (1991) Unusual diffuse pulmonary lymphatic proliferation in a young boy. Chest 100: 556

Kenny JD, Adams JM, Corbet AJS, Rudolph AJ (1976) The role of acidosis at birth in the development of hyaline membrane disease. Pediatrics 58: 184

Keszler M, Donn SM, Bucciarelli RL, Alverson DC, Hart M, Lunyong V et al. (1991) Multicenter controlled trial comparing high frequency jet ventilation and conventional mechanical ventilation in newborn infants with pulmonary interstitial emphysema. J Pediatr: 85–93

Khan AS, Ksiazek TG, Zaki SR, Nichol ST, Rollin PE, Peters CJ et al. (1995) Fatal hantavirus pulmonary syndrome in an adolescent. Pediatrics 95: 276

Khong TY, Keeling JW (1990) Massive congenital mesenchymal malformation of the lung: another case of non-immune hydrops. Histopathology 16: 609

Khong TY, Frappell JM, Steel HM, Stewart CM, Burke M (1986) Perinatal listeriosis. A report of six cases. Br J Obstet Gynaecol 93: 1083

Khorsand J, Tennant R, Gillies C, Phillipps AF (1985) Congenital alveolar capillary dysplasia: a developmental vascular anomaly causing persistent pulmonary hypertension of the newborn. Pediatr Pathol 3: 299

Kim KH, Suh JS, Han WS (1993) Leiomyoma of the bronchus treated by endoscopic resection. Ann Thorac Surg 56: 1164

Kimura H, Futamura M, Kito H, Ando T, Goto M, Kuzushima K et al. (1991) Detection of viral DNA in neonatal herpes simplex virus infections: frequent and prolonged presence in serum and cerebrospinal fluid. J Infect Dis 164: 289

Kinane BT, Mansell AL, Zwerdling RG, Lapey A, Shannon DC (1993) Folliculara bronchitis in the pediatric population. Chest 104: 1183

King TE Jr, Christopher KL, Schwarz MI (1982) Multiple pulmonary chondromatous hamartomas. Hum Pathol 13: 496

Kino T, Kohara Y, Tsuji S (1972) Pulmonary alveolar microlithiasis. A report of two young sisters. Am Rev Respir Dis 105: 105

Kitamura S, Maeda M, Kawashima Y, Masaoka A, Manabe Y (1969) Leiomyoma of the intrathoracic trachea – report of a case successfully treated by primary end-to-end anastomosis following circumferential resection of the trachea. J Thorac Cardiovasc Surg 57: 126

Kjellman B, Elinder G, Garwicz S, Svan H (1984) Idiopathic pulmonary haemosiderosis in Swedish children. Acta Paediatr Scand 73: 584

Klapholz A, Salomon N, Perlman DC, Talavera W (1991) Aspergillosis in the acquired immunodeficiency syndrome. Chest 100: 1614

Klatt EC, Pavlova Z, Teberg AJ, Yonekura ML (1986a) Epidemic perinatal listeriosis at autopsy. Hum Pathol 17: 1278

Kleinclaus I, Floquet J, Chamapigneulle J, Perrin C, Simon C, Vignaud JM (1993) Les esthésioneuromes (esthésioneuroblastomes) oflactifs. Etude anatomopathologique à propos de 7 observations. Ann Pathol 13: 241

Klingebiel T, Pickert A, Dopfer R, Ranke MB, Siedner R (1989) Unusual course of a *Chlamydia* pneumonia in an infant with IgG2/IgG4-deficiency. Eur J Pediatr 148: 431

Knox EWF, Hooton VN, Barson AJ (1987) Pulmonary vascular cadidiasis and use of central venous catheters in neonates. J Clin Pathol 40: 559

Kobayashi T, Shido A, Nitta K, Inui S, Ganzuka M, Robertson B (1990) The critical concentration of surfactant in fetal lung liquid at birth. Resp Physiol 80: 181

Kobler E, Ammann RW (1977) Accessory lung arising from the upper esophagus. A rare congenital anomaly in the adult. Respiration 34: 236

Kondepudi A, Johnson A (1993) Cytokines increase neutral endopeptidase activity in lung fibroblasts. Am J Respir Cell Mol Biol 8: 43

Korppi M, Katila ML, Jööskelöainen J, Leinonen M (1992a) Role of *Moraxella (Branhamella) catarrhalis* as a respiratory pathogen in children. Acta Paediatr 81: 993

Korppi M, Katila ML, Jööskelöainen J, Leinonen M (1992b) Role of non-capsulated *Haemophilus influenzae* as a respiratory pathogen in children. Acta Paediatr 81: 989

Korvick JA, Yu VL (1987) Legionnaires' disease: an emerging surgical problem. Ann Thorac Surg 43: 341

Koss MN, Hochholzer L, O'Leary T (1991) Pulmonary blastomas. Cancer 67: 2368

Kovacs A, Frederick T, Church J, Eller A, Oxtoby M, Mascola L (1991) CD4 T-lymphocyte counts and *Pneumocystis carinii* pneumonia in pediatric HIV infection. JAMA 265: 1698

Kuan S-F, Persson A, Parghi D, Crouch E (1994) Lectin-mediated interactions of surfactant protein D with alveolar macrophages. Am J Respir Cell Mol Biol 10: 430

Kuhn JP, Lee SB (1973) Pneumatoceles associated with *Escherichia coli* pneumonias in the newborn. Pediatrics 51: 1008

Kulhanjian JA, Soroush V, Au DS, Brozan RN, Yasukawa L, Weylman LE et al. (1992) Identification of women at unsuspected risk of primary infection with Herpes simplex virus type 2 during pregnancy. N Engl J Med 326: 916

Kumagami H (1991) Testosterone and estradiol in juvenile angiofibroma tissue. Acta Otolaryngol 111: 569

Kung ITM, Loke SL, So SY, Lam WK, Mok CK, Aung Khin M (1985) Intrapulmonary thymoma: report of two cases. Gut 40: 471

Kuroki Y, Gasa S, Ogasawara Y, Makita A, Akino T (1992) Binding of pulmonary surfactant protein A to galactosylceramide and asialo-Gm2. Arch Biochem Biophys 299: 261

Kuroki Y, Mason RJ, Voelker DR (1988) Alveolar type II cells express a high-affinity receptor for pulmonary surfactant protein A. Proc Natl Acad Sci USA 85: 5566

Kuroki Y, Shiratori M, Ogasawara Y, Tsuzuki A, Akino T (1991) Characterization of pulmonary surfactant protein D: its copurification with lipids. Biochim Biophys Acta 1086: 185

Kurotaki H, Kamata Y, Kimura M, Nagai K (1993) Multiple papillary adenomas of type II pneumocytes found in a 13-year-old boy with von Recklinghausen's disease. Virchows Archiv A [Pathol Anat] 423: 319

Kurup VP, Kumar A (1991) Immunodiagnosis of aspergillosis. Clin Microbiol Rev 4: 439

Kuruvilla A, Wenig BM, Humphrey DM, Heffner DK (1990) Leiomyosarcoma of the sinonasal tract. Arch Otolaryngol Head Neck Surg 116: 1278

Kurzner SI, Garg M, Bautista DB, Bader D, Merritt RJ, Warburton D et al. (1988) Growth failure in infants with bronchopulmonary dysplasia: nutrition and elevated resting metabolic expenditure. Pediatrics 81: 379

Kuwano K, Bosken CH, Par PD, Bai TR, Wiggs BR, Hogg JC (1993) Small airways dimensions in asthma and in chronic obstructive pulmonary disease. Am Rev Respir Dis 148: 1220

Kwittken J, Reiner L (1962) Congenital cystic adenomatoid malformation of the lung. Pediatrics 30: 759

Kyllonen KEJ (1964) Intralobar pulmonary sequestration and theory as to its etiology. Acta Chir Scand 127: 307

La Salle AJ, Andrassy RJ, Steeg KV, Ratner I (1979) Congenital tracheoesophageal fistula without esophageal atresia. J Thorac Cardiovasc Surg 78: 583

Lagrange AM, Servais B, Wurtz A, Laffite JJ, Janin A, Ribet M et al. (1988) Liposarcome lipoblastique du poumon. Etude ultra-structurale d'un cas. Ann Pathol 8: 152

Laitinen L, Laitinen LA (1991) Cellular infiltrates in asthma and in chronic obstructive pulmonary disease. Am Rev Respir Dis 143: 1159

Landing BH (1957) Anomalies of the respiratory tract. Pediatr Clin North Am 4: 73

Landing BH, Dixon LG (1979) Congenital malformations and genetic disorders of the respiratory tract (larynx, trachea, bronchi, and lungs). Am Rev Respir Dis 120: 151

Landing BH, Shirkey HS (1957) A syndrome of recurrent infection and infiltration of viscera by pigmented lipid histiocytes. Pediatrics 20: 431

Landing BH, Wells TR (1973) Tracheobronchial anomalies in children. In: Rosenberg HS, Boland RP (eds) Perspectives in pediatric pathology. Year-Book Medical Publishers, Chicago, p 1

Landry ML, Fong CKY, Nedderman K, Solomon L, Hsiung GD (1987) Disseminated adenovirus infection in an immunocompromised host. Am J Med 83: 555

Langston C (1991) Case 2. Misalignment of pulmonary veins and alveolar capillary dysplasia. Pediatr Pathol 11: 163

Laraya-Cuasay LR, Deforest A, Palmer J, Huff DS, Lischner HW, Huang NN (1974) Chronic pulmonary complications of early influenza virus infection. Am Rev Respir Dis 109: 703

Lauweryns JM (1969) The body lymphatics in neonatal hyaline membrane disease. Pediatrics 44: 126

Lauweryns JM (1970) "Hyaline membrane disease" in newborn infants. Macroscopic, radiographic and light and electron microscopic studies. Hum Pathol 1: 175

Lauweryns J, Deleersnyder M, Boussauw L (1971) A morphometrical study of the aeration of the pulmonary parenchyma in neonatal hyaline membrane diseases. Beitr Pathol 144: 344

Lawson RM, Ramanathan L, Hurley G, Hinson KW, Lennox SC (1976) Bronchial adenoma: review of an 18-year experience at the Brompton Hospital. Thorax 31: 245

Lebecque P, Lapierre JG, Brochu P, Spier S, Lamarre A (1987) Pulmonary plasma cell granuloma. Eur J Pediatr 146: 174

Lebrun D, Avni EF, Goolaerts JP, Rocmans P, Tondeur M, Ardichvili D (1985) Prenatal diagnosis of a pulmonary cyst by ultrasonography. Eur J Pediatr 144: 399

Lee DA, Rao BR, Meyer JS, Prioleau PG, Bauer WC (1980) Hormonal receptor determination in juvenile nasopharyngeal angiofibromas. Cancer 46: 547

Leighton SEJ, Gallimore AP (1994) Extranodal sinus histiocytosis with massive lymphadenopathy affecting the subglottis and trachea. Histopathology 24: 393

Leong KH, Boey ML, Feng PH (1991) Coexisting *Pneumocystis carinii* pneumonia, cytomegalovirus pneumonitis and salmonellosis in systemic lupus erythematosus. Ann Rheum Dis 50: 811

Levene MI, Wigglesworth JS, Desai R (1980) Pulmonary fat accumulation after intralipid infusion in the preterm infant. Lancet ii: 815

Levine PA, McLean WC, Cantrell RW (1986) Esthesioneuroblastoma: the University of Virginia experience 1960–1985. Laryngoscope 96: 742

Leviton A, Gilles F, Strassfeld R (1977) The influence of route of delivery and hyaline membranes on the risk of neonatal intracranial haemorrhages. Ann Neurol 2: 451

Leviton A, Kuban KC, Pagano M, Allred EN, Van Marter L (1993) Antenatal corticosteroids appear to reduce the risk of postnatal germinal matrix hemorrhage in intubated low birth weight newborns. Pediatrics 91: 1083

Li EP (1977) Second malignant tumours after cancer in childhood. Cancer 40: 1899

Lieberman J (1969) Pulmonary plasminogen-activator activity in hyaline membrane disease. Pediatr Res 3: 11

Liebner EJ (1976) Embryonal rhabdomyosarcoma of head and neck in children: correlation of stage, radiation dose, local control and survival. Cancer 37: 2777

Liebow AA, Hubbell DS (1956) Sclerosing hemangioma (histiocytoma, xanthoma of the lung). Cancer 9: 53

Liebow AA, Carrington CRB, Friedman PJ (1972) Lymphomatoid granulomatosis. Hum Pathol 3: 457

Lilien LD, Yeh TF, Novak GM, Jacobs NM (1978) Early onset *Haemophilus* sepsis in newborn infants: clinical roentgenographic and pathologic features. Pediatrics 62: 299

Limper AH, Offord KP, Smith TF, Martin WJ II (1989) *Pneumocystic carinii* pneumonia. Differences in lung parasite number and inflammation in patients with and without AIDS. Am Rev Respir Dis 140: 1204

Lin-Chu M, Lee Y-J, Ho MY (1989) Malignant mesothelioma in infancy. Arch Pathol Lab Med 113: 409

Lincoln JCR, Stark, J, Subramanian S, Aberdeen E, Bonham-Carter RE, Berry CL, Waterston DJ (1971) Congenital lobar emphysema. Ann Surg 173: 55

Lindsay ML Jr, Hermann EC Jr, Morrow GW Jr, Brown AL Jr (1970) Hong Kong influenza. Clinical, microbiologic and pathologic features in 127 cases. JAMA 214: 1825

Lipscomb MF, Lyons CR, Nunez G, Ball EJ, Stastny P, Vial W, Lem V, Weissler J, Miller LM, Toews GB (1986) Human alveolar macrophages: HLA-DR-positive macrophages that are poor stimulators of a primary mixed leukocyte reaction. J Immunol 136: 497

Liston SL, Gehz RC, Siegel LG, Tilelli J (1983) Bacterial tracheitis. Am J Dis Child 137: 764

Lloreta J, Mackay B, Troncoso P, Ribalta–Farres T, Smith T, Khorana S (1992) Neuroendocrine tumours of the nasal cavity: an ultrastructural and morphometric study of 24 cases. Ultrastruct Pathol 16: 165

Loire R, Tabib A, Bastien O (1993) Complications aspergillaires mortelles après transplantation cardiaque. Ann Pathol 13: 157

Loyd JE, Tillman BF, Atkinson JB, Des Prez RM (1988) Mediastinal fibrosis complicating histoplasmosis. Medecine 67: 295

Lundemose AG, Lundemose JB, Birkelund S, Christiansen G (1989) Detection of *Chlamydia* in postmortal formalin-fixed tissue. APMIS 97: 68

Lutsky I, Livni N, Mor N (1986) Retrospective confirmation of mycoplasma infection by the immunoperoxidase technique. Pathology 18: 390

MacGregor FB, Geddes NK (1993) Nasal dermoids: the significance of a midline punctum. Arch Dis Child 68: 418

Machin GA (1975) A perinatal mortality survey in south-east London, 1970–73: the pathological findings in 762 necropsies. J Clin Pathol 28: 428

Madan E, Meyer MP, Amortegui AJ (1988) Isolation of genital mycoplasms and *Chlamydia trachomatis* in stillborn and neonatal autopsy material. Arch Pathol Lab Med 112: 749

Maeda A, Sata T, Sato Y, Kurata T (1994) A comparative study of congenital and postnatally acquired human cytomegalovirus infection in infants: lack of expression of viral immediate early protein in congenital cases. Virchows Arch 424: 121

Maesen FPV, Santana B, Lamers J, van den Bnekel B (1983) A supernumerary bronchus of the right upper lobe. Eur J Respir Dis 64: 473

Maesen FPV, Geraedts WH, Goei R (1993) Agenesis of the right upper lobe. Chest 103: 1612

Maeta T, Fujiwara Y, Ohizumi T, Kato E, Kakizaki G, Ishidate T, Fujiwara T (1977) Pathological study of tracheal and pulmonary lesions in autopsy cases of congenital esophageal atresia. Tohoku J Exp Med 123: 23

Mahut B, Delacourt C, de Blic J, Mani TM, Schleinmann P (1993) Bronchiectasis in a child after acrolein inhalation. Chest 104: 1286

Maisel RH, Ogura JH (1974) Neurofibromatosis with laryngeal involvement. Laryngoscope 84: 132

Malm G, Berg U, Forsgren M (1995) Neonatal herpes simplex: clinical findings and outcome in relation to type of maternal infection. Acta Paediatr 84: 256

Malm G, Forsgren M, el Azazi M, Persson A (1991) A follow-up study of children with neonatal herpes simplex virus infections with particular regard to late nervous disturbances. Acta Paediatr Scand 80: 226

Manivel JC, Priest JR, Watterson J, Steiner M, Woods WG, Wick MR et al. (1988) Pleuropulmonary blastoma. The so-called pulmonary blastoma of childhood. Cancer 62: 1516

Marchau FE, van Roy BC, Parizel PM, Lambert JR, de Canck I, Leroy JG et al. (1993) Tricho–rhino–phalangeal syndrome type I (TRP I) due to an apparently balanced translocation involving 8q24. Am J Med Genet 45: 450

Mardini MK, Nyhan WL (1985) Agenesis of the lung. Report of four patients with unusual anomalies. Chest 87: 522

Margraf LR, Paciga JE, Balis JU (1990) Surfactant-associated glycoproteins accumulate in alveolar cells and secretions during reparative stage of hyaline membrane disease. Hum Pathol 21: 392

Margraf LR, Tomashefski JF Jr, Bruce MC, Dahms BB (1991) Morphometric analysis of the lung in bronchopulmonary dysplasia. Am Rev Respir Dis 143: 391

Marinopoulos GC, Huddle KRL, Wainwright H (1991) Obliterative bronchiolitis: virus induced? Chest 99: 243

Mark PH, Turner JAP (1968) Lung abscess in childhood. Thorax 23: 216

Mark EJ, Matsubara O, Tan-Liu NS, Fienberg R (1988) The pulmonary biopsy in the early diagnosis of Wegener's (pathergic) granulomatosis: a study based on 35 open lung biopsies. Hum Pathol 19: 1065

Mark Y, Rogers BB, Oyer CE (1993) Diagnosis and incidence of fetal parvovirus infection in an autopsy series: II. DNA amplification. Pediatr Pathol 13: 381

Marrie TJ (1993) *Chlamydia pneumoniae*. Thorax 48: 1

Martensson G, Larsson S, Zettergren L (1984) Malignant mesothelioma in two pairs of siblings: is there a hereditary predisposing factor? Eur J Respir Dis 65: 179

Martin WJ (1993) Pathogenesis of *Pneumocystis carinii* pneumonia. Am J Respir Cell Mol Biol 8: 356

Martin WJ, Howard DM (1986) Paraquat-induced neutrophil alveolitis: reduction of the inflammatory response by pretreatment with endotoxin and hyperoxia. Lung 164: 107

Martin JJ, Philippart M, Van Hauwaert J, Callahan JW, Deberdt R (1972) Niemann–Pick disease (Crocker's group A) – late-onset and pigmentary degeneration resembling Hallervorden–Spatz syndrome: Arch Neurol 27: 45

Martin JR, Holt RK, Langston C, Gilden DH, Richardson EP Jr, Manz HJ et al. (1991) Type-specific identification of herpes simplex and varicella–zoster virus antigen in autopsy tissues. Hum Pathol 22: 75

Mascie-Taylor BH, Wardman AG, Madden CA, Page RL (1985) A case of alveolar microlithiasis: observation over 22 years and recovery of material by lavage. Thorax 40: 952

Massaro D, Kayz S, Matthews MJ, Higgins G (1965) Von Recklinghausen's neurofibromatosis associated with cystic lung disease. Am J Med 38: 233

Massimo M, Gasparini M, Ballerini E, Del-Bo R (1995) Primary thyroid carcinoma in children: a retrospective study of 20 patients. Med Pediatr Oncol 24: 13

Massumi RA, Legier JF (1966) Rheumatic pneumonitis. Circulation 33: 417

Matsumoto A, Bessho H, Uehira K, Suda T (1991) Morphological studies of the association of mitochondria with chlamydial inclusions and the fusion of chlamydial inclusions. J Electron Microsc 40: 356

Matters GL, Scandalios JG (1986) Effect of the free radical-generating herbicide paraquat on the expression of the superoxide dismutase (Sod) genes in maize. Biochim Biophys Acta 882: 29

Matthews TJ, Hornall D, Sheppard MN (1993) Comparison of the use of antibodies to "a" smooth muscle actin and desmin in pulmonary lymphangioleiomyomatosis. J Clin Pathol 46: 479

Mayer GJ (1979) Pulmonary paragonimiasis. J Pediatr 95: 75

McAdams AJ, Coen R, Kleinman LI, Tsang R, Sutherland J (1973) The experimental production of hyaline membranes in premature Rhesus monkeys. Am J Pathol 70: 277

McBride DE, Koenig JQ, Luchtel DL, Williams PV, Henderson WR Jr (1994) Inflammatory effects of ozone in the upper airways of subjects with asthma. Am J Respir Crit Care Med 149: 1192

McDonnell T, Kyriakos M, Roper C, Mazoujian G (1988) Malignant fibrous histiocytoma of the lung. Cancer 61: 137

McGinnis M, Jacobs G, El-Naggar A, Redline RW (1993) Congenital peribronchial myofibroblastic tumour (so-called "congenital leiomyosarcoma"). A distinct neonatal lung lesion associated with nonimmune hydrops fetalis. Mod Pathol 6: 487

McLauchlin J (1990a) Distribution of serovars of Listeria monocytogenes isolated from different categories of patients with listeriosis. Eur J Clin Microbiol Infect Dis 9: 210

McLauchlin J (1990b) Human listeriosis in Britain, 1967–85. A summary of 722 cases. 2. Listeriosis in non-pregnant individuals, a changing pattern of infection and seasonal incidence. Epidemiol Infect 104: 191

McLelland J, Broadbent V, Yeomans E, Malone M, Pritchard J (1990) Langerhans' cell histiocytosis: the case for conservative treatment. Arch Dis Child 65: 301

Meacham LR, Winn KJ, Culler FL, Parks JS (1991) Double vagina, cardiac, pulmonary, and other genital malformations with 46,XY karyotype (see comments). Am J Med Genet 41: 478

Mendoza A, Voland J, Wolf P, Benirschke K (1986a) Supradiaphragmatic liver in the lung. Arch Pathol Lab Med 110: 1085

Mendoza A, Wolf P, Edwards DK, Leopold GR, Voland JR, Benirschke K (1986b) Prenatal ultrasonographic diagnosis of congenital adenomatoid malformation of the lung. Arch Pathol Lab Med 110: 402

Merlier M, Rochainzanir, Rojas-Miranda A, Levasseur P, Sulzer JD, Verley JM, Langlois J, Binet JP, LeBrigand H (1970) Les aspects anatomo-cliniques des séquestrations pulmonaires. A propos de 46 observations. Ann Chir Thorac Cardiovasc 9: 511

Messina MS, O'Riordan TG, Smaldone GC (1991) Changes in mucociliary clearance during acute exacerbations of asthma. Am Rev Respir Dis 143: 993

Meyers WM, Neafie RC, Connor DH (1977) Onchocerciasis: invasion of deep organs by Onchocerca volvulus. Autopsy findings. Am J Trop Med Hyg 26: 650

Micheau C (1986) What is new in histological classification and recognition of naso-pharyngeal carcinoma (NPC). Pathol Res Pract 181: 249

Micheau C, Luboinski B, Sancho H, Cachin Y (1975) Modes of invasion of cancer of the larynx. A statistical, histological and radioclinical analysis of 120 cases. Cancer 38: 346

Michels VV, Driscoll DJ, Ferry GD, Duff DF, Beaudet AL (1979) Pulmonary vascular obstruction associated with cholesteryl ester storage disease. J Paediatr 94: 621

Midulla F, Villani A, Panuska JR, Dab I, Kolls JK, Merolla R et al. (1993) Respiratory syncytial virus lung infection in infants: immunoregulatory role of infected alveolar macrophages. J Infect Dis 168: 1515

Miettinen M, Lehto VP, Virtanen I (1982) Nasopharyngeal lymphoepithelioma. Histological diagnosis as aided by immunohistochemical demonstration of keratin. Virchows Arch [B] 40: 163

Mihatsch MJ, Ohnacker H, Just M, Nars PW (1972) Lethal measles giant cell pneumonia after live measles vaccination – a case of thymic alymphoplasia Gitlin. Helv Paediatr Acta 27: 143

Millard PR, Heryet AR (1988) Observations favouring Pneumocystis carinii pneumonia as a primary infection: a monoclonal antibody study on paraffin sections. J Pathol 154: 365

Miller RP, Myer CM III, Gray SD, Cotton RT (1989) Imaging case study of the month. Posterior subglottic cyst. Ann Otol Rhinol Laryngol 98: 411

Miller RR (1990) Bronchioloalveolar cell adenomas. Am J Surg Pathol 14: 904

Miller FC, Sacks DA, Yeh SY, Paul RH, Schifrin BS, Martin CB Jr, Hon EH (1975) Significance of meconium during labor. Am J Obstet Gynecol 122: 573

Miller RW, Salcedo JR, Fink RJ, Murphy TM, Magilavy DB (1986) Pulmonary hemorrhage in pediatric patients with systemic lupus erythematosus. J Pediatr 108: 576

Miller WT Jr, Sais GJ, Frank I, Gefter WB, Aronchick JM, Miller WT (1994) Pulmonary aspergillosis in patients with AIDS. Clinical and radiographic correlations. Chest 105: 37

Mills J, Masur H (1990) AIDS-related infections. Sc Am 262: 50

Mistchenko AS, Lenzi HL, Thompson FM, Mota EM, Vidaurreta S, Navari C et al. (1992) Participation of immune complexes in adenovirus infection. Acta Paediatr 81: 983

Miyamura K, Malhotra R, Hoppe H-J, Reid KBM, Phizackerley PJR, Macpherson P et al. (1994) Surfactant proteins A (SP-A) and D (SP-D): levels in human amniotic fluid and localization in the fetal membranes. Biochim Biophys Acta 1210: 303

Moch H, Oberholzer M, Christen H, Buser M, Dalquen P, Wegmann W et al. (1993a) Diagnostic tools for differentiating pleural mesothelioma from lung adenocarcinoma in paraffin embedded tissue. II. Design of an expert system and its application to the diagnosis of mesothelioma. Virchows Archiv A [Pathol Anat] 423: 493

Moch H, Oberholzer M, Dalquen P, Wegmann W, Gudat F (1993b) Diagnostic tools for differentiating between pleural mesothelioma and lung adenocarcinoma in paraffin embedded tissue. Part I: Immunohistochemical findings. Virchows Archiv A [Pathol Anat] 423: 19

Moler FW, Palmisano JM, Green TP, Custer JR (1993) Predictors of outcome of severe respiratory syncytial virus-associated respiratory failure treated with extracorporeal membrane oxygenation. J Pediatr 123: 46

Monday LA, Cornut G, Bouchayer M, Roch JB (1983) Epidermoid cysts of the vocal cords. Ann Otol Rhinol Laryngol 92: 124

Montefort S, Lai CKW, Kapahi P, Leung J, Lai KN, Chan HS et al. (1994) Circulating adhesion molecules in asthma. Am J Respir Crit Care Med 149: 1149

Moore TC, Cobo JC (1985) Massive symptomatic cystic hygroma confined to the thorax in early childhood. J Thorac Cardiovasc Surg 89: 459

Moorthy AV, Chesney RW, Segar WE, Groshong T (1977) Wegener granulomatosis in childhood: prolonged survival following cytotoxic therapy. J Pediatr 91: 616

Moran TJ (1955) Experimental aspiration. IV. Inflammatory and reparative changes produced by introduction of autologous gastric juice and hydrochloric acid. Arch Pathol 60: 122

Morgan D, Bailey M, Phelps P, Bellman S, Grace A, Wyse R (1993) Ear–nose–throat abnormalities in the CHARGE association. Arch Otolaryngol Head Neck Surg 119: 49

Morgenstern B, Klionsky B, Doshi N (1981) Yellow hyaline membrane disease. Identification of the pigment and bilirubin binding. Lab Invest 44: 514

Morimitsu T, Matsumoto I, Okada S, Takahashi M, Kosugi T (1981) Congenital cricoid stenosis. Laryngoscope 91: 1356

Morisot C, Kacet N, Bouchez MC, Rouland V, Dubos JP, Gremillet C et al. (1990) Risk factors for fatal pulmonary interstitial emphysema in neonates. Eur J Pediatr 149: 493

Mortola JP (1987) Dynamics of breathing in newborn mammals. Physiol Rev 67: 187

Moskaluk CA, Pogrebniak HW, Pass HI, Gallin JI, Travis WD (1994) Surgical pathology of the lung in chronic granulomatous disease. Am J Clin Pathol 102: 684

Motomatsu K, Adachi H, Uno T (1979) Two infant deaths after inhaling baby powder. Chest 75: 448

Moyland FMB, Shannon DC (1979) Preferential distribution of lobar emphysema and atelectasis in bronchopulmonary dysplasia. Pediatrics 63: 130

Mroueh S, Spock A (1994) Allergic bronchopulmonary aspergillosis in patients with cystic fibrosis. Chest 105: 32

Muder RR, Yu VL, Woo AH (1986) Mode of transmission of *Legionella pneumophila*. A critical review. Arch Intern Med 146: 1607

Muldoon RL, Jaecker DL, Kiefer HK (1981) Legionnaires' disease in children. Pediatrics 67: 329

Müller H (1918) Uber Lappungsanomalien der Lungen, insbesondere über einen Fall von trachealer Nebenlunge. Virchows Arch 225: 284

Murata Y, Kuroki Y, Akino T (1993) Role of the C-terminal domain of pulmonary surfactant protein A in binding to alveolar type II cells and regulation of phospholipid secretion. Biochem J 291: 71

Murayama J-I, Yoshizawa Y, Ohtsuka M, Hasegawa S (1993) Lung fibrosis in hypersensitivity pneumonitis. Association with CD4+ but not CD8+ cell dominant alveolitis and insidious onset. Chest 104: 38

Murguia de Sierra T, Kumar ML, Wasser TE, Murphy BR, Subbarao EK (1993) Respiratory syncytial virus-specific immunoglobulins in preterm infants. J Pediatr 122: 787

Murray JF, Mills J (1990) Pulmonary infectious complications of human immunodeficiency virus infection. Part I. Am Rev Respir Dis 141: 1356

Murry CE, Schmidt RA (1992) Tissue invasion by *Pneumocystis carinii*: a possible cause of cavitary pneumonia and pneumothorax. Hum Pathol 23: 1380

Muthuswamy PP, Alrenga DP, Marks P, Barker WL (1986) Granular cell myoblastoma: rare localization in the trachea. Report of a case and review of the literature. Am J Med 80: 714

Myers JL, Katzenstein A-LA (1986) Microangiitis in lupus-induced pulmonary hemorrhage. Am J Clin Pathol 85: 552

Nagata N, Dairaku M, Sueishi K, Tanaka K (1987) Sclerosing hemangioma of the lung. Am J Clin Pathol 88: 552

Nakamura Y, Fukuda S, Hashimoto T (1990) Pulmonary elastic fibers in normal human development and pathological conditions. Pediatr Pathol 10: 689

Nakamura Y, Saitoh Y, Yamamoto I, Fukuda S, Hashimoto T (1988) Regenerative process of hyaline membrane disease. Electron microscopic, immunohistochemical, and biochemical study. Arch Pathol Lab Med 112: 821

Nasser WY, Keogh PF, Doshi R (1970) Myoblastoma of the larynx. J Laryngol 84: 751

Natale R, Nasello-Paterson C, Connors G (1988) Patterns of fetal breathing activity in the human fetus at 24 to 28 weeks of gestation. Am J Obstet Gynecol 158: 317

Nathrath WDJ, Remberger K (1986) Immunohistochemical study of granular cell tumours. Demonstration of neurone specific release S100 protein luminin and α_1-antichymetrypsin. Virchows Arch [A] 408: 421

Naughton M, Fahy J, FitzGerald MX (1993) Chronic eosinophilic pneumonia. A long-term follow-up of 12 patients. Chest 103: 162

Naylor JC, Wagner KR (1985) Neonatal sepsis due to *Streptococcus pneumoniae*. Can Med Assoc J 133: 1019

Neagos GR, Feyssa A, Peters-Golden M (1993) Phospholipase A2 in alveolar type II epithelial cells: biochemical and immunologic characterization. Am J Physiol 264: L261

Neijens HJ, Frenkel J, de Muinck Keizer–Schrama SMPF, Dzoijic-Danilovic G, Meradji M, van Dongen JJM (1989) Invasive aspergillus infection in chronic granulomatous disease: treatment with itraconazole. J Pediatr 115: 1016

Neilson DB (1958) Primary intrapulmonary neurogenic sarcoma. J Pathol 76: 419

Neldam S (1982a) Fetal respiratory movements: relationship to postnatal respiratory capacity. Am J Obstet Gynecol 142: 862

Neldam S (1982b) Fetal respiratory movements: a nomogram for fetal thoracic and abdominal respiratory movements. Am J Obstet Gynecol 142: 867

Nelson (1984) Gastroesophageal reflux and pulmonary disease. J Allergy Clin Immunol 73: 547

Nespoli L, Duse M, Vitiello MA, Perinotto G, Fiocca R, Giannetti A, Colombo A (1979) A rapid unfavorable outcome of Wegener's granulomatosis in early childhood. Eur J Pediatr 131: 277

Nezelof C, Meyer B, Dalloz JC, Joly P, Paupe J, Vialatte J (1970) La bronchiolite oblitérante: à propos de deux observations anatomocliniques infantiles. Ann Pediatr 17: 534

Nguyen K-L, Corbett ML, Garcia DP, Eberly SM, Massey EN, Le HT et al. (1993) Chronic sinusitis among pediatric patients with chronic respiratory complaints. J Allergy Clin Immunol 92: 824

Nicholls S, Yuille TD, Mitchell RG (1975) Perinated infections caused by *Haemophilus influenzae*. Arch Dis Child 50: 739

Nicolini V, Fisk NM, Rodeck CH, Talbert DG, Wigglesworth JS (1989) Low amniotic pressure in oligohydramnios. Is this the cause of pulmonary hypoplasia? Am J Obstet Gynecol 161: 1098

Nicoll JAR, Love S, Burton PA, Berry PJ (1994) Autopsy findings in two cases of neonatal herpes simplex virus infection: detection of virus by immunohistochemistry, in situ hybridization and the polymerase chain reaction. Histopathology 24: 257

Niedobitek G, Young LS (1994) Epstein–Barr virus persistence and virus-associated tumours. Lancet 343: 333

Nielson KA, Yunis EJ (1990) Demonstration of respiratory syncytial virus in an autopsy series. Pediatr Pathol 10: 491

Niitu Y, Kubota H, Hasegawa S, Horikawa M, Komatsu S, Suetake T, Fujimura S, Nagashima Y (1974) Lung cancer (squamous cell carcinoma) in adolescence. Am J Dis Child 127: 108

Nikolaizik WH, Warner JO (1994) Aetiology of chronic suppurative lung disease. Arch Dis Child 70: 141

Nilsson R, Grossmann G, Robertson B (1978) Lung surfactant and the pathogenesis of neonatal bronchiolar lesions induced by artificial ventilation. Pediatr Res 12: 249

Nishioka H, Furusho K, Yasunaga T, Tanaka K, Yamanouchi A, Yokota T et al. (1988) Congenital malignant mesothelioma. A case report and electron-microscopic study. Eur J Pediatr 147: 428

Noguchi M, Kodama T, Morinaga S, Shimosato Y, Saito T, Tsuboi E (1986) Multiple sclerosing hemangiomas of the lung. Am J Surg Pathol 10: 429

Northcutt AD, Tio FO, Chamblin SA Jr, Britton HA (1985) Massive metastatic pulmonary calcification in an infant with aleukemic monocytic leukemia. Pediatr Pathol 4: 219

Northway WH Jr (1990) Bronchopulmonary dysplasia: then and now. Arch Dis Child 85: 1076

Northway WH Jr, Moss RB, Carlisle KB, Parker BR, Popp RL, Pitlick PT et al. (1990) Late pulmonary sequelae of bronchopulmonary dysplasia. N Engl J Med 323: 1793

Nouri L, Al-Rahim K (1970) Kerosene poisoning in children. Postgrad Med J 46: 71

Novak RW (1981) Laryngotracheoesophageal cleft and unilateral pulmonary hypoplasia in twins. Pediatrics 67: 732

Nussbaum E, Maggi JC (1990) Laryngomalacia in children. Chest 98: 942

Oddo D, Etchart M, Thompson L (1990) *Histoplasmosis duboisii* (African histoplasmosis). An African case reported from Chile with ultrastructural study. Pathol Res Pract 186: 514

O'Halloran LR, Lusk RP (1994) Amyloidosis of the larynx in a child. Ann Otol Rhinol Laryngol 103: 590

Ohlms L, Jones DT, McGill TJI, Healy GB (1994) Interferon α_{2A} therapy for airway hemangiomas. Ann Otol Rhinol Laryngol 103: 1

Ohlms LA, McGill T, Healy GB (1994) Malignant largngeal tumors in children: a 15-year experience with four patients. Ann Otol Rhinol Laryngol 103: 686

Ohori NP, Yousem SA, Sonmez–Alpan E, Colby TV (1991) Estrogen and progesterone receptors in lymphangioleiomyomatosis, epithelioid hemangioendothelioma, and sclerosing hemangioma of the lung. Am J Clin Pathol 96: 529

Okeda R (1978) Heterotopic brain tissue in the submandibular region and lung. Report of two cases and comments about pathogenesis. Acta Neuropathol 43: 217

Oliver TK Jr, Smith B, Clatworthy HW Jr (1959) Staphylococcal pneumonia, pleural and pulmonary complications. Pediatr Clin North Am 6: 1043

Ollikainen J, Hiekkaniemi H, Korppi M, Sarkkinen H, Heinonen K (1993) *Ureaplasma urealyticum* infection associated with acute respiratory insufficiency and death in premature infants. J Pediatr 122: 756

Olmedo G, Rosenberg M, Fonseca R (1982) Primary tumours of the trachea. Clinicopathologic features and surgical results. Chest 81: 701

Olson JL, Mendelsohn G (1978) Congenital cystic adenomatoid malformation of the lung. Arch Pathol Lab Med 102: 248

Olson KD, Carpenter RJIII, Kern EB (1979) Nasal septal trauma in children. Pediatrics 64: 32

Onadeka BO, Beetlestone CA, Cooke AR, Abioye AA, Adetuyibi A, Sofowora EO (1977) Pulmonary alveolar microlithiasis. Postgrad Med J 53: 165

Oomen LCJM, Ten Have-Opbroek AAW, Hageman PC, Oudshoorn-Snoek M, Egberts J, van der Valk MA et al. (1990) Fetal mouse alveolar type II cells in culture express several type II cell characteristics found in vivo, together with major histocompatibility antigens. Am J Respir Cell Mol Biol 3: 325

Oppenheim EH, Rosenstein BJ (1979) Differential pathology of nasal polyps in cystic fibrosis and atopy. Lab Invest 40: 445

Orton HB (1947) Carcinoma of the larynx: clinical report of case – age $13\frac{1}{2}$ years. Laryngoscope 57: 299

Osamura RY (1977) Ultrastructure of localized fibrous mesothelioma of the pleura. Report of a case with histogenetic considerations. Cancer 39: 139

Otto-Verberne CJM, Ten Have-Opbroek AAW, De Vries ECP (1990) Expression of the major surfactant-associated protein, SP-A, in type II cells of human lung before 20 weeks of gestation. Eur J Cell Biol 53: 13

Pabst R (1992) Is BALT a major component of the human lung immune system? Immunol Today 13: 119

Page DV, Stocker JT (1982) Anomalies associated with pulmonary hypoplasia. Am Rev Respir Dis 125: 216

Pai SH, Cameron CTM, Lev R (1971) Accessory lung presenting as juxtagastric mass. Arch Pathol 91: 569

Papadopoulos T, Ionescu L, Dämmrich J, Toomes H, Müller-Hermelink HK (1990) Type I and type IV collagen promote adherence and spreading of human type II pneumocytes in vitro. Lab Invest 62: 562

Papageorgiou A, Bauer CR, Fletcher BD, Stern L (1973) *Klebsiella* pneumonia with pneumatocele formation in a newborn infant. Can Med Assoc J 109: 1217

Pappa A, Shenker N, Hack M, Redline RW (1994) Extensive intraalveolar pulmonary hemorrhage in infants dying after surfactant therapy. J Pediatr 124: 621

Pappin AL, Shenker N, Hack N, Redline R (1994) Differing patterns of pulmonary hemorrhage in infants dying after surfactant

therapy. J Pediatr 124: 621

Paradis IL, Grgurich WF, Dummer JS, Dekker A, Dauber JH (1988) Rapid detection of cytomegalovirus pneumonia from lung lavage cells. Am Rev Respir Dis 138: 697

Parto K, Svedström E, Majurin M-L, Hërkënen R, Simell O (1993) Pulmonary manifestations in lysinuric protein intolerance. Chest 194: 1176

Passwell J, Katz D, Frank Y, Spirer Z, Cohen BE, Ziprkowski M (1976) Fatal disseminated BCG infection. An investigation of the immuno-deficiency. Am J Dis Child 130: 433

Pastorino U, Gasparini M, Valente M, Tavecchio L, Azzarelli A, Mapelli S et al. (1992) Primary childhood osteosarcoma: the role of salvage surgery. Ann Oncol 3, Suppl 2: S43

Patten BM (1968) Human embryology, 3rd edn. McGraw-Hill New York, p 358

Patterson K, Kapur S, Chandra RS (1986) "Nasal gliomas" and related brain heterotopias: a pathologist's perspective. Pediatr Pathol 5: 353

Pattishall EN, Strope GL, Spinola SM, Denny FW (1986) Childhood sarcoidosis. J Pediatr 108: 169

Paulli M, Rosso R, Kindl S, Boveri E, Marocolo D, Chioda C et al. (1992) Immunophenotypic characterization of the cell infiltrate in five cases of sinus histiocytosis with massive lymphadenopathy (Rosal–Dorfman disease). Hum Pathol 23: 647

Perlman EJ, Dickman PS, Askin FB, Grier HE, Miser JS, Link MP (1994) Ewing's sarcoma – routine diagnostic utilization of MIC_2 analysis: a pediatric oncology group/children's cancer group intergroup study. Hum Pathol 25: 304

Perlman EJ, Moore GW, Hutchins GM (1989) The pulmonary vasculature in meconium aspiration. Hum Pathol 20: 701

Perlman JM, Volpe JJ (1989) Movement disorder of premature infants with severe bronchopulmonary dysplasia: a new syndrome. Pediatrics 84: 215

Perzin KH, Fu YS (1980) Non-epithelial tumors of the nasal cavity, paranasal sinuses and nasopharynx. A clinicopathologic study. XI. Fibrous histiocytomas. Cancer 45: 2616

Perzin KH, Lefkowitch JH, Hui RM (1981) Bilateral nasal squamous carcinoma arising in papillomatosis. Report of a case developing after chemotherapy for leukemia. Cancer 48: 2375

Pettersson T, Stenström R, Kyrönseppa H (1974) Disseminated lung opacities and cavitation associated with *Strongyloides stercoralis* and *Schistosoma mansoni* infection. Am J Trop Med Hyg 23: 158

Pettinato G, Manivel JC, Saldana MJ, Peyser J, Dehner LP (1989) Primary bronchopulmonary fibrosarcoma of childhood and adolescence: reassessment of a low-grade malignancy. Hum Pathol 20: 463

Pfenninger J, D'Apuzzo V (1977) Powder aspiration in children. Report of two cases. Arch Dis Child 52: 157

Phelps DS, Floros J (1991) Localization of pulmonary surfactant proteins using immunohistochemistry and tissue in situ hybridization. Exp Lung Res 17: 985

Pick T, Maurer HM, McWilliams NB (1974) Lymphoepithelioma in childhood. J Pediatr 84: 96

Pinar H, Makarova N, Ruben L, Singer DB (1993) Pathology of the lung in surfactant treated neonates. Pediatr Pathol 13: 105

Pinon JM, Poirriez J, Leroux B, Dupouy D, Quereux C, Garin JP (1987) Diagnostic précoce et surveillance de la toxoplasmose congénitale. Méthode des profils immunologiques comparés. Presse Med 16: 471

Pison U, Lopez FA, Heidelmeyer CF, Rossaint R, Falke KJ (1993) Inhaled nitric oxide reverses hypoxic pulmonary vasoconstriction without impairing gas exchange. J Appl Physiol 74: 1287

Polak MJ, Donnelly WH, Bucciarelli RL (1989) Comparison of airway pathologic lesions after high frequency jet or conventional ventilation. Am J Dis Child 143: 228

Pollak ER, Naunheim KS, Little AG (1985) Fibromyxoma of the trachea. A review of benign tracheal tumors. Arch Pathol Lab Med 109: 926

Polos PG, Wolfe D, Harley RA, Strange C, Sahn SA (1992) Pulmonary hypertension and human immunodeficiency virus infection. Chest 101: 474

Poole JB, Marcial-Rojas PA (1971) Echinococcosis. In: Marcial-Rojas PA (ed) Pathology of protozoal and helminthic diseases with clinical correlation. Williams & Wilkins, Baltimore, p 635

Popek EJ, Strain JD, Neumann A, Wilson H (1993) In utero development of pulmonary artery calcification in monochorionic twins: a report of three cases and discussion of the possible etiology. Pediatr Pathol 13: 597

Popow-Kraupp T, Kern G, Binder C, Tuma W, Kundi M, Kung C (1986) Detection of respiratory syncytial virus in nasopharyngeal secretions by enzyme linked immunosorbent assay, indirect immunofluorescence, and virus isolation: a comparative study. J Med Virol 19: 123

Popper H, Kakse R, Loidolt D (1985) Problems in the differential diagnosis of Kartagener's syndrome and ATPase deficiency. Pathol Res Pract 180: 481

Porter HJ, Heryet A, Quantrill AM, Fleming KA (1990) Combined non-isotopic in situ hybridisation and immunohistochemistry on routine paraffin wax embedded tissue: identification of cell type infected by human parvovirus and demonstration of cytomegalovirus DNA and antigen in renal infection. J Clin Pathol 43: 129

Possmayer F (1988) Pulmonary perspective. A proposed nomenclature for pulmonary surfactant-associated proteins. Am Rev Respir Dis 138: 990

Potter EL (1962) Pathology of the fetus and infant, 2nd edn. Year Book Medical Publishers, Chicago, p 492

Powell DA, Schuit KE (1979) Acute pulmonary blastomycosis in children: clinical course and follow-up. Pediatrics 63: 736

Powell HC, Elliott ML (1977) Congenital lobar emphysema. Virchows Arch [Pathol Anat] 374: 197

Pramanik AK, Holtzman RB, Merritt TA (1993) Surfactant replacement therapy for pulmonary diseases. Pediatr Clin North Am 40: 913

Pratt LW (1965) Medline cysts of the nasal dorsum: embryologic origin and treatment. Laryngoscope 75: 968

Präuer HW, Mack D, Babic R (1983) Intrapulmonary teratoma 10 years after removal of a mediastinal teratoma in a young man. Thorax 38: 632

Preblud SR (1986) Varicella: complications and costs. Pediatrics 78 (suppl): 728

Press E, Adams WC, Chittenden RF, Christian JR, Grayson R, Stewart CC, Everist BW (1962) Co-operative kerosene poisoning study. Evaluation of gastric lavage and other factors in the treatment of accidental ingestion of petroleum distillate products. Pediatrics 29: 648

Primhak RA, Tanner MS, Spencer RC (1993) Pneumococcal infection in the newborn. Arch Dis Child 69: 317

Pruksananonda P, Breese Hall C, Insel RA, McIntyre K, Pellett PE, Long CE et al. (1992) Primary human herpesvirus 6 infection in young children. N Engl J Med 326: 1445

Pryce DM (1946) Lower accessory pulmonary artery with intralobar sequestration of lung: report of 7 cases. J Pathol Bacteriol 58: 457

Pryce DM (1948) The lining of healed but persistent abscess cavities in the lung with epithelium of ciliated columnar type. J Pathol 60: 259

Pryce DM, Sellors TM, Blair LG (1947) Intralobar sequestration of lung associated with an abnormal pulmonary artery. Br J Surg 35: 18

Puchhammer-Stäckl E, Kunz C, Wagner G, Enders G (1994) Detection of varicella zoster virus (VZV) DNA in fetal tissue by polymerase chain reaction. J Perinat Med 22: 65

Pulpeiro JR, Lopez I, Sotelo T, Ruiz JC, Garcia-Hidalgo E (1987) Congenital cystic adenomatoid malformation of the lung in a young adult. Br J Radiol 60: 1128

Pysher TJ, Newstein WB (1984) Ciliary dysmorphology. Perspect Pediatr Pathol 8: 101

Qazi QH, Kanchanapoomi R, Beller E, Collins R (1982) Inheritance of posterior choanal atresia. Am J Med Genet 13: 413

Raafat F, Salman WD, Roberts K, Ingram L, Rees R, Mann JR (1986) Carney's triad: gastric leiomyosarcoma, pulmonary chondroma and extra-adrenal paraganglioma in young females. Histopathology 10: 1325

Radoycich GE, Zuppan CW, Weeks DA, Krous HF, Langston C (1992) Patterns of measles pneumonitis. Pediatr Pathol 12: 773

Rais-Bahrami K, MacDonald MG, Eng GD, Rosenbaum KN (1994) Persistent pulmonary hypertension in newborn infants with congenital myotonic dystrophy. J Pediatr 124: 634

Raju TNK, Langenberg P (1993) Pulmonary hemorrhage and exogenous surfactant therapy: a metaanalysis. J Pediatr 123: 603

Ramani P, Rampling D, Link M (1993) Immunocytochemical study of 12E7 in small round-cell tumours of childhood: an assessment of its sensitivity and specificity. Histopathology 23: 557

Ramani P, Shah A (1993) Lymphangiomatosis. Histologic and immunohistochemical analysis of four cases. Am J Surg Pathol 17: 329

Ramos CD, Londero AT, Gal MCL (1981) Pulmonary paracoccidioidomycosis in a nine year old girl. Mycopathologia 74: 15

Raney RB Jr, D'Angio GT (1989) Langerhans' cell histiocytosis (histiocytosis X): experience in the children's hospital of Philadelphia, 1970–1984. Med Pediatr Oncol 17: 20

Rayner CFJ, Rutman A, Dewar A, Cole PJ, Wilson R (1995) Ciliary disorientation in patients with chronic upper respiratory tract inflammation. Am J Respir Crit Care Med 151: 800

Ratech H, Burke JS, Blayney DW, Sheibani K, Rappaport H (1989) A clinicopathologic study of malignant lymphomas of the nose, paranasal sinuses, and hard palate, including cases of lethal midline granuloma. Cancer 64: 2525

Redington AN, Raine J, Shinebourne EA, Rigby ML (1990) Tetralogy of Fallot with anomalous pulmonary venous connections: a rare but clinically important association. Br Heart J 64: 325

Redjaee B, Rohatgi PK, Herman MA (1990) Multicentric endobronchial granular cell myoblastoma. Chest 98: 945

Reid LM (1986) Structure and function in pulmonary hypertension. New perceptions. Chest 89: 279

Ricci C, Patrassi N, Massa R, Benedetti-Valentini F Jr, Mineo TC (1973) Carcinoid syndrome in bronchial adenoma. Am J Surg 126: 671

Rice DH, Batsakis JG, Headington JT (1974) Fibrous histiocytomas of the nose and paranasal sinuses. Arch Otolaryngol 100: 398

Rifkin RH, Blocker SH, Palmer JO, Ternberg JL (1986) Multiple granular cell tumors. A familial occurrence in children. Arch Surg 121: 945

Risco C, Romero C, Asuncion Bosch M, Pinto Da Silva P (1994) Type II pneumocytes revisited: intracellular membranous systems, surface characteristics, and lamellar body secretion. Lab Invest 70: 407

Roberts JD Jr, Shaul PW (1993) Advances in the treatment of persistent pulmonary hypertension of the newborn. Pediatr Clin North Am 40: 983

Robertson B (1987) Pathology of neonatal surfactant deficiency. Perspect Pediatr Pathol 11: 6

Robinson PC, Watters LC, King TE, Mason RJ (1988) Idiopathic pulmonary fibrosis. Abnormalities in bronchoalveolar lavage fluid phospholipids. Am Rev Respir Dis 137: 585

Roenspies U, Morin D, Gloor E, Hochstetter AR von, Saegesser F, Senning A (1978) Bronchopulmonale Hamartome, Chondrome, Fibrome und Myxome. Schweiz Med Wochenschr 108: 332

Rogers BB, Mark Y, Oyer CE (1993) Diagnosis and incidence of fetal parvovirus infection in an autopsy series: 1 Histology. Pediatr Path 13: 371

Rontal M, Duritz G (1977) Proboscis lateralis – case report and embryonic analysis. Laryngoscope 87: 996

Rosan RC (1975) Hyaline membrane disease and a related spectrum of neonatal pneumopathies. Perspect Pediatr Pathol 2: 15

Rosen N, Gaton E (1975) Congenital bronchiolitis obliterans. Beitr Pathol 155: 309

Rosenak D, Ariel I, Arnon J, Diamant YZ, Chetrit AB, Nadjari M et al. (1991) Recurrent tetraamelia and pulmonary hypoplasia with multiple malformations in sibs. Am J Med Genet 38: 25

Rosenberg HS, Vogler C, Close LG, Warshaw HE (1981) Laryngeal fibromatosis in the neonate. Arch Otolaryngol 107: 513

Rosenblum ND, Colvin RB (1993) Case records of the Massachusetts General Hospital. Case 16-1993. N Engl J Med 328: 1183

Rosenfeld SJ, Young NS (1991) Viruses and bone marrow failure. Blood Rev 5: 71

Rosenthal AF, Vargas MG, Schiff SV (1974) Comparison of four indexes of fetal pulmonary maturity. Clin Chem 20: 486

Rothschild MA, Catalano P, Urken M, Brandwein M, Som P, Norton K et al. (1994) Evaluation and management of congenital cervical teratoma. Arch Otolaryngol Head Neck Surg 120: 444

Rottem M, Fauci AS, Hallahan CW, Kerr GS, Lebovics R, Leavitt RY et al. (1993) Wegener granulomatosis in children and adolescents: clinical presentation and outcome. J Pediatr 122: 26

Roy V, Veys P, Jackson F, Ryan J, Lowdell M, Newland AC (1989) Adult respiratory syndrome following autologous bone marrow transfusion. Bone Marrow Transplant 4: 711

Royall JA, Levin DL (1988) Adult respiratory distress syndrome in pediatric patients. I. Clinical aspects, pathophysiology, pathology, and mechanisms of lung injury. J Pediatr 112: 169

Ruben FL, Talamo TS (1986) Secondary pulmonary alveolar proteinosis occurring in two patients with acquired immune deficiency syndrome. Am J Med 80: 1187

Rubinstein I, Brandon J, Mullen M, Hoffstein V (1988) Morphologic diagnosis of idiopathic pulmonary alveolar lipoproteinosis – revisited. Arch Intern Med 148: 813

Ruiz-Palomo F, Calleja JL, Fogue L (1990) Primary liposarcoma of the lung in a young woman. Thorax 45: 298

Rupp ME, Schwartz ML, Bechard DE (1993) Measles pneumonia. Treatment of a near-fatal case with corticosteroids and vitamin A. Chest 103: 1625

Rusch VW, Shuman WP, Schmidt R, Laramore GE (1989) Massive pulmonary hemangiopericytoma. An innovative approach to evaluation and treatment. Cancer 64: 1928

Russler S, Tapper MA, Knox KK, Liepins A, Carrigan DR (1991) Pneumonitis associated with coinfection by human herpesvirus 6 and *legionella* in an immunocompetent adult. Am J Pathol 138: 1405

Rutledge JC, Jensen P (1986) Acinar dysplasia: a new form of pulmonary maldevelopment. Hum Pathol 17: 1290

Ryan RM, Morris RE, Rice WR, Ciraolo G, Whitsett JA (1989) Binding and uptake of pulmonary surfactant protein (SP-A) by pulmonary type II epithelial cells. J Histochem Cytochem 37: 429

Ryland D, Reid L (1971) Pulmonary aplasia – a quantitative analysis of the development of the single lung. Thorax 26: 602

Sabin AB (1977) Mortality from pneumonia and risk conditions during influenza epidemics. High influenza morbidity during nonepidemic years. JAMA 237: 2823

Saito F, Yutani C, Imakita M, Ishibashi–Ueda H, Kanzaki T, Chiba Y (1989) Giant cell pneumonia caused by varicella zoster virus in a neonate. Arch Pathol Lab Med 113: 201

Salvaggio JE, de Shazo RD (1986) Pathogenesis of hypersensitivity pneumonitis. Chest 89: 1905

Sanchez PJ (1993) Perinatal transmission of *Ureaplasma urealyticum*: current concepts based on review of the literature. Clin Infect Dis 17: S107

Sandstrom RE, Proppe KH, Trelstad RL (1978) Fibrous histiocytoma of the trachea. Am J Clin Pathol 70: 429

Sankaran K, Bhagirath CP, Bingham WT, Hjertaas R, Haight K (1983) Tracheal atresia, proximal esophageal atresia and distal tracheoesophageal fistula: report of two cases and review of literature. Pediatrics 71: 821

Satoh Y, Tsuchiya E, Weng S-Y, Kitagawa T, Matsubara T, Nakagawa K et al. (1989) Pulmonary sclerosing hemangioma of the lung. A type II pneumocytoma by immunohistochemical and immunoelectron microscopic studies. Ann Otol Rhinol Laryngol 64: 1310

Savic B, Birtel FJ, Tholan W, Funke HD, Knoche R (1979) Lung sequestration: report of seven cases and review of 540 published cases. Thorax 34: 96

Sawyer SM, Johnson PDR, Hogg GG, Robertson CF, Oppedisano F, MacIness SJ et al. (1994) Successful treatment of epiglottitis with two doses of ceftriaxone. Arch Dis Child 70: 129

Sax CM, Flannery DB (1986) Craniofrontal dysplasia: clinical and genetic analysis. Clin Genet 29: 508

Say B, Carpenter NJ, Giacoia G, Jegathesan S (1980) Agenesis of the lung associated with a chromosome abnormality (46,XX,2p+). J Med Genet 17: 477

Scattini CM, Orsi A (1973) Multiple bilateral fibromas of the pleura. Thorax 28: 782

Schapiro RL, Evans ET (1972) Surgical disorders causing neonatal respiratory distress. AJR Am J Roentgenol 114: 305

Scheidemandel HE, Page RS (1975) Special considerations in epiglottis in children. Laryngoscope 85: 1738

Schiff M, Gonzalez AM, Ong M, Baird A (1992) Juvenile nasopharyngeal angiofibroma contains an angiogenic growth factor: basic FGF. Laryngoscope 102: 940

Schlech WF (1986) Listeriosis. New pieces to an old puzzle. Arch Intern Med 146: 459

Schlegel RJ (1975) Chronic granulomatous disease 1974. JAMA 231: 615

Schlesinger AE, Tucker GF Jr (1986) Elliptical cricoid cartilage: a unique type of congenital subglottic stenosis. Am J Radiol 146: 1133

Schmitt FC, Filho CZ, Bacchi MM, Castilho ED, Bacchi CE (1989) Adenoid cystic carcinoma of trachea metastatic to the placenta. Hum Pathol 20: 193

Schneider P (1912) Die Missbildungen der Atmungsorgane. In: Schwalbe E (ed) Die Morphologie der Missbildungen des Menschen und der Tiere, Bd III. Fischer, Jena, p 763

Schroeder SA, Shannon DC, Mark EJ (1992) Cellular interstitial pneumonitis in infants. A clinicopathologic study. Chest 101: 1065

Schwartz DA, Ogden PO, Blumberg HM, Honig E (1990) Pulmonary malakoplakia in a patient with the acquired immunodeficiency syndrome. Differential diagnostic considerations. Arch Pathol Lab Med 114: 1267

Schwartz RM, Luby AM, Scanlon JW, Kellogg RJ (1994) Effect of surfactant on morbidity, mortality and resource use in newborn infants weighing 500 to 1500 g. N Engl J Med 330: 1476

Scott JE, Yang S-Y, Stanik E, Anderson JE (1993) Influence of straini on [3H]thymidine incorporation, surfactant-related phospholipid synthesis, and cAMP levels in fetal type II alveolar cells. Am J Respir Cell Mol Biol 8: 258

Scott RJ, Peat D, Rhodes CA (1994) Investigation of the fetal pulmonary inflammatory reaction in chorioamnionitis, using an in situ Y chromosome marker. Pediatr Pathol 14: 997

Scowden EB, Schaffner W, Stone WJ (1978) Overwhelming strongyloidiasis: an unappreciated opportunistic infection. Medicine 57: 527

Scully RE, Mark EJ, McNeely WF, McNeely BU (1992) Case records of the Massachusetts General Hospital. Case 13-1992. N Engl J Med 326: 875

Sears MR, Chang AR, Taylor AJ (1971) Pulmonary alveolar microlithiasis. Thorax 26: 704

Seballos RM, Klein RL (1994) Pulmonary blastoma in children: report of two cases and review of the literature. J Pediatr Surg 29: 1553

Sedano HO, Cohen MM Jr, Jirasek J, Gorlin RJ (1970) Frontonasal dysplasia. J Pediatr 76: 906

Seider MJ, Cleary KR, van Tassel P, Alexanian R, Schantz SP, Frias A et al. (1991) Plasma cell granuloma of the nasal cavity treated by radiation therapy. Cancer 67: 929

Self JT (1969) Biological relationships of the Pentastomida: a bibliography on the Pentastomida. Exp Parasitol 24: 63

Selman M, Gonzale G, Bravo M, Sullivan-Lopez J, Ramos C, Montano M et al. (1990) Effect of lung T lymphocytes on fibroblasts in idiopathic pulmonary fibrosis and extrinsic allergic alveolitis. Thorax 45: 451

Semenzato G, Trentin L, Zambello R, Agostini C, Cipriani A, Marcer G (1988) Different types of cytotoxic lymphocytes recovered from the lungs of patients with hypersensitivity pneumonitis. Am Rev Respir Dis 137: 70

Seo S, Gillin SE, Mirkin LD (1990) Hyaline membranes in postmature infants. Pediatr Pathol 10: 539

Sepkowitz KA, Brown AE, Telzak EE, Gottlieb S, Armstrong D (1992) Pneumocystis carinii pneumonia among patients without AIDS at a cancer hospital. JAMA 267: 832

Seppälä M, Aho I (1975) Physiological role of meconium during delivery. Acta Obstet Gynecol Scand 54: 209

Sessions RB, Zarin DP, Bryan RN (1981) Juvenile nasopharyngeal angiofibroma. Am J Dis Child 135: 535

Shabot JM, Patterson M (1978) Amebic liver abscess: 1966–1976. Am J Dig Dis 23: 110

Shanklin DR (1959) Cardiovascular factors in development of pulmonary hyaline membrane. Arch Pathol 68: 49

Sheffield LJ, Danks DM, Hammond JW, Hoogenradd NJ (1976) Massive pulmonary hemorrhage as a presenting feature in congenital hyperammonemia. J Pediatr 88: 450

Shenai JP, Chytil F (1990) Effect of maternal vitamin-A administration on fetal lung vitamin-A stores in the perinatal rat. Biol Neonate 58: 318

Sherrier RH, Chiles C, Roggli V (1989) Pulmonary lymphangioleiomyomatosis CT findings. AJR Am J Roentgenol 153: 937

Sheth KJ, Leichter HE, Kishaba G, Cohen AH (1992) Focal segmental glomerulosclerosis in desquamative interstitial pneumonia. Child Nephrol Urol 12: 43

Shi SR, Goodman ML, Bhan AK, Pilch BZ, Chen LB, Sun TT (1984) Immunohistochemical study of nasopharyngeal carcinoma using monoclonal keratin antibodies. Am J Pathol 117: 53

Shikes RH, Ryder JW (1989) Case 5. Adenovirus pneumonia in a newborn. Pediatr Pathol 9: 199

Shimizu H, Miyamura K, Kuroki Y (1991) Appearance of surfactant proteins, SP-A and Sp-B, in developing rat lung and the effects of in vivo dexamethasone treatment. Biochim Biophys Acta 1081: 53

Shulman RJ, Langston C, Schanler RJ (1987) Pulmonary vascular lipid deposition after administration of intravenous fat to infants. Pediatrics 79: 99

Shurbaji MS, Dumler JS, Gage WR, Pettis GL, Gupta PK, Kuhadja FP (1990) Immunohistochemical detection of chlamydial antigens in association with cystitis. Am J Clin Pathol 93: 363

Shvero J, Hadar T, Segal K, Abraham A, Sidi J (1987) Laryngeal carcinoma in patients 40 years of age and younger. Cancer 60: 3092

Sie KCY, McGill T, Healy GB (1994) Subglottic hemangioma: ten years' experience with the carbon dioxide laser. Ann Otol Rhinol Laryngol 103: 167

Sigurs N, Bjarnason R, Sigurgergsson F, Kjellman B, Björkstén B (1995) Asthma and immunoglobulin E antibodies after respiratory syncytial virus bronchiolitis: a prospective cohort study with matched controls. Pediatrics 95: 500

Silver MM, Thurston WA, Patrick JE (1988) Perinatal pulmonary hyperplasia due to laryngeal atresia. Hum Pathol 19: 110

Silver MM, Vilos GA, Milne KJ (1988) Pulmonary hypoplasia in neonatal hypophosphatasia. Pediatr Pathol 8: 483

Simmonds EJ, Littlewood JM, Hopwood V, Evans EGV (1994) Aspergillus fumigatus colonisation and population density of place of residence in cystic fibrosis. Arch Dis Child 70: 139

Simon M, Kahn T, Schneider A, Pirsig W (1994) Laryngeal carcinoma in a 12-year-old child. Association with human papillomavirus 18 and 33. Arch Otolaryngol Head Neck Surg 120: 277

Simpson GT, Healy GB, McGill T, Strong MS (1979) Benign tumors and lesions of the larynx in children. Surgical excision by CO_2 laser. Ann Otol Rhinol Laryngol 88: 479

Simpson W, Hacking PM, Court SDM, Gardner PS (1974) The radiological findings in respiratory syncytial virus infection in children. II. The correlation of radiological categories with clinical and virological findings. Pediatr Radiol 2: 155

Sing KP, Pahor AL (1977) Congenital syst of nasopharynx. J Laryngol Otol 91: 75

Singh W, Ramage C, Best P, Angus B (1980) Nasal neuroblastoma secreting vasopressin. A case report. Cancer 45: 961

Singer AD, Thibeault DW, Hobel CJ, Heiner DC (1976) α_1-Antitrypsin in amniotic fluid and cord blood of preterm infants with the respiratory distress syndrome. Pediatrics 88: 87

Sinniah D, Landing BH, Siegel SE, Laug WE, Gwinn JL (1986) ˙.lmonary alveolar septal calcinosis causing progressive respiratory failure in acute lymphoblastic leukemia in childhood. Pediatr Pathol 6: 439

Sir G (1962) Bronchiolitis obliterans connata. Zentralbl Allg Pathol 103: 129

Siwersson V, Kindblom LG (1984) Oncocytic carcinoid of the nasal cavity and carcinoid of the lung in a child. Pathol Res Pract 179: 562

Skillrud DM, Martin WJ (1984) Paraquat-induced injury of type II alveolar cells. An in vitro model of oxidant injury. Am Rev Respir Dis 129: 995

Slack MPE, Mayon-White RT (1978) Group B streptococci in pharyngeal aspirates at birth and the early detection of neonatal sepsis. Arch Dis Child 53: 540

Sladen A, Zanca P, Hadnott WH (1971) Aspiration pneumonitis – the sequelae. Chest 59: 448

Smith H, Congdon P (1985) Neonatal systemic candidiasis. Arch Dis Child 60: 365

Smith LJ, Lawrence JB, Katzenstein A-LA (1983) Vascular sarcoidosis: a rare cause of pulmonary hypertension. Am J Med Sci 285: 38

Smith RJH, Smith MCF, Glossop LP, Bailey CM, Evans JNG (1984) Congenital vascular anomalies causing tracheoesophageal compression. Arch Otolaryngol 110: 82

Smith SB, Schwartzman M, Mencia F, Blum EB, Krogstad D, Nitzkin J, Healy GR (1977) Fatal disseminated strongyloidiasis presenting as acute abdominal distress in an urban child. J Pediatr 91: 607

Smith JD, Cotton R, Meyer CM (1990a) Subglottic cysts in the premature infant. Arch Otolaryngol Head Neck Surg 116: 479

Smith C, Feldman C, Levy H, Kallenbach JM, Zwi S (1990b) Cryptogenic fibrosing alveolitis. A study of an indigenous African population. Respiration 57: 364

Smyth RL, Carty H, Thomas H, van Velzen D, Heaf D (1994) Diagnosis of interstitial lung disease by a percutaneous lung biopsy sample. Arch Dis Child 70: 143

Sobonya RE, Quan SF, Fleishman JS (1985) Pulmonary lymphangioleiomyomatosis: quantitative analysis of lesions producing airflow limitation. Hum Pathol 16: 1122

Soler P, Kambouchner M, Valeyre D, Hance AJ (1992) Pulmonary Langerhans cell granulomatosis (histiocytosis X). Annu Rev Med 43: 105

Som PM, Nagel BD, Feuerstein SS, Strauss L (1979) Benign pleomorphic adenoma of the larynx. A case report. Ann Otol Rhinol Laryngol 88: 112

Sotomayor JL, Godinez RI, Borden S, Wilmott RW (1986) Large-airway collapse due to acquired tracheobronchomalacia in infancy. Am J Dis Child 140: 367

Spagnolo DV, Papadimitriou JP, Archer M (1984) Postirradiation malignant fibrous histiocytoma arising in juvenile nasopharyngeal angiofibroma and producing α_1-antitrypsin. Histopathology 8: 339

Speer M, Rosan RC, Rudolph AJ (1978) Hemophilus influenzae infection in the neonate mimicking respiratory distress syndrome. J Pediatr 93: 295

Speich R, Jenni R, Opravil M, Pfab M, Russi EW (1991) Primary pulmonary hypertension in HIV infection. Chest 100: 1268

Spencer H (1961) Pulmonary blastoma. J Pathol Bactriol 82: 161

Spencer H (1977a) Congenital abnormalities of the lung, pulmonary vessels and lymphatics. In: Spencer H (ed) Pathology of the lung, vol I. Pergamon, Oxford, p 71

Spencer H (1977b) Congenital abnormalities of the lung, pulmonary vessels and lymphatics. In: Spencer H (ed) Pathology of the lung, vol. I. Pergamon, Oxford, p 87

Spencer H, Dail DH, Arneaud J (1980) Non-invasive bronchial epithelial papillary tumors. Cancer 45: 1486

Spickard A III, Hirschmann JV (1994) Exogenous lipoid pneumonia. Arch Intern Med 154: 686

Stahl RS, Jurkiewicz MJ (1985) Congenital posterior choanal atresia. Pediatrics 76: 429

Stallmach T, Karolyi L (1994) Augmentation of fetal granulopoiesis with chlorioamnionitis during the second trimester of gestation. Hum Pathol 25: 244

Stanley RJ, Scheithauer BW, Weiland LH, Neel HB III (1987) Neural and neuroendocrine tumors of the larynx. Ann Otol Rhinol Laryngol 96: 823

Stark AR, Mark EJ (1992) A Full-Term Newborn Boy with Chronic Respiratory Distress. N.E.J.M. 326: 875

Statz T, Lynch J, Ortmann M, Roth B (1989) Tracheal agenesis: a case report. Eur J Pediatr 149: 203

Steinkamp G, Müller KM, Schirg E, von der Hardt H (1990) Fibrosing alveolitis in childhood. A long-term follow-up. Acta Paediatr Scand 79: 823

Stell PM, Maran AGD (1975) Laryngocele. J Laryngol Otol 89: 915

Stephanopoulos C, Catsaras H (1963) Myxosarcoma complicating a cystic hamartoma of the lung. Thorax 18: 44

Stocker JT (1986) Pathologic features of long-standing "healed" bronchopulmonary dysplasia: A study of 28 3- to 40-month-old infants. Hum Pathol 17: 943

Stocker JT (1987) Case 6 postinfarction peripheral cysts of the lung. Pediatr Pathol 7: 111

Stocker JT (1994) Congenital and Development Diseases. In Dail DH and Hammar SP Eds: Pulmonary Pathology 2ed p 155 Springer Verlag

Stocker JT, Kagan-Hallet K (1979) Extralobar pulmonary sequestration. Analysis of 15 cases. Am J Clin Pathol 72: 917

Stocker JT, Madewell JE, (1977) Persistent interstitial pulmonary emphysema: another complication of the respiratory distress syndrome. Pediatrics 59: 847

Stocker JT, Madewell JE, Drake RM (1977) Congenital cystic adenomatoid malformation of the lung. Classification and morphologic spectrum. Hum Pathol 8: 155

Stocker JT, Drake RM, Madewell JE (1978) Cystic and congenital lung disease in the newborn. Perspect Pediatr Pathol 4: 93

Stone FJ, Churg AM (1977) The ultrastructure of pulmonary hamartoma. Cancer 39: 1064

Straumann Kunz U, Pospischil A, Paccaud MF (1991) Immunohistochemical detection of chlamydiae in formalin-fixed tissue sections: comparison of a monoclonal antibody with yolk derived antibodies (IgY). J Vet Med B38: 292

Strauss RG, Bove KE (1975) Fever, shock and hepatomegaly in a 13-month-old boy. J Pediatr 87: 819

Strauss M, Widome MD, Roland PS (1981) Nasopharyngeal hemangioma causing airway obstruction in infancy.

Laryngoscope 91: 1365

Stringer JR (1993) The identity of Pneumocystis carinii: not a single protozoan, but a diverse group of exotic fungi. Infect Agents Dis 2: 109

Strunge P (1972) Infantile lobar emphysema with lobar agenesis and congenital heart disease. Acta Paediatr Scand 61: 209

Strunk RC, Eidlen DM, Mason RJ (1988) Pulmonary alveolar type II epithelial cells synthesize and secrete proteins of the classical and alternative complement pathways. J Clin Invest 81: 1419

Sturgess JM, Turner JAP (1984) Ultrastructural pathology of cilia in the immotile cilia syndrome. Perspect Pediatr Pathol 8: 133

Sturgess JM, Chao J, Turner JAP (1980) Transposition of ciliary microtubules. Another cause of impaired ciliary motility. N Engl J Med 303: 318

Sturgess JM, Thompson MW, Czegledy-Nagy E, Turner JAP (1986) Genetic aspects of immotile cilia syndrome. Am J Med Genet 25: 149

Sueishi K, Watanabe T, Tanaka K, Shin H (1974) Intrauterine bronchiolitis obliterans: report of an autopsy case and review of the literature. Virchows Arch [Pathol Anat] 362: 223

Suissa S, Ernst P, Boivin J-F, Horwitz RI, Habbick B, Cockroft D et al. (1994) A cohort analysis of excess mortality in asthma and the use of inhaled β-agonists. Am J Respir Crit Care Med 149: 604

Sulayman R, Thilenius O, Replogie R, Arcilla RA (1975) Unilateral emphysema in total anomalous pulmonary venous return. J Pediatr 87: 433

Sun B, Curstedt T, Robertson B (1993) Surfactant inhibition in experimental meconium aspiration. Acta Paediatr 82: 182

Sun C-C J, Duara S (1985) Fatal adenovirus pneumonia in two newborn infants, one case caused by adenovirus type 30. Pediatr Pathol 4: 247

Sundar B, Guine EJ, O'Donnell M (1975) Congenital H-type tracheo-oesophageal fistula. Arch Dis Child 80-862

Svare J, Andersen LF, Langhoff-Roos J, Madsen H, Bruun B (1991) Maternal – fetal listeriosis: 2 case reports. Gynecol Obstet Invest 31: 179

Swaminathan S, Quinn J, Stabile MW, Bader D, Platzker ACG, Keens TG (1989) Long-term pulmonary sequelae of meconium aspiration syndrome. J Pediatr 114: 356

Synder R, Perzin K (1972) Papillomatosis of the naval cavity and paranasal sinuses (inverted papilloma, squamous papilloma). A clinico-pathologic study. Cancer 30: 668

Szalay GC, Bledsoe RC (1972) Congenital dermoid cyst and fistula of the nose. Am J Dis Child 124: 392

Takahashi T, Takahashi Y, Nio M (1994) Remodeling of the alveolar structure in the paraquat lung of humans: a morphometric study. Hum Pathol 25: 702

Tan-Liu NS, Matsubara O, Grillo HC, Mark EJ (1989) Invasive fibrous tumor of the tracheobronchial tree: clinical and pathologic study of seven cases. Hum Pathol 20: 180

Taxy JB (1977) Juvenile nasopharyngeal angiofibroma. An ultrastructural study. Cancer 39: 1044

Taxy, JB (1990) Meningioma of the paranasal sinuses. A report of two cases. Am J Surg Pathol 14: 82

Taxy JB, Bharani NK, Mills SE, Frierson HF, Gould VE (1986) The spectrum of olfactory neural tumors. A light-microscopic immunohistochemical and ultrastructural analysis. Am J Surg Pathol 10: 687

Taylor BW, Erich JB (1967) Dermoid cysts of the nose. Mayo Clin Proc 42: 488

Tazelaar HD, Yousem SA (1988) The pathology of combined heart–lung transplantation: an autopsy study. Hum Pathol 19: 1403

Telzak EE, Cote RJ, Gold JWM, Campbell SW, Armstrong D (1990) Extrapulmonary Pneumocystis carinii infections. Scand J Infect Dis 12: 380

Templer J, Hast M, Thomas JR, Davis WE (1981) Congenital laryngeal stridor secondary to flaccid epiglottis, anomalous accessory cartilages and redundant aryepiglottic folds. Laryngoscope 91: 394

Tenner AJ, Robinson SL, Borchelt J, Wright JR (1989) Human pulmonary surfactant protein (SP-A), a protein structurally homologous to Clq, can enhance FcR- and CRl-mediated phagocytosis. J Biol Chem 264: 13923

Thaller S, Fried MP, Goodman ML (1985) Symptomatic solitary granular cell tumor of the trachea. Chest 88: 925

Tharrington CL, Bossen EH (1992) Nasopharyngeal teratomas. Arch Pathol Lab Med 116: 165

Thawley SE, Osborn DA (1974) Granular cell myoblastoma of the larynx. Laryngoscope 84: 1545

Thompson EN, Soothill JF (1970) Chronic granulomatous disease: quantitative clinico-pathological relationships. Arch Dis Child 45: 24

Thompson AB III, Spurzem JR, Rennard SI (1992) Idiopathic pulmonary fibrosis. Immunol Allergy Clin North Am 12: 401

Thornton CM, Halliday HL, O'Hara MD (1994) Surfactant replacement therapy in preterm neonates – a comparison of post mortem pulmonary histology in treated and untreated infants. Paediat Pathol 14: 945–953

Thorpe-Beeston JG, Nicolaides KH (1994) Cystic adenomatoid malformation of the lung: prenatal diagnosis and outcome. Prenatal Diagnos 14: 677

Thulliez P, Daffos F, Forestier F (1992) Diagnosis of Toxoplasma infection in the pregnant woman and the unborn child: current problems. Scand J Infect Dis 84: 18

Tizzano EF (1993) Recent advances in cystic fibrosis research. J Pediatr 122: 985

Tizzano EF, Buchwald M (1992) Cystic fibrosis: beyond the gene to therapy. J Pediatr 120: 337

Tomashefski JF Jr, Abramowsky CR, Chung Park M, Wisniewska J, Bruce MC (1992) Immunofluorescence studies of lung tissue in cystic fibrosis. Pediatr Pathol 12: 313

Tomashefski JF Jr, Butler T, Islam M (1989) Histopathology and etiology of childhood pneumonia: an autopsy study of 93 patients in Bangladesh. Pathology 21: 71

Toran N, Ruiz de Miguel C, Reig J, Garcia-Bonaf M (1989) Lobar emphysema associated with patent ductus arteriosus and pulmonary obstructive vascular disease. Pediatr Pathol 9: 163

Toriello HV, Bauserman SC (1985) Bilateral pulmonary agenesis: association with the hydrolethalus syndrome and review of the literature from a development field perspective. Am J Med Genet 21: 93

Toriello HV, Higgins JV, Jones AS, Radecki LL (1985) Pulmonary and diaphragmatic agenesis: report of affected sibs. Am J Med Genet 21: 87

Torikata C, Kawai T, Nogawa S, Ikeda K, Shimizu K, Kijimoto C (1991) Nine Japanese patients with immotile–dyskinetic cilia syndrome: an ultrastructural study using tannic acid-containing fixation. Hum Pathol 22: 830

Torriani R, Zimmermann A, Morell A (1979) Die BCG-Sepsis als letale Komplikation der BCG-Impfung. Schweiz Med Wochenschr 109: 708

Tos M, Mogensen C, Thomsen J (1977) Nasal polyps in cystic fibrosis. J Laryngol Otol 91: 827

Townsend GL, Neel HB III, Weiland LH, Devine KD, McBean JB (1973) Fibrous histiocytoma of the paranasal sinuses. Report of a case. Arch Otolaryngol 98: 51

Travis WD, Borok Z, Roum JH, Zhang J, Feuerstein I, Ferrans VJ et al. (1993) Pulmonary Langerhans' cell granulomatosis (histiocytosis X). A clinicopathologic study of 48 cases. Am J Surg Pathol 17: 971

Travis WD, Carpenter HA, Lie JT (1987) Diffuse pulmonary hemorrhage. An uncommon manifestation of Wegener's granulomatosis. Am J Surg Pathol 11: 702

Travis WD, Colby TV, Lombard C, Carpenter HA (1990) A clinicopathologic study of 34 cases of diffuse pulmonary hemorrhage with lung biopsy confirmation. Am J Surg Pathol 14: 1112

Travis WD, Pittaluga S, Lipschik GY, Ognibene FP, Suffredini AF, Masur H et al. (1990) Atypical pathologic manifestations of Pneumocystis carinii pneumonia in the acquired immune deficiency syndrome. Am J Surg Pathol 14: 615

Travis WD, Fox CH, Devaney KO, Weiss LM, O'Leary T, Ognibene FP et al. (1992) Lymphoid pneumonitis in 50 adult patients infected with the human immunodeficiency virus: lymphocytic interstitial pneumonitis versus nonspecific interstitial pneumonitis. Hum Pathol 23: 529

Trinca M, Rey C, Breviere GM, Vaksmann G, Francart C, Dupuis C (1993) Familial scimitar syndrome. Arch Mal Coeur Vaiss 86: 635

Trompeter R, Yu VYH, Aynsley-Green A, Roberton NRC (1975) Massive pulmonary haemorrhage in the newborn infant. Arch Dis Child 50: 123

Tsokos M (1992) Peripheral primitive neuroectodermal tumors. Diagnosis, classification, a prognosis. Perspect Pediatr Pathol 16: 27

Turkel SB, Mapp JR (1983) A ten-year retrospective study of pink and yellow neonatal hyaline membrane disease. Pediatrics 72: 170

Tyler DC (1985) Laryngeal cleft: report of eight patients and a review of the literature. Am J Med Genet 21: 61

Ucan ES, Keyf AI, Aydilek R, Yalcin Z, Sebit S, Kudu M et al. (1993) Pulmonary alveolar microlithiasis review of Turkish reports. Thorax 48: 171

Ueda K, Gruppo R, Unger F, Martin L, Bove K (1977) Rhabdomyosarcoma of lung arising in congenital cystic adenomatoid malformation. Cancer 40: 383

Ulbright TM, Katzenstein ALA (1980) Solitary necrotizing granulomas of the lung. Differentiating features and etiology. Am J Surg Pathol 4: 13

Umene K, Nunoue T (1993) Partial nucleotide sequencing and characterization of human parvovirus B19 genome DNAs from damaged human fetuses and from patients with leukemia. J Med Virol 39: 333

Unger L (1952) The recognitioin of nonallergic asthma. Dis Chest 22: 671

Usui Y, Takayama S, Nakayama M, Miura H, Kimula Y (1992) Case report of desquamative interstitial pneumonia: documentation of preserved pulmonary function after twelve clinical relapses. Respiration 59: 112

Uyama T, Monden Y, Harada K, Sumitomo M, Kimura S (1988) Pulmonary leiomyomatosis showing endobronchial extension and giant cyst formation. Chest 94: 644

Valderrama E, Saluja G, Shende A, Lanzkowsky P, Berkman J (1978) Pulmonary blastoma. Report of two cases in children. Am J Surg Pathol 2: 415

Valdes-Dapena MA, Arey JB (1967) Pulmonary emboli of cerebral origin in the newborn: a report of two cases. Arch Pathol 84: 643

Valdes-Dapena MA, Nissim JE, Arey JB, Godleski J, Schaaf HD, Haust MD (1976) Yellow pulmonary hyaline membranes. J Pediatr 89: 128

Vale JA, Meredith TJ, Buckley BM (1987) Paraquat poisoning: clinical features and immediate general management. Hum Toxicol 6: 41

Valli M, Fabris GA, Dewar A, Hornall D, Sheppard MN (1994) Atypical carcinoid tumour of the lung: a study of 33 cases with prognostic features. Histopathology 24: 363

Van Asperen PP, Seeto I, Cass DT (1986) Acquired tracheo–oesophageal fistula after ingestion of a mercury button-battery. Med J Anat 145: 413

Van Dijk C, Wagenvoort CA (1973) The various types of congenital adenomatoid malformation of the lung. J Pathol 110: 131

Van Golde LMG, Batenburg JJ, Robertson B (1988) The pulmonary surfactant system: biochemical aspects and functional significance. Physiol Rev 68: 374

Van Klaveren RJ, Hassing HHM, Wierama-van Tilburg JM, Lacquet LK, Cox AL (1994) Mesenchymal cystic haematoma of the lung: a rare cause of relapsing pneumothorax. Thorax 49: 1175

van Kreel BK (1991) Estimation of fetal lung maturity by assessment of lamellar body particle concentration. Ann Clin Biochem 28: 574

Van Lierde S, Corbeel L, Eggermont E (1989) Clinical and laboratory findings in children with adenovirus infections. Eur J Pediatr 148: 423

Van Lierde S, Cornelis A, Devlieger H, Moerman P, Lauweryns J, Eggermont E (1991) Different patterns of pulmonary sequelae after hyaline membrane disease: heterogeneity of bronchopulmonary dysplasia? Biol Neonate 60: 152

Van Maarsseven AC MTh, Mullink H, Alons CL, Stam J (1986) Distribution of T-lymphocyte subsets in different portions of sarcoid granulomas: immunohistologic analysis with monoclonal antibodies. Hum Pathol 17: 493

Vassilopoulou-Sellin R, Klein MJ, Smith TH, Samaan NA, Frankenthaler RA, Goepfert H et al (1993) Pulmonary metastases in children and young adults with differentiated thyroid cancer. Cancer 71: 1348

Veliath AJ, Khanna KK, Subhas BS, Ramakrishnan MR, Aurora AL (1977) Primary lymphosarcoma of the lung with unusual features. Thorax 32: 632

Venkatesh VC, Iannuzzi DM, Ertsey R, Ballard PL (1993) Differential glucocorticoid regulation of the pulmonary hydrophobic surfactant proteins SP-B and SP-C. Am J Respir Cell Mol Biol 8: 222

Vera–Roman JM, Sobonya RE, Gomez–Garcia JL, Sanz–Bondia JR, Paris–Romeu F (1983) Leiomyoma of the lung. Literature review and case report. Cancer 52: 936

Verbeken EK, Demedts M, Vanwing J, Deneff G, Lauweryns JM (1989) Pulmonary phospholipid accumulation distal to an obstructed bronchus. Arch Pathol Lab Med 113: 886

Verlaat CWM, Peters HM, Semmekrot BA, Wiersma-van Tilburg JM (1994) Congenital pulmonary lymphangiectases presenting as a unilateral hyperlucent lung. Eur J Pediatr 153: 202

Verra F, Fleury-Feith J, Boucherat M, Pinchon M-C, Bignon J, Escudier E (1993) Do nasal ciliary changes reflect bronchial changes? An ultrastructural study. Am Rev Respir Dis 147: 908

Viale G, Codecasa L, Bulgheroni P, Giobbi A, Madonissi E, Dell'Orto P, Coggi G (1986) T-cell subsets in sarcoidosis: an immunocytochemical investigation of blood, bronchoalveolar lavage fluid, and prescalemic lymphnodes from eight patients. Hum Pathol 17: 476

Vincent A, Vodoz JF, Lenenberger P (1987) Pulmonary lymphangiomyomatosis and angiomyolipoma. A proposal of 2 cases. Schweiz Med Wochenschr 117: 958

Vitale VJ, Saiman L, Haddad J Jr (1993) Herpes laryngitis and tracheitis causing respiratory distress in a neonate. Arch Otolaryngol Head Neck Surg 119: 239

Vohr BR, Coll CG, Lobato D, Yunis KA, O'Dea C, Oh W (1991) Neurodevelopmental and medical status of low-birthweight survivors of bronchopulmonary dysplasia at 10 to 12 years of age. Dev Med Child Neurol 33: 690

Volk MS, Tucker GF Jr (1987) Congenital laryngeal anomalies associated with tracheal agenesis. Ann Otol Rhinol Laryngol 96: 505

Volk BW, Adachi M, Schneck L (1975) The gangliosidoses. Hum Pathol 6: 555

Voorhout WF, Veenendaal T, Haagsman HP, Verkleij AJ, von Golde LMG, Geuze HJ (1991) Surfactant protein A is localized at the corners of the pulmonary tubular myelin lattice. J Histochem Cytochem 39: 1331

Wailoo MP, Emery JL (1979) The trachea in children with tracheo-oesophageal fistula. Histopathology 3: 329

Waites KB, Crouse DT, Cassell GH (1993) Systemic neonatal infection due to Ureaplasma urealyticum. Clin Infect Dis 17: S131

Waites KB, Crouse DT, Philips JB III, Canupp KC, Cassell GH (1989) Ureaplasmal pneumonia and sepsis associated with persistent pulmonary hypertension of the newborn. Pediatrics 83: 79

Wall CP, Goff AM, Carrington CB, Gaensler EA (1979) Lymphomatoid granulomatosis. Case report from the thoracic services. Boston University Medical School. Respiration 38: 332

Walsh WF, Stanley S, Lally KP, Stribley RE, Treece DP, McCleskey F et al. (1991) Ureaplasma urealyticum demonstrated by open lung biopsy in newborns with chronic lung disease. Pediatr Infect Dis J 10: 823

Walsh-Sukys M, Stork EK, Martin RJ (1994) Neonatal ECMO: iron lung of the 1990s? J Pediatr 124: 427

Walti H, Tordet C, Gerbaut L, Saugier P, Moriette G, Relier JP (1989) Persistent elastase/proteinase inhibitor imbalance during prolonged ventilation of infants with bronchopulmonary dysplasia: evidence for the role of nosocomial infections. Pediatr Res 26: 351

Walton JC, Silver M, Chance GW, Vilos GA (1985) Laryngeal atresia, pleurodesis, and diaphragmatic hypertrophy in a newborn infant with findings relevant to fetal lung development. Pediatr Pathol 5: 1

Walzer PD (1991a) Pneumocystis carinii – new clinical spectrum? N Engl J Med 324: 263

Walzer PD (1991b) Immunopathogenesis of Pneumocystis carinii infection. J Lab Clin Med 118: 206

Wang NS, Huang SN, Thurlbeck WM (1970) Combined Pneumocystis carinii and cytomegalovirus infection. Arch Pathol 90: 529

Wang EEL, Cassell GH, Sanchez PJ, Regan JA, Payne NR, Liu PP (1993a) Ureaplasma urealyticum and chronic lung disease of prematurity: critical appraisal of the literature on causation. Clin Infect Dis 17: S112

Wang LT, Wilkins EW Jr, Bode HH (1993b) Bronchial carcinoid tumors in pediatric patients. Chest 103: 1426

Ward KN, Gray JJ (1994) Primary human herpesvirus-6 infection is frequently overlooked as a cause of febrile fits in young children. J Med Virol 42: 119

Warter A, Satge D, Roeslin N (1987) Angioinvasive plasma cell granulomas of the lung. Cancer 59: 435

Wayoff M, Labaeye P (1973) Sarcome botryoide du larynx chez un garcon de 10 ans. J Fr Otorhinolaryngol 22: 349

Weaver TE (1991) Surfactant proteins and SP-D. Am J Respir Cell Mol Biol 5: 4

Webb JK, Job CK, Gault EW (1968) Tropical eosinophilia: demonstration of microfilariae in lung, liver and lymph nodes. Lancet i: 835

Webber S, Wilkinson AR, Lindsell D, Hope PL, Dobson SRM, Isaacs D (1990) Neonatal pneumonia. Arch Dis Child 65: 207

Weber AL, Grillo HC (1978) Tracheal tumours. A radiological, clinical and pathological evaluation of 84 cases. Radiol Clin North Am 16: 227

Weber TR, Connors RH, Tracy TF Jr (1991) Acquired tracheal stenosis in infants and children. J Thorac Cardiovasc Surg 102: 29

Weis JW, Winter MW, Phylikiy RL, Bonke PM (1986) Peripheral T-cell lymphomas: histologic immunohistologic and clinical characterization. Mayo Clin Proc 61: 411

Weiss LM, Yousem SA, Warnke RA (1985) Non-Hodgkin's lymphomas of the lung. A study of 19 cases emphasizing the utility of frozen section immunologic studies in differential diagnosis. Am J Surg Pathol 9: 480

Weiss LM, Movahed LA, Berry GJ, Billingham ME (1990) In situ hybridization studies for viral nucleic acids in heart and lung allograft biopsies. Am J Clin Pathol 93: 675

Wellons HA Jr, Eggleston P, Golden GT, Allen MS (1976) Bronchial adenoma in childhood. Two case reports and review of literature. Am J Dis Child 130: 301

Wells TR, Landing BH, Shamszadeh M, Thompson JW, Bove KE, Caron KH (1992) Association of Down syndrome and segmental tracheal stenosis with ring tracheal cartilages: a review of nine cases. Pediatr Pathol 12: 673

Wenig BM, Hyams VJ, Heffner DK (1988) Nasopharyngeal papillary adenocarcinoma. A clinicopathologic study of a low-grade carcinoma. Am J Surg Pathol 12: 946

Westgren LMR, Malcus P, Svenningsen NW (1986) Intrauterine asphyxia and long-term outcome in preterm fetuses. Obstet Gynecol 67: 512

Whalen TV, Albin DM, Woolley MN (1987) Esophageal atresia and tracheoesophageal fistula in the twin. Anatomic variants. Ann Surg 205: 322

Wheat LJ, French MLV, Wass JL (1989) Sarcoidlike manifestations of histoplasmosis. Arch Intern Med 149: 2421

White CW, Sondheimer HM, Crouch EC, Wilson H, Fan LL (1989) Treatment of pulmonary hemangiomatosis with recombinant interferon α_{2a}. N Engl J Med 320: 1197

Whitewell F, Scott J, Grimshaw M (1977) Relationship between occupations and asbestos-fibre content of the lungs in patients with pleural mesothelioma, lung cancer and other diseases. Thorax 32: 377

Wigglesworth JS, Keith IH, Girling DJ, Slade SA (1976) Hyaline membrane disease, alkali and intraventricular haemorrhage. Arch Dis Child 51: 755

Wigglesworth JS, Desai R, Hislop AA (1987) Fetal lung growth in congenital laryngeal atresia. Pediatr Pathol 7: 515

Wigglesworth JS, Hislop AA, Desai R (1991) Biochemical and morphometric analyses in hypoplastic lungs. Pediatr Pathol 11: 537

William CL, Busque L, Griffith B, Favara BE, McClain KL, Duncan MH et al. (1994) Langerhans cell histiocytosis (histiocytosis X) – a clonal proliferative disease. N Engl J Med 331: 154

Williams RI (1960) Modern concepts in the clinical management of allergy in otolaryngology. Ann Otol 76: 1389

Williams HL, Williams RI (1969) The therapeutic implications of the hypothesis of allergic hypersensitivity as a dysfunction of the intracellular immune mechanisms. Ann Allergy 27: 434

Williams A, Vawter G, Reid L (1979) Increased muscularity of the pulmonary circulation in victims of sudden infant death syndrome. Pediatrics 63: 18

Williams A, Baskerville A, Dowsett AB, Conlan JW (1987) Immunocytochemical demonstration of the association between Legionella pneumophila, its tissue-destructive protease, and pulmonary lesions in experimental legionnaires' disease. J Pathol 153: 257

Winestock DP, Burtlett PC, Sondheimer FK (1978) Benign nasal polyps causing bone destruction in the nasal cavity and paranasal sinuses. Laryngoscope 88: 675

Winn RE, Kollef MH, Meyer JI (1994) Pulmonary involvement in the hypereosinophilic syndrome. Chest 105: 656

Winther LK (1978) Congenital choanal atresia. Anatomic, physiological and therapeutic aspects, especially the endonasal approach under endoscopic vision. Arch Otolaryngol 104: 72

Wirtz H, Schmidt M (1992) Ventilation and secretion of pulmonary surfactant. Clin Invest 70: 3

Wiswell TE, Clark RH, Null DM, Kuehl TJ, deLemos RA, Coalson JJ (1988) Tracheal and bronchial injury in high-frequency oscillatory ventilation and high-frequency flow interruption compared with conventional positive-pressure ventilation. J Pediatr 112: 249

Wiswell TE, Bent RC (1993) Meconium staining and the meconium aspiration syndrome. Unresolved issues. Pediatr Clin N Amer 40: 955

Wiswell TE, Turner BS, Bley JA, Fritz DL, Hunt RE (1989) Determinants of tracheobronchial histologic alterations during conventional mechanical ventilation. Pediatrics 84: 304

Witwer JP, Tampas JP (1973) Tracheal fibroxanthoma in a child. Postgrad Med 54: 228

Wohl MEB, Chernick V (1978) Bronchiolitis. Am Rev Resper Dis 118: 759

Wollner N, Burchenal JH, Lieberman PH, Exelby PR, D'Angio GJ, Murphy ML (1976) Non-Hodgkin's lymphoma in children. Med Pediatr Oncol 1: 235

Wood NL, Coltman CA Jr (1973) Localized primary extranodal Hodgkin's disease. Ann Intern Med 78: 113

Woodruff AW (1975) Diseases of travel with particular reference to tropical diseases. Postgrad Med J 51: 825

Wreghitt TG, Gandy GM, King A, Sutehall G (1984) Fatal neonatal Echo 7 virus infection. Lancet ii: 465

Wright DH (1970) Microscopic features, histochemistry, histogenesis and diagnosis. In: Burkitt DP, Wright D (eds) Burkitt's lymphoma. Livingstone, Edinburgh, p 82

Wright JE, Butt HL (1994) Perinatal infection with beta haemolytic streptococcus. Arch Dis Child 70: 145

Wright JR, Clements JA (1987) Metabolism and turnover of lung surfactant. Am Rev Respir Dis 135: 426

Wu JP, Gilbert EF, Pellett JR (1974) Pulmonary liposarcoma in a child with adrenogenital syndrome. Am J Clin Pathol 62: 791

Yamaguchi M, Oshima Y, Hosokawa Y, Ohashi H, Tsugawa C, Nishijima E et al. (1990) Concomitant repair of congenital tracheal stenosis and complex cardiac anomaly in small children (see comments). Chest 98: 510

Yeoh GPS, Bale PM, de Silva M (1989) Nasal cerebral heterotopia: the so-called nasal glioma or sequestered encephalocele and its variants. Pediatr Pathol 9: 531

Yoshimura N, Matsubara O, Tamura A, Kasuga T, Mark EJ (1992) Wegener's granulomatosis associated with diffuse pulmonary hemorrhage. Acta Pathol Jpn 42: 657

Young LW, Kim KS, Sproles ET III (1978) Radiological case of the month. Am J Dis Child 132: 311

Yousem SA, Colby TV, Carrington CB (1985) Follicular bronchitis/bronchiolitis. Hum Pathol 16: 700

Yousem SA, Flynn SD (1988) Intrapulmonary localized fibrous tumor. Intraparenchymal so-called localized fibrous mesothelioma. Am J Clin Pathol 89: 365

Yousem SA, Hochholzer L (1986) Alveolar adenoma. Hum Pathol 17: 1066

Yousem SA, Hochholzer L (1987) Malignant fibrous histiocytoma of the lung. Cancer 60: 2532

Yousem SA, Hochholzer L (1994) Mucoepidermoid tumors of the lung. Cancer 60: 1346

Yousem SA, Wick MR, Randhawa P, Manivel JC (1990) An immunohistochemical analysis with comparison with fetal lung in its pseudoglandular stage. Am J Clin Pathol 93: 167

Yousem SA, Wick MR, Singh G, Katyal SL, Manivel JC, Mills SE et al. (1988) So-called sclerosing hemangiomas of lung. An immunohistochemical study supporting a respiratory epithelial origin. Am J Surg Pathol 12: 582

Youssem SA (1993) Lymphocytic bronchitis/bronchiolitis in lung allograft recipients. Am J Surg Pathol 17: 491

Yow MD, Demmler GJ (1992) Congenital cytomegalovirus disease – 20 years is long enough. N Engl J Med 326: 702

Zangwill BC, Stocker JT (1993) Congenital cystic adenomatoid malformation within an extralobar pulmonary sequestration. Pediatr Pathol 13: 309

Zapol WM, Rimar S, Gillis N, Marletta M, Bosken CH (1994) Nitric oxide and the lung. Am J Respir Crit Care Med 149: 1375

Zelefsky MN, Janis M, Bernstein R, Blatt C, Lin A, Meng CH (1971) Intralobar bronchopulmonary sequestration with bronchial communication. Chest 59: 266

Zerella JT, Finberg FJ (1990) Obstruction of the neonatal airway from teratomas. Surg Gynecol Obstet 170: 126

Ziegels-Weissman J, Nadji M, Penneys NS, Morales AR (1984) Prekeratin immunohistochemistry in the diagnosis of undifferentiated carcinoma of the nasopharyngeal type. Arch Pathol Lab Med 108: 588

Zijlstra FJ, Vincent JE, van den Berg B, Hoogsteden HC, Neyens HJ, van Dongen JJM (1987) Pulmonary alveolar proteinosis: determination of prostaglandins and leukotrienes in lavage fluid. Lung 165: 79

Zinserling A (1972) Peculiarities of lesions in viral and mycoplasma infections of the respiratory tract. Virchows Arch [Pathol Anat] 356: 259

8 · Kidney and Lower Urinary Tract

R. Anthony Risdon

Embryology

The kidneys develop from an intermediate mass of mesoderm (the nephrogenic cord) situated on the posterior wall of the intraembryonic coelom between the dorsal somites and the lateral plate mesoderm. Three successive excretory organs develop in the early human embryo – the pronephros, the mesonephros and the metanephros. These three "kidneys" form sequentially and progressively, and more caudally, but there is considerable overlap both chronologically and topographically. The pronephros and mesonephros are transient vestigial structures, and the definitive kidney forms from the metanephros. The mesonephric (or Wolffian) duct persists in male embryos as the duct of the epididymis, the vas deferens and the ejaculatory duct.

The metanephros develops in two parts: the nephrons (glomeruli and tubules) from the nephrogenic cord caudal to the mesonephros (the metanephric blastema); and the excretory system (the ureter, pelvis, calcyces and collecting ducts) from the ureteric bud, which develops as a branch of the Wolffian duct near its distal end at the fifth week (5 mm stage). During early development the ureteric bud grows cranially and impinges on the metanephric blastema, where it begins a process of rapid dichotomous branching. Our understanding of the differentiation of the metanephros has been greatly extended by the microdissection studies of human fetal kidneys by Osthanondh and Potter (1963a–c, 1966a, b). These authors recognized two parts of the ureteric bud and each of its branches:

1. The dilated tips, or ampullae, which are capable of dichotomous branching and the induction of nephron formation in the related metanephric blastema
2. Tubular, or interstitial, portions behind the ampullae, which are capable of growth by elongation.

Rapid branching of the ureteric bud on reaching the metanephric blastema results in a large number of ampullae with short interstitial portions. Nephron formation and subsequent urine secretion cause their dilatation and coalescence to form the renal pelvis and calyces. The renal pelvis and major calyces are derived from the first three to five branches and the minor calyces from the next three to five branches of the ureteric bud. Urine production causes dilatation and coalescence of the generations of branches forming the minor calyces, but the differentiation of nephrons around the calyces limits the dilatation of adjoining calyces and results in the invagination of overlying parenchyma to produce the renal papillae surrounded by flask-shaped calyces.

During the early phase of nephron production, branching of the ureteric bud continues. Condensations of metanephric blastema, from which the nephrons develop, become related to the ampullae. As the nephrons form they quickly become attached to the ampullae, which in turn develop into collecting ducts. This rapid attachment to the growing tips of the ureteric bud ensures that the nephrons are carried outwards as the ureteric bud grows and branches. Figure 8.1 illustrates the process of nephron formation. Subsequently (from about the 14th week of gestation onwards) branching of the ureteric bud ceases and each ampulla becomes capable of inducing the formation of a number of new nephrons. Each of these becomes attached in turn to the previously formed nephrons, to form a chain or nephron arcade. The inner members of the arcade are formed first, and

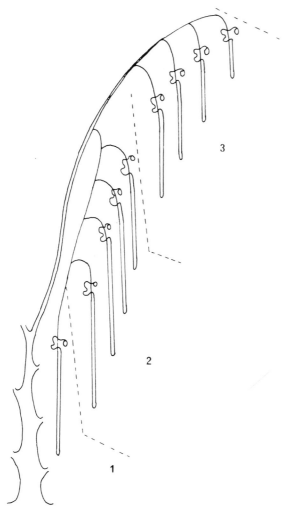

3

2

1

lumen of the developing nephron rapidly connects with the lumen of the ureteric bud. The proximal part of the S-shaped nephron becomes concave around the capillaries that form the glomerular tuft, which are derived from capillary sprouts arising from arteriovenous shunts adjacent to the glomeruli. The walls of the proximal limb of the developing nephron become stretched over the tuft to form the epithelial cells covering the glomerular tuft capillaries (the podocytes) and the lining cells of Bowman's capsule, with the lumen between them forming the urinary space. The rest of the curved tubular portions of the developing nephron elongate and differentiate into the various parts of the nephronic tubules (proximal and distal convoluted tubules and the loop of Henle).

Congenital Anomalies

The commoner congenital abnormalities of the kidneys can conveniently be divided into anomalies of position and form, and parenchymal maldevelopments.

Renal Ectopia

Renal ectopia is defined as the permanent malposition of the kidney outside its normal lumbar site; it is seen in about 1 in 800 radiological examinations of the kidney, and may affect one or both kidneys, or a solitary kidney in unilateral renal agenesis. It is slightly more common in females and on the left side.

During its development, the metanephros ascends to its ultimate level (between the 12th thoracic and 3rd lumbar vertebrae). This apparent upward migration is largely due to differential growth of the caudal part of the embryo, and is accompanied by medial rotation of the kidney so that the hilus and renal pelvis, which are at first located anteriorly, come to lie on the anteromedial aspect. Interference with, or arrest of, this process results in an abnormal position and often in an abnormal shape of one or both kidneys, or to their fusion across the midline. Rarely, ectopic kidneys undergo reversed rotation so that the renal pelvis is located on the outer (lateral) border of the kidney, and exceptionally rotation through 180° occurs so that the pelvis points posteriorly. There are reports of ectopic kidneys located higher than normal, even in the thorax in association with a diaphragmatic defect (Hill and Bunts 1960).

Ectopic kidneys are most commonly found at the pelvic brim or in the pelvic cavity. They are usually

the innermost nephron in the chain is one of those formed during the first phase when the ureteric bud was branching.

After about 22 weeks' gestation, the ampullae advance outwards beyond the point where nephron arcades are formed, and subsequently new nephrons are added singly. At this stage the nephrons become attached just behind the zone of active ampullary growth, and are not, therefore, carried outwards as the ampullae advance. By 36 weeks, ampullary growth and new nephron induction cease (Fig. 8.2).

Individual nephrons form from oval condensations of metanephric blastema, which rapidly develop a lumen that elongates and becomes S-shaped. The

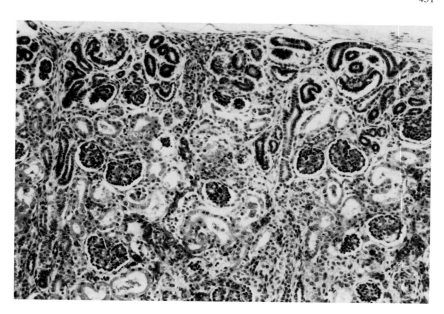

Fig. 8.2. Subcapsular "nephrogenic zone" in the outer cortex of a premature infant. (H&E, × 80)

malrotated with the renal pelvis pointing forward, are rounded or lobulated rather than reniform, and have an ectopic blood supply. Commonly a number of small arteries supply the kidney rather than a single large renal artery; these arise from the aorta near the bifurcation, or from the iliac arteries. It is not uncommon for ectopic kidneys to exhibit parenchymal maldifferentiation (renal dysplasia), and distortion or kinking of the renal pelvis may cause hydronephrosis predisposing to renal infection. Pelvic ectopia is sometimes associated with anorectal anomalies, particularly rectal atresia, or with congenital absence or atresia of the vagina in females (Dretler et al. 1971).

Crossed Ectopia

Occasionally, ectopic kidneys occur on the opposite side to the ureteric orifice, the ureter crossing the midline. Both kidneys are thus located on the same side of the body and may be fused. This is a rare anomaly, with an incidence of approximately 1 in 8000. The displaced kidney may lie behind the aorta or vena cava.

"Horseshoe" and "Doughnut" Kidney

Fusion of the two kidneys across the midline can be regarded as a form of renal ectopia. Most commonly fusion of the lower poles occurs to produce the horseshoe kidney (Fig. 8.3); the incidence of this condition on radiological examination is about 1 in 600. Ring or doughnut kidneys fused at both poles are much rarer. The fused mass of renal tissue may be palpable as an apparently pulsatile mass on account of the underlying aorta, thus giving rise to a mistaken diagnosis of an aneurysm. There is an elevated incidence of renal fusion in Turner's syndrome and in association with other congenital urogenital anomalies. In the horseshoe kidney the renal pelves are generally sited anteriorly with high ureteropelvic junctions that may give rise to hydronephrosis. Occasionally there is associated ureteric duplication or ectopia, and rarely part or all of the horseshoe kidney is dysplastic.

Renal Agenesis

Complete absence of the kidney may be unilateral or bilateral. In the latter case the lesion is incompatible with life, although the affected infant may live for a few days after birth. Bilateral agenesis is associated with a syndrome of defects (Potter 1946), including pulmonary hypoplasia, bow legs, low-set ears, receding chin and a beak-like nose (Fig. 8.4) attributed to the oligohydramnios associated with this condition (Fantel and Shepard 1975). By consideration of the other congenital abnormalities in the lower end of the body that may accompany it, renal agenesis is seen as a developmental field defect of varying extent. Anomalies may be confined to the kidney and ureter, usually together with those of mesonephric and paramesonephric derivatives (absence of vas deferens and seminal vesicles, and maldevelopment of testis in

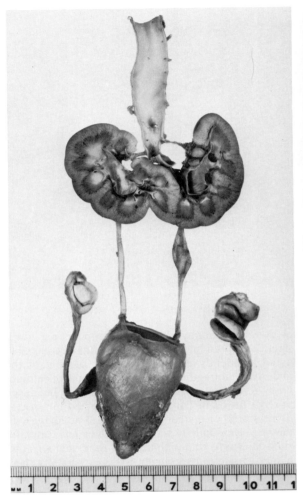

Fig. 8.3. Horseshoe kidney with fusion of the lower poles.

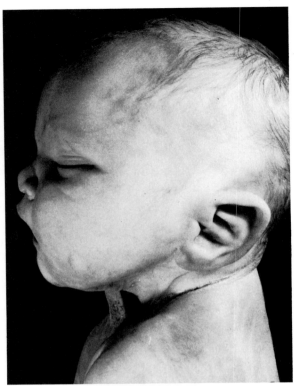

Fig. 8.4. Potter facies. Note the low-set ears, slightly receding chin and beak-like nose.

males; abnormalities or absence of Fallopian tubes, uterine horns and upper vagina in females; Fig 8.5). In these instances associated renal agenesis is more commonly unilateral, but if the field defect is more extensive, renal agenesis is usually bilateral. Associated abnormalities may then include anomalies of the hind-gut and cloacal membrane, and in the most extreme examples the field defect involves the whole caudal end of the embryo (sirenomelia or the caudal regression syndrome). In the former there is fusion of the posterior limb buds and in the latter absence of the hind-gut, sacrum, urethra and external genitalia; accompanying renal agenesis is invariably bilateral. In a proportion of such cases, the bladder, urethra and external genitalia fail to develop. The adrenals are disc-shaped because of the lack of moulding by the kidney, and in a small number of cases the gland fails

to develop. Major anomalies of other systems are common, and in unilateral agenesis are the usual reason for clinical presentation.

Based on autopsy studies, bilateral renal agenesis has an incidence of about 1 in 4000, and unilateral agenesis of about 1 in 1000 births. Males are affected about twice as often as females. The corresponding ureter and trigonal area of the bladder are usually absent, but occasionally a short stump of a lower ureter can be identified. Studies of arsenate-induced renal agenesis in the rat (Burk and Beaudoin 1977) indicate that the lesion is caused by failure of the mesonephric duct to give rise to the ureteric bud, with subsequent failure of induction of the meta-nephric blastema.

Hereditary Renal Adysplasia

Renal adysplasia is a term used to describe unilateral renal agenesis combined with dysplasia of the con-

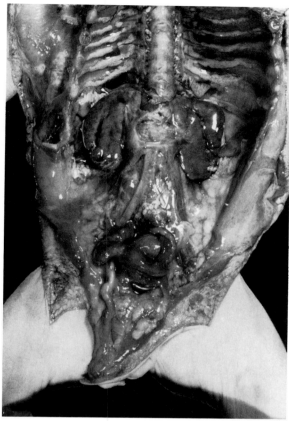

Fig. 8.5. Renal agenesis. Note the disc-shaped adrenals, absent kidneys and ureters and the anomaly of the female genital tract (bicornuate uterus).

tralateral kidney. Hereditary renal adysplasia has a slightly different connotation and refers to renal agenesis and renal dysplasia (unilateral or bilateral) together with renal adysplasia in any combination, affecting different members of the same family (Delver et al. 1974; Schimke and King 1980).

A familial tendency for bilateral renal agenesis has been recognized for many years (Rizza and Dowling 1971), and more recently for hereditary adysplasia (as described above). In this condition, the index case usually has bilateral renal agenesis discovered at necropsy. Other family members are then shown to have unilateral agenesis or dysplasia. Other siblings or different generations of the family may be affected. Bilateral agenesis as part of familial adysplasia is not associated with sirenomelia or caudal regression; dysplastic kidneys are usually tiny and rudimentary (renal aplasia) or occasionally multicystic (Squiers et al. 1987). Unilateral involvement in females is often associated with absence of the ipsilateral ovary or Fallopian tube. The mode of inheri-

tance in familial adysplasia has been reported as autosomal dominant (Buchta et al. 1973), but cases of agenesis/dysplasia affecting siblings with normal parents indicate that other types of inheritance may be involved.

Supernumerary Kidneys

"Extra" kidneys are extremely rare, and precise diagnosis requires complete separation of two kidneys on the affected side of the body with separate pelvicalyceal systems. The draining ureters may fuse or join the bladder separately.

Renal Hypoplasia and Dysplasia

Normally, renal growth is allometric, i.e. there is a close correlation between body size and renal weight. Table 8.1 shows the mean normal kidney weights at various ages up to 12 years, derived from the studies of Coppoletta and Wolbach (1933), whose findings are in striking agreement with those of Landing and Hughes (1962). Similar correlations exist between renal mass and body surface area (Risdon 1975).

Renal hypoplasia can thus be defined as a condition in which the kidney is congenitally small (i.e. more than 2 SD below the expected mean). In practice, however, this definition may be very difficult to apply: kidneys may be shrunken as a result of acquired disease, and congenitally small kidneys may be prone to acquired injuries, such as pyelonephritis or hydronephrosis, which will mask the underlying developmental anomaly.

The majority of congenitally small kidneys also show microscopic evidence of anomalous metanephric differentiation, often associated with cyst formation. These are currently described as dysplastic kidneys. The term renal hypoplasia should thus be retained for cases where the kidney is abnormal only in terms of its overall size, number of nephrons and perhaps its number of lobules (reniculi). Boissonnat (1962) has shown that normal kidneys possess ten or more lobes, whereas hypoplastic kidneys usually have five or fewer, and occasionally only one (so-called unirenicular hypoplasia). Reduced renal size has also been ascribed to hypoplasia on the basis of finding a small narrow (hypoplastic) main renal artery. This is not a reliable criterion, because atrophy of the renal artery may occur in any long-standing disease, causing marked reduction in parenchymal mass. However, Portsman (1970) has suggested that, when the renal artery is narrowed in acquired disease, it retains a wide funnel-shaped

Table 8.1. Mean normal kidney weights at various ages from birth to 12 years

Age	Renal weight (g)		
	Right	Left	Combined
Birth to 3 days	13	14	27
3– 7 days	14	14	28
1– 3 weeks	15	15	30
3– 5 weeks	16	16	32
5– 7 weeks	19	18	37
7– 9 weeks	19	18	37
9–13 weeks	20	19	39
– 4 months	22	21	43
– 5 months	25	25	50
– 6 months	26	25	51
– 7 months	30	30	60
– 8 months	31	30	61
– 9 months	31	30	61
–10 months	32	31	63
–11 months	34	33	67
–12 months	36	35	71
–14 months	36	35	71
–16 months	39	39	78
–18 months	40	43	83
–20 months	43	44	87
–22 months	44	44	88
–24 months	47	46	93
– 3 years	48	49	97
– 4 years	58	56	114
– 5 years	65	64	129
– 6 years	68	67	135
– 7 years	69	70	139
– 8 years	74	75	149
– 9 years	82	83	165
–10 years	92	95	187
–11 years	95	96	189
–12 years	95	96	191

Data from Coppoletta and Wolbach (1933).

segment near its origin from the aorta as an indication of its previously normal overall calibre.

Simple hypoplasia is very rare and usually bilateral. Extreme degrees of bilateral renal hypoplasia are encountered in the condition *oligoméganéphronie* (oligonephronic hypoplasia) described by Royer et al. (1962). The kidneys are extremely small (with combined weights of as little as 20 g) and are usually unirenicular or birenicular. The number of nephrons in the kidneys is greatly reduced, and those present are enlarged and hypertrophied. Cross-sectional areas of glomeruli are increased some 12 times, and microdissection studies show marked hypertrophy and hyperplasia of the proximal convoluted tubules, whose mean length is four times the normal length and whose mean volume is approximately 17 times normal (Fetterman and Habib 1969). Children with oligonephronic hypoplasia suffer from impaired renal function with polyuria, polydipsia, dehydration, anaemia and growth failure. The ureters and lower urinary tract are usually normal in reported cases, and familial incidence has not been observed. Royer et al.

(1962) have described the gradual development of segmental and global glomerulosclerosis, tubular atrophy and interstitial fibrosis in oligonephronic hypoplasia, and McGraw et al. (1984) have noted the development of increasing proteinuria with the development of renal failure. These clinical and histological findings parallel in many respects those seen experimentally in the remnant kidney model (Hostetter et al. 1981; Olson et al. 1982; Rennke 1984; Shimamura and Morrison 1975).

Much less severe degrees of bilateral hypoplasia have been described in association with congenital anomalies or with long-standing disease of the central nervous system (Bernstein and Meyer 1964; Roosen-Runge 1949).

Unilateral simple hypoplasia (i.e. without evidence of dysplasia) is extremely rare, and one of the few acceptable cases in the literature is that described by Bernstein and Meyer (1972). However, ectopic kidneys may be smaller than expected even in the absence of dysplasia; this may be related to their abnormal blood supply.

Segmental Hypoplasia (Ask-Upmark Kidney)

The term "segmental hypoplasia" refers to a particular type of small kidney associated with hypertension in childhood (Ask-Upmark 1929). The condition may be unilateral or bilateral and is characterized by reduced renal size and the presence of a transverse groove on the capsular surface, classically near the upper pole, overlying an area of marked parenchymal thinning and an elongated calyx-like recess arising from the renal pelvis (Fig. 8.6a). In the area of parenchymal thinning glomeruli are very sparse or absent and tubules are markedly atrophic (Fig. 8.6b). Meshes of thick-walled blood vessels are apparent in the atrophic area, and Ljungqvist and Largergren (1963) describe the vascular arrangement as both cortical and medullary in type, although the medullary portion is greatly reduced. Interpretations of this lesion have varied. Although Royer et al. (1971) consider the segmental areas to be developmental abnormalities, it is difficult to exclude the possibility of acquired disease. Differences in the reported incidence of the condition in different countries (it appears to be much commoner in France than in the UK and the USA) also suggests differences in interpretation. It is of interest that vesicoureteric reflux is a relatively commonly associated abnormality, and it is highly likely that many cases previously interpreted as segmental hypoplasia are in fact examples of reflux nephropathy (see chronic pyelonephritis, p. 493).

In the reported cases of Ask-Upmark kidney, severe arterial hypertension has been the chief clin-

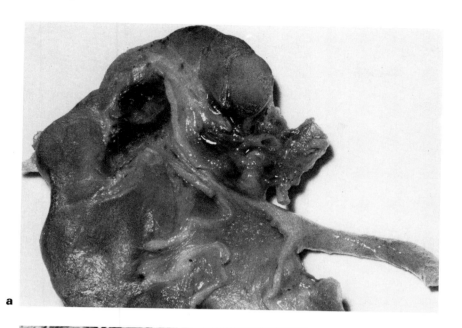

a

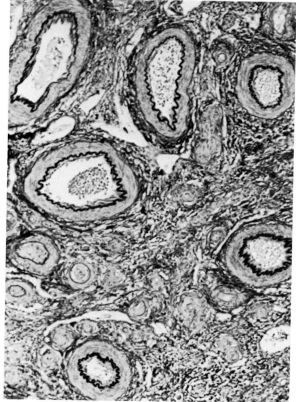

b

Fig. 8.6. The Ask-Upmark kidney in a 10-year-old girl with a history of vesicoureteric reflux, urinary infection and hypertension. **a** Club-shaped upper pole calyx with thinning of the overlying cortex. **b** Tubular loss and glomerular sclerosis with prominent thick-walled arteries. (Elastin/van Gieson, × 300) (Reproduced from Risdon et al. 1975, by permission of the Editor of *Pediatric Radiology*.)

ical abnormality. In unilateral cases, nephrectomy occasionally relieves hypertension, but often fails to do so.

Renal Dysplasia

Renal dysplasia is a developmental abnormality of the kidney resulting from anomalous metanephric differentiation (Risdon 1971a, b). The condition is recognized histologically by disorganization of the renal parenchyma, by the presence of abnormally developed immature nephronic and ductal structures resembling those found during fetal life, and sometimes by cyst formation. These changes may involve the whole kidney, or they may affect the organ only focally or segmentally, so that part of the parenchyma is normal (Risdon 1971a, b). Affected kidneys may be distorted, and if cyst formation is marked they can be larger than expected. A wide variety of macroscopical appearances is thus encountered, and simple hypoplasia and cystic disease of the kidneys may have to be considered in the differential diagnosis.

It is clear that a precise diagnosis of renal dysplasia can only be made on histological grounds, by recognizing the various immature structures that suggest embryonic maldevelopment. The most important of these are *primitive ducts* (Ericsson and Ivemark 1958a, b), which are tubular structures lined with columnar and sometimes ciliated epithelium, surrounded by mantles of cellular mesenchyme in which

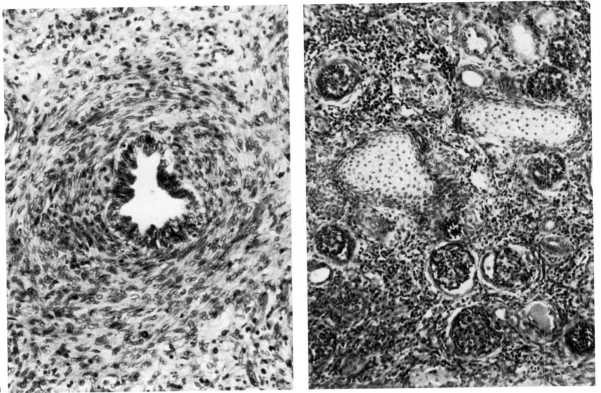

a
b

Fig. 8.7. Renal dysplasia. **a** Primitive duct lined by columnar epithelium and surrounded by mesenchymal cells. (H&E, × 300) **b** Primitive glomeruli and bars of metaplastic cartilage. (H&E, × 100) (Reproduced from Risdon 1971a, by permission of the Editor of the *Journal of Clinical Pathology.*)

smooth muscle can sometimes be demonstrated (Fig. 8.7a). These are regarded as persistent derivatives of the ureteric bud. Bars of metaplastic cartilage, thought to represent aberrant differentiation of the metanephric blastema (Bigler and Killingworth 1949), are also important markers of renal dysplasia (Fig. 8.7b). Other immature nephronic and tubular structures are encountered, including primitive glomeruli with prominent layers of cuboidal cells enveloping the tuft and primitive tubules lined with low cuboidal epithelial cells with darkly basophilic nuclei. Multiple, often fibrous-walled, cysts are present in variable numbers, but these are not confined to renal dysplasia and are a frequent finding in other congenital and some acquired conditions of the kidney (Ekström 1955; Baxter 1961; Elkin and Bernstein 1969; Bernstein 1971). Immature glomeruli and tubules may also occur in acquired renal disease, e.g. infections, ischaemia, or in scars resulting from renal biopsy (Bernstein 1968). It follows that the findings of primitive ducts and metaplastic cartilage are the only features peculiar to renal dysplasia, and a histological diagnosis of this condition should be

confined to cases in which one or other of these elements is recognized.

The diagnosis of renal dysplasia is helped by the recognition that the renal parenchymal maldevelopment is almost always associated with other congenital abnormalities of the ureter or of the lower urinary tract – ureteric reduplication, ureteric ectopia, and ureterocele or posterior urethral valves (Rubenstein et al. 1961). For this reason, dysplasia is best regarded as an anomaly of the whole urinary tract and not solely of the kidney. Classification of the various types of dysplasia can then be based not just on the presence or extent of any renal parenchymal maldevelopment, but rather on the pattern of the coexisting urinary tract abnormalities (Risdon et al. 1975). This is important because the clinical outcome, in terms both of likely complications, such as infection and hydronephrosis, and of the probable success of surgical treatment, depends largely on the type of urinary tract abnormality present. It is also true that in a minority of individual examples of complex dysplastic anomalies, such as ectopic ureterocele, definite dysplastic markers in the kidney may be inapparent

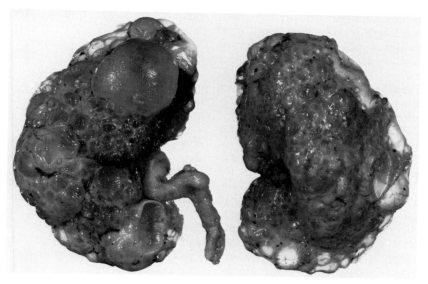

Fig. 8.8. Multicystic dysplastic kidney with atretic ureter.

or masked by acquired disease. However, because these cases are indistinguishable in other respects, separate classification of them appears illogical.

The frequent coexistence of renal dysplasia with other urinary tract anomalies has led to the concept that the metanephric maldevelopment results from urinary obstruction or vesicoureteric reflux operating from the early phases of organogenesis (Bialestock 1965). Microdissection studies of grossly cystic dysplastic kidneys (Osthanondh and Potter 1964) reveal diminished branching of the ureteric bud, often with failure of nephron induction and cystic dilatation of the ureteric bud branches. However, it is apparent that severe bilateral dysplasia can occur in the absence of urinary obstruction as occurs, for example, in diffuse cystic dysplasia associated with syndromes of multiple congenital abnormalities; in these cases other factors are clearly important. It is also possible that ureteric atresia accompanying multicystic renal dysplasia may be a secondary consequence of a lack of urine flow from a non-functioning kidney, rather than a primary obstructive event. Stephens and coworkers (Heneberry and Stephens 1980; Mackie and Stevens 1975; Schwarz et al. 1981) have produced an alternative hypothesis relating renal maldevelopment (dysplasia) to the position of the ureteric orifice on the bladder trigone as an indication of ectopic origin of the ureteric bud from the mesonephric duct. These authors consider that normal metanephric differentiation occurs only when the ureteric bud impinges on the metanephric blastema at the correct point of contact. Should it arise too far caudally (ectopic orifice in the bladder neck, urethra or vagina) or too far cranially (laterally ectopic orifice in the bladder), anomalous metanephric differentiation may occur.

Renal dysplasia can be classified as follows:

1. Multicystic and aplastic dysplasia
2. Hypodysplasia (hypoplastic dysplasia)
3. Dysplasia in duplex systems:
   a) Ectopic ureterocele
   b) Lower pole dysplasia
4. Dysplasia with congenital lower urinary tract obstruction:
   a) Posterior urethral valves
   b) Urethral atresia
   c) Prune belly and megacystis – megaureter syndromes
5. Diffuse cystic dysplasia:
   a) In hereditary and multiple anomaly syndromes
   b) Sporadic
6. Hereditary renal adysplasia (see p. 452)
7. Dysplasia with vesicoureteric reflux

Multicystic and Aplastic Dysplasia. Multicystic and aplastic dysplastic kidneys form a continuum. The multicystic kidney is the best recognized clinically; it is enlarged, sometimes weighing several hundred grams, and is grossly cystic with an irregular outline (Fig. 8.8). The largest cysts are usually immediately beneath the capsule, and the renal pelvis and calyces are absent or severely attenuated. Aplastic kidneys are extremely small, functionless, rudimentary organs consisting of a tiny cluster of cysts or a small nubbin of grossly dysplastic renal tissue. In both varieties the draining ureter is atretic for part (usually the upper part) or all of its length, or less commonly it is absent. In some cases vesicoureteric reflux occurs into the distal patent segment of the ureter, which can then appear dilated.

Renal dysplasia of these types may be unilateral or bilateral. In bilateral multicystic or aplastic kidneys the renal maldevelopment is so gross as to be incompatible with life, and the clinical presentation is like that of renal agenesis. Although ureteric atresia has been considered to be universal in multicystic kidneys, it is not uncommon in bilateral disease for the ureters to be patent although hypoplastic. Distinction from polycystic disease is important in such cases, because the genetic implications are quite different. Unilateral multicystic and aplastic kidneys are slightly more common in males than in females, and the left kidney is slightly more frequently affected than the right. Standard intravenous urography shows no excretion of contrast medium on the affected side, although occasionally the lower ureter is visualized by reflux of contrast from the bladder. High-dose excretion urography may demonstrate opacification of the more solid portions of the kidney with outlining of the cysts (Warshawsky et al. 1977).

On the whole, unilateral multicystic or aplastic kidneys have a good prognosis. However, Pathak and Williams (1963) have emphasized that unilateral multicystic kidneys are not uncommonly associated with stenosis of the contralateral ureter, either at the pelviureteric junction or elsewhere along its length. This may be associated with hydronephrosis or infection of the remaining functioning kidney, so that early radiological recognition and surgical treatment of this condition are imperative. A similar association with contralateral ureteric stenosis may occur in unilateral small dysplastic and aplastic kidneys. Unilateral multicystic kidneys presenting as a loin mass in a young infant or neonate may be misdiagnosed as a congenital nephroblastoma. In fact congenital Wilms' tumours are extremely rare, if they occur at all (see p. 879), and with this presentation the multicystic kidney is a far more likely diagnosis.

The introduction of fetal ultrasonography as a means of diagnosis in utero has led to some interesting insights into these conditions. Serial examinations in fetuses with unilateral multicystic kidneys have shown that the size and configuration of the cysts may alter (Hashimoto et al. 1986; Avni et al. 1987) and occasionally the whole cystic mass may apparently disappear (Pedicelli et al. 1986). It is unlikely that the whole kidney really regresses, so it seems likely that what appears to be an aplastic kidney postnatally may, in some cases at least, be a multicystic kidney in utero. This further supports the concept that multicystic and aplastic kidneys are closely related

and are similar expressions of gross dysplastic renal development.

With these varieties of dysplasia there is a greater-than-chance association with major anomalies in other systems. These include ventricular septal defect, preductal aortic coarctation, duodenal, oesophageal and rectal atresia, the Arnold–Chiari malformation and meningomyelocele.

Hypoplastic Dysplasia (Hypodysplasia). Hypoplastic dysplastic kidneys have a variety of appearances and associated ureteric abnormalities. They are small, their weights falling in the hypoplastic range of less than 2 SD below the expected mean, and they may be misshapen or partly cystic. The distinguishing feature is that at least some normally differentiated parenchyma is present, and so, at least initially, some functional activity and ability to excrete urine is retained. Some degree of normal lobation and corticomedullary demarcation is visible, and dysplastic development is generally more apparent in the medulla. This often contains primitive ducts that radiate from poorly differentiated papillae in a "delta-like" fashion. Cortical dysplasia is variable, although primitive ducts, immature nephronic structures and sometimes metaplastic cartilage may be seen. Sometimes dysplastic development may be minimal, and it is these kidneys that in the past have been labelled merely "hypoplastic". Cystic change is variable in extent, but when marked may lead to confusion with the multicystic kidney, particularly now that some such kidneys are first recognized by fetal ultrasonography. The important distinctions are that in hypoplastic dysplasia the ureter is patent, some pelvicalyceal development is seen and some functional parenchyma is present.

The associated ureteric abnormalities include ureteric dilatation and tortuosity, ectopic insertion of the ureter and sometimes a ureterocele. Infrequently the ureter may be normal. The pelvicalyceal system is usually poorly formed but may be dilated.

When the ureter is dilated vesicoureteric reflux may be present (see Renal Dysplasia and Vesicoureteric Reflux, p. 460).

Because the ureteric anomalies may be obstructive or associated with reflux, hydronephrosis and chronic pyelonephritis are frequent complications and the resulting inflammatory and regressive changes in the kidney may mask or overshadow evidence of dysplastic development. Primitive delta-like medullary ducts are useful in confirming dysplasia in these cases, although when hydronephrosis is marked confirmation may be difficult. In pure hydronephrosis, however, medullary thinning is generally more extreme than cortical thinning, whereas the reverse is usually true in hypodysplasia.

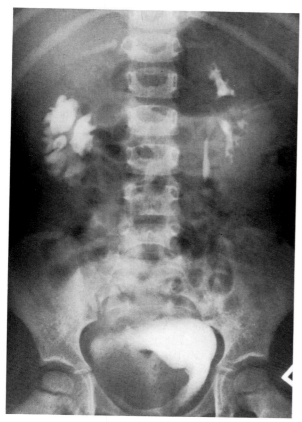

Fig. 8.9. Intravenous urogram from a child with ectopic uretero-cele. Note the absence of excretion by the dysplastic right upper pole, the filling defect in the bladder, caused by ureterocele, and the dilatation of the right lower pole calyces caused by obstruction of the lower pole ureter by a ureterocele. (Reproduced from Risdon et al. 1975, by permission of the Editor of *Pediatric Radiology*.)

Dysplasia in Duplex Systems. Duplex kidney with ectopic ureterocele (Fig. 8.9) is a complex anomaly in which the dysplastic upper pole of a double kidney is drained by a separate renal pelvis and ureter inserted ectopically at its lower end. Here it forms a cystic swelling, or ureterocele, which bulges into the bladder. The upper pole ureteric orifice is usually beneath the internal sphincter at the bladder neck or in the upper urethra; the lower pole ureter is inserted separately in the normal position in the trigone. The upper pole ureter is nearly always obstructed, tortu-ous and dilated, and the dysplastic upper pole of the kidney is hydronephrotic. The ureterocele at the insertion of the upper pole ureter is not invariably present.

The lesion can be unilateral or bilateral; in the former instance there is a tendency for the right side to be affected more often than the left. In about 10% of cases the double kidney is bilateral, but in most cases the ureters on the contralateral side join together and have a single, normal insertion. The full ectopic ureterocele is seldom bilateral. Ectopic urete-rocele is six times commoner in females than in males. Patients with this condition usually present with recurrent urinary tract infections, and sometimes with dribbling incontinence resulting either from the ectopic ureter or from cystitis. Occasionally the urete-rocele obstructs both the lower pole and the upper pole ureters. The results of surgery are generally good.

Much less commonly a duplex kidney exhibits dysplasia of the lower rather than the upper pole. Such kidneys have double ureters, both of which are inserted into the trigone. The lower pole ureter, which is tortuous, dilated and subject to vesi-coureteric reflux, is inserted *above* the upper pole ureter in the trigone (Williams 1962).

Renal Dysplasia and Lower Urinary Tract Ob-struction. Congenital lower urinary tract obstruction occurs most commonly in infant boys with posterior urethral valves (Fig. 8.10). Other causes include urethral atresia, the prune belly syndrome (Duckett 1980) and the megacystis–megaureter syndrome (Paquin et al. 1960), in which bilateral hydronephro-sis with gross vesicoureteric reflux and bladder dis-tension occur in the absence of anatomical bladder outlet obstruction. With posterior urethral valves, obstruction produces bilateral hydronephrosis, hydroureters and bladder hypertrophy. Renal dyspla-sia is common in individuals with severe obstruction who present in the neonatal period, but is not seen in patients whose obstruction is less complete and who present later. Dysplastic changes and cyst formation are often most prominent in the outer cortex and involve the nephrons that develop last.

Cystic change, when present, is usually confined to the outer cortex, but can be more extensive. In these instances the macroscopic appearances resemble those in diffuse cystic dysplasia. Renal papillae are poorly formed or completely effaced and medullary dysplasia with a delta-like radiating configuration of primitive ducts is usual.

The ureters are thick walled, tortuous and often have laterally displaced, open ureteric orifaces subject to vesicoureteric reflux in about 80% of cases.

Often the extent of hydronephrotic atrophy and dysplastic development varies on the two sides, and this appears to relate to the degree of vesicoureteric reflux that is correspondingly asymmetrical. Hoover and Duckett (1982) described patients with posterior urethral valves and unilateral vesicoureteric reflux in whom renal dysplasia was confined to the refluxing side. Posterior urethral valves are now frequently diagnosed in utero by fetal ultrasonography that

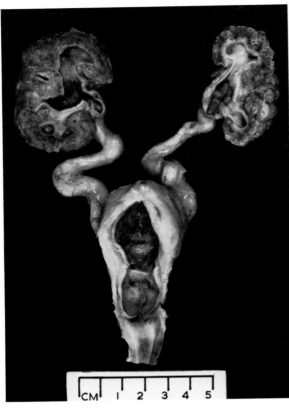

Fig. 8.10. Bilateral hydronephrosis and hydroureters with cysts in the outer renal cortex caused by posterior urethral valves. A staghorn calculus is visible in the renal pelvis on the left side. (Reproduced from Risdon 1971b, by permission of the Editor of the *Journal of Clinical Pathology*.)

demonstrates bilateral hydronephrosis and bladder distension which persists in serial scans.

In patients with the "prune belly" syndrome (congenital absence of the anterior abdominal wall musculature with wrinkling of the overlying skin; Williams and Burkholder (1967), similar bilateral hydroureters and bladder hypertrophy may occur, although mechanical lower urinary tract obstruction can seldom be demonstrated. These patients are almost exclusively male; their kidneys commonly exhibit severe renal dysplasia and the testes fail to descend.

Diffuse Cystic Dyplasia. In this condition both kidneys are symmetrically enlarged with diffuse parenchymal cystic change. The whole cortex is replaced by small rounded cysts of a few millimetres diameter. Nephronic structures are extremely sparse, but some cysts can be identified as dilated glomeruli or tubules. Connective tissue between the cysts is increased, but metaplastic cartilage is distinctly

uncommon. The medullary pyramids are poorly formed and dysplastic with scanty primitive ducts radially orientated. The pelvicalyceal system is not defined, but the ureter is patent though thin and the bladder often hypoplastic.

Diffuse cystic dysplasia is distinguished from bilateral multicystic kidneys by the uniform and generally smaller size of the cysts and the patency of the ureters. Separation from autosomal recessive polycystic kidneys is easily achieved by microscopic examination and by the retention of a reniform shape and renal lobation, together with the tendency of kidneys to collapse on cutting as fluid drains from the cysts in the latter condition.

Although distinctly rare and occasionally sporadic, the importance of diffuse cystic dysplasia lies in its association with multiple hereditaary syndromes of multiple congenital abnormalities (Bernstein and Kissare 1973; Bernstein et al. 1974). The best known of these are Meckel's syndrome (Opitz and Howe 1969) of microcephaly and posterior encephalocele associated with polydactyly, cleft palate and lip, and genital anomalies, together with its variants (Bernstein 1976). Others include the Zellweger (Smith et al. 1976), Jeune (Bernstein 1976), oral–facial–digital (Stapleton et al. 1982) and trisomy D (Mottet and Jensen 1965) syndromes.

Renal Dysplasia and Vesicoureteric Reflux. The close association between vesicoureteric reflux and renal scarring is encompassed by the term "reflux nephropathy" (Bailey 1973), and is further discussed on p. 493. Much of the research on this subject has centred on the concept that vesicoureteric reflux and the associated phenomenon of intrarenal reflux are vital factors in the development of acquired segmental renal scarring either by the introduction of pathogenic organisms into the kidney or by hydrodynamic effects alone. However, it is important to recognize that both vesicoureteric reflux and renal dysplasia represent aspects of abnormal development of the urinary tract and, therefore, commonly coexist. Thus some 10% of scarred kidneys associated with vesicoureteric reflux also exhibit histological evidence of dysplastic maldevelopment. The advent of fetal ultrasonography has allowed earlier recognition of some cases of vesicoureteric reflux by demonstrating hydronephrosis in utero and confirming the presence of vesicoureteric reflux in the early postpartum period. Reflux nephropathy identified in infancy is often bilateral and associated with gross vesicoureteric reflux; unlike cases diagnosed later, the incidence in males is much higher and a substantial portion of cases have evidence of renal dysplasia (Risdon et al. 1993). Whether vesicoureteric reflux and renal dysplasia are separate, causally unrelated expressions of abnormal development, remains to be elucidated.

Cystic Diseases of the Kidney

Renal cysts occur under a wide variety of circumstances. They may be unilateral or bilateral, affect part or all of the kidney, and involve the renal cortex, medulla or both.

Particularly when multiple, cysts are often regarded as evidence of anomalous development, but it is now recognized that cystic dilatation is frequently a secondary change, which can occur in any part of a normally differentiated nephron or collecting duct. Renal cysts occur under a wide variety of circumstances and the cause is usually unknown. The concept that cystic change is merely a manifestation of what is vaguely described as polycystic disease is evidently an oversimplification. A number of different varieties of cystic kidney can be distinguished by their clinical presentations and pathological characteristics, and as some types are heritable their accurate diagnosis is important for genetic counselling purposes. Renal cystic disease can be classified as follows:

1. Polycystic disease:
   a) Autosomal dominant polycystic kidney disease (ADPKD):
      i) In adults and older children (classic form)
      ii) In infants (glomerulocystic disease)
   b) Autosomal recessive polycystic kidney disease (ARPKD):
      i) In newborn and young infants (classic form)
      ii) In older children and adults with congenital hepatic fibrosis
2. Simple cysts
3. Acquired cystic disease
4. Localized cystic disease
5. Medullary cystic disease:
   a) Medullary sponge kidney
   b) Familial nephronophthisis – medullary cystic disease (FN-MCD)
6. Renal dysplasia (see p. 455)
7. Glomerulocystic disease
8. Renal cysts in hereditary syndromes:
   a) Tuberose sclerosis
   b) Von Hippel–Lindau syndrome
   c) Diffuse cystic dysplasia (see p. 460)
9. Multilocular renal cysts

Renal Dysplasia

Cystic change is common in renal dysplasia and may be the dominant pathological finding. The multicystic dysplastic kidney is the variety of renal dysplasia most likely to be confused with polycystic disease. Unilateral multicystic dysplasia should present no problems, because true polycystic disease is invariably bilateral. Bilateral multicystic kidneys are recognized histologically by the presence of dysplastic elements (see p. 455).

Polycystic Disease

Polycystic kidney diseases encompass two genetically distinct disorders in which cystic change involves both kidneys diffusely. The more common, autosomal dominant polycystic kidney disease (ADPKD), generally affects adults (adult polycystic disease) and the less common, autosomal recessive polycystic kidney disease (ARPKD), usually affects infants (infantile polycystic disease). Because the infantile form may be recognized in older children and even adults, and the adult form may be diagnosed occasionally in infants, the older terms of "adult" and "infantile" polycystic disease are being superseded by the less committed terms ADPKD and ARPKD, which are more specific in terms of inheritance.

Autosomal Dominant Polycystic Kidney Disease

ADPKD has an incidence of about 1 in 1000 of the general population (Iglesias et al. 1983) and is said to be less common in blacks than in Caucasians (Torres et al. 1985). Its autosomal dominant inheritance was confirmed by Cairns (1925) and Dalgaard (1957). Hatfield and Pfister (1972) noted that the expected family history was not obtained in over 25% of cases; varied explanations for this have been offered, such as inadequate communication between family members, failure to diagnose the condition in asymptomatic individuals and variable expressivity of the disease. Cam et al. (1989) have shown that asymptomatic patients represent a significant proportion of those with ADPKD; in many of these lifespan may be normal.

The abnormal gene associated with ADPKD has been found to be closely linked with the α-globin gene cluster and the phosphoglycolate phosphatase gene on the short arm of chromosome 16 (Reeders et al. 1985, 1986; Breuning et al. 1987). However, in some kindreds with ADPKD, linkage of the mutant gene to chromosome 16 has not been identified (Kimberling et al. 1988; Romeo et al. 1988) so that at

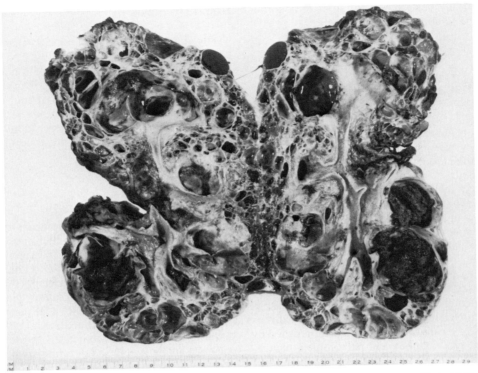

Fig. 8.11. Adult polycystic disease. The kidney weighed 800 g. Note the irregularly sized cysts, some filled with blood clot.

least two mutant genes exist for ADPKD, that on chromosome 16 being called *PCK1* and the less frequent one, unlinked to chromosome 16, being designated *PCK2*.

Typically, ADPKD presents clinically in the third, fourth or fifth decade with bilateral palpable loin masses, progressive renal failure, hypertension and a positive family history. Gross or microscopic haematuria is common. Without renal transplantation or dialysis, symptomatic patients rarely survive more than 3 years after diagnosis. In younger or asymptomatic patients the condition may be recognized by intravenous urography, ultrasonography or computed axial tomography, the latter being probably the best method (Levine and Grantham 1981). It has been claimed that a completely normal ultrasound examination in patients more than 20 years old virtually excludes the diagnosis (Bear et al. 1984). Ultrasonographic prenatal diagnosis has been reported (Zerres et al. 1982), and DNA analysis of a chorionic villous sample has confirmed the diagnosis in a 9 week fetus by demonstrating the same gene linkage as in other affected family members (Reeders et al. 1986).

In typical examples of ADPKD in adults the kidneys are enlarged (often grossly so) and their reniform shape is lost because of diffuse cystic change (Fig. 8.11). The cysts are usually spherical, unilocular and vary between a few millimetres and several centimetres in diameter. Haemorrhage within the cysts is common and renal infection may be a complication, particularly terminally. The development of new cysts seems unlikely, but gradual enlargement of those present is an integral part of disease progression. Quantitative studies such as those of Grantham et al. (1987) indicate that only 1% or 2% of nephrons are cystic, but microdissection (Osthanondh and Potter 1964) and lectin binding studies (Faraggiana et al. 1985) show that the cysts can arise in any part of the nephron or collecting system and usually retain luminal continuity with their tubules of origin. Histologically the cysts are generally lined by a single layer of epithelium, but focal hyperplasia and polypoid projections may be a feature (Gregoire et al. 1987). The largest cysts tend to be subcapsular and often have fibrous walls. Normal or atrophic renal parenchyma is present adjacent to the cysts.

In those unusual examples presenting at birth or in infancy, the kidneys are variably enlarged and glomerular cysts with dilatation of Bowman's space usually dominate the histological picture. ADPKD accounts for about half the cases of glomerulocystic disease seen in infancy (see p. 468).

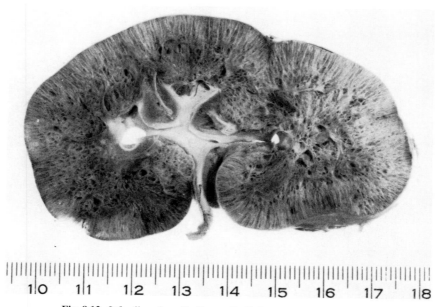

Fig. 8.12. Infantile polycystic disease: Radially aligned, fusiform cysts.

Cysts may be present in organs other than the kidneys in ADPKD. Cysts in the liver were demonstrated in 44% of patients with ADPKD in a study using computed tomography (Levine et al. 1985). These arise in portal tracts; they have thin fibrous walls and are lined by a single layer of flattened epithelium, but do not contain bile or communicate with bile ducts. Even when cysts are sufficiently extensive to cause hepatic enlargement, they do not interfere with liver function. They are uncommon in childhood but their frequency increases with age and these are almost always present in patients coming to renal transplantation. Cysts occur in the pancreas in about 10% of cases, and rare examples of cysts in the spleen, thyroid and seminal vesicles are recorded.

Vascular anomalies may also accompany ADPKD – most notably berry aneurysms of the cerebral arteries. Rupture of a berry aneurysm, particularly in hypertensive patients, is a common cause of death. Dissecting aneurysms, aortic root dilatation and mitral valvular disease are also reported. Diverticular disease of the colon is very common in ADPKD.

Autosomal Recessive Polycystic Kidney Disease

Although ARPKD is of more relevance in children, the overall incidence of this form of cystic disease is much less than that of the adult variety, affecting between 1 in 6000 and 1 in 14 000 live births.

Classically, the condition presents in infants who are stillborn or die in the neonatal period. Both kidneys are grossly enlarged, sometimes to a degree that causes difficulty during delivery. Despite their often huge size the kidneys retain their reniform shape, and fetal lobation is usually exaggerated. The pelvis, calyces and ureter are normal. The smooth renal surface is studded with innumerable small cysts of uniform size, which on cutting the kidney are seen as radially orientated fusiform or cylindrical dilatations throughout the cortex and medulla (Figs. 8.12 and 8.13a). Microdissection (Osthanondh and Potter 1964) and lectin-binding studies (Faraggiana et al. 1985) suggest that the disease is attributable to dilatation and hyperplasia of the interstitial portions of the branches of the ureteric bud, which form the collecting ducts. These branches retain their ability to induce nephron formation, and the number of nephrons appears to be normal.

Abnormalities of other systems are confined to the liver. In every case the intrahepatic bile ducts are increased in number in every portal tract and exhibit a curious angulated branching and occasionally cystic dilatation. This is associated with a varying degree of portal fibrosis, and the lesion is referred to as congenital hepatic fibrosis (Fig. 8.13b). Reconstructions of the bile duct anomaly in serial sections (Jørgensen 1972, 1973, 1974) show that the ducts form a ring of interconnecting sacs and cisterns at the edges of the portal zones, a configuration seen during develop-

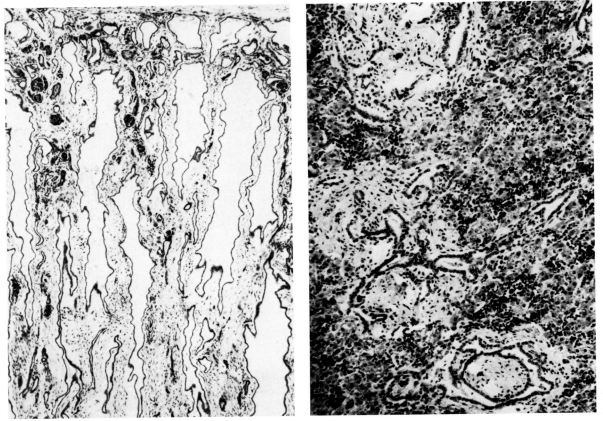

Fig. 8.13. a Infantile polycystic disease. The renal cysts are seen as a fusiform dilatation of collecting ducts. (H&E, × 25) **b** Liver in infantile polycystic disease. Note the angulated branching of bile ducts, which appear to run in the plane of the section, and the increase in portal fibrous tissue. (H&E, × 250)

ment of the bile duct system. The appearances seen in ARPKD are thus an apparent arrest of normal differentiation.

In the classic form of the disease, affected infants are usually anuric. This is difficult to explain, as there is no anatomical obstruction, and it is increasingly recognized that a minority of affected infants may survive into childhood with varying degrees of renal functional impairment.

Since the 1970s forms of ARPKD associated with congenital hepatic fibrosis occurring in older children and even adults have been documented. As the age of presentation increases, the relative degree of renal enlargement tends to be less, and cystic change less diffuse. In the liver, on the other hand, portal fibrosis tends to be more pronounced. Where it is marked, it may be accompanied by portal hypertension, splenomegaly and oesophageal varices, bleeding from which may be fatal. Sometimes there is non-obstructive cystic dilatation of the bile duct elements (so-called Caroli's disease), which may be compli-

cated by ascending cholangitis (Caroli et al. 1958; Mall et al. 1974). When hepatic fibrosis dominates, renal cystic change may be confined to ectasia of collecting ducts, giving a radiological appearance on intravenous urography indistinguishable from that of medullary sponge kidney (see p. 466; Reilly and Neuhauser 1960; Kerr et al. 1962).

Intermediate degrees of renal involvement are characterized by irregularly distributed, cystically dilated collecting ducts that are often rounded in shape and have fibrous walls. The intervening parenchyma may be partly normally differentiated or show interstitial fibrosis, glomerular obsolescence and tubular atrophy. The kidneys are often palpably enlarged and show a superficial resemblance to those seen in ADPKD, but are distinguished by the accompanying hepatic fibrosis and the degree of medullary duct ectasia.

Current concepts of ARPKD present a continuum of phenotypical expressions. At one end is the classic form, originally designated as infantile polycystic disease, in infants who are stillborn or die in the post-natal period from renal failure and pulmonary insufficiency. At the other end are older children or adults with portal hypertension and only mild renal involvement. Morphometric studies of the liver in ARPKD show that the degree of portal fibrosis is nearly twice as severe in patients presenting after the first year of life (Helczynski et al. 1984). Whether these differences reflect genetic distinctions, or whether relatively mild renal involvement and preservation of renal function allows gradual progression of the hepatic fibrosis until portal hypertension supervenes, remains unclear. The study of Blyth and Ockendon (1971) indicated that within a particular family the relative renal and hepatic involvement appeared to be constant, and on this basis the authors suggested that a number of mutant genes may operate. However, later studies (Chilton and Cremin 1981; Gang and Herrin 1986; Kaplan et al. 1988) suggest that the distinction is less clear, and that siblings do not necessarily express the same hepatic and renal involvement, or present at the same age.

It is important to realize that congenital hepatic fibrosis may occasionally accompany other types of autosomal recessive renal cystic disease, notably Meckel's syndrome, juvenile nephronophthisis (Delaney et al. 1978) and Jeune's thoracic dystrophy. It may even occur as an isolated, though probably familial, anomaly in as many as 50% of cases (Kissane 1976). However, mild degrees of accompanying renal cystic disease may be difficult to exclude.

Recently, the increasing use of fetal ultrasound has allowed prenatal diagnosis of ARPKD by the demonstration of enlarged hyperechogenic kidneys. However, the sonographic appearances may be impossible to distinguish from other forms of bilateral renal cystic disease (Habif et al. 1982) unless other siblings have been affected.

Simple Renal Cysts

One or more cysts can be found in the kidneys at necropsy in up to 50% of patients over the age of 50 years. Their comparative rarity in younger adults and children strongly supports the concept that they are acquired lesions. The cysts are usually cortical, often solitary, and they vary in size from a few millimetres to several centimetres in diameter. They can be unilocular or, less commonly, multilocular; they have a fibrous wall with a single lining layer of flattened epithelial cells.

Because of their frequency in arteriosclerotic or otherwise scarred kidneys, they have been thought to arise from local blockage of tubules or collecting ducts by local cicatrization. However, Fetterman (1970) noted small diverticula to arise on renal tubules with increasing frequency with advancing age. Baert and Steg (1977a, b) suggest that simple cysts may arise by closure of the connection between a diverticulum and its parent tubule, followed by gradual expansion of the diverticulum by fluid accumulation to form a cyst.

Occasionally simple cysts are sufficiently numerous and bilateral to pose problems of differentiation from ADPKD. Usually, the extent of the intervening solid parenchyma, the lack of a family history and the absence of hepatic cysts by ultrasonography or computed tomography in multiple simple cysts allow the distinction to be made, and advances in the development of markers for the ADPKD gene will probably solve the problem where doubt remains.

Acquired Cystic Disease

Dunnill et al. (1977) first drew attention to the fact that cystic change occurs in end-stage kidney disease in patients on long-term maintenance dialysis, and this finding has been amply confirmed in other studies (Grantham and Levine 1985; Hughson et al. 1986; Jabour et al. 1987). The frequency of this complication has varied widely in different reports, probably depending on the number of cysts a particular author requires to make the diagnosis. Thomson et al. (1986) noted an incidence of 63% when more than one cyst was present, of 39% when five or more cysts were seen and of 15% when more than 15 cysts were required.

Acquired cystic disease is also reported in patients on chronic peritoneal dialysis (Truong et al. 1988), and the frequency of this complication increases with the length of time on dialysis (Thomson et al. 1986). However, it is also seen in patients with end-stage renal disease who have not been dialysed (Narasimham et al. 1986), so that it is likely that the total duration of uraemia is the factor determining the development of cystic change.

The kidneys involved may be enlarged, of normal size or, more frequently, smaller than expected. The cysts are more frequent in the cortex but may involve the medulla. They vary in size from a few millimetres to 1–2 cm. They may arise from any portion of the tubules or collecting ducts and contain clear fluid, although sometimes haemorrhage occurs. They are lined generally by flattened epithelial cells, but occasionally epithelial hyperplasia and papillary infolding may occur. It is probable that this epithelial cell proliferation is a basis of the neoplastic changes that sometimes complicate acquired cystic disease (Hughson et al. 1980, 1986; Konishi et al. 1980). As well as the cystic changes, the kidneys exhibit glomerulosclerosis, tubulointerstitial changes, arterial intimal hyperplasia and crystalline oxalate deposits consistent with end-stage disease. Cyst formation may be a result of tubular blockage, interstitial scarring or epithelial hyperplasia. Saccular tubular diverticula have been demonstrated, so that mechanisms similar to those described in simple cyst formation (see above) may also operate.

Localized Cystic Disease

Cho et al. (1979) described three patients with renal cystic disease localized to part of one kidney. Two of the patients were adult males and the third a 3-year-old girl; all presented with haematuria and hypertension. There was no family history of renal cystic disease. Pathological examination revealed cysts of glomerular, tubular and collecting duct origin, superficially resembling ADPKD but distinguished by their confinement to part of only one kidney. The cystic areas showed no sharp demarcation or evidence of a capsule separating them from the normal parenchyma. Areas of compressed or normal-appearing parenchyma were present within the cystic zones, and there was no histological evidence of dysplastic development. These features clearly distinguished the condition from cystic nephroma (see below) and cystic renal dysplasia. The condition is probably commoner than the one report in the literature; I have seen three further examples, all in male children, none of whom had a family history of renal cystic disease. One of these was a neonate, indicating the probable developmental nature of the condition.

It is also possible that descriptions of ADPCK confined to one kidney (Sellers et al. 1972; Lee et al. 1978; Kossow and Meek 1982) may be examples of localized cystic disease. It is recognized that cystic change in ADPCK may rarely be strikingly asymmetrical so that the possibility of unilateral involvement may be raised, particularly during life, when detailed pathological examination is impossible. Equally, localized cystic disease may conceivably involve the whole of one kidney rather than just a part. From a practical viewpoint, the diagnosis of unilateral involvement in ADPKD would be hard to accept without a confirmatory positive family history, perhaps the demonstration of hepatic cysts and evidence of a mutant gene by genetic probes.

Medullary Cystic Disease

Cystic changes confined to, or occurring predominantly in, the renal medulla are found in two distinct conditions – medullary sponge kidney and familial nephronophthisis–medullary cystic disease complex.

Medullary Sponge Kidney

Medullary sponge kidney has a reported incidence of between 1 in 5000 and 1 in 20 000 of the general population. It is diagnosed at intravenous urography by the presence of dilated medullary collecting ducts that fill with contract medium ("ductal ectasia") (Ekström et al. 1959). Flecks of medullary calcification may also be evident radiologically. Patients with this condition are often asymptomatic, and the diagnosis is ordinarily made in adult life. The radiological findings are commonly incidental to the investigation of other disease, and renal function is unimpaired apart from a urinary concentration defect. Nephrolithiasis occurs in about half the patients with medullary sponge kidney and may be complicated by haematuria or renal colic (Yendt 1982). Many of these patients have hypercalciuria (Ekstrom et al. 1959; O'Neill et al. 1981). Urinary infection may also complicate medullary sponge kidney, although it is unclear whether this is merely a complication of nephrolithiasis (Huland et al. 1976). A family history is not usually obtained (Habib et al. 1965), although it has occasionally been reported (Morris et al. 1965). The condition may affect all the pyramidal ducts in both kidneys, but occasionally there is involvement of only one or two pyramids or only one kidney. The sex incidence is equal and the anomaly is usually sporadic, but it has been recorded in siblings and even in one report in three generations of the same family (Kuiper 1971).

Associations with the Ehlers–Danlos (Levine and Michael 1967) and Weidemann–Beckwith (Charro Salgado et al. 1977) syndromes, as well as with hemihypertrophy (Harrison and Rose 1979) are reported. It is probable, however, that in hemihypertrophy and Weidemann–Beckwith syndrome the renal lesion is a form of medullary dysplasia.

Association with congenital hepatic fibrosis is best regarded as a part of the ARPKD spectrum (see p. 463).

Macroscopically, medullary sponge kidneys are of normal size or slightly enlarged. In the absence of infection and nephrolithiasis the renal surfaces are smooth. The ectatic or cystic medullary ducts are largely confined to the papillary tips, which appear flattened. They may contain inspissated material and calcified concretions. The lining epithelium may be ulcerated or exhibit squamous metaplasia, particularly if calculi are present. Inflammation of the papillary tip is usual.

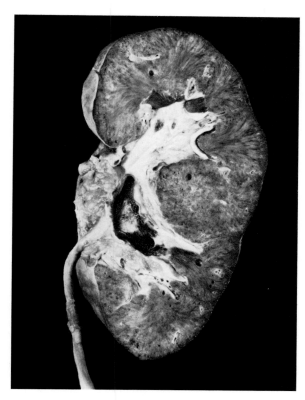

Fig. 8.14. Juvenile nephronophthisis. The kidney, from a 6-year-old girl, weighed 45 g (about half the expected weight). It is diffusely contracted and a few tiny cysts are visible, mainly at the corticomedullary junction. Photographed in ultraviolet light. (Reproduced from Jones et al. 1973, by permission of the Editor of *Pediatric Radiology*.)

The Familial Nephronophthisis–Medullary Cystic Disease (FN-MCD) Complex

Medullary cystic disease and juvenile nephronophthisis were first described as separate entities (Smith and Graham 1948; Fanconi et al. 1951), the former characterized pathologically by the presence of prominent medullary cysts, and the latter as a hereditary nephropathy, apparently with an autosomal recessive mode of inheritance, causing polyuria and renal failure in children. The realization that the two conditions have many clinical and pathological features in common (Strauss and Sommers 1967) and the fact that the two conditions may occur in the same family (Sworn and Eisinger 1972) have led to the idea that they are identical even though their aetiology is unknown. The spectrum of juvenile nephronophthisis and medullary cystic disease is not entirely homogeneous, however, and in particular there is growing evidence of *genetic* heterogeneity with apparent auto-

somal recessive, autosomal dominant and sporadic forms. Cases presenting in childhood, when by common usage the condition is called juvenile nephronophthisis, usually exhibit an autosomal recessive inheritance, whereas cases presenting in adult life, when the term usually applied is medullary cystic disease, are either sporadic or inherited as an autosomal dominant trait. A further complication is the occurrence of a third group, in which juvenile nephronophthisis/medullary cystic disease is associated with extrarenal anomalies, predominantly, tapetoretinal degeneration and retinitis pigmentosa (Bois and Royer 1970; Waldherr et al. 1982), congenital hepatic fibrosis (Boichis et al. 1973; Proesmans et al. 1975; Delaney et al. 1978) and cone-shaped phalangeal epiphyses (Robins et al. 1976; Steele et al. 1980). These examples show an autosomal recessive inheritance.

The pathological features of juvenile nephronophthisis/medullary cystic disease are fairly constant. Both kidneys are uniformly contracted, and both cortex and medulla are involved (Fig. 8.14). There is widespread periglomerular fibrosis, glomerular sclerosis, tubular atrophy and interstitial fibrosis with focal interstitial chronic inflammation (Fig. 8.15). Typically, tubular and interstitial changes are more prominent than glomerular alterations, particularly in the early stages of the disease, which are sometimes encountered in biopsy specimens. Thickening and lamination of tubular basement membranes is often marked. Cysts occur in both the cortex and medulla; large and macroscopically obvious medullary cysts are the distinguishing features of cases that have been labelled medullary cystic disease. Microdissection studies (Sherman et al. 1971) show the cysts as diverticula normally limited to the distal convoluted tubules. The medullary cysts are most prominent near the corticomedullary junction, a feature that contrasts with the medullary sponge kidney, where cysts occur near the papillary tips.

In cases of juvenile nephronophthisis presenting in childhood the clinical features are characteristic. There is marked growth retardation and the main complaints are usually of polyuria, nocturia, polydipsia and craving for salt. The urine in dilute, proteinuria is trivial or absent, and there is no excess of cells in the urine deposit. A normochromic, normocytic anaemia is present and may be disproportionate to the degree of renal failure. Salt wasting is a further characteristic feature. In the later stages symptoms due to renal failure develop and renal osteodystrophy is apparent. Without renal transplantation death usually occurs towards the end of the first decade. Juvenile nephronophthisis is now recognized as the second commonest cause of chronic renal failure in child-

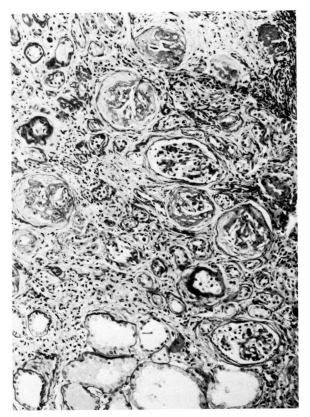

Fig. 8.15. Juvenile nephronophthisis. Note the widespread tubular atrophy and loss and glomerulosclerosis. (PAS, × 200) (Reproduced from Jones et al. 1973, by permission of the Editor of *Pediatric Radiology*.)

hood (Betts and Forrest-Hay 1973; Anonymous 1979). The clinical features in adult cases are similar. They may develop a salt-wasting syndrome, which is clinically not unlike Addisons disease except that there is no response to mineralocorticoid therapy (Thorn et al. 1944).

Glomerulocystic Disease

This term, first used by Taxy and Filmer (1976), describes a heterogeneous group of conditions with the common feature of dilatation of Bowman's spaces (Joshi and Kaszina 1984; Bernstein and Landing 1989). In infants and young children, early-onset ADPKD is the most common cause of glomerulocystic disease, accounting for about half the recorded cases (Fellows et al. 1976; Proesmans et al. 1982; Rapola and Kääriänen 1988). Glomerular cysts are also a feature in some examples of a wide variety of inherited and sporadic disorders, including

the Zellweger cerebrohepatorenal syndrome (Joshi and Kaszina 1984), tuberose sclerosis (Rolfes et al. 1985), trisomy 13 syndrome, Majewski short rib – polydactyly syndrome (Joshi and Kaszina 1984), oro-faciodigital syndrome (Stapleton et al. 1982) and brachymesomelia – renal syndrome (Langer et al. 1983). It is also an occasional feature in renal dysplasia, although except in small biopsy specimens this is unlikely to produce diagnostic difficulties.

Renal Cysts and Multiple Malformation Syndromes

Familial forms of renal dysplasia (hereditary renal adysplasia and diffuse cystic dysplasia) and of glomerulocystic disease associated with multiple malformation syndromes have been covered under the appropriate sections (see above).

Multiple renal cortical cysts developing in glomeruli, convoluted tubules and collecting ducts are not uncommon in a number of syndromes of multiple malformations, notably the autosomal trisomy 13 and 18 syndromes, Jeunes thoracic dystrophy and Zellweger cerebrohepatorenal syndrome (Bernstein and Kissane 1973).

The cysts are generally small and widely spaced, and are not usually associated with any functional impairment. Very occasionally the cystic change is associated with histological evidence of dysplasia, i.e. with evidence of metanephric maldifferentiation, but usually such changes are absent. There may be focal tubular and glomerular sclerosis associated with the cysts, so it is probable that, in these cases at least, the cystic change is a secondary phenomenon occurring in normally differentiated nephrons.

In Jeune's asphyxiating thoracic dystrophy (a familial disorder of chest wall development), renal cystic change is often more marked and there is an associated hepatic lesion resembling closely that of the congenital hepatic fibrosis seen in ARPKD and Meckel's syndrome. Special mention needs to be made of the renal cystic disease in the tuberose sclerosis complex and Von Hippel–Lindau disease.

Tuberose Sclerosis

This systemic disorder inherited as an autosomal dominant trait is characterized by hamartomatous malformations affecting singly, or in combination, the skin, kidney, brain, eye, liver, lung and bone.

Renal involvement is seen in 50% of affected patients, the most common lesions being angiomyolipomas. Renal cystic lesions are common, a feature better appreciated with improvements in diagnostic imaging techniques.

Microscopically, the cysts, which occur in both cortex and medulla and vary in size, are distinctive. They are lined by large hyperplastic epithelial cells with acidophilic cytoplasm, which often form multiple layers and sometimes fill cyst lumina. Despite their superficial resemblance to proximal tubular epithelial cells, microdissection studies indicate that they can develop from any portion of the nephron (Potter 1972). Occasionally glomerular cysts are the predominant feature, so that tuberose sclerosis may constitute one form of glomerulocystic disease (see p. 468).

As well as angiomyolipomas and renal cysts, distinctive microhamartomatous glomerular lesions composed of compact collections of lipid-containing large clear cells confined within the glomerular basement membrane have been described in tuberose sclerosis (Nagashima et al. 1988).

Von Hippel–Lindau Disease

This autosomal dominant condition is characterized by angiomatous cysts in the cerebellum, retinal angiomas, and cysts or tumours of abdominal organs.

Renal lesions occur in about two-thirds of affected patients and include renal cell carcinomas and cysts of varying size. These may be solitary or multiple and are sometimes sufficiently numerous to mimic ADPKD. The cysts are lined by flattened or hyperplastic epithelium, and sometimes renal cell carcinomas appear to arise within cysts (Christenson et al. 1982).

Multilocular Renal Cysts

Multilocular cyst (also known as cystic nephroma, multilocular cystic nephroma, renal cystadenoma, cystic mesoblastic nephroma, polycystic nephroblastoma and cystic differentiated nephroblastoma) is a rare condition currently considered, as the synonyms suggest, as a cystic neoplasm.

Powell et al. (1951) identified the following morphological characteristics:

1. There is a solitary, well demarcated, multilocular cystic lesion, usually several centimetres in diameter, which replaces most of the kidney.
2. The lesion is unilateral.
3. The cysts are filled with fluid and are discrete, i.e. they communicate neither with each other nor with the collecting system of the kidney.

4. The cysts are lined with flattened epithelium and the septa between them contain only nondescript mesenchyme and no differentiated renal elements.

Some of these characteristics require modification, because multilocular cysts are occasionally bilateral (Chatten and Bishop 1977) and, particularly in children, the cyst septa contain tubular structures, smooth muscle and even cartilage or bone (Gonzales-Crussi et al. 1982).

The suggestion that the multilocular cyst is a neoplasm related to Wilms' tumour (nephroblastoma) stems from the recognition of a spectrum of tumours with typical multilocular cysts at one end, nephroblastoma at the other, and intermediate forms macroscopically indistinguishable from the multilocular cyst in which cyst septa contain tubular elements and blastema indistinguishable from nephroblastoma (the so-called cystic partially differentiated nephroblastoma, Joshi et al. 1977; Joshi and Beckwith 1989). Sometimes all parts of the spectrum can be recognized with a single tumour (Domizio and Risdon 1991).

Multilocular cysts have a biphasic age distribution, with one peak under 2 years in which the sex distribution is equal and another peak in middle age when females are more often affected (Baldauff and Shulz 1976). The condition is sporadic, with no reports of familial cases. Grossly the multilocular cyst is generally large, spherical and clearly encapsulated, although prolapse of daughter cysts into the pelvicalyceal system is not uncommon and may cause obstruction. On section, the individual non-communicating spherical cysts are separated by delicate pale fibrous trabeculae and the whole lesion is surrounded by a thick capsule.

Microscopically the cysts are lined by single layers of nondescript cuboidal or occasionally pegged epithelial cells. The cells are said to have ultrastructural features of collecting duct epithelium (Coleman 1980), but immunochemical and lectin-binding studies (Domizio and Risdon 1991) do not support this interpretation. The thin intercystic septa consist of fibrovascular tissue, but in children usually contain more cellular mesenchyma as well as smooth muscle cells or even striated muscle, cartilage or bone. Occasional epithelial tubules may also occur, but the presence of tubular structures and particularly blastemal areas like those seen in nephroblastoma are indicative of the cystic partially differentiated nephroblastoma (see above).

A typical multilocular cyst occurring in a child or adult can be regarded as a wholly benign neoplasm curable by surgical excision alone. The cystic partially differentiated nephroblastoma is at least potentially malignant, but there are no reports of metastatic spread, so that nephrectomy and follow-up seem appropriate therapy. Rarely, in adults, histologically malignant and mitotically active sarcomatous elements are seen in the cyst walls (Madewell et al. 1983), and these tumours should be regarded as truly malignant.

Renal Diseases Principally Affecting the Glomeruli

Glomerular disease can be classifed as:

1. Acquired:
    a) Primary:
        i) Acute postinfective glomerulonephritis (including poststreptococcal glomerulonephritis)
        ii) Glomerulonephritis with crescents
        iii) Minimal change disease
        iv) Focal segmental glomerulosclerosis
        v) Diffuse mesangial hypercellularity (including IgM nephropathy)
        vi) Membranoproliferative (mesangiocapillary) glomerulonephritis
        vii) Membranous nephropathy
        viii) Bergers IgA nephropathy
    b) Secondary:
        i) Schönlein–Henoch purpura
        ii) Lupus nephritis
        iii) Diabetic nephropathy
        iv) Renal amyloidosis
2. Congenitial – hereditary nephropathies, including Alports syndrome, thin basement membrane nephropathy and congenital nephrotic syndrome.

Glomerulonephritis

Much clinical and experimental evidence indicates that many forms of inflammatory glomerular disease are immunologically mediated. Although the exact pathogenic mechanisms in humans are far from clear, earlier experimental studies (Unanue and Dixon 1967; Dixon 1968) have suggested two basic patterns:

1. Fixation of antiglomerular basement membrane (anti-GBM) antibodies to the GBM (anti-GBM disease)
2. Deposition of immune (antibody–antigen) complexes in the glomerulus (immune complex disease)

In clinical practice these two mechanisms have been distinguished by immunofluorescence or immunohistochemical staining. Deposition of immunoglobulins and complement show a continuous linear staining along the GBM in the one form of human anti-GBM nephritis recognized, namely Goodpasture's syndrome. In immune complex disease, by far the commonest form of human glomerulonephritis, deposition is in a granular pattern in the mesangium or along glomerular capillary walls.

Goodpasture's syndrome has been well characterized as an autoimmune disease in which circulated autoantibodies to a component of the GBM are formed. The antigen responsible has been identified as a component of the α_3-chain of the non-collagenous (NC1) domain of type IV collagen (Hudson et al. 1989).

The situation with immune complex disease is more complicated. Original concepts suggested that complexes were formed exclusively in the circulation and were then entrapped within the glomeruli to initiate glomerulonephritis. It is now believed that complexes can also form in situ within the glomerulus. Circulating antibodies can initiate in situ complexes either by interaction with native antigenic constituents of the glomerulus or by their combination with nonglomerular antigens planted in the glomerulus. Experimental evidence of in situ complex formation by antibodies to a glomerular constituent has been verified in the rat model of Heyman nephritis, where the antigen involved is gp 330, a glycoprotein found on the apical plasmalemmal domain of proximal tubular cells as well as on glomerular podocytes (Kerjaschki and Farguhar 1983). In other models exogenous antigens planted in the glomeruli have been complexed with specific antibodies introduced into the circulation, the complexes generally forming on the subepithelial aspect of the GBM (Wilson 1981; Vogt et al. 1982; Vogt 1984).

Whatever the mechanism initiating primary deposition of complexes in the glomeruli, they are significantly modified before the appearance of aggregates recognized as granular immunofluorescene patterns or on electron microscopy. These alterations may include aggregation, or enlargement by the addition of circulating reactants such as free antibody or free antigen, further immune complexes, complement components and autoantibodies to immunoglobulins, or complement. Immune complexes may also be engulfed by infiltrating neutrophils or mesangial cells, and may be redistributed within the glomerulus.

Factors influencing the glomerular deposition and distribution of circulating complexes include their size (Germuth and Rodrigues 1972) and charge (Gallo et al. 1981; Kanwar et al. 1986). Older experimental studies (Germuth 1953; Dixon et al. 1958, 1961) using the acute and chronic serum sickness models identified soluble complexes formed in conditions of antigen excess as particularly important in eliciting glomerulonephritis, but later evidence (Cameron and Clark 1982) suggests that insoluble complexes may also have a role; current concepts indicate that high levels of large precipitating complexes containing high-avidity antibodies produce mild disease with mainly mesangial deposits, whereas lower levels of smaller complexes containing low-avidity antibodies produce severe glomerular changes with deposits located on glomerular capillary walls.

Host factors are also important in determining glomerular complex deposition. This may be facilitated by deficiencies in the complement system, which, through the erythrocyte complement receptor 1 (CR1) mechanism (Waxman et al. 1986) have a role in clearing circulating complexes in conjunction with the mononuclear phagocyte system; complement also has a role in inhibiting precipitation and promoting solubilization of immune complexes.

Immunologically mediated glomerular damage can result through the activation of the complement system with associated release of enzymes from polymorphonuclear leucocytes and sometimes the initiation of blood-clotting mechanisms (Unanue and Dixon 1967). Recent research has also implicated T-cell mechanisms (Bhan et al. 1978, 1979) in glomerular damage, and other mediators of tissue injury such as cytokines (Camussi et al. 1990), oxygen metabolites (Shah 1989) and eicosanoids (Rahman et al. 1987) may also be involved.

In addition, antineutrophil cytoplasmic antibodies (ANCA) have been identified in some forms of necrotizing and crescentic glomerulonephritis in humans. These patients have scanty or no immune deposits (pauci-immune) demonstrable in renal biopsy specimens (Niles et al. 1993).

Acute Postinfective Glomerulonephritis

This type of glomerulonephritis follows infections – most commonly streptococcal throat or skin infections, but rarely those caused by other organisms including bacteria, viruses and fungi. In addition, this form of glomerulonephritis may accompany infected ventriculoatrial shunts inserted for the relief of hydrocephalus (shunt nephritis), or may complicate infective endocarditis or deep abscesses. Classical acute poststreptococcal glomerulonephritis follows infections by group A, β-haemolytic streptococci, usually of types 12, 4 or 1 in throat infections and types 49, 42 or 2 in skin infections. Characteristically there is a latent period between the infection and the development of nephritic symptoms of 1–2 weeks with throat and 3–6 weeks with skin infections. Nephritis is characterized by the abrupt onset of haematuria, proteinuria, oliguria and facial oedema. This is due to salt and water retention, which is also responsible for a transient dilutional anaemia and hypertension in some cases.

Acute poststreptococcal glomerulonephritis may occur sporadically or in epidemics, particularly following skin infections, such as those in the Red Lake Indian Reserve in Minnesota in 1953 and 1956 (Kleinman 1954; Anthony et al. 1967). It usually affects children and young adults (especially in the epidemic forms), but may occur at all ages. Males are affected about twice as commonly as females (Baldwin et al. 1974; Rodriquez-Iturbe 1984). Acute poststreptococcal glomerulonephritis is increasingly rare in Europe and North America but remains common in Africa, the Caribbean and South America.

The evidence that the nephritis is immunologically mediated is compelling. The latent period between the infection and the onset of nephritis is compatible with the time required to develop antibodies. The kidney, blood and urine are sterile, indicating that the renal lesion is not a direct result of infection. Serum complement levels are low during the episode of acute nephritis, implying the involvement of the complement system as a mediator of an immune response. Titres of ASOT and anti-DNAase-B (Farmer 1985) are often raised, suggesting that an immune reaction to streptococcal antigens occurs, although these particular antibodies have not been implicated in the pathogenesis of the nephritis.

Current evidence suggests that the acute poststreptococcal glomerulonephritis is mediated by immune complexes possibly formed in the circulation or in the glomeruli following in situ planting of antigen. Streptococcal antigens have proved extremely difficult to identify within presumed complexes in the glomeruli or circulating blood, but some investigations have demonstrated such antigens and others have identified mesangial and GBM antigens in the serum of patients during the acute phase of the disease (Seegal et al. 1965; Andres et al. 1966; Michael et al. 1966; Lange 1983; Kefalides et al. 1986).

On light microscopy during the acute phase all the glomerular tufts appear swollen and hypercellular, virtually filling the urinary spaces (Fig. 8.16). There is a proliferation of intracapillary (mesangial and endothelial) cells, which virtually obliterate the tuft capillary lumina, and infiltration by polymorphonuclear leucocytes and monocytes. The tubular epithelium is usually well preserved, but there is a variable

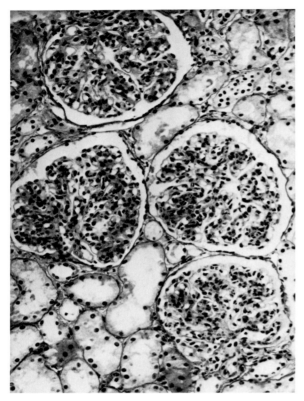

Fig. 8.16. Acute diffuse (post streptococcal) glomerulonephritis in a 10-year-old boy. Note the diffuse glomerular involvement, the marked hypercellularity of glomerular tufts and the presence of numerous polymorphs within the tufts. (MSB, × 400)

degree of interstitial oedema and mononuclear cell infiltration. In some patients there is a variable degree of capsular crescent formation. The relative contribution of the various cell types to glomerular hypercellularity has been debated at length. Comparison with animal models, the use of electron microscopy and the application of cell markers (histochemical staining for non-specific esterase and α_1-antitrypsin) suggest that much of the early glomerular hypercellularity is due to an influx of blood-borne mononuclear cells and sometimes polymorphs, but at a later stage proliferation of intrinsic glomerular (particularly mesangial) cells is more prominent (Magil et al. 1981; Magil and Wadsworth 1981).

On electron microscopy, electron-dense deposits (presumed to be complexes) are seen to occur predominantly on the epithelial side of the GBM, and especially large deposits (termed "humps") are characteristic (Fig. 8.17). Deposits may also be seen beneath the endothelium and occasionally within the GBM.

Immunofluorescence or immunohistochemical staining usually demonstrates fine granular deposition of IgG and often C3 along glomerular capillary walls in the acute stage. Sometimes deposits assume a near-linear pattern because of their confluence. Sorger et al. (1982) describe three different appearances: the "garland" pattern with discrete and dense deposition of C3 in glomerular capillary walls, associated with numerous humps ultrastructurally, and seen in patients with acute nephritis and heavy (sometimes

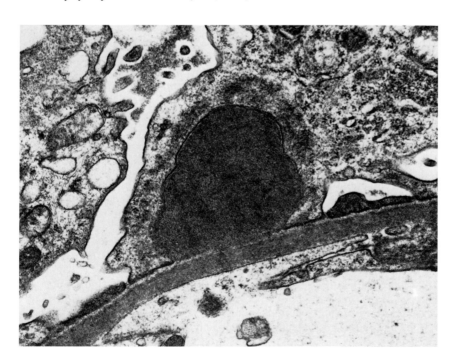

Fig. 8.17. Acute post streptococcal glomerulonephritis: electron micrograph showing an electron-dense hump on the epithelial side of the glomerular basement membrane and surrounded by epithelial cell cytoplasm. (× 10 000)

nephrotic) proteinuria; the "starry sky" pattern with smaller granular deposits often on the GBM overlying the mesangium, and the mesangial pattern in which granular deposits are mainly within the mesangium, usually seen in the resolving phase. Smaller deposits of other immunoglobulins may also occur, usually in the mesangium, and fibrin may also be demonstrated in the mesangium or in crescents if present.

In the great majority of cases (probably 90% of children and some 60% of adults) the disease is not progressive and the glomerular lesion completely resolves or leaves a minimum of glomerular scarring. This implies that the circulation and glomerular trapping of soluble immune complexes is usually short-lived. Certainly deposits can no longer be seen with the electron microscope in biopsies taken more than 6 weeks after the onset of disease from patients who subsequently recover completely. Increased mesangial hypercellularity may persist for some months, however, and may be accompanied clinically by proteinuria.

In a minority of patients glomerular abnormalities persist for more than a year and the disease is said to have entered a latent phase (Jennings and Earle 1961). In an unknown percentage of such patients chronic glomerulonephritis develops (Schacht et al. 1976). Progressive hyalinization and scarring of glomeruli with secondary tubular and interstitial changes develop, and there is a gradual diminution of renal function ending in chronic renal failure. Hypertension may also supervene, and the accompanying vascular changes add a component of ischaemic damage to the kidneys.

A very small minority of patients die in the acute phase of the disease from such complications as acute left ventricular failure with pulmonary oedema or cerebral haemorrhage.

With a diminishing incidence of poststreptococcal glomerulonephritis (Meadow 1975), it is becoming clear that by no means all cases of acute diffuse proliferative glomerulonephritis follow streptococcal infections. From these cases it is evident that other antigens, possibly of bacterial or viral origin, may precipitate this type of immune complex disease (Hyman et al. 1975; Rainford et al. 1978; Ronco et al. 1982; Maher et al. 1984).

A histologically similar form of glomerulonephritis (or more usually a mesangiocapillary glomerulonephritis) may rarely complicate infection (generally by coagulase-negative staphylococci) of ventriculoatrial shunts inserted for the relief of hydrocephalus (Narchi et al. 1988). Acute immune-complex-mediated glomerulonephritis is a rare complication of deep-seated visceral abscesses (Beaufils 1981) and may accompany infective endocarditis.

Glomerulonephritis with Crescents

In "glomerulonephritis with crescents", a prominent histological feature is the proliferation of cells outside the glomerular tuft and within Bowman's capsule. These cells often produce crescentic masses (capsular crescents), which fill and obliterate the urinary space (Fig. 8.18). Until recently the cells forming capsular crescents were considered to be

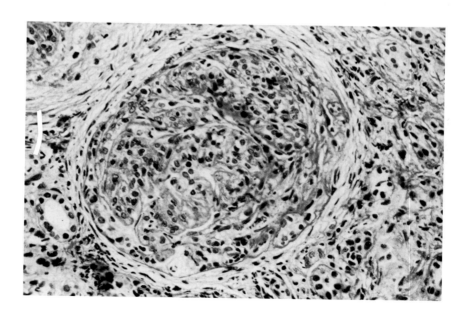

Fig. 8.18. Proliferative glomerulonephritis with capsular crescent formation. (MSB, × 500)

derived from epithelial cells covering the glomerular tufts or lining Bowmans capsule. However, experimental (Kondo et al. 1972; Atkins et al. 1976, 1980) and clinical (Ferrario et al. 1985; Bolton et al. 1987) studies indicate that many of the cells are derived from circulating monocytes. The stimulus to crescent formation is leakage of fibrin from the vascular compartment, probably through breaks in the glomerular basement membrane which can be demonstrated ultrastructurally. Associated changes within the glomerular tufts include hypercellularity and necrotizing or sclerotic lesions; tuft compression by the crescents may make their recognition difficult without careful examination.

Crescent formation may be a feature in occasional examples of well defined varieties of glomerulonephritis such as poststreptococcal, membranous, IgA, hereditary (Alport's syndrome) and mesangiocapillary glomerulonephritis (particularly dense deposit disease). It may also occur in glomerulonephritides that are expressions of systemic diseases such as mixed essential cryoglobulinaemia, systemic lupus erythematosus, Schönlein–Henoch syndrome, polyarteritis nodosa and Wegener's granulomatosis. Occasional crescents are not uncommon in most varieties of glomerulonephritis, and definitions for inclusion under the heading of glomerulonephritis with crescents vary with different authors from 30% of glomeruli affected (Cohen et al. 1981) to more than 50% (Whitworth et al. 1976). In general, the presence of significant numbers of crescents imparts a poor prognosis and often a rapidly progressive course. This accounts for the older term for cresentic glomerulonephritis of "rapidly progressive glomerulonephritis". Histological features related to a poor outcome include an increasing proportion of glomeruli exhibiting crescents (Morrin et al. 1978), necrotizing changes in the glomerular tufts (Neild et al. 1983) and significant tubulointerstitial damage (Striker et al. 1973).

Excluding those examples secondary to well defined varieties of glomerulonephritis or systemic diseases described above, primary crescentic glomerulonephritis is of three main types (Heptinstall 1992). A minority have antiglomerular basement membrane disease, sometimes accompanied by pulmonary haemorrhage (Goodpasture's syndrome). These are recognized by immunofluorescence microscopy, which displays linear deposition of IgG along glomerular capillary tuft walls sometimes accompanied by granular C3. The second type is an immune-complex nephritis in which immunoglobulins and C3 are distributed in a granular pattern along glomerular capillary walls and in the mesangium. In such cases, careful evaluation of the clinical and pathological features, including the ultrastructural findings, is important to exclude specific entities such as IgA nephropathy and membranous or mesangiocapillary glomerulonephritis. In the third type there is little or no glomerular immunoglobulin or complement deposition, although fibrin may be demonstrated in the crescents (pauci-immune type). There are no electron-dense deposits on electron microscopy. This type is more frequent in males; it has a number of features in common with the cresentic glomerulonephritis accompanying polyarteritis nodosa, including the frequent finding of antineutrophil cytoplasmic antibodies (ANCA) in the serum.

Minimal Change Disease

As has long been recognized (Dunn 1934), the majority of children (some 80%) presenting with the nephrotic syndrome show no, or only minor, glomerular changes on renal bipsy ("minimal change" disease). In some patients a mild increase in mesangial matrix or slight mesangial hypercellularity is evident (see below). The tubules often contain hyaline droplets or protein casts, and cytoplasmic lipid may be evident on frozen sections as a reflection of the derangement in lipid metabolism that occurs in the nephrotic syndrome. Immunofluorescence microscopy is generally completely negative, although small deposits of immunoglobulin (IgG and IgM) and complement are seen in the glomeruli in a minority (20%–30%). In untreated cases, the major ultrastructural abnormality is a loss or effacement of epithelial cell (podocyte) foot processes.

Minimal change nephrotic syndrome in children has a peak incidence between 2 and 4 years, and 80% present before the age of 6 years. It is commoner in males than in females (2: 1). Microscopic haematuria occurs in about one-third of patients, but macroscopic haematuria is distinctly rare. Proteinuria in children is usually selective, i.e. molecules of the size of albumin or smaller are excreted preferentially in the urine (Cameron and White 1965).

The distinctive clinical feature of minimal change nephrotic syndrome is its favourable response to steroid therapy, 95% of patients achieving complete remission of proteinuria within 2 weeks of treatment with prednisolone in a dose of 60 mg/m² per day. About 20% of patients never relapse after one course of steroids, but of the remainder 30% relapse infrequently and 70% frequently. Among patients who experience frequent relapses, a minority relapse while steroids are being withdrawn or within 2 weeks of completion of the course, and are described as steroid dependent. In these patients, more sustained remission can sometimes be obtained with cyclophosphamide or chlorambucil (Barratt and Soothill 1970).

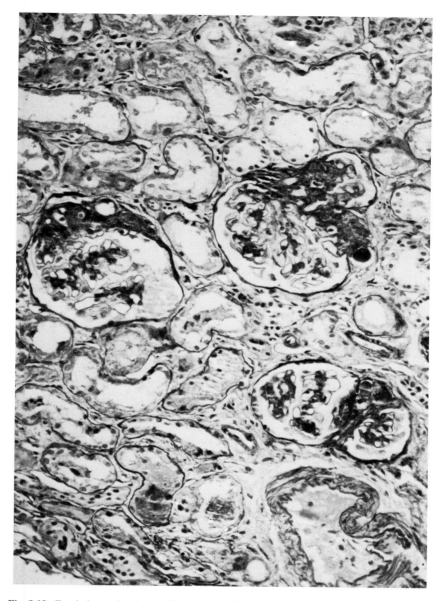

Fig. 8.19. Focal glomerulosclerosis. Three glomeruli showing segmental hyalinosis. (PAS, × 300)

Whatever the initial response to steroid therapy, the ultimate prognosis in minimal change disease is good. Although a small minority (less than 3%) die of renal failure or intercurrent infection, over 85% ultimately go into permanent remission (Trompeter et al. 1985).

Focal Segmental Glomerulosclerosis

This lesion is characterized by sclerosing lesions, often with hyaline inclusions, affecting one or more segments of some but not all glomeruli (Churg et al. 1970; Habib and Gubler 1971) (Fig. 8.19). Of the remaining glomeruli, some may be globally sclerosed; they may appear normal by light microscopy or exhibit mild mesangial hypercellularity.

Segmental sclerotic lesions occur most commonly near the glomerular hilus, but may also affect the periphery of the glomerular tuft. The fully developed lesion occupies a glomerular lobule which is collapsed and shows increased mesangial matrix and thickening of the glomerular capillary wall. The capillary lumen may be destroyed or contain a mass of

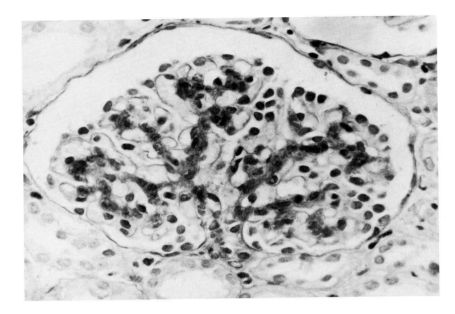

Fig. 8.20. Mesangial proliferative glomerulonephritis. Note the widely patent glomerular capillary loops, mild centrilobular hypercellularity and increase in mesangial matrix. (PAS, × 1000)

proteinaceous material (hyalinosis) best distinguished by its poor argyrophilia on silver methenamine staining. Foam cells are seen occasionally within the residual capillary lumina.

Immunofluorescence microscopy usually demonstrates staining with IgM and C3 confined to sclerotic lesions in the affected glomerular tufts.

Tubules associated with focally or globally sclerosed glomeruli are usually atrophic. In early lesions focal sclerotic glomeruli may be sparse, and their distribution is not random, the deep juxtamedullary glomeruli being affected first (Rich 1957). Both these factors may result in failure to recognize the condition in renal biopsy specimens, and a mistaken diagnosis of minimal change disease. Particularly in children, the presence of focal tubular atrophy is a useful pointer and should elicit a careful search for focal sclerotic glomerular lesions that may require serial sections for their demonstration.

Focal segmental glomerulosclerosis affects both children and adults, and presents insidiously with proteinuria or the nephrotic syndrome. Of children with the nephrotic syndrome, about 10% have focal segmental glomerulosclerosis (White et al. 1970). These are more commonly males, but unlike in minimal change disease the age distribution in childhood is more even. Microscopic haematuria is more common in focal segmental glomerulosclerosis, affecting more than 50% of patients. In children with focal segmental glomerulosclerosis, proteinuria is usually non-selective.

The distinctive features of focal segmental glomerulosclerosis are its generally poor response to steroid therapy (only about 20% respond initially, but many of these relapse and become resistant) and its tendency towards a progressive course to chronic renal failure, although the speed with which this occurs varies widely from case to case (with a range of about 3–20 years). Non-response to steroids and accompanying haematuria appear to be bad prognostic factors (Habib and Gubler 1973, 1975).

Diffuse Mesangial Proliferative Glomerulonephritis

In about 3% of children presenting with idiopathic nephrotic syndrome, renal biopsy shows an increase in mesangial cells and an excess of mesangial matrix affecting most or all the glomeruli (Fig. 8.20). Glomerular capillary walls are unthickened and capillary lumina are widely patent (Glasgow et al. 1970; White et al. 1970). This appearance, termed mesangial proliferative glomerulonephritis, may also occur in other clinical settings, notably in resolving poststreptococcal glomerulonephritis (Jennings and Earle 1961), Bergers (1969) IgA nephropathy (p. 480), lupus nephritis and Schönlein–Henoch purpura (p. 481).

Nephrotic children with mesangial proliferative glomerulonephritis are slightly more commonly male than female, tend to be older than those with minimal change disease, have a higher incidence of microscopic haematuria (45%) and more often have non-selective proteinuria; about half fail to respond to steroid therapy (International Study of Kidney Disease in Childhood 1978).

The morphological distinction of mesangial proliferative glomerulonephritis from minimal change disease in the context of childhood nephrotic syndrome is clearly somewhat subjective, particularly if one recognizes a histological variant of minimal change disease with mild mesangial hypercellularity. The International Study of Kidney Disease in Childhood (1981) attempted to resolve this issue by defining 3 cells/area in some peripherial mesangial areas as indicating mild mesangial hypercellularity (1 or 2 cells/area being "normal"), and ≥ 4 cells/area as indicating mesangial proliferative glomerulonephritis. However, these definitions clearly depend on factors such as section thickness, and remain subjective. The problem is complicated by two further factors. Firstly, some patients with focal segmental glomerulosclerosis show mild mesangial hypercellularity or even mesangial proliferative glomerulonephritis of "background" glomeruli not affected by sclerosis. Secondly, diffuse mesangial deposits of IgM and C3 may be found on immunofluorescence microscopy in some patients with minimal change, mild mesangial hypercellularity or mesangial proliferative glomerulonephritis. The significance of the latter finding, referred to by some as IgM nephropathy, is controversial. Some authorities claim an increased tendency for steroid dependence or resistance and a poorer prognosis (Cohen et al. 1982; Gonzalo et al. 1985); others report no differences (Allen et al. 1982; Vilches et al. 1982). Some of this confusion relates to different diagnostic criteria for IgM nephropathy, some accepting minimal IgM deposition on immunofluorescence microscopy, others requiring diffuse prominent mesangial IgM and C3 deposition, coupled with mesangial hypercellularity and mesangial deposits on electron microscopy.

Membranoproliferative (Mesangiocapillary) Glomerulonephritis

Although uncommon, this type of proliferative glomerulonephritis, which is usually accompanied by hypocomplementaemia, has sinister clinical implications and is an important cause of progressive renal failure, usually accompanied by hypocomplementaemia, in children and young adults (West et al. 1965; Cameron et al. 1970; Bohle et al. 1974).

Light microscopy reveals uniform involvement of all glomeruli, which are enlarged and show prominent lobulation of the glomerular tufts. A variable degree of proliferation of mesangial cells and an increase in mesangial matrix is associated with diffuse thickening of glomerular capillary walls (Fig. 8.21a). Infiltration of the glomerular tufts by monocytes and neutrophil polymorphs is frequent, and cap-

sular crescents may be present. Ultrastructural studies reveal three types of glomerular capillary wall thickening, of which two (types I and III) are probably variants of the same process, but the third (type II) is distinctly different (Berger and Galle 1963; Burkholder et al. 1973; Habib et al. 1973; Levy et al. 1979).

Type I: Double-contour Variety. Thickening of the capillary wall is caused by the extension of mesangial cell cytoplasm and matrix around the circumference of the capillary loop between the GBM and the lining endothelium. A second layer of basement-membrane-like material is seen between the mesangial layer and the endothelium; this can be seen by light microscopy if silver methenamine staining methods are used, producing a "tramline" or "double-contour" effect (Fig. 8.21b). Electron-dense deposits are seen both along the endothelial aspect of the GBM and in the mesangium. Immunofluorescence microscopy reveals immunoglobulins (generally IgG and IgM) and C3 in a granular pattern along peripheral glomerular capillary walls and sometimes in the mesangium. Less commonly, C3 alone is deposited in the mesangium and to a lesser extent on capillary walls.

This variety of mesangiocapillary glomerulonephritis is usually primary, but may be seen occasionally in association with many other disorders, including shunt nephritis, hepatitis B antigenaemia, α_1-antitrypsin deficiency and hereditary deficiencies of complement components.

Type II: Linear Dense-deposit Variety. Thickening is caused by ribbon-like electron-dense deposits within the basement membrane. These deposits extend diffusely along the capillary walls and often involve the basement membrane of Bowman's capsule and the renal tubules. The deposits are particularly well seen on light microscopy in plastic-embedded sections stained with toluidine blue, for which they have a high affinity (Fig. 8.22). They are not argyrophilic, and in paraffin sections stained with methenamine silver the paucity of silver staining of the thickened glomerular capillary walls is a useful pointer to this diagnosis. On immunofluorescence microscopy, deposits of C3 (but not C1q) and the absence of immunoglobulin deposition are characteristic findings. With C3, bright granules in the mesangium are associated with weaker linear deposits on the basement membrane.

Type III. This variety (Burkholder et al. 1970) has features of type I such as double contours, mesangial interposition and subendothelial deposits. In addition, there are subepithelial deposits that may be numerous

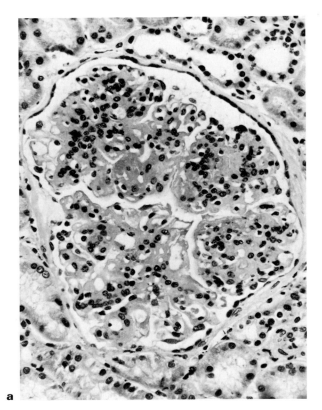
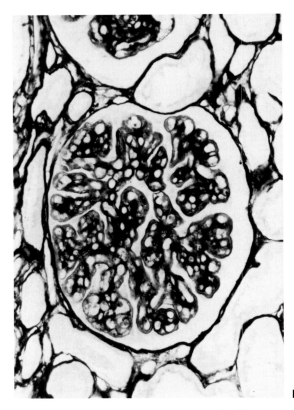

a
b

Fig. 8.21. Membranoproliferative (mesangiocapillary) glomerulonephritis. **a** Note the lobulation of the glomerular tuft with marked hypercellularity and thickening of capillary walls. (H&E, × 800) **b** Silver methenamine stain to show double contouring of capillary walls. (× 600)

and can be associated with epithelial "spikes" (see Membranous Glomerulonephritis). By light microscopy, glomerular enlargement and hypercellularity is less marked than in type I (Anders et al. 1977). Strife et al. (1977) described in type III deposits within the GBM, focal replication of the lamina densa, and occasional continuity between subendothelial and subepithelial deposits. By immunofluorescence microscopy, finely granular C3 deposits (and in some cases IgG and IgM) are seen along glomerular capillary walls and occasionally in the mesangium.

Clinically, type I is more frequent than types II and III. Both types I and III usually present with a nephrotic syndrome often accompanied by haematuria; type II more often presents with an acute nephritic syndrome or recurrent macroscopic haematuria. All three varieties have a progressive course to end-stage renal failure, often accompanied by hypertension; progression is usually more rapid in type II. Persistent hypocomplementaemia is characteristic and is almost invariable in type II. In some cases this appears at least partly to result from the presence of an IgG autoantibody (termed C3 nephritic factor) that

initiates complement consumption by the alternative pathway (Schreiber et al. 1976). However, C3 nephritic factor is not always present in patients with mesangiocapillary glomerulonephritis, occurring in up to 70% of patients with type II and up to 30% of those with type I; it is noticeably absent in type III.

Mesangiocapillary glomerulonephritis, almost always the linear dense-deposit variety, may also occur in association with partial lipodystrophy (Peters et al. 1973; Peters and Williams 1975). In this condition there is a symmetrical loss of subcutaneous fat from the face and sometimes from the arms, trunk and hips. The lower extremities, however, show a normal or even increased deposition of fat. Males are affected four times as frequently as females. Patients with partial lipodystrophy and mesangiocapillary glomerulonephritis are usually hypocomplementaemic and often have C3 nephritic factor. Occasionally, lipodystrophy and hypocomplementaemia occur in the absence of demonstrable renal disease, and this has been taken as further evidence that the association between hyocomplementaemia and mesangioglomerulonephritis is indirect.

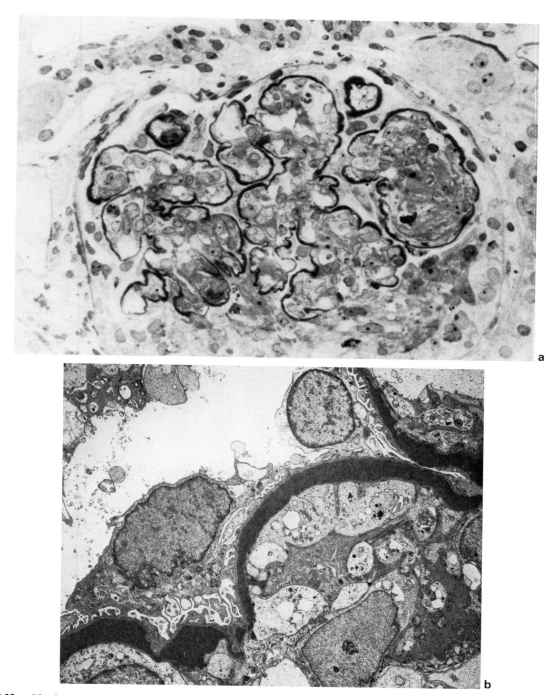

Fig. 8.22. a Membranoproliferative (mesangiocapillary) glomerulonephritis of the dense-deposit type. Note the linear deposits in the glomerular basement membrane. (Epon section, toluidine blue, × 800) **b** Electron micrograph of the same case. (× 10 000)

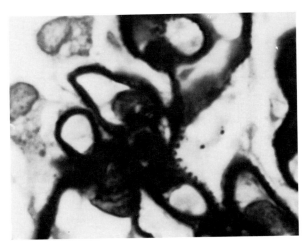

Fig. 8.23. Membranous (epimembranous) nephropathy. Note the argyrophilic spikes on the epithelial aspect of the basement membrane. (Jones' silver methenamine stain, × 1500)

Membranous Nephropathy

The glomerular lesion in membranous nephropathy is characterized histologically by a diffuse thickening of the walls of all the glomerular capillaries (Fig. 8.23), without significant cellular proliferation (Ehrenreich and Churg 1968).

Special staining techniques (trichrome stains and silver methenamine methods) for light microscopy, and electron microscope examination reveal that the glomerular capillary thickening is caused by discrete deposits closely applied to the outer (epithelial) aspect of the GBM. As the lesion progresses, spike-like extensions of the GBM protrude between the deposits like the teeeth of a comb (Fig. 8.22). Immunofluorescence microscopy demonstrates the deposits, which contain both IgG and C_3, as a beaded array following the same distribution along the epithelial aspect of the GBM as seen on electron microscopy.

Further progression of the glomerular capillary wall thickening results from the deposition of more basement membrane material around the deposits, which gradually become less distinct and are finally incorporated in the now greatly thickened GBM. Collapse and obliteration of capillary loops by this process leads to a gradual hyalinization of whole glomeruli.

Clinically, membranous nephropathy is usually recognized in patients with the nephrotic syndrome or persistent proteinuria. It is the commonest cause of nephrotic syndrome in adults and has a peak incidence in middle age, but occurs much less frequently in children. Its representation as a chronic progres-

sive form of glomerulonephritis, with a protracted course leading gradually to renal failure over many years, is probably a considerable oversimplification. In many patients it is clear that spontaneous resolution of membranous glomerulonephritis occurs, and this may be particularly true in children (Habib and Kleinknecht 1975). The likelihood of spontaneous remission appears to relate inversely to the degree of proteinuria and to any impairment of renal function. Patients with heavy proteinuria and some degree of renal failure are more likely to be symptomatic and come to renal biopsy. They represent the more severe end of the spectrum of membranous glomerulonephritis, but many cases are probably subclinical and may resolve without biopsy confirmation of their disease. When diagnosis is based on widespread population screening for haematuria and proteinuria, a significant proportion of patients with membranous nephropathy, both children and adults, are found not to be nephrotic (Beregi and Varga 1974; Kida et al. 1986).

Membranous glomerulonephritis is usually a primary disease, but secondary forms occur in autoimmune diseases such as systemic lupus erythematosus and rheumatoid arthritis, in chronic infections such as hepatitis B, following drug therapy (with, for example, penicillamine or gold salts) and accompanying conditions such as sarcoidosis, Sjögren's syndrome and some malignant tumours.

Berger's IgA Nephropathy

The cardinal feature of IgA nephropathy, first recognized by Berger (1969), is the presence of diffuse mesangial IgA deposition in all or most of the glomeruli. Some IgA deposition can occur in a wide variety of glomerulonephritides, but in most cases the staining intensity is less than for other immunoglobulins or complement. In addition, strong IgA staining may be seen in glomerular lesions of diseases such as systemic lupus erythematosus, Schönlein–Henoch purpura or chronic liver disease. Thus, primary IgA nephropathy can be defined as the presence of dominant or codominant glomerular mesangial IgA deposition in the absence of clinical or laboratory evidence of other diseases such as those cited above.

By light microscopy, a wide variety of histological changes may be recognized. The most common patterns are: apparently normal glomeruli; diffuse mesangial proliferative glomerulonephritis; or focal and segmental proliferative glomerulonephritis with focal necrotizing or sclerotic lesions. However, many other patterns also occur, including focal segmental sclerosis and mesangiocapillary, crescentic or even membranous glomerulonephritis.

By immunofluorescence microscopy, strong granular or clumped IgA staining of the mesangium is required for the diagnosis. IgA may occasionally extend to glomerular capillary walls, and this finding has been suggested as an indicator of more serious disease (Andreoli et al. 1986). C3 deposition is almost invariable; IgG staining is seen in about 60% of biopsies and IgM in about 30%.

By electron microscopy, usually numerous discrete electron-dense deposits are present in the mesangial matrix or in the paramesangial regions. Occasionally subendothelial, subepithelial or intramembranous deposits are evident, generally confined to the capillary wall adjacent to the mesangium.

Clinically, IgA nephropathy affects children and young adults (Clarkson et al. 1977) with a striking male predominance (Sissons et al. 1975). It is recognized throughout the world, and in many countries is the most common glomerular disease now recognized (D'Amico et al. 1985). Presentation is usually with recurrent episodes of gross haematuria in children or with persistent microhaematuria and proteinuria in older patients. Episodes of gross haematuria commonly follow upper respiratory tract infections by 24–48 h (Clarkson et al. 1977). Less commonly, presentation may be with nephrotic syndrome, hypertension or an acute nephritic syndrome, all of which indicate a poorer prognosis (Levy et al. 1985). Until recently, IgA nephropathy was regarded as a usually benign condition, but long-term follow-up studies indicate progression to renal failure in up to 50% after 20 years (Woodroffe et al. 1982; Droz et al. 1984).

Schönlein–Henoch Purpura

This condition is a form of systemic vasculitis, mainly affecting children between the ages of 5 and 15 years, that classically involves the skin, gastrointestinal tract and joints. This gives rise to a purpuric skin rash, colicky abdominal pain and migratory arthritis. Schönlein–Henoch purpura is commonly preceded by an upper respiratory tract infection, and in some patients repeated attacks occur. Renal involvement is common, usually indicated by microscopic haematuria with or without proteinuria, or sometimes by gross haematuria (Meadow 1978).

The pathology of the renal lesions associated with Schönlein–Henoch purpura are strikingly similar to those of IgA nephropathy (see p. 480), although clinically the systemic features serve to distinguish Schönlein–Henoch purpura. In both conditions IgA deposition in the walls of superficial capillary vessels in the skin may be demonstrated by immunofluorescence microscopy.

In the glomeruli IgA deposition, as in IgA nephropathy, is dominant or codominant. In Schönlein–Henoch nephritis mesangial deposition of IgA and C3 is prominent, but extension of IgA around peripheral capillary walls is usual. IgG and IgM deposition occurs in about 10% of biopsies, but is less abundant than IgA.

Progression to end-stage renal failure occurs in about 5% of children with Schönlein–Henoch nephritis. This usually occurs early in the course of the disease, but late progression is also reported (Counahan and Cameron 1977). Such patients are usually older, and there is little risk of developing end-stage disease in those presenting under the age of 6 years. Heavy proteinuria and particularly nephrotic syndrome are poor prognostic indicators. Crescentic nephritis in an initial biopsy, particularly when crescents affect more than 50% of the glomeruli, is also indicative of progressive disease (Goldstein et al. 1992).

Lupus Nephritis

Systemic lupus erythematosus (SLE) is a multisystem disorder of apparent "autoimmune" origin, which may occur during childhood. A number of circulated antibodies may be found, including antibodies to double-stranded DNA, to individual histones (41, 42A, 42B and 44), to histone complexes and to nonhistone proteins. Low levels of haemolytic complement, circulating immune complexes and high titres of anti-DNA antibodies are indicative of active disease and renal involvement. The nephritis of SLE appears to be an immune complex disease associated with a wide variety of glomerular lesions (McCluskey 1975). Class I lesions show no or only minor glomerular abnormalities with (or sometimes without) immunoglobulin and C3 deposition by immunofluorescence microscopy. Class II lesions are characterized by mild or moderate mesangial cell proliferation with immune deposits and ultrastructural electron-dense deposits confined to the mesangium. Class III lesions are characterized by segmental or diffuse proliferation with or without scattered necrotizing or sclerosing lesions, usually superimposed on mesangial proliferative changes as seen in Class II. Leucocytic infiltration and nuclear debris may be present in the tufts, and capsular crescents may be seen. Class IV lesions are similar to Class III but are more diffuse. Sometimes the appearances resemble those in acute postinfectious glomerulonephritis, but more often variable degrees of segmental necrosis and sclerosis are seen. Focal thickening of individual capillary loops caused by

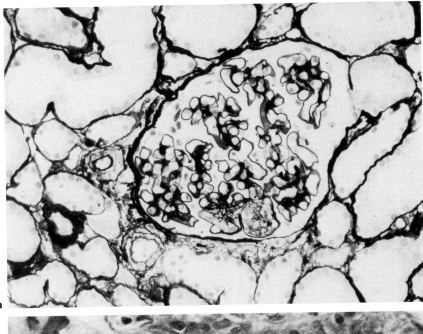

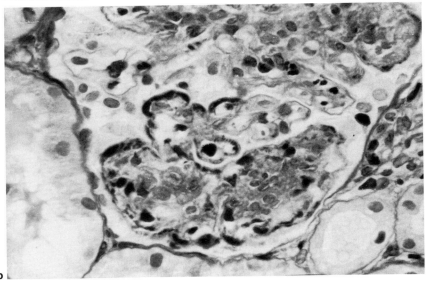

Fig. 8.24. Lupus nephritis.
a Focal glomerular lesion. (Jones' silver methenamine stain, × 600)
b Wire loop lesion. (MSB, × 1500)

subendothelial deposits (wire-loops, Fig. 8.24) may be prominent, and fragmented altered nuclear debris (haematoxyphil bodies) may occur. In both Class III and IV lesions, immune deposits and electron-dense deposits are generally numerous in the mesangium and extend to peripheral capillaries both beneath the endothelium and epithelium and sometimes within the GBM. Class V lesions resemble those seen in membranous nephropathy, and Class VI lesions indicate an end-stage advanced sclerosing glomerulonephritis. Mixed pictures and transformations from one class to another in individual patients is common.

It has been suggested that the various glomerular lesions indicate differences in the immune response in individual patients. Class II lesions with mesangial involvement alone are related to deposition of small amounts of stable intermediate-sized complexes with high-avidity antibodies. The capacity of the mesangium to accomodate and clear macromolecules is overloaded, and they then accumulate beneath the endothelium (Class III and IV lesions). When the immune response produces small unstable circulating complexes with low-avidity antibodies in conditions of antigen excess, the complexes may dissociate and reform in situ on the glomerular capillary wall (Class V lesions) (Hayslett and Hardin 1982).

The pattern of pathological changes shows some correlation with the clinical manifestations and response to treatment in lupus nephritis (Table 8.2).

Table 8.2. Pathological changes and clinical manifestations in different forms of lupus nephritis

Class	Clinical manifestation
I	May have little or no clinical evidence of renal involvement
II	Mild proteinuria and haematuria, Renal insufficiency rare, but disease can be progressive
III and IV	Heavy proteinuria (often nephrotic) Haematuria and active urinary sediment Rapidly progressive disease
V	Proteinuria, often nephrotic Relatively indolent clinical course
VI	End-stage renal failure

Diabetic Nephropathy

A number of renal diseases, including pyelonephritis, necrotizing papillitis and nephrosclerosis, can complicate diabetes mellitus. The term "diabetic nephropathy" is usually reserved for a more distinctive glomerular lesion occurring in patients with long-standing diabetes. It is characterized clinically by persistent proteinuria and sometimes by the nephrotic syndrome, and pathologically by nodular or diffuse glomerular lesions, which may occur separately or together in any individual case. The nodular, or Kimmelsteil–Wilson, lesion consists of rounded, homogeneous, eosinophilic, hyaline deposits situated in the peripheries of the glomerular tuft lobules in the axial regions. These nodules, which vary in size, often affect more than one lobule in a single tuft. The diffuse lesion consists of widespread mesangial thickening in all glomeruli, accompanied by thickening of tuft capillary walls. In both patterns the hyaline material has ultrastructural characteristics resembling basement membrane material. Characteristically severe arteriolar sclerosis with hyaline thickening of the arteriolar walls accompanies diabetic nephropathy. The pathogenesis of the lesion is unknown, but the deposits have been interpreted as accumulations of fibrin-derived products altered by ageing, which originally seep from the glomerular capillaries as a result of the increased capillary permeability associated with diabetes, or, alternatively, as a reflection of abnormal basement membrane synthesis resulting from deranged carbohydrate metabolism.

Although clinical evidence of diabetic nephropathy is rare in children, pathological involvement of the renal glomeruli has been described on a number of occasions in this age group (Urizar et al. 1969; Balodimos et al. 1970; Westberg and Michael 1972). In general, the incidence of significant renal involvement increases with the duration of the diabetes (White 1956).

Renal Amyloidosis

Detailed discussion of renal amyloidosis here is inappropriate; the condition is rare in children and differs in no significant way from the adult disease. Occasional cases of secondary amyloidosis with renal involvement occur in this age group, but are uncommon with modern treatment of the causative disorders. Familial forms of amyloidosis, such as Mediterranean fever, may develop renal manifestations during childhood (Sohar et al. 1967).

Hereditary Nephropathy

A number of uncommon or very rare, and usually progressive, forms of renal disease of unknown aetiology are distinguished by their familial incidence. They can be classified to a limited extent by their clinical associations, pathological features and mode of inheritance, but in most cases information on all these points is sparse and often conflicting. Only the more familiar varieties are dealt with here and the reader is referred to Kissane (1973) for detailed consideration of the topic.

Alport's Syndrome

This disease, named after Alport (1927), is a progressive familial renal disease associated with deafness in which males are affected more severely than females. End-stage renal disease occurs in nearly all affected males, although the rate of progression is variable. In females the course is generally more benign and life expectancy is rarely affected, although there are some exceptions, and progressive disease is occasionally seen in females.

Most patients present with haematuria, which can be present from birth. Usually haematuria is persistent and microscopic, but many patients have episodic gross haematuria that may be precipitated by upper respiratory infections. Proteinuria is generally absent in early childhood, but increases progressively in affected males and may reach nephrotic proportions (Gubler et al. 1981). Hypertension is another

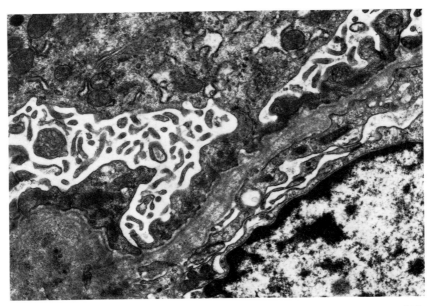

Fig. 8.25. Alport's syndrome. Electron micrograph showing foot process fusion, irregular basement membrane thickening, and distortion and splitting of the lamina densa. (× 9000)

feature in males that increases in frequency and severity with age.

The hearing defect in Alport's syndrome is always accompanied by evidence of renal disease and, though absent in childhood, usually develops by the age of 15 years in affected males. At first its detection requires audiometry and is confined to frequencies in the 2000–8000 Hz range. With progression of the deafness, other frequencies are eventually involved. Progressive hearing loss in affected females is unusual, and is predictive that progressive renal disease will also occur (Grünfeld et al. 1985). Occular abnormalities, particularly anterior lenticonus, occur in about 15%–30% of affected patients. Epstein et al. (1972) has also described two families with Alport's syndrome who had megathrombocytopathia.

The mechanism of inheritance in Alport's syndrome has not been completely elucidated. Current evidence (Evans et al. 1980; Feingold et al. 1985) suggests that an X-linked dominant transmission is most common, but that autosomal dominant and autosomal recessive inheritance also occur.

The histological features of Alport's syndrome on renal biopsy are variable and, by light microscopy, non-specific. Early in the disease the appearances may be normal or there may be focal thickening of occasional glomerular capillary loops or of Bowman's capsule, sometimes mild mesangial expansion and occasionally some mesangial hypercellularity. Tubules, apart from occasional erythrocytes, are normal. With progression the glomerular

changes become more marked and segmental (particularly at the vascular pole) and focal global glomerulosclerosis is seen, together with interstitial fibrosis and tubular atrophy. Collections of interstitial foam cells are a useful pointer to the diagnosis. Similar collections may be seen in any nephrotic patient, but with lesser degrees of proteinuria are suggestive of Alport's syndrome. Capsular crescents are an occasional feature.

The important diagnostic morphological features are seen by electron microscopy (Fig. 8.25). These include a variable thickening and thinning of the GBM, with multilayering of the lamina densa, typically in a "basket weave" pattern. Electron-dense dots are seen in the clear electron-lucent lucunae between the layers of the lamina densa. Sometimes, particularly in young children and females, there is diffuse thinning of the GBM without the changes noted above.

An important observation, reported by Olson et al. (1980), is that the glomeruli in Alport's syndrome fail to bind the anti-GBM antibodies present in the serum of patients with Goodpasture's syndrome. As noted previously (p. 470), the epitope recognized by this antibody is a component of the α_3-chain of the non-collagenous domain of type IV collagen (Hudson et al. 1989). This raises the possibility that Alport's syndrome represents a defect in type IV collagen the (predominant collagenous component of basement membranes), perhaps due to deletion or derangement of a gene on the X chromosome.

This might also explain the different severity of the disease in males and females, at least in Alport's syndrome inherited as an X-linked dominant trait. Affected males would have a single X chromosome harbouring the defective gene and so would synthesize only abnormal glomerular basement membrane. In heterozygous females, following the Lyon principle (Lyon 1972), basement-membrane-producing cells would have either the normal or the abnormal gene so that both normal and abnormal glomerular basement membrane would result. Recently a further abnormality of the GBM in Alport's syndrome has been recognized by immunofluorescence microscopy, namely the absence of amyloid P (Melvin et al. 1986).

Thin Glomerular Basement Membrane Nephropathy

In children and adults presenting with persistent microscopic or sometimes episodic gross haematuria, the only abnormality on renal biopsy may be a diffuse thinning of the GBM on electron microscopy (thin glomerular basement membrane nephropathy). In many of these patients the condition is familial and, because there is generally no tendency to progressive renal disease, the term "benign familial haematuria" has been applied.

Although many cases are familial, sporadic cases are not uncommon (Yoshikawa et al. 1984). In familial cases, inheritance is usually autosomal dominant, but autosomal recessive transmission is also recorded (Eisenstein et al. 1979). It is notable that some patients with apparently benign familial haematuria exhibit no GBM attenuation (Waldherr et al. 1982). Because some patients with early Alport's syndrome show only diffuse glomerular basement membrane thinning, without the more specific ultrastructural features of that condition (Habib et al. 1982), careful evaluation of other family members is important. The use of antisera against the Goodpasture antigen may also be helpful in distinguishing such cases. Despite the name "benign familial nephropathy", the development of significant proteinuria, hypertension and renal failure does occur in a minority of patients (Dische et al. 1985).

In children the diagnosis may be complicated by the fact that the GBM is normally thinner in childhood, particularly in the very young, and confirmation may require morphometric measurement (Lang et al. 1990). Thin glomerular basement membrane nephropathy is probably commoner than generally realized, the frequency in the series reported by Lang et al. (1990) being similar to that of IgA nephropathy.

Hereditary Multifocal Osteolysis with Nephropathy

Hereditary osteolysis is a rare disorder in which sclerosis, gradual lysis and collapse affect the carpal and tarsal bones. Osseous involvement commences in early childhood and the disease becomes static by adult life, when deformity may be marked. Inheritance is usually described as autosomal dominant in type, with variable expressivity.

Some patients with hereditary osteolysis develop progressive renal disease with hypertension. Most of the few pathological descriptions of the renal lesion have indicated chronic glomerulonephritis. This has usually been reported in adult patients (Marie et al. 1963), but it also occurs in children (Counahan et al. 1976).

Hereditary Onycho-osteodysplasia (Nail–Patella Syndrome)

The nail–patella syndrome is a curious disorder inherited as an autosomal dominant trait with variable expressivity closely allied to that for ABO blood groups and characterized by abnormal development of the finger and toe nails and hypoplasia or absence of the patellae. Malformations of the radii and asymptomatic osseous spurs projecting from the ilium may also be seen. About one-third of the patients affected have evidence of renal disease with proteinuria, sometimes accompanied by haematuria. Renal insufficiency develops very slowly and late in the course of the disease. The morphological changes in the kidney are non-specific and usually mild, with focal thickening of glomerular capillary walls, irregular glomerular sclerosis, and areas of tubular atrophy by light microscopy.

Ultrastructurally, the GBM appears "moth eaten", with multiple mottled and lucent areas (Angelov et al. 1981). Within these spaces are coarse fibrils that appear to be cross-banded collagen.

Congenital Nephrotic Syndrome

Two main varieties are recognized, the commoner "Finnish" type and the less common "French" type, also termed diffuse mesangial sclerosis. The Finnish type is inherited as an autosomal recessive trait; the nephrotic syndrome is recognized at or soon after birth, and the affected infant is often premature and of low birth weight. As well as proteinuria, hypoalbuminaemia and oedema, microscopic haematuria is often present. The placenta is large and oedematous, frequently constituting 25%–60% of the birth weight

(Kouvalainen et al. 1962). The nephrotic syndrome is resistant to both steroids and immunosuppressive agents. Survival beyond the first year is unusual because of intercurrent infection, but the prognosis has improved as renal transplantation has become an option in this age group.

Histologically, on renal biopsy the glomeruli are immature and may exhibit mild to moderate mesangial hypercellularity and increase in mesangial matrix. Tubules may be cystically dilated. As the disease progresses, glomerular sclerosis and tubular atrophy develop. Immunofluorescent microscopy is generally negative, and electron microscopy reveals diffuse podocyte foot process fusion. This change can sometimes be seen in fetal kidneys and may allow a presumptive diagnosis following therapeutic abortion for raised α-fetoprotein levels in the amniotic fluid and maternal blood (for which congenital nephrotic syndrome is a cause).

Diffuse mesangial sclerosis (Habib and Bois 1975) also present with nephrotic syndrome in the first year of life, sometimes in the first few weeks but usually later than the Finnish type. Although there are reports of diffuse mesangial sclerosis in siblings, its autosomal recessive inheritance is less securely documented than in the Finnish variety. The disease progresses to renal failure at between 1 and 3 years. Histologically the glomerular lesion is characterized by mesangial sclerosis with a marked increase in mesangial matrix and obliteration of most capillary lumina. The process transforms the glomerular tuft to a rounded mass covered by hypertrophied and sometimes vacuolated epithelial cells. Tuft cells nuclei are surprisingly well preserved in view of the degree of the mesangial sclerosis, and in the contracted tufts give an impression of hypercellularity. This change, together with the sometimes prominent "double contouring" of residual peripheral capillary loops has led to erroneous descriptions of this disease as a mesangiocapillary glomerulonephritis. Capsular adhesions and crescents are uncommon. Examinations of sections of the whole kidney reveal that the more advanced glomerular lesions are in the mid or outer cortex; juxtamedullary glomeruli may be only slightly affected, or even normal. In the subcapsular cortex a rim of small and partly sclerosed glomeruli with a simplified lobular structure associated with atrophic tubules may form a distinct layer. Tubulointerstitial changes are generally severe. Atrophic tubules are admixed with hypertrophied, and often cystically dilated tubules containing proteinaceous casts.

Immunofluorescence microscopy commonly demonstrates IgM and C3 in the expanded mesangial areas and along capillary loops. Ultrastructurally, mesangial sclerosis is confirmed, with occasional mesangial interposition around capillary loops, corresponding to the double contours seen by light microscopy. Focally the GBM outside the lamina densa may be thickened with an undulating subepithelial contour. Strands of lamina-densa-like material surrounding clear lacunae may be seen in the thickened outer GBM, to give an appearance superficially resembling that in Alport's syndrome.

An exactly similar glomerular disease of diffuse mesangial sclerosis to that seen in congenital nephrotic syndrome is also a feature of the Drash syndrome of male pseudohermaphroditism, nephropathy and Wilms' tumour (nephroblastoma). In Drash syndrome, the nephrotic syndrome and progressive renal failure develop in early childhood. Incomplete forms without Wilms' tumour, or occurring in genotypic females, are also described.

Renal Vascular Disease

Arterial Hypertension

Essential hypertension is rarely diagnosed in children, and for this reason secondary forms are of greater practical importance than in adults. However, concepts regarding the nature of hypertension are currently changing. The practical importance of a raised arterial blood pressure, apart from its direct effects, lies in the increased risk of complications such as cerebrovascular accidents and ischaemic heart disease. However, hypertension is not a disease in the generally accepted sense. Among individuals in a particular population arterial pressure is normally distributed, and although the risk of complications increases as blood pressure rises further beyond the mean, there is no arbitrary level that defines the "normal" value. Recent work suggests that an individual becomes fixed on a particular blood pressure centile for the population as a whole early in life, perhaps even in infancy (see Berry 1978 for discussion). Genetic factors are undoubtedly important, as pressures tend to be higher in infants of whom one or both parents are hypertensive (Zinner et al. 1971; Beresford and Holland 1975). Because blood pressure tends to increase with age, a child with an arterial pressure significantly above the mean will tend to become hypertensive as an adult, even though his or her pressure in early life may be below that usually associated with an increased risk of complications. The practical implications of these ideas, particularly whether treatment with hypotensive agents is justified in children with persistent arterial pressures significantly above average, have yet to be clarified.

In both essential and secondary forms of hypertension, persistent elevation of the arterial blood pressure may be associated with changes in arterial vessels throughout the body, including those in the kidneys. The nature of these changes depends on the rapidity with which hypertension develops and on the degree of elevation of the arterial pressure. In general, changes in vessels in children with hypertension are not different from those in adults, but complicating factors (atherosclerosis and age-related changes) are absent. Essential hypertension-related renal damage takes many years to develop and is seldom evident in childhood, but in malignant hypertension secondary nephrosclerosis is marked and proliferative changes, even capsular crescent formation and focal necroses, may be apparent in the glomerular tufts. Malignant hypertension may give rise to renal failure, or an increase in intracranial pressure, which can be recognized clinically by the presence of papilloedema.

Causes of Secondary Hypertension in Children

Glomerulonephritis is the commonest cause of hypertension in children. In acute poststreptococcal glomerulonephritis hypertension is usually transient, and most reports suggest that it results from overload of the extracellular fluid space or an imbalance in the normal homornal regulatory mechanisms. Persistent hypertension may be a feature of any chronic glomerulonephritis, particularly when chronic renal failure develops. Allen et al. (1960) found hypertension in about a quarter of patients with nephritis following Schönlein–Henoch purpura, and it is a prominent feature in about half of all children with haemolytic uraemic syndrome (p. 489). Hypertension may also occur in children subjected to renal transplantation either immediately following transplantation or during rejection episodes.

The pathology of chronic pyelonephritis and reflux nephropathy is considered in detail on p. 493 Hypertension is sometimes present, particularly in patients with severe bilateral disease. It is rarely present in children without evidence of renal failure, but is occasionally seen in patients without azotaemia and in those with unilateral involvement. The mechanisms involved are disputed (see Heptinstall 1974b), and it is probable that a number of different factors are involved in individual cases.

Segmental renal hypoplasia (the Ask-Upmark kidney) commonly presents with hypertension, which is often severe and may occur with unilateral or bilateral disease. As discussed on p. 454, there is some confusion about the exact nature of this condition. The fact that "segmental hypoplasia" is not uncommonly associated with vesicoureteric reflux raises the possibility that it is an acquired disease rather than a congenital anomaly, and may be just a form of reflux nephropathy (Johnson and Mix 1976). The separation of cases of segmental hypoplasia may merely represent clinical selection of those cases presenting with hypertension. The associated vesicoureteric reflux may be regarded as insignificant; it may be overlooked if not specifically looked for; or it may have ceased by the time the patient is investigated, because vesicoureteric reflux resolves in a majority of children (see p. 493).

Both renal dysplasia and polycystic disease (see pp. 455 and 461) may be accompanied by hypertension. As with pyelonephritis, renal dysplasia is seldom complicated by hypertension except where severe bilateral involvement has led to renal failure. Superadded chronic infection is common in these instances. Hydronephrosis may also be accompanied by hypertension, and a few cases of unilateral hydronephrosis with ureteric obstruction are on record in which complicating hypertension was relieved by surgical removal of the obstruction (Belman et al. 1968; Palmer et al. 1970).

Children with renal tumours may develop hypertension. Nephroblastoma, according to some reports, is commonly associated with a raised arterial blood pressure (Campbell 1951), and occasionally hypertension can be severe (Mitchell et al. 1970). Renal tumours may cause hypertension by perirenal compression of the kidney, or distortion of the renal arteries causing a renovascular type of hypertension. In addition, some renal tumours, including some examples of nephroblastoma, produce a pressor substance with renin-like activity (Robertson et al. 1967; Mitchell et al. 1970).

Hypertension may follow irradiation of the kidneys, usually following treatment of nephroblastoma or, less commonly, adrenal neuroblastoma.

A number of renovascular lesions, particularly renal artery dysplasia (Harrison and McCormack 1971), may cause hypertension in childhood. In renal artery dysplasia, changes usually affect the media of the main renal artery. The most common type (*medial fibroplasia with aneurysms*) is characterized by multiple stenotic segments formed by fibromuscular ridges that alternate with thinned, dilated, aneurysmal segments in which the internal elastic lamina is lost. This change produces a string-of-beads deformity on angiography. Other forms of medial renal artery stenosis are *perimedial fibroplasia*, in which stenosis is due to replacement of the outer media by collagen, and *medial hyperplasia*, in which a usually short, but severely stenotic, segment is produced by localized medial muscular thickening. Medial renal artery dysplasias are commonly bilateral, may affect segmental as well as main renal arteries and occur predominantly in young women. Much less frequent forms of renal artery dysplasia are due to *intimal* or *adventitial fibroplasia*.

Hypertension may also occur in children with von Recklinghausen's neurofibromatosis. This may be due to renal artery dysplasia (Devaney et al. 1991), aneurysm formation, stenosis of the main renal artery through extrinsic compression by an adjacent neurofibroma, or a more generalized narrowing of intrarenal arteries by proliferation of spindle-celled myofibroblasts, mainly in the outer part of the intima. Hypertension due to the association of phaeochromocytoma with von Recklinghauser's disease is very rare in childhood.

Arterial hypertension is commonly seen in regions of the body proximal to a coarctation of the aorta. It may also be due to the hormonal effects of functioning adrenal or extra-adrenal chromaffin tumours, congenital hyperplasia of the adrenal cortex, or mineralocorticoid-producing tumours of the adrenal cortex.

Renal vein thrombosis following umbilical artery catheterization may lead to rapidly progressive hypertension and death in the neonate (Buchi and Seigler 1986), and persistent hypertension may also follow this lesion.

Some causes of hypertension in childhood are:

1. Renal:
   a) Glomerulonephritis (all forms)
   b) Pyelonephritis and reflux nephropathy
   c) Ask-Upmark kidney
   d) Renal dysplasia
   e) Hydronephrosis
   f) Polycystic disease
   g) Renal tumours
   h) Renal parenchymal damage following irradiation
2. Vascular:
   a) Coarctation of the aorta
   b) Renal artery anomalies (stenosis, dysplasia, arteritis, aneurysms, neurofibromatosis)
3. Other:
   a) Adrenal tumours (neuroblastoma, phaeochromocytoma)
   b) Adrenogenital syndrome
   c) Cushing's syndrome
   d) Primary aldosteronism

Renal Hypoperfusion

Circulatory failure may result in acute renal failure, which may be rapidly reversed without structural damage to the kidney if the underlying circulatory disturbance can be corrected. More prolonged renal hypoperfusion can cause renal injuries that do not recover immediately on restoration of a normal circulation. These lesions include renal tubular necrosis, renal cortical necrosis, renal medullary necrosis and renal vein thrombosis, and in infants and young children suffering from renal hypoperfusion a combination of these lesions is often present. In such patients the underlying cause of the circulatory failure may be a cardiac abnormality, reduction in blood volume from haemorrhage, reduction of plasma volume from hypoalbuminaemia, loss of extracellular fluid (as in severe burns or sodium depletion), crushing injuries, or severe bacterial infection.

Acute tubular necrosis following hypoperfusion usually affects both the proximal and distal convoluted tubules and the loops of Henle. Tubular necrosis may also follow direct poisoning by heavy metals such as mercury and arsenic, organic solvents such as carbon tetrachloride, and drugs such as sulphonamides and methoxyflurane. Toxic damage of this type is usually confined to the proximal convoluted tubules. With successful clinical management, regeneration of the necrotic tubular epithelial cells can be anticipated.

In infancy, and particularly during the first 2 months of life, renal vein thrombosis is likely to complicate renal hypoperfusion. Clinically this is recognized by the development of an enlarged firm renal mass in a sick infant with oliguria and haematuria. Disseminated intravascular coagulation and thrombocytopenia may also be present. Dehydration following gastrointestinal disturbances is a common underlying cause. Involvement may be unilateral or bilateral, and the thrombus may occlude the main renal vein and all its tributaries, or merely some of the tributaries. Depending on the degree of thrombosis and other factors, part or all of the kidney may undergo venous infarction. Sometimes venous infarction is confined to the renal medulla.

Medullary and cortical necrosis frequently coexist, and etiological factors giving rise to these lesions in the newborn include severe anaemia, asphyxia, severe haemolytic disease and disseminated intravascular coagulation. Haemorrhagic infarction of the renal medullae and inner adrenal cortex has been described in infants dying from echovirus II infections (Nagington et al. 1978). In older infants and young children, severe gastroenteritis with vomiting and diarrhoea leading to marked dehydration, other severe bacterial infections, postoperative shock, diabetic ketosis, or haemolytic–uraemic syndrome may also cause these lesions. Unilateral or bilateral renal involvement occurs and the kidneys may show patchy or diffuse changes. The deep juxtamedullary cortex and a thin rim of subcapsular cortex are generally spared even in severe bilateral symmetrical cortical necrosis. In the acute phase of the disease the kidneys are swollen and enlarged, but in patients who survive for several weeks the kidneys become shrunken and show marked nodularity because of the hypertrophy of the surviving parenchyma. Calcification of the necrotic cortical tissue occurs and may be visible on radiological examination. When there is accompanying medullary necrosis, pelvicalyceal deformities are present, giving rise to a radiological picture on intravenous urography that closely resembles that seen in chronic pyelonephritis (Chrispin 1972).

Renal Infarction

Obstruction of the renal arterial blood supply may produce infarction of the whole kidney or of a segment. Extreme venous engorgement following venous obstruction may also give rise to infarction.

Arterial occlusion is usually the result of thromboembolism, the emboli arising, for example, from vegetation on heart valves or a coarcted aortic segment. Thrombosis of the renal artery is a rare complication of polyarteritis nodosa and other forms of arteritis during childhood.

Nephropathy in Sickle Cell Anaemia

Diffuse intravascular sickling with agglutination of distorted red cells characteristically occurs in haemolytic crises in patients with sickle cell anaemia. Patchy ischaemic lesions may then develop in various organs including the kidneys. In patients who survive a number of such crises, widespread renal scarring is not unusual and may result in renal failure. Ischaemic medullary fibrosis is the probable underlying cause of the diminished ability to concentrate the urine, which is an almost invariable feature of sickle cell anaemia.

Haemolytic–Uraemic Syndrome

This term describes a form of thrombotic microangiopathy associated with a haemolytic anaemia, thrombocytopenia and acute renal failure. Classically, it affects infants and young children under the age of 2 years, but all ages may be affected. The sex incidence is equal and there is a seasonal variation, the disease being more common in the summer and autumn in the northern hemisphere. The disease tends to be more severe in older patients and is usually preceded by a prodromal episode of diarrhoea and vomiting, or less commonly a respiratory tract infection. Within a few days this is followed by the abrupt onset of acute renal failure jaundice, anaemia, bleeding tendency and sometimes central nervous system and hypertension disturbances. Renal manifestations include haematuria, proteinuria, oliguria, and sometimes haemoglobinuria or anuria (Gianantonio et al. 1973; Habib et al. 1982). Hyperkalaemia and raised urea and creatinine levels are present. A blood film shows deformity (burr cells) and fragmentation of red blood cells. The Coombs' test is negative and platelet numbers are decreased. Central nervous system manifestations include irritability, tremor, ataxia and convulsions. Sometimes colitis is present.

The pathological changes in the kidney are variable. Cortical necrosis may be present, particularly in acutely ill patients who die. Glomerular changes reflect the stage of the disease. Early manifestations include endothelial swelling, with red blood cells and fibrin and platelet thrombi in tuft capillary lumina. There may be mesangial expansion and hypercellularity, and occasionally fragmented red blood cells are seen. Foci of tuft necrosis and occasional capsular crescents are sometimes a feature. As the lesion evolves, the glomeruli may show a solidification of the tufts which have a fibrillar appearance and a decrease in the number of tuft nuclei. Immunofluorescence microscopy demonstrates fibrin in glomerular thrombonecrotic foci and sometimes slight immonoglobin and complement deposition in the glomerular tufts. Ultrastructurally the glomerular capillary walls are thickened due to the deposition of granular fibrillary electron-dense material in the widened subendothelial space. This may give rise to double contours seen by light microscopy in silver preparations. Damage to endothelial cells is an early manifestation, and sometimes endothelial cells are detached from the GBM. Fibrin thrombi with platelets and fragmented red cells may occlude tuft capillaries.

In the arteries and arterioles, early changes include fibrin infiltration of arteriolar walls (fibrinoid necrosis), fibrin and platelet thrombi, and endothelial cell swelling. Later there is intimal proliferation by myointimal cells that may occlude vascular lumina. When severe, the vascular changes are associated with glomerular shrinkage and sclerosis, and with tubular atrophy and interstitial fibrosis.

The pathogenesis of haemolytic–uraemic syndrome probably involves two basic abnormalities; endothelial damage and blood coagulation and its sequelae. Endothelial damage may be due to bacterial or viral toxins associated with the prodromal illness. Verotoxin-producing *Escherichia coli* are emerging as an important precipitating agent (Konowalchuk et al. 1977), and other infective agents such as *Shigella dysenteriae* have also been incriminated. Neuraminidase, produced by some bacterial and viral agents, may not only damage endothelial cells, but may also affect red blood cells and cause haemolysis (Paschmann et al. 1976). Damaged endothelial surfaces are probably important in eliciting coagulation and activating platelets. Certain drugs, particularly cyclosporin A and mitomycin have also been associated with haemolytic–uraemic syndrome (Atkinson et al. 1983; Proia et al. 1984). As well as the possible effects of neuraminidase, red cell damage may be partly mechanical, their disruption due to traversing fibrin meshworks.

As well as classic probably postinfective haemolytic–uraemic syndrome, some cases appear hereditary and recurrent. In some familial cases, particularly when different family members are affected simultaneously or over a short time span, the explanation may lie in prodromal infection with same organism (Kaplan et al. 1975). In other families, where this is not the case, hereditary factors may be important, and an autosomal dominant transmission has been suggested (Farr et al. 1975; Karlsberg et al. 1977). In some familial cases, disorders of the complement system are recorded (Carreras et al. 1981; Gonzalo et al. 1981). In both familial and recurrent haemolytic–uraemic syndrome, histological changes are often particularly severe in renal arteries and arterioles, hypertension is common, and the disease, which occurs at any age, is generally severe.

Interstitial Nephritis

A number of disease processes of widely differing aetiologies produce renal parenchymal damage that affects predominantly the tubules and interstitial tissues (and in some cases the blood vessels), rather than the glomeruli. A varying degree of interstitial inflammation is also often present. Because it is impossible to tell on microscopic examination of the kidney alone whether the primary lesion is of tubules, interstitial tissues or blood vessels, the non-committal term "interstitial nephritis" has proved useful to describe these parenchymal changes. The fact that this description is vague is valuable, as it emphasizes the need for careful clinicopathological evaluation to seek a possible underlying cause. Not uncommonly, even after thorough investigation the aetiology remains obscure, but gradually more and more factors producing this type of renal damage are becoming recognized.

Renal infection, particularly chronic pyelonephritis, is a significant cause of interstitial nephritis in paediatric practice, and this will be discussed below. In the past, however, it has not been sufficiently appreciated that a number of other types of interstitial nephritis can produce a very similar histological picture to that seen in chronic pyelonephritis. This label has been attached indiscriminately to cases where renal infection is either not involved in the pathogenesis or is merely a complication of another underlying renal lesion.

Traditionally, interstitial nephritis is divided into acute and chronic forms, the former characterized by an acute clinical course and pathologically by interstitial oedema, active tubular damage and an interstitial infiltrate. Although this is predominantly of activated lymphocytes, it may include granulocytes. The chronic form has a more protracted clinical course and the changes on biopsy include interstitial fibrosis and tubular atrophy. The interstitial infiltrate includes lymphocytes, histiocytes and plasma cells; granulomas may be seen in some varieties.

In childhood, some of the more common forms include drug reactions, immunologically mediated tubulointerstitial disease and those secondary, to systemic disease (such as sarcoidosis and Sjögren's syndrome) as well as rare hereditary forms.

Renal Infection

Infection of the urinary tract may be serious particularly in the neonate, because of the risks both of spread of infection and of septicaemia, but the usual clinical concern is the possibility of involvement of the renal parenchyma (pyelonephritis). It is important to recognize, however, that renal involvement is by no means invariable or even particularly common in urinary tract infections.

Pyelonephritis occurs in both acute and chronic forms and may or may not be associated with obstructive lesions of the urinary tract. In following sections the mechanisms whereby urinary infection may spread to the renal parenchyma are discussed and the pathology of acute and chronic pyelonephritis is considered.

The pathophysiological events following the introduction of pathogenic organisms to the renal parenchyma have been studied extensively by Roberts and coworkers (Roberts et al. 1982, 1983, 1986; Kaack et al. 1986; Roberts 1991), who indicate that ischaemia and reperfusion injury due to the release of superoxide are important mechanisms.

Spread of Infection to the Kidneys

Pyelonephritis usually follows established lower urinary tract infection, and this sequence may be influenced by a number of factors.

Theoretically, organisms gain access to the kidneys by three routes:

Lymphatic Spread

There is little or no clinical or experimental evidence that this mechanism is important.

Haematogenous Spread

This undoubtedly occurs in some instances. The kidney may be infected in humans in the course of septicaemia following staphylococcal infections such as boils, carbuncles, osteomyelitis or endocarditis. Haematogenous spread of gram-negative organisms to the kidney sometimes complicates instrumentation or surgical operations on the urethra (Scott 1929; Barrington and Wright 1930).

Direct Ascent from the Lower Urinary Tract

This is widely accepted as the most frequent route by which infection of the kidneys occurs, although infections of the bladder and urethra are usually confined to the lower urinary tract. The long intramural and submucosal segment of the ureter at the vesicoureteric junction provides an efficient valvular mechanism, which normally prevents the return of the bladder urine and any organisms it might contain into the ureter and upper tract. In some patients, however, congenital or acquired defects of the vesicoureteric junction render it likely to permit reflux of urine during detrusor contraction at micturition. A congenital lack of obliquity of the intramural and submucosal ureter may render the vesicoureteric junction incompetent. This defect can occur as an isolated lesion, which sometimes has a familial incidence (Bredin et al. 1975; Dwoskin 1976; de Vargas et al. 1978), and also in combination with other urinary tract anomalies, such as posterior urethral valves, megacystis–megaureter, ectopic ureter and ectopic ureterocele. Acquired incompetence of the vesicoureteric junction leading to vesicoureteric reflux can occur in patients with a "neurogenic" bladder, and even bladder infection can produce sufficient mucosal inflammation and oedema to convert the submucosal segment of the ureter into a rigid tube, resulting in reflux.

During micturition intravesical pressure rises, and in patients with incompetence of the vesicoureteric junction the increased pressure is transmitted directly to the renal pelvis. This results in reversal of the normal pressure gradient between the tubular system of the kidney and the renal pelvis. Thus refluxed urine may pass retrogradely into the papillary ducts and renal tubules in the kidney parenchyma. This process of *intrarenal reflux* (Hodson et al. 1975) provides a mechanism whereby any organisms in the bladder urine may be carried directly to the renal substance, where infection can become established. This explains many of the features of pyelonephritic scarring and is dealt with in more detail in the section on chronic pyelonephritis (see below).

When vesicoureteric reflux is gross the ureters become dilated and tortuous. Urine that refluxed into such capacious ureters during micturition returns to the bladder when voiding is complete. This residual urine provides a suitable medium in which organisms can multiply. This predisposes to urinary infection and helps to perpetuate established infection.

Progressive Bacterial Colonization

An alternative mechanism for ascending infection independent of vesicoureteric reflux relates to the ability of some strains of *E. coli* to adhere to wet mucosa surfaces by attachment (type 1) fimbriae ("pili"), which are hair-like structures projecting from the surface of the bacterial cell. Progressive colonization of the ureteric mucosa by these "sticky" fimbriated *E. coli* has been proposed by Roberts et al. (1985) as a means of ascent of infection to the kidney.

Urinary Tract Obstruction

Obstructive lesions anywhere in the urinary tract are associated with a 20-fold increase in the incidence of pyelonephritis (Campbell 1951). In infants and children, urinary obstruction is most commonly caused by congenital anomalies such as posterior urethral valves, congenital ureteric stenosis, ureterocele, etc., but may result from acquired lesions such as urolithiasis. A neurogenic bladder complicating spina bifida, for example, may produce functional obstruction. The normal bladder is relatively resistant to colonization with microorganisms. Voiding during micturition empties the bladder efficiently and flushes out any organisms that may be present. In addition, the bladder mucosa has a number of antibacterial protective mechanisms, which help to maintain the sterility of the urine. However, abnormalities such as outflow obstruction leading to stagnant residual urine provide a medium in which organisms can multiply. It is now recognized that even a healthy urethra often harbours

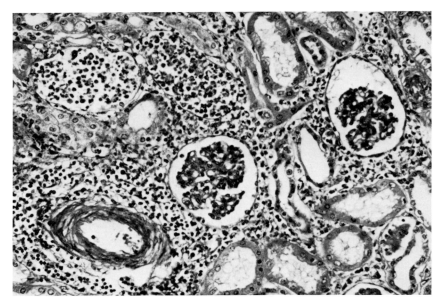

Fig. 8.26. Acute pyelonephritis. Note acute interstitial inflammation and oedema with acute inflammatory tubular destruction. (H&E, × 250)

microorganisms; these may be a source of urinary infection, particularly following trauma during urethral instrumentation such as catheterization. The mechanism whereby organisms gain access to the kidney in urinary obstruction uncomplicated by vesicoureteric reflux is not clear-cut. There is evidence, based on mathematical considerations, that they can ascend within the lumen of the ureter against the flow of urine (Shapiro 1967), but spread to involve the renal parenchyma is more difficult to explain. Severe pyogenic inflammation of the upper tract occurring with, for example, pyelonephrosis or infective urolithiasis can probably extend into the renal substance directly. It is probable, however, that lower urinary tract infection in the presence of urinary obstruction often involves the kidney via the haematogenous route. Obstruction slows the passage of urine through the kidneys, and any organisms filtered from the blood will therefore become established more easily in the renal parenchyma. Transient bacteraemia certainly occurs with lower urinary tract infections, particularly during catheterization.

Renal Factors

It is old experimental observation that infection within the kidney tends to localize in areas of pre-existing damage (de Navasquez 1956). Histological evidence of parenchymal infection (the presence of pus cells within tubules) is not infrequently found at necropsy in the diseased kidneys of patients dying with chronic glomerulonephritis, diabetic glomerulosclerosis or cystic kidneys. Renal infections of this nature are usually a terminal event and are probably the result of haematogenous infection. Pyelonephritis is a common complication of renal dysplasia and this too has been attributed to an abnormal susceptibility of the malformed kidney to infection (Marshall 1953; Ericsson and Ivemark 1958a, b). However, as previously emphasized, renal dysplasia is almost invariably associated with other urinary tract anomalies, with are either obstructive or accompanied by vesicoureteric reflux. It is probable that these factors are the principal predisposing causes of parenchymal infection in renal dysplasia (Risdon 1971a, b).

Acute Pyelonephritis

Descriptions of the pathology of acute pyelonephritis usually relate to cases seen at necropsy with severe fulminating infection, associated with urinary obstruction or staphylococcal septicaemia (the "pyaemic kidney"). This condition is illustrated in Fig. 8.26.

Grossly the kidney is swollen, and small yellow abscesses are usually visible through the capsule. On section, the bulging cut surface is discoloured by wedge-shaped areas of cortical congestion and pallor and by yellowish radial streaks. In cases with urinary obstruction the pelvicalyceal system is dilated, and the lining mucosa is congested, oedematous and covered with pus. Sometimes the renal papillae are yellow and necrotic (necrotizing papillitis).

It is important to recognize that this severe and diffuse inflammation may not be typical of the much commoner milder cases of acute upper tract infection seen clinically. It is quite possible that many patients with urinary infections and symptoms of upper tract involvement, such as loin pain, may have infection confined to the ureter and renal pelvis (acute pyelitis) without renal parenchymal involvement (Heptinstall 1974a).

Chronic Pyelonephritis (Reflux Nephropathy)

Recent observations would suggest that the spectrum of reflux nephropathy is wider than previously envisaged, with at least two clinically distinct groups (Lancet leader 1992; Risdon 1993; Risdon et al. 1993). In the first, renal scarring is recognized during childhood or sometimes not until adolescence or adult life. Presentation may be with recurrent urinary infection or, in older patients, with renal insufficiency or hypertension. The renal scarring is segmental and is probably acquired through infected vesicoureteric reflux in early childhood (as described above), the kidneys being normally developed. Vesicoureteric reflux may be demonstrated at presentation or may have remitted spontaneously. In the second group renal damage is recognized in infancy, vesicoureteric reflux is frequently gross and bilateral, and there may be significant renal impairment. In these infants, it is likely that at least some damage has occurred in utero, and there is usually an element of dysplastic renal maldevelopment as well as scarring in the affected kidneys. This subject is addressed in the section on renal dysplasia and vesicoureteric reflux (see pp. 460, 504).

On gross examination the kidney affected by chronic pyelonephritis is smaller than expected and coarsely scarred. Renal involvement is usually, but by no means invariably, bilateral. When both kidneys are affected the degree of reduction in renal size is usually unequal, and it is common for one kidney to be appreciably smaller than the other. Characteristically the scarred segments of parenchyma directly overlie a renal calyx that is misshapen and dilated ("clubbed"). The scarred areas tend to be wedge-shaped, the parenchyma in these zones is thinned, and corticomedullary demarcation is blurred. In cases with urinary obstruction or severe vesicoureteric reflux the pelvicalyceal system is generally dilated; calyceal clubbing results partly from scarring and contraction of the renal papilla. With longstanding obstruction or reflux, generalized parenchymal

atrophy accompanies pelvicalyceal dilatation and the segmental nature of the scarring is much less easy to appreciate. The mucosa lining the renal calyces and pelvis is thickened and its surface is granular.

Microscopically, there is considerable interstitial fibrosis and chronic inflammation accompanied by tubular atrophy and loss. There is infiltration by lymphocytes, together with some histiocytes and plasma cells, and well formed lymphoid follicles are often present (Fig. 8.27). Sometimes aggregates of atrophic tubules lined with homogeneous eosinophilic material give a thyroid-like appearance. Glomerular damage is variable but is usually less conspicuous than the tubular and interstitial changes. The glomeruli in the scarred zones usually appear crowded together as a result of tubular loss and interstitial fibrosis. Some glomeruli are totally destroyed and converted to rounded acellular scars. Others appear relatively normal or show concentric periglomerular fibrosis. The overall number of glomeruli is frequently diminished, suggesting that some destroyed glomeruli are subsequently absorbed. Vascular changes, particularly fibroelastic intimal thickening of arteries and arterioles, are prominent in the scarred areas even in cases uncomplicated by arterial hypertension. Luminal narrowing of these vessels may be extreme, and it is likely that some of the parenchymal damage is due to, or augmented by, ischaemia. Chronic inflammatory cell infiltration of the subepithelial tissues in the renal calyces, pelvis and ureter is present (Fig. 8.27b). The intensity of this chronic inflammatory infiltrate varies, but when marked is often accompanied by lymphoid follicle formation.

The pathogenesis of chronic pyelonephritis is far from being completely understood.

In children, urinary obstruction, usually attributable to congenital anomalies, and vesicoureteric reflux are the most important associated conditions. Intrarenal reflux accompanying vesicoureteric reflux provides a convincing mechanism whereby pathogenic organisms present in the urine could gain access to the renal parenchyma, and also explains some of the pathological features of the segmental pyelonephric scar (its wedge shape, its often sharp demarcation from surrounding normal parenchyma, and its relation to the renal papilla). These associations are confirmed by clinical radiological and experimental observations (Rolleston et al. 1974; Hodson et al. 1975; Ransley and Risdon 1978). Vesicoureteric reflux in children, particularly when severe, shows a significant correlation with segmental scar formation.

Anatomical studies of the renal papillae in both piglets and young children have demonstrated two distinct forms (Ransley and Risdon 1975a, b). One is

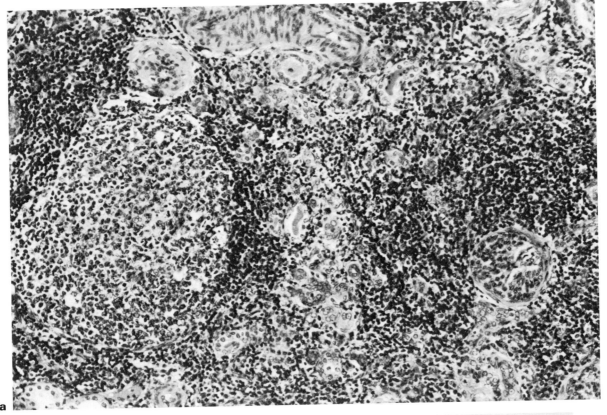

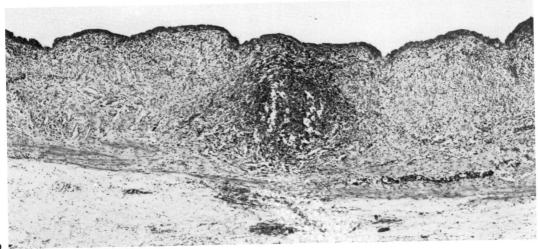

Fig. 8.27. Chronic pyelonephritis. **a** Chronic interstitial inflammation with lymphoid follicle formation. (H&E, × 150) **b** Chronic inflammation of the subepithelial connective tissue in the renal pelvis. (H&E, × 25) (Reproduced from Risdon et al. 1975, by permission of the Editor *Pediatric Radiology*)

a simple conical structure resembling the classic description of the renal papilla in anatomical textbooks. Papillary ducts open obliquely into its convex tip in a way that causes them to close when the intra-

calyceal pressure around the tip of the papillar rises (Fig. 8.28). Thus the papillary duct openings possess a check-valve mechanism, which protects them from intrarenal reflux during an episode of vesicoureteric

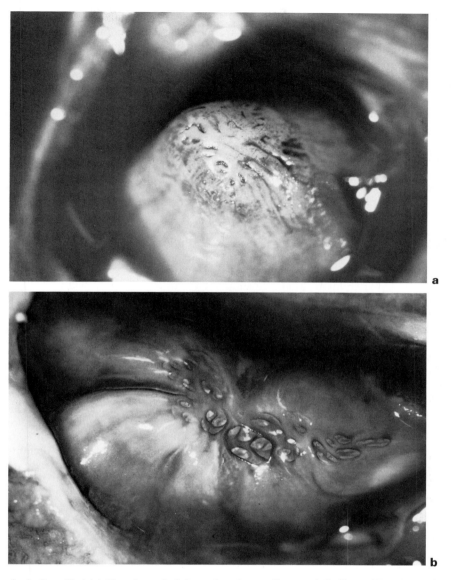

Fig. 8.28. a "Non-refluxing" papilla (pig). Note the conical shape, domed area cribrosa and slit-like papillary duct orifices. This type of papilla is not associated with intrarenal reflux. **b** "Refluxing" papilla (pig). Note the compound structure with a concave area cribrosa and wide open papillary duct orifices. This type of papilla is associated with intrarenal reflux. (Reproduced from Ransley and Risdon 1978, by permission of the Editor of the *British Journal of Radiology*)

reflux. These simple non-refluxing papillae occur principally in the mid-zones of the kidney, where segmental scar formation is relatively uncommon.

The other type of papilla is a compound structure formed by the fusion of a number of papillary units. The calyceal surface is flattened, concave or deeply indented, and the papillary ducts open directly onto this surface (Fig. 8.28b). Thus there is no protective check-valve mechanism, so that such papillae are freely susceptible to intrarenal reflux in the presence of vesicoureteric reflux. Segmental pyelonephritic scarring is most common in the polar regions of the kidney in areas of parenchyma drained by these refluxing papillae.

The suggestion has been made that intrarenal reflux of sterile urine may cause segmental scarring by its hydrodynamic effects alone. This hypothesis has been advanced as an explanation of segmental renal scarring in children who have no clinical evidence of urinary infection (Bailey 1973, 1977).

However, experimental studies indicate that intra-renal reflux of infected urine may cause segmental scarring with dramatic speed in the course of only a few days (Ransley and Risdon 1978). Thus the lack of clinical documentation of renal infection is not evidence that is has never occurred. Clinical observations indicate that renal scarring usually occurs very early in life when for a variety of reasons urinary infection may be difficult to detect. In most children with renal scars the scars are already present when the child is first seen, and the development of new scars is relatively rare. Changes in the radiological appearances can usually be attributed to growth of the surrounding normal parenchyma. This strongly supports the concept advanced by Ransley in Risdon (1978) that scarring usually occurs in the very young, probably in infancy in association with episodes of urinary infection that may not be detected clinically (Anonymous 1978).

It is also true that some children do not develop scars even in the presence of vesicoureteric reflux and after repeated urinary infections. Anatomical studies of the kidneys from infants and young children indicate that about one-third do not possess any refluxing papillae (Ransley and Risdon 1975b). Such kidneys would be immune from intrarenal reflux, and this presumably explains the lack of scars in such cases.

Renal scars are also relatively frequently detected in older children who have sterile urine and no vesicoureteric reflux. Clinical studies on vesicoureteric reflux indicate, however, that in a high proportion of cases reflux ceases spontaneously. Thus the absence of reflux in an older child does not necessarily mean that it has never occurred (Ransley 1978).

There are also studies documenting a lack of new scars or deterioration in renal function during long-term follow-up of patients with vesicoureteric reflux (Fritjoffson and Sundin 1966; Stephens 1972; Smellie et al. 1975). In addition Ransley et al. (1987) and Godley et al. (1989) demonstrated no deleterious effects of sterile reflux, even with raised voiding pressures, on the glomerular filtration rate, plasma creatinine level, dimercaptosuccinic acid (DMSA) uptake or renal growth in scarred kidneys in a experimental pig model.

However, both Hodson et al. (1975) and Ransley et al. (1984) were able to produce scarring experimentally with sterile vesicoureteric reflux under certain circumstances. This was achieved in the studies of Ransley et al. only in the presence of extreme urethral obstruction sufficient to produce detrusor decompensation. Because of the unphysiological conditions required, these authors were unwilling to ascribe much clinical significance to their observations.

It is also recognized that progressive renal damage occurs after a period of years in some patients with segmental scarring. Various mechanisms have been postulated, including ischaemic changes following alterations in renal blood vessels, particularly in patients who become hypertensive, and secondary immunological damage. Experimental studies based on fluorescence microscopy have occasionally demonstrated residual bacterial antigens in pyelonephrotic scars (Cotran 1969), but the evidence linking this with progressive renal destruction is tenuous. Kincaid-Smith (1979) reported significant proteinuria in some patients with reflux nephropathy progressing to renal failure. The majority of such patients exhibit glomerular lesions of focal sclerosis and hyalinosis (Bhathena et al. 1979).

Renal Tuberculosis

Tuberculous infection of the kidney is considered separately from other renal infections. The infection is invariably blood-borne, usually from a primary source in the lungs, less commonly from other sites. The primary source of infection may heal and disappear, leaving the renal lesion as the dominant site of tuberculosis ("isolated-organ renal involvement").

Renal tuberculosis may be part of a generalized systemic haemategenous spread (miliary tuberculosis), when numerous small discrete tubercles are scattered throughout the renal parenchyma, or may involve massive nodular areas of conglomerate caseous necrosis affecting both cortex and medulla. There is often cavitation and sloughing of renal pyramids, with considerable calcification and fibrosis, and tuberculous ulceration into the pelvicalyceal system. Spread to the mucosa lining the renal pelvis and ureter may cause stricture formation. The dilated pelvicalyceal system becomes filled with caseous material and the renal parenchyma is reduced to thin surrounding shell (*tuberculous pyonephrosis*). Histologically the appearance is that of a typical tuberculous reaction, and acid-fast bacilli can usually be demonstrated.

Renal tuberculosis may be unilateral or bilateral and may involve one or several segments of the kidney. In all forms of renal involvement there is usually associated tuberculous cystitis, which is clinically significant because it is more likely to give rise to symptoms than is renal tuberculosis.

Urolithiasis

Calculi can form at any level in the urinary tract and the incidence at the various sites differs in different parts of the world. In the UK they are commonest in the pelvicalyceal system.

Stones are composed of crystalloid bound by a complex mucoprotein matrix, usually arranged in concentric layers around a nucleus of organic or crystalloidal material. Common crystalloid constituents are calcium oxalate, calcium phosphate, triple phosphates and uric acid; less frequent components are the amino acids cystine and xanthine. Stones can occur in pure forms, but are much more commonly mixed.

Phosphate stones are off-white or grey in colour, smooth, and often crumbly. Large phosphate stones may fill the pelvicalyceal system to form "stag-horn" calculi.

Oxalate stones are much harder and have a spiny exterior ("mulberry" stone). They are usually dark brown or black because of blood staining caused by trauma.

Uric acid stones are moderately hard and yellow-brown in colour.

Cystine stones are usually multiple and small. They are smooth and rounded, yellowish in colour, and waxy in consistency.

The mechanisms leading to stone formation are incompletely understood. Urine is a complex mixture of many substances, including crystalloids, which are present in concentrations that in ordinary aqueous solution would be supersaturated. It is believed that various colloid constituents of urine help to maintain the crystalloids in solution, and factors that disturb this balance may influence stone formation.

Changes in urine pH are important in this respect. Uric acid and cystine stones form in acid urine, and both these substances are much less soluble at low pH. Phosphate stones form in alkaline solution, and urinary infection with urea-splitting organisms such as *Proteus*, which keep the urinary pH high, are particularly associated with stones of this kind. Dehydration may also be important in stone formation, by increasing the concentrations of crystalloids.

Calculus formation is a recognized complication of various conditions in which there is increased urinary excretion of the various constituent crystalloids.

Hypercalciuria may occur without obvious predisposing cause (idiopathic hypercalciuria) or as a complication of hyperparathyroidism, sarcoidosis, Cushing's syndrome, prolonged immobilization as a result of illness, primary renal tubular acidosis, or milk-alkali syndrome, all of which can occur in childhood. In some patients with these conditions deposits of calcium are also present in the kidneys (nephrocalcinosis).

The condition of *primary hyperoxaluria* is associated with oxalate stone formation and deposits of calcium oxalate in organs throughout the body,

including the kidneys, but most oxalate stones are not associated with increased urinary oxalate excretion.

Cystine and xanthine stones are rare and occur almost exclusively in the metabolic disorders cystinuria and xanthinuria, when urinary excretion of these amino acids is high.

Local factors are also probably involved in stone formation. A nucleus of organic or crystalloidal material can usually be found at the centre of a calculus, which presumably acts as a nidus around which aggregates of crystals can form. Tiny blood clots, fibrin, cellular debris or collections of bacteria have been suggested as possible foreign bodies that could initiate stone formation. Small areas of calcification (*Randall's plaques*) can sometimes be found in the collecting ducts near the apices of the renal pyramids, and these have been suggested as a possible focus for crystal deposition leading to calculus formation. However, they are fairly common even in individuals who do not form stones, and are often absent when stones are present.

Hereditary Abnormalities of Renal Tubular Transport

A number of hereditary disorders of renal tubular transport are described, but the pathological changes produced in the kidney are seldom of great help in making a specific diagnosis. For this reason a brief account only is given in the table form (Table 8.3). The classification used is based on that of Kisane (1973).

Bartter's Syndrome

Bartter's syndrome is an uncommon disorder, usually occurring in children and characterized by profound hypokalaemia, hypocholaemic alkalosis, hyperaldosteronism, hyperreninaemia and normal blood pressure. Renal biopsy shows marked hyperplasia of the juxtaglomerular apparatus.

Symptoms may develop shortly after birth but diagnosis is occasionally delayed, sometimes until early adult life. Early symptoms include failure to thrive, polyuria, polydipsia, constipation, muscular weakness and craving for salt. Growth retardation is common in children, and many are mentally retarded.

The syndrome has been reported in siblings, including twins. It occurs in both sporadic and familial forms, and in the latter appears to be inherited as an autosomal recessive trait (Pereira and van Wersch 1983).

Table 8.3. Familial abnormalities of tubular transport

Disorder	Inheritance	Functional abnormality	Morphological changes in kidneys	Clinical effects
Specific disorders of amino-acid transport				
Cystinuria	Autosomal recessive	Proximal tubular defect→ increased urinary excretion of cystine, lysine, arginine and ornithine	–	Cystine calculi in the urinary tract
Hartnup disease	Autosomal recessive	Proximal tubular defect→ increased urinary excretion of alanine, glutamine, asparagine, nistidine, serine, theonine, phenylalanine, tyrosine and tryptophan	–	Pellagra-like skin rash Attacks of cerebellar ataxia
Iminoglycinuria	Autosomal recessive	Proximal tubular defect→ increased urinary excretion of glycine, proline and hydroxyproline	–	Urinary tract calculi
Non-specific disorders of amino-acid transport				
Cystinosis (de Toni-Faconi–Lignan–Debre syndrome) Childhood form	Autosomal recessive	Proximal tubular defect→ aminoaciduria, hyperphosphaturia, acidosis and hypokalaemia May be proteinuria	Deposition of cystine crystals in tubules, glomerular epithelial cells and interstitium (as well as elsewhere in the body) Swan-neck deformity of nephrons on microdissection	Vomiting, fever, polyuria, Vitamin D-resistant rickets Occasionally pitressin-resistant diabetes insipidus Renal failure
Idiopathic form	Autosomal recessive and dominant described	Proximal tubular defect→ glycosuria, aminoaciduria, hypophosphaturia	No cystine deposition	Milder disease than the childhood form Usually affects adults but may be present in childhood
Lowe's syndrome	Sex-linked recessive	Proximal tubular defect→ aminoaciduria, hypophosphaturia Acidosis, proteinuria and inability to concentrate the urine	Tubular atrophy and glomerulosclerosis	Congenital glaucoma, cataracts, mental retardation, rickets and renal failure
Tubular defects due to endogenous poisons				
Galactosaemia	Autosomal recessive	Galactose-1-phosphate uridyl transferase deficiency→ galactose retention Effect on proximal tubules→ aminoaciduria and proteinuria	–	Cataracts, mental deficiency and hepatic cirrhosis
Wilson's disease	Autosomal recessive	Defect of copper metabolism associated with reduced serum caeruloplasmin and deposition of copper Effect on proximal tubules→ aminoaciduria	–	Extrapyramidal symptoms, Kayser–Fleischer rings, hepatic cirrhosis
Disorders of other transport mechanisms				
Renal glycosuria	Autosomal dominant	Prominent tubular defect→ glycosuria	–	–
Vitamin D-resistant rickets	Sex-linked dominant	Increased clearance of phosphate due to reduced reabsorption in the proximal tubules	–	Rickets refractory to therapy with vitamin D

Table 8.3. (*continued*)

Disorder	Inheritance	Functional abnormality	Morphological changes in kidneys	Clinical effects
Vasopressin-resistant diabetes insipidus	Probably sex-linked dominant with variable expressivity	Distal tubular defect resulting in unresponsiveness to vasopressin	Microdissection indicates diminution in proximal tubule convolutions	Vasopressin-resistant diabetes insipidus
Primary renal acidosis Infantile form	Autosomal recessive	Distal tubular defect→ inability to acidify urine	Reduction in renal size and nephro calcinosis in some cases	Vomiting, failure to thrive, dehydration and hypotonia Complete recovery following treatment usual Failure in maturation of tubular function
Late form	Autosomal dominant with increased penetration in females	As in the infantile form increased potassium loss in urine may occur	May be cortical scarring and urolithiasis	More serious disorder than the infantile form May develop periodic paralysis, rickets and renal stones

The principal morphological abnormality in the kidney is marked hyperplasia and increased granularity of the juxtaglomerular apparatus (JGA) (Fig. 8.29). The macula densa is usually prominent. The glomeruli exhibit varying degrees of mesangial cell hypercellularity and some increase in the amount of mesangial matrix. Focally, glomeruli with an immature appearance similar to that seen in the fetal kidney may be present. Tubular lesions associated with potassium deficiency are sometimes seen. Hyperplasia of renal medullary interstitial cells has also been described (Donker et al. 1977).

The pathogenesis is unknown. The mechanism initially suggested (Bartter et al. 1962) was a primary resistance of peripheral arterioles to the pressor action of angiotensin, leading to inappropriate stimulation of the renin/angiotensin system with hyperplasia of the JGA, promoting increased adrenal

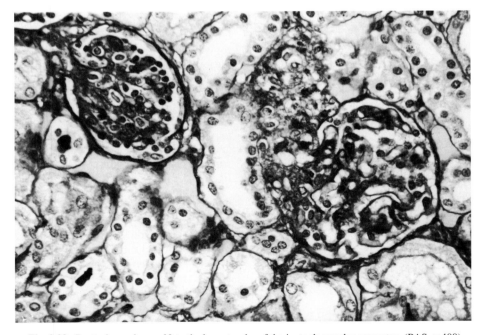

Fig. 8.29. Bartter's syndrome. Note the hypertrophy of the juxtaglomerular apparatus. (PAS, × 400)

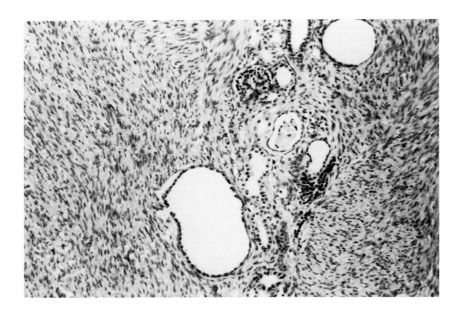

Fig. 8.30. Congenital mesoblastic nephroma. Interlacing sheets of spindle-shaped cells with entrapped glomerular and tubular structures. (H&E, × 80)

production of aldosterone and consequent urinary potassium loss. However, total adrenalectomy fails to correct the potassium wastage. It has also been suggested that impaired chloride transport across the tubular epithelium might lead to urinary sodium and potassium loss (Gill and Bartter 1978).

An increased urinary excretion of prostaglandins, their increased synthesis in the kidney and the beneficial effects of indomethecin in patients with Bartter's syndrome have also been noted (Fichman et al. 1976; Donker et al. 1977; Richards et al. 1978).

Renal Tumours

Malignant nephroblastoma (Wilms' tumour), which is described in Chapter 17 (see p. 867), is the commonest solid (i.e. non-leukaemic) malignant tumour outside the central nervous system occurring in children. Other renal tumours and hamartomas are rare, and a description of the more important entities is included in the following sections.

Benign Tumours and Hamartomas

Congenital Mesoblastic Nephroma

Congenital mesoblastic nephroma, usually recognized clinically in the neonatal period or in early infancy, has been separated from nephroblastoma (Bolande et al. 1967). This distinction is important because, the majority of congenital mesoblastic nephromas reported have behaved as benign neoplasms, cured by surgery. The previous confusion of these tumours with Wilms' tumour probably accounts, at least in part, for the unexpectedly good prognosis in some series of malignant nephroblastomas diagnosed during the first year of life. In addition, vigorous treatment consisting in surgery followed by radiotherapy and chemotherapy carries an appreciable morbidity and mortality rate, particularly in very young children, and though necessary for Wilms' tumour it is inappropriate for congenital mesoblastic nephroma (Hilton and Keeling 1973).

Macroscopically, the congenital mesoblastic nephroma is a bulky, usually spherical tumour mass up to 5 cm in diameter, but occasionally exceeding 10 cm, replacing part of the kidney, from which it appears fairly well demarcated. The surface is smooth and covered by the expanded renal capsule. The cut surface presents a white whorled appearance very like that of a myometrial fibroid.

Microscopically, the tumour is composed of interlacing bands of closely packed spindle cells with eosinophilic cytoplasm and round or oval vesicular nuclei. A characteristic finding is the presence of foci of glomeruli and tubules throughout the tumour (Fig. 8.30). These often have an immature appearance and appear to represent normal nephronic structures trapped within the expanding tumour. The margin of the neoplasm extends to incorporate parenchymous elements adjacent to it and the tumour is not encapsulated. Within the tumour mass mitotic figures may be frequent, although this is not an indication of malignant transformation. These lesions are generally regarded as hamartomatous developmental anomalies (Kay et al. 1966). The cell of origin is uncertain, and ultrastructural studies have identified cells which have been regarded as of smooth muscle origin and as undifferentiated mesenchyme. Marsden and Newton (1986) have recently reviewed 38 mesoblastic nephromas occurring in children up to 18 months of age. In all cases the behaviour of the tumours was benign. In addition to the features noted above, these authors described islands of cartilage in six tumours, extensive subcapsular extension of the tumour in two, and squamous epithelial islands in three. In the adjacent renal tissue, vacuolated and dysplastic tubules, cysts and epithelial tumourlets were occasional features, suggesting some common aspects between mesoblastic nephroma and both real dysplasia and nephroblastoma.

Although some of these tumours are reported to recur after surgical excision, mitotic activity has proved to be a poor indicator of this risk. Very few deaths have been regarded as due to aggressive tumours, and the vast majority of mesoblastic nephromas are entirely benign. The few recurrent tumours described have been in children more than 3 years old.

Angiomyolipoma

Angiomyolipomas are hamartomatous lesions that can be single or multiple and occur in the renal cortex, usually immediately beneath the renal capsule. They are rounded, sharply circumscribed but unencapsulated swellings often forming nodular projections from the renal surface. They are usually only 2–3 cm in diameter or less, but occasionally larger lesions have been described (Moolten 1942).

Microscopically, they consist of a disorderly arrangement of smooth muscle cells, abnormal thick-walled blood vessels, and adipose tissue, in varying proportions. A few renal parenchymal elements may be incorporated at the margins of the lesion.

Their importance lies in their frequent association with tuberous sclerosis, particularly when they are multiple, and they are usually regarded as part of the tuberous sclerosis complex. About 80% of patients with tuberous sclerosis have renal tumours, and about 50% of patients with renal angiolipomas have other stigmata of tuberous sclerosis.

Another renal cortical hamartoma consisting of nodular collections of cells with abundant eosinophilic cytoplasm resembling enlarged renal tubular epithelial cells is also occasionally encountered in tuberous sclerosis, and very rarely with other phakomatoses. A feature of this lesion is that the centres of the nodules sometimes break down to give a pseudocystic appearance.

Other Primary Renal Tumours

Renal cortical adenomas similar to those seen in adults occur in children but are extemely rare.

Connective tissue tumours such as haemangiomas, lipomas, liposarcomas, leiomyomas, osteomas and chondromase occurring in or adjacent to the kidney have been described in children, but are also rare. Benign teratomas have also been described in the kidney (Walker 1897), but need to be distinguished carefully from retroperitoneal teratomas, which merely compress the adjacent kidney.

Although Wilms' tumour is by far the most important malignant renal tumour in children, renal cell carcinomas also occur very occasionally in this age group. In 1961 Scruggs and Ainsworth collected 51 reports of renal cell carcinoma in children. These tumours have the same histological appearances as those in adults and behave in a similar fashion.

Clear-cell Sarcoma

This is a rare malignant tumour constituting about 3% of childhood renal tumours. It occurs more commonly in male than in female children, with a peak incidence between 2 and 3 years and a range from infancy to 14 years.

Clear-cell sarcoma is a bulky, usually spherical, tumour with a grey-tan or pinkish-white homogeneous or occasionally lobulated cut surface. Metastatic spread to regional lymph nodes is common, and a particular feature of clear-cell sarcoma is its propensity to skeletal metastases, which occur in 42%–76% of cases. This accounts for its original description as the "bone-metastasizing renal tumour" (Marsden and Lawler 1978).

Microscopically, the tumour is composed of ill-defined spindle or stellate cells with "clear" or vacuolated cytoplasm and round or oval nuclei with finely granular chromatin. The cells are aggregated in nests or cords separated by a delicate arborizing network of small blood vessels (Fig. 8.31). Lateral branches of these vessels often arise almost at right angles, a distinctive and diagnostically useful feature on reticulin staining. Mitotic activity is usually sparse, giving a deceptively benign appearance. Microscopic infiltration at the tumour edge is, however, usually apparent.

Clear-cell sarcoma is a highly malignant tumour, which together with the anaplastic variety of

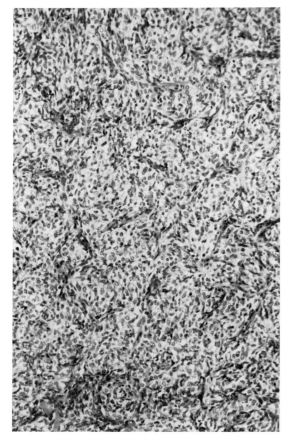

Fig. 8.31. Clear-cell sarcoma. Note the packeted appearance of the tumour cells and the prominent vascular stroma. (H&E, × 80)

nephroblastoma and malignant rhabdoid tumour (see below) is included in the "unfavourable histology" varieties of malignant renal tumours of childhood. In the National Wilms' Tumour Studies in the United States, 31 clear-cell sarcomas were included. Of these 20 (65%) relapsed, and there were 15 (48%) tumour-related deaths.

Malignant Rhabdoid Tumour

This is another rare, highly malignant renal tumour of childhood, accounting for about 2% of kidney tumours in this age group. Males are affected slightly more commonly than females. In the National Wilms' Tumour Studies 21 malignant rhabdoid tumours were identified in children aged between 3 months and $3\frac{1}{2}$ years (mean 13 months); of these 19 died, reflecting the extreme malignant potential of this neoplasm.

Malignant rhabdoid tumours generally form large spherical masses with homogeneous pale cut surfaces, in which areas of necrosis are common. The tumour margins, even macroscopically, are ill-defined, and infiltrative growth is usually evident. Extension to the renal vein is common, and metastatic spread may be evident at diagnosis. Regional lymph nodes are often involved, and distant spread to lung and liver is frequent. Cerebral metastases are also common.

Microscopically, the tumour is composed of solid sheets of round or polygonal cells with round or oval nuclei, which have distinct nuclear membranes, sparse chromatin and prominent single nucleoli. The cells often have abundant acidophilic cytoplasm, giving a superficial resemblance to rhabdomyoblast, from which the description "rhabdoid" is derived. However, cross-striations are never present, and immunostaining for desmin is consistently absent. Many cells contain rounded hyaline PAS-positive diastase-resistant globules in the cytoplasm. These globules stain immunohistochemically for vimentin, and ultrastructurally are composed of concentric whorled arrays of 6–10 mm intermediate filaments. Positive immunostaining for S-100 protein, neuron-specific enolase, neurofilaments, α_1-antichymotrypsin, lysosome and 54 kD cytokeratin in tumour cells have all been reported, but the results are inconsistent and many tumours stain for vimentin alone.

Hypercalcaemia has occasionally been described in patients with malignant rhabdoid tumours, presumably a result of secretion of a parathormone-like substance by the tumour. In addition, there are occasional reports of second primary intracranial neuroectodermal tumours in the midline of the posterior fossa.

There are also a number of reports of extrarenal tumours arising in various sites such as the brain, bladder, liver and subcutaneous tissues that appear histologically and ultrastructurally identical to malignant rhabdoid tumours of the kidney. These extrarenal tumours are even rarer than their renal counterparts; the age at presentation is more variable, with some occurring in adults, and the prognosis, although still poor, is better than that of renal rhabdoid tumours.

Metastatic Tumours

The most frequent metastatic involvement of the kidney during childhood occurs in leukaemia. The kidneys are often diffusely enlarged, producing easily palpable bilateral loin masses. Renal function is rarely impaired even with massive involvement, but leukaemic cells may be demonstrated in the urine deposit.

Embryology of the Renal Pelvis, Ureter, Bladder and Urethra

The ureter and renal pelvis develop from the metanephric duct, itself formed as an offshoot with a cranial course from the lower end of the mesonephric (Wolffian) duct. The ureter is formed by the caudal (unbranched) portion of the metanephric duct, and the renal pelvis and calyces are derived by coalescence of the first generations of dichotomous divisions of its cranial portion, which occur when the advancing tip impinges on the metanephric blastema (see p. 449).

Distally, the metanephric duct joins with the terminal portion of the mesonephric duct to form a short common excretory duct that drains into the cloaca. The cloaca is continuous with three endodermal tubes: the hind-gut, the allantois and the blind-ending diverticulum of the tail-gut. It is marked externally by a shallow depression covered by the cloacal membrane. At about the 5 mm stage, a septum (the urogenital septum) develops above, in the angle between the allantois and the hind-gut. This septum gradually extends caudally until it reaches and fuses with the cloacal membrane at about the 16 mm stage. The cloaca is thus divided into a smaller dorsal portion (the primitive rectum) and a larger ventral part (the primitive urogenital sinus).

The common excretory ducts from each side join the urogenital sinus, dividing it into an upper portion above the ducts (the vesicourethral canal from which the bladder and upper urethra develop) and a lower portion below the ducts (the definitive urogenital sinus).

The vesicourethral canal is an elongated cylinder, slightly flattened dorsoventrally, which is continuous cranially with the allantois. With the growth of the anterior abdominal wall below the umbilicus, the bladder segment of the vesicourethral canal enlarges and the definitive urogenital sinus becomes flattened from side to side and elongated dorsoventrally.

Probably as a result of dilatation of the common excretory duct and its subsequent absorption into the wall of the vesicourethral canal, the mesonephric and metanephric ducts come to drain separately into the vesicourethral canal. With further development, the ureteric orifices move progressively cranially and laterally in relation to the mesonephric duct openings, which remain close together near the midline. In the male the mesonephric duct persists as the epididymis, vas deferens, seminal vesicle and common ejaculatory duct. In the female the mesonephric duct generates, starting at about the 30 mm stage, and, apart from the vestigial epoöphoron and Gärtner's ducts,

disappears. The triangular zone between the ureteric orifices and the mesonephric duct openings forms the trigone of the bladder. Unlike the rest of the bladder, which is an endodermal structure, the trigone is a mesodermal derivative. The upper part of the bladder is continuous with the allantois, which regresses early and is replaced by a solid fibrous cord (the urachus).

In the female, the primitive urethra, which is derived from the lower part of the vesicourethral canal, forms almost all the definitive urethra. In the male, however, the primitive urethra forms only the upper part of the prostatic urethra. The lower portion of the prostatic urethra and the membranous urethra are derived from the upper (pelvic) portion of the urogenital sinus. The penile urethra is formed by fusion of the urethral folds on each side of the ventral surface of the developing phallus. The groove between these folds (the urethral groove) is formed by a plate of cells (the urethral plate), which extends from the lower (phallic) portion of the urogenital sinus. Fusion of the urethral folds in the midline occurs from behind forwards, and posteriorly it is marked externally by the median raphe. This process of fusion extends distally only as far as the circular coronary sulcus, which delineates the glans penis. A cord of ectodermal epithelial cells grows through the glans to reach the distal closed tip of the urethra. This later becomes canalized and its lumen becomes continuous with that of the urethra, thus forming its terminal (glandular) portion and the urethral meatus.

The prostate gland in the male develops at about the 55 mm stage as a series of buds from the primitive urethra and from the adjacent upper portion of the urogenital sinus.

Renal Pelvis and Ureter

Congenital Abnormalities

Duplications

Duplications of the renal pelvis and ureter are common, some degree of pelviureteric duplication being present in about 5% of unselected necropsies. The extent of duplication varies from a mere bifurcation of the extrarenal portion of the renal pelvis draining into a single ureter to complete duplication of the whole system, with separate lower ureteral openings into the bladder. Females are more commonly affected than males. Rare instances of triplication or even quadruplication of the ureters occur. The usual type of duplication is the conjoint ureter (Stephens

1956), in which the upper part of the ureter is divided, the two arms joining to form a single lower ureter that drains normally into the trigone of the bladder. In the great majority of cases the upper system is the smaller, the majority of the renal calyces draining into the lower system. In a small minority of instances (less than 1%), and usually with complete duplications, the ureter is ectopic (see below).

Only 20% of duplications are bilateral. Clinically the condition is usually entirely asymptomatic, but in rare cases obstruction occurs, usually as the result of stenosis of the upper system in conjoint ureters. Complicating hydronephrosis or urinary infection may bring the condition to light.

Ureteral Ectopia

An ectopic ureter drains to a site other than the trigone of the bladder. In females an ectopic ureter may open into the urethra, the vagina or the rectum. In males it may drain into the urethra, the seminal vesicle or the rectum. In females ureteral ectopia is usually associated with dribbling incontinence of urine. In males, when the ectopic ureter drains into the urethra or seminal vesicle urinary continence is unaffected, because the insertion of the ureter is almost always above the verumontanum and contraction of the urethral sphincter prevents incontinence.

Ureterocele

A ureterocele is a saccular expansion of the lower end of the ureter about its orifice, involving the intramural segment in the bladder wall and the submucosal portion that extends beneath the bladder mucosa immediately above the orifice. Ureteroceles are usually associated with upper tract obstruction and hydronephrosis. Radiologically, the kidney drained by a ureter with a ureterocele may not excrete contrast medium, but the diagnosis can be made by the presence of a globular filling defect in the bladder caused by the ureterocele. Sometimes the ureterocele obstructs the bladder neck and causes bilateral hydronephritis.

Ureteroceles may occur with a normally sited ureteric orifice, but are more commonly associated with ureteral ectopia and ureteral duplication. The term "ectopic ureterocele" (Berdon et al. 1968) is usually applied to a complex anomaly, which consists of a duplex kidney with two separate ureters. The ureter draining the lower part of the double kidney is inserted normally in the trigone of the bladder. The ureter draining the upper pole is inserted ectopically

and is associated with a ureterocele. The insertion is below and medial to that of the lower pole ureter, usually into the upper urethra. The ectopic ureter is dilated and tortuous as a result of obstruction, and the upper pole of the kidney, apart from showing changes secondary to obstruction, is very commonly dysplastic (see p. 459). Ectopic ureterocele is much commoner in females. There is often duplication of the contralateral ureter, but this is usually of the conjoint type, and the full ectopic ureterocele is only rarely bilateral. Symptoms are variable. Recurrent urinary infection is the usual presentation, but in girls there may be dribbling incontinence; occasionally the ureterocele prolapses into the urethra and may be visible externally. Surgical excision of the ectopic ureter, ureterocele and upper pole of the kidney usually gives excellent results.

Vesicoureteric Reflux

The importance of vesicoureteric reflux in the pathogenesis of pyelonephritis and renal scarring is well recognized and has already been discussed (see p. 493). The clinical aspects of this complication, and the other consequences of vesicoureteric reflux in childhood, for example its possible effects on renal growth, have led to considerable controversy regarding appropriate management. These topics are expertly discussed by Ransley (1978).

Vesicoureteric reflux does not occur under normal conditions. An abnormality of the vesicoureteric junction producing reflux may be isolated ("primary" reflux) or may occur in association with other abnormalities, such as posterior urethral valves, ureteral duplication or a neuropathic bladder ("secondary" reflux). There is a tendency for primary vesicoureteric reflux to disappear as the affected child grows, a change most marked in children with milder degrees of reflux (assessed by the degree of ureteral dilatation on micturating cystography), 80% of whom eventually stop refluxing spontaneously.

The abnormality of the vesicoureteric junction associated with vesicoureteric reflux is often recognizable on cystoscopy, particularly when the degree of reflux is gross. The ureteric orifice appears as a rounded hole ("golf-hole" orifice) rather than the normal semilunar slit. Direct inspection is not a reliable method of diagnosing or assessing vesicoureteric reflux; however, this is usually done radiologically by micturating cystography.

The great majority of children with vesicoureteric reflux present as a result of urinary infection. Conversely, about 50% of infants, and about 30% of older children with urinary tract infections, can be shown to have vesicoureteric reflux (Shannon 1970).

In a proportion of cases, particularly of those considered to have gross reflux judged by the degree of upper tract dilatation on micturating cystography, the kidney may be dysplastic. This has led to the suggestion of a developmental abnormality in cases involving the whole upper tract (Bialestock 1965). It is of interest that some infants with renal dysplasia and vesicoureteric reflux also have an abnormal urethra with a smooth symmetrical narrowing at the level of the external sphincter. The consequent urinary obstruction is freely communicated to the upper tract, which acts like a bladder diverticulum. It can be assumed that this process occurs in utero and probably accounts for the dysplastic renal development (Beck 1971).

Although vesicoureteric reflux is relatively uncommon, affecting less than 0.5% of the general population, there is a much higher incidence (between 8% and 26%) in families in which one member is known to be affected (Bredin et al. 1975; Dwoskin 1976; de Vargas et al. 1978). This suggests that screening for vesicoureteric reflux, which is impractical on a population basis, would be of value in affected families.

Retrocaval Ureter

In the rare anomaly of retrocaval ureter the upper ureter passes behind the inferior vena cava and descends into the pelvis medial to it. The malformation results from the formation of the distal inferior vena cava from the lateral cardinal veins rather than from the posterior cardinal veins, which is the normal pattern. Incomplete obstruction of the ureter results from its retrocaval course.

Hydronephrosis

The term "hydronephrosis" describes a dilatation of the renal pelvis and calyces and the secondary effects on the renal parenchyma. The usual cause is a localized narrowing in the ureter, most commonly at the pelviureteric junction. Stenosis may also occur at the vesicoureteric junction and, less commonly, elsewhere in the ureter. Such ureteral narrowings may be congenital or acquired defects. Rarer causes of hydronephrosis in infancy and childhood include anomalous inferior segmental renal arteries (White and Wyatt 1942) and uteric valves (Wall and Wachter 1952).

The degree of upper tract dilatation and renal parenchymal atrophy depends partly on the degree of stenosis and partly on the duration of obstruction. Macroscopic changes in the kidney include blunting of the renal papillae and parenchymal thinning.

Microscopically, there is dilatation of collecting ducts, which run tangentially rather than radially in the medulla, and varying degrees of tubular atrophy and interstitial fibrosis. Atrophy is most marked in the medulla rather than the renal cortex, except in the extreme examples, when the whole parenchyma is reduced to a thin rim composed largely of fibrous tissue surrounding the grossly dilated collecting system. Renal infection and stone formation are common complications, particularly in cases of long standing.

Occasionally hydronephrosis may develop in utero, when it is usually associated with obstruction at the pelviureteric junction. This may be due to an intrinsic abnormality of the ureteric musculature producing a narrow aperistaltic segment, to kinks, fibrous bands or adhesions producing abnormal angulation of the ureter against the renal pelvis, or rarely to mucosal folds or polyps. Aberrant segmental arteries crossing the pelviureteric junction have also been implicated, but even when these occur an intrinsic narrowing of the junction is usually also present.

The condition is usually unilateral, but is bilateral in some 20% of cases. Boys are more commonly affected than girls. Sometimes extreme hydronephrosis ("giant" hydronephrosis) producing an easily palpable loin mass is encountered. In these cases hydronephrotic renal atrophy is extreme and may be associated with dysplastic changes.

Bladder

Congenital Abnormalities

Agenesis

Absence of the bladder is an extremely rare anomaly; it is usually associated with other severe congenital abnormalities and is generally found in stillborn infants. Glen (1959) described a case of bladder agenesis in a 3-year-old girl and collected less than ten previously reported cases. As in Miller's case (Miller 1948), also a girl, the urethra was blind and the ureters were inserted into the vagina. Lepoutre (1939/40) reported a male child with absence of the bladder, in whom the ureters were inserted into the rectum.

Urachal Anomalies

During embryonic life the urachus extends from the umbilicus to the dome of the bladder. Persistence of the urachus results in a fistula opening at the umbilicus. Partial persistence results in a urachal diverticulum, which is usually asymptomatic but may be associated with stone formation (Dreyfuss and Fliess 1941).

Occasionally the mid-part of the urachus persists, with obliteration of the two ends to produce a urachal cyst, which may occasionally become infected.

Duplications

A review of the bladder duplication has been made by Abrahamson (1961).

Duplications of the bladder may be classified as complete or incomplete. In complete duplication two separate bladders lie side by side in a common adventitial sheath. Each bladder has a separate urethra with a separate external meatus. Duplications of the hindgut is almost always present, and a rectourethral fistula involving one side is present in over half the reported cases. Other associated rectal and genital anomalies are common.

In incomplete duplication there are two bladders side by side. These are joined at the base and have a single urethra and external meatus.

Septation

When a *complete sagittal septum* is present the bladder appears either normal or bilobed from the outside. The complete sagittal septum is found on opening the bladder. If a ureter drains into the obstructed side, hydronephrosis is present on that side. Sometimes the obstructed half may also obstruct the half draining into the urethra, and bilateral hydronephrosis then results.

If the *sagittal septum* is *incomplete* no obstruction occurs, but other anomalies frequently coexist.

In the presence of an *incomplete frontal septum* the bladder is incompletely divided into anterior and posterior cavities by a septum.

Kohler (1940) describes a case of *multiseptate bladder* with complete obstruction of both upper tracts in an infant dying of uraemia.

In the *hourglass bladder* the shape probably reflects a partial persistence of the urachus.

Exstrophy

Bladder exstrophy is the commonest manifestation of a series of congenital abnormalities resulting from a failure of midline fusion of the mesodermal elements in the anterior abdominal wall below the umbilicus, involving the anterior wall of the bladder and urethra, the genital tubercle, and the pubis. This spectrum of anomalies ranges from minor degrees of epispadias, involving the penis with exposure of the terminal urethra, to a gross abnormality in which there is ectopia vesicae and vesicointestinal fistula, with gross bowel anomalies accompanying the bladder lesion.

In bladder exstrophy the infraumbilical abdominal wall is shortened and a midline defect is present. The size of this varies from a small hole through which the bladder trigone protrudes on straining to an extensive defect through which the entire posterior wall of the bladder protrudes. Some degree of diastasis of the pubis and epispadias are invariably present.

Secondary changes (squamous metaplasia, cystitis cystica, cystitis glandularis) invariably occur in the exposed bladder mucosa, and squamous carcinoma or adenocarcinoma may develop in patients who survive childhood. Vesicoureteric reflux is common in patients with exstrophy of the bladder following surgical reconstruction.

In *cloacal exstrophy*, the extrophied bladder is in two separate halves, each with a ureteric orifice. The two hemibladders are separated by extrophied bowel that has two openings – an upper orifice communicating with the terminal ileum (which often prolapses as a tube covered by intestinal mucosa), and a lower orifice continuous with a blind-ending segment of colon. The anus is imperforate and there may be a separate appendicular orifice (or sometimes two if the appendix is duplicated). A large exomphalos above the exstrophy is present, and may contain liver as well as intestine. An episadic penis is present in males and is frequently duplicated. The testes are undescended and the scrotum is absent. In females the uterus is duplicated, the vagina septate and the external genitalia fail to develop.

Covered exstrophy is characterized by delayed closure of the abdominal wall followed by formation of an exstrophy. The umbilicus is low, and the abdominal wall below is paper thin. Epispadias is present in males and the pubes are separated.

Diverticula

Bladder diverticula appear as herniations of the bladder mucosa through the detrusor muscle and generally occur at a weak point 1–2 cm behind and lateral to the ureteric orifice. In children they are usually small and single, but larger examples may cause ureteric obstruction. Focal cystitis and stone formation are commoner complications (Forsthe and Smyth 1959).

Outflow Obstruction

Obstruction of the bladder outflow may have mechanical causes, such as posterior urethral valves, congenital urethral stenosis and ectopic ureterocele, or may be associated with a neurogenic bladder. Posterior urethral valves in infant boys are the commonest cause of congenital urethral obstruction. The various types are described in the classic work of Young and McKay (1929), who identified the commonest variety as an accentuation of a pair of folds normally present in the male urethra extending from the verumontanum down laterally to the urethral wall. Wigglesworth (1984) illustrates a diaphragmatic obstruction with a pinhole orifice at the level of the verumontanum dividing the distended upper from the lower urethra. He regarded this as the commonest variety he encountered in perinatal necropsies and suggested that it might be converted to the type described by Young and McKay by passage of a catheter, which would split the diaphragm, or by opening the urethra anteriorly with scissors at necropsy. When such obvious causes are excluded, many cases remain in which difficulty in voiding, incontinence and recurrent urinary infection are associated with hypertrophy and trabeculation of the bladder. Vesicoureteric reflux can often be demonstrated radiologically, and progressive dilatation of the bladder and ureters may develop (megacystic–megaureter). Ureteric peristalsis can be demonstrated at first, but with increasing dilatation this may fail and gross hydronephrosis with abundant residual urine results. The underlying cause is obscure. Early reports (Andreassen 1953) suggested deficiencies in the autonomic innervation of the bladder, analogous in Hirschsprung's disease of the intestine, but other authors (Winkelman 1967) describe a normal bladder innervation. Bodian (1957) performed extensive histological studies of the bladder neck and urethra in a number of these patients, and demonstrated elongation of the prostatic urethra with increased amounts of fibroelastic tissue in a submucosa of the bladder neck. Urethral fibroelastosis is accepted as a cause of bladder outflow obstruction in some cases, but it is likely that other lesions are also responsible, and it must be admitted that their pathology has been inadequately studied.

Prune Belly Syndrome

A combination of "absence" of the muscles of the anterior abdominal wall, undescended testes with bilateral hydronephrosis and hydroureter has been called the "prune belly syndrome" (Wigger and Blanc 1977) because of the appearance of the flaccid, col-

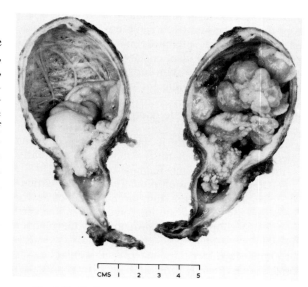

Fig. 8.32. Embryonal rhabdomyosarcoma of the bladder.

lapsed abdomen in affected infants. Obstruction may or may not be found, although functional obstruction has been demonstrated clinically. The pathogenesis of the syndrome has been determined by studying aborted fetuses; lower urinary tract obstruction causes intrauterine abdominal distension with ischaemic necrosis of the abdominal musculature (Berry et al. 1982). Obstruction may be associated with changes in the upper tract, including dysplasia.

Tumours

Benign bladder tumours are rare in children. Neurofibromas, usually multiple, may occur as an isolated lesion or as part of generalized neurofibromatosis (von Recklinghausen's disease). Haemangiomas and leiomyomas (Williams and Schistad 1961) also occur.

The most frequent bladder tumour in childhood is the embryonal rhabdomyosarcoma. Macroscopically, this consists of a translucent, grape-like, lobulated mass, which partially or almost completely fills the bladder (sarcoma botryoides) and often originates from the region of the trigone. The tumour often extends to involve the urethra and the lower ureters, which may become obstructed. Embryonal rhabdomyosarcoma of the bladder usually presents in the first few years of life and is commoner in boys. Histologically the tumour is composed of small spindle cells with hyperchromatic nuclei, set in an often abundant myxoid stroma (Fig. 8.32). The cellularity often varies in different parts of the tumour, and a compacted layer immediately beneath the intact overlying urothelium (the "cambium" layer) is characteristic. Cellular pleomorphism may occur and some cells with abundant eosinophillic cytoplasm or strap-like cells, some with cross-striations, may be apparent. Immunostaining for vimentin, and usually with desmin, is positive.

A lack of cellular pleomorphism and relatively sparse cellularity may give a deceptively benign appearance, particularly in small biopsy specimens where immunohistochemistry may be particularly useful in establishing the diagnosis.

The application of multimodality therapy, particularly irradiation of the tumour bed and effective chemotherapy to eradicate micrometastases has very significantly improved the prognosis of the bladder rhabdomyosarcoma.

Epithelial bladder tumours (transitional-cell carcinomas) are extremely rare, but have been reported in children (Waller and Roll 1957).

Urethra

Congenital Abnormalities

Atresia

Ureteral atresia is a very rare anomaly, usually occurring at the level of the membranous urethra. Drainage of the bladder may be affected via a coexisting rectourethral or urachal fistula. In some cases there is a concomitant prune belly syndrome (congenital absence of the anterior abdominal wall muscles), and rectal agenesis may also coexist.

Duplication

Complete duplications of the urethra are usually found in association with complete duplication of the bladder or diaphallus. Occasionally, in males, the urethra divides and has one normally situated urethral meatus and a second meatus opening at the perineum.

Valves and Strictures

Congenital urethral stenosis may result from strictures resulting from faulty coaptation of the genital tubercles (in males) or from membranous mucosal diaphragms; in either case they can be single or multiple. Meatal stenosis is the most common variety.

Urethral valves in infant boys are the commonest cause of congenital urethral obstruction. These are usually situated in the posterior urethra, and the three varieties described by Young and McKay (1929) are shown diagrammatically in Fig. 8.33.

Acquired strictures of the posterior urethra are almost always the result of urethral rupture following fracture of the pelvis.

Anterior Urethral Diverticulum

Wide-mouthed (saccular) or narrow-mouthed (globular) diverticula are occasionally seen in males at any point from the membranous to the mid-penile urethra.

Hypospadias

This congenital anomaly of the male urethra is characterized by an ectopic urinary meatus sited on the underside of the penis proximal to its normal site at the tip of the glans. The condition is classified on the meatal position as glandular, coronal, distal, mid or proximal shaft, penoscrotal, scrotal or perineal. The ventral foreskin is deficient, the penis is often short and is usually bent downwards by tethering connective tissue bands (ventral chordee).

Prostatic Utricle (Müllerian Duct) Cyst

Developmental cysts of Müllerian origin situated posteriorly in the urethra just above the prostate and below the bladder are encountered occasionally in males.

Polyp of Verumontanum

Connective tissue polyps covered by urothelium may arise from the floor of the prostatic urethra near the verumontanum in males.

Disorders of Differentiation of the Genital Tract

This account presents a simplified view of the anomalies of genital tract differentiation. They are sometimes extremely complex, and for a more extensive review and bibliography the texts of Shapiro (1982) and Warkany (1971) should be consulted.

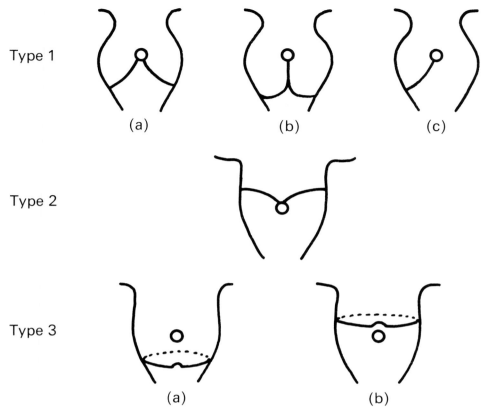

Type 1   (a)   (b)   (c)

Type 2

Type 3   (a)   (b)

Fig. 8.33. Congenital urethral valves. (After Young and McKay 1929)

Anomalies of Genetic Origin

Alterations in the sex chromosomes may be transmitted by one parent (gonadal dysgenesis) or may occur in the embryo although the initial stages of fertilization were normal (true hermaphroditism).

Gonadal dysgenesis results from non-disjunction of the sex chromosomes during gametogenesis, and may result in Klinefelter's syndrome (XXY) or Turner's syndrome (XO) with ovarian agenesis, or other genetically complex anomalies. True hermaphroditism is associated with failure of disjunction of sex chromosomes during the first cleavage mitoses of the egg, leading to XY/XX or XY/XO mosaicism. The relative proportions of the components of the mosaic greatly affect the phenotypic expression of the anomaly.

Sexual Anomalies of Hormonal Origin

Hormone-conditioned sexual anomalies may occur in individuals with normal genetic constitution. Primary and secondary characteristics may be ambiguous, depending on the degree of exposure to endogenous or exogenous androgen.

Male Pseudohermaphroditism

In a normal XY male pseudohermaphroditism may occur because of deficient androgen production. The abnormalities produced will depend on the stage of development at which the deficiency becomes manifest; in the later stages a small penis, hypospadias, and vulviform appearance of the scrotum may be evident, but severe deficiency in early stages may permit the persistence of a Müllerian system; in this case a vagina and uterus coexist with normal vasa deferentia. The external genitalia are female and the testes ectopic.

Female Pseudohermaphroditism

Virilization of a female fetus with normal ovaries and an XX karyotype results in female pseudohermaphroditism. Changes may be caused by androgen produc-

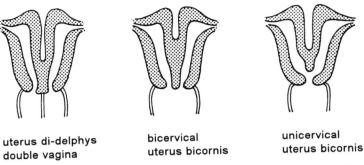

uterus di-delphys
double vagina

bicervical
uterus bicornis

unicervical
uterus bicornis

(a) Partial or complete fusion of lower part of Müllerian ducts

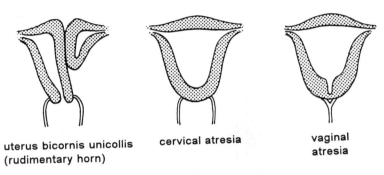

uterus bicornis unicollis
(rudimentary horn)

cervical atresia

vaginal
atresia

(b) Partial or total atresia of the lower part of one or both Müllerian ducts

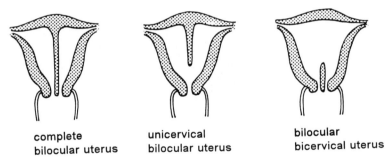

complete
bilocular uterus

unicervical
bilocular uterus

bilocular
bicervical uterus

(c) Persistant utero-vaginal septum after fusion of Müllerian ducts

Fig. 8.34. Abnormalities of Müllerian development. (After Tuchman-Duplessis and Haegel 1974)

tion by the fetal adrenal, or by administration of progestagens or anabolic steroids with androgenic effects.

The Müllerian system develops normally, but the Wolffian system, which would normally involute in the female, persists to varying degrees due to the influence of androgen, which also causes changes in the external genitalia, with clitoral hypertrophy, a tendency to closure of the urogenital sinus and fusion of the labia majora.

Malformations of the Uterus and Vagina

In uterine and vaginal malformations the Müllerian system develops as bilaterally symmetrical elements that fuse in their lower parts, giving rise to the upper part of the vagina, the cervix uteri and body of the uterus, and the Fallopian tubes. Various abnormalities of fusion occur, and atresia of all or part of the primordia may also occur (Fig. 8.34).

Morphological Abnormalities of the Male Genital Tract

Penis

Absence of the penis is usually associated with complex urogenital malformations (Campbell 1951). Duplication of the penis is extremely rare and is also associated with other anomalies. In the severe forms of anorectal agenesis abnormalities of the genitalia are common.

Failure of fusion of the urogenital groove at around the 11th or 12th week of gestation results in the production of hypospadias, which may result in balanic (simple ectopia of the urethral meatus), penile/scrotal (where the urethra opens on the shaft of the penis or scrotum) or perineal. In these severe forms there is an associated abnormality of the scrotal swellings, which coalesce giving rise to a vulviform appearance, and the penis is usually small.

Testes

Absence. Absence of the testis, unilateral or bilateral, may accompany renal agenesis, but is extremely rare as an isolated abnormality. There are less than 100 reports in the literature, most of which were published more than 40 years ago and are not accompanied by chromosome studies. Supernumerary and fused testes are also very rare.

Incomplete Descent. Incomplete descent of the testis is a manifestation of imperfect coordination of the development of the posterior abdominal wall and the various derivatives of the mesonephros and metanephros. The elongation of the parietes and the active descent of the testis and appendages becomes asynchronous, and although hormonal mechanisms are known to be involved (pituitary gonadotrophins have a significant effect) their precise role is far from clear. The testis normally reaches the orifice of the inguinal canal by the 6th month, descends through it during the 7th, and reaches its definitive intrascrotal position towards the end of the 8th month.

The undescended testis may be in the inguinal canal (80%) or in an intra-abdominal situation (20%). Occasionally a presumed intra-abdominal testis is absent. Non-descent is commoner in the right but can

be bilateral. An ipsilateral inguinal hernia is found in most instances.

Histological changes have been described by Farrington (1969). The normal sequence of events in testicular development, with a static phase (0–4 years), a growth phase (4–10 years), and maturation (10 years to puberty) is not well defined in undescended testes, which have fewer germinal cells by the time the age of 6 years is reached, although the tubules may continue to grow normally. Interstitial fibrosis may also occur, with peritubular hyalinization of the older testis.

There are a number of possible complications of cryptorchidism. The inguinal testis is more susceptible to trauma, the intra-abdominal testis to torsion. Fertility may be impaired, and bilaterally cryptorchid males are likely to be sterile if orchiopexy is delayed. Secondary sexual characteristics develop normally. Cryptorchidism is undoubtedly associated with neoplasia and, although estimates vary widely, risks between 15 and 40 times the normal are given. There is no evidence to suggest that this risk is modified by orchiopexy, however early this is performed, but earlier diagnosis is practicable with an intrascrotal testis. The subject is discussed in detail by Whitaker (1976).

Ectopic Testis. Ectopic testes do not follow the normal course of testicular descent. The classification of Wattenburg et al. (1949) is generally used. The testis may be:

1. Superficial, inguinal or interstitial, i.e. lodged superficially in the inguinal region or at the base of the scrotum
2. Pubopenile, i.e. lodged at the base of the penis
3. Femoral, i.e. lodged subcutaneously in the superomedial aspect of the thigh
4. Transverse, i.e. lodged high in the scrotum but lying transversely
5. Perineal, i.e. posterior to the scrotum in the subcutaneous tissue (Wattenburg et al. 1949).

References

Abrahamson J (1961) Double bladder and related anomalies, clinical and embryologic aspects and a case report. Br J Urol 33: 195

Allen DM, Diamond LK, Howel DA (1960) Anaphylactoid purpura in children (Schönlein–Henoch syndrome): review with a follow-up of the renal complications. Am J Dis Child 99: 833

Allen WR, Travis LB, Cavallo T, Brouhard BH, Cunningham RT (1982) Immune deposits and mesangial hypercellularity in minimal change nephrotic syndrome: clinical relevance. J Pediatr 100: 188

Alport AC (1927) Hereditary familial congenital haemorrhagic nephritis. Br Med J i: 504

Anders D, Agricola B, Suppel M, Thoenes W (1977) Basement membrane changes in membranoproliferative glomerulonephritis. II. Characterization of a third type by silver impregnation of ultrathin sections. Virchows Arch A Pathol Anat 376: 1

Andreassen M (1953) Vesical neck obstruction in children. Acta Chir Scand 105: 398

Andreoli SP, Yum MN, Bergstein JM (1986) IgA nephropathy in children: significance of basement membrane deposition of IgA. Am J Nephrol 6: 28

Andres GA, Accinni L, Hsu KC, Zabriskie JB, Seegal BC (1966) Electron microscopic studies of human glomerulonephritis with ferritin conjugated antibody: localization of antigen–antibody complexes in glomerular structures of patients with acute glomerulonephritis. J Exp Med 123: 399

Angelov A, Boykinov B, Dragiev M (1981) Electron microscope study of renal lesions in the nail patella syndrome. Folia Med (Plovdiv) 23: 41

Anonymous (1978) (V.U.R. + I.R.R.) + U.T.I.=C.P.N. Lancet ii: 301 (leading article)

Anonymous (1979) Nephronophthisis – just a pretty name? Lancet i: 141 (leading article)

Anthony BF, Kaplan EL, Chapman SS, Oyie PG, Wannamaker LW (1967) Epidemic acute nephritis with reappearance of type-49 streptococcus. Lancet ii: 787

Ask-Upmark E (1929) Über juvenile maligne Nephrosklerose und ihr Verhältnis zu Störungen in der Nierenentwicklung. Acta Pathol Microbiol Scand 6: 383

Atkins RC, Holdsworth SR, Glasgow EF, Matthews EF (1976) The macrophage in human rapidly progressive glomerulonephritis. Lancet i: 830

Atkins RC, Glasgow EF, Holdsworth SR, Thomson NM, Hancock WW (1980) Tissue culture of isolated glomeruli from patients with glomerulonephritis. Kidney Int 17: 515

Atkinson K, Biggs JC, Hayes J, Ralston M, Dodds AJ (1983) Cyclosporin A associated nephrotoxicity in the first 100 days after allogeneic bone marrow transport: three distinct syndromes. Br J Haematol 54: 59

Avni EF, Thoua Y, Lalmand B, Didier F, Droulle P, Schulman CC (1987) Multicystic dysplastic kidney: natural history from in utero diagnosis and postnatal follow-up. J Urol 138: 1420

Baert L, Steg A (1977a) On the pathogenesis of simple renal cysts in the adult. A microdissection study. Urol Res 5: 103

Baert L, Steg A (1977b) Is the diverticulum of the distal and collecting tubules a preliminary stage of the simple cyst in the adult? J Urol 118: 707

Bailey RR (1973) The relationship of vesico-ureteric reflux to urinary tract infection and chronic pyelonephritis – reflux nephropathy. Clin Nephrol 1: 132

Bailey RR (1977) The relationship of vesico-ureteric reflux. Arch Dis Child 52: 804 (letter)

Baldauff MC, Shulz DM (1976) Multilocular cyst of the kidney. Report of three cases with review of the literature. Am J Clin Pathol 65: 93

Baldwin DS, Gluck MC, Schacht RG, Gallo G (1974) The long-term course of poststreptococcal glomerulonephritis. Ann Intern Med 80: 342

Balodimos MC, Legg MA, Bradley RF (1970) Diabetic glomerulosclerosis in children. Diabetes 20: 622

Barratt TM, Soothill JF (1970) Controlled train of cyclophosphamide in steroid-sensitive relapsing nephrotic syndrome of childhood. Lancet ii: 479

Barrington FJF, Wright HD (1930) Bacteraemia following operations on the urethra. J Pathol Bacteriol 33: 871

Bartter FC, Pronove P, Gill JR Jr, MacCardle RC (1962) Hyperplasia of the juxtaglomerular complex with hyperaldosteronism and hypokalemic alkalosis: a new syndrome. Am J Med 33: 811

Baxter TJ (1961) Morphogenesis of renal cysts. Am J Pathol 38: 721

Bear JC, McManamon P, Morgan J, Payne RH, Lewis H, Gault MH, Churchill DN (1984) Age at clinical onset and at ultrasonographic detection of adult polycystic kidney disease: data for genetic counselling. Am J Med Genet 18: 45

Beaufils M (1981) Glomerular disease complicating abdominal sepsis (Clinical Conference). Kidney Int 19: 609

Beck AD (1971) Effects of intro-uterine obstruction upon the development of the fetal kidney. J Urol 105: 784

Belman AB, Kropp KA, Simon NM (1968) Renal-pressor hypertension secondary to unilateral hydronephrosis. N Engl J Med 278: 1133

Berdon WE, Baker DH, Becker JA, Uson AC (1968) Ectopic ureterocele. Radiol Clin North Am 6: 205

Beregi E, Varga I (1974) Analysis of 260 cases of membranous glomerulonephritis in renal biopsy material. Clin Nephrol 2: 215

Beresford SAA, Holland WW (1975) Levels of blood pressure in children: a familial study. Proc R Soc Med 66: 1009

Berger J (1969) IgA glomerular deposits in renal disease. Transplant Proc 1: 939

Berger J, Galle P (1963) Dépôts denses au sein des membranes basales du rein. Presse Med 49: 2351

Bernstein J (1968) Developmental abnormalities of the renal parenchyma – renal hypoplasia and dysplasia. Pathol Annu 3: 213

Bernstein J (1971) Heritable cystic disorders of the kidney. Pediatr Clin North Am 18: 435

Bernstein J (1976) A Classification of renal cysts. In: Gardner KD Jr (ed) Cystic diseases of the kidney. Wiley, New York, p 7

Bernstein J, Kissane JM (1973) Hereditary disorders of the kidney. In: Rosenberg H, Bolande RP (eds) Perspectives in paediatric pathology, vol 1. Year Book Medical Publishers, Chicago, p 435

Bernstein J, Landing BH (1989) Glomerulocystic kidney diseases. Prog Clin Biol Res 305: 27

Bernstein J, Meyer R (1964) Some speculations on the nature and significance of developmentally small kidneys (renal hypoplasia). Nephron 1: 137

Bernstein J, Meyer R (1972) Parenchymal maldevelopment of the kidney. In: Kelley V (ed) Brennemann's practice of pediatrics, vol 3, chap 26. Harper & Row, Hagerstown

Bernstein J, Brough AJ, McAdams AJ (1974) The renal lesion in syndromes of multiple congenital malformations. Birth Defects 10: 35

Berry CL (1978) Hypertension and arterial development: long-term considerations. Br Heart J 40: 709

Berry CL, Pinto T, Baitham SI, Giwam YAM (1982) The prunebelly syndrome – a possible pathogenesis. Diag Histopathol 5: 195

Betts PR, Forrest-Hay I (1973) Juvenile nephronophthisis. Lancet ii: 475

Bhan AK, Collins AB, Schneeberger EF, McCluskey RT (1979) A cell mediated reaction against glomerular-bound immune complexes. J Exp Med 150: 1410

Bhan AK, Schneeberger EF, Collins AB, McCluskey RT (1978) Evidence for a pathogenic role of cell mediated immune mechanism of experimental glomerulonephritis. J Exp Med 148: 246

Bhathena DB, Weiss JH, Holland NH, McMorrow RG, Curtis JJ, Lucas BA, Luke RC (1979) Focal and segmental glomerulosclerosis in reflux nephropathy (chronic pyelonephritis). Am J Med 63: 886

Bialestock D (1965) Studies of renal malformations and pyelonephritis in children, with and without associated vesicoureteral reflux and obstruction. Aust N Z J Surg 35: 120

Bigler JA, Killingworth WP (1949) Cartilage in the kidney. Arch Pathol 47: 487

Blyth H, Ockendon BG (1971) Polycystic disease of the kidneys and liver presenting in childhood. J Med Genet 8: 257

Bodian M (1957) Some observations on the pathology of congenital "idiopathic bladder-neck obstruction" (Marion's disease). Br J Urol 29: 393

Bohle A, Gärtner HV, Fishback H, Bock KD, Edel HH, Frötscher U, Kluth R, Mönninghoff W, Scheler F (1974) The morphological and clinical features of membranoproliferative glomerulonephritis in adults. Virchows Arch A Pathol Anat 363: 213

Boichis H, Passwell J, David R, Miller H (1973) Congenital hepatic fibrosis and nephronophthisis. A family study. Q J Med 165: 221

Bois E, Royer P (1970) Association de néphropathie tubulo-interstitielle chronique et de dégénérescence tapéto-rétinienne. Etude génétique. Arch Fr Pédiatr 27: 471

Boissonnat P (1962) What to call hypoplastic kidney? Arch Dis Child 37:142

Bolande RP, Brough AJ, Izant RJ (1967) Congenital mesoblastic nephroma of infancy. Paediatrics 40: 272

Bolton WK, Innes DJ Jr, Sturgill BC, Kaiser DL (1987) T-cells and macrophages in rapidly progressive glomerulonephritis: clinicopathologic correlations. Kidney Int 32: 869

Bredin HC, Winchester P, McGovern JH, Degnan M (1975) Family study of vesico-ureteral reflux. J Urol 113: 623

Breuning MH, Reeders ST, Brunner H (1987) Improved early diagnosis of adult polycystic kidney disease with flanking DNA markers. Lancet ii: 1359

Buchi KF, Seigler RL (1986) Hypertension in the first month of life. J Hypertens 4: 525

Buchta RM Viseskul C, Gilbert EF, Sarto GE, Optiz JM (1973) Familial bilateral renal agenesis and hereditary renal adysplasia. Z Kinderheilk 115: 111

Burk D, Beaudoin AR (1977) Aresenate-induced renal agenesis in rats. Teratology 16: 247

Burkholder PM, Marchand A, Krueger RP (1970) Mixed membranous and proliferative glomerulonephritis: a correlative light, immunofluorescence and electron microscopy study. Lab Invest 23: 459

Burkholder PM, Hyman LR, Krueger RP (1973) Characterization of mixed membranous and proliferative glomerulonephritis: recognition of three varieties. In: Kincaid-Smith P, Mathew TH, Becker EL (eds) Glomerulonephritis: morphology, natural history and treatment. Wiley, New York, p 557

Cairns HWB (1925) Hereditary in polycystic disease of the kidney. Q J Med 18: 359

Cam G, Simon P, Ang KS (1989) Prevalence of symptomatic forms of adult polycystic kidney disease (APKD). Program and Abstracts of American Society of Nephrology, p 59A

Cameron JS, Clark WF (1982) A role for insoluble antibody–antigen complexes in glomerulonephritis? Clin Nephrol 18: 55

Cameron JS, White RHR (1965) Selectivity of proteinuria in children with the nephrotic syndrome. Lancet i: 463

Cameron JS, Glasgow EF, Ogg CS, White RHR (1970) Membranoproliferative glomerulonephritis and persistent hypocomplementaemia. Br Med J 4: 7

Campbell MF (1951) Clinical paediatric urology. Saunders, Philadelphia, p 698

Camussi G, Tetla C, Bussolindo F, Turello E, Brentjens J, Baglioni C, Andreas G (1990) The effect of leukocyte stimulation on rabbit immune complex glomerulonephritis. Kidney Int 38: 1047

Caroli J, Covinaud C, Soupault R, Porcher P, Etévé J (1958) Une affection nouvelle, sans doute congénitale, des voies biliaires: la dilatation kystique unilobaire des canaux hépatiques. Sem Hop Paris 34: 496

Carreras L, Romero R, Requesens C, Oliver AJ, Carrera M, Clavo M, Alsina J (1981) Familial hypocomplementemic hemolytic uremic syndrome with HLA-A3, B7 haplotype. JAMA 245: 602

Chatten J, Bishop HC (1977) Bilateral multilocular cysts of the kidney. J Pediatr Surg 12: 749

Charro Salgado AL, Lopez Marcia A, Freire A, Paramo P, Fernandez-Cruz A (1977) Beckwith–Wiedemann syndrome with medullary sponge kidneys, agonadism and persistent testosterone production. Eur Urol 3: 108

Chilton SJ, Cremin BJ (1981) The spectrum of polycystic disease in children. Pediatr Radiol 11: 9

Cho KJ, Thornbury JR, Bernstein J, Heidelberger KP, Walter JF (1979) Localized cystic disease of the kidney: angiographic–pathologic correlation. Am J Radiol 132: 891

Chrispin AR (1972) Medullary necrosis in infancy. Br Med Bull 18: 233

Churg J, Habib R, White RHR (1970) Pathology of the nephrotic syndrome in children: a report for the International Study of Kidney Disease in Children. Lancet i: 1299

Christenson PJ, Craig JP, Bibro MC, O'Connell KJ (1982) Cysts containing renal cell carcinoma in von Hippel–Lindau disease. J Urol 128: 798

Clarkson AR, Seymour AE, Thompson AJ, Haynes WDG, Chan Y-L, Jackson B (1977) IgA nephropathy: a syndrome of uniform morphology, diverse clinical features, and uncertain prognosis. Clin Nephrol 8: 459

Cohen AH, Border WA, Fong H, Glassock RJ, Trygstad C (1982) Glomerulonephritis with mesangial IgM deposits. Kidney Int 21: 147

Cohen AH, Border WA, Shankel E, Glassock RJ (1981) Crescentic glomerulonephritis: immune vs nonimmune mechanisms. Am J Nephrol 1: 78

Coleman M (1980) Multilocular renal cyst. Case report ultrastructure and review of the literature. Virchows Arch A Pathol Anat 387: 207

Coppoletta JM, Wolbach SB (1933) Body length and organ weights of infants and children: study of body length and normal weights of more important organs of the body between birth and 12 years of age. Am J Pathol 9: 55

Cotran RS (1969) The renal lesion in chronic pyelonephritis: immunofluorescence and ultrastructural studies. J Infect Dis 120: 109

Counahan R, Cameron JS (1977) Henoch–Schönlein nephritis. Contrib Nephrol 7: 143

Counahan R, Simmons MJ, Charlwood GJ (1976) Multifocal osteolysis with nephropathy. Arch Dis Child 51: 717

Dalgaard OZ (1957) Bilateral polycystic disease of the kidneys. a follow-up study of 284 patients and their families. Acta Med Scand 158 (suppl 328): 1

D'Amico G, Imbasciati E, Barbiano di Belgioioso G, Bertoli S, Fogazzi G, Ferrario F, Fellin G, Ragni A, Colasanti G, Minetti L, Ponticelli C (1985) Idiopathic IgA mesangial nephropathy: clinical and histological study of 374 patients. Medicine (Baltimore) 64: 49

de Navasquez S (1956) Further studies in experimental pyelonephritis produced by various bacteria with special reference to renal scarring as a factor in pathogenesis. J Pathol 71: 27

de Vargas A, Rosenberg A, Barratt TM, Ransley PG, Williams DI, Carter CO (1978) Vesico-ureteric reflux – a family study. J Clin Genet 15: 85

Delaney V, Mullaney J, Bourke E (1978) Juvenile nephronophthisis congenital hepatic fibrosis and retinal hypoplasia in twins. Q J Med 186: 281

Delver R, Griggs D, Lackey DA, Kagan BM (1974) Familial renal agenesis and total dysplasia. Am J Dis Child 128: 377

Devaney K, Kapur SP, Patterson MD, Chandra RS (1991) Paediatric renal artery dysplasia: a morphometric study. Pediatr Pathol 11: 609

Dische FE, Weston MJ, Parsons V (1985) Abnormally thin glomerular basement membrane associated with hematuria, proteinuria or renal failure in adults. Am J Nephrol 5: 103

Dixon FJ (1968) The pathogenesis of glomerulonephritis. Am J Med 44: 493

Dixon FJ, Vazquez JJ, Weigle WO, Cochrane CG (1958) Pathogenesis of serum sickness. AMA Arch Pathol 65: 18

Dixon FJ, Feldman JD, Vazquez JJ (1961) Experimental glomerulonephritis: the pathogenesis of a laboratory model resembling the spectrum of human glomerulonephritis. J Exp Med 113: 899

Domizio P, Risdon RA (1991) Cystic renal neoplasms of infancy and childhood: a light microscopical, lectin histochemical and immunohistochemical study. Histopathology 19: 199

Donker AJM, de Jong PE, Statius van Eps LW, Berentjens JRH, Bakker K, Doorenbos H (1977) Indomethacin in Bartter's syndrome: does the syndrome represent a state of hyperprostaglandinism? Nephron 19: 200

Dretler SP, Olsson C, Pfister RC (1971) The anatomic, radiologic and clinical characteristics of the pelvic kidney: an analysis of 86 cases. J Urol 105: 623

Dreyfuss ML, Fliess M (1941) Patient urachus with stone formation. J Urol 46: 77

Droz D, Kramar A, Nawar T, Noel LH (1984) Primary IgA nephropathy: prognostic factors. Contrib Nephrol 40: 202

Duckett JW Jr (1980) The prune belly syndrome. In: Holder TM, Aschroft KW (eds) The surgery of infants and children. Saunders, Philadelphia, p 802

Dunn JS (1934) Nephrosis or nephritis? J Pathol Bacteriol 39: 1

Dunnill MS, Millard PR, Oliver D (1977) Acquired cystic disease of the kidneys: a hazard of long-term intermittent maintenance haemodialysis. J Clin Pathol 30: 868

Dwoskin JY (1976) Sibling uropathology. J Urol 115: 726

Ehrenreich T, Churg J (1968) Pathology of membraneous nephropathy. Pathol Annu 3: 145

Einsenstein B, Stark H, Goodman RM (1979) Benign familial hematuria in children from Jewish families in Israel. J Med Genet 16: 369

Ekström T (1955) Renal hypoplasia. A clinical study of 179 cases. Acta Chir Scand [Suppl] 203

Ekström T, Engfeldt B, Lagergren C, Lindvall N (1959) Medullary sponge kidney. Almqvist & Wicksell, Stockholm

Elkin M, Bernstein J (1969) Cystic disease of the kidney. Clin Radiol 20: 65

Epstein CJ, Sahud MA, Piel CF, Goodman JR, Bernfield MR, Kushner JH, Albin AR (1972) Hereditary macrothrombocytopathia, nephritis and deafness. Am J Med 52: 299

Ericsson NO, Ivemark BI 1958a) Renal dysplasia and urinary tract infection. Acta Chir Scand 115: 58

Ericsson NO, Ivemark BI (1958b) Renal dysplasia and pylonephritis in infants and children. 2. Primitive ductules and abnormal glomeruli. Arch Pathol 66: 264

Evans SH, Erickson RP, Kelsch R, Pierce JC (1980) Apparently changing patterns of inheritance of Alport's hereditary nephritis: genetic heterogeneity versus altered diagnostic criteria. Clin Genet 17: 285

Fanconi G, Hanhart E, von Albertini A, Euhlinger R, Dohvo E, Prader A (1951) Die familiäre juvenile Nephronopthise Helv Paediatr Acta 6: 1

Fantel AG, Shepard RH (1975) Potter syndrome: nonrenal features induced by oligoamnios. Am J Dis Child 129: 1346

Faraggiana T, Bernstein J, Strauss L, Churg J (1985) Use of lectins in the study of histogenesis of renal cysts. Lab Invest 53: 575

Farmer SG (1985) Immunology of bacterial infections. In: Lennette EH, Balows A, Hausler WJ, Shadomy HJ (eds) Manual of clinical microbiology, 4th ed. American Society for Microbiology, Washington, p 898

Farr MJ, Roberts S, Morley AR, Dewar PJ, Roberts DF, Undall PR (1975) The haemolytic uraemic syndrome. A family study. Q J Med 44: 161

Farrington GH (1969) Histologic observations in cryptorchidism: the congenital germinal-cell deficiency of the undescended testis. J Pediatr Surg 4: 606

Feingold J, Bois E, Chompret A, Broyer M, Gubler MC, Grüfeld JP (1985) Genetic heterogeneity of Alport's syndrome. Kidney Int 27: 672

Fellows RA, Leonidas JC, Beatty EC Jr (1976) Radiologic features of "adult type" polycystic kidney disease in the neonate. Pediatr Radiol 4: 87

Ferrario F, Castiglione D, Colasanti G, Barbiano DI, Belgioioso G, Bertolis S, D'Amico G (1985) The detection of monocytes in the human glomerulonephritis. Kidney Int 28: 513

Fetterman GH (1970) Microdissection in the study of normal and abnormal renal structure and function of Pathol Annu 5: 173

Fetterman GH, Habib R (1969) Congenital bilateral oligonephronic renal hypoplasia with hypertrophy of nephrons (oligomeganephronie): studies by microdissection. Am J Clin Pathol 52: 199

Fichman MP, Telfer N, Zia P, Speckart P, Gollub M, Rude R (1976) Role of prostaglandins in the pathogenesis of Bartter's syndrome. Am J Med 60: 785

Forsythe IW, Smyth BT (1959) Diverticulum of the bladder in children: a study of 13 cases. Pediatrics 24: 322

Fritjoffson A, Sundin T (1966) Studies of renal function in vesicoureteric reflux. Br J Urol 38: 445

Gallo GR, Caulin-Glaser T, Lamm ME (1981) Charge of circulating immune complexes as a factor in glomerular basement membrane localization in mice. J Clin Invest 67: 1305

Gang DL, Herrin JT (1986) Infantile polycystic disease of the liver and kidneys. Clin Nephrol 25: 28

Germuth FG Jr (1953) Comparative histologic and immunologic study in rabbits of induced hypersensitivity of serum sickness type. J Exp Med 97: 257

Germuth FG Jr, Rodriquez E (1972) Immunopathology of the renal glomerules: immune complex deposit and antibasement membrane disease. Little Brown, Boston

Gianantonio CA, Vitacco M, Mendilaharzu F, Gallo GE, Sojo ET (1973) The hemolytic–uremic syndrome. Nephron 11: 174

Gill JR Jr, Bartter FC (1978) Evidence for a prostaglandin-independent defect in chloride reabsorption in the loop of Henle as a proximal cause of Bartter's syndrome. Am J Med 65: 766

Glasgow EF, Moncrieff MW, White RHR (1970) Symptomless haematuria in childhood. Br Med J ii: 687

Glen JF (1959) Agenesis of the bladder. JAMA 169: 2016

Godley ML, Risdon RA, Ransley PG (1989) Effects of unilateral vesicoureteric reflux on renal growth and the uptake of 99m Tc DMSA by the kidney. An experimental study in the minipig. Br J Urol 63: 340

Goldstein AR, White RHR, Akuse R, Chantler C (1992) Long-term follow-up of childhood Henoch–Schönlein nephritis. Lancet 339: 280

Gonzalez-Crussi F, Kidd JM, Hernandez RJ (1982) Cystic nephroma. Morphologic spectrum and implications. Urology 20: 88

Gonzalo A, Mampaso F, Gallego N, Bellas C, Sequi J, Ortune J (1981) Hemolytic–uremic syndrome with hypocomplementemia and deposits of IgM and C3 in the involved renal tissue. Clin Nephrol 16: 193

Gonzalo A, Mampaso F, Gallego N, Quereda C, Fierro C, Ortuno J (1985) Clinical significance of IgM mesangial deposits in the nephrotic syndrome. Nephron 41: 246

Grantham JJ, Levine E (1985) Acquired cystic disease: replacing one kidney disease by another. Kidney Int 28: 99

Grantham JJ, Geiser JL, Even AP (1987) Cyst formation and growth in autosomal dominant polycystic kidney disease. Kidney Int 31: 1145

Gregoire JR, Torres VE, Holley KE, Farrow GM (1987) Renal epithelial hyperplastic and neoplastic proliferation in autosomal dominant polycystic kidney disease (ADPKD). Am J Kidney Dis 9: 27

Grünfeld JP, Noël LH, Hafez S, Droz D (1985) Renal prognosis in women with hereditary nephritis. Clin Nephrol 23: 267

Gubler MC, Levy M, Broyer M, Naizot C, Gonzales G, Perrin D, Habib R (1981) Alport's syndrome: a report of 58 cases and a review of the literature. Am J Med 70: 493

Habib R, Bois E (1975) Congenital and infantile nephrotic syndrome. In: Strauss J (ed) Pediatric nephrology, vol 2. Stratton Intercontinental Medical, New York, p 335

Habib R, Gubler MC (1971) Les lésions glomérulaires focales des syndromes néphrotiques idiopathiques de l'enfant: á propos de 49 observations, Nephron 8: 382

Habib R, Gubler MC (1973) Focal sclerosing glomerulonephritis. In: Kincaid-Smith P, Mathew TH, Becker EL (eds) Glomerulonephritis. Wiley, New York, p 263

Habib R, Gubler MC (1975) Focal glomerulosclerosis, associated with idiopathic nephrotic syndrome. In: Rubin MI, Barratt TM (eds) Paediatric nephrology. Williams & Wilkins, Baltimore, p 499

Habib R, Kleinknecht C (1975) Membranous nephropathy (extramembranous glomerulonephritis). In: Rubin MI, Barratt TM (eds) Paediatric pathology. Williams & Wilkins, Baltimore, p 515

Habib R, Mouzet Massa MT, Coutecuisse V, Royer P (1965) L'ectasie tubulaire précalicielle chez l'enfant. Ann Pediat 12: 288

Habib R, Kleinknecht C, Gubler MC, Maiz HB (1973) Idiopathic membranoproliferative glomerulonephritis: morphology and natural history. In: Kincaid-Smith P, Mathew TH, Becker EL (eds) Glomerulonephritis: morphology, natural history and treatment. Wiley, New York, p 491

Habib R, Levy M, Gagnadoux MF, Broyer M (1982a) Prognosis of the hemolytic uremic syndrome in children. Adv Nephrol 11: 99

Habib R, Gubler MC, Hinglais M, Nöel LH, Droz D, Levy M, Mathieu P, Foidart JM, Perrin D, Bois E, Grünfeld JP (1982b) Alport's syndrome: experience at Hospital Necker. Kidney Int 21: 520

Habif DV Jr, Berdon WE, Yeh MN (1982) Infantile polycystic disease. In utero sonographic diagnosis. Radiology 142: 475

Harrison EG, McCormack LJ (1971) Pathologic classification of renal arterial disease in renovascular hypertension. Mayo Clin Proc 46: 161

Harrison AR, Rose GA (1979) Medullary sponge kidney. Urol Res 7: 197

Hashimoto BE, Filly RA, Callen PW (1986) Multicystic dysplastic kidney in utero: changing appearance on US. Radiology 159: 107

Hatfield PM, Pfister RC (1972) Adult polycystic disease of the kidneys (Potter type 3). JAMA 222: 1527

Hayslett JP, Hardin JH (1982) Advances in systemic lupus erythematosus. Am J Kidney Dis 11: 97

Helczynski L, Wells TR, Landing BH, Lipsey AI (1984) The renal lesion of congenital hepatic fibrosis: pathologic and morphometric analysis with comparison to the renal lesion of infantile polycystic disease. Pediatr Pathol 2: 441

Henneberry MO, Stephens FD (1980) Renal hypoplasia and dysplasia in infants with posterior urethral valves. J Urol 123: 912

Heptinstall RH (1974a) Pyelonephritis: pathologic features. In: Pathology of the kidney. 2nd edn. Little Brown, Boston, p 878

Hepinstall RH (1974b) Pyelonephritis: pathologic features. In: Pathology of the kidney. 2nd edn. Little Brown, Boston, p 913

Heptinstall RH (1992) Crescentic glomerulonephritis. In: Heptinstall RH (ed) Pathology of the kidney. 4th edn. Little Brown, Boston, p 627

Hill JE, Bunts RC (1960) Thoracic kidney: case reports. J Urol 84: 460

Hilton C, Keeling JW (1973) Neonatal renal tumours. Br J Urol 46: 157

Hodson CJ, Maling TMJ, McMamamon PJ, Lewis MG (1975) The pathogenesis of reflux nephropathy (chronic atrophic pyelonephritis). Br J Urol Suppl 13

Hoover DL, Duckett JW Jr (1982) Posterior urethral valves, unilateral reflux and renal dysplasia: a syndrome. J Urol 128: 994

Hostetter T, Olson JL, Rennke HG, Venkatachalam MA, Brennar BM (1981) Hyperfiltration in remnant nephrons: a potential adverse response to renal ablation. Am J Physiol 241: F 85

Hudson BG, Wieslander J, Wisdom BJ Jr, Noelken ME (1989) Biology of disease. Goodpasture syndrome: molecular architecture and function of basement membrane antigen. Lab Invest 61: 256

Hughson MD, Buchwald D, Fox M (1986) Renal neoplasia and acquired cystic disease in patients receiving long-term dialysis. Arch Pathol Lab Med 110: 592

Hughson MD, Hennigar GR, McManus JFA (1980) Atypical cysts, acquired renal cystic disease and renal cell tumours in end stage dialysis kidneys. Lab Invest 42: 475

Huland H, Lewin K, Stamey TA (1976) Unilateral medullary sponge kidney. Cause of persistent bacteriuria. Urology 8: 373

Hyman LR, Jenis EH, Hill GS, Zimmerman SW, Burkholder PM (1975) Alternative C3 pathway activation in pneumococcal glomerulonephritis. Am J Med 58: 810

Iglesias CG, Torres VE, Offord KP, Holley KE, Beard CM, Kurland LT (1983) Epidemiology of adult polycystic kidney disease, Olmstead county, Minnesota: 1935–1980. Am J Kidney Dis 2: 630

International Study of Kidney Disease in Childhood (1978) Nephrotic syndrome in children: prediction of histopathology from clinical and laboratory characteristics at time of diagnosis. Kidney Int 13: 159

International Study of Kidney Disease in Childhood (1981) Primary nephrotic syndrome in children: clinical significance of histopathologic variants of minimal change and of diffuse mesangial hypercellularity. Kidney Int 20: 765

Jabour BA, Rals PW, Tang WW, Boswell WD Jr, Colletti PM, Feinstein EI, Massry SG (1987) Acquired cystic disease of the kidneys: computed tomography and ultrasonography appraisal in patients on peritoneal and haemodialysis. Invest Radiol 22: 728

Jennings RB, Earle DP (1961) Post-streptococcal glomerulonephritis: histopathologic and clinical studies of the acute, subsiding acute and early chronic latent phases. J Clin Invest 40: 1525

Johnson HL, Mix LW (1976) The Ask-Upmark kidney: a form of ascending pyelonephritis? Br J Urol 48: 393

Jones DN, Risdon RA, Hayden K, Barratt TM, Crispin AR (1973) Juvenile nephronophthisis: clinical radiological and pathological correlationships. Paediatr Radiol 1: 164

Joshi VV, Beckwith JB (1989) Multilocular cyst of the kidney (cystic nephroma) and cystic partially differentiated nephroblastoma. Terminology and criteria for diagnosis. Cancer 64: 466

Joshi VV, Kaszina J (1984) Clinicopathologic spectrum of glomerulocystic kidneys: report of two cases and a brief review of literature. Pediatr Pathol 2: 171

Joshi VV, Banerjee AK, Krishna Y, Pathak IC (1977) Cystic partially differentiated nephroblastoma. Cancer 40: 489

Jørgensen M (1972) Three-dimensional reconstruction of intrahepatic bile ducts in case of polycystic disease of the liver in an infant. Acta Pathol Microbiol Scand 80: 201

Jørgensen M (1973) A stereological study of intrahepatic bile ducts. 3. Infantile polycystic disease. Acta Pathol Microbiol Scand 81: 670

Jørgensen M (1974) A stereological study of intrahepatic bile ducts. 4. Congenital hepatic fibrosis. Acta Pathol Microbiol Scand 82: 21

Kaack MB, Dowling KJ, Patterson GM, Roberts JA (1986) Immunology of pyelonephritis. VIII. E. coli causes granulocyte aggregation and renal ischemia. J Urol 136: 1117

Kanwar YS, Caulin-Glaser T, Gallo GR, Lamm ME (1986)

Interaction of immune complexes with glomerular heparan sulphate-proteoglycans. Kidney Int 30: 842

Kaplan BS, Chesney RW, Drummond KN (175) Hemolytic uremic syndrome in families. N Engl J Med 292: 1090

Kaplan BS, Kaplan P, de Chadarevian JP, Jequier S, O'Regan S, Russo P (1988) Variable expression of autosomal recessive polycystic kidney disease and congenital hepatic fibrosis within a family. Am J Med Genet 29: 639

Karlsberg RP, Lacher JW, Bartecchi E (1977) Adult hemolytic-uremic syndrome: familial variant. Arch Intern Med 137: 1155

Kay S, Pratt CB, Salzberg AM (1966) Hamartoma (leiomyomatous type) of the kidney. Cancer 19: 1825

Kefalides NA, Pegg MT, Ohno N, Poon-King T, Zabriskie J, Fillit H (1986) Antibodies to basement membrane collagen and to laminin are present in sera from patients with poststreptococcal glomerulonephritis. J Exp Med 163: 588

Kerjaschki D, Farquhar MG (1983) Immunocytochemical localization of the Heymann nephritis antigen (gp 330) in glomerular epithelial cells of normal Lewis rats. J Exp Med 157: 667

Kerr DNS, Warrick CK, Hart-Mercer JA (1962) A lesion resembling medullary sponge kidney in patients with congenital hepatic fibrosis. Clin Pathol 13: 85

Kida H, Asamoto T, Yokoyama H, Tomosugi N, Hattori (1986) Long-term prognosis in membranous nephropathy. Clin Nephrol 25: 64

Kimberling WJ, Fain PR, Kenyon JB, Goldgar D, Sujansky E, Gabow PA (1988) Linkage heterogeneity of autosomal dominant polycystic kidney disease. N Engl J Med 319: 913

Kindcaid-Smith P (1979) Glomerular lesions in atrophic pyelonephritis (PN). In: Hodson CJ, Kincaid-Smith P (eds) Reflux nephropathy. Masson, New York, p 268

Kissane JM (1973) Hereditary disorders of the kidney. II. In: Rosenberg HS, Bolande RP (eds) Perspectives in pediatric pathology, vol 1. Year Book Medical Publishers, Chicago, p 117

Kissane JM (1976) The morphology of renal cystic disease. In Gardner KD Jr (ed) Cystic diseases of the kidney. Wiley, New York

Kleinman H (1954) Epidemic acute glomerulonephritis at Red Lake. Minn Med 37: 479

Kohler HH (1940) Multiseptate bladder. J Urol 44: 63

Kondo Y, Shigematsu H, Kobayashi Y (1972) Cellular aspect of rabbit Masugi nephritis. II. Progressive glomerular injuries with crescent formation. Lab Invest 27: 620

Konishi F, Mukawa A, Kitada H (1980) Acquired cystic disease of the kidney and renal cell carcinoma on long term haemodialysis. Four surgical cases of young adults in Japan. Acta Pathol Jpn 30: 847

Konowalchuk J, Speirs JI, Stavric S (1977) Vero response to cytotoxin of Escherichia coli. Infect Immun 18: 775

Kossow AS, Meek JM (1982) Unilateral adult polycystic kidney disease. J Urol 127: 297

Kouvalainen K, Hjelt L, Hallman N (1962) Placenta in congenital nephrotic syndrome. Ann Paediatr Fenn 8: 181

Kuiper JJ (1971) Medullary sponge kidney. In: Gardner KD Jr (ed) Cystic diseases of the kidney. Wiley, New York, p 151

Lancet Leader (1992) Vesicoureteric reflux and nephropathy. Lancet 339: 398

Landing BH, Hughes ML (1962) Analysis of weights of kidneys in children. Lab Invest 11: 452

Lange K (1983) Evidence for the in situ origin of post-streptococcal GN: glomerular localization of endostreptosin. Clin Nephrol 19: 3

Lang S, Stevenson B, Risdon RA (1990) Thin basement membrane nephropathy as a cause of recurrent haematuria in childhood. Histopathology 16: 331

Langer LO Jr, Nishino R, Yamaguchi A, Ito Y, Ueke T, Togari H, Kato T, Opitz JM, Gilbert EF (1983) Brachymesomelia-renal

syndrome. Am J Med Genet 15: 57

Lee JKT, McCleannan BL, Kissane JM (1978) Unilateral polycystic kidney disease. Am J Radiol 130: 1165

Lepoutre C (1939/40) Sur un cas d'absence congénital de la vessie (persistence du cloaque). J Urol Med Chir 48: 334

Levine E, Grantham JJ (1981) The role of computed tomography in the evaluation of adult polycystic kidney disease. Am J Kidney Dis 1: 99

Levine AS, Michael AF (1967) Ehlers–Danlos syndrome with renal tubular acidosis and medullary sponge kidney. J Pediatr 71: 107

Levine E, Cook LT, Grantham JJ (1985) Liver cysts in autosomal-dominant polycystic kidney disease: clinical and computed tomographic study. Am J Radiol 145: 229

Levy M, Loirat C, Haibb R (1973) idiopathic membranoproliferative glomerulonephritis in children (correlations between light, electron, immunofluorescent microscopic appearances and serum C_3 and C_3 levels). Biomedicine [Express] 19: 447

Levy M, Gonzales-Burchard C, Broyer M, Dommergues JP, Foulard M, Sorez JP, Habib R (1985) Berger's disease in children: natural history and outcome. Medicine (Baltimore) 64: 157

Levy M, Gubler MC, Habib R (1979) New concepts in membranoproliferative glomerulonephritis. In: Kincaid-Smith P, d'Apice AJF, Arkins RC (eds) Progress in glomerulonephritis. Wiley, New York, p 177

Ljungqvist A, Largergren C (1963) The Ask-Upmark kidney: a congenital renal anomaly studied by micro-angiography and histology. Acta Pathol Microbiol Scand 56: 277

Lyon MF (1972) X-chromosome inactivation and developmental patterns in mammals. Biol Rev 47: 1

McCluskey RT (1975) Lupus nephritis. In: Summers SC (ed) Kidney pathology: decennial. Appleton and Lange, New York, p 456

McGraw M, Poucell S, Sweet J, Baumal R (1984) The significance of focal glomerulo-sclerosis in oligomeganephronia. Int J Pediatr Nephrol 5:67

Mackie GG, Stephens FD (1975) A correlation of renal dysplasia with position of ureteral orifice. J Urol 114: 274

Madewell JE, Goldman SM, Davis CJ Jr, Hartman DS, Feigin DS, Lichtenstein JE (1983) Multilocular cystic nephroma: a radiologic–pathologic correlation of 58 patients. Radiology 146: 309

Magil AB, Wadsworth LD, Loewen M (1981) Monocytes and human renal glomerular disease: a quantitative evaluation. Lab Invest 44: 27

Magil AB, Wadsworth LD (1981) Monocytes in human glomerulonephritis. An electron microscopic study. Lab Invest 45: 77

Maher ER, Hamilton DV, Thiru S, Wheatley T (1984) Acute renal failure due to glomerulonephritis associated with staphylococcal infection. Postgrad Med J 60: 433

Mall JC, Ghahremani GG, Boyer JL (1974) Caroli's disease associated with congenital hepatic fibrosis and renal tubular ectasia. Gastroenterology 66: 1029

Marie J, Lévêque R, Lyon G, Bêbe M, Watchi J-M (1963) Acro-ostéolyse essentielle compliquée d'insuffisance rénale d'évolution fatale. Presse Med 71: 249

Marsden HB, Lawler W (1978) Bone metastasising renal tumour of childhood. Br J Cancer 38: 437

Marsden HB, Newton WA (1986) New look at mesoblastic nephroma. J Clin Pathol 39: 508

Marshall AG (1953) Persistence of foetal structures in pyelonephritic kidneys. Br J Surg 41: 38

Meadow SR (1975) Post-streptococcal glomerulonephritis – a rare disease. Arch Dis Child 50: 379

Meadow SR (1978) The prognosis of Henoch–Schönlein nephritis. Clin Nephrol 9: 87

Melvin T, Kim Y, Michael AF (1986) Amyloid P component is not present in the glomerular basement membrane in Alport-type familial nephritis. Am J Pathol 125: 460

Michael AF, Drummond KN, Good RA, Vernier RL (1966) Acute poststreptococcal glomerulonephritis: immune deposit disease. J Clin Invest 45: 237

Miller HL (1948) Agenesis of the urinary bladder and urethra. J Urol 59: 1156

Mitchell JD, Baxter TJ, Blair-West JR, McCredie DA (1970) Renin levels in nephroblastoma (Wilms' tumour). Report of a renin-secreting tumour. Arch Dis Child 45: 376

Moolten SE (1942) Hamartial nature of tuberous sclerosis complex and its bearing on the tumour problem: a report of a case with tumour anomaly of the kidney and adenoma sebaceum. Arch Intern Med 69: 589

Morris RC, Yamacuchi H, Pulubinskas AJ, Howenstein J (1965) Medullary sponge kidney. Am J Med 38: 883

Mottet NK, Jensen H (1965) The anomalous embryonic development associated with trisomy 13–15. Am J Clin Pathol 43: 334

Morrin PAF, Hinglais N, Nabarra B, Kreis H (1978) Rapidly progressive glomerulonephritis: a clinical and pathologic study. Am J Med 65: 446

Nagashima Y, Yoshihara O, Tanaka Y, Misugi K, Horiuchi M (1988) A case of renal angiomyolipomas associated with multiple and various hamartomatous microlesions. Virchows Arch A Pathol Anat 413: 177

Nagington J, Wreghitt TG, Gandy G, Roberton NRC, Berry PJ (1978) Fatal echovirus II infections in outbreak in special care baby unit. Lancet ii: 725

Narashimhan N, Golper TA, Wolfson M, Rahatzad M, Bennett WM (1986) Clinical characteristics and diagnostic considerations in acquired renal cystic disease. Kidney Int 30: 748

Narchi H, Taylor R, Azmy AF, Murphy AV, Beattie TJ (1988) Shunt nephritis. J Pediatr Surg 23: 839

Neild GH, Cameron JS, Ogg CS, Turner DR, Williams DG, Brown CB, Chantler C, Hicks J (1983) Rapidly progressive glomerulonephritis with extensive glomerular crescent formation. Q J Med 52: 395

Niles JL, Pan GL, Collins AB, Shannon T, Skates S, Fienberg R, Arnaout MA, McCluskey RT (1993) Value of antigen-specific radioimmunoassays for measuring antineutrophil cytoplasmic antibodies (ANCA) in the differential diagnosis of rapidly progressive glomerulonephritis. J A Soc Nephrol (in press)

O'Neill M, Breslau NA, Pak CYC (1981) Metabolic evaluation of nephrolithiasis in patients with medullary sponge kidney. JAMA 245: 1233

Olson DL, Anand SK, Landing BH, Heuser E, Grushkin CM, Lieberman E (1980) Diagnosis of hereditary nephritis by failure of glomeruli to bind anti-glomerular basement membrane antibodies. J Pediatr 96: 697

Olson JL, Hostelter TH, Rennke HG, Brenner BM, Venkatachalam MA (1982) Altered glomerular permeselectivity and progressive sclerosis following extreme ablation of renal mass. Kidney Int 22: 112

Optiz JM, Howe JJ (1969) The Meckel syndrome (dysencephalia splanchnocystica, the Gruber syndrome). Birth Defects 5: 167

Osthanondh V, Potter EL (1963a) Development of human kidneys as shown by microdissection. I. Preparation of tissue with reasons for possible misinterpretation of observations. Arch Pathol 76: 271

Osthanondh V, Potter EL (1963b) Development of human kidneys as shown by microdissection. II. Renal pelvis, calyces and papillae. Arch Pathol 76: 277

Osthanondh V, Potter EL (1963c) Development of human kidneys as shown by microdissection. III. Formation and interrelationships of collecting tubules and nephrons. Arch Pathol 76: 290

Osthanondh V, Potter EL (1964) Pathogenesis of polycystic kidneys: historical survey; type 1 due to hyperplasia of interstitial portions of collecting tubules; type 2 due to inhibition of ampullary activity; type 3 due to multiple abnormalities of development; type 4 due to urethral obstruction; survey or results of microdissection. Arch Pathol 77: 459

Osthanondh V, Potter EL (1966a) Development of human kidneys as shown by microdissection. IV. Development of tubular portions of nephrons. Arch Pathol 82: 391

Osthanondh V, Potter EL (1966b) Development of human kidneys as shown by microdissection. V. Development of vascular glomerulus. Arch Pathol 82: 403

Palmer JM, Zweiman RG, Assay Keen TA (1970) Renal hypertension secondary to hydronephrosis with normal plasma renin activity. N Engl J Med 283: 1032

Paquin A, Marshall VF, McGovern JH (1960) The megacystis syndrome. J Urol 83: 634

Paschmann A, Fischer K, Grundmann A, Vongjirad A (1976) Neuraminidase-induzierte Hämolyse: experimentelle und klinische Untersuchungen. Monatsschr Kinderheilkd 124: 15

Pathak IG, Williams DI (1963) Multicystic and cystic dysplastic kidneys. Br J Urol 36: 318

Pedicelli G, Jequier S, Bowen A, Boisvert J (1986) Multicystic dysplastic kidneys. Spontaneous regression demonstrated with US. Radiology 160: 23

Pereira RR, van Wersch J (1983) Inheritance of Bartter's syndrome. Am J Med Genet 15: 79

Perkoff GT, Nugent CA Jr, Dolowitz DA, Stephens FE, Carnes WH, Tyler FH (1958) A follow-up study of hereditary chronic nephritis. Arch Intern Med 102: 733

Peters DK, Williams DG (1975) Pathogenic mechanisms in glomerulonephritis. In: Jones NF (ed) Recent advances in renal disease. Churchill Livingstone, Edinburgh, p 90

Peters DK, Williams DG, Charlesworth JA, Boulton-Jones JM, Sissons JGP, Evans DJ, Kourilsky O, Morel-Maroger L (1973) Mesangiocapillary nephritis, partial lipodystrophy and hypocomplementaemia. Lancet ii: 535

Portsman W (1970) Renal angiography in children. Prog Pediatr Radiol 3: 51

Potter EL (1946) Facial characteristics of infants with bilateral renal agenesis. Am J Obstet Gynecol 51: 885

Potter EL (1972) Normal and Abnormal Development of the kidney. Year Book Medical Publishers, Chicago

Powell T, Schackmann R, Johnson HD (1951) Multilocular cysts of the kidney. Br J Urol 23: 142

Proesmans W, van Damme B, Macken J (1975) Nephronophthisis and tapetoretinal degeneration associated with liver fibrosis. Clin Nephrol 3: 160

Proesmans W, van Damm B, Caeser P, Marchal G (1982) Autosomal dominant polycystic kidney disease in the neonatal period. Association with cerebral ateriovenous malformation. Pediatr 70: 971

Proia AD, Harden EA, Silberman HR (1984) Mitomycin-induced hemolytic–uremic syndrome. Arch Pathol Lab Med 108: 959

Rahman MA, Stork JE, Dunn MJ (1987) The roles of eicosanoids in experimental glomerulonephritis. Kidney Int 32: S40

Rainford DJ, Woodrow DF, Sloper JC, de Wardener HE, Griffiths I (1978) Post-meningococcal acute glomerular nephritis. Clin Nephrol 9: 249

Ransley PG (1978) Vesico-ureteric reflux: continuing surgical dilemma. Urology 12: 246

Ransley PG, Risdon RA (1975a) Renal papillary morphology and intrarenal reflux in the young pig. Urol Res 3: 105

Ransley PG, Risdon RA (1975b) Renal papillary morphology in infants and young children. Urol Res 3: 111

Ransley PG, Risdon RA (1978) Reflux and renal scarring. Br J Radiol Suppl 14

Ransley PG, Risdon RA, Godley ML (1984) High pressure sterile vesico-ureteral reflux and renal scarring: an experimental study in the pig and minipig. Contr Nephrol 39: 320

Ransley PG, Risdon RA, Godley ML (1987) Effects of vesicoureteric reflux on renal growth and function as measured by

GFR, plasma creatinine and urinary concentrating ability. An experimental study in the minipig. Br J Urol 60: 193

Rapola J, Kääriäinen H (1988) Morphologic diagnosis in recessive and dominant polycystic kidney disease in infancy and childhood. Acta Pathol Microbiol Scand 96: 68

Reeders ST, Bruening MH, Davies KE, Nicholls RD, Jarman AP, Higgs DR, Peason PL, Weatherall DJ (1985) A highly polymorphic DNA marker linked to adult polycystic kidney disease on chromosome 16. Nature 317: 542

Reeders ST, Gal A, Propping P, Waldherr R, Davies KE, Zerres K, Hogenkamp T, Schmidt W, Dolata MM, Weatherall DJ (1986) Prenatal diagnosis of autosomal dominant polycystic kidney disease with a DNA probe. Lancet ii: 6

Reilly BJ, Neuhauser EBD (1960) Renal tubular ectasia in cystic disease of the kidney and liver. AJR Am J Roentgenol 84: 546

Rich AR (1957) Hitherto undescribed vulnerability of juxtamedullary glomeruli in lipoid nephrosis. Bull Johns Hopkins Hosp 100: 173

Rennke HG (1984) Hemodynamically mediated glomerular damage following reduction of functioning nephron units. In: Losse H, Asscher AW, Lison AE, Andriole VT (eds) Pyelonephritis, vol 5. Urinary tract infections. Thieme-Verlag, Stuttgart, p 66

Richards CJ, Mark AL, van Orden DE, Kaloyanides GJ (1978) Effects of indomethacin on the vascular abnormalities of Bartter's syndrome. Circulation 58: 544

Richart R, Benirschke K (1960) Penile agenesis: report of a case, review of the world literature and discussion of pertinent embryology. Arch Pathol 70: 252

Risdon RA (1971a) Renal dysplasia. Part I: A clinicopathological study of 76 cases. J Clin Pathol 24: 57

Risdon RA (1971b) Renal dysplasia. Part II: A necropsy study of 41 cases. J Clin Pathol 24: 65

Risdon RA (1975) Gross anatomy of the kidney. In: Rubin MI, Barratt TM (eds) Pediatric nephrology. Williams & Wilkins, Baltimore, p 2

Risdon RA (1993) The small scarred kidney in childhood. Pediatr Nephrol 7: 361

Risdon RA, Young LW, Crispin AR (1975) Renal hypoplasia and dysplasia. A radiological and pathological correlation. Pediatr Radiol 3: 213

Risdon RA, Yeung CK, Ransley PG (1993) Reflux nephropathy in children submitted to unilateral nephrectomy: a clinicopathological study. Clin Nephrol 40: 308

Rizza JM, Dowling SE (1971) Bilateral renal agenesis in two female siblings. Am J Dis Child 121: 60

Roberts JA (1991) Etiology and pathophysiology of pyelonephritis. Am J Kidney Dis 17: 1

Roberts JA, Roth JK Jr, Domingue G, Lewis RW, Kaack B, Baskin G (1982) Immunology of pyelonephritis in the primate model. V. Effect of superoxide dismutase. J Urol 129: 1394

Roberts JA, Roth JK Jr, Domingue G, Lewis RW, Kaack B, Baskin G (1983) Immunology of pyelonephritis in the primate model. VI. Effect of complement depletion. J Urol 129: 193

Roberts JA, Suarez GM, Kaack B, Kallenius G, Svenson SB (1985) Experimental pyelonephritis in the money. VII. Ascending pyelonephritis in the absence of vescoureteral reflux. J Urul 133: 1068

Roberts JA, Kaack MB, Fussel EF, Baskin G (1966) Immunology of pyelonephritis. VII. Effect of Allopurinol. J Urol 136: 960

Robertson PW, Klidjian A, Harding LK, Walters G, Lee MR, Robb-Smith AHT (1967) Hypertension due to a renin-secreting tumour. Am J Med 43: 963

Robins DC, French TA, Chakera TMH (1976) Juvenile nephronophthisis associated with skeletal abnormalities and hepatic fibrosis. Arch Dis Child 51: 799

Rodriguez-Iturbe B (1984) Poststreptococcal glomerulonephritis. In: Robinson RR (ed) Nephrology. Springer-Verlag, New York, p 623

Rolfes DB, Towbin R, Bove KE (1985) Vascular dysplasia in a child with tuberous sclerosis. Pediatr Pathol 3: 359

Rolleston GL, Mailing TMJ, Hodson CJ (1974) Intrarenal reflux and the scarred kidney. Arch Dis Child 49: 531

Romeo G, Devoto M, Costa G, Roncuzzi L, Catizone L, Succhelli P, Germino GG, Keith T, Weatherall DJ, Reeders ST (1988) A second genetic locus for autosomal dominant polycystic kidney disease. Lancet ii: 8

Ronco P, Verroust P, Morel-Maroger L (1982) Viruses and glomerulonephritis. Nephron 31: 91

Roosen-Runge EC (1949) Retardation of postnatal development of kidneys in persons with early cerebral lesions. Am J Dis Child 77: 185

Royer P, Habib R, Mathieu H, Courtevuisse V (1962) L'hypoplasie rénale bilatérale congénitale avec reduction du nombre et hypertrophie des néphrons chez l'enfant. Ann Pediatr 9: 1330

Royer P, Habib R, Broyer M, Nauaille Y (1971) Segmental hypoplasia of the kidney in children. In: Advances in nephrology, vol 1. Year Book Medical Publishers, Chicago, p 145

Rubenstein M, Meyer R, Bernstein J (1961) Congenital abnormalities of the urinary system. I. A postmortem survey of development anomalies and acquired congenital lesions in a children's hospital. J Pediatr 58: 536

Schacht RG, Gluck MC, Gallo GR, Baldwin DS (1976) Progression to uremia after remission of acute post-streptococcal glomerulonephritis. N Engl J Med 295: 977

Schimke RN, King CR (1980) Hereditary urogenital adysplasia. Clin Genet 18: 417

Schorer CG (1956) Incidence of incomplete descent of the testicle at birth. Arch Dis Child 31: 198

Schreiber RD, Götze O, Müller-Eberhard HJ (1976) Nephritic factor: its structure and function and its relationship to initiating factor of the alternative pathway. Scand J Immunol 5: 705

Schwarz RD, Stephens FD, Cussen LJ (1981) The pathogenesis of renal dysplasia. III. Complete and incomplete urinary obstruction. Invest Urol 19: 101

Scott WW (1929) Blood stream infections in urology: a report of 82 cases. J Urol 21: 527

Scruggs CD, Ainsworth T (1961) Renal cell carcinoma in children: review of the literature and report of two cases. J Urol 86: 728

Seegal B, Andres GA, Hsu KC, Zabriskie JB (1965) Studies on the pathogenesis of acute and progressive glomerulonephritis in man by immunofluorescein and immunoferritin techniques. Fed Proc 24: 100

Sellers AL, Winfield A, Rosen V (1972) Unilateral polycystic kidney disease. J Urol 107: 527

Shah SV (1989) Role of reactive oxygen metabolites in experimental glomerular disease. Kidney Int 35: 1093

Shannon FT (1970) The significance and management of vesicoureteric reflux in infancy. In: Kincaid-Smith PE, Fairley KF (eds) Renal infection and renal scarring. Mercedes, Melbourne, p 241

Shapiro AH (1967) Pumping and retrograde diffusion in peristaltic waves. In: Glen JF (ed) Proceedings of a workshop in ureteral reflux in children. National Academy of Sciences–National Research Council, Washington, p 109

Shapiro LR (1982) Disorders of female sex differentiation. In: Blaustein A (ed) Pathology of the female genital tract, 2nd edn. Springer, New York, p 479

Sherman FE, Studnicki FM, Felterman GH (1971) Renal lesions of familial juvenile nephronophthisis examined by microdissection. Am J Clin Pathol 55: 391

Shimamura T, Morrison AB (1975) A progressive glomerulosclerosis occurring in partial five-sixths nephrectomy. Am J Pathol 79: 95

Sissons JGP, Woodrow DF, Curtis JR, Evans DJ, Gower PE, Sloper JC, Peters DK (1975) Isolated glomerulonephritis with mesangial IgA deposits. Br Med J iii: 611

Smellie JM, Edwards D, Hunter N, Normand ICS, Prescod N (1975) Vesicoureteric reflux and renal scarring. Kidney Int (Suppl) 4: S65

Smith CH, Graham JB (1948) Congenital medullary cysts of the kidney in severe refractory anemia. Am J Dis Child 69: 369

Smith DR (1969) Critique on the concept of vesical neck obstruction in children. JAMA 207: 1686

Smith DW, Opitz JM, Inhorn SL (1976) A syndrome of multiple developmental defects including polycystic kidneys and intrahepatic biliary dysgenesis in two siblings. J Pediatr 67: 617

Sohar E, Gatni J, Pras M, Heller H (1967) Familial Mediterranean fever: a survey of 470 cases and review of the literature. Am J Med 43: 227

Sorger K, Gessler U, Hübner FK, Köhler H, Olbing H, Schultz W, Thoenes W (1982) Subtypes of acute postinfectious glomerulonephritis: synopsis of clinical and pathological features. Clin Nephrol 17: 114

Squiers EC, Modern RS, Bernstein J (1987) Renal multicystic dysplasia: an occasional manifestation of hereditary renal adysplasia syndrome. Am J Med Genet (Suppl 3): 279

Stapleton FB, Johnson D, Kaplan GW, Griswold W (1982) The cystic renal lesion in tuberose sclerosis. J Pediatr 97: 574

Stephens FD (1972) Urological aspects of recurrent urinary tract infection in children. J Pediatr 80: 725

Stapleton FB, Bernstein J, Koh G, Roy S III, Wilroy RS (1982) Cystic kidneys in a patient with oral–facial–digital syndrome type I. Am J Kidney Dis 1: 288

Steele BT, Lirenman DS, Battie CW (1980) Nephronophthisis. Am J Med 68: 531

Stephens FD (1956) Double ureter in the child. Aust N Z J Surg 26: 81

Strauss MB, Sommers SC (1967) Medullary cystic disease and familial juvenile nephronophthisis. N Engl J Med 277: 863

Strife CF, McEnery PT, McAdams AJ, West CD (1977) Membranoproliferative glomerulonephritis with disruption of the glomerular basement membrane. Clin Nephrol 7: 65

Striker GE, Cutler RE, Huang TW, Benditt EP (1973) Renal failure, glomerulonephritis and glomerular epithelial cell hyperplasia. In: Kincaid-Smith P, Mathew TH, Becker EL (eds) Glomerulonephritis: morphology, natural history and treatment. Wiley, New York, p 657

Sworn MJ, Eisinger AJ (1972) Medullary cystic disease and juvenile nephronophthisis in separate members of the same family. Arch Dis Child 47: 278

Taxy JB, Filmer RB (1976) Glomerulocytic disease. Report of a case. Arch Pathol Lab Med 100: 186

Thomson BJ, Jenkins DAS, Allan PL, Elton RA, Winney RJ (1986) Acquired cystic disease of the kidney in patients with end stage chronic renal failure: a study of prevalence and aetiology. Nephrol Dial Transport 1: 38

Thorn G, Koepf GF, Clinton M Jr (1944) Renal failure simulating adrenocortical insufficiency. N Engl J Med 231: 76

Torres VE, Holley KE, Offord KP (1985) General features of autosomal dominant polycystic kidney disease. A epidemiology. In: Grantham JJ, Gardner KD (eds) Problems in the diagnosis and management of polycystic kidney disease. Proceedings of the First International Workshop on Polycystic Kidney Disease. PKR Foundation, Kansas City, p 49

Trompeter RS, Llyod BW, Hicks J, White RHR, Cameron JS (1985) Long-term outcome for children with minimal change nephrotic syndrome. Lancet i: 368

Truong LD, Ansari MQ, Ansari SJ, Wheeler TM, Mattioli CM, Gillum D (1988) Acquired cystic kidney disease: occurrence in patients on chronic peritoneal dialysis. Am J Kidney Dis 11: 192

Tuchmann-Duplesis H, Haegel P (1974) In: Illustrated human embryology, vol 2. Organogenesis. Springer, New York, p 102

Unanue ER, Dixon FJ (1967) Experimental glomerulonephritis: immunological events and pathogenic mechanisms. Adv Immunol 6: 1

Urizar RE, Schwartz A, Top F, Vernier RL (1969) The nephrotic syndrome in children with diabetes mellitus of recent origin. N Engl J Med 281: 173

Vilches AR, Turner DS, Cameron JS, Oggs CS, Chantler C, Williams DG (1982) Significance of mesangial IgM deposition in "minimal change" nephrotic syndrome. Lab Invest 46: 10

Vogt A (1984) New aspects of the pathogenesis of immune complex glomerulonephritis: formation of subepithelial deposits. Clin Nephrol 21: 15

Vogt A, Rohrbach S, Shimizu F, Takamiya H, Batsford S (1982) Interaction of cationized antigen with rat glomerular basement membrane: in situ immune complex formation. Kidney Int 22: 27

Waldherr R (1982) Familial glomerular disease. Contrib Nephrol 33: 104

Waldherr R, Lennert T, Weber HP, Födisch HJ, Schärer K (1982) The nephronophthisis complex. A clinicopathologic study in children. Virchows Arch A Pathol Anat 394: 235

Walker EW (1897) A floating kidney containing three dermoid cysts and several serous cysts: laparotomy; recovery. Trans Am Surg Assoc 15: 591

Wall B, Wachter HE (1952) Congenital ureteral valve. Its role as a primary obstructive lesion: classification of the literature and report of an authentic case. J Urol 68: 684

Waller JF, Roll WA (1957) Bladder carcinoma in teenage girl. J Urol 78: 764

Warkany J, Passarge E, Smith LB (1966) Congenital malformations in autosomal trisomy syndromes. Am J Dis Child 112: 502

Warshawsky AB, Miller KE, Kaplan GW (1977) Urographic visualization of multicystic kidneys. J Urol 117: 94

Wattenberg CA, Rape MG, Beare JB (1949) Perineal testicle. J Urol 62: 858

Waxman FJ, Hebert LA, Cosio FG, Smead WL, Van-Aman ME, Taguiam JM, Birmingham DJ (1986) Differential binding of immunoglobulin A and immunoglobulin G, complexes to primate erythrocytes in vivo: immunoglobulan A complexes bind less well to erythrocytes and are preferentially deposited in glomeruli. J Clin Invest 77: 82

West CD, McAdams AJ, McConville JM, Davies MC, Holland NH (1965) Hypocomplementemic and normocomplementemic persistent (chronic) glomerulonephritis: clinical and pathological characteristics. J Pediatr 67: 1089

Westberg NG, Michael AF (1972) Immunohistopathology of diabetic glomerulosclerosis. Diabetes 21: 163

Whitaker RG (1976) Congenital disorders of the testicle. In: Blandy J (ed) Urology. Blackwell Scientific, Oxford, p 1157

White P (1956) Natural course and diagnosis of juvenile diabetes. Diabetes 5: 445

White RHR, Glasgow EF, Mills RJ (1970) Clinicopathological study of nephrotic syndrome in childhood. Lancet ii: 1353

White RR, Wyatt GM (1942) Surgical importance of the aberrant renal vessel in infants and children. Am J Surg 58: 48

Whitworth JA, Morel-Maroger L, Mignon F, Richet G (1976) The significance of extracapillary proliferation: clinicopathological review of 60 patients. Nephron 16: 1

Wigger HJ, Blanc WA (1977) The prune belly syndrome. Pathol Annu 12: 17

Wigglesworth JS (1984) Perinatal pathology. Saunders, Philadelphia, p 365

Williams DI (1962) Reflux in double ureters. Proc R Soc Med 55: 423

Williams DI (1968) Renal dysplasia. In: Williams DI (ed) Paediatric urology. Butterworths, London, p 36

Williams DI, Burkholder GF (1967) The prune belly syndrome. J Urol 98: 244

Williams DI, Schistad G (1961) Lower urinary tract tumours in children. Br J Urol 36: 51

Wilson CB (1981) Nephritogenic antibody mechanisms involving antigens within the glomerulus. Immunol Rev 55: 257

Winkelman J (1967) Coexistent megacolon and megaureter: report of a case with normal vesical autonomic innervation. Paediatrics 39: 258

Woodroffe AJ, Clarkson AR, Seymour AE, Lomas-Smith JD (1982) Mesangial IgA nephritis. Springer Semin Immunopathol 5: 321

Yoshikawa N, Hashimoto H, Katayama Y, Yamada Y, Matsgo T, Okada S (1984) The thin basement membrane in children with haematuria. J Pathol 142: 253

Young HH, McKay RW (1929) Congenital valvular obstruction of the prostatic urethra. Surg Gynecol Obstet 48: 509

Yendt ER (1982) Medullary sponge kidney and nephrolithiasis. N Engl J Med 306: 1106

Zerres K, Weiss H, Bulla M, Roth B (1982) Prenatal diagnosis of an early manifestation of autosomal dominant adult-type polycystic kidney disease. Lancet ii: 988

Zinner SH, Levy PS, Kass EH (1971) Familial aggregation of blood pressure in childhood. N Engl J Med 284: 401

9 · Bones and Joints

Peter A. Revell

Normal Development of the Skeletal System

The skeleton is mesenchymal in origin. Most of its components pass through membranous and cartilaginous stages of development before becoming ossified, although in some parts there is only a membranous stage. These processes of endochondral and intramembranous ossification are well described in standard textbooks of histology. A detailed account of normal bone, its development and the structure and function of bone cells is available in Revell (1986).

Vertebral Column

The paraxial mesoderm of the developing embryo becomes segmented into somites at the end of the 3rd or beginning of the 4th week. The cells in the ventromedial parts of the somites make up the sclerotomes from which the axial skeleton is derived. Cells from the sclerotomes form the mesenchymal vertebral column around the framework provided by the notochord, each cell mass becoming a rudimentary vertebral body. Paired concentrations of mesenchyme extend dorsally from the body to surround the neural tube and establish the rudimentary neural arch, while lateral extensions form the rib precursors.

The mesenchymal tissue of the centrum, neural arches and ribs is converted to cartilage after the appearance of chondrification centres at about 7 weeks. Ossification centres appear in the vertebral body and neural arches and are well developed by 13 weeks (see p. 5). They advance posteriorly and laterally from the arches to surround the spinal cord and form the transverse processes.

Segments of notochord encased within the ossified vertebral bodies disappear, but those between the bones persist in the nucleus pulposus of the intervertebral discs. All the vertebrae consist of osseous tissue at birth, but cartilage persists at the junction of the neural arch with the body, in the transverse and spinous processes, and as plates analogous to epiphyseal plates at the upper and lower ends of each vertebral body. Longitudinal growth of the vertebral body and the processes is by way of endochondral ossification, and circumferential increase by way of subperiosteal intramembranous ossification. Union of the osseous parts of each vertebra commences in early childhood, and fusion of the cartilage plates of the bodies is completed by 14–15 years of age.

Skull

The brain is covered by a sheath of mesenchyme in the 4th and 5th weeks of development. The skull is formed in two distinct parts: a basal chondrocranium and the vault or calvaria, which is intramembranous in its ossification. The frontal bone is intramembranous in its ossification. It is formed in two halves, each with its own ossification centre, and centres of each parietal bone appear soon after those of the frontal bones. When osteogenesis is established, trabeculae of bone are formed and the intervening spaces become filled with bone marrow. The frontal and parietal bones are in close apposition at the time of birth, except for the anterior fontanelle, which is filled with fibrous tissue. A smaller fibrous space between the parietal and occipital bones forms the posterior fontanelle. The fontanelles are closed by ossification of the fibrous tissue, the posterior about 2 months after birth and the anterior during the second postnatal year. The skull vault further increases in

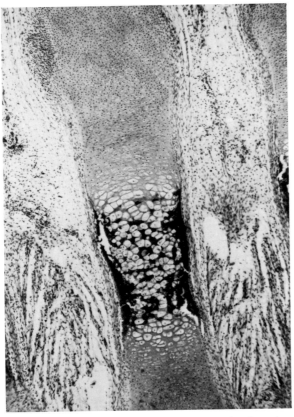

Fig. 9.1. Digital phalanx of a 10-week fetus, showing formation of cartilage in the mid-shaft region of the precartilage model and surrounding perichondrium. (H&E, × 200)

The mesenchymal cells proliferate in a way that brings about lengthening of the limb bud in a proximo distal direction until a certain length has been reached. Differentiation of a pentadactyl pattern then occurs by transformation of mesenchyme into precartilage and cartilage so that models of the future bones are formed, each surrounded by perichondrium (Fig. 9.1). The cartilage is avascular, but vascularization of the periochondrium leads to development of a ring of osseous tissue around the middle of the cartilage model, vasoformative tissue entering the degenerating and calcified cartilage from the surface in the process of endochondral ossification. The cuff of bone forming the cortex advances towards the ends of the bone ahead of the ossification in the shaft, in which some of the trabecular bone is resorbed and the marrow cavity is formed. Delineation of a transverse band of cartilage towards the end of the bone results in the formation of the epiphyseal plate, the principal site of longitudinal growth in developing long bones.

Epiphyses develop from the ends of the cartilage model beyond the epiphyseal plate. The cartilage of the epiphyses is penetrated by canals carrying small blood vessels derived from the perichondrium, a development occurring in most epiphyses by 3 months of intrauterine life. A variable amount of time elapses, depending on the particular bone, between vascularization and the appearance of an ossification centre in an epiphysis. After its appearance, the epiphyseal ossification centre grows centrifugally by endochondral bone formation, and at the same time the size of the epiphysis is increased by further cartilage formation surrounding the newly developing bone. Fusion of the ossified ephiphysis with the shaft is associated with disappearance of the intervening cartilage plate as it is replaced by bone. When external pressures are applied to the end of the bone up to this time (e.g. traumatic epiphyseal avulsion) the epiphyseal plate remains attached to the epiphysis and not the shaft.

size to accommodate the brain by new bone deposition at the pericranial surface, which becomes compacted to form the outer table. The surface area of the vault is increased by the addition of bone along the lines of the sutures – a process that continues for the first 7 years of life.

The chondrocranium develops as a parachordal part, in which notochordal remnants are embedded, and a prechordal part lying anterior to the notochord. Accounts of the development of these parts of the skeleton are available in anatomy and embryology textbooks and further details will not be given here.

Limbs

The limbs arise as outgrowths from the side of the embryo and comprise a mesenchymal core covered by ectoderm. The upper limb buds appear on the 26th day opposite somites 8–12, and the lower limb buds on the 28th day, opposite somites 24–29.

Joints

The sites of synovial joints appear as well defined zones of undifferentiated mesenchyme between the cartilaginous rudiments of the developing limb bud. Centrally, this interzonal mesenchyme becomes loose-meshed, whereas the general mesenchyme over the bone ends becomes vascularized. Synovial mesenchyme is made up of the interzonal tissue and the adjacent general mesenchyme, part of which is condensed to form the joint capsule. The joint space forms peripherally in the synovial mesenchyme and a single space is formed by the confluence of several small spaces, proceeding centrally. Synovial mesenchyme gives rise to the synovial membrane, ligaments and menisci.

Practically all synovial joints are well demarcated by 10 weeks of intrauterine development. Full differentiation of joints does not occur until postnatal life.

In the development of intervertebral discs, mesenchyme between developing vertebral bodies is converted into fibrous tissue and this subsequently becomes the fibrocartilage of the intervertebral disc. The semigelatinous nucleus pulposus of the disc contains notochordal remnants.

Postnatal Ossification of Bones

A fetus can be assumed to be full-term if there are centres of ossification present for the calcaneus, the talus and the lower femoral epiphysis. Postnatal ossification centres in the epiphyses show a regularity in sequence and time of appearance, and sets of normal values (standards) have been established for large numbers of carefully repeated radiological examinations in children from socioeconomic backgrounds that ensure well balanced diets and thus optimal developmental conditions. The chronology of skeletal development as a whole can be assessed by radiological examination of the limbs, and general skeletal status is well reflected in the hand and wrist alone. The age rating of a child in skeletal terms is based on the demonstration of the most recently ossified centre. Alterations in the ossification of the hand and wrist are likely to be present in children suffering severe illness or prolonged nutritional defects. Protracted illness during childhood disturbs the sequence of appearance of ossification centres, the delay in ossification being proportional to the duration and intensity of the illness. Endocrine disturbances such as hypothyroidism and hypopituitarism delay the appearance and retard the growth of postnatal ossification centres; accelerated endochondral ossification at the epiphyseal plates results in initial acceleration of growth in precocious puberty and is followed by premature epiphyseal fusion, the final height being below average.

A further factor that should be borne in mind when assessing skeletal status is the sex of the subject. Girls are in advance of boys in the time of appearance of ossification centres even at full term, and by 5 years of age they are up to 1 year ahead (Table 9.1). Fusion of many epiphyses occurs 2–3 years earlier in girls than in boys (Table 9.2). The data given in Table 9.1 and 9.2 represent approximate values obtained from several sources. Readers wishing to obtain more precise information or details relating to other bones should refer to the book by Jaffe (1972) or the papers by Francis and Werle (1939), Francis

Table 9.1. Time of appearance of some ossification centres in children aged up to 10 years

	Girls	Boys
Calcaneus	Birth	Birth
Talus	Birth	Birth
Distal femur	Birth	Birth
Proximal femur	Birth	Birth
Humeral head	Birth to 1 month	Birth to 1 month
Capitate	2–3 months	2–3 months
Hamate	2–3 months	3–4 months
Lateral cuneiform	3–4 months	4–5 months
Femoral head	3–4 months	4–5 months
Distal tibia	3–4 months	4 months
Distal fibula	9 months	12 months
Distal radius	9–10 months	12–13 months
Medial cuneiform	15–16 months	20–24 months
Patella	$2\frac{1}{2}$–3 years	4 years
Greater trochanter	$2\frac{1}{2}$ years	$3\frac{1}{2}$ years
Proximal radius	4 years	5 years
Distal ulna	4–5 years	7 years
Calcaneus, epiphysis	5 years	7 years
Olecranon	7–8 years	9–10 years
Talus, epiphysis	7–8 years	8–9 years
Lesser trochanter	8–9 years	9–11 years
Tibial tubercle	9–10 years	11–12 years

Table 9.2. Times of fusion of epiphyses of limb bones (years)

	Girls	Boys
Upper humerus	16–17	16–18
Lower humerus	13	15–16
Proximal radius	14	14–16
Distal radius	16–18	17–19
Proximal femur	13–14	14–17
Greater trochanter	14	16
Distal femur	14–17	16–19
Proximal tibia	14–15	16–18
Distal tibia	13–14	15–17
Calcaneus, apophysis	13–14	15–17

(1940), Flecker (1942) and Acheson (1957). The atlas by Wynne-Davies et al. (1985) gives examples of the radiographic appearances of various parts of the skeleton at different ages in normal childhood.

Abnormal Development

Teratogenic Agents and Limb Development

A large number of chemical agents have been demonstrated to alter limb development, although their effects are usually not specific just to the limbs. Some teratogens can selectively cause limb defects if administered over a limited period of time in preg-

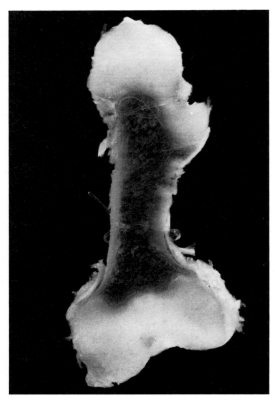

Fig. 9.2. Left femur of a full-term stillborn achondroplastic, showing a widened irregular lower metaphysis and widening of the lower epiphysis.

nancy. The limb is not equally sensitive at all stages of development, susceptibility beginning at the start of limb bud elongation and ending when the rudimentary skeleton is formed in cartilage. The stages in development of the fore-limb precede those of the hind-limb by 2–3 days, so that there is a cephalo caudal sensitivity gradient as well as a proximo distal one. Specific effects of teratogens on the skeleton have been reviewed by Berry (1978).

Dwarfism

Shortness of stature may be present at birth or may develop during childhood. Dwarfism is classified into certain broad categories.

In achondroplasia, there is a pronounced shortening of the extremities with minimal changes in the trunk. There are several rarer forms of short-limbed (micromelic) dwarfism. These disorders, together with even rarer abnormalities, are sometimes collectively termed the osteochondrodystrophies or chon-

drodysplasias. A complete list of constitutional disorders of bone is available in the revised international nomenclature (Beighton et al. 1983a, 1992). This classification is much too long to reproduce here. Certain disorders were regrouped in 1992; for example, thanatophoric dysplasia with or without clover-leaf skull, achondroplasia and hypochondroplasia are now put together in the achondroplasia group. There are 24 groups, which encompass well over two hundred separate disorders.

Dwarfism may be related to inborn errors of metabolism, most notably in the mucopolysaccharidoses, a group of disorders in which further subtypes are always being defined.

Two other types are the *ateliotic* dwarf, who remains infantile in appearance, and the subject with *progeria*, whose appearance becomes that of a shrivelled old person even when young. Neither of these shows skeletal disproportion.

Short stature may also be present in certain endocrine disorders (hypopituitarism, hypothyroidism, cretinism, pseudopseudohypoparathyroidism), and renal disease in childhood sometimes results in dwarfism.

Achondroplasia

The commonest of the chondrodysplasias is achondroplasia. It is considered to result from a primary disturbance of endochondral ossification in early fetal life, which has become well established by the time of birth. Severely affected fetuses die towards the end of gestation. Achondroplastics surviving the neonatal period normally grow to adulthood, and such milder cases are usually of normal intelligence.

The achondroplastic neonate shows well marked abnormalities, and those born dead have very severe shortening of the limbs. Pathological examination of achondroplastic neonates reveals long bones as little as half the normal length with considerable enlargement of epiphyses, which may extend up to half the length of the bone. The intervening shaft widens to surround the enlarged epiphysis at either end of the bone (Fig. 9.2). The most notable skull changes occur in the sphenoid and basal part of the occipital bone near the foramen magnum, which may be narrowed. The vertebral bodies are cartilaginous, containing underdeveloped ossification centres. The costochondral junctions are increased in diameter (beading) and shifted towards the axilla because of the shortness of the ribs.

Histologically, deficiency in cartilage cell proliferation is best seen at epiphyseal–diaphyseal junctions of long bones.

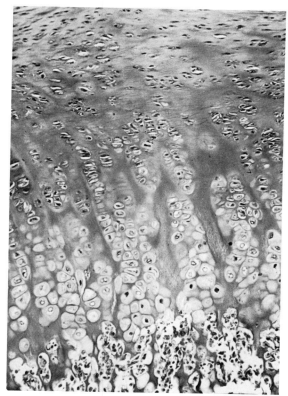

Fig. 9.3. Well organized endochondral ossification in the lower epiphysis of the femur of a stillborn achondroplastic. (H&E, × 400)

There have been few pathological studies of the changes present in achondroplastic children and adults. Biopsy studies in some typical achondroplastics have shown apparently regular and well organized endochondral ossification (Rimoin et al. 1976; Sillence et al. 1979a) (Fig. 9.3), and it has been suggested that the defect is a quantitative decrease in the rate of endochondral ossification. Maynard et al. (1981) showed a decrease in the hypertrophic zone of the growth plate and described columnar-cell and clustered-cell areas. A cluster-like arrangement of enlarged chondrocytes, vacuolization and premature calcification have been noted in a newborn heterozygous achondroplastic male (Briner et al. 1991). Periosteal ossification is normal and thus increased compared with endochondral bone formation. Periosteal overgrowth results in the cupping at bone ends seen on radiological examination (Rimoin et al. 1976).

The following features may be present in the achondroplastic. Apart from the shortening of the limbs, the ends of the long bones are enlarged and the cortices thickened. There may be coxa vara and genu varum. The position of the fibula relative to the tibia distinguishes the achondroplastic, the head of the fibula reaching to the level of the upper surface of the tibia. The skull is increased in circumference and there is frontal protuberance. Shortness of the base of the skull gives rise to the abnormal pug-shaped nose, and there may be prognathism. Lordosis and dorsolumbar kyphosis are often present in the spine. The ribs are abnormally broad, and the most important pelvic abnormality is anteroposterior flattening at the inlet, which gives rise to obstetric problems.

Achondroplasia shows autosomal dominant inheritance. More than 80% of achondroplastics, however, are sporadic cases with normal parents (Scott 1976) and therefore represent new mutations.

There continues to be a problem in the misdiagnosis of other chondrodysplasias as being achondroplasia, for example, thanatophoric dysplasia, another form of lethal neonatal dwarfism. Achondroplasia usually not lethal, is the most common of the skeletal dysplasias and is seen in those surviving into full adulthood.

Some of the confusion between lethal and non-lethal achondroplasia has been clarified because homozygous achondroplasia and lethal achondroplasia are now classified as disorders related to thanatophoric dysplasia, which has also itself been divided into two types (Spranger and Maroteaux, 1990).

Other Osteochondrodysplasias

Brief accounts of some of the other osteochondrodysplasias are given below.

The osteochondrodysplasias have been divided into two groups by Beighton (1978), according to the presence or absence of spinal involvement:

1. Osteochondrodysplasia without significant spinal involvement:
   a) Achondroplasia
   b) Hypochondroplasia
   c) Achondrogenesis
   d) Thanatophoric dwarfism
   e) Asphyxiating thoracic dysplasia
   f) Chondroectodermal dysplasia
   g) Multiple epiphyseal dysplasia
   h) Chondrodysplasia punctata
   i) Metaphyseal chondrodysplasia
   j) Mesomelic dwarfism
   k) Rhizomelic dwarfism
   l) Campomelic dwarfism
2. Osteochondrodysplasia with significant spinal involvement:
   a) Pseudoachondroplasia
   b) Spondyloepiphyseal dysplasia
   c) Spondylometaphyseal dysplasia

Table 9.3. Some conditions resulting in dwarfism

Type	Features	Inheritance
Incompatible with life Thanatophoric dwarfism	Severe micromelia Long narrow thorax Large cranial vault with depressed base Short ribs Reduced height of vertebral bodies	Mutation
Achondrogenesis	Severe micromelia Ossification defects in various bones, notably vertebral bodies not ossified, wide metaphyses in limbs	Autosomal recessive

Short-rib polydactyly syndromes	Various types
	Features include thoracic narrowing, polydactyly,
	    micromelia, congenital heart disease, anomalies in
	    genitourinary and gastrointestinal tracts, cleft lip and palate
		Autosomal recessive

Compatible with life Achondroplasia	Micromelia, dwarfism Craniofacial changes Small foramen magnum (see text for description)	Autosomal dominant Many sporadic
Spondyloepiphyseal dysplasia	Dwarfism with short trunk Delays in ossification and fragmented epiphyseal ossification centres Platyspondyly, talipes equinovarus Kyphoscoliosis and thoracic deformity develop in childhood	Autosomal dominant
Chondroectodermal dysplasia (Ellis–van Creveld syndrome)	Micromelia Polydactyly with hypoplasia or absence of nails Congenital heart disease Ectodermal dysplasia Normal intelligence (see text for description)	Autosomal recessive
Asphyxiating thoracic dysplasia (Jeune's syndrome)	Short limbs Long narrow thorax, short ribs with costochondral beading Head and spine normal Polydactyly in some (resemble Ellis–van Creveld) Respiratory difficulties, pneumonia, etc. Majority die in infancy	Autosomal recessive
Diastrophic dwarfism (dysplasia)	Micromelic dwarfism Club foot Posterior cleft palate Contractures of many joints External ear deformity (at 1 or 2 months of age) Later develop changes in epiphyses, genuvalgum, scoliosis (but spine may be deformed at birth)	Autosomal recessive

Metatropic dwarfism (dysplasia)	Micromelic dwarfism with trumpet-shaped metaphyses
	Skull and face usually normal
	Kyphoscoliosis with reduced height of
	    vertebral bodies (more marked in childhood)
	Pigeon chest (childhood)
		Autosomal recessive
		(In infancy, differentiate
		    from achondroplasia; in
		    childhood, differentiate
		    from Morquio's disease)

Mesomelic dwarfism (dysplasia)	Severe micromelia selective to the forearm
	    and leg
	Curved radius, fibular aplasia, genu valgum,
	    club foot etc., in different types
		Autosomal dominant
		    and autosomal recessive
		    types

Chondrodysplasia punctata	Micromelic dwarfism
	Cataract
	Skin manifestations
	Spotty calcification of epiphyses and vertebrae
	    (see text for description)
		Autosomal dominant
		    and autosomal recessive
		    types

Campomelic dysplasia	"Bent limbs" – bowing of tubular bones, especially legs Calcaneovalgus or equinovarus Flat face, low ears, micrognathia, cleft palate Platyspondyly, hypoplastic scapulae Death from respiratory insufficiency	Sporadic

d) Schwartz syndrome
e) Metatropic dwarfism
f) Kniest syndrome
g) Diastrophic dwarfism
h) Dyggue–Melchior–Clausen syndrome
i) Parastremmatic dwarfism

The reader wishing to obtain further clinical, radiological and genetic details about these disorders is referred to the book by Beighton (1978) and the radiological atlases by Cremin and Beighton (1978) and Wynne-Davies et al. (1985). Reviews by Gilbert et al. (1987) and Spranger and Maroteaux (1990) describe the infantile and lethal osteochondrodysplasias respectively.

The differential diagnosis of short-limbed stillborn and newborn dwarfism can be summarized as follows:

1. Stillborn (lethal):
   a) Achondrogenesis
   b) Thanatophoric dwarfism
   c) Achondroplasia (homozygous form)
   d) Asphyxiating thoracic dysplasia
   e) Short-rib polydactyly syndromes
   f) Chondroectodermal dysplasia
   g) Chondrodysplasia punctata (some)
   h) Campomelic dwarfism
   i) Osteogenesis imperfecta
   j) Hypophosphatasia
   k) Platyspondylic chondrodysplasia
2. Newborn (non-lethal – survival usual):
   a) Achondroplasia
   b) Mesomelic dwarfism
   c) Rhizomelic dwarfism
   d) Spondyloepiphyseal dysplasia
   e) Spondylometaphyseal dysplasia
   f) Metatropic dwarfism
   g) Diastrophic dwarfism

Some of these disorders are described briefly in the following account and in Table 9.3. Some of the terms used may be a source of confusion. "Micromelia" is used to mean shortening of all segments of the limbs. "Rhizomelia" denotes shortening of the proximal segment. "Mesomelia" and "acromelia" describe shortening of the middle (i.e. forearm and leg) and distal segments, respectively. More detailed pathological descriptions are available in Revell (1986) and Spranger and Maroteaux (1990).

Histological and Ultrastructural Studies of the Chondrodystrophies

Recent studies are beginning to throw light on the pathology of the chondrodystrophies. Adequate

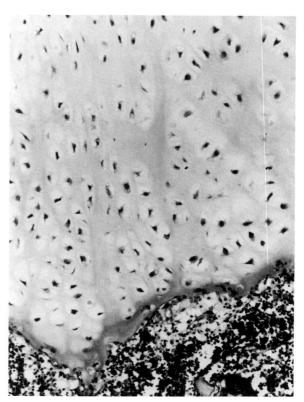

Fig. 9.4. Abnormality of the growth plate in achondrogenesis showing lack of regular column formation, hypercellularity with large chondrocytes having dark nuclei, and relatively little intervening matrix. (Azan, × 447)

histopathological examination of the skeleton in lethal chondrodysplasia requires sectioning of ribs, vertebral bodies, femur or humerus. Ribs, iliac crest and other limb bones could also be added (Revell 1986; Yang et al. 1986). The histopathological abnormalities appear to be characteristic in achondrogenesis, diastrophic dwarfism and thanotophoric dwarfism (Fig. 9.4). In other disorders (e.g. spondyloephiphyseal dysplasia) there is considerable heterogeneity, and no clear correlations are yet possible. Cartilage is relatively normal in achondroplasia, hypochondroplasia and multiple epiphyseal dysplasia, so that histological examination is of little diagnostic value. However, in thanatophoric dysplasia the resting cartilage is hypocellular with normal-sized cells, and the growth plate shows poor columnization and some fibrosis. The changes in platyspondylic chondrodysplasia depend on the subtype, there being hypercellularity of slightly larger resting zone cells and normal columnization (Torrance type), normal cellularity with large resting zone cells and poor columnization (San Diego type) or hypercellularity with large resting zone cells and focal disruption of columnization (Luton type) (Spranger and Maroteaux 1990). Ultrastructural studies show differences between some of the chondrodysplasias. The reader is referred to the articles by Rimoin et al. (1976), Hwang et al. (1979), Sillence et al. (1979a), Stanescu et al. (1984) and van der Harten (1987) for further details. Spranger and Maroteaux (1990) give details of the clinical and radiological features as well as mentioning the histological appearances of the growth plate in various disorders. The salient points on the features of the growth plates are summarized in Table 9.4.

Chondroectodermal Dysplasia (Ellis–van Creveld Syndrome)

Abnormal cartilage development, ectodermal dysplasia and polydactyly are the main features of the disorder first described by Ellis and van Creveld (1940). Other malformations, including congenital heart disease, may be present. In the newborn, the diagnosis can be made by the presence of short extremities, polydactyly with the extra digit on the ulnar side, and absence or hypoplasia of the nails. Small peg-shaped teeth may be present at birth or appear prematurely. Bronchial defects and hypoplasia of the lungs may

Table 9.4. Histological features of lethal osteochondrodysplasias

Type	Histological features of growth plate
Chondrodysplasia punctata	
Rhizomelic	Degenerate fibroblast-like chondrocytes Loss of cells Mucoid degeneration but well preserved growth zones
Lethal, X-linked	Chondrocyte clusters in resting cartilage with calcification and penetration by vascular channels
Achondrogenesis	
IA (Houston–Harris)	A few hypertrophied chondrocytes in growth zone, not aligned in columns Intracytoplasmic vacuoles with inclusions in resting cells
IB (Fraccaro)	Sparse matrix Collagen rings around chondrocytes
II (Langer–Saldino)	Hypercellular cartilage with large canals containing fibrous tissue Enlarged vacuolated chondrocytes Matrix deficient
Thanatophoric dysplasia	
Type 1	Decreased numbers of chondrocytes not aligned in columns Irregular provisional calcification zone
Type 2 (with clover-leaf skull)	Abundance of vascular channels penetrating growth plate
Platyspondylic lethal chondrodysplasias	
Torrance	Hypercellular resting cartilage, normal columnization
San Diego	Normal cellularity of resting cartilage, large cells, poor columnization
Luton	Hypercellular resting zone, large cells, focal disruption of growth plate
Short rib (–polydactyly) syndromes	
Type I (Saldino–Noonan)	Absence of columnization and of vascular penetration at the growth plate Tongues of cartilage reaching deep into metaphysis
Type II (Verma–Naumiff)	Short chondrocyte columns with a few hypertrophic cells Columnization absent and bone directly deposited in matrix in areas
Type III (Le Marec)	Cartilage tongues extend from growth plate into metaphysis
Asphyxiating thoracic dysplasia (Jeune)	Patchy endochondral ossification, islands of cartilage in metaphysis Proliferating and hypertrophic chondrocytes decreased in number and arranged in groups
Short rib–polydactyly syndrome	
Type VI (Majewski)	Irregular, poor columnization with haphazardly arranged small hypertrophic chondrocytes
Lethal metatrophic dysplasia (hyperchondrogenesis)	Hypertrophic chondrocytes in clusters without columnization Focal independent ossification due to focal vascularization
Fibrochondrogenesis	Fibrous strands in matrix Fibroblast-like chondrocytes
Kniest dysplasia (and related disorders)	Poorly staining spaces in resting cartilage give a Swiss-cheese-like appearance

After Spranger and Maroteaux (1990).

contribute to early respiratory death. Babies with severe heart disease die soon after birth. A large series of cases has been described by McKusick et al. (1964).

Chondrodysplasia Punctata (Stippled Epiphyseal, Chondrodystrophia Calcificans Congenita, Dysplasia Epiphysealis Punctata)

The rare disorder chondrodysplasia punctata is characterized by the presence of multiple punctate foci of calcification in the cartilaginous parts of the neonatal and infant skeleton. The presence of stippled epiphyseal is a striking feature on radiography but is not wholly diagnostic.

Many affected infants are stillborn or die soon after birth. The head and trunk are enlarged, the extremities are short with a proportionally greater reduction in length of proximal parts, and there may be flexion deformities of the hips, knees and shoulders. Localized skeletal abnormalities include unilateral micromelia, club foot and dislocation of the hip. Cataracts may be a feature, and skin manifestations (dyskeratosis, seborrhoeic dermatosis, hyperkeratosis or icthyosis) may occur.

Irregular focal calcification (stippling) is seen both in the epiphyseal of the femur, tibia, humerus and iliac crest, and in the posterior ends of the ribs and vertebral bodies on radiological examination. Pathological examination has been performed in a number of cases. Endochondral bone formation is markedly abnormal. The chondrocytes are not organized into columns and there is diminished mineralization of matrix associated with decreased vascularization of the cartilage. Resting cartilage contains areas of mucoid degeneration, with calcification and fragmentation (Rimoin et al. 1976).

Similar changes have been described in warfarin embryopathy (see p. 58).

Stippled epiphyses in the neonatal and infantile skeleton are a radiological feature also seen in mucolipidoses, mucopolysaccharidoses, trisomy 18, trisomy 21, thyroid disorders, fetal hydantoin syndrome and congenital infections with cytomegalovirus and rubella (Sheffield et al. 1976; Revell 1986).

Multiple Epiphyseal Dysplasia

Multiple epiphyseal dysplasia is inherited as a dominant trait. Characteristically, there are abnormalities in the growth of ossification centres with resultant shortness of stature. Growth abnormalities become apparent during the second or third years of life rather than at birth, and include knock knees, bow legs, short stubby digits, and minor wedge or biconcave deformities of the vertebral bodies.

Ossification centres are delayed in appearance and irregular in outline, appearing fragmented when present. The fragments eventually coalesce to form a single centre with an irregular outline. Alterations in structure are likely to be detectable in the hip, ankle and shoulder joints on radiography. Little is known of the detailed pathological features in the human because the condition is not lethal. The epiphyses of the femoral head are nearly always involved so that the femoral head becomes flattened. The similarity of intracytoplasmic inclusions in chondrocytes seen at electron microscopy in multiple epiphyseal dysplasia and pseudoachondroplasia has recently been noted (Stanescu et al. 1993). Prematurely developing osteoarthrosis is a frequent complication. The study by Rasmussen (1975) of multiple epiphyseal dysplasia in the dog is of some interest, because it followed the development of pathological changes. Initially, there was an accumulation of abnormal cartilage matrix in relation to chondrocytes. This was followed by liquefaction and cyst formation, and later by focal calcification.

Metaphyseal Chondrodysplasia

A disturbance of the metaphyses of long bones occurs in the group of conditions known collectively as metaphyseal dysplasia, which are rare. In the commonest form, the affected persons are of small stature and have coxa vara and genu vara. The changes may be mild, or severe and deforming. In young children, cupping of the metaphyses of long bones and expansion of the anterior ends of the ribs reflect the presence of large amounts of calcifying and ossifying cartilage. The chief problem is in differential diagnosis from rickets, where similar expansions of the ends of bones occurs.

The epiphyses, skull and trunk are essentially normal. Several types of metaphysical chondrodysplasia that have associated abnormalities have been described, e.g. cartilage-hair hypoplasia, malabsorption and neutropenia, thymolymphopenia, and asymptomatic hypercalcaemia. The reader is referred to specialist accounts for further details.

Histological examination shows disorganization of the growth plate and extension of cartilage into the metaplysis. Larger than normal chondrocytes are arranged in clusters instead of columns, and the intervening matrix has a fibrillar appearance. There is irregularity of vascular invasion resulting in irregular spicules of calcified cartilage and bone (see Rimoin et al. 1976).

Cleidocranial Dysplasia

Cleidocranial dysplasia is inherited as an autosomal dominant, but occasional sporadic cases occur. Although the principal abnormalities occur in the clavicles and calvaria, anomalies in bones formed in cartilage have been noted, including deficient ossification or even absence of parts of the pubic bones, hip-joint deformities, spina bifida occulta and abnormalities in dentition.

The clavicles are incompletely formed in typical cases. They are composed of fragments, which articulate normally with the sternum but have non-articulating lateral ends. They are either freely mobile or joined by fibrous bands to the choranoid process, acromion, first rib or glenoid cavity. In some cases, the clavicles may consist of lateral and medial ends separated by a wide gap containing fibrous tissue. They may be completely absent.

The defective calvaria has wide fontanelles and greatly separated sutures. These are gradually closed in later life by irregular islands of bone, but a large frontal defect often persists. The calvaria comprises a mosaic of small bones representing unfused ossification centres. There are large frontal bosses and the skull is flattened laterally.

Neurospinal Dysraphism

The various forms of neurospinal dysraphism involve defects in the closure of the neural tube and its surroundings to different degrees. The primary fault occurs in the neural tube and not in the related mesoderm. The severest deformity is total myeloschisis, in which all the vertebral arches are deficient and the whole spinal cord is laid open to the exterior. The number of vertebrae is often reduced and there may be a lordosis in the cervical region. In some cases even the vertebral bodies themselves may be divided.

In localized myeloschisis or myelocele, one or more vertebral arches are defective and other local spinal anomalies may coexist.

Congenital Dislocation of the Hip

Typical congenital dislocation of the hip does not exist at birth, and almost all examples of the disorder are the result of hip-joint anomalies that predispose to dislocation (see Hass 1951).

True congenital dislocation of the hip, with bilateral displacement, is rarer and is often known as atypical congenital dislocation of the hip. In this form, the hip-joint socket is diminished in size and flattened by the accumulation of cartilaginous connective tissue. The femoral neck is shortened. Other abnormalities that may be associated include torticollis, spina bifida, agenesis of the sacrum, knee contractures, fibular and femoral hypoplasia, and club foot.

The common form of congenital dislocation of the hip occurs more frequently in some families than in the general population (see p. 46). In the predisposed neonate, the cartilaginous portions of the joint are almost intact but there is hypoplasia of the osseous nuclei, especially those of the acetabulum. The obliquity of the acetabular roof is increased, the socket is flattened, and anteversion of the femoral head is increased in the stage before luxation. Ossification of the femoral head is retarded, the centre appearing later on the affected side.

In subluxation, the femoral head may still remain in contact with the original articular surface but protrudes from the acetabulum. The flattened acetabular roof becomes elongated and has a depression at the site where the femoral head rests. The femoral head is flattened and at a later stage moves over the rim of the acetabulum, losing contact with the original socket. Displacement is always upwards but may in addition be anterior, posterior or lateral. A secondary socket is formed opposite the dislocated femoral head, which is itself reduced in size. The direction of the femoral neck may be altered, resulting in coxa vara or coxa valga deformities. Newly formed fibrocartilage formed in the fat pad around the ligamentum teres fuses with the hyaline cartilage of the original socket, which is flattened. Further information on the growth of the acetabulum in the normal child and the changes in congenital hip dysplasia is available in the publications of Ponseti (1978a,b). Although the relationship between acetabular dysplasia and osteoarthritis in adulthood has been debated, a recent study of over 1500 cases has suggested that there may be a relationship in some cases (Croft et al. 1991).

Catterall (1984) has recently stressed the importance of precision in diagnosis of true dislocation and severe dysplasia, from a range of milder dysplastic changes, when congenital dislocation of the hip is under discussion. A recent interesting finding comes from Japan (Yamamuro and Ishida 1984). Traditionally the legs of infants in that country have been maintained in an extended position in a "swathing diaper". A national campaign to avoid this prolonged hip and knee extension in the early postnatal period has resulted in a change in incidence of dislocation of the hip from 1.1%–3.5% to less than 0.2%.

Club Foot (Talipes Equinovarus)

Any foot deformity involving the talus is called "talipes". Club foot (talipes equinovarus) is one of the most frequent skeletal malformations present at birth. About 20% of affected neonates are not viable because of associated malformations, especially neurospinal dysraphism. Club foot is a composite deformity in which the sole is turned medially so that the lateral margin of the foot touches the ground (varus) and the toes are held lower than the heel (equinus). The talus and calcaneus show the most marked changes. The talus is thickened, with its body turned forward and its elongated neck deflected inward and downward. The calcaneus is in a position of plantar flexion and the heel elevated.

Congenital Talipes Calcaneovalgus

In congenital talipes calcaneovalgus the foot is dorsiflexed and everted. The dorsum readily touches the antero-lateral surface of the leg and plantar flexion ceases at mid-position. It may be mistakenly diagnosed where there is congenital vertical talus, especially in very young babies. Vertical talus is distinguishable because there is subtalar rigidity and the heel is in equinus.

Skeletal Abnormalities Developed Later in Childhood or Adolescence

Juvenile Kyphosis (Preadolescent and Adolescent Kyphosis)

Juvenile kyphosis is not an uncommon condition, and it affects males and females equally. The abnormality is usually first recognized between 13 and 17 years of age, and is either asymptomatic or causes backache. On examination, there is lower thoracic or thoracolumbar kyphosis often associated with scoliosis. The main radiological and pathological features may be a mild increase in the normal thoracic curvature of the spine, with anterior narrowing of the intervertebral spaces. In more advanced cases the vertebral bodies show marked anterior narrowing in the affected region and disc protrusion cause indentations of the vertebral bodies so that the margin between disc and bone is irregular or there are Schmorl's nodes.

The cartilaginous growth plates of the vertebral bodies on either side of the affected intervertebral disc are subjected to undue pressure by the discs, causing changes in endochondral bone formation in the vertebral bodies, which may undergo extensive destruction. Changes in the disc result in a tendency to narrowing of the intervertebral space, but because the bodies are held posteriorly by the apophyseal joints only the anterior parts of the vertebral bodies move closer together. Inhibition of growth resulting from pressure on the anterior parts of the vertebral body results in the progressive development of a wedge-shaped vertebra. Areas of prolapsed disc in the vertebral bodies are eventually surrounded by osseous tissue and vascular fibrous tissue extends into the disc, so that an immobile fibrous union between adjacent vertebral bodies results.

Osteochondritis Dissecans

"Osteochondritis dissecans" is the term used to describe a condition in which a small piece of articular cartilage with related subcondral bone becomes detached and is found free in the joint space as an osteochondral body. It affects mainly males aged between 15 and 20 years and has a familial tendency.

The knee is affected in 90% of cases, usually on the lateral surface of the medial femoral condyle. The elbow, hip, ankle and shoulder may occasionally be involved. Radiological examination may show irregularity of the bone at the joint surface, a well delineated lesion that is partly attached, or a completely free body, usually lying in the anterior compartment when the knee joint is affected.

In early cases there are cracks and fissures in the involved cartilage on macroscopic examination. An osteochondral body loosely attached to cartilage or lying free in the joint space is elliptical. The surface cartilage of the body is normal or increased in thickness and the related subchondral bone is necrotic (Fig. 9.5).

Perthes' Disease

Perthes' disease is a condition in which there is partial or complete aseptic necrosis of the ossification centre of the femoral head. Males are affected four times more often than females, 90% of cases are unilateral, and the usual age of presentation is 5–9 years. Alterations in the femoral head are associated with certain changes in the femoral neck and acetabulum almost from the time of onset, and although the changes regress with appropriate treatment, the morphology of all three components may not be normal by the end of the growth period.

Necrosis of the capital ossification centre probably takes place over a short period of time. The contour

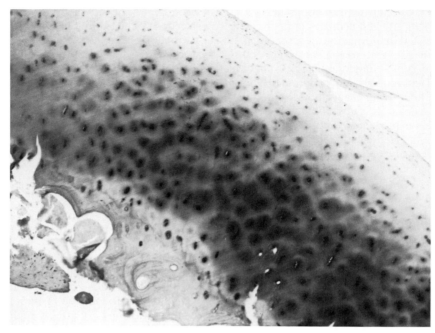

Fig. 9.5. Loose body from the knee of a 20-year-old male with osteochondritis dissecans, showing normal viable hyaline cartilage and necrotic subchondral bone. (H&E, × 150)

of the femoral head remains unaltered for a while, after which there is collapse of areas of bone, with amorphous debris present in the intertrabecular spaces. The area of infarction is segmental and situated superior to the fovea and axial to the anteroposterior line (Ferguson 1985). Curetings from the femoral head in Perthes' disease show necrotic bone and fibrous replacement of the bone marrow. The occurrence of Perthes' disease in active, healthy gymnastic and althletic males as a unilateral condition suggests that trauma may play some part, and the relationship of this and stress patterns in the developing femoral head are discussed by Ferguson (1985). The cartilaginous part of the femoral head remains completely viable because it receives its nutrition from the synovial fluid. With revascularization of the epiphysis (by vessels from the femoral neck, bone marrow and ligamentum teres), there is appositional new bone formation on the necrotic trabeculae. The femoral head may be flattened and the neck shorter and broader than normal when remodelling is completed (Fig. 9.6). Deformity of the femoral head and acetabulum predispose to the development of secondary osteoarthrosis, a common sequel of Perthes' disease.

An ultrastructural study suggests that there is a change in chondrocyte metabolism in this condition (Ippolito et al. 1989).

Slipped Capital Femoral Epiphysis

Gradual slipping of the femoral head off the neck occurs a little more commonly in males and presents at age 10–16 years in boys, a year or so earlier in girls. Many of the patients are taller and heavier than is normal for their age. The slipping of epiphyses may be unilateral or bilateral, although it is rarely synchronously bilateral. Subsequent involvement of the opposite side is more likely with unilateral disease.

The epiphysis itself is not altered in an uncomplicated case. The epiphyseal cartilage plate shows fragmentation, reduplication and folding, with occasional islands of cartilage being displaced into the epiphysis. Slipping of the epiphysis thus follows disruption of the epiphyseal cartilage plate (Sutro 1935; Ponseti and McClintock 1956). Increased vascularity with fibrous tissue and new bone formation are seen in the region of the plate. Reunion (synostosis) eventually occurs with the femoral head and neck malaligned. Complications include ischaemic necrosis of the slipped capital epiphysis and, more rarely, necrosis of the femoral and acetabular articular cartilages, which presumably results from altered synovial fluid formation. Secondary osteoarthrosis may develop. A long-term follow up study of a large number of cases shows the natural history of malunited slipped epi-

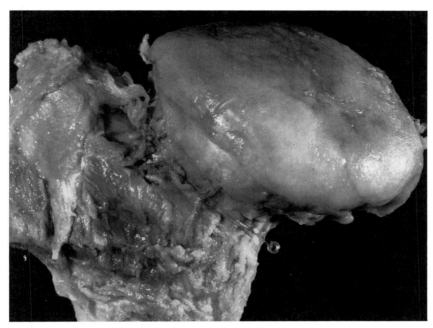

Fig. 9.6. Femoral head from an adult male with a history of Perthes' disease in childhood, showing typical flattening of the femoral head to a mushroom shape and shortening of the femoral neck.

physes (Boyer et al. 1981). An autopsy study of nine adults with untreated slipped capital femoral epiphyses showed retroversion of the femora or true varus deformities with severe osteoarthritis in eight cases (Cooperman et al. 1992).

Osteogenesis Imperfecta

Osteogenesis imperfecta is now recognized as a group of disorders in which there is an abnormality in type I collagen synthesis and, clinically, a marked tendency for the bones to fracture. Formerly, classification was into a severe "congenita" or "fetalis" type and a less pronounced "tarda" form. This has now been replaced by division into four types, as suggested by Sillence and his colleagues (Sillence and Rimoin 1978; Sillence et al. 1979b), although there is still heterogeneity within these groups (Smith 1984). Immunohistochemical studies have shown nests of cartilage in the bone, with types II and III collagen present in osteogenesis imperfecta type II, III and IV (Nerlich et al. 1993). The biochemical changes, mode of inheritance and chief clinical features are summarized in Table 9.5. Blue sclerae

are present in most cases, although a particularly severe form of bone disease occurs in some individuals with white sclerae (osteogenesis imperfecta type III) (Ibsen 1967; King and Bobechko 1971). Although blue sclerae are present in all types, the intensity remains throughout life in osteogenesis imperfecta type I, whereas in types III and IV the blueness fades so that by adult life the sclerae are of normal hue (Table 9.5). There may be dentinogenesis imperfecta. The skeletal complications in different main types of osteogenesis imperfecta have been reviewed in a large number of cases by Beighton et al. (1983b). Further details and references to the collagen abnormalities may be found in Shapiro and Rowe (1983), Pope et al. (1984), Smith (1984) and Barsh et al. (1985). Recombinant DNA technology indicates deletion in the genes for type I collagen in lethal perinatal osteogenesis imperfecta II (osteogenesis imperfecta congenita).

Descriptions of the histopathology of osteogenesis imperfecta differ considerably and this is a reflection of the heterogeneity of the disorder. The position should become clearer in the future as pathological changes are related to specific biochemical defects. The "congenita" type of the older descriptions is the most severe form of the disease and coincides with osteogenesis imperfecta II. However, even this is divided into broad-boned and thin-boned variants,

Table 9.5. Main clinical features, biochemical data and inheritance of osteogenesis imperfecta

	Type I	Type II	Type III	Type IV
Clinical features	Largest group Bone fragility Deafness Severe long-bone deformity uncommon	Stillborn or die in neonatal period Most frequent form OI in newborn Short bowed limbs Concertina femora beaded ribs, poor cranial ossification in radiographs	Progressive long bone and spinal deformity into adult life Fractures at birth or in early years Severe osteoporosis Usually not ambulatory	Clinically heterogeneous Moderate to severe deformities and osteoporosis Scoliosis Usually ambulatory
Sclerae	Blue	Blue	Bluish in infancy, white in adolescence and adult life	Blue, may lighten with age
Dentinogenesis imperfecta (prevalence)	25%	Unknown	25%	25%
Biochemical abnormality	Marked decrease in type I collagen synthesis $\alpha 1 : \alpha 2(I)$ ratio normal	Failure to secrete type I collagen $\alpha 1(I)$ and $\alpha 2(I)$ deletions and insertions	Normal type I collagen synthesis $\alpha 1 : \alpha 2$ ratio normal	Variable decrease in type I collagen synthesis $\alpha 1 : \alpha 2$ ratio elevated, two chain deletions Failure to process $\alpha 2(I)$ chains
Frequency	50%	5%	20%	–
Inheritance	Dominant (sporadic)	Recessive	Recessive	–

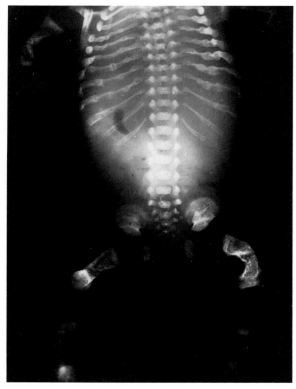

Fig. 9.7. Radiograph of a stillborn girl with osteogenesis imperfecta showing a fractured left femur and right humerus and multiple healed fractures of the ribs.

making interpretation of older studies difficult. (Further details of the osteogenesis imperfecta subtypes IIA, IIB and IIC are available elsewhere (Spranger and Maroteaux 1990).) Broad-boned osteogenesis imperfecta shows marked osteoporosis, severe crippling deformities and early death. Most reports describe the bone in the congenital form of disease as having a woven bone pattern, whereas it is lamellar in the other types (Falvo and Bullough 1973; Bullough et al. 1981). Generalized osteoporosis, a caput membranaceum, short stature with micromelia and bowing of long bones and multiple fractures are features of osteogenesis imperfecta type II (osteogenesis imperfecta congenital) (Fig. 9.7). The cellular characteristics of bone appear to vary considerably according to Falvo and Bullough (1973). Osteoid seams were more prominent than normal in osteogenesis imperfecta tarda (Doty and Matthews 1971; Falvo and Bullough 1973; Bullough et al. 1981). The appearances at the growth plate have been described by Bullough et al. (1981) and Marian et al. (1993). Healing fractures in osteogenesis imperfecta show differences from normal callus, often containing metaplastic cartilage (Spencer 1962; Revell 1986), and hyperplastic callus, which forms in some cases, comprises fibromucoid cartilage-like tissue resembling a tumour (King and Bobechko 1971; Lehmann et al. 1992; Stoss et al. 1993). Most ultrastructural studies have failed to detect changes in bone collagen (Bretlau et al. 1970; Doty and Matthews 1971; Riley and Brown 1971; Riley et al. 1973), although thinner collagen fibres than normal have been described in osteogenesis imperfecta congenita by scanning electron microscopy (Teitelbaum et al. 1974) and in osteogenesis imperfecta type I by transmission electron microscopy (Jones et al. 1984).

Hyperostosis (Osteosclerosis)

"Hyperostosis" and "osteosclerosis" are terms used to indicate an abnormal increase in skeletal ossification, not related to adaptive changes, due, for example, to increased mechanical work. Increased bone density occurs in osteopetrosis and other forms of bone disease in childhood.

Osteopetrosis (Albers–Schönberg Disease; Marble Bone Disease)

Increased density of bone on radiological examination is the characteristic feature of osteopetrosis, which often becomes apparent during infancy and has occasionally been diagnosed in utero. It may not present until late childhood, or even adult life in milder cases. The condition is sometimes subdivided into a severe infantile form (osteopetrosis fetalis) and a less severe type (osteopetrosis tarda).

In the severe neonatal form there may be hydrocephalus, anaemia, hepatosplenomegaly, lymphadenopathy, blindness, fractures and growth retardation. Fracture, usually of a long bone, is often the first manifestation. Anaemia is related to displacement of bone marrow by dense bone, and, when it is severe, extramedullary haematopoiesis is responsible for the hepatomegaly and superficial lymphadenopathy. Cranial nerve injury occurs and most often this takes the form of optic nerve atrophy owing to narrowing of the optic foramen, although any nerve can be similarly involved.

Bony encroachment of the sella turcica upon the pituitary may result in hypopituitarism, which in turn explains the short stature and sexual underdevelopment of some patients with osteopetrosis. The increased density and thickening of bones, together with the features of bony encroachment in the skull, are all visible on radiographs. Radiological examination of the spine shows increased density with horizontal more radiolucent bands in the mid-zone of the vertebral bodies. The radiodensity of the long bones may be so increased that the medullary cavity cannot be distinguished.

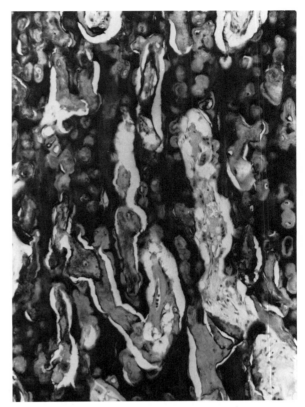

Fig. 9.8. Dense bone in the interior of the shaft of the femur in the severe infantile form of osteopetrosis, showing replacement of the myeloid tissue. (von Kossa, × 400)

Examination of bones from severe cases forms the basis of knowledge of the pathological processes. The cut surfaces of the long bones may show complete merging of the cortices, with dense bone in the interior replacing all myeloid tissue (Fig. 9.8). The cortex may be thickened externally by appositional periosteal bone. The vertebrae show similar changes and there is beading at the costochondral junctions. Postnatal ossification centres are retarded in development and made up of compact bone. Microscopic examination of areas of endochondral ossification show abnormally wide zones of proliferating cartilage. Areas of calcified cartilage are present in the intramedullary region, and confluent masses of non-lamellar bone in relation to this show sparse cellular (osteoblastic and osteoclastic) activity.

Attention has been paid to the osteoclasts in osteopetrosis at the light and electron microscopic levels (Bonucci et al. 1975; Shapiro et al. 1980). Although numbers of these cells are present, they lack ruffled borders, suggesting that they are functionally defective (Shapiro et al. 1980). There are lethal forms of osteopetrosis in rodents (Milhaud and Labat 1978; Loutit and Nesbit 1979) and in these animals the basic defect appears to be a failure of endosteal bone resorption. Injection of bone marrow cells from normal littermates into osteopetrotic rats (Milhaud et al. 1975) and mice (Walker 1975) has proved an effective way of restoring resorptive activity. Bone marrow transplantation has been applied recently with some success to the treatment of the lethal form of osteopetrosis in human infants (Ballet et al. 1977; Coccia et al. 1980).

Other Forms of Hyperostosis

Other conditions in which there is increased density of the skeleton include pycnodysostosis, melorheostosis, osteopoikilosis, osteopathia striata, endosteal hyperostosis, sclerosteosis and infantile cortical hyperostosis. Descriptions are available elsewhere (Jaffe 1972; Beighton and Cremin 1980; Revell 1986), but the features will be summarized here.

Pycnodysostosis

Pycnodysostosis, an autosomally recessive disorder, becomes apparent in early childhood when shortness of stature, small face with receding chin, persistently patent anterior fontanelle and osteosclerosis with increased bone fragility are among the main features. The main differential diagnosis is the separation from osteopetrosis (Elmore 1967; Roth 1976; Revell 1986).

Melorheostosis

Melorheostosis clinically presents in late childhood with indurated skin lesions overlying affected bones, bony swelling around joints, and contractures, particularly of the palms and soles. Radiological examination shows sclerotic linear streaks along the medullary surface of the affected bone with encroachment into medullary cavity a particular feature of childhood melorheostosis (Younge et al. 1979). Pathological examination shows thickening of cortical and medullary bone (Campbell et al. 1968).

Osteopoikilosis

Osteopoikilosis is a rare condition with autosomally dominant inheritance in which there are characteristic skin lesions and dermatofibrosis lenticularis disseminata, and which may occasionally cause problems of differentiation from melorheostosis (Green et al. 1962). Radiological examination shows patchy sclerosis mainly towards the ends of the affected limb bones, and pathological studies reveal small foci of compact bone within the trabecular bone of the medullary region (Jaffe 1972).

Osteopathia Striata

"Osteopathia striata" is a term used to describe the radiological appearance of bone striation seen in various conditions, including osteopetrosis, osteopoikilosis and melorheostosis. Some individuals may have striated bone in the pelvis, spine and long bones and sclerotic changes in the skull – the "osteopathia striata/cranial stenosis complex".

Endosteal Hyperostosis

Progressive asymmetrical enlargement of the mandile starting in late childhood is one of the features of endosteal hyperostosis. There may be thickening of the diaphyseal part of the limb bones and the skull, with cranial nerve encroachment in one of the two forms of this condition. Mandibular prognathism and thickening of the skull are features of sclerostosis which usually manifests itself by the age of 5 years. Affected children are taller than normal, and most subjects have partial or total syndactyly of the second and third fingers. Nerve compression may particularly affect the seventh, auditory and optic nerves, and death sometimes results from impaction of the medulla oblongata in the foramen magnum. Hyperostosis is seen radiologically in the skull, spine, ribs, limb girdles and long bones, and progresses until the third decade.

Infantile Cortical Hyperostosis

Infantile cortical hyperostosis (Caffey's disease) usually presents in the first few months of life, later regressing completely. Hyperostosis of the skull, limb girdles and long bones is accompanied by soft tissue swelling and pyrexia with leucocytosis. The enlargement of bones is subperiosteal, asymmetrical and uneven within the same limb. Histological examination shows an acute inflammatory subperiosteal infiltrate with accompanying new bone formation in the early stages; later the periosteum is thickened and fibrotic with an underlying layer of coarse bone.

Inborn Errors of Metabolism

The errors of metabolism affecting lipid and mucopolysaccharide will be dealt with under this heading. Other disorders that may have effects on the skeletal system include alkaptonuria, in which pigmentation of cartilages, disc calcification and premature development of arthritis occur. These changes are not a particular feature of the disease in childhood, although patients are of short stature in adult life because of the effects of the disease process on development.

The Mucopolysaccharidoses (see also p. 841)

Classification of the mucopolysaccharidoses is becoming more complicated, and the number of deficiencies recognized increases as biochemical investigations are carried out. The mucopolysaccharidoses comprise a group in which there is excessive intracellular storage of mucopolysaccharide (glycosaminoglycan). The biochemical basis of this group of disorders is considered briefly below, followed by descriptions of individual disease entities. Individual disorders are known by eponymous names or designated by Roman numerals (MPS I, II, etc.) (McKusick 1969). Scheie's syndrome was originally separated because it showed a distinct phenotype, but has been found to be biochemically similar to Hurler's syndrome and so is designated MPS I-S.

Biochemical Abnormalities

All the classified mucopolysaccharidoses, with the exception of Morquio's syndrome, involve a disturbance in the lysosomal catabolism of dermatan sulphate and heparan sulphate, either singly or together. Both are polymers made up of alternating sulphated hexosamine (glucosamine or galactosamine) and uronic acid (glucuronic or L-iduronic acid), and the major pathways for their degradation involve lysosomal glycosidases and sulphatases acting sequentially. A distinct enzyme is required to remove each chemical group, and several enzymes are needed to degrade each chain. If any one enzyme is missing the degradative sequence is interrupted, and breakdown by hyaluronidase to large fragments of the chains is the only method of catabolism available. Storage of these large fragments in cells is responsible for the pathological changes. The lysosomal defects and the primarily affected metabolites are summarized in Table 9.6, which also gives some clinical features of the disorders and their modes of inheritance. Further details of the biochemical disorders present in the mucopolysaccharidoses are available in the articles by Neufeld (1974) and Neufeld et al. (1975).

Hurler's Syndrome (Gargoylism)

Features of Hurler's syndrome become manifest in the early years of life, although affected individuals are considered normal for some months after birth. The clinical features comprise skeletal abnormalities, corneal opacities, hepatosplenomegaly and progressive mental retardation. The face becomes altered in appearance, with wide-set eyes, depressed nose, bulging cheeks, large mouth and thick lips. Subsequently bowing deformities of the limbs, shortness of the neck, dorsolumbar kyphosis, stubbiness of the fingers and limitation of joint movement develop. Retardation of growth, the spinal changes and the bowing of the lower limbs all contribute to dwarfism.

Radiological features include generalized rarefaction of tubular bones with widening of their metaphyseal ends, delay in the appearance of epiphyseal ossification centres, and later cortical thinning with rounded or tapered ends to long bones. The kyphosis is the result of failure of ossification of the anterior half of at least one vertebral body (usually D-12 or L-1), which gives rise to a conspicuous "beak-like" appearance on radiological examination. Sagittal section of the lumbar vertebral bodies reveals oval and irregular outlines and the presence of cartilage, not bone, in the upper anterior part of each of the beaked dorsolumbar vertebrae. The skull is thickened, sutures close prematurely, and there are osteophyte-like protrusions on the floor of the middle and posterior fossae, with narrowing of the foramen magnum. The ends of tubular bones show widened irregular epiphyseal plates and discoloured gelatinous articular cartilage, which is abnormally thick in places.

Histologically, marked disturbances of endochondral ossification are present, with loss of height in the cartilage proliferation zone at the ends of long bones and reduction in the amount of cartilage bordering epiphyseal ossification centres. Osseous tissue is present next to the epiphyseal plate and the cartilage of the epiphyseal ossification centres, there being no intermediate stages of capillary ingrowth and cartilage calcification. Collections of glycosaminoglycan-containing macrophages fill the bone-marrow spaces, and similar collections in periosteal connective tissue cells may produce cortical defects. Chondrocytes are larger than normal and have a granular cytoplasm, which on electron microscopy is found to represent lysosomal vacuoles containing apparently undegraded proteoglycan (Rimoin et al. 1976; Silveri et al. 1991). The cells seen in Sanfilippo's and

Table 9.6. Clinical features, inheritance and biochemical defects of the mucopolysaccharides

Disorder	Features	Inheritance	Enzyme defect	Metabolite affected

Hurler's syndrome MPS I-H	Dwarfism
	Mental retardation
	Hepatosplenomegaly
	Corneal opacities
	Altered facies
	Skeletal changes, including
	  bowed limbs and kyphosis
	  (see text)
		Autosomal recessive	α-L-Iduronidase	Dermatan sulphate
				Heparan sulphate

Hunter's syndrome MPS II	Dwarfism Mental retardation Hepatosplenomegaly Altered facies Cardiac abnormalities, deafness Corneal changes *not* present (see text) (Slower course than Hurler's)	Sex-linked recessive	Iduronate sulphatase	Dermatan sulphate Heparan sulphate
Sanfilippo's syndrome MPS III	Severe mental deficiency Deafness Altered facies Few skeletal changes	Autosomal recessive	Heparan *N*-sulphatase or *N*-acetyl- α-glucosaminidase (two subtypes)	Heparan sulphate
Scheie's syndrome MPS I-S	Normal stature Normal intelligence Corneal opacities Hepatosplenomegaly Claw hands, hypertrichosis Variable skeletal changes	Autosomal recessive	α-L-Iduronidase	Dermatan sulphate Heparan sulphate
Maroteaux–Lamy syndrome MPS IV	No mental retardation Growth retardation Altered facies Lumbar kyphosis, short limbs Corneal and auditory involvement variable	Autosomal recessive	*N*-Acetylgalactosamine sulphatase	Dermatan sulphate
Morquio's syndrome	Dwarfism Kyphoscoliosis, flat vertebrae No limb shortening Hip deformity Mental retardation not usually present	Autosomal recessive	*N*-Acetylhexosaminase 6-sulphate sulphatase	Keratan sulphate

Morquio's syndromes show similar changes (Silberberg et al. 1972). The usefulness of ultrastructural studies in the diagnosis of lysosomal storage diseases and the investigation of experimental models has recently been reviewed (Iancu 1992). That bone marrow transplantation can bring about a marked improvement in mucopolysaccharidoses I in dogs has been shown by Breider et al. (1989), who included ultrastructural and electrophoretic methods in their assessment.

Hunter's Syndrome

Onset of symptoms is delayed in Hunter's syndrome, but abnormal behaviour, feeding problems and mental retardation are usually manifest by the age of 3 years. The features include growth retardation, coarse facial features, enlargement of the head, hepatosplenomegaly, stiffness and contractures of the joints, cardiac abnormalities and deafness. Corneal changes are not present.

Sanfilippo's Syndrome

Skeletal and visceral lesions are less marked in Sanfilippo's syndrome, which is characterized by severe mental retardation, deafness, altered facies, clumsy gait, contractures, and respiratory and feeding difficulties.

Maroteaux–Lamy Syndrome (Polydystrophic Dwarfism)

Lack of growth between the ages of 2 and 3 years and development of the facial features of Hurler's syndromes are present in the Maroteaux–Lamy syndrome. Indeed, the lumbar kyphosis, with a wedge-shaped deformity of the dorsolumbar vertebrae (D-12 and L-1) seen on radiological examination, is similar to that present in Hurler's syndrome. The limbs and the trunk are short and there is platyspondyly. Corneal and auditory involvement are variable.

Morquio's Syndrome

The most marked abnormalities in Morquio's syndrome occur in the vertebral column, in which there is kyphoscoliosis, most marked in the dorsolumbar region. It is this change that is mostly responsible for the shortness of stature of the patients, although knock knees, dislocation of the hip, and the holding of the hips in semi-flexion all contribute, as does general growth retardation. The hands reach down to mid-thigh level, so that patients resemble rachitic rather than micromelic dwarfs.

Platyspondyly is a marked feature of the vertebral column and is more pronounced in the dorsal region. The flattened vertebral bodies are increased in diameter anteroposteriorly and transversely and have irregular upper and lower borders, which slope towards each other anteriorly. Centres of ossification are delayed in appearance and development. They may resemble multiple epiphyseal dysplasia on radiological examination.

Gaucher's Disease (see also p. 843)

Gaucher's disease is characterized by the presence of cerebroside-laden histiocytes in the lymphoreticular system and bone marrow. The enzyme deficiency is one of β-glucosidase, and the accumulated metabolite is glucosylceramide. The clinical course of the disease varies. Three variants have been recognized. Infantile and juvenile forms are lethal and show no evidence of skeletal involvement. The "adult" type (non-neuronopathic) Gaucher's disease has been described in young children by Hodson et al. (1979), and it is this type of involvement that affects the skeleton. The mutations in the glucocerebroside gene have recently been identified. The rare infantile and juvenile types, known as type III and type II respectively, involve the central nervous system. Type I ("adult" type) Gaucher's disease is not neuronopathic and is the commonest of all the lysosomal storage diseases. It particularly affects Ashkenazi jews. Further references to Gaucher's disease in childhood are available in Revell (1986). Magnetic resonance imaging to examine the bone changes in Gaucher's disease has been described by Cremin et al. (1990) and DeGasperi et al. (1990).

In the skeletal system, accumulation of Gaucher's cells in the bone marrow (Fig. 9.9) may show necrosis and accompanying fibrosis. Thinning of the bone cortex in relation to the collections of Gaucher's cells may be present. The use of a series of lectins to iden-

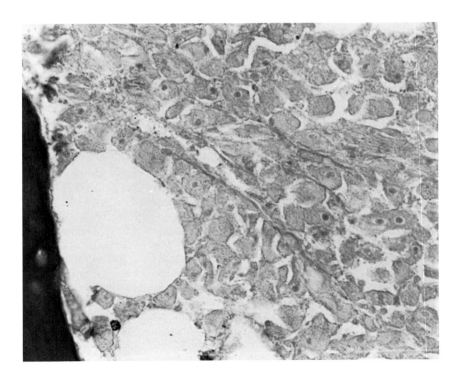

Fig. 9.9. Replacement of the bone marrow by Gaucher cells, with necrosis of adjacent bone. (Azan, × 1000)

tify the carbohydrates in the cytoplasm of cells in Gaucher's disease has been described by DeGasperi et al. (1990). The diploic spaces of the skull and medullary cavity of long bones may be replaced, and vertebral bodies so severely involved as to become collapsed. Necrosis of Gaucher's cells in the femoral head with accompanying partial collapse and deformity may simulate Perthes' disease.

Niemann–Pick Disease (see also p. 844)

Abnormal accumulation of phospholipid (sphingomyelin) occurs in histiocytes in the lymphoreticular system. Little information is available on the pathological appearances of the bones in this condition. Accumulation of lipid-laden cells in the bone marrow causes this to show yellow-coloured areas, and thinning of cortical and trabecular bone is seen. The appearance of secondary ossification centres is delayed, but this is related to general poor health rather than to specific bone effects. Collapse of the femoral head has not been described, and localized areas of bone marrow infiltration are not seen, in distinction from Gaucher's disease.

Hypophosphatasia

In hypophosphatasia, a group of inborn errors of metabolism, there is a deficiency in alkaline phosphatase in both the blood and the tissues. It is likely that there are autosomal recessive and autosomal dominant types (Moore et al. 1990; Caswell et al. 1991; Macfarlane et al. 1992). These conditions are fatal in infancy when severe, but milder cases survive into adult life. The current state of knowledge concerning the biochemical abnormalities is discussed by Gorodischer et al. (1976).

Extensive skeletal involvement is present at birth in the affected neonate, which has a globular head, soft calvaria, shortening and bowing of the limbs, and costochondral beading. Externally, clinical features may suggest a diagnosis of achondroplasia, but radiological examination shows poorly mineralized underdeveloped bones, sometimes with fractures and deformities in long bones. Widened growth plates and metaphyses with radiolucent bands resemble rickets. Streaking of the metaphysis is seen also in congenital syphilis and with intrauterine rubella infection, but the combination of this with an unossified skull and the limb bone changes is characteristic of hypophosphatasia (Cremin and Beighton 1978). The growth plates show a disorderly arrange-

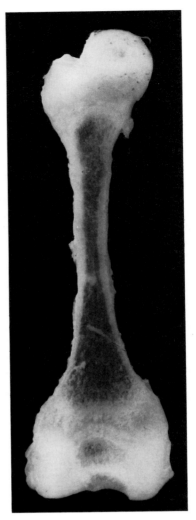

Fig. 9.10. Femur from a young child with hypophosphatasia, showing widening of the lower epiphysis.

ment of cells and failure of mineralization of cartilage matrix on histological examination. Wide osteoid seams and expansions of growth plates, such as a bead-like appearance at the costochondral junction, resemble rickets (Revell 1986; Shohat et al. 1991). Nephrocalcinosis is related to the hypercalcaemia present.

When the underlying defect is less severe, skeletal changes are not evident until some time after birth. In older infants and young children there may be only slight widening of epiphyseal cartilage plates (Fig. 9.10). The cortices of the long bones are thinner and more porotic than normal, and the epiphyses more radiolucent. Histological examination has shown changes similar to those occurring in rickets.

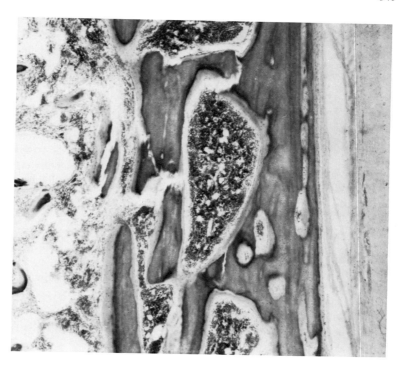

Fig. 9.11. Frontal bone of a 5-month-old boy with rickets, showing wide osteoid seams on the bone of the outer table. (von Kossa, × 150)

Metabolic Disorders Related to Bones

Rickets

Rickets is a disorder affecting endochondral ossification in growing long bones and membranous ossification in some bones. Its pathogenesis varies and includes renal and intestinal causes. Nutritional rickets principally affects infants and young children (6 months to 3 years), who may have insufficient exposure to sunlight, or pigmented skin in areas of moderate sunshine, concomitant low vitamin D intake, and dietary calcium and phosphorus deficiency, all favouring the development of the disease.

Widening of calvarial sutures and the anterior fontanelles may be the only manifestations at 3 or 4 months of age. Progressive development of deformities occurs, so that by the age of 2 years many of the following clinicopathological features may be present:

1. Craniotabes, parietal bossing, depressed anterior fontanelle, which may remain open until age 3 or 4 years
2. Pigeon-breasted appearance
3. Rickety rosary at costochondral junctions
4. Enlargement of ends of long bones (especially at wrists, ankles, elbows, and knees)
5. Bow legs or knock knees
6. Pelvic changes giving rise to serious problems in childbirth

The long bones show enlargement of epiphyseal–metaphyseal junctions, which on histological examination show a zone of disorganized and intermingled bone and cartilage. The changes consist of:

1. Deficient calcification of the proliferating cartilage
2. Disordered vascular penetration of cartilage with impaired chondrocyte proliferation
3. Abnormal amounts of cartilage accumulation
4. Deposition of osteoid in the metaphysis by osteoblasts

Increased osteoid formation in the calvaria of an infant with rickets is shown in Fig. 9.11. Increased curvature of the shaft of long bones results from the effects of weight-bearing, there is tilting of epiphyses with misdirection of growth, and greenstick fractures are found. Bow legs (genu varum) and knock knees (genu valgum) are the most typical deformities.

Enlargement of the costochondral junction (rickety rosary) has the same pathological basis as the widening at epiphyseal–metaphyseal junctions seen in long bones. These changes at the costochondral junction initiate anterior protrusion of the sternum to give a pigeon-breast deformity.

Disorders Giving Rise to Rickets

Apart from nutritional deficiency, rickets may result from any one of a series of disease processes. Briefly, malabsorption from whatever cause may result in sufficient lack of vitamin D absorption to cause bone disease. Gluten-sensitive enteropathy and cystic fibrosis of the pancreas (fibrocystic disease) are two important conditions in this respect. Disordered renal function, including Fanconi's syndrome, may result in rickets, and renal failure in children may cause dwarfism, rickets or the bone changes related to hyperparathyroidism, the latter more frequently in older children. An update on rickets and osteomalacia in association with renal disease has been provided by Mankin (1990). A rare cause of rickets in infants and young children is congenital biliary atresia.

A full list of causes is available elsewhere (Revell 1986) and also includes neonatal rickets (Felton and Stone 1966), impaired 25-hydroxylation of vitamin D in the liver and immaturity (Hillman and Haddad 1975) and neonatal hepatitis (Yu et al. 1971). The biochemical, hormonal and bone histomorphometric changes in hereditary hyperphosphataemic rickets with hypercalciuria are described by Gazit et al. (1991).

Endocrine Disorders and the Skeleton (see also Chapter 13, p. 681)

Primary Hyperparathyroidism

Primary hyperparathyroidism is extremely rare in children, and a detailed description of the related bone changes, known rather unsatisfactorily as "osteitis fibrosa cystica", need not be given here. Reference should be made to any of the standard texts on pathology for details.

The bone lesions of hyperparathyroidism may be focal, simulating an osteoclastoma radiologically and histologically, or diffuse. The pathological process characteristically shows proliferation of spindle cell masses, with fibrosis on bone surfaces and increased numbers of osteoclastic giant cells. Osteoblastic activity is unimpaired, so that evidence of bone regeneration may also be seen.

Secondary Hyperparathyroidism

The skeletal changes of hyperparathyroidism secondary to chronic renal disease may be conspicuous in children, and hyperparathyroidism in a child of less than 10 years is much more likely to be secondary than primary.

The changes are usually relatively mild and comprise increased resorptive activity on trabecular surfaces with fibrosis. Biochemical evidence (hypercalcaemia, hypophosphataemia, raised serum alkaline phosphatase) and radiological changes of hyperparathyroidism may be entirely lacking in patients with histological changes present on bone biopsy. In cases with protracted renal insufficiency, bone changes may be indistinguishable from those of primary hyperparathyroidism. Bone growth will usually be stunted in these patients and there may be coexisting changes of rickets.

Hyperpituitary Gigantism

Hyperpituitarism due to an eosinophil adenoma of the adenohypophysis results in gigantism in young patients, as growth hormone has a direct stimulatory effect at the epiphyseal cartilage plates. Growth hormone-producing tumours are rare in childhood, and little is known of the detailed histopathology of the condition.

Hypopituitary Dwarfism

Hypopituitary dwarfs have normal skeletal proportions and grow at a normal rate during the first years of life. The primary causes are intracranial lesions damaging either the adenohypophysis or the hypothalamohypophyseal system:

1. Craniopharyngioma
2. Gliomas of the optic chiasm
3. Hand–Schüller–Christian disease
4. Pituitary chromophobe adenoma
5. Basal meningitis, fracture or haemorrhage
6. Maldevelopment of the pituitary or pituitary fossa

There is delay in the appearance of postnatal ossification centres and arrest or retardation of ossification at the epiphyseal plates, which persist beyond the ages at which they would normally disappear. Because epiphyseal growth is retarded, the bone age of the child is less than the chronological age. The ossification centres are not abnormal in form, in contrast to hypothyroid dwarfism.

Hyperthyroidism

Accelerated bone growth may occur in hyperthyroidism in childhood and adolescence. Osteoporosis may develop where hyperthyroidism is longstanding.

Hypothyroid Dwarfism

Babies with cretinism show evidence of stunted physical development and mental retardation from the very first months of life. The effects of hypothyroidism on the skeleton of a child are similar to those of hypopituitarism, namely, delayed appearance and retarded growth of postnatal ossification centres, retarded growth at epiphyseal cartilage plates, and persistence of these plates and calvarial sutures beyond the age at which they would normally disappear. The skull develops a brachycephalic appearance because growth retardation is more severe at the base than at the vault. Postnatal ossification centres show areas of cystic degeneration of the epiphyseal cartilage, and differentiation from "stippled epiphyses" and Perthes' disease may be difficult. Collins (1966) believed it possible that some cases of stippled epiphyses described as dysplasia epiphysealis punctata represented cases of unrecognized hypothyroidism.

Cushing's Syndrome

Osteoporosis is one of the features of Cushing's syndrome, the spine and other cancellous bone being prominently affected. Decreased osteoblastic activity with no increase in osteoclastic resorption is the basis of the abnormality. Detailed pathological changes need not be described here and are available in standard textbooks of pathology. There are no other special features to the osteoporosis occurring in Cushing's syndrome or induced by steroid treatment in childhood. The administration of glucocorticoids to children has growth-inhibiting effects on the skeleton (Maassen 1952; Sissons and Hadfield 1955).

Eunuchism and Gonadal Dysgenesis

Males castrated in childhood grow tall, with a slender gracile skeletal structure. Excess growth tends to be greatest in the femur. The pelvis develops a female configuration. Epiphyseal cartilage plates persist longer than in normal development and, in contrast to hypopituitarism and hypothyroidism, are functionally active.

Patients with gonadal dysgenesis tend to be of short stature, with radiological changes resembling dysplasia epiphysealis multiplex. Features said to be helpful in the diagnosis include hyperplasia of the first cervical vertebra, tibia vara, wrist changes and shortening of the fourth metacarpal bone. There may be no skeletal abnormalities in some cases of gonadal dysgenesis in girls.

Adrenogenital Syndrome

Adrenal virilization associated with precocious puberty in young children is usually seen in boys. If the underlying tumour is not malignant, accelerated initial growth is followed by premature closure of epiphyseal cartilage plates, so that the patient eventually fails to reach average height.

Diabetes Mellitus

Children with diabetes mellitus of recent onset may have postnatal ossification centres present slightly ahead of the normal chronological age and be of above average height. Postnatal ossification centres are less well developed in longstanding childhood diabetes. Growth-arrest (Harris's) lines are often present in the metaphyses of long bones. Diabetics show evidence of detectable osteopenia within 5 years of the onset of disease (Levin et al. 1976; McNair et al. 1978).

Skeletal Changes in Haematological Disorders

Bone changes occur in sickle cell anaemia, thalassaemia and haemophilia. Each is dealt with briefly below.

Sickle Cell Anaemia

The pathological features of sickle cell anaemia may be considered under three main headings:

1. Erythroid hyperplasia of the bone marrow, resulting in local bone resorption, widening of the trabecular bone area, and thinning of the related cortical bone.
2. Blockage of small blood vessels by masses of sickle cells, giving rise to infarction in the territory supplied. Such ischaemic bone necrosis may

occur in any bone and at any site. The shaft or articular ends of long bones are frequent sites of necrosis, especially the femoral head (Chung and Ralston 1969). This may resemble that seen in Perthes' disease on radiographs. Fibrous tissue replaces necrotic bone marrow and there is new bone formation.

3. Osteomyelitis, usually involving bone in which there has been infarction. The organism is frequently of the *Salmonella* group and the route of infection is via the blood. In one large series of childhood cases of salmonella osteomyelitis from Nigeria, 90% of cases were HbS homozygotes (Adeyokunna and Hendrickse 1980). In a more recent study, *Staphylococcus aureus* predominated slightly over *Salmonella* in a series of sickle cell disease sufferers having chronic osteomyelitis (Epps et al. 1991). In those less than 2 years old, the small bones of the hands and feet were more commonly affected whereas older children showed limb long-bone involvement.

The radiological changes reflect marrow encroachment on bone, with increased radiolucency in the mandible, widening of the diploic region of the calvaria, and rarefaction of the vertebral bodies with cup-shaped outlines to their upper and lower surfaces, caused by expansion of the discs into the thinned bone.

Thalassaemia

Thalassaemia results from abnormal synthesis of either the α- or the β-chains of haemoglobin. The severity of the disease is related to whether the patient is homozygous (thalassaemia major) or heterozygous (thalassaemia minor).

Thalassaemia major is seen mainly in infants and young children who have progressive anaemia with evidence of haemolysis and hepatosplenomegaly. There may be changes in the facial bones to give a mongoloid appearance. The affected child often dies in early life. Severe cases of long duration show retarded skeletal maturation and growth.

Pathological examination of the thickened skull shows deep red hyperplastic bone marrow with thinning of the outer table. The amount of bone marrow is also increased at many other sites, including ribs, vertebrae, femora and iliac bones. The vertebrae are porotic and show concave cup-shaped superior and inferior surfaces with thinned cortical shells like those seen in sickle cell disease. Histological examination shows bone atrophy with hyperplastic bone marrow containing islands of foam cells and iron-laden macrophages.

The pathological changes are reflected in the radiological appearances as rarefaction of bones. The skull of the child with thalassaemia major shows thickening of the calvaria with a "hair on end" appearance, comprising radially arranged striations and poorly defined outer table. The development of rickets and scurvy-like lesions in patients with β-thalassaemia major receiving treatment with desferrioxamine has recently been described and the suggestion made that the changes result from long-term chelation therapy (Orzincolo et al. 1990).

Haemophilia

Haemorrhages may occur at any site of trauma in haemophilia, and in the skeletal system the main results are arthropathy and the relatively uncommon haemophilic pseudotumour.

The overall incidence of arthropathy in haemophilia is high. First evidence of joint involvement is unusual before 2 years of age but the incidence increases with increasing age and arthropathy is notable by 8–14 years. The knee is most commonly affected, followed by the elbow, ankle, hip, shoulder and wrist. Initially there are simple haemarthroses, but after several episodes in a given joint chronic haemophilic arthritis develops. The pathological findings depend on the severity and chronicity of the haemorrhages. The thickened synovial membrane is discoloured brown when repeated haemorrhages have occurred, and there is marked proliferation reactive inflammation with formation of numerous vascular pigment-stained synovial villi. Haemosiderin pigment is concentrated in the superficial layers of the synovium. The articular surface is also discoloured and may have defects filled with pigmented fibrous tissue, areas of cartilage loss down to subchondral bone and eburnation – changes that indicate progression to osteoarthrosis.

Haemophilic pseudotumour is a haematoma that appears radiologically as a large radiolucent area expanding the affected bone. It is important because it can be mistaken for a true bone neoplasm. The local bone cortex may undergo resorption because of pressure from the haematoma, which also causes periosteal elevation. There may be an accompanying pathological fracture.

Christmas Disease

The clinical and pathological features of Christmas disease in bones and joints are essentially the same as those of haemophilia.

Chronic Polyarthritis

Juvenile chronic polyarthritis (called juvenile rheumatoid arthritis in the USA) is a condition that presents, by definition, before the age of 16 years. There is arthritis (manifested as any two of pain, swelling and limitation of movement) present for a minimum period of 3 months, and the following diseases causing arthritis must have been excluded:

1. Infections:
   a) Bacterial arthritis (including tuberculosis)
   b) Viral and fungal arthritides
2. Other connective tissue disorders:
   a) Systemic lupus erythematosus
   b) Polymyositis and dermatomyositis
   c) Sjögren's syndrome
   d) Vasculitides (Schönlein–Henoch purpura, serum sickness, mucocutaneous lymph node syndrome, infantile polyarteritis)
   e) Progressive systemic sclerosis
   f) Mixed connective-tissue disorder
   g) Polyarteritis nodosa
   h) Arthritis in ulcerative colitis, regional enteritis, psoriasis, Reiter's and Behçet's syndromes
   i) Rheumatic fever
3. Neoplastic disease:
   a) Leukaemia
   b) Lymphoma
   c) Neuroblastoma
4. Haematological disorders:
   a) Haemophilia
   b) Sickle cell disease
5. Other bone and joint conditions:
   a) Gout and pyrophosphate arthropathy
   b) Osteochondritis
   c) Slipped femoral capital epiphysis
   d) Trauma: battered child syndrome, fractures, soft-tissue injuries
   e) Chondromalacia patellae
   f) Villonodular tenosynovitis
   g) Bone tumours (osteoid osteoma, osteosarcoma, etc.)

Classification within this definition is into three main subgroups according to the type of presentation:

1. Systemic illness
2. Polyarthritis
3. Pauciarticular disease (four or fewer joints affected)

The age of onset, sex incidence and subsequent natural history of these differ, as outlined below.

The eponym Still's disease is often used interchangeably with juvenile chronic arthritis, rather than in its original and more specific sense of polyarthropathy, splenomegaly and leukopenia.

Detailed recent information on this group of disorders may be obtained in the published proceedings of a symposium of the American Rheumatism Association (1977). A briefer account is that by Schaller (1977).

Ninety-five percent of juvenile arthritis is seronegative (Schaller 1979). Pauciarticular disease may be associated with sacroiliitis and HLA-B27 histocompatibility group, particularly in males. Associations with HLA-D molecules are complicated, and recognition of subgroups difficult. HLA-DW4 and DR-4 are much less common in juvenile arthritis than in adult rheumatoid arthritis (Stastny and Fink 1979).

Systemic-onset Chronic Arthritis

Systemic-onset chronic arthritis is the main subgroup of childhood chronic arthritis and has the feature of originally described by Still. Systemic involvement consists of fever, skin rashes, lymphadenopathy, hepatosplenomegaly and pericarditis. Lymphadenopathy is a much more prominent feature of juvenile chronic polyarthritis than of classic adult rheumatoid arthritis. Classical Still's disease occurs in children and in adults. It has a poor prognosis, proceeding to severe joint destruction and ankylosis of the cervical spine (Cabane et al. 1990).

The patients are seronegative, and two-thirds are aged under 5 years at onset. Boys are affected more frequently than girls. The joints especially involved are those of the wrist and ankle, often with small joints of the toes. Hip-joint involvement and tenosynovitis of some of the flexor tendons of the hand also often occur. The cervical spine is affected fairly frequently. The earlier the onset of the disease, the more likely are erosive joint changes and alterations in growth to develop.

Polyarticular Chronic Arthritis

The subgroup of polyarticular chronic arthritis is similar to adult rheumatoid arthritis. Girls are affected more often than boys, and, although the onset may be as early as 5 years of age, most patients are aged 10 years or more. The presence of IgM rheumatoid factor is usually noted soon after onset, and about one-fifth of cases have rheumatoid nodules at the elbow. The polyarthritis is symmetrical and involves distal limb joints (hands, feet, wrists, ankles, and knees) more than proximal. Persistent activity in

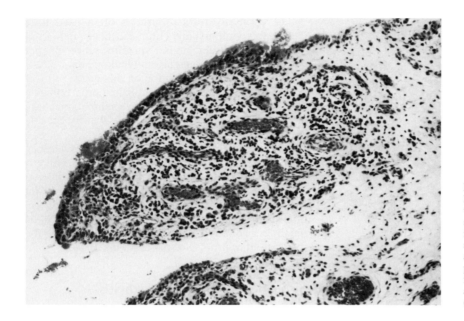

Fig. 9.12. Synovium from the knee of an 8-year-old presenting with monarticular arthritis, showing non-specific chronic inflammatory cell infiltrate, synovial lining cell hyperplasia and surface fibrin deposition. This patient subsequently developed features of ankylosing spondylitis and was HLA-B27 positive. (Courtesy of Dr A.I.D. Prentice)

joints with erosive changes and joint destruction within a year of onset is common.

Pauciarticular Chronic Arthritis

Pauciarticular arthritis usually occurs in young children (age 1–5 years) and affects girls more frequently than boys. Chronic iridocyclitis, a common feature in these patients, may lead to blindness or severe visual impairment. Tests for rheumatoid factor are negative, but 80% of cases have antinuclear antibody at the time of diagnosis.

The ankles, knees and elbows are the joints chiefly involved and the hips are rarely affected. Sacroiliitis does not develop (juvenile ankylosing spondylitis). Patients developing chronic iridocyclitis have a high incidence of HLA histocompatibility group HLA-DR5.

Juvenile Ankylosing Spondylitis

Pauciarticular arthritis in older children may be ankylosing spondylitis. Boys are affected about five times more often than girls and the age of onset is usually 8–12 years. The lower limb joints (hips, knees and ankles) are most commonly affected, and approximately half of all cases subsequently develop sacroiliitis. Atlantaxial subluxation may occur in the late teens or early twenties. Acute iridocyclitis is seen in about 20% of cases. A quarter of these patients have a family history of ankylosing spondylitis, and 90% are of the HLA-B27 histocompatibility group.

Children with this disorder satisfy the criteria for a childhood chronic arthritis early in its course, and only subsequently do the features of ankylosing spondylitis become apparent (Fig. 9.12).

Pathological Appearances in Juvenile Chronic Arthritis

On macroscopic examination, the joints in juvenile chronic arthritis resemble those of rheumatoid arthritis, with pannus formation in established cases. The articular cartilage of childhood and juvenile joints is thicker than that of adults and this may have some protective effect, i.e. the joints are destroyed more slowly and the stage of reversibility of the changes is prolonged. The histological features of the synovitis are indistinguishable from those of adult rheumatoid arthritis (Fig. 9.12). Marginal erosions, eburnation and the development of secondary osteoarthrosis are features in the late stage, but osteophyte formation is much less pronounced than in adults. Fibrous ankylosis is fairly common where there is hip- and knee-joint involvement.

Growth arrest may occur, with premature ossification of epiphyses and changes at the epiphyseal cartilage plates. The resultant "rheumatic dwarfism" must be distinguished from the arrest of growth brought about by long-term corticosteroid treatment.

Nodules over bony pressure points and in tendons show the classic features of rheumatoid nodules in seropositive cases, with central necrosis and palisaded surrounding histocytes. Seronegative cases

Table 9.7. Organisms causing septic arthritis in childhood

Organism	Percentage of cases affected	Age affected
H. influenzae	19	95% of cases age < 2 years
Staph aureus	18	69% of cases aged 2–10 years
Streptococci	9	Approx. 30% in each of the age ranges <2, 2–5 and 6–10 years
N. gonorrhoea	5	Unusual under 2 years
Staph. epidermidis	2	80% of cases aged 0–5 years
N. meningitidis	2	80% of cases aged 0–5 years
Enterobacter spp.	2	
Salmonella spp.	1	
Others	9	
Organism unknown	33	

After Fink et al. (1977).

have nodules that appear more like those found in rheumatic fever, with proliferating fibroblasts and irregular areas of fibrinous exudate.

There are often early indications of cervical spinal involvement, especially in the seronegative juvenile chronic arthritis group. The apophyseal joints are primarily affected and undergo ankylosis, especially at the second and third cervical vertebrae. Subsequent loss of movement and lack of growth of the vertebrae, with later fusion of vertebral bodies, may occur. Atlanto-occipital subluxation is rare in comparison with cervical subluxation in adult rheumatoid arthritis.

Infections of Bones and Joints

Bacterial Infections

Only special features of bone and joint infections as they occur in childhood will be described in this section. Reference should be made to standard textbooks of pathology for detailed accounts.

Septic Arthritis

Septic arthritis normally involves a single joint, most frequently the knee or hip, followed by the elbow and ankle. Infection of the hip joint in children has been reviewed by Petersen et al. (1980) and Allen and Ferguson (1985): *Staphylococcus aureus* was the most commonly found causative organism. Neonatal septic arthritis is caused predominantly by *Staphylococcus* followed by *Candida* and gram-negative enterobacteria in hospital-acquired cases,

whereas streptococci, then *Staphylococcus* and *Neisseria gonorrhoea* are responsible for community-acquired cases (Dan 1984). Small joints are only rarely affected. The incidence of infection with different organisms varies with age. *Haemophilus influenzae* accounts for the vast majority of cases aged 2 years and under. *Staph. aureus* is also an important organism, although it is less often involved in the young, most such infections occurring with increasing frequency from 3 years onwards, so that older children and adolescents are most often affected. A long list of other organisms could be included and a few are summarized in Table 9.7 Septic arthritis and osteomyelitis in children have been reviewed by Petty (1990).

Septic arthritis is one of the most common complications of osteomyelitis and is much more frequent in this form in infants and young children than in adults. The ends of long bones are the sites of predilection for osteomyelitis, and so nearby joints are likely to be affected by the direct spread of organisms. Joints are otherwise involved by direct synovial infection with blood-borne organisms.

Establishment of infection in a joint leads to acute inflammation of the synovial membrane with abundant polymorphs in the synovial fluid and destruction of the articular cartilage. Abscesses may develop, depending on the responsible organism. Necrotic fragments of cartilage become sequestrated in the joint space, and immobilization by fibrous adhesions and bony ankylosis may occur.

Osteomyelitis

Pyogenic osteomyelitis is due to *Staph. aureus* infection in the large majority of cases. Infection is usually blood-borne rather than direct from compound fractures or infected wounds. The haematogenously

Table 9.8. Organisms causing osteomyelitis in childhood

Organism	Percentage of cases affected	Age affected
Staph. aureus	59	All ages, but nearly 70% aged 2–10 years
Streptococci	9	70% of cases less than 5 years old
Staph. epidermidis	4	70% of cases less than 2 years old
H. influenzae	3	80% of cases less than 2 years old
Pseudomonas aeruginosa	2	
Others	8	Includes *Salmonella* spp., which accounts for 1% of cases
Organism unknown	15	

After Fink et al. (1977).

spread organisms lodge in the juxtaepiphyseal and metaphyseal regions of the bones.

Staphylococcal osteomyelitis is most frequent in the age range 3–15 years, although it is not rare in babies and infants. Osteomyelitis due to *Strep. pyogenes* occurs more often in babies and young children than older patients, and *H. influenzae* and *Strep. pneumoniae* infections, although less common, also occur in this age group. Children with sickle cell anaemia are especially likely to get salmonella osteomyelitis. The results recorded in a series by Fink et al. (1977) are summarized in Table 9.8.

Almost any bone may become infected, but the common sites are in the lower limb (75% in the femur or tibia at their proximal or distal ends). The lumbar region is the most frequent site of haematogenous infection of the vertebral column.

When organisms lodge in the bone marrow of the metaphysis abscess formation occurs, with death and fragmentation of trabecular bone. Extension of suppuration into haversian systems causes death of large areas of cortical bone, pieces of which become separated from living bone as sequestra, while increased osteoblastic activity of surviving living bone surrounds the necrotic bone with new bone (involucrum).

The complications of osteomyelitis include septicaemia, pathological fracture, sinus formation, and the development of septic arthritis in children.

Osteomyelitis may accompany middle ear infection, sinus infection or severe dental sepsis.

Brodie Abscess

A chronic bone abscess (Brodie abscess) is a sharply delineated infective focus occurring predominantly in those who have not yet completed skeletal growth. It is usually solitary, and a common site is the distal end of the tibia, although other bones, including the radius and femur, may be affected. The abscess contains fluid of variable consistency and appearance and has a wall lined with inflammatory granulation tissue surrounded by a connective tissue layer and sclerotic bone.

Tuberculosis

Skeletal tuberculosis in children occurs mostly in the age range 3–15 years, and is rare in the first year of life. Haematogenous dissemination to bones and joints occurs in children who have a primary lesion in the lung.

The main sites of involvement are the vertebral column, the hip and the knee. Detailed descriptions of the pathology of the disease in children will not be given here, as the histological changes are the same as in adults. Long bones tend to be involved at the epiphyseal ends near the articular surface, and the diaphysis is the site of infection in short bones. Spinal infection starts in the vertebral bodies and spreads from the marrow cavities through the bone to extend beneath the longitudinal ligaments to the margins of the intervertebral discs. Tuberculosis almost never starts in the discs, although this is theoretically possible because the discs still have blood vessels in children.

Collapse of vertebral bodies and discs gives rise to severe spinal deformities, and extension into the related soft tissues may give rise to a paravertebral abscess.

Radiologically, tuberculous involvement of the hip may be mistaken for Perthes' disease, and syphilitic arthritis (Clutton's joints) of the knee may resemble tuberculosis in children. Tuberculosis in the shaft of a long bone is often indistinguishable from pyogenic osteomyelitis.

Tuberculous involvement of synovial tissues occurs by two mechanisms, namely haematogenous and local spread, the latter from tuberculous osteomyelitis in the end of the neighbouring bone. The pathological appearances of tuberculous arthritis are variable, depending on the severity of involvement. The synovial fluid may vary from thin yellow fluid to thick purulent material. The synovial membrane may be only moderately thickened, with an inflamed injected appearance, or grossly thickened, with abundant surface fibrin. Histological examination shows typical tuberculoid granulomas, although the amount of caseation is variable. Cartilage destruction by tuberculous inflammatory tissue occurs and if it is present in a subchondral position there is undermining of the cartilage, which may become separated.

Lyme Arthritis

The multisystem disorder known as Lyme arthritis was characterized only recently. It affects both children and adults and shows close geographic clustering of cases in a small area of Connecticut (Steere et al. 1977a). Although early cases were thought to be a form of childhood arthritis (Steere et al. 1977b), the disease is now known to begin with a characteristic skin lesion, called erythema chronicum migrans. This is followed by neurological and cardiac changes and joint disease. The arthritis, which is typically intermittent and oligarticular, may proceed to chronic synovitis with erosive damage to the joint. Histopathological examination of the synovium shows villous hypertrophy, intimal cell hyperplasia and an infiltrate of lymphocytes and plasma cells, sometimes with lymphoid follicle formation (Johnston et al. 1985). The appearances closely resemble those of rheumatoid arthritis, except that obliterative microvascular changes are present in Lyme arthritis and not in rheumatoid synovia examined for comparison. The causation of Lyme disease is a spirochaete related to the genus *Borrelia*, which is transmitted by *Ixodes dammini* or related ixodid ticks (Steere et al. 1978, 1983; Steere and Malawista 1979; Burgdorfer et al. 1982; Johnston et al. 1985). The condition also occurs elsewhere in the USA, in Europe and in Australia (Wallis et al. 1978; Ackermann et al. 1980; Stewart et al. 1982).

Syphilis

Congenital syphilis has become rare in developed countries but still occurs commonly in parts of Africa (see p. 731). The pathological features in the skeleton of the fetus, newborn and young infant are osteochondritis, osteomyelitis of the diaphysis and periostitis.

Osteochondritis involves all sites of endochondral ossification, which show widening of the provisional calcification zone. Where there is severe involve-

ment, syphilitic inflammatory tissue may cause separation of the metaphysis from the epiphysis, and such epiphyseal separation occurs mostly in long bones of neonates and infants up to 3 months of age. Diaphyseal osteomyelitis arises independently or by extension of subchondral inflammation present in the late stages of osteochondritis. Foci of osteomyelitis with microscopic areas of bone necrosis result. In ossifying periostitis bone deposits are present along the shafts of lone bones and the surfaces of flat bones such as the ilium.

In patients with syphilitic infection that has been mild, unrecognized or inadequately treated during infancy, late manifestations of congenital syphilis occur, usually from 4 years of age onwards. The bone lesions are of two main types, namely gummatous and non-gummatous osteomyelitis and periostitis. A number of time-honoured descriptions exist for the changes, such as saddle-nose deformity and sabre tibia. Detailed descriptions of the changes can be found in the standard texts on pathology of bone.

Viral Infections

A small percentage of children surviving smallpox have been reported to have had osteomyelitis, and foci of bone-marrow necrosis have been noted in the long bones at autopsy in patients who die of disease. Shortening of long bones in adults who suffered from smallpox during childhood has been ascribed to changes in the epiphyses and epiphyseal–metaphyseal junctions. Bone involvement following smallpox vaccination is extremely rare (Jaffe 1972).

Rubella is well known to cause abnormalities in the developing fetus. As well as the congenital rubella syndrome, skeletal changes are evident radiologically in the metaphyseal region of long bones, where linear and ovoid areas of radiolucency appear. There is thickening of osteoid trabeculae, which are poorly mineralized (Singer et al. 1967). They disappear within a few months of birth.

Joint symptoms in viral infections are infrequent, usually acute, and self-limiting. True arthritis is unusual, arthralgia being the main manifestation. Children develop arthralgia with rubella infection or after vaccination, although less frequently than adults. Symptoms develop at about the time of appearance of circulating antibodies. Involvement is usually monarticular and symptoms last for 1–2 weeks. Histology of the synovial membrane is non-specific.

A serum sickness-like illness that includes polyarthralgia, and less often polyarthritis, occurs in some adults during the incubation period of type B viral hepatitis. This has also been recognized in children.

The synovial membrane shows non-specific vascular changes with a sparse inflammation reaction.

Certain arboviruses commonly cause arthritis in Africa and Australia, but not in the Western Hemisphere. Children are affected less frequently than adults. The viruses are mosquito-borne and cause Chikungunya and O'nyong nyong in Africa and Ross River (epidemic) polyarthritis in Australia.

Rare cases of arthritis have been reported in children with mumps and chickenpox. The reader is referred to the review of viral arthritis in children by Phillips (1977) for further details and references to these conditions.

Tumours and Tumour-like Conditions

Many tumours other than those described here occasionally affect children, but the majority of neoplasms seen in childhood fall into the categories described. Detailed descriptions of various bone tumours are available (Dahlin 1978; Huvos 1979; Mirra 1980; Schajowicz 1981), and a more generalized approach is given elsewhere (Revell 1986). Current trends in diagnosis and treatment are summarized by Schajowicz (1983) and Goorin et al. (1985). Skeletal tumours in children and adolescents have been reviewed by Spjut and Ayala (1983).

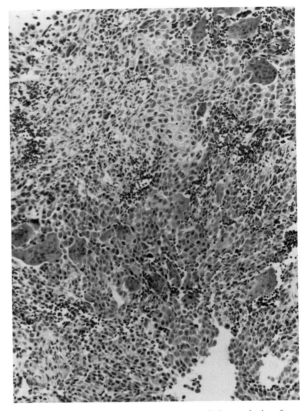

Fig. 9.13. Histological appearances of a radiolucent lesion from the region of the lower femoral epiphysis of a 15-year-old girl, showing polygonal and spindle-shaped chondroblasts, with intermingled giant cells. Chondroblastoma. (H&E, × 400)

Chondroblastoma

Chondroblastoma is a rare tumour, affecting males more often than females and usually occurring in the epiphyseal part of a bone. The femur, humerus and tibia are the most common sites. The age range is 10–20 years. Radiologically, there is a radiolucent defect in the epiphyseal region, which may extend into the metaphysis and be surrounded by a narrow margin of sclerosis. Macroscopically, this well demarcated lesion has a gritty blue-grey or grey-brown surface. Microscopy shows it to be composed of chondroblasts, which are polygonal, round or spindle-shaped, with oval nuclei (Fig. 9.13). Some chondroid matrix and giant cells are also present. Lace-like calcification is a helpful feature in the differential diagnosis (Spjut et al. 1970) but is not pathognomonic. A review of a large series also shows the immunohistochemical findings in chondroblastoma, the chondroblasts being S100 and vimentin positive and the matrix containing type II collagen

whereas the pericellular region is type VI collagen positive (Edel et al. 1992). Another shows that the cells additionally express CAM 5.2, EMA and cytokeratins 8, 18 and 19 (Semmelink et al. 1990).

Chondromyxoid Fibroma

Chondromyxoid fibroma is a localized benign tumour characterized by lobulated areas of spindle-shaped or stellate cells and abundant myxoid or chondroid intercellular matrix. These areas are separated by more cellular tissue with abundant spindle-shaped cells and variable numbers of giant cells.

Chondromyxoid fibroma occurs in the 10- to 30-year age group and the sexes are more or less equally affected. The metaphyseal region of a long bone, especially in the lower limb, is a common site (Spjut et al. 1970). It is a well circumscribed, lobulated, solid grey-white to tan mass that expands and erodes the cortex of the bone.

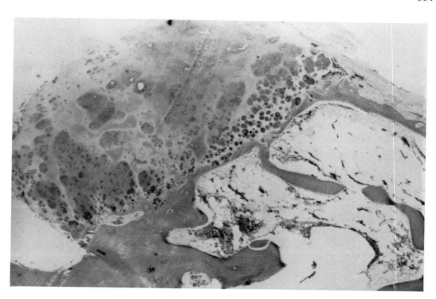

Fig. 9.14. Osteochondroma from the upper end of the humerus of a 15-year-old boy. (H&E, × 100)

Confusion with chondrosarcoma may occur when large pleomorphic tumour cells are present (Jaffe and Lichenstein 1948). This may be avoided by attention to the radiological features and histological recognition of the characteristic lobular pattern of chondromyxoid fibroma (Spjut and Ayala 1983).

Recurrence may occur after curettage, but cases with malignant change have been questioned as not being true examples (Dahlin 1967). Sarcomatous change, if it occurs, is a pathological rarity (Dahlin 1978).

Osteochondroma (Osteocartilaginous Exostosis)

Osteochondromas are cartilage-capped bony projections. They are the commonest benign bone tumours and occur most frequently in childhood; their growth usually ceases at the time of skeletal maturation. Osteochondromas are located on the external surface of the metaphyseal portions of long bones, commonly at the lower end of the femur upper tibia and upper humerus (Fig. 9.14) (Dahlin 1978). They may be solitary or multiple, multiple tumours occurring in the condition known as multiple osteocartilaginous exostosis (diaphyseal aclasis; hereditary deforming dyschondroplasia; hereditary multiple exostoses). Patients with this particular disorder may have bowing and shortening of the extremities and pelvic or pectoral girdle asymmetry (Spjut et al. 1970).

Malignant change is rare in solitary osteochondroma and occurs more frequently with multiple exostoses (Jaffe 1958; Dahlin 1978), although the

incidence may be fairly low even in these cases (Voutsinas and Wynne-Davies 1983). Cartilaginous exostoses have been described in children (usually less than 3 years of age) following radiotherapy for neuroblastoma, Wilms' tumour and eosinophilic granuloma. They occur within or near the field of radiation treatment (Murphy and Blount 1962; Cole and Darte 1963).

Chondroma

Chondromas are benign tumours of mature cartilage which are centrally placed in the affected bone and thus often called "enchondromas". The short tubular bones of the hands and feet are usually considered to be the most affected, although Spjut and Ayola (1983) found that long bones were most frequently involved and that there were few phalangeal lesions in their series of childhood cases. Radiological examination shows a central radiolucent, often lobulated, lesion with mottled calcification or ossification. A lobular grey-blue lesion resembling cartilage is seen macroscopically, and histological examination shows cartilage with small chondrocytes having regular nuclei. Occasionally, enlarged or atypical nuclei may be present; however, these are not a good indicator of malignancy in this type of tumour in a growing child in the absence of other features such as infiltration of adjacent bone, cortical destruction and extension into soft tissue. Multiple enchondromas are present in Ollier's disease and the Maffucci's syndrome, being accompanied in the latter by haemangiomas. Malignant transformation is well recognized

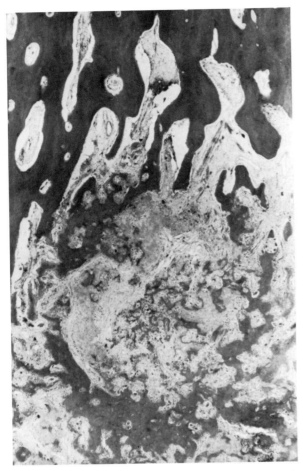

Fig. 9.15. Painful lesion from the mid-shaft region of the tibia of a 20-year-old male, showing the central nidus of an osteoid osteoma with surrounding sclerotic bone. (H&E, × 100)

cells, which may be mistaken for well differentiated chondrosarcoma. Periosteal chondroma affects the long bones and around half of all cases occur before the age of 20 years (Boriani et al. 1983; Spjut and Ayala 1983).

Chondrosarcoma

Chondrosarcoma is rare in children and adolescents. The distribution and appearances of these tumours are similar to those in adults. The diagnosis should be made with considerable caution in the young, and the possibility that an apparent chondrosarcoma is a chondroblastic osteosarcoma should be carefully excluded by consideration of the site, examination of multiple blocks for the presence of osteoid formation by malignant cells, and, if possible, staining of smears or frozen sections for alkaline phosphatase (Sanerkin 1980). A review in the French literature gives details of the incidence of different cartilaginous tumours in childhood and describes two cases of chondrosarcoma both dying with pulmonary metastases (Dumontier et al. 1989).

Osteoid Osteoma

Osteoid osteoma is a benign osteoblastic tumour, which is clearly demarcated, less than 1 cm in diameter (Byers 1968) and surrounded by new bone formation. Males are affected two or three times more often than females. The great majority of cases occur between the ages of 5 and 24 years (Byers 1968), and the diaphyses of long bones in the lower limb (tibia and femur) are most often involved. The lesions are generally painful.

A friable red-grey discrete "nidus" surrounded by sclerotic new bone is seen on macroscopic examination, and gives the radiologically classic appearance of a small central radiolucent or dense area with dense periphery. Histologically the nidus is composed of cellular, highly vascular, tissue containing islands of closely associated osteoid trabeculae, having irregular borders and surrounded by osteoblasts. Some calcification may be present and there is no evidence of cartilage formation. Well organized newly formed trabeculae make up the surrounding sclerotic bone (Spjut et at. 1970; Schajowicz et al. 1972) (Figs. 9.15 and 9.16).

Osteoblastoma

Osteoblastoma is related to osteoid osteoma and there are no specific histological criteria for their separa-

(Spjut et al. 1970) and occurs in the chondroid or vascular lesions in 15%–18% of cases of Maffucci's syndrome (Wynne–Davies et al. 1985). Malignant transformation in Ollier's disease is unusual but has been reported (Cannon and Sweetnam 1985; Wynne-Davies et al. 1985).

Recognition of periosteal chondroma is important because the radiological and histological features suggest malignancy and may therefore lead to over-treatment of what is a benign lesion (Rockwell et al. 1972; de Santos and Spjut 1981; Boriani et al. 1983). Radiological examination shows scalloping of the cortex related to the tumour with a well defined margin between tumour and bone, often peripheral lipping of the cortex, and associated calcification of the tumour. Light microscopy shows atypical chondrocytes with hyperchromatic nuclei and binucleate

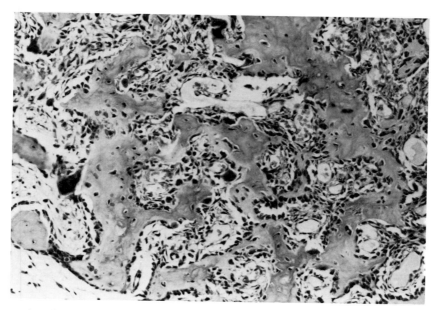

Fig. 9.16. High-power view of the nidus of an osteoid osteoma, showing vascular fibrous tissue containing irregular trabeculae of osteoid surrounded by osteoblasts. (H&E, × 400)

tion. The chief differences are the site, clinical presentation, radiological appearance, and changes in the surrounding bone. Reactive new bone is usually absent in relation to osteoblastomas.

The vertebrae, ilium, ribs and bones of the hand and foot are most commonly affected by osteoblastoma, and the patients are usually aged 10–35 years (Jaffe 1958; Lichtenstein 1965; Spjut et al. 1970). Three-quarters of the lesions in long bones were in the diaphysis in one series (McLeod et al. 1976). Some pain may be present but this is not as marked a feature as in osteoid osteoma. The radiological appearances lack specificity and may be mistaken for those of osteosarcoma, aneurysmal bone cyst, chondrosarcoma or osteoid osteoma (Pochaczevsky et al. 1960).

The lesions are usually over 1 cm in diameter, well circumscribed, and have a dark purple, red-grey or brown gritty cut surface. On histological examination the highly vascular osteoblastic stroma shows formation of osteoid and primitive bone, so that the tumour closely resembles osteoid osteoma (Jaffe 1958; Spjut et al. 1970). The existence of "malignant" or "aggressive" osteoblastoma has been suggested in recent years (Schajowicz and Lemos 1976; Revell and Scholtz 1979; Schajowicz 1983), and the question arises as to whether this is a separate entity or represents malignant transformation in a benign osteoblastoma (Dorfmann 1973; Merryweather et al. 1980). The whole question of the relationship between the various benign bone forming tumours has been

debated over recent years (Miyayama et al. 1993; Villanueva 1993).

The presence of cartilage in an apparent osteoblastoma raises the question of low-grade osteosarcoma in the view of some authors; others believe that this change occasionally occurs in osteoblastoma (Bertoni et al. 1993a, b).

Osteosarcoma (Osteogenic Sarcoma)

Osteosarcoma is a malignant tumour showing evidence of osteoid or bone formation by the tumour cells (Fig. 9.17). Most cases occur between the ages 10 and 20 years, and boys are affected more often than girls. Any bone can be affected but the metaphyseal ends of long bones (lower femur, upper tibia, upper femur and upper humerus) are the most frequently involved, especially in young patients (Table 9.9). The most common symptoms are pain and local swelling.

Radiological appearances usually include evidence of bone destruction, new bone formation in relation to cortical destruction, and subperiosteal new bone formation. These radiological appearances are often thought to be specific, but a large minority of cases have none of the characteristic features, and occasional cases have the appearances of a benign lesion.

Macroscopically, the tumour arises centrally and has usually penetrated the cortex and invaded soft tissues by presentation. The naked-eye appearances

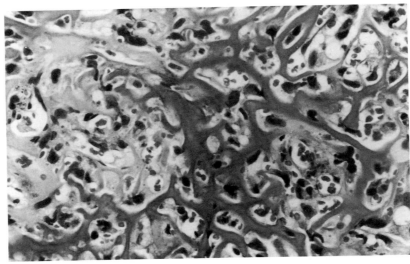

Fig. 9.17. Osteosarcoma, showing formation of osteoid trabeculae by pleomorphic osteoblastic tumour cells. (H&E, × 438)

Table 9.9 Site of involvement with osteosarcoma in five large series (percentage of cases)

	Hayles et al. (1960)[a]	Lindbom et al. (1961)	Weinfeld and Dudley (1962)	McKenna et al. (1966)	Dahlin and Coventry (1967)
Skull			1	<1	2
Jaw	2		7	5	
Vertebra	1		3		3
Sternum		3			
Clavicle	1	3		<1	<1
Ribs	1	2		2	2
Scapula		3		1	2
Humerus	10	13	11	13	11
Radius					1
Ulna		3	2	<1	<1
Wrist and hand		3			<1
Pelvis	4	5	5	3	9
Femur	58	39	45	52	46
Tibia	22	26	17	18	19
Fibula	1		4	3	6
Ankle and foot	1	2	1	1	1
Total number of cases	129	96	94	258	600

[a] Specifically children (aged <16 years)

vary with the amount of cartilaginous, fibrous or osseous tissue in the tumour. Some are highly vascular. The histological features are also variable, depending on the amount of tumour bone production, the pleomorphism of the tumour cells, and the extent to which fibrous, myxoid and cartilaginous elements are present (Spjut et al. 1970; Schajowicz et al. 1972). Classically, a malignant stroma of spindle-shaped and oval cells with variable numbers of mitoses and some multinucleate cells contains malignant osteoid or bone. The bone consists of islands of these osseous tissues surrounded by pleomorphic osteoblasts. Some tumours may contain vascular areas with numerous thin-walled vessels. Telangiectatic osteosarcoma having cystic spaces lined with anaplastic spindle cells has a poorer prognosis according to Matsuno et al. (1976). This is an unusual form of osteosarcoma, but important in that it may sometimes be confused with aneurysmal bone cyst (Ruiter et al. 1977; Revell 1986). Osteosarcomas may have large areas of malignant cartilage, foci with characteristics of malignant fibrous histiocytoma, epithelioid features, or small round-cell appearance (Unni and Dahlin 1989; Yoshida et al. 1992; Hasegawa et al. 1993; Kramer et al. 1993). The presence of low-grade tumours on the inside of the affected bone has recently been recognized (Kurt et al. 1990; Mirra et al. 1991; Bertoni et al. 1993). The lesions resembled parosteal osteosarcoma, fibrous dysplasia or desmoplastic fibroma, or had a mixed pattern. They recurred locally and in two of ten cases metastasized. Small-cell osteosarcoma has Ewing's-like lymphoma-like and spindle-celled histological patterns (Ayala et al. 1989).

Histochemical studies have demonstrated the presence of alkaline phosphatase in tumour cells (Jeffree and Price 1965), and if available, this method may help in the identification of osteosarcoma (Sanerkin 1980). Fine needle aspirate and cytological techniques are finding increased use in the diagnosis of bone tumours, including osteosarcoma (Kumar et al. 1993; Layfield et al. 1993).

Osteosarcoma metastasizes almost exclusively by the haematogenous route and 90% of cases die with secondary deposits in the lung. Metastases sometimes occur in other organs, other bones and lymph nodes.

Role of the Pathologist in the Diagnosis and Treatment of Osteosarcoma

The importance of accurate diagnosis in the management of bone tumours cannot be emphasized too highly, and the need to examine and discuss radiographs and clinical details with colleagues in these specialities has been stressed elsewhere (Spjut et al. 1970; Revell 1986). Recent changes in the management of osteosarcoma with the use of chemotherapy and limb-sparing surgery have added further responsibilities to the work of the histopathologist. Patients may have received a course of cytotoxic treatment before excision of the tumour, and it is now becoming important that the effects of this on tumour viability and morphology are assessed, so that changes in therapy can be made postoperatively if necessary. Details are available elsewhere (Rosen et al. 1982; Spjut and Ayala 1983; Ayala et al. 1984), and the effects of these methods of treatment are reviewed by Goorin et al. (1985).

Osteosarcoma Outside the Bone

A small percentage of osteosarcomas arise on the outside of the bone and may pose particular diagnostic problems. It is important to distinguish periosteal and parosteal osteosarcoma from each other and from conventional high-grade osteosarcoma occurring on the outside of the bone (Unni et al. 1976a, b; Campanacci et al. 1984; Wold et al. 1984). Periostal osteosarcomas are large fusiform or cauliflower-like projections, most commonly from the tibia or femur,

showing a predominantly lobulated chondrosarcomatous appearance on light microscopy, but with evidence of osteoid formation by malignant cells in areas (Unni et al. 1976b). Parosteal (juxtacortical) osteosarcomas are rare, affect adolescents or young adults, and are seen as dense lobulated masses on the outside of the metaphyseal part of a long bone. Macroscopically, these are hard osseous tumours, and histological examination shows a low-grade bone-forming sarcoma with irregular bone trabeculae covered by osteoblasts or spindle cells. Graduation from immature to more mature lesional bone is seen (Unni et al. 1976a; Campanucci et al. 1984). Confusion with myositis ossificans may occur radiologically, clinically and pathologically.

Ewing's Sarcoma

Ewing's sarcoma, an uncommon primary malignant bone tumour, arises in almost any bone, although the mid-shaft or metaphysis of the femur, humerus and tibia, the ilium and the ribs are the usual sites. Children and adolescents are most often affected, two-thirds of cases presenting before the age of 20 years (Dahlin et al. 1961; Spjut et al. 1970; Kissane et al. 1983). The radiological appearances are non-specific (see, e.g. Vohra 1967) and may be mistaken for those of osteosarcoma, chondrosarcoma, malignant lymphoma, osteomyelitis, or eosinophilic granuloma of bone. The presence of multiple layers of subperiosteal reactive new bone may give an "onion-skin" appearance.

Macroscopically, the tumour is situated in the medullary cavity, and is soft and grey-white in colour, with haemorrhagic areas sometimes present. On histological examination the tumour is found to be made up of small round cells (Figs. 9.18 and 9.19), which are larger than lymphocytes and present in sheets, cords and nests, characteristically, separated by fibrous septa. Diffuse lobular, filigree and pseudorosette patterns have been described by Kissane et al. (1983) (see Fig. 19.18). It is richly vascular and may show the presence of a rosette pattern due to the collection of tumour cells around vascular spaces. Recent immunohistochemical studies suggest a close relationship between Ewing's sarcoma and the neuroectodermally derived cells, so that these tumours are sometimes referred to now as primitive neuroectodermal tumours (PNET) of bone (Dehner 1993; Loizaga 1993; Shishikura et al. 1993). Neural markers (synaptophysin, neuron-specific enolase, glial fibrillary protein, neurofilament protein) and S100 are usually positive. The chief problems in the histological differential diagnosis are metastatic neuroblastoma, poorly differentiated lymphoma and

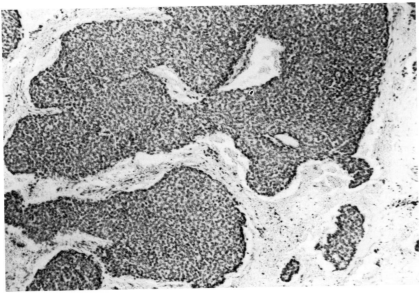

Fig. 9.18. Replacement of the bone marrow by sheets of small round cells in Ewing's sarcoma. The aggregates of tumour cells are separated by fibrovascular septa, giving a "lobular" pattern. (H&E, × 80)

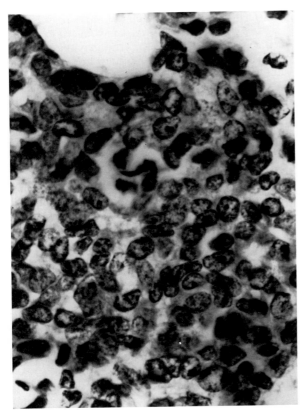

Fig. 9.19. High-power view of Ewing's sarcoma, showing cells with indistinct cytoplasmic outlines and well-defined nuclear membranes. (H&E, × 1500)

metastatic carcinoma, notably oat-cell carcinoma, although this usually occurs in a much older age group (Spjut et al. 1970).

Careful attention to the clinical details, especially the possible presence of an adrenal mass, is required in the differential diagnosis of neuroblastoma and Ewing's sarcoma. The determination of levels of catecholamine metabolites is a useful discriminant (Gitlow et al. 1970) and should be recommended to clinicians. The formation of rosettes in neuroblastoma is often quoted as a feature (e.g. Spjut et al. 1970). This may be true of primary neuroblastoma, but metastatic tumour is not likely to show this appearance (Jaffe 1958). The presence of glycogen granules in the cells of Ewing's sarcoma has been demonstrated by Schajowicz (1959) by light microscopy, and confirmed in an ultrastructural study by Friedman and Gold (1968). The demonstration of glycogen granules by electron microscopy is of limited value according to Llombart-Bosch et al. (1978). Malignant lymphoma of bone contains no glycogen (Schajowicz 1959) and there are PAS-positive granules present in neuroblastomas (Spjut et al. 1970). Llombart-Bosch et al. (1978) describe the ultrastructural features of Ewing's sarcoma and discuss the differentiation from reticulum-cell sarcoma and other round-cell sarcomas. Differentiation of Ewing's sarcoma from lymphoblastic lymphoma may be difficult. Lennert (1978) states that Ewing's sarcoma and metastatic neuroblastoma show cells tightly packed together, whereas the cells of lymphoblastic lymphoma of convoluted-cell type (see Chapter 11) are isolated from one another. Lymphoblastic lymphoma of Burkitt type may also be present in bone marrow. Convoluted-cell lymphoblastic lymphomas shows the presence of a diastase-resistant PAS-positive reaction in a single clumped pattern in the cytoplasm of tumour cells. The cells of Burkitt-type lymphoblastic lymphoma are not PAS-positive (Lennert 1978). Immunohistochemical staining using monoclonal antibodies that react with different lymphocyte populations, neuroblastoma and neuroectodermal-associated antigen promises to be a useful tool in discriminating between round-cell tumours of bone (Sugimoto et al. 1985).

More than a quarter of patients with Ewing's sarcoma have metastases at the time of presentation. Common sites are other bones (especially the skull), the lungs, lymph nodes and other viscera. Cases with soft tissue extension at the primary site have metastatic disease at the time of presentation more often than those with tumour confined to bone (Mendenhall et al. 1983).

Rarely, the tumour may present as an extraskeletal lesion.

Primary Malignant Lymphoma

Malignant lymphoma primarily affecting bone is a rare occurrence in childhood, especially under the age of 10 years. The classification of malignant lymphoma has changed over recent years and may do so again as more precise immunological methods are applied to the characterization of lymphoid cell populations. Reticulum cell sarcoma of bone in the old literature is probably synonymous with the poorly differentiated high-grade lymphomas.

Primary lymphoma of bone is a focally destructive tumour on radiological examination, although sometimes it may show sclerotic lesions (Sweet et al. 1981; Spagnoli et al. 1982). The femur, tibia, pelvis and humerus are the most common sites (Spjut and Ayala 1983), and the tumour has a homogeneous grey or reddish-grey appearance on naked-eye examination. Malignant lymphomas in bone have similar histological appearances to those occurring in lymph nodes. Primary skeletal involvement with Hodgkin's disease is rare. The major problem is the differentiation of bone lymphoma from other rounded-cell tumours of bone. This is aided by the use of stains for glycogen, enzyme histochemistry, immunohistochemistry and electron microscopy. For further details of the lymphoreticular neoplasms see Chapter 11 (p. 647).

Leukaemia

Most children with acute leukaemia have radiographic bone changes. Leukaemic infiltration results in a rounded osteolytic lesion seen on radiographs, and failure of normal bone formation with radiolucent lines near the epiphyses. There may be large areas of bone necrosis (Thomas et al. 1961).

Other Tumours of Bone

Other tumours of bone occurring in childhood are either themselves rare or uncommon in the younger patient. Fewer than 3% of adamantinomas of long bones have occurred in children less than 10 years old, and about 20% of these tumours present before 20 years of age. The most commonly involved bone is the tibia, and an association with fibrous dysplasia has been noted. Histological examination shows a tumour with squamoid, basaloid, angiomatoid and spindle-celled features present in varying degrees.

The vascular tumours are unusual in children, mainly situated in the skull or spine, and histologically like haemangiomas elsewhere in the soft tissues or skin. Most are cavernous haemangiomas (Dorfmann et al. 1971). Bone is lost in relation to the vascular spaces in these lesions. Massive osteolysis occurs in "disappearing bone disease", which presents in childhood and adolescence in most cases. The affected bone progressively disappears on radiological examination, whereas histology shows the features of a haemangioma and fibrous tissue replacement of bone. Angiosarcomas occasionally occur in the bones of children.

Giant-cell tumour (osteoclastoma) most affects patients aged 20–55 years, and only about 10% of all cases occur under the age of 10 years (Spjut and Ayala 1983). Most giant-cell tumours are located in the epiphyseal region of long bones, and although there are no specific radiological features, an eccentrically placed lytic lesion lacking a sclerotic margin is suggestive. The naked-eye appearance is heterogeneous, with solid yellow areas, grey-red vascular tissue and cystic or necrotic areas. There may be a pathological fracture. Numerous oval or spindle-shaped cells with interspersed osteoclast giant cells are seen on histological examination. The picture may be complicated by secondary changes, such as repair reaction in response to a pathological fracture. Care is required in excluding other giant-cell lesions before making a diagnosis of giant-cell tumour in a child. Non-ossifying fibroma, chondroblastoma, chondromyxoid fibroma, giant-cell reparative granuloma, aneurysmal bone cyst and brown tumour of hyperparathyroidism are among the lesions that may be confused with a giant-cell tumour.

Tumour-like Conditions

Histiocytic Disorders

The histiocytic disorders are non-neoplastic conditions characterized by the abnormal proliferation of the monocyte-macrophage (histiocyte) series. The histiocytic disorders have been reviewed by Cline and Golde (1973), Bokkerink and de Vaan (1980) and Favara et al. (1983). They include Letterer–Siwe disease, Hand–Schüller–Christian disease and eosinophilic granuloma, and are sometimes collectively known as "histiocytosis X". Bone lesions are a prominent feature of over three-quarters of cases of histiocytosis X. The skull and pelvis are the most frequently involved sites, followed by the femur, ribs, humerus, vertebrae and tibia. It will be noted that these are the bones in which there is haemopoietic tissue.

The unifying aspect of this group of disorders is the presence of histiocytes with no cytological features of malignancy, intermingled with variable numbers of eosinophils, giant cells, neutrophils, foamy macrophages and areas of fibrosis.The histiocytes contain intracytoplasmic granules of a characteristic appearance and similar to those seen in Langerhans' cells of the skin (Basset et al. 1972). The ultrastructural appearances have recently been described by Corrin and Basset (1979) and the enzyme histochemistry of the cells by Elema and Poppema (1978).

Letterer–Siwe Disease. Most cases of Letterer–Siwe disease present in infancy or early childhood (up to the age of 2 years), and occasional congenital cases have been described. Most affected infants die within weeks or months of onset; a few survive for 1 or 2 years. The clinical features are those of a febrile illness with a skin rash, hepatosplenomegaly, lymphadenopathy, a bleeding diathesis with purpura and "tumours" of bones. These tumours are destructive lesions present especially in the calvaria, mandible and basisphenoid regions of the skull.

The basic pathological finding is one of generalized increases in non-lipid-containing macrophages in the many affected organs, either as nodules or diffusely. Small numbers of lymphocytes, plasma cells and eosinophils are intermingled with the histiocytes. The histiocytes may contain phagocytosed material, including red cells or haemosiderin. Longstanding lesions may have fibrous scarring and foamy histio-

cytes resembling those seen in Hand–Schüller–Christian disease.

Hand–Schüller–Christian Disease. This is a rare histiocytic disorder of childhood, the great majority of cases occurring in the age group 4–10 years. In its classic form it comprises the triad of diabetes insipidus, exophthalmos and defects in bone, notably of the skull, but it is rare for all these features to be present in a single case. Radiologically, the common sites of the osteolytic lesions are the calvaria, petrous and mastoid bones, mandible and maxilla.

The histological features differ from those of Letterer–Siwe disease, although there is some similarity. The lesions consist of focal accumulations of histiocytes (Fig. 9.20), many with a foamy cytoplasm, and collagenous fibrous tissue. Some lymphocytes, plasma cells, neutrophils and eosinophils may be present.

Eosinophilic Granuloma. This bone lesion generally presents before the age of 10 years, usually as a single focus, but multifocal changes are not rare. Almost any bone can be affected, and common sites are:

1. Calvaria
2. Frontal and parietal bones
3. Mandible
4. Humerus
5. Proximal metaphysis of femur
6. Ribs
7. Pelvis
8. Vertebrae

The lesion nearly always occurs in the shaft when present in a long bone. Epiphyseal involvement is very rare (Ochsner 1966). Vertebral involvement may lead to collapse of vertebral bodies into a wedge-shape. Multifocal disease suggests an overlap with Hand–Schüller–Christian disease. The lesions are osteolytic on radiological examination and may be round and confined to the bone (e.g. in a long bone). There may be clinical and radiographic confusion with osteomyelitis and Ewing's sarcoma (Spjut et al. 1970).

The findings on histological examination are variable and depend on the age of the lesion, the presence of repair reactions, and whether there has been pathological fracture. In a typical case there are sheets of large histiocytes with which eosinophils and multinucleate giant cells are mixed (Fig. 9.21). The histiocytes have large single or double nuclei, and many contain phagocytosed red or white cells. Variable numbers of neutrophils, lymphocytes and plasma cells may be present. When there are few eosinophils

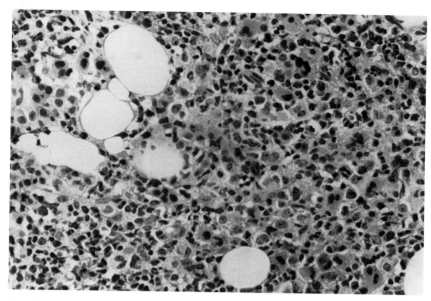

Fig. 9.20. Osteolytic lesion from the ilium comprising mainly histiocytes with small numbers of lymphocytes, neutrophils and eosinophils. Hand–Schüller–Christian disease (histiocytosis X). (H&E, × 1000)

and the histiocytes predominate, appearances may resemble those of Hodgkin's disease.

Other Histiocytic Disorders. There is a variety of other disorders affecting histiocytes, which it is not appropriate to describe in detail here. The reader is referred to Chapter 11. Recent references to these disorders, which include Langerhans' cell histiocytosis, haemophagocytic syndromes, Rosai–Dorfman disease, juvenile xanthogranuloma, multicentric reticulohistiocytosis and malignant histiocytosis, can be found in the articles by Kenik et al. (1990), Russo and

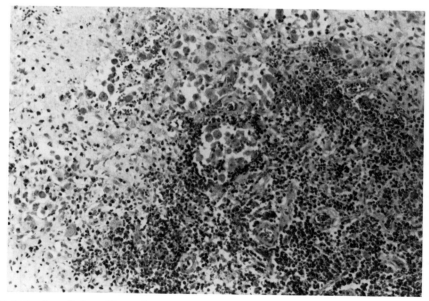

Fig. 9.21. Osteolytic lesion from the frontal bone of an 18-year-old male presenting with a palpable mass. There are numerous large histiocytes intermingled with eosinophils, some lymphocytes and neutrophils. Eosinophilic granuloma (histiocytosis X). (H&E, × 400)

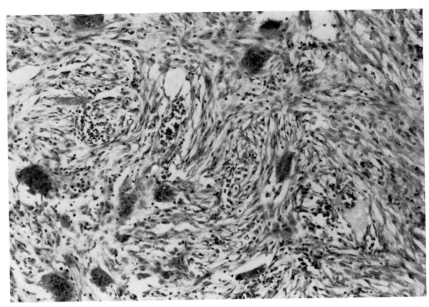

Fig. 9.22. Metaphyseal fibrous defect from the lower end of the radius of a 12-year-old girl, showing a whorled pattern of fibrous tissue and giant cells. (H&E, × 400)

Seidman (1990), Kodet et al. (1991) and Malone (1991). These disorders do not normally affect bone to any extent.

Fibrous and Cystic Defects

Metaphyseal Fibrous Defect (Non-ossifying Fibroma)

Metaphyseal fibrous defect is a non-neoplastic lesion occurring in the metaphyseal region of long bones of growing children and adolescents, the lower end of the femur or either end of the tibia being commonly affected. There may be pain or pathological fracture at presentation, but the lesions are often entirely asymptomatic. Selby (1961) found such fibrous cortical defects in 27% of apparently normal children.

Metaphyseal fibrous defects take the form of well localized osteolytic areas in the cortex or marrow space, containing fibrous tissue with a whorled appearance, multinucleate giant cells (Fig. 9.22), foamy macrophages and haemosiderin pigment. The giant cells are widely scattered or may be present in small nests. The lesion has sometimes been confused with giant-cell tumour of bone (Spjut et al. 1970). The interlacing and whorled pattern of the stroma is a helpful feature in this differential diagnosis.

Fibrous cortical defect is a small asymptomatic lesion confined to the cortex of the bone in the region of the metaphysis. Non-ossifying fibroma is considered by Jaffe (1958) to represent a more advanced form of this lesion, which is no longer confined to the cortex.

Fibrous Dysplasia

Fibrous dysplasia is a benign, relatively uncommon abnormality of unknown aetiology made up of fibrous tissue with a characteristic whorled pattern, which contains trabeculae of immature woven non-lamellar bone (Fig. 9.23). These islands of bone usually lack osteoblasts at the surface, and typically are formed into C and O shapes. Presentation is in childhood or adolescence; the condition can be monostotic or polyostotic, and is one of the commonest benign lesions of the ribs. The femur, tibia and facial skeleton are also often affected. Dysplastic lesions at the base of the skull or in the jaw are sometimes classified as ossifying fibromas, osteoid fibromas or fibro-osteomas. They are regarded as variants of fibrous dysplasia by Dahlin (1978). Radiological examination reveals a characteristic "ground glass" appearance.

Polyostotic lesions, which are predominantly unilateral, when combined with cutaneous pigmentation and, in girls, precocious puberty, form the complex known as Albright's syndrome (Albright et al. 1938; Harris et al. 1962). Osteogenic sarcoma developed in

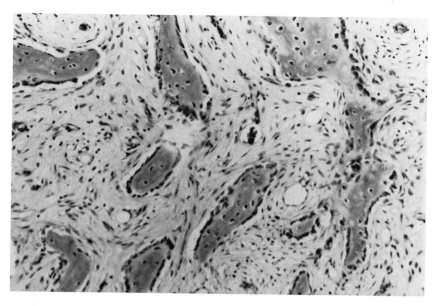

Fig. 9.23. Slowly growing lesion from the mandible of a 7-year-old male showing the presence of immature osseous trabeculae in fibrous tissue. The trabeculae show the presence of appositional osteoblasts. Fibro-osseous dysplasia (ossifying fibroma). (H&E, × 400)

one of the cases of Harris et al. The present author has seen one similar case.

Solitary Bone Cyst (Simple or Unicameral Bone Cyst)

Solitary bone cysts are benign and occur in children and adolescents, affecting boys three times more frequently than girls (Bosecker et al. 1968). They consist of a fluid-filled cavity most frequently situated in the metaphysis at the upper end of the humerus or femur, abutting the epiphyseal plate in many cases. Distal long bones are also sometimes affected. Fractures are present in approximately two-thirds of cases where the long bones are involved. Radiological examination is essential in the diagnosis of solitary bone cyst (Lodwick 1958).

The cyst is lined with loose vascular connective tissue, which forms a membrane of variable thickness and may contain giant cells, osteoid and bone trabeculae. Most of these cysts contain some granulation tissue and show evidence of previous haemorrhage, fibrin, calcified material and cholesterol clefts (Spjut et al. 1970; Schajowicz et al. 1972).

Aneurysmal Bone Cyst

Aneurysmal bone cyst usually presents in patients under 30 years of age and involves the metaphyseal region of long bones and the vertebral column, but involvement of almost all bones has been described. The distribution of lesions in one large series is shown in Table 9.10. It is an eccentrically placed osteolytic lesion consisting of blood-filled spaces of variable size outlined by fibrous septa containing osteoid, bone trabeculae or osteoclastic cells in granulation tissue. Parts of an aneurysmal small bone cyst may be solid, and the presence of osteoid may give rise to confusion with telangiectatic osteosarcoma. Differentiation from a giant-cell tumour of bone may be difficult or impossible, especially where curettings are submitted for a histological opinion. As with other bone tumours, the examination of adequate biopsy material and careful review of clinical and radiological features are essential for a correct diagnosis (Reed and Rothenberg 1964; Spjut et al. 1970; Dahlin 1978).

Over recent years, the concept of "solid" aneurysmal bone cyst has gained acceptance. Such lesions

Table 9.10. Distibution of aneurysmal bone cyst in 193 cases

	%
Lower limb	53
Vertebrae	27
Upper limb	18
Thorax	9
Pelvis	7
Skull and mandible	3

Data from Dabska and Buraczewski (1969).

have a spindle-celled stroma, giant cells and variable amounts of bone production, fibromyxoid areas and small aneurysmal spaces. Some authors consider them to be giant-cell reparative granulomas occurring in sites other than the jaw. They have been described in children as well as adults, and occur in the axial skeleton or long bones (Edel et al. 1992; Oda et al. 1992; Bertoni et al. 1993c).

References

Acheson RM (1957) The Oxford method of assessing skeletal maturity. Clin Orthop 10: 19

Ackermann R, Runne U, Klenk W, Dienst C (1980) Erythema Chronicum Migrans mit Arthritis. Dtsch Med Wochenschr 105: 1779

Adeyokunna AA, Hendrickse RG (1980) Salmonella osteomyelitis in childhood. A report of 63 cases seen in Nigeria of whom 57 had sickle cell anaemia. Arch Dis Child 55: 175

Albright F, Scoville B, Sulkowitch HW (1938) Syndrome characterized by osteitis fibrosa disseminata, areas of pigmentation and a gonadal dysfunction. Further observations including the report of two more cases. Endocrinology 22: 411.

Allen BL, Ferguson RL (1985) Topics of interest in pediatric orthopaedics. Pediatr Clin North Am 32: 1333

American Rheumatism Association (1977) [Proceedings of a symposium devoted to pediatric rheumatology]. Arthritis Rheum 20/2: [Suppl]

Ayala AG, Raymond AK, Jaffe N (1984) The pathologist's role in the diagnosis and treatment of osteosarcoma in children. Hum Pathol 15: 258

Ayala Ali, Ro JY, Raymond AK, Jaffe N, Chawla S, Carrasco H, Link M, Jimenez J, Edeiken J, Wallace S et al. (1989) Small cell osteosarcoma. A clinicopathologic study of 27 cases. Cancer 64: 2162

Ballet JP, Griscelli C, Coutris G, Milhaud G, Maroteaux P (1977) Bone marrow transplantation in osteopetrosis. Lancet ii: 1137

Barsh GS, Roush CL, Bonadio J, Byers PH, Gelinas RE (1985) Intron-mediated recombination may cause a deletion in an α_1 type I collagen chain in a lethal form of osteogenesis imperfecta. Proc Natl Acad Sci USA 82: 2870

Basset F, Escaig J, Le Crom M (1972) A cytoplasmic membranous complex in histiocytosis X. Cancer 29: 1380

Beighton P, Giedion A, Gorlin R, Hall J, Horton B, Kozlowski R, Lachman R, Langer LO, Maroteaux P, Poznanski A, Rimoin DL, Sillence D, Spranger J (1992) International classification of osteochondrodysplasias. Am J Med Genet 44 : 223

Beighton P (1978) Inherited disorders of the skeleton. Churchill Livingstone, Edinburgh (Genetics in medicine and surgery series)

Beighton P, Cremin BJ (1980) Sclerosing bone dysplasias. Springer, New York

Beighton P, Cremin B, Faure C, Finidor G, Giedion A, Jequier S, Kaufmann H, Labrune M, Lenzi L, Maroteaux P, Poznanski A, Spranger J, Sauvegrain J, Stanescu R, Stanescu V (1983a) International Nomenclature of Constitutional Diseases of Bone. Ann Radiol (Paris) 26: 457

Beighton P, Spranger, J, Versveld G (1983b) Skeletal complications in osteogenesis imperfecta. A review of 153 South African patients. S Afr Med J 64: 565

Berry CL (1978) Drugs and the developing skeleton. Invest Cell Pathol 1: 129

Bertoni F, Unni KK, Lucas DR, McLeod RA (1993a) Osteoblastoma with cartilaginous matrix. An unusual morphologic presentation in 18 cases. Am J Surg Pathol 17: 69

Bertoni F, Bacchini P, Fabbri N, Mercuri M, Picci P, Ruggieri P, Campanacci M (1993b) Osteosarcoma. Low-grade intraosseous-type osteosarcoma histologically resembling parosteal osteosarcoma, fibrous dysplasia and desmoplastic fibroma. Cancer 71: 338

Bertoni F, Bacchini P, Capanna R, Ruggieri P, Biagini R, Ferruzzi A, Betelli G, Picci P, Campanacci M (1993c) Solid variant of aneurysmal bone cyst. Cancer 71: 729

Bokkerink JPM, de Vaan GAM (1980) Histiocytosis X. Eur J Pediatr 135: 129

Bonucci E, Sartori E, Spina M (1975) Osteopetrosis fetalis. Report on a case with special reference to the ultrastructure. Virchows Arch A Pathol Anat 368: 109

Boriani S, Bruhimi P, Bertoni F, Campanacci M (1983) Periosteal chondroma. A review of twenty cases. J Bone Joint Surg [Am] 65: 205

Bosecker EH, Bickel WH, Dahlin DC (1968) A clinicopathologic study of simple unicameral bone cysts. Surg Gynecol Obstet 127: 550

Boyer DW, Mickelson MR, Ponseti IV (1981) Slipped capital femoral epiphysis. Long-term follow-up study of 121 patients. J Bone Jt Surg [Am] 63:85

Breider MA, Shull RM, Constantopoulos G (1989) Long-term effects of bone marrow transplantation in dogs with mucopolysaccharidosis. I. Am J Pathol 134: 677

Bretlau P, Jorgenson MB, Johansen H (1970) Osteogenesis imperfecta: light and electron microscopic studies of the stapes. Acta Otolaryngol 69:172

Briner J, Giedion A, Spycher MA (1991) Variation of quantitative and qualitative changes of enchondral ossification in heterozygous achondroplasia. Pathol Res Pract 187: 271

Bullough PG, Davidson D, Lorenzo J (1981) The morbid anatomy of the skeleton in osteogenesis imperfecta. Clin Orthop Rel Res 159:42

Burgdorfer W, Barbour AG, Hayes SF, Benach JL, Grunwaldt E, Davis JP (1982) Lyme disease – a tick-borne spirochetosis? Science 216: 1317

Byers PD (1968) Solitary benign osteoblastic lesions of bone. Osteoid osteoma and benign osteoblastoma. Cancer 22:43

Cabane J, Michon A, Ziza JM, Bourgeonis P, Bietry O, Godeau P, Kahn MF (1990) Comparison of long term evolution of adult onset and juvenile onset Still's disease, both followed up for more than 10 years. An Rheum Dis 49: 283

Campanacci M, Picci P, Gherlinzoni F, Guerra A, Bertoni F, Neff JR (1984) Parosteal osteosarcoma. J Bone Joint Surg [Br] 66:313

Campbell CJ, Papademetriou T, Bonfiglio M (1968) Melorheostosis: a report of the clinical, roentgenographic and pathological findings in 14 cases. J Bone Joint Surg [Am] 50: 1281

Cannon Sr, Sweetnam DR (1985) Multiple chondrosarcomas in dyschondroplasia (Ollier's disease). Cancer 55: 580

Caswell AM, Whyte MP, Russell RG (1991) Hypophosphatasia and the extracellular metabolism of inorganic pyrophosphate: clinical and laboratory aspects. Crit Rev Clin Lab Sci 28: 175

Catterall A (1984) What is congenital dislocation of the hip? J Bone Joint Surg [Br] 66: 469

Chung SMK, Ralston EL (1969) Necrosis of the femoral head associated with sickle cell anaemia and its genetic variants. J Bone Joint Surg [Am] 51: 33

Cline MJ, Golde DW (1973) A review of re-evaluation of the histiocytic disorders. Am J Med 55: 49

Coccia PF, Krivit W, Cervenka J, Clawson C, Kersey JH, Kim TH, Nesbit ME, Ramsay NKC, Warkentin PI, Teitelbaum SL, Kahn AJ, Brown DM (1980) Successful bone-marrow transplantation for infantile malignant osteopetrosis. N Engl J Med 302: 701

Cole ARC, Darte JMM (1963) Osteochondromata following irradiation in children. Pediatrics 32: 285

Collins DH (1966) Pathology of bone. Butterworths, London

Cooperman DR, Charles LM, Pathria M, Latimer B, Thompson GH (1992) Post-mortem description of slipped capital femoral epiphysis. J Bone Joint Surg [Br] 74: 595

Corrin B, Basset F (1979) A review of histiocytosis X with particular reference to eosinophilic granuloma of the lung. Invest Cell Pathol 2: 137

Cremin BJ, Beighton P (1978) Bone dysplasias of infancy. A radiological atlas. Springer, New York

Cremin BJ, Davey H, Goldblatt J (1990) Skeletal complications of type I Gaucher disease; the magnetic resonance features. Clin Radiol 41: 244

Croft P, Cooper C, Wickham C, Coggon D (1991) Osteoarthritis of the hip and acetabular dysplasia. Ann Rheum Dis 50: 308

Dabska M, Buraczewski J (1969) Aneurysmal bone cyst. Pathology, clinical course and radiologic appearances. Cancer 23: 371

Dahlin DC (1967) Chondromyxoid fibroma. In: Bone tumours, 2nd edn. Thomas, Springfield

Dahlin DC (1978) Bone tumours, 3rd edn. Thomas, Springfield

Dahlin DC, Coventry MB (1967) Osteogenic sarcoma. A study of six hundred cases. J Bone Joint Surg [Am] 49: 101

Dahlin DC, Coventry MB, Scanlon PW (1961) Ewing's sarcoma. A critical analysis of 165 cases. J Bone Joint Surg [Am] 43: 185

Dan M (1984) Septic arthritis in young infants: clinical and microbiological correlations and therapeutic implications. Rev Infect Dis 6: 147

de Santos LA, Spjut HJ (1981) Periosteal chondroma: a radiographic spectrum. Skeletal Radiol 6: 15

DeGasperi R, Alroy J, Richard R, Goyal V, Orgad U, Lee RE, Warren CD (1990) Glycoprotein storage in Gaucher disease: lectin histochemistry and biochemical studies. Lab Invest 63: 385

Dehner LP (1993) Primitive neuroectodermal tumor and Ewing's sarcoma. Am J Surg Pathol 17:1

Dorfmann HD (1973) Malignant transformation of benign bone lesions. Proc Natl Cancer Conf 7: 901

Dorfmann HD, Steiner GC, Jaffe HL (1971) Vascular tumours of bone. Hum Pathol 2: 349

Doty SB, Matthews RS (1971) Electron microscopic and histochemical investigation of osteogenesis imperfecta tarda. Clin Orthop 80: 191

Dumontier C, Rigault P, Padovani JP, Touzet P, Finidori G, Mallet JF (1989) Tumeurs cartilagineuses de l'enfant. Chir Pediatr 30: 91

Edel G, Ueda Y, Nakanishi J, Brinker KH, Roessner A, Blasius S, Vestring T, Muller-Miny H, Erlemann R, Wuisman P (1992) Chondroblastoma of bone. A clinical, radiological, light and immunohistochemical study. Virchows Arch A Pathol Anat Histopathol 421: 355

Edel G, Roessner A, Blasius S, Erlemann R (1992) "Solid" variant of aneurysmal bone cyst. Pathol Res Pract 188: 791

Elema JD, Poppema S (1978) Infantile histiocytosis X (Letterer-Siwe disease). Investigation with enzyme histochemical and sheep erythrocyte rosetting techniques. Cancer 42: 555

Ellis RWB, van Creveld S (1940) A syndrome characterised by ectodermal dysplasia, polydactyly, chondroplasia and congenital morbus cardis. Arch Dis Child 15: 65

Elmore SM (1967) Pycnodysostosis: a review. J Bone Joint Surg [Am] 49: 153

Epps CH, Bryant DD, Colers J, Castro O (1991) Osteomyelitis in patients who have sickle-cell disease. Diagnosis and treatment. J Bone Joint Surg [Am] 73: 1281

Falvo KA, Bullough PG (1973) Osteogenesis imperfecta: a histometric analysis. J Bone Joint Surg [Am] 55: 275

Favara BE, McCarthy RC, Mierau GW (1983) Histiocytosis X.

Hum Pathol 14: 663

Felton DJC, Stone WD (1966) Osteomalacia in African immigrants during pregnancy. Br Med J i: 1521

Ferguson AB (1985) Segmental vascular changes in the femoral head in children and adults. Clin Orthop 200: 291

Fink CW, Dick VQ, Howard J, Nelson JD (1977) Infection of bone and joints in children. Arthritis Rheum 20 [Suppl 2]: 578

Flecker H (1942) The time of appearance and fusion of ossification centres as observed by roentgenographic methods. Am J Roentgenol 47: 97

Francis CC (1940) The appearance of centres of ossification from 6 to 15 years. Am J Phys Anthropol 27: 127

Francis CC, Werle PP (1939) The appearance of centres of ossification from birth to 5 years. Am J Phys Anthropol 24: 273

Friedman AB, Gold H (1968) Ultrastructure of Ewing's sarcoma of bone. Cancer 22: 307

Gazit D, Tieder M, Liberman UA, Passi-Even L, Bab IA (1991) Osteomalacia in hereditary hypophosphatemic rickets with hypercalciuria; a correlative clinical–histomorphometric study. J Clin Endocrinol Metab 72: 229

Gilbert EF, Yang SS, Langer L, Opitz JM, Roskamp JO, Heidelberger KP (1987) Pathologic changes of osteochondrodysplasia in infancy. In: Rosen PP, Fechner RE (eds) Pathology annual, part 2. Appleton and Lange, Connecticut

Gitlow SE, Bertani LM, Rausen A, Gribetz O, Dziedzig SW (1970) Diagnosis of neuroblastoma by qualitative and quantitative determination of catecholamine metabolites in urine. Cancer 25: 1377

Goorin AM, Abelson HT, Frei E (1985) Osteosarcoma: 15 years later. N Engl J Med 313: 1637

Gorodischer R, Davidson RG, Mosovich LL, Yaffe SJ (1976) Hypophosphatasia: a developmental anomaly of alkaline phosphatase? Pediatr Res 10: 650

Green AE, Ellswood WH, Collins JR (1962) Melorheostosis and osteopoikilosis: with review of literature. Am J Roentgenol Radium Ther Nucl Med 87: 1096

Harris WH, Dudley GR, Barry RJ (1962) The natural history of fibrous dysplasia. An orthopedic, pathological and roentgeographic study. J Bone Joint Surg [Am] 44: 207

Hasegawa T, Shibata T, Hirose T, Seki K, Hizaura K (1993) Osteosarcoma with epithelioid features. An immunohistochemical study. Arch Pathol Lab Med 117: 295

Hass J (1951) Congenital dislocation of the hip. Thomas, Springfield

Hayles AB, Dahlin DC, Coventry MB (1960) Osteogenic sarcoma in children. JAMA 174: 1174

Hillman LS, Haddad JG (1975) Perinatal vitamins D metabolism. II. Serial 25-hydroxy-vitamin D concentrations in the sera of full term and premature infants. J Pediatr 86: 928

Hodson P, Goldblatt J, Beighton P (1979) Non-neuropathic Gaucher disease presenting in childhood. Arch Dis Child 54: 707

Horev G, Kornreich L, Hadar H, Katz K (1991) Hemorrhage associated with "bone crisis" in Gaucher's disease identified by magnetic resonance imaging. Skeletal Radiol 20: 479

Huvos AG (1979) Bone tumours: diagnosis, treatment and prognosis. Saunders, Philadelphia

Hwang WS, Tock EPC, Tan KL, Tan LKA (1979) The pathology of cartilage in chondrodysplasias. J Pathol 127: 11

Iancu TC (1992) The ultrastructural spectrum of lysosomal storage diseases. Ultrastruct Pathol 16: 231

Ibsen KH (1967) Distinct varieties of osteogenesis imperfecta. Clin Orthop 50: 279

Ippolito E, Bellocci M, Farsetti P, Tudiso C, Perugia D (1989) An ultrastructural study of slipped capital femoral epiphysis: pathogenetic considerations. J Orthop Res 7: 252

Jaffe HL (1958) Tumors and tumorous conditions of the bones and joints. Lea and Febiger, Philadelphia

Jaffe HL (1972) Metabolic, degenerative and inflammatory diseases of bones and joints. Lea and Febiger, Philadelphia

Jaffe HL, Lichtenstein L (1948) Chondromyxoid fibroma of bone. A distinctive benign tumor likely to be mistaken especially for chondrosarcoma. Arch Pathol 45: 541

Jeffree GM, Price CHG (1965) Bone tumours and their enzymes. A study of the phosphatases, non-specific esterases and beta-glucuronidase of osteogenic and cartilaginous tumours, fibroblastic and giant cell lesions. J Bone Joint Surg [Br] 47: 120

Johnston YE, Duray PH, Steere AC, Kashgarian M, Buza J, Malawista SE et al. (1985) Lyme arthritis. Spirochetes found in synovial microangiopathic lesions. Am J Pathol 118: 26

Jones CP, Cummings C, Ball J, Beighton P (1984) Collagen defect of bone in osteogenesis imperfecta (type I). An electron microscopic study. Clin Orthop 183: 208

Kenik GJ, Fok E, Huerter CJ, Hurley JA, Stanosheck JF (1990) Multicentric reticulohistiocytosis in a patient with malignant melanoma: a response to cyclophosphamide and a unique cutaneous feature. Arthritis Rheum 33: 1047

King JD, Bobechko WP (1971) Osteogenesis imperfecta. An orthopaedic description and surgical review. J Bone Joint Surg [Br] 53: 72

Kissane JM, Askin FB, Foulkes M, Stratton JB, Faulkner Shirley S (1983) Erwing's sarcoma of bone: clinicopathologic aspects of 303 cases from the intergroup Ewing's sarcoma study. Hum Pathol 14: 773

Kodet R, Elleder M, DeWolf-Peeters C, Mottl H (1991) Congenital histiocytosis. A heterogeneous group of diseases, one presenting as so-called congenital self healing histiocytosis. Pathol Res Pract 187: 458

Kramer K, Hicks DG, Palis J, Rosier RN, Oppenheimer J, Fallon MD, Cohen HJ (1993) Epithelioid osteosarcoma of bone. Immunocytochemical evidence suggesting divergent epithelial and mesenchymal differentiation in a primary osseous neoplasm. Cancer 71: 2977

Kumar RV, Rao CR, Hazarika D, Mukherjee G, Gowda BM (1993) Aspiration cytology of primary bone lesions. Acta Cytol 37: 83

Kurt AM, Unni KK, McLeod RA, Pritchard DJ (1990) Low-grade intraosseous osteosarcoma. Cancer 65: 1418

Layfield LJ, Armstrong K, Zaleski S, Eckardt J (1993) Diagnostic accuracy and clinical utility of fine needle aspiration cytology in the diagnosis of clinically primary bone lesions. Diagn Cytopathol 9: 168

Lehman HW, Nerlich A, Brenner RE, Bodo M, Muller PK (1992) Hyperplastic callus formation in osteogenesis imperfecta. Eur J Pediatr Surg 2: 281

Lennert K (1978) Malignant lymphomas. Springer, New York

Levin ME, Boisseau V, Avioli LV (1976) Effect of diabetes melitus on bone mass in juvenile and adult-onset diabetes. N Engl J Med 294: 241

Lichtenstein L (1965) Bone tumors, 3rd edn. Mosby, St Louis

Lindbom A, Söderberg G, Spjut HT (1961) Osteogenic sarcoma. A review of 96 cases. Acta Radiol 56: 1

Llombart-Bosch A, Blache R, Pedro-Olaya A (1978) Ultrastructural study of 28 cases of Ewing's sarcoma. Cancer 41: 1362

Lodwick GS (1958) Juvenile unicameral bone cyst. A roentgen reappraisal. AJR Am J Roentgenol 80: 495

Loizaga JM (1993) What's new in Ewing's tumour? Pathol Res Pract 189: 616

Loutit JF, Nesbit NW (1979) Resorption of bone.Lancet ii: 26

Maassen AP (1952) The effect of desoxycorticosterone acetate (Doca) on body growth and ossification. Acta Endocrinol (Copenh) 9: 291

Macfarlane JD, Kroon HM, van der Harten JJ (1992) Phenotypically dissimilar hypophosphatasia in two sibships. Am J Med Genet 42: 117

Malone M (1991) The histiocytosis of childhood. Histopathology 19: 105

Mankin H (1990) Rickets, osteomalacia, and renal osteodystrophy. An update. Orthop Clin North Am 21: 81

Marian MJ, Gannon FH, Fallon MD, Mennuti MT, Lodar RF, Kaplan FS (1993) Skeletal dysplasia in perinatal lethal osteogenesis imperfecta. Clin Orthop 293: 327

Matsuno T, Unni KK, McLeod RA, Dahlin DC (1976) Telangiectatic osteogenic sarcoma. Cancer 38: 2538

Maynard JA, Ippolito EG, Ponseti IV, Mickelson MR (1981) Histochemistry and ultrastructure of the growth plate in achondroplasia. J Bone Joint Surg [Am] 63: 969

McKenna RJ, Schwinn CP, Soong KY, Higinbotham NL (1966) Sarcomata of the osteogenic series (osteosarcoma, fibrosarcoma, chondrosarcoma, parosteal osteogenic sarcoma, and sarcomata arising in abnormal bone). An analysis of 552 cases. J Bone Joint Surg [Am] 48:1

McKusick VA (1969) The nosology of the mucopolysaccharidoses. Am J Med 471: 730

McKusick VA, Egeland JA, Eldridge R, Krusen DE (1964) Dwarfism in the Amish. The Ellis–van Creveld syndrome. Bull Johns Hopkins Hosp 115: 306

McLeod RA, Dahlin DC, Beabout JW (1976) The spectrum of osteoblastoma. Am J Roentgenol Radium Ther Nucl Med 126: 321

McNair P, Madsbad S, Christiansen C, Faber OK, Transbol I, Binder C (1978) Osteopenia in insulin treated diabetes melitus. Its relation to age at onset, sex and duration of disease. Diabetologia 15: 87

Mendenhall CM, Marcus RB, Enneking WF, Springfield DS, Thar TL, Million RP (1983) The prognostic significance of soft tissue extension in Ewing's sarcoma. Cancer 51: 913

Merryweather R, Middlemiss JH, Sanerkin NG (1980) Malignant transformation of osteoblastoma. J Bone Joint Surg [Br] 62: 381

Milhaud G, Labat M-L (1978) Thymus and osteopetrosis. Clin Orthop 135: 260

Milhaud G, Labat M-L, Graf B, Juster M, Balmain N, Moutier R, Toyama K (1975) Demonstration cinétique, radiographique et histologique de la guérison de l'ostéopétrose congénitale du rat. CR Acad Sci (Paris) [D] 280: 2485

Mirra JM (1980) Bone tumours: diagnosis and treatment. Lippincott, Philadelphia

Mirra JM, Dodd L, Johnson W (1991) Case report 700. Primary intracortical osteosarcoma of the femur, sclerosing variant, grade 1 or 2 anaplasia. Skeletal Radiol 20: 613

Miyayama H, Sakamoto K, Ide M, Ise K, Hirota K, Yasunaga T, Ishinhara A (1993) Aggressive osteoblastoma of the calcaneus. Cancer 71: 143

Moore CA, Ward JC, Rivas ML, Magill HL, Whyte MP (1990) Infantile hypophosphatasia: autosomal recessive transmission to two related sibships. Am J Med Genet 36: 15

Murphy FD, Blount WP (1962) Cartilaginous exostoses following irradiation. J Bone Joint Surg [Am] 44: 662

Nerlich AG, Brenner RE, Wiest I, Lehmann H, Yang C, Muller PK, van der Mark K (1993) Immunohistochemical localization of interstitial collagens in bone tissue from patients with various forms of osteogenesis imperfecta. Am J Med Genet 45: 258

Neufeld EF (1974) The biochemical basis for mucopolysaccharidoses and mucolipidoses. Prog Med Genet 10: 81

Neufeld EF, Lim TW, Shapiro LJ (1975) Inherited disorders of lysosomal metabolism. Annu Rev Biochem 44: 357

Ochsner SF (1966) Eosinophilic granuloma of bone; experience with 20 cases. AJR Am J Roentgenol 97: 719

Oda Y, Tsuneyoshi M, Shinohara N (1992) "Solid" variant of aneurysmal bone cyst (extragnathic giant cell reparative granuloma) in the axial skeleton and long bones. A study of its morphologic spectrum and distinction from allied giant cell lesions. Cancer 70: 2642

Orzincolo C, Castaldi G, DeSanctis V, Scutellari PN, Ciaccio L, Vullo C (1990) Rickets- and/or scurvy-like bone lesions in beta thalassemia major. Radiol Med 80: 823

Petersen S, Knudsen FU, Anderson EA, Egeblac M (1980) Acute haematogenous osteomyelitis and septic arthritis in childhood. A 10 year review and follow-up. Acta Orthop Scand 51: 451

Petty RE (1990) Septic arthritis and osteomyelitis in children. Curr Opin Rheumatol 2: 616

Philips PE (1977) Viral arthritis in children. Arthritis Rheum 20 [Suppl 2]: 584

Pochaczevsky R, Yen YM, Sherman RS (1960) The roentgen appearance of benign osteoblastoma. Radiology 75: 429

Ponseti IV (1978a) Growth and development of the acetabulum in the normal child. J Bone Joint Surg [Am] 60: 575

Ponseti IV (1978b) Morphology of the acetabulum in congenital dislocation of the hip. J Bone Joint Surg [Am] 60: 586

Ponseti IV, McClintock R (1956) The pathology of slipping of the upper femoral epiphysis. J Bone Joint Surg [Am] 38: 71

Pope FM. Cheah KSE, Nicholls AC, Price AB, Grosveld FG (1984) Lethal osteogenesis imperfecta congenita and a 300 base pair deletion for an α_1 (I)-like collagen. Br Med J 288: 431

Rasmussen PG (1975) Multiple epiphyseal dysplasia. II. Morphological and histochemical investigation of cartilage matrix, particularly in the pre-calcification state. Acta Pathol Microbiol Scand [A] 83: 493

Reed RJ, Rothenberg M (1964) Lesions of bone that may be confused with aneurysmal bone cyst. Clin Orthop 35: 150

Revell PA (1986) The pathology of bone. Springer, New York

Revell PA, Scholtz CL (1979) Aggressive osteoblastoma. J Pathol 127: 195

Riley FC, Brown DM (1971) Morphological and biochemical studies in osteogenesis imperfecta. J Lab Clin Med 78: 1000 (abstract)

Riley FC, Jowsey J, Brown DM (1973) Osteogenesis imperfecta: morphologic and biochemical studies of connective tissue. Pediatr Res 9: 757

Rimoin DL, Silberberg R, Hollister PW (1976) Chondro-osseous pathology in the chondrodystrophies. Clin Orthop 114: 137

Rockwell MA, Saiter ET, Enneking WF (1972) Periosteal chondroma. J Bone Joint Surg [Am] 54: 102

Rosen A, Caparros B, Huvos AG, Kosloff C, Nirenberg RN, Cacavio A, Marcove RC, Lane RM, Mehta B, Urban C (1982) Preoperative chemotherapy of osteogenic sarcoma: selection of postoperative adjuvant chemotherapy based on the response of the primary tumour to preoperative chemotherapy. Cancer 49: 1221

Roth VG (1976) Pycnodysostosis presenting with bilateral subtrochanteric fractures. A case report. Clin Orthop 117: 247

Ruiter DJ, Cornelisse CJ, van Rijssel ThG, van der Velde EA (1977) Aneurysmal bone cyst and telangiectatic osteosarcoma. A histopathological and morphometric study. Virchows Arch A Pathol Anat 377: 311

Russo PA, Seidman E (199) An unusual histiocytoid proliferation in infancy. Hum Pathol 21: 564

Sanerkin NG (1980) Definitions of osteosarcoma, chondrosarcoma and fibrosarcoma of bone. Cancer 46: 178

Schajowicz F (1959) Ewing's sarcoma and reticulum cell sarcoma of bone with special reference to the histochemical demonstration of glycogen as an aid to differential diagnosis. J Bone Joint Surg [Am] 41: 349

Schajowicz F (1981) Tumors and tumor-like lesions of bone and joints. Springer, New York

Schajowicz F (1983) Current trends in the diagnosis and treatment of malignant bone tumors. Clin Orthop 180: 220

Schajowicz F, Lemos C (1976) Malignant osteoblastoma. J Bone Joint Surg [Br] 58: 202

Schajowicz F, Ackerman LV, Sissons HA (1972) Histological typing of bone tumours. International histological classification of tumours, no. 6. World Health Organization, Geneva

Schaller JG (1977) Arthritis of childhood onset. Clin Rheum Dis 3: 333

Schaller JG (1979) The seronegative spondyloarthropathies of childhood. Clin Orthop 143: 76

Scott CI (1976) Achondroplastic and hypochondroplastic dwarfism. Clin Orthop 114: 18

Selby S (1961) Metaphyseal defects in the tubular bones of growing children. J Bone Joint Surg [Am] 43: 395

Semmelink HJ, Pruszcynski M, Wiersma-van Tilburg A, Smedts F, Ramaekers FC (1990) Cytokeratin expression in chondroblastomas. Histopathology 16: 257

Shapiro F, Glimcher MJ, Holtrop ME, Tashjian AH, Brickley-Parsons D, Kenzora JE (1980) Human osteopetrosis. J Bone Joint Surg [Am] 62: 284

Shapiro R, Rowe DW (1983) Collagen genes and brittle bones. Ann Intern Med 99: 700

Sheffield LJ, Danks DM, Mayne VM, Hutchinson LA (1976) Chondrodysplasia punctata: 23 cases of a mild and relatively common variety. J Pediatr 89: 916

Shishikura A, Ushigome S, Shimoda T (1993) Primitive neuroectodermal tumors of bone and soft tissue: histological subclassification and clinicopathologic correlations. Acta Pathol Jpn 43: 176

Shohat M, Rimoin DL, Gruber HE, Lachman RS (1991) Perinatal lethal pyrophosphatasia; clinical, radiologic and morphologic findings. Pediatr Radiol 21: 421

Silberberg R, Rimoin DL, Rosenthal R, Hasler M (1972) Ultrastructure of cartilage in the Hurler and Sanfillipo syndromes. Arch Pathol 94: 500

Sillence DO, Rimoin DL (1978) Classification of osteogenesis imperfecta. Lancet i: 1041

Sillence DO, Horton WA, Rimoin DL (1979a) Morphologic studies in the skeletal dysplasias. Am J Pathol 96: 813

Sillence DO, Senn A, Danks DM (1979b) Genetic heterogeneity in osteogenesis imperfecta. J Med Genet 16: 101

Silveri CP, Kaplan FS, Fallon MD, Bayever E, August CS (1991) Hurler syndrome with special reference to the histologic abnormalities of the growth plate. Clin Orthop 269: 305

Singer DB, Rudolph AJ, Rosenberg HS, Rawls WE, Boniuk M (1967) Pathology of the congenital rubella syndrome. J Pediatr 71: 665

Sissons HA, Hadfield GJ (1955) The influence of cortisone on the structure and growth of bone. J Anat 89: 69

Smith R (1984) Osteogenesis imperfecta 1984. Br Med J 289: 394 (leading article)

Spagnoli I, Gathoni F, Viganolti G (1982) Roentgenographic aspects of non-Hodgkin's lymphoma presenting with osseous lesions. Skeletal Radiol 8: 39

Spencer AT (1962) A histochemical study of long bones in osteogenesis imperfecta congenita. J Pathol Bacteriol 83: 423

Spjut HJ, Dorfman HD, Fechner RE, Ackerman LV (1970) Tumours of bone and cartilage. Armed Forces Institute of Pathology, Washington DC (Atlas of tumour pathology, 2nd ser, fasc 5)

Spjut HJ, Ayala AG (1983) Skeletal tumors in children and adolescents. Hum Pathol 14: 628

Spranger J, Maroteaux P (1990) The lethal osteochondrodysplasias. In: Harris H, Hirschhorn K (eds) Advances in human genetics, vol 19. Plenum, New York, p 1

Stanescu V, Stanescu R, Maroteaux P (1984) Pathogenic mechanisms in osteochondrodysplasias. J Bone Joint Surg [Am] 66: 817

Stanescu R, Stanescu V, Muriel M-P, Maroteaux P (1993) Multiple epiphyseal dysplasia: Fairbank type: morphologic and biochemical study of cartilage. Am J Med Genet 45: 501

Stastny P, Fink CW (1979) Different HLA-D associations in adult and juvenile rheumatoid arthritis. J Clin Invest 63: 124

Steers AC, Malawista SE (1979) Cases of Lyme disease in the United States: locations correlated with distribution of *Ixodes damini*. Ann Intern Med 91: 730

Steere AC, Malawista SE, Snydman DR, Shope RE, Andiman WA, Ross MR (1977a) Lyme arthritis: an epidemic of oligoarticular arthritis in children and adults in three Connecticut communities. Arthritis Rheum 20: 7

Steere AC, Malawista SE, Hardin JA, Ruddy S, Askenase PW, Andiman WA (1977b) Erythema chronicum migrans and Lyme arthritis: the enlarging clinical spectrum. Ann Intern Med 86: 685

Steere AC, Broderick TE, Malawista SE (1978) Erythema chronicum migrans and Lyme arthritis; epidemiologic evidence for a tick vector. Am J Epidemiol 108: 312

Steere AC, Grodzicki RL, Kornblatt AN, Craft JE, Barbour AG, Burgdorfer W et al. (1983) The spirochetal aetiology of Lyme disease. N Engl J Med 308: 733

Stewart A, Glass J, Patel A, Watt G, Cripps A, Clancy R (1982) Lyme arthritis in Hunter valley. Med J Aust 1: 139

Stoss H, Pontz B, Vetter U, Karbowski A, Brenner R, Spranger J (1993) Osteogenesis imperfecta and hyperplastic callus formation: light and electron microscopic findings. Am J Med Genet 45: 260

Sugimoto T, Sawada T, Arakawa S, Matsumara T, Sakamoto I, Takeuchi Y, Reynolds CP, Kemshead JT, Helson L (1985) Possible differential diagnosis of neuroblastoma from a rhabdomyosarcoma and Ewing's sarcoma by using a panel of monoclonal antibodies. Jpn J Cancer Res 76: 301

Sutro CJ (1935) Slipping of the capital epiphysis of the femur in adolescence. Arch Surg 31: 345

Sweet DL, Mass DP, Simon MH, Shapiro CM (1981) Histiocytic lymphoma (reticulum-cell sarcoma) of bone. J Bone Joint Surg [Am] 63: 79

Teitelbaum SL, Kraft WJ, Lange R, Avioli LV (1974) Bone collagen aggregation abnormalities in osteogenesis imperfecta. Calcif Tissue Res 17: 75

Thomas LB, Forkner CE, Frei E, Besse BE, Stabenau JR (1961) The skeletal lesions of acute leukaemia. Cancer 14: 608

Unni KK, Dahlin DC, Beabout JW, Ivins JC (1976a) Parosteal osteogenic osteosarcoma. Cancer 37: 2466

Unni KK, Dahlin DC, Beabout JW (1976b) Periosteal osteogenic osteosarcoma. Cancer 37: 2476

Unni KK, Dahlin DC (1989) Osteosarcoma: pathology and classification. Semin Radiol 24: 143

van der Harten JH (1987) The skeletal system. In: Keeling JW (ed) Fetal and neonatal pathology. Springer , New York, p 529

Villanueva J (1993) Osteoblastoma and osteoid osteoma. Clinical and morphological features of 162 cases. Pathol Res Pract 189: 33

Vohra VG (1967) Roentigen manifestations of Ewing's sarcoma. A study of 156 cases. Cancer 20: 727

Voutsinas S, Wynne-Davies R (1983) The infrequency of malignant change in diaphyseal aclasis and neurofibromatosis. J Med Genet 20: 345

Walker DG (1975) Bone resorption in osteopetrotic mice by transplants of normal bone marrow and spleen cells. Science 190: 784

Wallis RC, Brown SE, Kloter KO, Main AJ (1978) Erythema chronicum migrans and Lyme arthritis; field study of ticks. Am J Epidemiol 108: 322

Weinfeld MS, Dudley HR (1962) Osteogenic sarcoma. A follow up study of the ninety-four cases observed at the Massachussetts General Hospital from 1920–1960. J Bone Joint Surg [Am] 44: 269

Wold LE, Beabout JW, Unni KK, Pritchard DJ (1984) High-grade surface osteosarcomas. Am J Surg Pathol 8: 181

Wynne-Davies R, Hall M, Apley AG (1985) Atlas of skeletal dysplasias. Churchill Livingstone, Edinburgh

Yamamuro T, Ishida K (1984) Recent advances in the prevention, early diagnosis and treatment of congenital dislocation of the hip in Japan. Clin Orthop 184: 34

Yang SS, Kitchen E, Gilbert EF, Rimoin DL (1986) Histopathologic examination in osteochondrodysplasia. Arch Pathol Lab Med 110: 10

Yoshida H, Yumoto T, Minamizaki T (1992) Osteosarcoma with features mimicking malignant fibrous histiocytoma. Virchows Arch A Pathol Anat Histopathol 421: 229

Younge D, Drummond D, Herring J, Cruess RL (1979) Melorheostosis in children. Clinical features and natural history. J Bone Joint Surg [Br] 61: 415

Yu JS, Walker-Smith JA, Burnard ED (1971) Rickets, a common complication of neonatal hepatitis. Med J Aust I: 790

10 · Muscle and Peripheral Nerve

Michael Swash

The histological study of muscle and peripheral nerve forms a major part of paediatric pathology because neuromuscular disorders are common problems. Modern histopathological techniques have led to greater understanding of these disorders and thus to a more rational approach to diagnosis and treatment. Naturally, new problems and controversies have also arisen.

In this chapter a general account of the pathological reactions of muscle and nerve will be given, together with brief descriptions of the characteristic features of those disorders that occur in infancy and childhood. Neuromuscular pathology is mainly based on biopsy material, but some attention will also be given to autopsy findings.

Muscle Biopsy Techniques

Study of muscle and nerve specimens requires the use of unfixed frozen material so that enzyme and immunohistochemical techniques can be utilized. With these methods, subcellular organelles can be studied by light microscopy, and different muscle fibre types can be identified. In addition, the classic histological stains, adapted for frozen material, can still be used. Many of these techniques produce permanent results so that slides can be stored for future study. The blocks of frozen tissue can themselves be stored indefinitely in liquid nitrogen. Formol–saline fixation alone is not adequate for muscle and nerve biopsy work.

Techniques for snap-freezing muscle are well described in other texts (Dubowitz 1985; Swash and Schwartz 1991). To avoid artefacts it is important to take particular care to prepare small cylindrical blocks of tissue (3 × 2 mm) from the fresh biopsy specimen. The muscle should be kept moist in buffered saline or Ringer's solution to avoid any

drying artefact before freezing. It is preferable to freeze the tissue, attached to a small disc of cork by a blob of Tissue-Tek, in isopentane cooled to near its freezing point in a thermos of liquid nitrogen. When cutting sections in the cryostat sudden changes in temperature, such as would be caused by a warm cryostat knife or warm slides, must be avoided to prevent the development of ice-crystal artefact. This can sometimes be cleared from a block by allowing it to thaw at room temperature and then refreezing, although this manoeuvre usually results in the loss of some enzyme activity. A series of up to 12 transverse sections, each 5–8 μm thick, should be cut. Longitudinal sections, which are difficult to produce because of imperfect orientation of muscle fibres in most blocks, are also useful. In each case, small pieces of fresh tissue should be fixed in glutaraldehyde so that, if necessary, sections can be prepared for electron microscopy. Muscle is best examined in the relaxed state, and this can be achieved by the addition of procaine to the fixative. It is fundamental to all biopsy work that the tissue specimen should be taken by an experienced surgeon, handled carefully, and snap-frozen for light microscopy or fixed for ultrastructural studies immediately.

Histological Methods

The haematoxylin and eosin (H&E) method provides general information about the biopsy (Fig. 10.1). The elastin–van Gieson stain is sometimes useful, particularly in assessing connective tissue changes. The modified Gomori trichrome stain allows delineation of nuclei, fibrous tissue, myofibrillar material (bluish) and intermyofibrillar substance (red). Trichrome stains may also differentiate two muscle fibre types, the red and pale fibres of older workers, but this is not always very obvious.

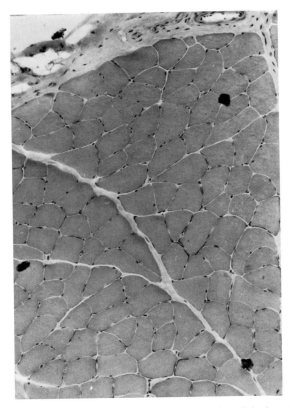

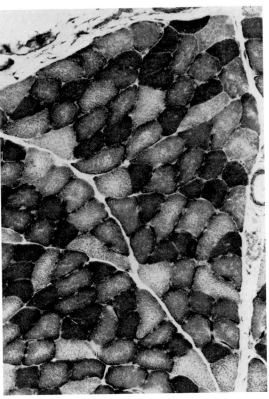

Fig. 10.1. In this transverse section the close interdigitation of normal muscle fibres is clearly seen. The muscle fibre nuclei are almost all subsarcolemmal. The muscle fibres are arranged in fascicles. Three "spots" represent tissue fragments superimposed on the section – a common artefact. Normal muscle. (H&E, × 140)

Fig. 10.2. A mosaic arrangement of fibres of various staining intensity is seen in this serial section. Type 1 fibres are darkly stained; type 2 fibres are relatively pale. Type 2A fibres tend to be darker than type 2B fibres. The intermyofibrillar substance has a finely granular appearance. Arteriolar walls also stain positively. (NADH tetrazolium reductase, × 140)

A variety of enzyme-histochemical reactions are available for histological work. In most laboratories a routine series is used to provide differentiation of fibre type and organelle-specific reaction products so that mitochondria, sarcoplasmic lipid droplets, myofibrils, cell membranes and sarcoplasmic glycogen, and perhaps also ribonucleic acid and acid phosphatase, can be identified by light microscopy. The nicotine adenine dinucleotide (NADH) tetrazolium reductase technique is particularly useful, as it produces a permanent preparation with good contrast (Fig. 10.2), which allows fibre type differentiation to be recognized approximately. The reaction product is localized in mitochondria and, non-specifically, in the tubular system of the intermyofibrillar sarcoplasm. Succinic dehydrogenase (SDH) is located only in mitochondria, but the reaction product is often less easily visualized.

Fibre typing is conventionally performed in myofibrillar adenosine triphosphatase (ATPase) preparations (Dubowitz and Brooke 1973; Swash and Schwartz 1991). This reaction produces different results depending on the pH of the preincubation (Figs. 10.3 and 10.4). Preincubations are carried out at pH 9.4, 4.5 and 4.3. In good preparations there should be a pattern reversal between the pH 9.4 and pH 4.3 preincubations, fibres which are dark in the former (type 2 fibres) being pale in the latter (Figs. 10.3 and 10.4). In the intermediate (pH 4.5) preincubation some type 2 fibres show an intermediate reaction-product density (type 2B fibres). Myophosphorylase, located at the cross-bridges of the active component of the myofilament, can also be demonstrated, but this method does not produce permanent results.

Neutral lipid droplets are most satisfactorily demonstrated by the oil red O method; a counter-stain of Ehrlich's haematoxylin enables basophilic fibres and sarcolemmal nuclei to be recognized. A number of other stains can be used for neutral lipid, e.g.

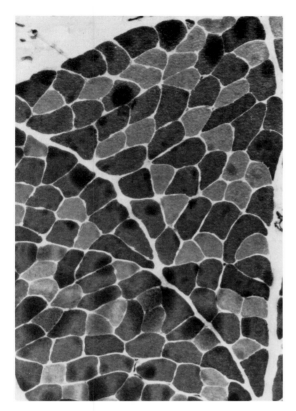

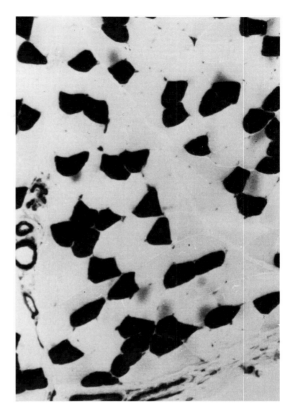

Fig. 10.3. In this reaction type 1 fibres are pale and type 2 fibres are dark. Serial section. (ATPase pH 9.4, × 140)

Fig. 10.4. The mosaic pattern has reversed: type 1 fibres are dark and type 2 fibres are very pale. Serial section. (ATPase pH 4.3, × 140)

Sudan black, but they are generally less satisfactory and less specific. Glycogen granules and cell membranes, together with other myofibrillar membranous structures, can be demonstrated by the periodic acid–Schiff (PAS) method. Predigestion with diastase allows proof of the presence of glycogen in the untreated sections. The sections should be fixed on the slides with alcohol for the most uniform results. Acid phosphatase, localized in lysosomes, can be demonstrated in abnormal fibres, particularly in those undergoing autolysis. A summary of the enzyme-histochemical reactions in fibres of different histochemical types is given in Table 10.1.

Type 1 fibres probably correspond to slow-contracting, oxidative fibres, type 2B to fast-contracting glycolytic fibres, and type 2A to fast-contracting oxidative/glycolytic fibres (Peter et al. 1972).

In addition to these routine histological and histochemical methods, the use of frozen tissue enables immunohistochemical techniques to be employed for demonstration of immunoglobulins and complement in blood vessels (Whitaker and Engel 1972). There are several well-tried methods for the demonstration

Table 10.1. Summary of the enzyme-histochemical reactions in fibres of different histochemical types

	Type 1	Type 2A	Type 2B
ATPase pH 9.4	Pale	Dark	Dark
ATPase pH 4.5	Dark	Pale	Dark
ATPase pH 4.3	Dark	Pale	Pale
NADH	Dark	Intermediate	Intermediate
Glycogen	Pale	Dark	Intermediate
Myophosphorylase	Pale	Dark	Intermediate
Neutral lipid	Plentiful	Sparse	Sparse

of cholinesterase at the synaptic folds of motor end-plates, one of which is combined with silver to show the nerve terminals themselves (Pestronk and Drachman 1978). In fresh unfrozen muscle, motor end-plates and the terminal innervation can be demonstrated by supravital methylene blue staining (Cöers and Woolf 1953) (Fig. 10.5).

Electron microscopy is useful in some instances to examine the ultrastructure of cellular abnormalities detected by light microscopy (for example, to study paracrystalline inclusions in mitochrondria in ragged-

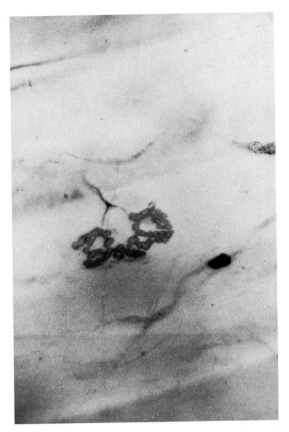

Fig. 10.5. The terminal axon branch innervates the ending, which consists of an arborization of subterminal expansions forming the neural part of the motor end-plate. Normal motor end-plate. (Supravital methylene blue, × 140)

red fibres, or to study tubular aggregates). It is not generally useful in routine diagnosis, although semi-thin sections of plastic-embedded muscle stained with toluidine blue or p-phenylenediamine provide a useful adjunct to light microscopy of frozen sections. The striations, mitochondria, triads of the sarcotubular system, and intermyofibrillar granular sarcoplasm are shown in longitudinal section in Fig. 10.6.

Histological Features of Neuromuscular Disease

Statistical Methods

The changes found in the distribution and size of type 1 and type 2 fibres can be described by simple statis-

tical methods. These descriptions give important information about selective involvement of fibre types (see W.K. Engel 1970; Swash and Schwartz 1996).

Fibre-type Predominance

The proportions of fibres of each histochemical type vary in different muscles (Brooke and Engel 1969a, b; Johnson et al. 1973). For example, extensor hallucis longus normally contains a majority of type 1 fibres. However, in the three muscles most commonly biopsied in clinical practice (quadriceps, biceps brachii and deltoid), type 2 fibres are found in greater numbers than type 1. A change in the proportion of either fibre type is termed "fibre type predominance"; type 1 fibre predominance is present when more than 55% of fibres in one of these three muscles are type 1 fibres, and type 2 predominance when more than 80% of fibres are type 2 (see Dubowitz and Brooke 1973).

Fibre Diameter

Atrophy and hypertrophy are difficult to assess subjectively, and it is useful to calculate the means of the lesser diameter of at least 100 fibres, including fibres of both fibre types, to compare these with normal values (Polgar et al. 1972; Dubowitz and Brooke 1973). Because muscle fibres in children are smaller than those of adults, and their diameters vary at different ages, these measurements are less important in paediatric practice, but selective atrophy of type 1 or type 2 fibres may occur in certain diseases and this may be important in diagnosis (Brooke and Engel 1969b). Fibre area measurements have been used in some laboratories.

Selective atrophy of type 2 fibres is common; it is a feature of disuse atrophy of any cause and can therefore occur in patients immobilized in bed for orthopaedic procedures, in cachexia, in corticospinal tract lesions, in myasthenia gravis, or in arthropathies of any cause. It may also occur in collagen-vascular diseases (Engel 1965) and in steroid myopathy and osteomalacia. Atrophy of type 1 fibres is less common. It is a particular feature of myotonic dystrophy (Engel and Brooke 1966), but also occurs in myotubular myopathy, nemaline myopathy and congenital fibre type disproportion (see below). In collagen-vascular disease, such as dermatomyositis of childhood (Banker and Victor 1966), selective atrophy of fibres of both histochemical types may occur at the periphery of the fascicles: this phenomenon is known as perifascicular atrophy. This is probably due to capillary shutdown from arteriolar or capillary involvement, leading to ischaemia of the

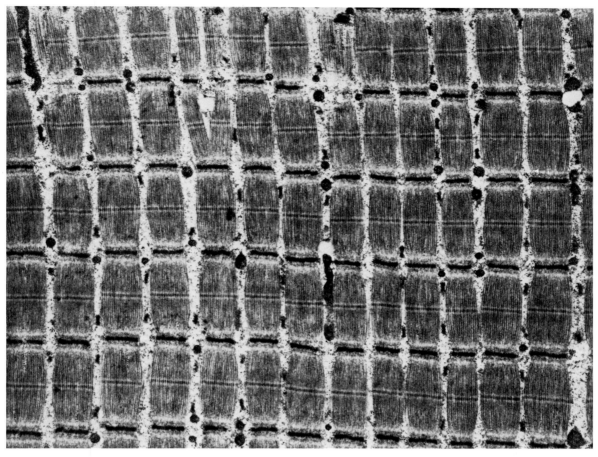

Fig. 10.6. Normal contracted muscle, longitudinal section. Mitochondria (*M*) and triads of the sarcotubular system (*T*) are located near the Z line (*Z*). (Electron micrograph, × 22 500)

periphery of the fascicle and so to atrophy or even necrosis of these fibres (Carpenter et al. 1976).

Central Nucleation

Centrally placed nuclei are found in less than 3% of fibres in normal muscle biopsies. Central nucleation occurs in hypertrophied fibres as a feature associated with fibre splitting (Fig. 10.7) and in regenerating fibres (Fig. 10.8) and is especially prominent in centronuclear myopathy and myotonic dystrophy.

Denervation and Reinnervation

Muscle fibres are normally arranged in a random mosaic distribution of fibre types within fascicles

(James 1971). Fibres supplied by a single motor axon (the motor unit) are widely dispersed within the muscle (Edstrom and Kugelberg 1968).

The findings of groups of fibres of similar histochemical type is evidence that reinnervation of denervated fibres has occurred, probably by collateral sprouting from nearby motor axons (Fig. 10.9). This is therefore evidence of effective functional compensation, indicating a neurogenic disorder of some chronicity. *Fibre-type grouping* is said to occur when two or more fibres of the same histochemical type are enclosed, at all points on their circumference, by other fibres of the same histochemical type. This usually means that there are at least ten fibres in the group, but this depends on the relative equality of fibre size. When fibre-type predominance exceeds about 80% enclosed fibres will become frequent (Johnson et al. 1973), without necessarily implying that fibre-type grouping is present. Fibre-type pre-

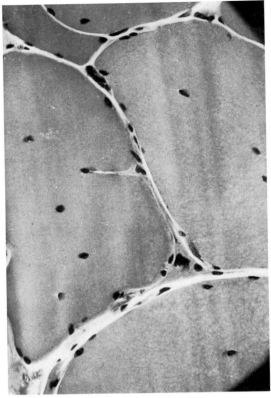

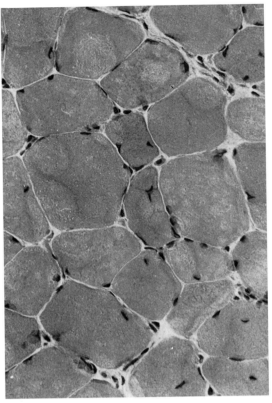

Fig. 10.7. Central nucleation, fibre splitting and small denervated fibres in a chronic neurogenic disorder. (H&E, × 360)

Fig. 10.8. Central nucleation in regenerating muscle fibres in acute polymyositis. The two fibres in the centre of the field are slightly basophilic. The slight variation in staining intensity in the other fibres are "architectural changes", which are commonly found in polymyositis. (H&E, × 360)

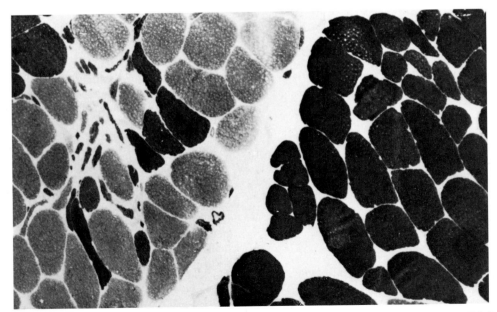

Fig. 10.9. Fibre-type grouping in juvenile-onset spinal muscular atrophy (Kugelberg–Welander disease). (ATPase pH 9.4), × 140)

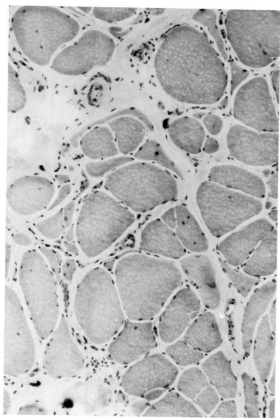

Fig. 10.10. Clusters of small pointed fibres in association with larger rounded fibres. Interstitial fibrosis has occurred. Spinal muscular atrophy. (H&E, × 140)

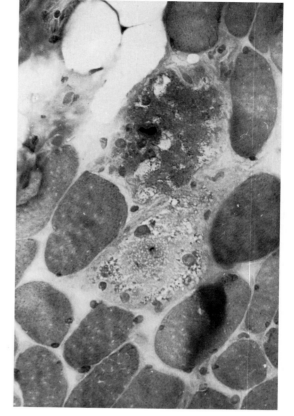

Fig. 10.11. Two necrotic fibres undergoing phagocytosis. (Modified Gomori trichrome, × 560)

dominance is a factor that should lead to the suspicion of a neurogenic disorder.

Groups of small pointed fibres indicate that irreversible denervation has occurred. When this is due to a chronic disorder, in which there has been opportunity for collateral reinnervation of isolated denervated fibres, the group of denervated fibres may be very large, even occupying whole fascicles (*grouped denervation atrophy*). Scattered narrow, atrophic fibres or clusters of three to six small angular narrow fibres (*disseminated neurogenic atrophy*) typically occur in more rapidly progressive, or poorly compensated, neurogenic disorders when collateral reinnervation has failed (Fig. 10.10).

Denervated fibres appear small, narrow and pointed, often with rather dark basophilic cytoplasm and with dark pyknotic nuclei. Neural cell adhesion molecule (NCAM) may be demonstrated on the cell surface as part of the process of reinnervation by axonal sprouting (Schubert et al. 1989). The denervated fibre expresses extrajunctional acetylcholine receptor (AChR) widely on the plasma membrane,

extending from the junctional area previously occupied by the motor end-plate.

Degenerative Changes

Necrotic fibres are a common feature in myopathies; they are also found, although far less frequently, in biopsies from patients with chronic neurogenic disorders (Cazzato 1970; Schwartz et al. 1976). They appear pale and hyaline. Later they lose their eosinophilic character, become pale and patchily stained, and begin to undergo phagocytosis (Fig. 10.11). Sometimes an endomysial cellular reaction occurs around them, composed of endothelial capillary nuclei and sarcolemmal nuclei. Necrotic fibres usually contain prominent acid phosphatase-positive material. If the blood supply to a region of fibre necrosis is impaired, the endomysial tubes and basal lamina scaffold may remain intact, producing an appearance of rings of empty endomysial tubes, i.e. subendomysial necrosis. This is seen particularly in polymyositis (Schmalbruch 1976) and in other acute necrotizing myopathies more usually found in adults (Urich and Wilkinson 1970). Large rounded hyaline fibres are particularly characteristic of Duchenne-type muscular dystrophy (see Fig. 10.29).

Regenerative Changes

Regeneration occurs after necrosis or injury in most tissues of the body, and muscle fibres, which are particularly susceptible to injury in everyday life, have considerable regenerative potential. After fibre necrosis, which may be limited to a segment of the muscle fibre, regeneration can occur either in continuity with the undamaged portions of the fibre (continuous repair) or from myoblast formation in the necrotic segment itself (discontinuous repair). Regeneration thus begins at a stage when phagocytosis of necrotic material is still incomplete, while mononucleated cells are abundant in the interstitium around the necrotic fibre.

Regenerating fibres are usually smaller than neighbouring normal fibres (see Fig. 10.12). Their sarcoplasm is basophilic and contains neutral lipid droplets. The nuclei are centrally located, large and vesicular, and contain prominent nucleoli.

During regeneration of muscle cells protein synthesis occurs. This can be shown by the presence of RNA in the cytoplasm, e.g. by the acridine orange technique and by the basophilic cytoplasm, in H&E stains. During the early phase of regeneration after muscle cell necrosis, vimentin synthesis is up-regulated (Thornell et al. 1980) even before the development of basophilia in the sarcoplasm. Vimentin is an intermediate filament protein which is an essential component of myoblasts and of the cytoskeleton of striated muscle fibres (Price and Sanger 1982). Vimentin expression, demonstrated using an immunoperoxidase sandwich technique based on a monoclonal mouse antivimentin antibody, may therefore be used as a marker for regeneration in muscle cells. Regenerating muscle cells express NCAM on their cell surface (Schubert et al. 1989). NCAM expression is primarily regarded as a marker for denervation, and regenerating muscle cells will often have been functionally denervated by necrosis, by separation from their innervation.

In discontinuous regeneration, repair proceeds from mononucleated myoblasts (Sloper and Pegrum 1967), which are probably themselves derived from activation of satellite cells (Reznik and Engel 1970), and these myoblasts form long basophilic multinucleated ribbon-like cells, which later fuse, forming a new fibre (Reznik 1973). Satellite cells are found in normal muscle fibres as a nucleus, surrounded by

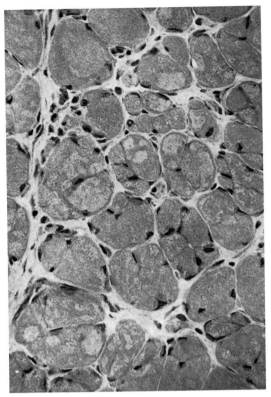

Fig. 10.12. Subendomysial regeneration. Individual endomysial tubes contain immature regenerating fibres. These muscle fibres stain irregularly. (H&E, × 560)

sparse granular sarcoplasm containing abundant free fibrosomes, Golgi apparatus, endoplasmic reticulum and mitochondria, but devoid of myofilaments. The satellite cell is limited by plasma membrane, and is situated beneath the basement membrane of the muscle fibre. The numbers of such cells in muscle are increased after injury (Reznik 1973) and after denervation (Ontell 1974). Reznik (1973) reviewed the ultrastructural sequence of changes found in these cells, giving rise to myoblast formation during regeneration after cold-induced injury.

Fig. 10.13. Ragged-red fibres, transverse section. **a** Gomori trichrome three fibres appear granular and show an irregular darkly staining (red) rim. **b** NADH. The pattern of intermyofibrillar reaction is disturbed in the ragged-red fibres. The rims of these fibres stain darkly, but not uniformly. **c** ATPase pH 4.3. The abnormal material does not stain. **d** Succinic dehydrogenase (SDH). This histochemical enzyme reaction delineates the distribution of the mitochondrial abnormality, which is largely restricted to type 1 fibres. (All × 403)

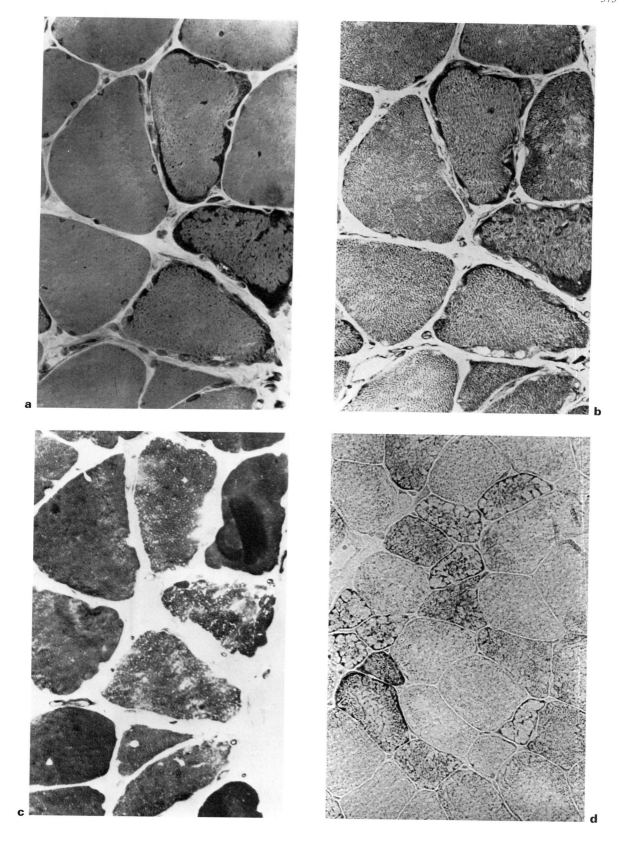

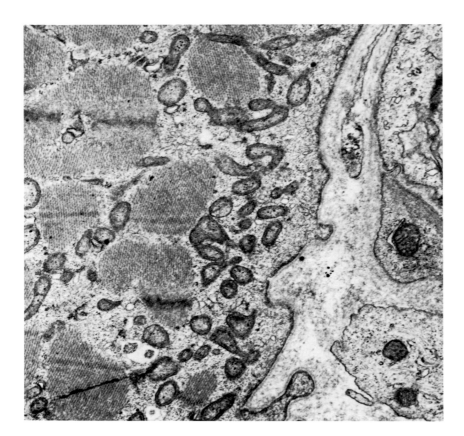

Fig. 10.14. Peripherally located aggregates of mitochondria. These show abnormal cristae and contain osmiophilic dense bodies. Deltoid biopsy from patient with progressive external ophthalmoplegia.
(Electron micrograph, × 150)

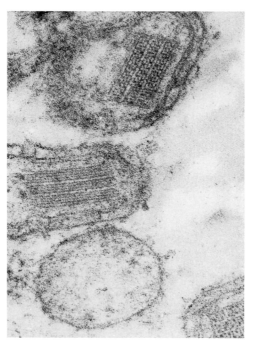

Fig. 10.15. Intramitochondrial paracrystalline material. (Electron micrograph, × 90 000)

Webb (1977) drew attention to the importance of programmed cell death of myotubes during embryonic myogenesis. The stimulus for cell death is unknown, but a similar phenomenon probably occurs during differentiation of myoblasts in regenerative repair, because several developing myotubes are found in the early stages of repair before fusion occurs and the single myofibre is reconstituted. It is possible that the achievement of functional reinnervation, which can occur only when the fibre is reconstituted across the necrotic segment, is important in this process (see Schmalbruch 1985).

Granular Fibres

Granular fibres (Brooke 1966) appear coarsely granular in H&E preparations. The granular material is faintly basophilic and is usually distributed in the sarcoplasm; it is particularly prominent at the periphery of the affected fibres. This material stains red in the Gomori trichrome preparation, is dark in NADH and SDH preparations, and does not stain in ATPase preparations (Fig. 10.13). Affected fibres are almost always type 1 fibres. In addition, this material is

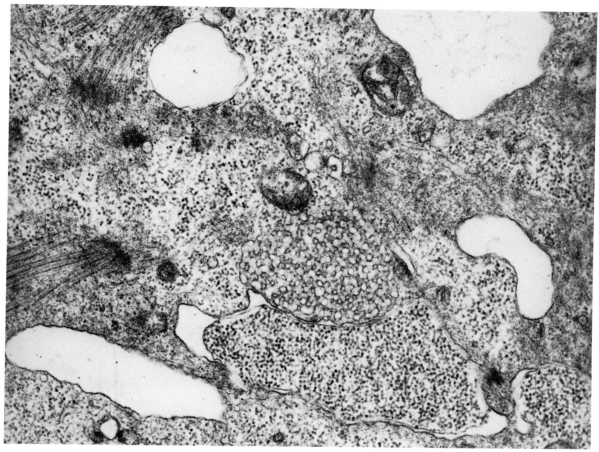

Fig. 10.16. Stacked tubules forming a tubular aggregate and dilated T tubules in a patient with hypokalaemic paralysis. (Electron micrograph, × 60 000)

usually faintly basophilic and is often associated with droplets of neutral lipid. These fibres, termed *ragged-red fibres* (Fig. 10.13) are a characteristic feature in myopathies and myoencephalopathies associated with defective mitochondrial oxidation (Engel 1971; Morgan-Hughes et al. 1978; Petty et al. 1986). Electron microscopy reveals that the granular appearance results from an accumulation of mitochondria (Fig. 10.14), which may show morphological abnormalities and which often contain osmiophilic bodies and paracrystalline material (Fig. 10.15).

Tubular Aggregates

Tubular aggregates may resemble ragged-red fibres; however, they do not usually produce a generally granular appearance, the abnormal red material being limited to a peripheral segment of affected fibres. Furthermore, they are found in type 2B fibres, and

although the abnormal zones are darkly stained in oxidative enzyme reaction they are negative in Succinic dehydrogenase (SDH) preparations. Electron microscopy demonstrates the characteristic stacked tubules (Fig. 10.16). Although in itself a highly characteristic finding, this change is not specific for any particular disorder (Dubowitz and Brooke 1973). Nevertheless, some patients with this abnormality have been reported as having myopathy with tubular aggregates.

Fibre Splitting

Fibre splitting is found particularly in chronic disorders. It is a feature of chronic neurogenic muscle disease, such as intermediate spinal muscular atrophy, when it particularly affects the hypertrophied type 1 fibres. Splitting usually begins from the periphery of affected fibres, the line of separation running into the centre of the fibre towards a centrally

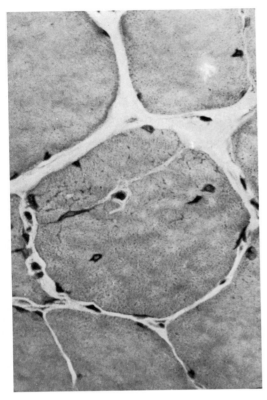

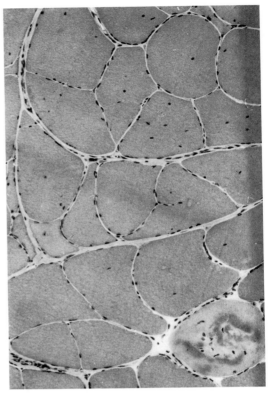

Fig. 10.17. Fibre splitting and its relation to a central nucleus. The cleft of incomplete splitting is basophilic. (H&E, × 560)

Fig. 10.18. Fibre splitting in hypertrophied fibres with prominent central nucleation. There are several narrow atrophic fibres, which are probably denervated. A large fibre is necrotic. These are the features of secondary myopathic change in a chronic neurogenic disorder: Kugelberg–Welander disease. (H&E, × 140)

placed nucleus (Fig. 10.17). The cleft is usually basophilic and the nuclei associated with it may be vesicular (Schwartz et al. 1976). Sometimes a fibre is split into multiple fragments, some of which can become separated from the "parent" fibre, resulting in denervation of the separated segment (Swash and Schwartz 1977). Splitting of this type is probably due to mechanical stress associated with functional overload of weakened muscles (Hall-Craggs 1972; Schwartz et al. 1976).

Similar splitting occurs in Duchenne-type dystrophy (Bell and Conen 1968), limb–girdle myopathies and polymyositis (Swash et al. 1978b). It may be important in functional compensation in these disorders (Swash and Schwartz 1977), and in chronic neurogenic disorders it can lead to an appearance of combined fibre necrosis and regeneration, with variability in fibre size and central nucleation (Fig. 10.18), called secondary "myopathic" change (Drachman et al. 1967; Schwartz et al. 1976). Fibre splitting is a normal phenomenon near musculotendinous insertions (Bell and Conen 1968). It must not be

confused with subendomysial regeneration (Fig. 10.12) occurring after fibre necrosis (Schmalbruch 1976; Swash et al. 1978a).

Target Fibres

Target fibres (Engel 1961) are best seen in ATPase and NADH preparations (Fig. 10.19). These fibres contain a central unstained zone, surrounded by a densely stained intermediate zone, and a third, relatively normal outer zone. Most affected fibres are type 1 fibres. Target fibres are usually associated with denervation, especially that associated with neuropathies, but they have been produced experimentally by tenotomy (Engel et al. 1966).

Central Cores

It is often difficult to distinguish central cores from target fibres. The core consists of a central zone of

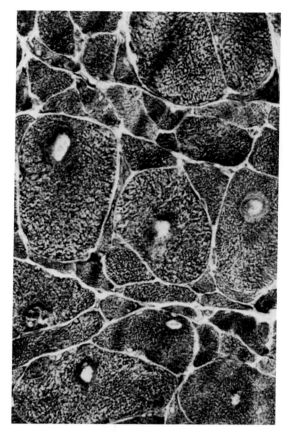

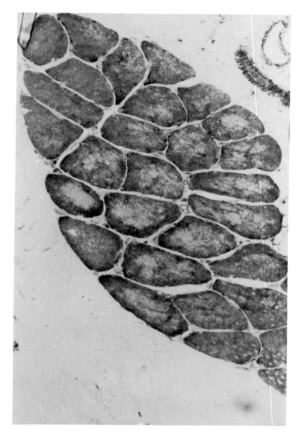

Fig. 10.19. Target fibres with grouped denervation atrophy after a peripheral nerve injury. (NADH, × 560)

Fig. 10.20. Moth-eaten fibres in dermatomyositis. (NADH, × 140)

myofibrillar disruption, non-reactive in NADH preparations, which extends the length of the fibre. A distinction has been drawn between fibres with structured (ATPase-positive) and unstructured (ATPase-negative) cores (Neville and Brooke 1971), but it is doubtful whether this is useful in practice. The latter are sometimes called core-targetoid fibres, a term that illustrates the difficulties.

Moth-eaten Fibres

Moth-eaten fibres (Brooke and Engel 1966) are fibres in which the normally regular intermyofibrillar network seen in the oxidative enzyme reactions is disturbed. Type 1 fibres are preferentially affected. The abnormality often consists of a whorled appearance, and areas of non-reactivity to NADH are often present near these whorls (Fig. 10.20). This change is not specific for any single disorder, but is particularly associated with inflammatory myopathies.

Rod Bodies

The Gomori preparation gives the best visualization of rod bodies. They consist of small red rod-like bodies, scattered in the sarcoplasm of affected fibres (Fig. 10.21). These rods are faintly visible as basophilic structures in H&E stains, and are derived from Z-band material (Fig. 10.22). They were first described in a familial non-progressive myopathy with hypotonia by Shy et al. (1963) and were termed nemaline myopathy by these authors. However, they have also been reported in adult limb–girdle myopathies, polymyositis (Sato et al. 1971) and a variety of other disorders.

Cytoplasmic Bodies

Cytoplasmic bodies, consisting of small eosinophilic PAS-positive zones within otherwise normal muscle fibres, have been particularly associated with colla-

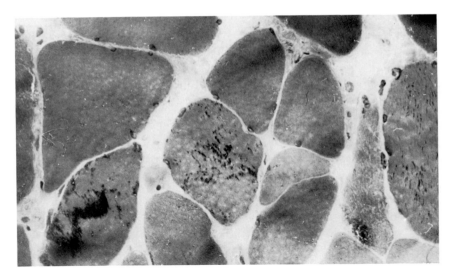

Fig. 10.21. Rod bodies. There is abnormal variability in fibre size with interstitial fibrosis. (Gomori trichrome, × 560)

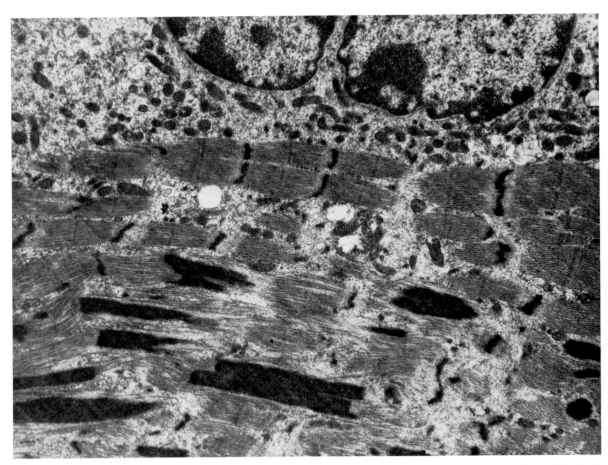

Fig. 10.22. Rod bodies in longitudinal section; their origin from Z-band material is evident. There are associated abnormalities in the organization of the structure of myofibrils. (Electron micrograph, × 22 500)

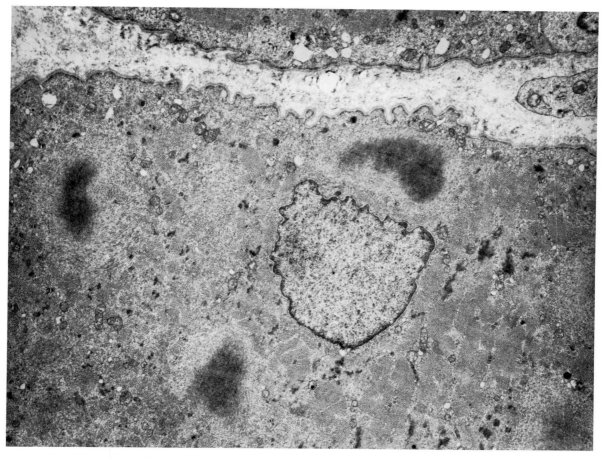

Fig. 10.23. Cytoplasmic bodies in dermatomyositis. (Electron micrograph, × 15 000)

gen vascular disease, such as dermatomyositis (Fig. 10.23), but when present in small numbers their significance is doubtful.

Ring Fibres

Although formerly associated with myotonic dystrophy, ring fibres (Fig. 10.24) can occur in many other chronic disorders. Nevertheless they are most frequently encountered in myotonic dystrophy and are then often associated with *sarcoplasmic masses*. Ring fibres (*Ringbinden*) consist of fibres in which a displaced myofibrillar strand has taken up a spiral position around the periphery of the fibre. Sarcoplasmic masses consist of peripheral zones of sarcoplasm, devoid of myofibrils and of other cell organelles (Klinkerfuss 1967).

Other Features

Motor End-plates

Motor end-plates (see Fig. 10.5) are seen occasionally in random biopsies, but can be studied more easily in motor point biopsies. Their morphology has been reviewed by Gauthier (1976) and by Brumback and Gerst (1984). Marked axonal sprouting occurs from the terminal axons, and the motor end-plate itself during reinnervation following partial denervation of muscle fibres.

Blood Vessels

Blood vessels, including arterioles, veins and capillaries, are found in all muscle biopsies. Abnormalities

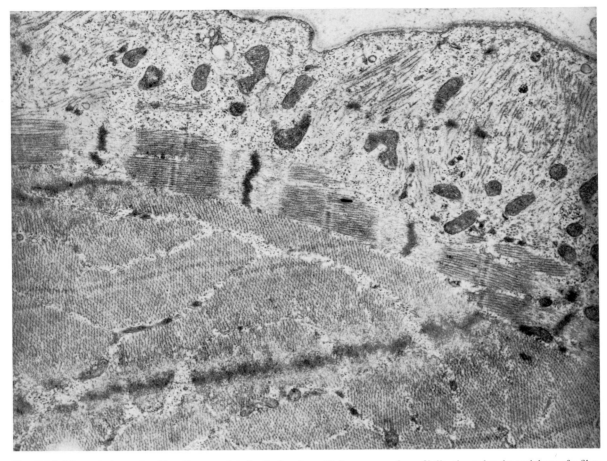

Fig. 10.24. Myotonic dystrophy. Ring fibres consist of a displaced myofibril, or group of myofibrils, situated at the periphery of a fibre. There are peripheral sarcoplasmic masses containing myofibrillar debris. (Electron micrograph, × 30 000)

in blood vessels are uncommon, except in polymyositis and polyarteritis, when necrosis of the arteriolar wall, hyaline change, thrombosis and, most frequently, infiltration by small round cells and plasma cells may occur. The capillaries have been little studied, although it has been suggested that the perifascicular atrophy found in inflammatory myopathies may be due to capillary necrosis or shutdown (Carpenter et al. 1976), and tubular inclusions have been reported in these endothelial cells in childhood dermatomyositis. In childhood dermatomyositis Whitaker and Engel (1972) found depositions of immune complexes in the walls of capillaries and arterioles.

Connective Tissue

The connective tissue in the endomysium is increased in any chronic neuromuscular disease, but marked fibrosis is an especially typical feature of Duchenne-type muscular dystrophy.

Small *nerve fascicles* are often found in muscle biopsies, and it is occasionally possible to recognize abnormalities such as demyelination, or congenital absence of myelination (Karch and Urich 1975), and the axonal change of "dying-back" neuropathies. Methylene blue impregnations performed by the supravital method (Cöers and Woolf 1953) are valuable in the assessment of such disorders, but they are time consuming and are rarely performed in routine laboratory practice (Harriman 1961).

Muscle Spindles

Muscle spindles (Fig. 10.25) are found fairly frequently in muscle biopsies (Swash 1983). Normal muscle spindles consist of a capsule of perineurial cells, fibrocytes and collagen enclosing a periaxial

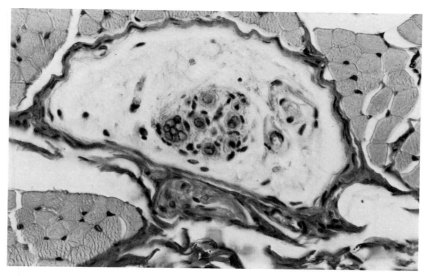

Fig. 10.25. Normal muscle spindle. The spindle consists of a capsule enclosing a mucopolysaccharide-filled periaxial space and a cluster of intrafusal muscle fibres. In this transverse section the nuclear bag and nuclear chain fibres can be recognized. In children, as in this illustration, extrafusal muscle fibres are not much larger than the intrafusal muscle fibres. (van Gieson, × 560)

space containing several small intrafusal muscle fibres, the nuclear bag and nuclear chain fibres, a bundle of small nerve fibres, and a few capillaries. There are normally at least two bag fibres (Fig. 10.25) and three to ten chain fibres. These fibres receive a complex motor and sensory innervation (Swash and Fox 1972). They undergo characteristic changes, consisting in fragmentation of intrafusal muscle fibres (Fig. 10.26) in myotonic dystrophy (Swash and Fox 1975a, b), and abnormalities also occur (Swash and Fox 1976) in Duchenne-type muscular dystrophy (Fig. 10.27) and in motor and sensory denervation (Fig. 10.28) (Swash and Fox 1974).

Classification of Neuromuscular Disorders

The classification of neuromuscular disorders introduced by the World Federation of Neurology (Walton et al. 1994) is comprehensive, but cumbersome because of the extreme rarity of many of the disorders included in it. Neuromuscular diseases are broadly classified into myopathic and neurogenic disorders:

A. *Myopathic disorders*
  1. *Muscular dystrophies*
    a) Duchenne-type muscular dystrophy

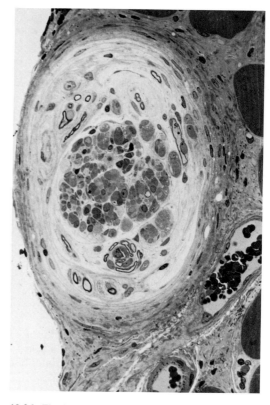

Fig. 10.26. The intrafusal muscle fibres are fragmented and the pattern of innervation is abnormal in this case of myotonic dystrophy. (Toluidine blue, semi-thin section, × 560)

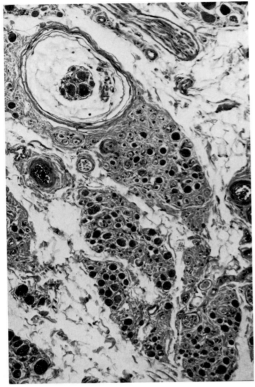

Fig. 10.27. Duchenne-type muscular dystrophy: autopsy specimen. There is dense fibrosis with fat replacement. Remaining muscle fibres are rounded. The muscle spindle shows fibrosis of the intrafusal muscle fibre bundle with dilatation of the periaxial space and capsular thickening. (van Gieson, × 140)

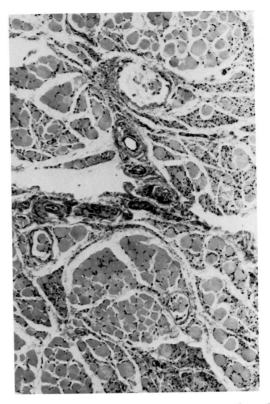

Fig. 10.28. Werdnig–Hoffman disease: autopsy specimen. The spindle at the *top* shows dilatation of the periaxial space. There is a slight increase in the number of intrafusal muscle fibres and these are smaller than normal. Atrophy of extrafusal muscle fibres has resulted in crowding and prominence of the spindle capsules. (van Gieson, × 140)

      b) Becker muscular dystrophy
      c) Limb–girdle muscular dystrophy
      d) Facioscapulohumeral muscular dystrophy
      e) Congenital muscular dystrophy
      f) Muscular dystrophy with external ophthalmoplegia
  2. *Benign congenital myopathies*
      a) Central-core and multicore disease
      b) Nemaline myopathy
      c) Myotubular myopathy
      d) Congenital fibre-type disproportion
      e) Other myopathies
  3. *Myotonic syndromes*
      a) Myotonic dystrophy (Steinert's disease)
      b) Myotonic congenita (Thomsen's disease)
      c) Paramyotonia congenita (Eulenburg's disease)
      d) Other myotonic syndromes
  4. *Metabolic and endocrine myopathies*
      a) Metabolic myopathies
        i) Glycogenoses

        ii) Mitochondrial myopathies
        iii) Periodic paralysis
        iv) Myopathies with myoglobinuria
        v) Malignant hyperpyrexia
      b) Endocrine myopathies
        i) Thyroid disorders
        ii) Parathyroid disorders and osteomalacia
        iii) Pituitary and adrenal disorders
  5. *Arthrogryposis multiplex* (This disorder also has neurogenic causes)
B. *Inflammatory myopathies*
      a) Dermatomyositis and polymyositis
      b) Infective myositis
C. *Disorders of neuromuscular transmission*
      a) Myasthenia gravis
      b) Congenital myasthenic syndromes
D. *Neurogenic disorders*
  1. *Spinal muscular atrophy*
      a) Severe (infantile) spinal muscular atrophy (Werdnig–Hoffmann disease)
      b) Intermediate spinal muscular atrophy

c) spinal muscular atrophy (Kugelberg–Welander disease)
2. Motor neuron disease
2. *Genetically determined neuropathies*
   a) Charcot–Marie–Tooth syndrome (hereditary motor and sensory neuropathies; HMSN)
   b) Hereditary sensory and autonomic neuropathies (HSAN)
   c) Hereditary amyloid neuropathies
   d) Others
3. *Genetically determined neuropathies with known metabolic defect*
   a) Porphyric neuropathy
   b) Refsum's disease
   c) Metachromatic leucodystrophy (sulphatide lipidosis)
   d) Tangier disease
   e) Bassen–Kornzweig's syndrome
   f) Krabbe's disease
   g) Fabry's disease
   h) Other lipid storage disease
4. *Acquired neuropathies* (see p. 614)

There are clearly recognizable differences in the histological changes found in the myopathies and neurogenic disorders (Table 10.2).

Myopathic Disorders

Muscular Dystrophies

The term "muscular dystrophy" refers to a group of genetically determined diseases characterized by progressive degenerative changes in muscle fibres without primary abnormality in the lower motor neuron. They are classified according to their clinical, morphological and genetic characteristics (see above).

The X-linked myopathies are listed in Table 10.3.

Xp21 Muscular Dystrophies

The Xp21 myopathies are membrane disorders. In the dystrophinopathies (Table 10.3) there is defective expression of dystrophin in the muscle cell membrane. McLeod syndrome is an abnormal phenotype characterized by disturbed red blood cell morphology (poikilocytes) and a mild myopathy, but with normal dystrophin expression. The genetic locus for McLeod phenotype is close to, but does not overlap with, that

Table 10.2. Changes found in myopathic and neurogenic disorders

Myopathic	Neurogenic
1. Prominent degenerative and regenerative changes in individual fibres	1. Fibre-type grouping
2. Increased variability in fibre size	2. Fibre-type atrophy
3. Fibrosis may be prominent	3. Clusters of small pointed fibres, often dark in NADH and non-specific esterase preparations
4. Architectural changes prominent	4. Type 1 fibre hypertrophy
5. Various specific morphological abnormalities	5. Only rare degenerative changes
6. Type 2 fibre atrophy	6. Rare architectural changes
7. Perifascicular atrophy	7. Little fibrosis
8. Blood vessels abnormal in inflammatory myopathies	8. Blood vessels normal
9. Fibre-type grouping uncommon	9. Target fibres or core fibres

Table 10.3. X-linked muscular dystrophies

	Affected gene basis
Dystrophinopathies	
Duchenne muscular dystrophy	Xp21.2
Becker muscular dystrophy	Xp21.2
Myalgia–cramp syndrome	Xp21.2
McLeod myopathy	Xp21 (1–2)
Emery–Dreifuss muscular dystrophy	Xq27.3–28
Centronuclear myopathy	Xq28
Scapuloperoneal myopathy	?

for Duchenne disease. It is sometimes associated with chronic granulomatous disease (Swash et al. 1983).

Duchenne-type Muscular Dystrophy

This is a progressive myopathy inherited in a sex-linked recessive pattern.

It presents in infancy with delay in the achievement of motor developmental milestones, especially walking, and is often characterized by hypertrophy and hardness of the calf and shoulder muscles on palpation. Weakness is principally proximal at first, but as the disease progresses weakness becomes generalized, although distal muscles are always relatively spared and the external ocular muscles are apparently never clinically affected. Scoliosis, dysphagia and cardiomyopathy develop and there is often a degree of mental retardation. Boys affected by the condition

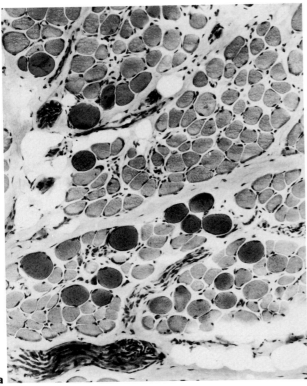

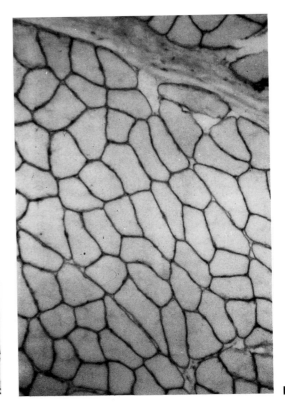

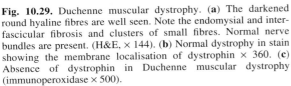

a

b

Fig. 10.29. Duchenne muscular dystrophy. (**a**) The darkened round hyaline fibres are well seen. Note the endomysial and interfascicular fibrosis and clusters of small fibres. Normal nerve bundles are present. (H&E, × 144). (**b**) Normal dystrophy in stain showing the membrane localisation of dystrophin × 360. (**c**) Absence of dystrophin in Duchenne muscular dystrophy (immunoperoxidase × 500).

never learn to run, and death occurs before the end of the third decade in almost all cases. The blood creatine kinase level is greatly raised, often to values several hundred times the normal range, and this abnormality is present before the disease is recognizable clinically. Female carriers of the gene for Duchenne dystrophy usually also show slightly raised levels of creatine kinase in their blood, both at rest and after exercise (Dreyfus et al. 1960).

Muscle biopsies show the typical features of myopathy, but these abnormalities vary in severity according to the stage of the disease and the muscle biopsied. In the early stages there is abnormal variation in fibre size, with prominent focal areas of small basophilic regenerating fibres. The muscle fibres usually appear abnormally rounded. Even at this stage of the disease there may be increased interfascicular and endomysial fibrous tissue (Fig. 10.29). Rounded, large, dark-staining fibres (hyaline fibres), which are markedly eosinophilic and stain red in trichrome preparations, are a prominent feature (Fig. 10.30). Scattered necrotic fibres undergoing phagocy-

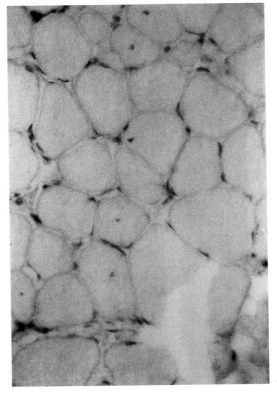

c

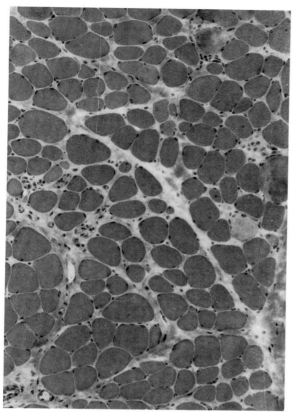

Fig. 10.30. Duchenne muscular dystrophy. The muscle fibres are unusually rounded. There is abnormal variability in fibre size. (Gomori trichrome, × 140)

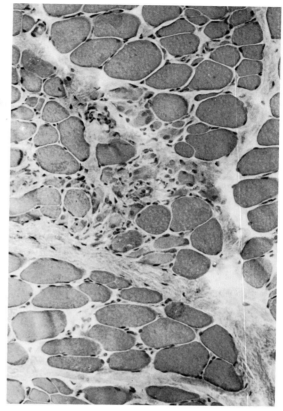

Fig. 10.31. Duchenne muscular dystrophy. Clusters of small regenerating fibres are a characteristic feature. (H&E, × 140

tosis and small clusters of regenerating fibres are also present (Fig. 10.31). Fibre splitting may be prominent at this early stage of the disease. As the disorder progresses fibrosis becomes more evident. In severely affected muscles the fascicular pattern of the muscle is destroyed, and the remaining muscle fibres become arranged in irregular bundles surrounded by adipose and fibrous tissue (see Fig. 10.27). Nerve fascicles are relatively spared, but muscle spindles are involved and are eventually destroyed (Swash and Fox 1976). In the early stages it is not uncommon for regenerating clumps of fibres to form small groups of fibres of similar histochemical type, but fibre-type grouping is not a feature of the disease (Schwartz et al. 1977a). Biopsies usually show type 1 fibres to be predominant (Fig. 10.32), and the normally clear differentiation of type 1 and type 2 fibres in the ATPase reaction at pH 9.4 is impaired, so that many fibres appear to be of intermediate histochemical type. These are type 2C fibres, normally uncommon in human muscle.

Electron microscopy shows degenerative and regenerative changes, which are not specific. However, electron microscopic studies show that plasma membranes of necrotic (Milhorat et al. 1966) and of apparently normal muscle fibres in Duchenne dystrophy are defective, allowing abnormal permeability and thus leading to swelling and focal necrosis of fibres (Mokri and Engel 1975). This abnormality explains the presence of focal "hypercontraction bands" in muscle fibres in this disorder, an abnormality that seems to underlie the formation of the darkly staining hyaline fibres.

At autopsy most of the proximal muscles are found to be replaced by fat and fibrous tissue. The peripheral nerves and spinal cord are normal and there is a normal number of anterior horn cells. However, in the brain, abnormal patterns of gyral development, pachygyria and microscopic heterotopias have been observed, and brains from boys with Duchenne dystrophy weigh less than those of age-matched controls (Rosman and Kalkulas 1966).

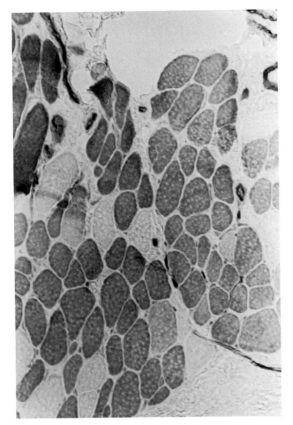

Fig. 10.32 Duchenne-type muscular dystrophy. The rounded fibres are well shown. There is quite prominent type 1 fibre predominance. (ATPase, pH 4.3, × 140)

In Duchenne muscular dystrophy there is a genetic defect on the X chromosome at the Xp21.2 locus. The normal product of this gene is dystrophin, a membrane protein which is particularly important in muscle. Dystrophin is located on the inner surface of the plasma membrane at the attachment of the I and M bands of myofilaments to the muscle fibre membrane. This site is co-localized with spectrin in the muscle membrane. The N-terminal end of the dystrophin molecule is attached to the subsarcolemmal actin cytoskeleton, and the C-terminal end to a 59 kDa protein that is itself linked to a transmembrane 156 kDa glycoprotein complex that binds to a component of laminin in the extracellular matrix. Dystrophin deficiency results in increased vulnerability to injury and less effective repair. Muscle cell destruction in the disease is probably caused by calcium-dependent protease activity, and absence of dystrophin is important in allowing this process to develop (Hoffman et al. 1987). The genetic defect in Duchenne muscular dystrophy results, in about 65%

of cases, from an out-of-frame deletion in the gene (Kunkel and Hoffman 1989). In others the mutation is an exon duplication or cannot yet be identified.

Carrier Detection. Formerly, detection of carrier females was accomplished by measurement of venous blood creatine kinase levels in three intermenstrual fasting samples drawn at weekly intervals, and an elevated creatine kinase level was taken as indicative of carrier status (Emery 1980). Sometimes, muscle biopsy was also used to detect minor myopathic features, representing variation in the degree of Lyonization of paternal or maternal X chromosomal material in the phenotype.

Genetic testing is now used. The first step is to identify the causative mutation in the proband. In 65% of cases this is a deletion in the dystrophin gene. In affected males this can be detected by polymerase chain reaction (PCR) amplification. A number of methods are used to detect deletions in one of the two X chromosomes of potential carriers, including polymorphic gene markers, multiplex PCR amplification, and other more specialized techniques. None is, as yet, entirely reliable (Abbs and Bobrow 1993).

Becker-type Muscular Dystrophy

Becker-type muscular dystrophy disorder is similar to Duchenne dystrophy but of lesser severity, so that survival into adult life with preservation of the ability to walk is a criterion for diagnosis. Many patients present in adult life, sometimes with cardiomyopathy. Like Duchenne dystrophy, it is inherited as an X-linked recessive disorder (Becker 1962). Muscle biopsy generally reveals similar features to those of Duchenne dystrophy, but the abnormalities may be less severe, and there are sometimes large numbers of small fibres, some of which appear pointed and resemble denervated fibres (Bradley et al. 1978). The dystrophin gene abnormality in Becker disease is an in-frame deletion causing synthesis of an abnormal dystrophin molecule.

Other X-linked Disorders

The pathology of other X-linked muscle disorders, of X-linked scapuloperoneal myopathy and Emery–Dreifuss syndrome is not generally distinctive (see Swash and Schwartz 1996).

Limb–girdle Muscular Dystrophy

Muscular dystrophy in a limb–girdle distribution, with proximal weakness affecting the legs more than the arms, is difficult to distinguish from Becker dystrophy. Limb–girdle dystrophy is inherited in an autosomal recessive pattern, but many cases are sporadic. A useful classification is that of Jerusalem and Sieb (1992):

1. Autosomal recessive muscular dystrophy of childhood
   a) Pelvifemoral type (Leyden–Moebius)
   b) Scapulohumeral type (Erb)
   c) Severe childhood type (North African)
   d) Bethlem myopathy
   e) Rigid spine syndrome
2. Autosomal dominant disorders
   a) Early-onset with contractures
   b) Late-onset (Nevin)
3. Others
   a) Desmin myopathy
   b) Fukuyama disease

The disease may progress rapidly or slowly. This pattern of muscular weakness does not represent a specific disease entity, but results from a number of different biochemical disorders. Indeed, several clinically similar syndromes within this description of limb–girdle weakness have been reclassified on the basis of recognized metabolic defects of glycogen storage disease. In the past, juvenile-onset spinal muscular atrophy (see p. 602) was often misclassified as limb–girdle dystrophy, but modern enzyme-histochemical methods have eliminated this problem. The creatine phosphokinase is usually slightly or moderately elevated in limb–girdle dystrophy.

Muscle biopsy shows fibres of varying size, with increased central nucleation, a few scattered necrotic or regenerating fibres, and striking hypertrophy of some fibres. Fibre-type grouping is absent. Oxidative enzyme preparations show fibres, particularly larger fibres, with a whorled appearance, indicating an abnormal distribution of lipid and mitochondria and therefore an abnormal pattern of myofibrils. PAS preparations show a similar abnormality. Electron microscopy shows no specific abnormality. No characteristic pathological features are found in this syndrome.

In the *pelvifemoral* and *scapulohumeral* types of autosomal recessive disease, no distinctive pathological changes occur other than those described above.

In *Bethlem myopathy*, an infantile-onset syndrome with contractures of fingers, elbows and ankles, the muscle biopsy shows fibre hypertrophy, muscle fibre splitting and central nucleation, but no necrosis or regeneration (Mohire et al. 1988).

In *rigid spine syndrome*, an infantile-onset disorder mainly affecting boys, the sternomastoids and

girdle muscles are weak and cardiomyopathy may be a feature, with complete heart block (Goebel et al. 1977a). The creatine kinase level is raised. The muscle biopsy shows hypertrophic and atrophic fibres, type 2 predominance, central nucleation and fibrosis (Goebel et al. 1977a; Poewe et al. 1985).

In the Mahgreb area of Tunisia, and uncommonly in other countries, a *severe autosomal recessive muscular dystrophy*, in many respects resembling Duchenne dystrophy except for its occurrence in girls, has been recognized. The biopsy shows type 1 fibre predominance, with myopathic change and fibrosis, but relatively few hyaline fibres (Ben Hamida et al. 1983). This disorder has been linked to a locus on chromosome 13q, and shown to be due to an absence of the 50 kDa dystrophin-associated membrane glycoprotein on the surface of muscle fibres (Othmane et al. 1992).

Fukuyama disease is a fatal progressive muscular dystrophy presenting in utero, by abortion or at birth. There is severe weakness and flaccid tone, and contractures are a feature. Seizures, mental retardation and anomalous gyration of the brain with hypercholesterolaemia and myoglobinuria are found. Expression of the 43 kDa dystrophin-associated glycoprotein in muscle is markedly reduced (Matsumora et al. 1993).

Desmin myopathy presents with weakness at birth and progressively worsens, with delayed motor milestones. The biopsy shows desmin inclusions in a subsarcolemmal location. These appear eosinophilic by light microscopy (Fardeau et al. 1978; Prelle et al. 1992).

Facioscapulohumeral Muscular Dystrophy

The shoulder girdle and facial muscles are principally affected in facioscapulohumeral muscular dystrophy, which is an autosomal dominant defect (chromosome 4q 35). The syndrome probably results from a number of different causes, including muscular dystrophy, myasthenia gravis, various congenital myopathies (especially myotubular myopathy), nemaline myopathy, central-core disease and mitochondrial myopathies (Van Wijngaarden and Bethlem 1971), polymyositis, and chronic denervating disorders. Cases resulting from idiopathic dystrophy are a minority in this list of causes, and in these cases changes found in biopsies of affected muscles are often surprisingly slight. Scapuloperoneal myopathy forms a rare subgroup of this disorder in which weakness principally affects periscapular and peroneal muscles; the extensor digitorum brevis muscles are strikingly spared. This latter disorder also has a neurogenic form (see Kaeser 1965).

Congenital Muscular Dystrophy

The syndrome of congenital muscular dystrophy presents from birth with hypotonia and generalized weakness. Contractures develop. There may be associated mental retardation. In some cases improvement occurs with increasing age. The muscle biopsy shows striking myopathic changes with marked endomysial fibrosis and accumulations of adipose tissue. The muscle fibres are often strikingly small, and fibre-type differentiation may be abnormal. This syndrome is one of the causes of arthrogryposis multiplex (see p. 598). Several of the myopathic causes are described in the preceding section of this chapter.

Muscular Dystrophy with Involvement of External Ocular Muscles

Cases of progressive external ophthalmoplegia with ptosis (Kiloh and Nevin 1951), oculopharyngeal myopathy, often associated with some skeletal muscular weakness (Victor et al. 1962; Barbeau 1966), and external ophthalmoplegia with limb–girdle weakness, sometimes associated with cerebellar ataxia, retinitis pigmentosa, heart block, elevated cerebrospinal fluid protein levels (Kearns and Sayre 1958) and other features (Drachman 1968; Berenberg et al. 1977), form a distinct group of syndromes.

In these syndromes with external ophthalmoplegia, biopsy of a proximal upper limb muscle may reveal a characteristic abnormality, consisting of lightly vacuolated fibres, rimmed with material stained red with the Gomori stain – "ragged red fibres" (see Fig. 10.13). This abnormality predominantly affects type 1 fibres. Other myopathic features, including slightly increased variability in fibre size, increased central nucleation and increased endomysial fibrous tissue, may be seen. Ultrastructural studies reveal mitochondrial abnormalities similar to those found in other *mitochondrial myopathies*.

It is striking that external ophthalmoplegia does not occur in other myopathies or dystrophies, although it is also a feature of myasthenia gravis.

"Benign" Myopathies of Childhood

These myopathic disorders present at birth or in early infancy as the floppy infant syndrome, or later in childhood as proximal or generalized muscular weakness. In most instances these disorders are non-progressive or only very slowly progressive, and the creatine kinase level is often normal.

Central-core Disease

Shy and Magee (1956) defined *central-core disease* as a non-progressive congenital myopathy beginning shortly after birth, but more recently cases have been described that are apparently of later onset (Bethlem et al. 1966), and some have been associated with congenital dislocation of the hip (Armstrong et al. 1971). Hypotonia is a prominent feature, and weakness is not severe. The disorder is usually dominantly inherited. The muscle biopsy shows type 1 fibre predominance or, sometimes, poorly differentiated fibres with a core of tissue devoid of enzyme reactivity in oxidative enzyme preparations, e.g. NADH preparations. Most cores occur in type 1 fibres. Electron microscopy shows that these cores contain few mitochondria and little sarcoplasmic reticulum; various myofibrillar abnormalities, including streaming of the Z-line, occur in this region (Seitelberger et al. 1961). The cores have a predilection for type 1 fibres (Dubowitz and Roy 1970) and must be distinguished from target fibres (Swash and Schwartz 1981), an abnormality found in denervated muscle. Cores may be "structured", retaining their myofibrillar pattern and thus being demonstrable in ATPase preparations, or "unstructured", losing their myofibrillar and intermyofibrillar structure (Neville and Brooke 1973).

In *multicore (minicore) disease*, similar but sporadic or autosomal recessive disorder, muscle biopsy shows multiple areas of focal decrease in mitochondrial oxidative enzyme activity, usually associated with focal degenerative changes in myofibrils. These areas (Fig. 10.33), unlike the cores of classic central-core disease, do not extend throughout the length of affected fibres but are relatively sharply circumscribed (Currie et al. 1974). Central nucleation is usually prominent. *Focal loss of cross-striations* is a less common but related abnormality in which linear transverse zones (Fig. 10.33) resembling short unstructured cores are found extending only through several sarcomeres (Van Wijngaarden et al. 1977; Swash and Schwartz 1981). This abnormality is associated with a non-progressive myopathy in which external ocular muscles may be involved. Improvement may occur during adolescence.

Nemaline Myopathy (Rod-body Myopathy)

Shy and Magee (1956) and Gonatas et al. (1966) described rod-like structures in the muscle biopsies of several infants that had been floppy since birth and showed weakness of the arms more than of the legs. Other workers (Hopkins et al. 1966) have recognized that this disorder was the same as had previously

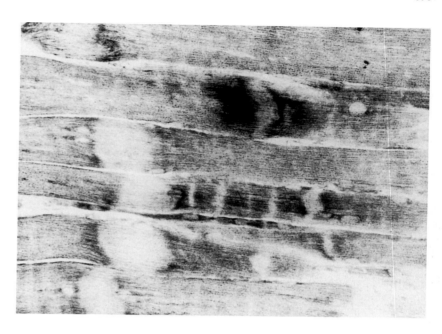

Fig. 10.33. Central cores and focal loss of cross-striations. (NADH, ×448)

been termed "Krabbe's universal muscular atrophy". The disease is probably inherited as an autosomal dominant characteristic. Respiratory difficulties are common in infancy. The severity of the disorder varies widely from case to case, and the nosological position of nemaline myopathy is made particularly controversial by reports of the occurrence of similar nemaline bodies in a variety of other disorders, including denervation, psychosis, myotonic dystrophy, polymyositis and Adie's syndrome, and after experimental tenotomy (see Dubowitz and Brooke 1973; Swash and Fox 1976). Late-onset cases also occur (Engel and Resnick 1966).

In some cases of nemaline myopathy the biopsy has been normal, apart from the presence of the rods, but in many instances there is increased variability in fibre size (the rod bodies being more prominent in the smaller fibres) and increased central nucleation. In oxidative enzyme preparations whorled fibres are sometimes seen. The rod bodies are difficult to recognize in H&E preparations, but in Gomori stains (Figs. 10.21 and 10.22) they appear as short bright-red masses and are usually predominantly subsarcolemmal in location. Aggregates of rods appear as negatively stained areas in ATPase preparations. Either or both fibre types may be affected. Electron microscopy reveals that the rods are derived from Z-band material (Figs. 10.14 and 10.27), and Shafiq et al. (1967) have suggested that they are derived from tropomyosin, a protein devoid of tryptophan. Rod bodies have been reported to coexist with central cores (Afifi et al. 1965) and with failure of fibre type differentiation (Nienhuis et al. 1967), and there may

thus be similarities between these apparently dissimilar disorders.

Myotubular Myopathy

Myotubular myopathy (Spiro et al. 1966), also known as centronuclear myopathy (Sher et al. 1967), is a disorder characterized by hypotonia with delayed motor developmental milestones in infancy, followed by a slowly progressive myopathy involving facial and sometimes external ocular musculature. Adult-onset examples have also been reported (Bethlem et al. 1968). These have usually affected females, and in one family there was an association with diabetes mellitus (Swash et al. 1970). Central nucleation is found in nearly all the fibres in the biopsy and the term "centronuclear myopathy" is sometimes preferred to that of myotubular myopathy. In the central regions of affected fibres oxidative enzyme activity is absent or abnormally intense, and myofibrillar ATPase is absent in these regions. In some cases type 1 fibre hypertrophy has been described (Bethlem et al. 1969).

Congenital Fibre-type Disproportion

The characteristic feature of congenital fibre-type disproportion is evident only on muscle biopsy (Brooke 1973). Clinically, affected infants have been floppy or even very weak from birth, but after 2 years of age there is usually some improvement. The disorder is associated with congenital dislocation of the hip, low body weight and short stature, kyphoscoliosis, a high-arched palate and foot deformities (Cavanagh et al. 1979). The biopsy shows small type 1 fibres and normal or enlarged type 2 fibres. No other abnormality is present (Fardeau et al. 1975). The differential diagnosis must include severe infantile spinal muscular atrophy (which has a much poorer prognosis), congenital myotonic dystrophy and myotubular myopathy with type 1 fibre hypotrophy. The pattern of inheritance is variable, and the prognosis uncertain.

Other Congenital Myopathies

In a number of reports, individual patients or families have been described in whom myopathies beginning in infancy have been associated with muscle fibre abnormalities that are, as yet, difficult to classify. These include myopathies with subsarcolemmal "fingerprint" inclusions (Engel et al. 1972), myopathies with abnormal sarcotubular systems, zebra-body myopathy (Lake and Wilson 1975), and myopathies with cytoplasmic bodies or tubular aggregates. Dubowitz (1978) has proposed the term "minimal change myopathy" to describe cases such as these, in which the muscle biopsy shows only minimal myopathic abnormalities without more specific features.

Myotonic Syndromes

The group of myotonic syndromes involves patients in whom myotonia, a state of delayed relaxation or of sustained contraction of muscle fibres, occurs alone or in association with myopathic muscular weakness. Myotonia, although recognizable clinically, must be differentiated by electromyographic criteria from other forms of persistent contraction of muscle fibres. It is due to an abnormality in ionic conductance in the muscle fibre membrane (Barchi 1975) as a result of specific genetic defects in ion channels in the muscle fibre membrane (Table 10.4).

Myotonic Dystrophy

In myotonic dystrophy, myotonia is typically associated with muscular weakness and wasting, frontal baldness, testicular atrophy, ptosis, dysphagia and cataract. Cardiomyopathy and diabetes mellitus and some degree of mental retardation are common. The disease usually begins in adult life or in adolescence, and the weakness is most evident in facial,

Table 10.4. Genetic classification of the myotonias

	Affected gene locus
Chloride channel disorders	Ch 17q
Myotonia congenita	
Dominant (Thomsen)	
Recessive (Becker)	
Sodium channel disorders	Ch 7q
Hyperkalaemic periodic paralysis	
Paramyotonia congenita	
Potassium-sensitive myotonia congenita	
Protein kinase-related myotonia	Ch 19q
Myotonic dystrophy	
Other myotonic syndromes	
Schwartz–Jampel disease	
Andersen's syndrome	
Drug-induced myotonia	

From Ptacek et al. (1992, 1993).

sternomastoid, neck extensor and distal limb muscles. The tendon reflexes are usually absent. In childhood the disease can also present with these features, but in the congenital form of myotonic dystrophy the clinical manifestations are somewhat different. There is hypotonia and failure to thrive, with respiratory difficulties in the perinatal period. Facial weakness is very prominent but myotonia is usually absent. If the infant survives, cardiomyopathy and mental retardation become evident. This form of disease is particularly common in children of mothers with the disease (Harper 1975). Myotonic dystrophy is inherited as a Mendelian dominant characteristic; the gene defect consists of a CTG trinucleotide repeat in the coding region on chromosome 19q13.3 (Harley et al. 1992). Genetic anticipation is explained by an increased number of CTG repeats in the gene. The gene codes a protein kinase, but the specific protein disorder underlying the phenotype is unknown.

In both adult-onset and congenital-onset cases the creatine kinase level is usually normal. Abnormalities in IgG and IgM concentration and metabolism have been reported (Wochner et al. 1966; Bundey et al. 1970). In the adult type of the disease muscle biopsies show marked changes. There is increased variability in fibre size, with type 1 fibre atrophy, and some degenerative changes in single fibres, consisting both in fibre necrosis and in patchy myofibrillar degeneration, often with the formation of peripherally placed masses of granular sarcoplasm free of myofibrils (see Fig. 10.24) (Klinkerfuss 1967). Fibrosis is a feature only in very wasted muscles. There may be a number of other abnormalities, including fibres with a moth-eaten appearance in the NADH preparation, and a variety of inclusions are seen in ultrastructural studies. Rod bodies have also been reported in myotonic dystrophy. A striking feature is central migration and proliferation of muscle fibre nuclei, resulting in the occurrence of long chains of centrally placed vesicular nuclei in longitudinal sections. Displaced myofibrils, forming *Ringbinden* (see Fig. 10.24), are also common in this disease.

The muscle spindles show a characteristic abnormality consisting of fragmentation of intrafusal muscle fibres (see Fig. 10.26), which is more marked in their polar than their equatorial regions, with proliferation of the motor and sensory innervation (Swash and Fox 1972, 1975a, b). The muscle spindle abnormality is not uniformly distributed, some spindles being more severely affected than others.

Small pointed fibres that are strongly positive for NADH and for non-specific esterase and contain pyknotic nuclei are commonly found in myotonic dystrophy, suggesting that denervation occurs in the disease. The innervation of the extrafusal muscle fibres in myotonic dystrophy is abnormal. Motor endplates show proliferative changes, with extensive subterminal axonal branching and expansion of the end-plate zone, but there is some doubt as to whether these abnormalities are primary or secondary to the dystrophic changes in the muscle fibres themselves (Allen et al. 1969).

In the less common congenital form of myotonic dystrophy the muscle biopsy shows similar abnormalities, but the main feature is the presence of small round fibres with central nuclei and atrophy of type 1 fibres.

Other Myotonic Syndromes (Table 10.4)

These are rare. They are usually diagnosed clinically and by electromyography. Confusion with myotonic dystrophy should no longer arise, given the availability of genetic markers for the specific channel defects identified (Ptacek et al. 1993).

Muscle pathology is not contributory to diagnosis. Hypertrophy of muscle fibres is most marked in recessive generalized myotonia, with increased central nucleation. In this disorder scattered necrotic and regenerating fibres may be detected, and type 2B fibres may be absent. In hyperkalaemic periodic paralysis, vacuolar change, tubular aggregates and a mild myopathy are prominent. Other abnormalities in these syndromes are non-specific.

Metabolic Myopathies

Metabolic myopathies are a group of myopathies of varying severity associated with biochemical defects. In some a fixed or progressive myopathy develops, but in others there are recurrent episodes of muscular weakness, often associated with transient myoglobinuria and muscular pain.

Glycogenoses

The glycogen storage diseases are all uncommon, and muscular involvement does not occur in all of them. Myopathy is prominent, among other manifestations, in acid maltase deficiency (type 2 glycogenosis), amylo-1,6-glucosidase deficiency (type 3 glycogenosis), myophosphorylase deficiency (type 5 glycogenosis: McArdle's disease) and phosphofructokinase deficiency (type 7 glycogenosis), but only in the last two are muscular symptoms the only manifestation.

Acid Maltase Deficiency. This disorder (type 2 glycogenosis) occurs in infantile-onset and adult-onset forms, inherited as an autosomal recessive disorder on chromosome 17q 23.

In the infantile autosomal recessive variety, proximal weakness, often associated with enlargement of the heart, liver and tongue, develops. Death usually occurs from cardiorespiratory failure before the age of 1 year. A milder form of the disease, leading to death in the second decade, resembles Duchenne dystrophy in its clinical manifestations. An adult-onset form has also been reported (Engel et al. 1973).

The creatine kinase level is slightly raised and, muscle biopsy shows a marked vacuolar myopathy (Fig. 10.34). The normal histological pattern of the muscle is destroyed by glycogen-containing PAS-positive vacuoles. These vacuoles are also strongly reactive for acid phosphatase (A.G. Engel 1970a). The autophagic nature of the vacuoles is confirmed by electron microscopy, which reveals glycogen granules packed free in the sarcoplasm, in whorled membrane-bound glycogen bodies, and in autophagic vacuoles (A.G. Engel 1970a; Swash et al. 1985).

Debranching Enzyme Deficiency. Type 3 glycogenosis involves liver and muscle. Although muscular involvement is relatively slight, the muscle biopsy shows a prominent vacuolar myopathy (Fig. 10.35). The vacuoles contain glycogen, but unlike those found in type 2 glycogenosis these vacuoles are not lysosomal in origin and are negative in stains for acid phosphatase (Illingworth et al. 1956; Brunberg et al. 1971).

Myophosphorylase and Phosphofructokinase Deficiencies. In myophosphorylase deficiency (type 5 glycogenosis) (McArdle 1951; Schmid and Mahler 1959) and phosphofructokinase deficiency (type 7 glycogenosis) (Tarui et al. 1965), easy fatiguability is

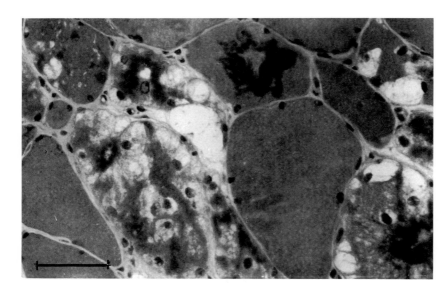

Fig. 10.34. Acid maltase deficiency. Vacuolar myopathy: the disorder is virtually limited to type 1 fibres. (H&E, × 574) (Reproduced from Swash et al. 1985)

followed, in late childhood or adolescence, by severe muscular cramps with weakness on exertion. Transient myoglobinuria may occur in these episodes. Later mild permanent proximal weakness may develop.

Although an autosomal recessive pattern of inheritance (chromosome 11q13) is usual, McArdle's syndrome (type 5 glycogenosis) is commoner in boys than in girls. The blood creatine kinase levels are raised after exertion in both syndromes, and during ischaemic exercise the venous lactate level fails to rise (Mellick et al. 1962). The muscle biopsy shows only minor histological changes. There are some small PAS-positive subsarcolemmal vacuoles and PAS staining shows an excess of sarcoplasmic glycogen. Necrotic or small fibres occur and internal nucleation is common. A fatal infantile form has been recorded (Miranda et al. 1979). Histochemical stains for phosphorylase demonstrate no reaction in McArdle's disease, and an absence of phosphofructokinase has been demonstrated in type 7 glycogenosis (Tarui et al. 1965). Ultrastructurally, glycogen deposition is prominent both in intermyofibrillar sarcoplasm and in the subsarcolemmal vacuoles.

Phosphoglycerate mutase deficiency, phosphoglycerate kinase deficiency and lactate dehydrogenase deficiency are rare glycogenoses that may present with exercise intolerance and myoglobinuria (see Swash and Schwartz 1996 for a review).

Mitochondrial Myopathies

Primary mitochondrial disorders are associated with a number of different clinical syndromes including mitochondrial myopathies, e.g. Luft's syndrome of hypermetabolism, myopathy with progressive external ophthalmoplegia (PEO) and exertional weakness, myopathy alone, and myopathy with associated central nervous system disorders including ataxia, deafness, myoclonus, seizures and dementia (Morgan-Hughes et al. 1982; Petty et al. 1986). Several major clinical syndromes are recognizable (Table 10.5).

Ragged-red fibres in these disorders are associated with defective mitochondrial oxidation due to substrate transport defects, substrate utilization defects, respiratory chain defects or energy transduction defects (Morgan-Hughes 1982). Similar histological

Table 10.5. Mitochondrial disorders involving muscle

Disorder	Mitochondrial genetics	Occurrences
Kearns Sayre syndrome (KSS)	Large mitochondrial deletion	Sporadic
Mitochondrial encephalopathy, myopathy, lactic acidosis, stroke-like syndrome (MELAS)	Point mutations	Maternal inheritance
Myoclonic epilepsy with ragged red fibres (MERRF)	Point mutations of mitochondrial DNA	Maternal inheritance
Mitochondrial myopathy	Deletions of mitochondrial DNA	Maternal inheritance
Progressive external ophthalmoplegia	Deletions of mitochondrial DNA	Sporadic

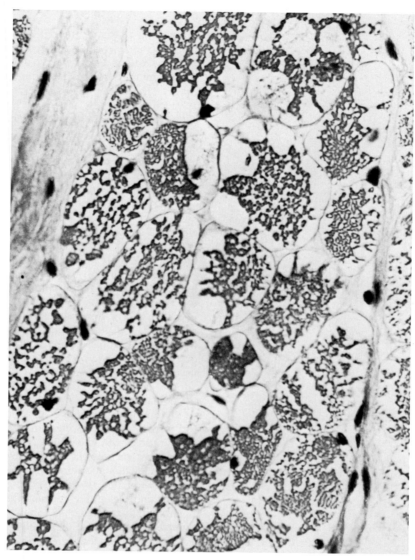

Fig. 10.35. Glycogen storage disease, type 3 rectus abdominis muscle. The vacuoles are filled with glycogen, which is invisible with this stain. (H&E, × 950)

abnormalities occur in Kearns–Sayre syndrome.

In carnitine deficiency and carnitine palmityl transferase deficiency there is probably a primary defect of mitochondrial oxidation; the characteristic morphological abnormality is found in muscle mitochondria in the former, but not in the latter disorders (see p. 575). Weakness and myoglobinuria, with muscular pain, occur after exercise. In carnitine deficiency, plasma, muscle and hepatic carnitine levels are low and there is sometimes hypoglycaemia. There is gross wasting and cachexia. In carnitine palmityl transferase deficiency cachexia is not a feature.

Fasting can induce attacks of weakness and myoglobinuria, together with a rise in blood triglycerides. The muscle biopsy in carnitine palmityl transferase deficiency is usually normal, but in carnitine deficiency there is a severe destructive myopathy with prominent lipid-containing acid-phosphatase-positive vacuoles (Bank et al. 1975; Karpati et al. 1975). Diagnosis of these disorders rests on demonstration of the primary biochemical disorder by quantitative biochemical studies, although it may be possible to suggest the likely defect from the clinical, biochemical and histological features.

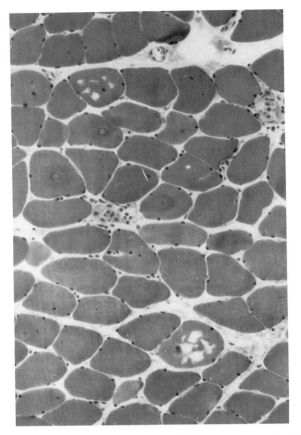

Fig. 10.36. Hypokalaemic periodic paralysis, transverse section of muscle. Several fibres contain large vacuoles; two others have undergone necrosis with phagocytosis. These are the features of longstanding periodic paralysis, with a recent acute attack. (H&E, × 140)

Other Causes of Myoglobinuria

Myoglobinuria can occur whenever there is acute necrosis of muscle, as in polymyositis, acute toxic myopathies, etc. (Table 10.6).

Table 10.6. Classification of myoglobinuric myopathies

	Example
Metabolic	Glycogenoses, lipid storage myopathies, malignant hyperpyrexia
Toxic	Carbon monoxide poisoning, alcohol, drugs
Traumatic	Major injuries
Ischaemic	Anterior tibial compartment syndrome
Idiopathic rhabdomyolysis	

Periodic Paralyses

Periodic paralyses are inherited as autosomal dominant traits and are characterized by attacks of flaccid paralysis of varying severity associated with low, normal or high serum potassium levels during the attacks. The term "adynamia episodica hereditaria" has been used to describe the normokalaemic variety (Gamstorp 1956), and in some patients attacks of weakness have been observed with normal and with raised serum potassium levels. The clinical features of these three forms of periodic paralysis overlap. In hypokalaemic periodic paralysis, weakness often begins during sleep, although, as in hyperkalaemic periodic paralysis, a period of rest after vigorous exercise may also induce attacks. Weakness may be provoked in the hypokalaemic variety by a heavy carbohydrate meal, cold, anxiety or a glucose load. Insulin will also induce an attack. The attacks of weakness are usually more severe and more prolonged in hypokalaemic paralysis than in the other forms of periodic paralysis, but death in an attack is uncommon. The disease usually begins in infancy or childhood, and after several attacks of severe weakness it may become apparent that there is some fixed or even progressive proximal weakness. This is often asymmetrical. Myoglobinuria is obvious only in severe attacks. In oriental races a form of hypokalaemic paralysis may be a presenting feature of thyrotoxicosis (Cheah et al. 1975).

Biopsies taken between attacks of weakness may show little or no abnormality, but in attacks there are often large vacuoles in muscle fibres (Fig. 10.36). In severe attacks some fibres become necrotic, and the typical sequence of necrosis, ingestion by macrophages and basophilic regeneration, usually subsarcolemmal, then occurs. Although the vacuoles appear empty in H&E stains they usually contain traces of PAS-positive material. However, electron microscopy reveals that the vacuoles are membrane bound (Fig. 10.37) and continuous with the sarcoplasmic reticulum and T-tube system (Howes et al. 1966; Engel 1970b). Other, non-specific, tubular abnormalities have also been described (Bradley 1969). Weller and McArdle (1971) demonstrated calcium salts (hydroxyapatite) in the vacuoles and in the muscle fibres themselves in biopsies from patients with longstanding periodic paralysis. The fixed myopathy found in some patients with these syndromes is associated with typical but non-specific histological features of a myopathy, including variability in fibre size, central nucleation, single-fibre necrosis and regeneration, and increased endomysial fibrous tissue (see Fig. 10.36). However, even in these cases there is sometimes vacuolation of fibres, and this can be an important clue in diagnosis.

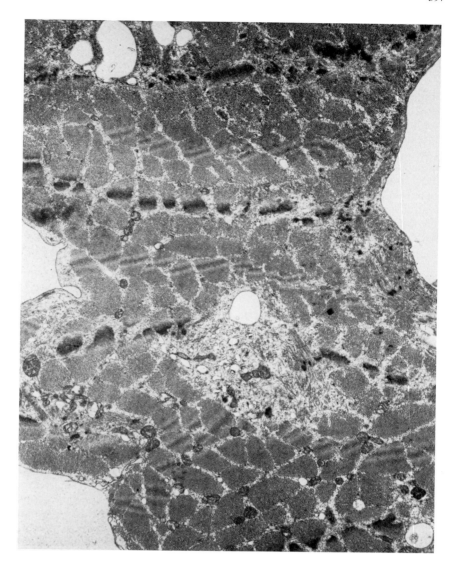

Fig. 10.37. Hypokalaemic periodic paralysis. The vacuoles are continuous with tubules of the sarcoplasmic reticulum and T-tube system, and are therefore bound by a single-layered membrane. Myofibrils near these vacuoles have become disrupted. (Electron micrograph, × 15 000)

Other Forms of Hypokalaemic Paralysis

Severe hypokalaemia of any cause can induce muscular weakness with typical vacuolar changes in the muscle biopsy. For example, hypokalaemia resulting from diuretic therapy, renal disease or liquorice ingestion may occasionally be sufficiently severe to induce weakness.

Malignant Hyperpyrexia

In malignant hyperpyrexia a mild or even subclinical myopathy, dominantly inherited, is associated with a tendency for fatal hyperpyrexia to develop during general anaesthesia. It is one of the major causes of death associated with anaesthesia. The hyperpyrexia results from heat produced by intense and generalized muscular rigidity with tachycardia, tachypnoea, cyanosis and severe metabolic acidosis. Extensive muscular necrosis follows, with myoglobinuria, a very high serum creatine kinase level and sometimes renal failure. Recovery is usually complete in patients who survive the hyperpyrexia, hyperkalaemia and acidosis. The underlying metabolic disorder is ill-defined, but it has been suggested that certain anaesthetic drugs, especially halothane and depolarizing muscle relaxant drugs such as succinylcholine, release sarcoplasmic and sarcotubular calcium ions, causing muscular contraction. The primary defect is in calcium-induced channels in skeletal muscle (the ryanodine receptor). The gene for this receptor protein has been mapped to chromosome 19q13.1 (Gillard et al. 1992). Susceptibility can be recognized by provocation tests on muscle tissue obtained by biopsy in an in vitro test (Moulds and Denborough 1972; Ellis et al. 1973).

Muscle biopsies taken after an attack of hyperpyrexia show extensive muscle fibre necrosis, followed by regeneration. Biopsies taken from susceptible subjects who are otherwise not affected show minor abnormalities consisting of slightly increased variability in fibre size with increased central nucleation. The serum creatine kinase level may be slightly raised in these patients (Isaacs and Barlow 1970).

Endocrine Myopathies

Muscular weakness may complicate thyrotoxicosis, hypothyroidism, hyperparathyroidism, osteomalacia, acromegaly and Cushing's disease. In these disorders, myopathy is rarely severe, and histological changes may be very slight. Atrophy of type 2 fibres occurs, especially in steroid myopathy and in osteomalacia, and in acromegaly there may also be hypertrophy of type 1 fibres. Myopathy due to steroid therapy may be clinically severe, but the histological features resemble those of Cushing's disease.

Arthrogryposis Multiplex

Arthrogryposis is a syndrome of varying causation. The term refers to a complex clinical deformity, usually due to a progressive disorder, consisting of muscular wasting, and joint and skeletal deformities. The child is usually unable to stand or walk. The onset is in infancy. This syndrome may occur in a number of progressive congenital myopathies, in spinal muscular atrophy, or in chronic infantile polyneuropathies.

Floppy Infant Syndrome

The floppy infant syndrome is a syndrome of weakness and hypotonia in infancy, caused by any of a number of congenital or acquired myopathies, neurogenic disorders or brain diseases of infancy. It is not a disease entity. This syndrome may also be caused by disorders of elastic tissue, such as Ehlers–Danlos disease.

Inflammatory Myopathies

The inflammatory myopathies are less common in adults than in children. They are:

1. Idiopathic
   a) Polymyositis
   b) Dermatomyositis; childhood and adult forms
   c) Associated with connective tissue disease
   d) Inclusion body myositis (of adults)
2. Paraneoplastic polymyositis (of adults)
3. Myositis due to viral or bacterial infection
4. Drug-induced polymyositis
5. Polymyositis associated with other disorders, e.g. sarcoidosis
6. Eosinophilic polymyositis

Dermatomyositis of childhood

This is a distinct but uncommon disorder, presenting with muscular weakness, skin lesions and systemic symptoms. Muscular weakness is usually proximal, sometimes very severe, and usually also involves facial muscles. The skin lesion, as in adult polymyositis/dermatomyositis, may be florid or quite inconspicuous. It is more prominent in exposed skin. There is usually muscular pain and tenderness, with fever and weight loss, hepatosplenomegaly, fleeting polyarthropathy, cardiac involvement, and calcification of the muscle and skin (Cook et al. 1963); ulceration of skin and gastrointestinal tract also occurs in some cases (Banker and Victor 1966). Both the creatine kinase level and the erythrocyte sedimentation rate are usually, but not always, raised, and in patients with widespread muscular damage the creatine kinase level may be raised to as much as several hundred times the normal value.

The muscle biopsy shows increased variability in fibre size, with atrophy of both fibre types. Fibre hypertrophy is uncommon, but in chronic cases there may be some hypertrophy of type 1 fibres. In these patients fibre splitting may occur (Swash et al. 1978a). Scattered small angular fibres that are intensely reactive for NADH are usually present, indicating the presence of denervation, which results either from damage to the peripheral nerves, as in polyarteritis nodosa or, in most cases, from infarction of small nerve twigs in the muscles themselves. Fibre-type grouping is seen in some biopsies, but the numbers of fibres within these groups are small compared with the numbers in biopsies from neurogenic disorders. Necrotic, and basophilic regenerating, fibres are common, especially in patients with a suba-

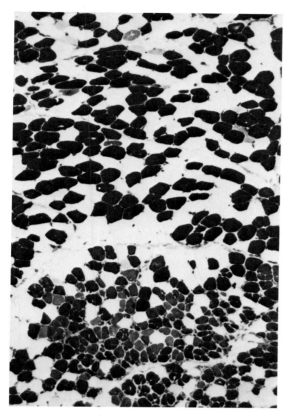

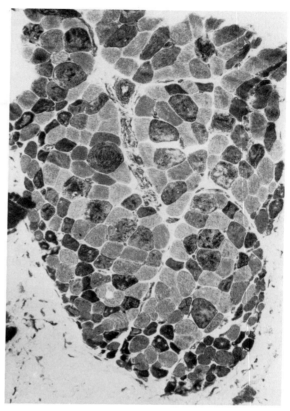

Fig. 10.38. Childhood form of dermatomyositis. Subendomysial necrosis and regeneration is limited by the fascicular planes of the muscle, suggesting a vascular causation. Many of the regenerating fibres are intermediate in histochemical type. (ATPase, pH 4.3, × 140)

Fig. 10.39. Childhood form of dermatomyositis. Perifascicular atrophy with prominent architectural change, and whorled and moth-eaten fibres. (NADH, × 140)

cute course, and central nucleation is frequent. In patients with an acute onset there may be patchy but widespread subendomysial necrosis of fibres, often in a fascicular distribution (Fig. 10.38), suggesting a vascular causation (Banker and Victor 1966; Swash et al. 1978a). Architectural changes in individual fibres are common, particularly in those at the periphery of a fascicle (Fig. 10.39). These changes include loss of ATPase reaction in the centre of a fibre, patchy loss, and accentuation of the NADH and PAS reactions, causing a pronounced moth-eaten appearance or even a "ghost" fibre that is unreactive in all enzyme preparations (see Fig. 10.38). Cytoplasmic bodies and ring fibres also occur. Inflammatory changes, often predominantly perivascular, occur in about 75% of biopsies (Dubowitz and Brooke 1973). Fibrosis occurs as the disease progresses.

Banker has emphasized the vascular origin of the childhood forms of dermatomyositis (Banker and Victor 1966), suggesting that the muscular and systemic features of the disorder are due to a vasculitis

affecting arterioles, small veins and capillaries in affected muscles and other organs. The finding of extensive perifascicular atrophy and architectural changes supports this concept. Whitaker and Engel (1973) found deposits of immunoglobulin and complement in small blood vessels, particularly in veins, in childhood dermatomyositis. In addition, cell-mediated mechanisms have gained some support in hypotheses on the pathogenesis of the disorder (Dawkins and Mastaglia 1973). Nevertheless, the finding that muscle capillary endothelial cells contain undulating tubular cytoplasmic inclusions, and evidence that these cells are thicker than normal and are often surrounded by reduplicated basal lumina (Jerusalem et al. 1974; Banker 1975), have led Carpenter et al. (1976) to suggest that capillary necrosis is the primary lesion in the childhood form of dermatomyositis, leading to the characteristic perifascicular distribution of the changes in muscle fibres in the disease. Undulating tubules and evidence of capillary necrosis have not been reported as characteristic features of the adult form of polymyositis, but capillary damage does occur in adult-onset polymyositis and in polymyositis associated with connective tissue disorders, such as rheumatoid arthritis (Carpenter et al. 1976).

The earliest change in dermatomyositis is probably deposition of complement C_5b-9 membrane attack complex in arterioles and capillaries (Kissel et al. 1993). Endomysial cellular infiltration, consisting of B cells with an increased CD4/CD8 ratio, and macrophages, is characteristic. There is an excess of cases with HLA B8 DR3 haplotype.

Although a viral aetiology has been suggested, only a few cases associated with high antibody titres, especially for Coxsackie B virus (Chou and Gutmann 1970) and myxovirus (Chou 1968) have been reported. It is possible, however, that the disease may be triggered as an allergic response to a preceding viral infection, because muscular symptoms commonly follow banal "influenzal" symptoms (see Schwartz et al. 1978). Human retroviral infection (HIV or HTLV-1) has been associated with inflammatory myopathy (Chad et al. 1990).

Myasthenia Gravis

Myasthenia gravis is characterized by fluctuating weakness, particularly affecting cranial muscles but consisting principally in abnormal fatiguability after sustained activity, with improvement after rest. The disease is commonest in young adults, affecting women three times more frequently than men, but two childhood forms exist: juvenile myasthenia, a disorder similar to the adult disease; and transient neonatal myasthenia in infants born to myasthenic mothers.

Juvenile myasthenia gravis is an uncommon condition. Although a quarter of patients with myasthenia gravis present before the age of 20 years, less than 5% present before the age of 10 years (Bundey 1972). Myasthenia beginning before the age of 2 years is usually termed congenital myasthenia. Although the clinical features of congenital and juvenile myasthenia may be similar, patients with congenital myasthenia tend to have a benign, non-progressive course (Namba et al. 1971) and ocular manifestations may be prominent (Whiteley et al. 1976). This disorder is due to one of several congenital defects in the postsynaptic or presynaptic acetylcholine receptor system and is thus not related to the commoner acquired myasthenia gravis. Shillito

et al. (1993) have reviewed the pathogenesis of these syndromes, which are of interest because of the information they give regarding the molecular mechanism of acetylcholine release and uptake at the neuromuscular junction.

The term "infantile myasthenia" is better reserved for cases of *severe* myasthenia beginning before the age of 2 years (Whiteley et al. 1976), because this disorder may present with bulbar and respiratory problems (Conomy et al. 1975). In both congenital and infantile myasthenia siblings are also commonly affected, an uncommon feature in adult or juvenile myasthenia (Bundey 1972), but the association of myasthenia with HLA-B1, HLA-B8 and HLA-DW3 haplotypes found in about 70% of patients with juvenile or adult myasthenia (Behan et al. 1973; Pirskanen 1976) is not found in the congenital form (Whiteley et al. 1976). Neonatal myasthenia is a transient disorder. About 15% of infants born to myasthenic mothers are floppy and weak, requiring anticholinesterase therapy during the first month after birth (Osserman 1958; Stern et al. 1964). Finally, myasthenia is occasionally associated with thyrotoxicosis and with polymyositis.

In juvenile myasthenia lymphoid hyperplasia and an increase in the number and size of germinal centres occurs in the thymus in about two-thirds of patients, but thymoma in infants and children is very rare (Namba et al. 1978). In infantile myasthenia the thymus is usually normal. Muscle biopsies in myasthenia of any type reveal little abnormality in most cases. Lymphorrhages, usually related to blood vessels, are common (Russell 1953), but are not specific for myasthenia, having been reported in neurogenic disorders and in polymyositis (Dubowitz and Brooke 1973). Engel and McFarlin (1966) found atrophy of type 2 fibres in about half their patients, and lymphorrhages in only a quarter. Dubowitz and Brooke (1973) noted that type 2 fibre atrophy was often irregularly distributed within the biopsy, suggesting that it was not necessarily a non-specific phenomenon. Scattered small pointed fibres, and even fibre-type grouping, have also been reported, which suggests that denervation and reinnervation occur during the course of the disease (Fenichel and Shy 1963; Brownell et al. 1972). Denervation has usually been attributed to myasthenic damage to motor endplates, but it has been shown that treatment with anticholinesterase drugs itself causes morphological and functional changes in motor end-plates (Schwartz et al. 1977b).

Cöers and Desmedt (1959) described characteristic abnormalities in the motor innervation in myasthenia gravis (Fig. 10.40), consisting of elongated motor endings without evidence of axonal sprouting (dysplastic pattern) and increased collateral ramification

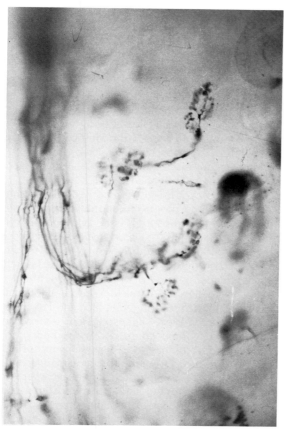

Fig. 10.40. Myasthenia gravis. The motor end-plates show sprouting and elongation. (Supravital methylene blue impregnation, ×350)

plates, is reduced (Engel et al. 1977), as is the total amount of α-bungarotoxin bound at an end-plate (Fambrough et al. 1973). In myasthenia gravis this loss of functioning acetylcholine receptors is due to an interaction between the receptor protein itself and a circulating acetylcholine-receptor antibody found within the IgG fraction of the serum proteins. Such antibodies to extracted human acetylcholine receptor protein can be demonstrated in 90% of patients with myasthenia gravis (Lindstrom et al. 1976). This antibody does not occupy the acetylcholine-binding site of the receptor moiety; rather its effect is to cause loss of acetylcholine receptor protein from the postsynaptic membrane (Lindstrom and Lambert 1978). Receptor degradation is thus accelerated in this condition (Drachman et al. 1978). The site of synthesis of acetylcholine-receptor antibody in myasthenia gravis, and the role of the thymus or thymus-dependent lymphocytes in this humoral disorder, are uncertain. Vincent et al. (1978) demonstrated that cells from one of four thymus glands and three of five thymic lymphocyte preparations synthesized the acetylcholine-receptor antibody.

Passive transfer of IgG from myasthenic patients to the mouse (Toyka et al. 1977) causes myasthenic weakness in the recipient mouse, and neonatal myasthenia, shown to be associated with gradually declining levels of acetylcholine receptor antibody in the serum of affected infants (Keesey et al. 1977), may result from a similar passive transfer mechanism. However, the severity of myasthenic weakness in juvenile myasthenia does not correlate readily with levels of circulating acetylcholine receptor antibody. Furthermore, in congenital myasthenia acetylcholine-receptor antibody is not demonstrable, and this disorder is due to one or more of several different congenital defects of the postsynaptic membrane. These newer concepts of myasthenia gravis have led to rationalization of the role of anticholinesterase drugs, of immunosuppressant therapy, and of thymectomy in the management of the disease.

of motor axons (dystrophic pattern) with the formation of multiple end-plates (Cöers and Telerman-Toppet 1976). Cöers (1975) has suggested that the dystrophic pattern is a feature of older patients and the dysplastic pattern of younger patients. In patients with a dystrophic pattern the terminal innervation ratio may be increased (Cöers and Telerman-Toppet 1976), an observation suggesting that denervation has occurred. Schwartz et al. (1977b) considered that this might be due to the effect of prolonged anticholinesterase therapy, rather than to the myasthenia itself. Ultrastructural studies of motor end-plates in myasthenia have shown that the postsynaptic region is smaller than normal, with loss (simplification) of the postsynaptic folds. The mean nerve terminal area is also smaller in myasthenic end-plates, but the numbers of synaptic vesicles are normal (Santa et al. 1972).

The area of postsynaptic membrane capable of binding α-bungarotoxin, a snake venom with specific affinity for acetylcholine receptors at motor end-

Neurogenic Disorders

Neurogenic disorders are caused by diseases of the motor unit, which is composed of the lower motor neuron (anterior horn cell, motor nerve fibre, motor end-plates) and the individual muscle fibres innervated by these structures. These disorders can be grouped into those due to disease of the anterior horn cells themselves (the *spinal muscular atrophies*) and those in which the motor nerve fibres are primarily affected (the *motor neuropathies*). In the latter group of diseases there can be damage to axons or to Schwann cells, and in many there is associated involvement of sensory nerve fibres. These peripheral neuropathies are discussed later (see p. 610)

Spinal Muscular Atrophies

The spinal muscular atrophies, which affect only the lower motor neuron, are probably the commonest of the neuromuscular disorders of childhood. Subclassification of these cases into severe infantile, intermediate and mild types is at best arbitrary, because the age of onset of all three groups overlaps and classification can only be finally determined by the outcome (Fried and Emery 1971). However, there are pathological differences between them.

The three common forms are inherited as an autosomal recessive trait; the same genetic locus is implicated for each, on chromosome 5q11–13. The reason for phenotypic variation in this disorder is not yet understood, and the gene product is unknown.

The *severe infantile form* (*Werdnig–Hoffmann disease*) has a well defined genetic basis, being inherited as an autosomal recessive trait, but sporadic cases also occur. Severe generalized weakness with hypotonia becomes evident during the first few days of life, or may even be noticed by the mother before birth, because fetal movements become progressively weakened in some cases. Bulbar palsy develops and death usually occurs before the age of 1 year, although survival to about 3 years occurs in a somewhat milder form of the disorder. In a rare variant of spinal muscular atrophy the bulbar nuclei may be selectively involved, causing a progressive bulbar paralysis (Fazio–Londé syndrome).

In *intermediate spinal muscular atrophy* disability is less marked, but the child is usually unable to walk or stand unaided. Weakness is symmetrical and is accompanied by marked wasting of affected muscles. Proximal muscles are almost always predominantly affected. Fasciculation is not a usual feature, but the tendon reflexes are usually absent. The disorder usually begins between 3 and 15 months of age. It is only slowly progressive, and survival into adolescence is common; some patients improve a little. Cardiac muscle is not involved. Both autosomal recessive and dominant forms occur.

The commonest form of spinal muscular atrophy (*Kugelberg–Welander disease*) begins in adolescence or in early adult life. The course is only very slowly progressive, and the ability to stand and walk is retained. Weakness is predominantly proximal and the presentation may be similar to that of muscular dystrophy. Occasionally, a neurogenic disorder, due

either to a sensorimotor neuropathy or to a form of spinal muscular atrophy, presents in a scapuloperoneal distribution. In this syndrome, the scapular weakness and the characteristic sparing of the extensor digitorum brevis muscles excludes Charcot–Marie–Tooth syndrome. Scapuloperoneal weakness can also be myopathic in origin.

There are a number of other syndromes, with specific associations (e.g. deafness, or involvement of one limb) but these are uncommon (see Swash and Schwartz 1995 for a review).

Motor neuron disease (amyotrophic lateral sclerosis) is very rare in childhood.

Muscles biopsies in spinal muscular atrophy show similar features in the severe and intermediate varieties. There is atrophy of both type 1 and type 2 fibres, and atrophic fibres are usually arranged in large groups, even affecting whole fascicles (Fig. 10.41; see also Figs. 10.9 and 10.28). Some fascicles contain smaller groups of hypertrophied fibres of uniform histochemical type. In Werdnig–Hoffmann disease atrophic fibres can retain their mosaic pattern of histochemical type, suggesting that denervation has occurred without compensatory reinnervation. Interpretation of atrophy of this type is very difficult without fibre-type grouping or hypertrophy in a biopsy. It has been suggested that these sheets of small rounded atrophic and poorly differentiated fibres are persistent fetal or immature fibres that have never reached their motor innervation, the disorder having begun in utero. Because atrophy can be very severe, the muscle spindles, which show changes due to denervation only in more chronic disorders (Swash and Fox 1974), may be unusually conspicuous in severe spinal muscular atrophy.

Degenerative changes in single muscle fibres are not a primary feature of this disease, but in chronic milder forms, especially in Kugelberg–Welander syndrome, such changes are common. These consist of increased interstitial fibrosis, degenerative and regenerative changes in single muscle fibres, fibre hypertrophy (especially affecting type 1 fibres), fibre splitting, increased central nucleation, and fibres with cores, whorls or a moth-eaten myofibrillar pattern in NADH preparations (Schwartz et al. 1976). In H&E-stained sections these secondary myopathic changes may be so prominent (see Fig. 10.17) that an erroneous diagnosis of primary myopathy may be suggested unless ATPase preparations show fibre-type grouping.

Clusters of narrow pointed fibres are relatively uncommon in spinal muscular atrophies, although this is a characteristic feature of other acquired forms of denervation. In mild spinal muscular atrophy, supravital methylene blue stains will reveal terminal axonal branching and sprouting, illustrating the effec-

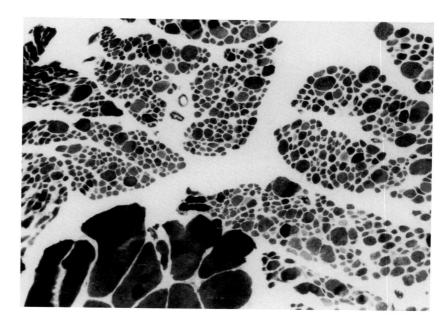

Fig. 10.41. Werdnig–Hoffmann (type 1) spinal muscular atrophy. There is fascicular atrophy, with a nearby fascicle containing hypertrophied fibres. The abnormal fibres are rounded and vary in size. (ATPase, pH 9.4, × 288)

tiveness of the collateral reinnervation associated with fibre type grouping. In the central nervous system anterior horn cells are lost, and remaining anterior horn cells and somatic motor neurons in the bulbar nuclei show degenerative changes, consisting of chromatolysis, pyknosis, neuronophagia and gliosis.

Diseases of Peripheral Nerve

Anatomy

Peripheral nerves consist of bundles of myelinated and unmyelinated axons, arranged in fascicles surrounded by connective tissue, collagen and perineurial cells (Fig. 10.42). The endoneurial space contains small blood vessels. The peripheral nerves tend to be associated with arteries and veins, forming neurovascular bundles. Even small nerve branches situated in muscles show this relationship. Almost all peripheral nerves contain both motor and sensory fibres. During development there is a close interdependence between motor and sensory nerves, growing out from anterior horn cells of the spinal cord and from posterior root ganglia respectively, in the 4th to 6th weeks of intrauterine life. Mesodermal–neural interactions are also important; if the limb nerves are damaged experimentally or fail to grow during this time the appropriate mesodermal somites do not develop

properly, leading to congenital anomalies of the limbs.

The *epineurial sheath*, consisting of an outer layer of connective tissue, binds the nerve fascicles together. Each nerve fascicle is surrounded by concentric layers of flattened cells separated by collagen. Each thin cellular layer is surrounded by a layer of basement membrane, and tight junctional complexes and pinocytotic vesicles are prominent features of these cells. These *perineurial* cells form a permeability barrier between the endoneurial space and blood and other extracellular tissue compartments. In the nerve roots the perineurial layer is continuous with the arachnoid cellular layer that surrounds the central nervous system. The cerebrospinal fluid and the endoneurial space are thus potentially in continuity. The *endoneurial space* contains nerve fibres, Schwann cells and blood vessels. Thin cellular septa, fibroblasts and longitudinally orientated collagen fibrils (Fig. 10.43), together with bundles of randomly orientated collagen fibrils, fibroblasts and acid mucopolysaccharide ground substance called Renaut bodies, are also found in the endoneurial space. The function of Renaut bodies is obscure (Asbury 1973).

The proportions, diameters and numbers of myelinated and unmyelinated nerve fibres vary in different peripheral nerves, but normal values are available for several human nerves, including the sural nerve, which is the one most commonly biopsied (Ochoa and Mair 1969; Dyck 1975). In this nerve unmyelinated fibres (30 000/mm^3) are four times more numerous than myelinated fibres (8000/mm^3). Unmyelinated fibres in this nerve range from 0.5 to

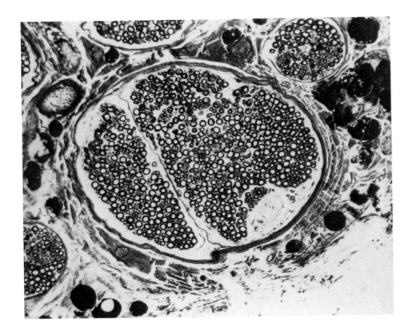

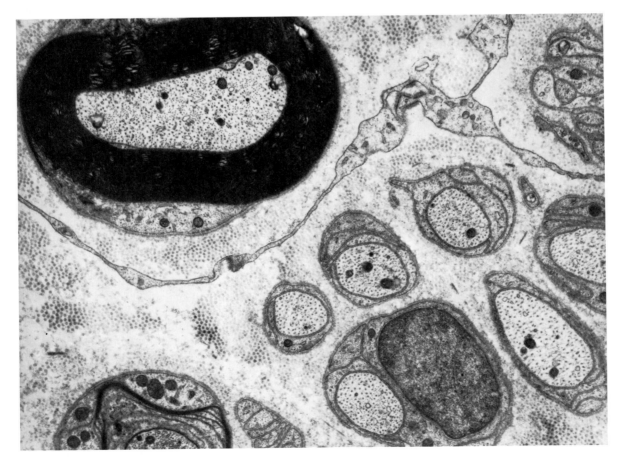

Fig. 10.42. Normal median nerve, transverse section. The normal distribution of myelinated nerve fibres in fascicles in the nerve can be seen. Osmium method for myelin.

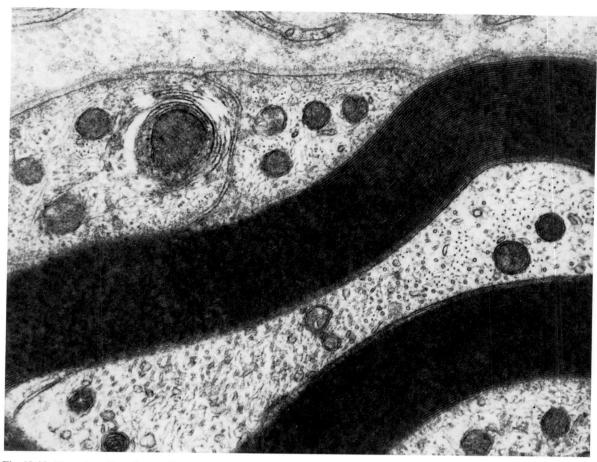

Fig. 10.44. Normal myelinated nerve fibre, transverse section. The axon contains neurofilaments and neurotubules, with small mitochondria. The myelin lamellae and the Schwann cell covering surrounded by a layer of basement membrane can be clearly seen. (× 60 000)

0.3 μm in diameter, and myelinated fibres range from 2.0 to 17.0 μm in diameter, with bimodal peaks of diameter at 5.0 μm and 13.0 μm. There are slight variations from these figures for very young children and elderly subjects.

Myelinated nerve fibres can be demonstrated in sectioned material or in teased preparations of single

Fig. 10.43. Normal sural nerve, transverse section. There is a large thickly myelinated nerve fibre. The internal and external mesaxon of its Schwann cell, and the dot-like neurofilaments, peripherally situated neurotubules, mitochondria and lipid droplets of its axon can be seen. Collagen filaments and part of a fibroblast separate this nerve fibre from an adjacent fibre sectioned through a node of Ranvier. Note the dense axonal membrane. Unmyelinated nerve fibres surrounded by thin layers of Schwannian cytoplasm occupy the remainder of the field. (Electron micrograph, × 22 500)

nerve fibres. Myelin is formed by layers of Schwannian membranes wrapped concentrically around the axon. The numbers of Schwann cells associated with individual nerve fibres are determined in fetal life; during development these cells elongate to take account of increasing axonal length. The gap between individual Schwann cells, called the node of Ranvier, is specialized to allow electrolyte exchange during the process of saltatory conduction of the nervous impulse. The thickness of the myelin sheath is related to axonal diameter.

Axons of myelinated nerve fibres can be shown up for light microscopy by silver impregnation. On electron microscopy they are seen as lucent cytoplasm containing dot-like neurofilaments and more peripherally located neurotubules, surrounded by a layer of plasma membrane (Fig. 10.44). Mitochondria and

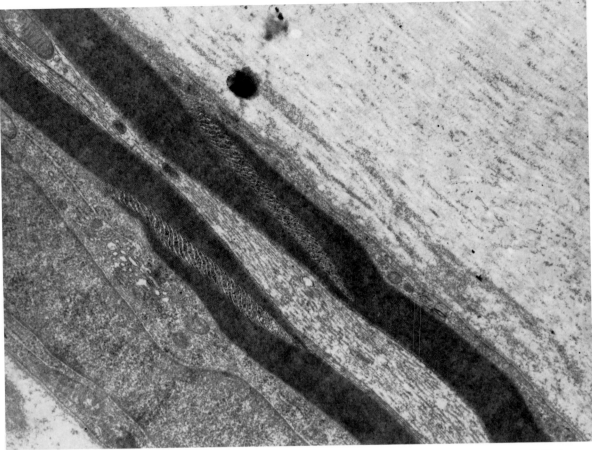

Fig. 10.45. Normal myelinated nerve fibre. Schmidt–Lantermann incision. This normal structure consists of Schwann-cell-filled separations of the myelin lamellae.

smooth endoplasmic reticulum can usually be recognized (Figs. 10.43 and 10.44). The Schwann cells are closely invested by a layer of basement membrane, which enables them to be distinguished from fibroblasts in sectioned material; several axons can be myelinated by a single Schwann cell. The ultrastructure of Schwann cells, with their nodes of Ranvier and Schmidt–Lanterman incisures, is complex (Fig. 10.45). Detailed descriptions of the structure of myelinated nerve fibres are available elsewhere (Thomas et al. 1993).

Unmyelinated nerve fibres (Fig. 10.43) are also associated with Schwann cells, but myelin lamellae are not present (see Ochoa 1976). Typically, Schwann cells are associated with groups of unmyelinated axons (Fig. 10.46). Motor end-plates and sensory receptors in skin and muscle, including muscle spindles (Swash and Fox 1972, 1974), have also been studied in peripheral neuropathies, but they are not routinely evaluated.

Peripheral Nerve Biopsy

The sural nerve is usually selected for biopsy. This nerve is distally located, and thus likely to show abnormalities in patients with peripheral neuropathy. It is superficially located just lateral to the Achilles region, near the ankle, and is thus easily approached surgically, and it is purely sensory, supplying a small area of skin on the dorsolateral surface of the foot near the ankle. Occasionally, in very severe chronic neuropathies, it may be justifiable to biopsy other nerves, such as the median nerve. The superficial branch of the radial nerve, near the dorsal surface of the base of the thumb, may also be selected for biopsy. During biopsy it is important not to squeeze or apply tension to the nerve, because this leads to artefactual folding, tearing and even disruption or myelin lamellae. Even cutting the nerve with scissors may result in significant artefact. A short length of nerve is removed, and this can be prepared for light

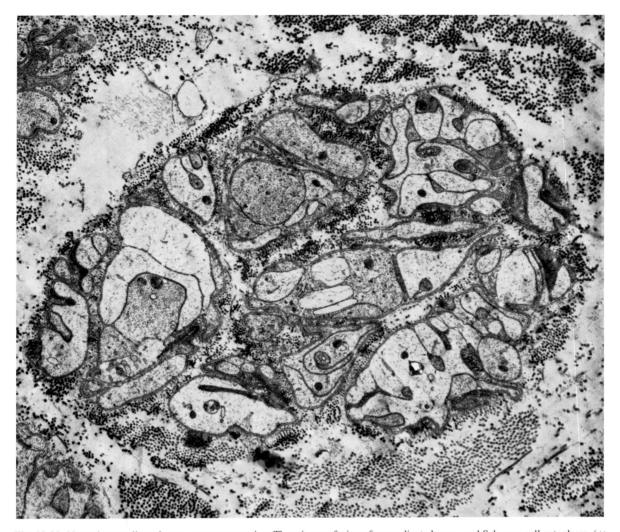

Fig. 10.46. Normal unmyelinated axon, transverse section. There is a profusion of unmyelinated axons and Schwann cell cytoplasm. (× 22 500)

and electron microscopy after fixation in glutaraldehyde and embedding in epoxy resin. Toluidine blue staining of semi-thin sections is particularly useful. It is helpful to soak a small piece of the nerve biopsy in isopentane–liquid nitrogen so that histochemical stains for amyloid, and sometimes for complement and immunoglobulins, can be employed. A full discussion of the biopsy technique has been given by Stevens et al. (1975).

Pathological Reactions of Nerve Fibres

The pathological reactions of peripheral nerve fibres are grouped broadly into axonal and demyelinating neuropathies. In the former the axon is damaged and in the latter the Schwann cell is affected. Degeneration of an axon may lead to Wallerian changes in its Schwann cell covering.

Axonal Degeneration

Axonal degeneration is the consequence of failure of the metabolic machinery of the neuron itself, resulting in impaired transport of metabolites and proteins along the axon to the periphery. If the neuronal cell body dies axonal degeneration occurs along the length of the axon, with resultant *Wallerian changes* (Figs. 10.47 and 10.48). Such a process will be selec-

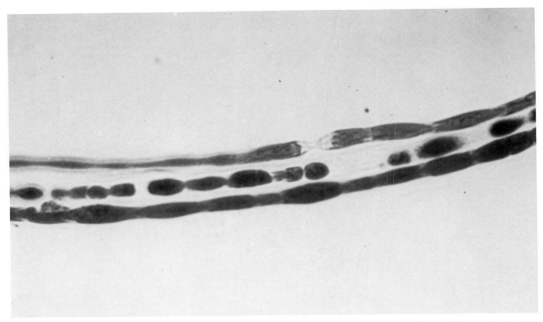

Fig. 10.47. Teased osmicated nerve fibres. One fibre has undergone Wallerian degeneration, with myelin ovoid formation. (× 160)

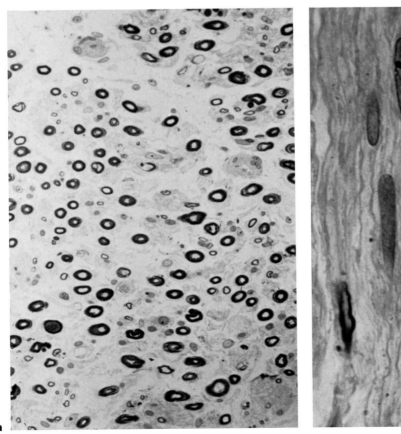

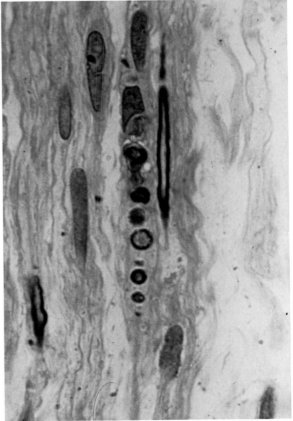

a

b

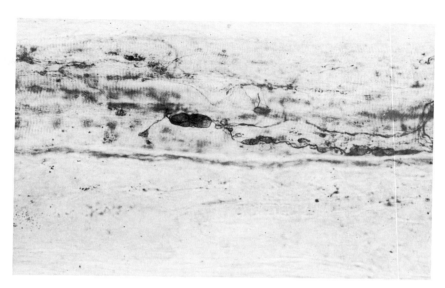

Fig. 10.49. Axonal degeneration, longitudinal section. In this muscle spindle, in a patient with tabes dorsalis, a sensory ending shows degenerative changes, with the terminal axonal swelling and constriction typical of a dying-back process. (Barker and Ip teased preparation, × 950)

tive, affecting only certain populations of neurons and their axons.

Distal Axonal Degeneration

Distal axonal degeneration (dying-back neuropathy) occurs when metabolism of the distal parts of certain axons fails (Cavanagh 1964). It is thought that this usually results from impaired metabolism of the perikaryon of the nerve cell itself, but local abnormalities in distal axonal metabolism could also produce the change. Myelin breakdown, often segmental in character, occurs in the region of the axonal degeneration, which takes the form of irregularities in axonal size and shape (Fig. 10.49) and of degeneration of axoplasmic constituents and of the axonal terminations themselves, e.g. sensory receptors and motor end-plates (Fig. 10.47). Recovery from this process is possible if the metabolic abnormality can be corrected, e.g. by replacement of vitamin deficiency or cessation of exposure to neurotoxic drugs or industrial chemicals. Distal axonal atrophy also occurs in inherited neuropathies.

The cell body proximal to a sectioned axon undergoes *chromatolysis*, a reversible change that is probably part of the regenerative response. The cell body becomes rounded and enlarged, the nucleus and nucleolus enlarge, and the nucleus displaced towards

the side of the cell away from the axon hillock. The Golgi apparatus moves away from the nucleus towards the cell periphery, and slightly cytoplasmic agyrophilia develops. The light microscopic changes correspond to the ribosomal dispersion, proliferation of endoplasmic reticulum, and increase in numbers of mitochondria and neurofilaments seen in electron microscopic studies of chromatolysis.

Segmental Demyelination

Segmental demyelination occurs in neuropathies, including those caused by diphtheria toxin or lead poisoning, in which the Schwann cells are selectively damaged. Myelin breakdown occurs and may be restricted to individual Schwann cells so that degeneration is limited by the nodes of Ranvier. This abnormality is particularly easily recognized in teased osmicated preparations, but it can usually also be discerned in longitudinal sections of plastic-embedded material (Fig. 10.50). During the process of remyelination, shortened "intercalated" nodes are formed, a characteristic finding indicating that segmental demyelination and remyelination "onion bulbs" (Fig. 10.51) are formed. This term refers to the presence of circumferential leaflets of Schwann cell processes surrounding an axonal core. The outer leaflets are interspersed with collagen fibrils and fibroblasts. This proliferation of interstitial elements may result in palpable enlargement of affected nerves (hypertrophic neuropathy).

Compression of a nerve that is sufficient to produce segmental demyelination at the site of injury usually produces Wallerian degeneration in some

Fig. 10.48. a Axonal neuropathy, transverse section. There is a reduction in the number of myelinated axons. (Toluidine blue, × 500.) **b** Wallerian degeneration secondary to axonal degeneration, longitudinal section. (Toluidine blue, × 1800)

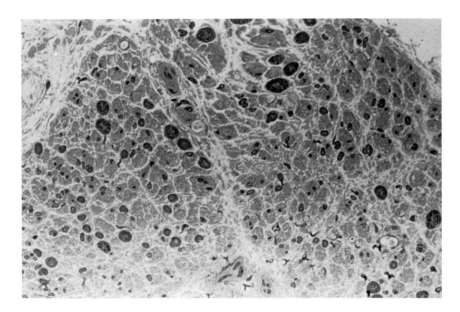

Fig. 10.50. Segmental demyelination, transverse section. There is a marked absence of myelin rings, although the axons can still be seen. (Toluidine blue, × 400)

fibres. There is controversy concerning the role of increased pressure within nerves, e.g. in amyloidosis, ischaemic swelling, or the inflammatory polyneuropathies, as a factor leading to axonal or Schwann cell injury.

Genetically Determined Neuropathies

Hereditary Motor and Sensory Neuropathies (Charcot–Marie–Tooth Diseases)

Heredofamilial sensorimotor neuropathies have been classified by Dyck and Lambert (1968a,b) according to clinical, genetic and electrophysiological criteria. Because of their variety, no clinical classification is entirely satisfactory. They can be broadly classified as:

1. Hereditary motor and sensory neuropathies (HMSN). Synonym: Charcot–Marie–Tooth syndromes (CMT)
2. Hereditary sensory neuropathies (HSN)
3. Hereditary neuropathies with specific metabolic defects

The CMT syndromes have become better understood with the advent of a genetic classification based not only on gene localization, but on gene product. The

CMT syndromes can be classified in such a way that the underlying defect can be recognized:

A. Type 1 CMT (hypertrophic form):
   1. Autosomal dominant:
      Type 1a (Ch17p11.2–12) (PMP22 disease)
        Duplication of PMP22 gene
        Point mutation of PMP22 gene
        Hereditary liability to pressure palsies
        PMP22 deletion
        Other genetic defects
      Type 1b (Ch1q21–23) (Po disease)
   2. Autosomal recessive
B. Type 2 CMT (neuronal form):
   1. Autosomal dominant
   2. Autosomal recessive:
      Adult onset
      Severe childhood type
C. Type 3 CMT (Dejerine–Sottas disease):
   1. Autosomal recessive – congenital hypomyelinating neuropathy
D. X-linked dominant CMT (ChXq12–13)
E. Complex unclassified syndromes with deafness, optic atrophy or spastic paraparesis

Myelin contains several major structural proteins. The protein Po and proteolipid protein (PLP) together constitute about 50% of peripheral myelin protein. Myelin basic protein (MBP) makes up 10%, and peripheral myelin protein 22 (PMP22) about 5% (Suter et al. 1993). In CMT 1a there is duplication of the gene for PMP22 so that there are three copies of the gene present. Some individuals with four copies

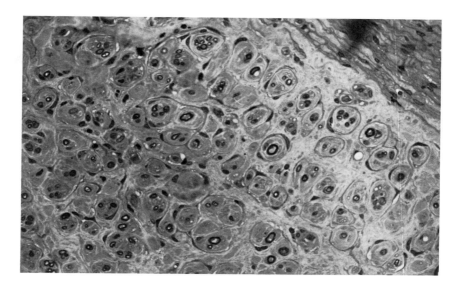

Fig. 10.51. "Onion bulbs" in burnt-out leprosy, semi-thin section. Single axon or small clusters of axons are surrounded by rings of hypertrophied Schwann cells and fibrous tissue. (Toluidine blue, × 350)

of this gene, i.e. with a double dose received from each parent, present with a severe childhood form of CMT 1a. The Trembler mouse model has a mis-sense mutation at 17p11.2–12, and human homologues of this mutation have been recognized. Deletion of the PMP22 gene on one chromosome results in hereditary liability to pressure palsies (Hoogendjik et al. 1992; Hallam et al. 1992). However, this syndrome is not genetically homogenous, and other causes exist that have not yet been characterized. Type 1b CMT is due to a separate Po protein gene mutation, although the phenotype of this disorder is clinically indistinguishable from the CMT 1a syndrome. This mutation is linked to the Duffy blood group locus on chromosome 1q21–23 (Guiloff et al. 1982: Hiyasaki et al. 1993).

In all of them there is progressive distal weakness and wasting, beginning in early childhood. Pes cavus or curling of the toes (hammer toes) may be the first abnormality noticed. Sensory impairment is usually present in the feet before the hands and may be slight. Distal tendon reflexes are lost. The type 1 CMT disorder is associated with hypertrophied peripheral nerves, and nerve conduction velocities are usually less than half normal. The cerebrospinal fluid protein level is raised. This phenotype is similar to type 2 CMT, but in the latter symptoms usually begin later, the peripheral nerves are *not* enlarged, distal atrophy is not so marked (although weakness may be more severe), and nerve conduction velocities are usually normal, indicating that axonal degeneration is the primary abnormality. The onset of the type 2 disorder may be delayed into adult life.

Dejerine–Sottas disease (type 3) is inherited as an autosomal recessive trait. Motor milestones are delayed, but the ability to walk is retained into adult life. There is mild distal sensory loss, and ataxia may be a feature.

In Type 1 CMT, the peripheral nerves are enlarged and the nerve conduction velocity is slowed indicating segmental demyelination, a suggestion confirmed by pathological studies.

It is likely that PMP22 is a nerve cell adhesion molecule. Abnormalities in this protein lead to discompaction of myelin and unravelling of the myelin lamellae following disaggregation of the axon–myelin junction.

Nerve biopsies in these hypertrophic neuropathies show enlargement of the diameter of the nerve fascicle, which contains excess collagen fibrils. The perineurium is thickened, owing to extra layers of perineurial cell cytoplasm and fibrosis. There is only a slight loss of nerve fibres. Large axons may be unmyelinated or surrounded by only thin myelin rings, an appearance suggesting that remyelination is occurring. Furthermore, clusters of axons, or single axons, become enveloped in multiple rings of Schwannian cytoplasm – the onion bulbs seen on light microscopy (Fig. 10.51). Sometimes Schwann cell cytoplasm envelops a few collagen fibrils, forming collagen pockets. Teased fibre preparations confirm that segmental demyelination is present in these cases (Gutrecht and Dyck 1966). In Refsum's disease (type 4), small sudanophilic droplets have been found in the endoneurial spaces, Schwann cells, meninges and glia, and there is loss of Purkinje cells.

In all the axonal neuropathies or neuronal disorders in the classification of Dyck and Lambert (19688a, b), an axonal reaction occurs in anterior horn cells and there is degeneration in the posterior columns secondary to the peripheral lesions. Nerve biopsy in the neuronal type of peroneal muscular atrophy (type 2) shows loss of larger axons, with relative preservation of smaller myelinated axons and of unmyelinated fibres. Wallerian change occurs and this can readily be recognized by light microscopy (see Figs. 10.48 and 10.49). Cardiomyopathy may be a feature of some of these disorders. The myocardium shows focal scarring and fibrosis similar to that found in Friedreich's ataxia.

Other Syndromes

Hereditary spastic paraplegia is sometimes associated with a mild sensorimotor neuropathy. The scapuloperoneal syndrome, consisting of proximal weakness in the upper limbs and distal weakness in the legs, with a predominantly scapular and peroneal distribution, respectively, is a heterogeneous syndrome due either to a primary myopathy (Thomas et al. 1972) or to a neurogenic disorder resembling spinal muscular atrophy (Kaeser 1965). Davidenkow (1939) described a group of cases with neurogenic scapuloperoneal atrophy and distal sensory loss (Schwartz and Swash 1975).

Muscle biopsies in these disorders show the typical features of neurogenic disorders. In the type 2 disorder, thought to be neuronal in origin, these changes are pronounced (Haase and Shy 1960), with fibre-type atrophy and fibre-type grouping affecting both type 1 and type 2 fibres. Clusters of small narrow angulated fibres, darkly stained in the NADH preparations, are common, and there may be compensatory fibre hypertrophy with mild secondary "myopathic" change in the more chronic cases (Schwartz et al. 1976). Terminal axonal sprouting can be demonstrated in methylene blue preparations (Cöers and Woolf 1953), but degenerative and end-plate changes, including axonal expansions and fusion of end-plate expansions into ill-formed masses, also occur (Harriman 1976). By contrast, in types 1 and 3 HMSN, neurogenic atrophy is less prominent in muscle biopsies. In the latter form the neuropathy results from an abnormality in the Schwann cells, leading to a demyelinating neuropathy with relative preservation of the axis cylinders themselves.

A number of very rare neuropathies due to metabolic disorders may present in infancy and childhood:

1. Refsum's disease
2. Infantile polyneuropathy with defective myelination
3. Metachromatic leucodystrophy (sulphatidosis)
4. Krabbe's disease (globoid-cell leucodystrophy)
5. Fabry's disease (angiokeratoma corporis diffusum)
6. Tangier disease (α-lipoprotein deficiency)
7. Bassen–Kornzweig's disease (β-lipoprotein deficiency)
8. Acute intermittent porphyria
9. Chediak–Higashi syndrome
10. Late infantile and juvenile amaurotic idiocy
11. Cockayne's syndrome
12. Congenital insensitivity to pain

Detailed reviews of the pathology of these disorders are available elsewhere.

Refsum's Disease

This is a hypertrophic sensorimotor neuropathy, usually beginning insidiously in childhood or adolescence, associated with ataxia and other cerebellar signs, night blindness, retinitis pigmentosa, neural deafness, cardiomyopathy, cataracts, pupillary abnormalities, dry scaly skin and epiphyseal abnormalities. The neuropathy may undergo sudden periods of deterioration, and the protein level is raised (Refsum 1946). The disease is associated with inability to metabolize dietary phytanic acid, resulting in storage of this material in affected tissues (Steinbert et al. 1966) and in high blood levels of phytanic acid.

Infantile Polyneuropathy

Infantile polyneuropathy with defective myelination (Karch and Urich 1975) is a disorder that was first reported by Lyon (1969), in which hypotonia is noted from early infancy, with absent tendon jerks, distal wasting and delayed motor milestones. Death may occur in infancy. Biopsies of sural nerve reveal preservation of axons, but absence of myelin sheaths. There is mild endoneurial fibrosis. Electron microscopy in one case revealed concentric whorls or reduplicated basal laminae, with scanty Schwann cell processes resembling onion bulbs. Similar findings have been described in an autopsied case (Karch and Urich 1975). The relation of this disorder to hypertrophic neuropathy beginning in infancy (type I HMSN) is uncertain (Dyck 1966; Joosten et al. 1974). These disorders form part of the spectrum of diseases responsible for the floppy infant syndrome.

Metachromatic Leucodystrophy

Metachromatic leucodystrophy (sulphatidosis) occurs in two forms: arylsulphatase A deficiency and multiple sulphatase deficiency (mucosulphatidosis). In both these variants motor signs are prominent, but epilepsy and mental retardation are also features, as in other leucodystrophies. The onset is usually at about 2 or 3 years of age, but juvenile-onset and adult-onset forms have also been described. In the central nervous system there is demyelination, loss of oligodendroglia, and accumulation of metachromatic sulphatide lipid granules within neurones. In the peripheral nervous system metachromatic granules are found in Schwann cells and endoneurial macrophages. Large-diameter myelinated fibres are usually lost, with very extensive segmental demyelination. Ultrastructurally, the sulphatide deposits consist of groups of rounded inclusions about 1 µm in diameter, often situated near a myelinated nerve fibre. Metachromatic lipid can also be found in desquamated renal tubular cells in the urine. Diagnosis can thus be established by examination of the urine, or by sural nerve biopsy. The underlying biochemical defect can be confirmed in cultures of skin fibroblasts (Kamensky et al. 1973).

Other Rare Neuropathies

Segmental demyelination is also a feature of the peripheral nerve abnormality (Bischoff 1975) found in *Krabbe's globoid cell leucodystrophy* (cerebroside sulphotransferase deficiency). The Schwann cell cytoplasm contains crystalline deposits and increased acid phosphatase activity (Dunn et al. 1969), and posterior root ganglia may show degenerative changes (Sourander and Olsson 1968).

In *Fabry's disease (angiokeratoma corporis diffusum)* sural nerve biopsy may show reduction of myelinated nerve fibres with lamellated glycolipid (ceramide trihexoside) deposits in the perineurium (Kocen and Thomas 1970). However, the diagnosis is more easily made by skin biopsy.

Two inherited lipoprotein disorders are associated with neuropathy. *Tangier disease*, due to absence of high-density α-lipoproteins in the blood with low blood cholesterol levels, presents in childhood with tonsillar enlargement due to accumulation of cholesterol ester producing an orange-flecked tonsillar surface. The viscera may also be enlarged, and a progressive sensorimotor neuropathy with moderately slowed nerve conduction velocities develops. Histologically this neuropathy is characterized by loss of myelinated and unmyelinated nerve fibres without segmental demyelination but with accumulations of cholesterol esters in the Schwann cells (Kocen et al. 1973). In *β-lipoproteinaemia (Bassen–Kornzweig's disease)* a variety of other clinical manifestations occur besides peripheral neuropathy,

including acanthocytosis, retinitis pigmentosa, progressive posterior column degeneration, loss of anterior horn cells, mental retardation, steatorrhoea and hypocholesterolaemia (Mars et al. 1969). The peripheral neuropathy in this disorder probably results partly from axonal damage and partly from segmental demyelination.

Late infantile and juvenile variants of amaurotic idiocy, including Bassen–Bielschowsky syndrome, some cases of Niemann–Pick disease and Spielmeyer–Vogt disease, may be diagnosed by a combination of biochemical and ultrastructural studies or sural nerve biopsies. Diagnosis is usually made more easily by biochemical examination of blood and other tissues. Pompe's disease can also be recognized in sural nerve biopsies by glycogen deposition in both cytoplasm and lysosomes in macrophages, fibroblasts and Schwann cells (Goebel et al. 1977b).

In *acute intermittent porphyria* and in *porphyria variegata*, acute spontaneous or drug-induced attacks of mainly motor neuropathy are a characteristic manifestation. The disease usually presents in adolescence. Porphobilinogen and δ-aminolaevulinic acid are excreted in the urine in attacks. The lower limbs are particularly affected and wasting can be very severe. The ankle jerks are sometimes unexpectedly preserved (Ridley 1969). Recovery is often slow and incomplete (Hierons 1957). This neuropathy is a typical example of a selective axonal neuropathy. The distal portions of large motor fibres are predominantly affected, especially in proximal muscles (Cavanagh and Mellick 1965), suggesting that the neuropathy is attributable to a dying-back process (Cavanagh 1964), although the largest motor fibres are unexpectedly spared in most cases of this disease. Wallerian degeneration is a prominent feature and there is central chromatolysis in anterior horn cells of the spinal cord. The biochemical disorder has been reviewed by Sweeney et al. (1970) and by Ridley (1975).

In *Chediak–Higashi syndrome*, a disorder characterized by partial albinism, hepatosplenomegaly, and peroxidase-positive granules in polymorphonuclear leucocytes (see p. 638), cranial and peripheral neuropathy can be associated with spinocerebellar degeneration and mental retardation. Intracytoplasmic inclusions are found in neurons and axons, and perivascular infiltrates are sometimes found in both the central and the peripheral nervous systems (Sheramata et al. 1971).

Cockayne's syndrome of mental and physical retardation, with dwarfism, deafness, retinitis pigmentosa and other defects may be complicated by peripheral neuropathy (Moosa and Dubowitz 1970).

Congenital indifference to pain, a disorder in which normal pain sensation is absent, may be due to an HMSN, but the nosological position of this syndrome is dubious. It has also been reported in patients with familial dysautonomia (*Riley–Day syndrome*) and in the *Lesch–Nyhan syndrome*. These neuropathies usually present in adult life.

The *familial amyloid neuropathies* have been reported only in adults (see Swash and Schwartz 1996 for a review).

Acquired Neuropathies

There are many acquired neuropathies:

1. Traumatic neuropathies
2. Entrapment and compressive neuropathies
3. Toxic neuropathies (e.g drug-induced neuropathies, lead poisoning)
4. Inflammatory polyradiculoneuropathy (Guillain–Barré syndrome)
5. Viral infections (Herpes zoster, poliomyelitis)
6. Leprosy
7. Neuropathies associated with arteritis
8. Metabolic neuropathies (diabetes, uraemia, vitamin deficiencies)

Traumatic Neuropathies

Traumatic neuropathies commonly occur after penetrating trauma, but may also be caused by excessive stretching during injury. Several grades of severity of nerve injury have been described, on the basis of the varying degree of recovery expected (Sunderland 1978):

1. The nerve may be severed, in which case there will be axonal discontinuity, resulting in Wallerian degeneration in the distal stump and denervation atrophy of muscles supplied by the nerve. Regeneration occurs by axonal sprouting from the proximal end of the severed nerve (Fig. 10.49); the effectiveness of this regeneration depends on the presence of empty perineurial tubes and the absence of a fibrous barrier (scar formation). Without surgical apposition of the cut ends or insertion of an autogenous graft, the prognosis for functional recovery is poor (Tallis et al. 1978).
2. If the nerve is stretched or crushed, resulting in axonal severance, but continuity of the perineurial tissues, or even of Schwann tubes, is maintained, more effective regeneration is possible. Axon

regeneration occurs at a rate of about 1–2 mm per day (Young 1942).
3. Transient failure of function may occur after acute compressive injury without anatomical disruption of tissue. Recovery usually occurs within about 3 weeks. The neurological disorder is probably due to the disruption of myelin lamellae (Ochoa et al. 1971).

Traumatic lesions occur most commonly in superficially placed nerves, e.g. the ulnar nerve at the olecranon groove on the medial side of the elbow and the common peroneal nerve at the head of the fibula. The radial nerve can be damaged by supracondylar fractures of the humerus or by injury in the spiral groove, and the median nerve is susceptible during arterial or venous puncture in the antecubital fossa. The sciatic nerve is occasionally injured by injection into the buttock. Trauma, especially in road accidents, can cause stretch injury or even rupture of anterior or posterior nerve roots. The posterior roots are more commonly affected and the lower cervical roots are most vulnerable, usually during sudden torsional injuries to the neck.

Entrapment and Compressive Neuropathies

In many respects the pathogenesis of entrapment and compressive neuropathies is similar to that described above. The classic example, the carpal tunnel syndrome, is scarcely found in childhood, except occasionally in children with rheumatoid arthritis or mucopolysaccharidosis, in which the transverse carpal ligaments sometimes become thickened. Entrapment can also occur at the intervertebral foramina, by protruded disc material after injury. In these neuropathies there is compression with intussusception of myelin lamellae in the paranodal regions, leading to paranodal demyelination and conduction block (Ochoa et al. 1971). The underlying lesion, therefore, is segmental demyelination, but in severe examples axonal degeneration occurs. Repeated stretching probably plays a role in the pathogenesis of the lesion (McLellan and Swash 1976).

Toxic and Drug-induced Neuropathies

Neuropathies occur after exposure to a variety of compounds, including organic solvents, drugs, heavy metals and bacterial toxins. Most drugs and many organic and non-organic substances used in solvents and in industry cause an axonal degeneration of the dying-back type discussed by Cavanagh (1964). The morphological changes are those most obvious in intramuscular nerve fibres and motor end-plates, and in sensory receptors in skin and muscle. Segmental demyelination occurs after exposure to diphtheria toxin and in lead poisoning. The earliest changes occur in the paranodal regions. Full discussions of these neuropathies and of the substances that cause them are available elsewhere (Dyck et al. 1975; Argov and Mastaglia 1979; Schaumberg and Spencer 1979).

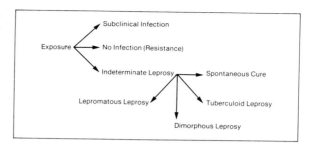

Fig. 10.52. Possible consequences of exposure to *M. leprae*.

Inflammatory Polyradiculoneuropathy

Inflammatory polyradiculoneuropathy, or the Guillain–Barré syndrome, is an acute disorder characterized by weakness, paraesthesiae, muscle tenderness, absent tendon reflexes and a raised cerebrospinal fluid protein level, with a normal cell count (Guillain et al. 1916). The disease is often preceded by an ill-defined febrile illness, and relapsing and chronic varieties, some with central manifestations, are also recognized (Arnason 1975; Swash 1979). Cranial nerves, especially the facial nerves, are often affected, and there may be autonomic involvement. A similar subacute type of polyneuritis occurs after specific virus infections, such as mumps, measles, vaccinia, herpes zoster and infectious mononucleosis, and after rabies vaccination (see Swash 1979). Pathologically, the characteristic feature of the acute disorder is segmental demyelination, which affects the nerves throughout their length, even involving nerve roots, accompanied by perivascular lymphocytic infiltration. The latter is particularly prominent near demyelinated nerve. Macrophages and plasma cells also infiltrate affected nerve fascicles. Axonal degeneration occurs in some of these areas, resulting in denervation atrophy in some muscles. In most cases recovery is rapid, disrupted myelin being rapidly reconstituted, but in severe cases recovery is delayed. Electron microscopy has shown that macrophages penetrate basement membranes of affected nerve fibres and displace Schwann cell cytoplasm from the myelin sheath, leading to separation of axons from their myelin envelopes (Prineas 1972). In relapsing and chronic cases nerve hypertrophy, with typical Schwannian onion bulbs surrounding demyelinated and remyelinated axons and a sparser inflammatory cell infiltrate, is found. This histological appearance is similar to that found in experimental allergic neuritis, an experimental demyelinating neuropathy induced by treatment with peripheral nerve protein (Thomas et al. 1969).

Autonomic neuropathy sometimes complicates Guillain–Barré syndrome, perhaps accounting for sudden death, which occurs in a small proportion of patients. A few cases of subacute autonomic neuropathy occurring without motor or sensory abnormalities, but similar in other respects to subacute Guillain–Barré syndrome, have been reported in childhood (Thomashefsky et al. 1972).

Virus Infections

Two viruses, poliomyelitis and herpes zoster, can invade the peripheral nervous system, although others, especially herpes simplex virus and rabies virus, may enter the nervous system by passing along endoneurial or perineurial tissues from distal sites of entry. Herpes zoster is uncommon in childhood, although it does occur in children with debilitating disorders and during chemotherapy for malignant disease. The poliomyelitis virus causes a form of leptomeningitis with perivascular lymphocytic cuffing in the spinal cord and brain stem and phagocytosis of infected dead anterior horn cells. Axonal degeneration and neurogenic muscular atrophy follow.

Leprosy

Leprosy is widespread in tropical and subtropical zones, and cases occur in temperate climates among immigrant populations. The disease is acquired only after prolonged contact in overcrowded conditions. Many people appear not to be susceptible to the disease, perhaps because of previous exposure to *Mycobacterium tuberculosis*. The factors leading to susceptibility are complex and largely determine the course and clinical type of the disease in individual patients. Nutritional and immunological factors are particularly important, but children are generally more susceptible than adults. Infection can occur through the skin or upper respiratory tract. Clinical manifestations of leprosy vary (Cochrane and Davey 1964; Sabin and Swift 1975), and several different types of the disease are recognized. Figure 10.52

shows the various possible outcomes of exposure to *M. leprae*.

Indeterminate

Indeterminate leprosy is an early lesion most commonly found in children. There is an indolent, hypopigmented skin lesion, which may be anaesthetic. Biopsy of this lesion shows a few inflammatory cells near neurovascular bundles, and *M. leprae* may be present in small cutaneous nerves.

Lepromatous

In lepromatous leprosy there is little immunological check to bacterial proliferation, and the skin and peripheral nervous system are extensively involved, particularly in cooler body areas such as the nose, exposed areas of the limbs, the cheeks and the pinna. Skin lesions are often difficult to see, even when very extensive. Large numbers of bacilli can be seen in acid-fast stains of skin biopsies. The bacilli are usually located within histiocytes, which may be distended by masses of bacilli. Nasal or skin scrapings usually reveal abundant bacilli in acid-fast stains.

The peripheral nerve trunks are grossly enlarged by fusiform rather than nodular swellings, and small cutaneous nerves are usually similarly palpably enlarged. Affected nerves are often tender. Histologically these nerves are oedematous, with relative preservation of their fascicular architecture. The perineurium is infiltrated by foamy histiocytes, and bacilli, oriented longitudinally to the nerve trunk, are prominent. Teased preparations of single nerve fibres show demyelinated or thinly myelinated axons, with short intercalcated segments, consistent with segmental demyelination. This lepromatous form represents the later uncontrolled stage of the infection.

Tuberculoid

In tuberculoid leprosy the cutaneous nerves are enlarged by firm nodules, often in association with a nearby skin lesion. The affected nerves show extensive destructive changes with loss of the fascular pattern, prominent axonal changes, and epithelioid and giant cell granulomas. Onion bulb formation may be prominent (Fig. 10.51). Only sparse bacilli are found in the nerves, and almost none in the skin in tuberculoid leprosy. There is a hyperimmune state to the antigenic stimulus of the disease.

Other Forms

Dimorphous leprosy represents an intermediate disorder between the lepromatous and tuberculoid forms. Clinically, dimorphous leprosy is unstable, and reversion to either of the major forms may occur. Histologically there are features of both forms, depending on the immunological state of the patient.

Diabetic Neuropathy

Neuropathy has been recognized as a complication of diabetes mellitus for more than 100 years. It is common only in adult diabetic patients, however, and its incidence increases with increasing age. The incidence in childhood is probably about 2%, but a higher incidence has been recorded (Lawrence and Locke 1963). Symmetrical, predominantly sensory, and mononeuropathic types occur. The last group includes isolated cranial nerve palsies and diabetic amyotrophy. Only the symmetrical sensory neuropathy is recorded in paediatric practice. Autonomic neuropathy may complicate this disorder. Pathologically, features of both axonal neuropathy and segmental demyelination are present (Greenbaum et al. 1964; Thomas and Lascelles 1966). These degenerative changes are most marked peripherally, but the spinal roots, particularly the posterior roots, may be involved (Olsson et al. 1968), and loss of posterior root ganglion cells and anterior horn cells has also been observed (Greenbaum et al. 1964). There is some evidence that diabetic polyneuropathy may be due to intraneural hypoxia from capillary disease.

Lead Poisoning

In children lead poisoning causes anaemia, convulsions and encephalopathy far more commonly than neuropathy. When it occurs in childhood lead neuropathy usually presents as foot drop, unlike the more familiar wrist drop of adults. The neuropathy, which remits when blood lead levels fall with treatment, is due to segmental demyelination.

Others

Neuropathies associated with arteritis and with various acquired metabolic disorders, such as uraemia and hepatic disease, are rare in childhood and will not be discussed here. They have been reviewed by Dyck et al. (1975) and by Swash and Schwartz (1995).

References

Abbs S, Bobrow M (1993) Workshop report: carrier diagnosis of Duchenne and Becker muscular dystrophy. Neuromusc Disord 3: 241

Afifi AK, Smith JW, Zellweger H (1965) Congenital nonprogressive myopathy: central core and nemaline myopathy in one family. Neurology (Minneap) 15: 371

Allen DE, Johnson AG, Woolf AL (1969) The intramuscular nerve endings in dystrophia myotonica: a biopsy study by vital staining and electron microscopy. J Anat 105: 1

Anonymous (1986) Molecular biology of the DMD locus. Lancet ii: 1135 (editorial)

Argov Z, Mastaglia FL (1979) Drug-induced peripheral neuropathies. Br Med J i: 663

Armstrong RM, Königsberger R, Mellinger J, Lovelace RE (1971) Central core disease with congenital hip dislocation: a study of two families. Neurology (Minneap) 21: 369

Arnason BGW (1975) Inflammatory polyradiculoneuritis. In: Dyck PJ, Thomas PK, Lambert EH (eds) Peripheral neuropathy, vol 2. Saunders, Philadelphia, p 1110

Asbury AK (1973) Renaut bodies: a forgotten endoneurial structure. J Neuropathol Exp Neurol 32: 334

Bank WJ, DiMauro S, Bonilla E, Capcizzi DM, Rowland LP (1975) A disorder of lipid metabolism and myoglobinuria. N Engl J Med 292: 443

Banker BQ (1975) Dermatomyositis of childhood: ultrastructural alternations of muscle and intramuscular blood vessels. J Neuropathol Exp Neurol 34: 46

Banker BQ, Victor M (1966) Dermatomyositis (systemic angiopathy) of childhood. Medicine (Baltimore) 45: 261

Barbeau A (1966) The syndrome of hereditary late-onset ptosis and dysphagia in French Canada. In: Kuhn E (ed) Symposium über progressive Muskeldystrophie. Springer, New York, p 102

Barchi RL (1975) Myotonia: an evaluation of the chloride hypothesis. Arch Neurol 32: 175

Becker PE (1962) Two new families of benign sex-linked recessive muscular dystrophy. Rev Can Biol 21: 551

Behan PO, Simpson JA, Dick JP (1973) Immune response genes in myasthenia gravis. Lancet ii: 1033

Bell CD, Conen PE (1968) Histopathological changes in Duchenne muscular dystrophy. J Neurol Sci 7: 529

Ben Hamida M, Fardeau M, Attia N (1983) Severe childhood muscular dystrophy affecting both sexes and frequent in Tunisia. Muscle Nerve 6: 469

Berenberg RA, Pollock JM, DiMauro S, Schotland DL, Bonilla E, Eastwood A, Hays A, Vicale CT, Behrens M, Chutarian A, Rowland LP (1977) Lumping or splitting? Ophthalmoplegia plus or Kearns–Sayre syndrome. Ann Neurol 1: 37

Bethlem J, van Gool J, Hülsmann WC, Meijer AEFH (1966) Familial non-progressive myopathy with muscle cramps after exercise: a new disease associated with cores in the muscle fibres. Brain 89: 569

Bethlem J, Meijer AEFH, Schellens JPM, Uvran JJ (1968) Centronuclear myopathy. Eur Neurol 1: 325

Bethlem J, van Wijngaarden GK, Meijer AEFH, Hülsmann WC (1969) Neuromuscular disease with type 1 fibre atrophy, central nuclei and myotube-like structures. Neurology (Minneap) 19: 705

Bischoff A (1975) Neuropathy in leucodystrophies. In: Dyck PJ, Lambert EH, Thomas PK (eds) Peripheral neuropathy. Saunders, Philadelphia, p 891

Bohan A, Peter JB (1975) Polymyositis and dermatomyositis. N Engl J Med 292: 344 and 403

Bradley WG (1969) Ultrastructural changes in adynamia episodica hereditaria and normokalaemic periodic paralysis. Brain 92: 379

Bradley WG, Jones MZ, Mussini J-M, Fawcett PRW (1978) Becker-type muscular dystrophy. Muscle Nerve 1: 111

Brooke MH (1966) The histological reaction of muscle to disease. In: Buskey EJ, Cassens R, Trautman J (eds) The physiology and biochemistry of muscle as a food. University of Wisconsin Press, Madison, p 151

Brooke MH (1973) A neuromuscular disease characterized by fibre type disproportion. In: Kakulas PA (ed) Clinical studies in myology. Excerpta Medica, Amsterdam, p 147 (ICS no. 295)

Brooke MH, Engel WK (1966) The histologic diagnosis of neuromuscular diseases: a review of 79 biopsies. Arch Phys Med Rehabil 47: 99

Brooke MH, Engel WK (1969a) The histographic analysis of human muscle biopsies with regard to fibre types. 1. Adult male and female. Neurology (Minneap) 19: 221

Brooke MH, Engel WK (1969b) The histographic analysis of human muscle biopsies with regard to fibre types. 4 children's biopsies. Neurology (Minneap) 19: 591

Brooke MH, Kaiser KK (1970) Muscle fibre types: how many and what kind? Arch Neurol 23: 369

Brownell B, Oppenheimer DR, Spalding JMK (1972) Neurogenic muscle atrophy in myasthenia gravis. J Neurol Neurosurg Psychiatry 34: 311

Brumback RA, Gerst J (1984) The neuromuscular junction. Futura, Mount Kisco, p 354

Brunberg JA, McCormick WF, Schochet SS Jr (1971) Type 3 glycogenosis: an adult with diffuse weakness and muscle wasting. Arch Neurol 25: 171

Bundey S (1972) Genetic study of infantile and juvenile myasthenia gravis. J Neurol Neurosurg Psychiatry 35: 41

Bundey S, Carter CO, Soothill JF (1970) Early recognition of heterozygotes for the gene of dystrophia myotonica. J Neurol Neurosurg Psychiatry 33: 279

Carpenter S, Karpati G, Rothman S, Watters G (1976) The childhood type of dermatomyositis. Neurology (Minneap) 26: 952

Cavanagh JB (1964) The significance of the 'dying back' process in experimental and human neurological disease. Int Rev Exp Pathol 7: 219

Cavanagh JB, Mellick RS (1965) On the nature of the peripheral nerve lesions associated with acute intermittent porphyria. J Neurol Neurosurg Psychiatry 28: 320

Cavanagh NBC, Lake BD, McManiman P (1979) Congenital fibre type disproportion myopathy: a histological diagnosis with an uncertain clinical outlook. Arch Dis Child 54: 735

Cazzato G (1970) Myopathic changes in denervated muscle: a study of biopsy material in various neuromuscular diseases. In: Walton JN, Canal N, Scarlato G (eds) Muscle disease. Excerpta Medica, Amsterdam, p 392 (ICS no. 199)

Chad DA, Smith TW, Blumenfeld A et al. (1990) Human immunodeficiency virus (HIV)-associated myopathy: immunocytochemical identification of an HIV antigen (gp 41) in muscle macrophages. Ann Neurol 28: 579

Cheah JS, Tock EPC, Tan SP (1975) The light and electron microscopic changes in the skeletal muscles during paralysis in thyrotoxic periodic paralysis. Am J Med Sci 269: 365

Chou SM (1968) Myxovirus-like structures and accompanying nuclear changes in chronic polymyositis. Arch Pathol 86: 649

Chou SM, Gutmann L (1970) Picornavirus-like crystals in subacute polymyositis. Neurology (Minneap) 20: 205

Cochrane RG, Davey TF (eds) (1964) Leprosy in theory and practice, 2nd edn. Wright, Bristol

Cöers C (1975) Motor innervation of myasthenic muscles related to age. Lancet ii: 55

Cöers C, Desmedt JE (1959) Mise en évidence d'une malformation caractéristique de la jonction neuromusculare dans la myasthenie. Acta Neurol Belg 59: 539

Cöers C, Telerman-Toppet N (1976) Morphological and histological changes of motor units in myasthenia. Ann NY Acad Sci F274: 6

Cöers C, Woolf AL (1953) The innervation of muscle. Blackwell, Oxford

Cook CD, Rosen FS, Banker BQ (1963) Dermatomyositis and focal scleroderma. Pediatr Clin North Am 10: 979

Conomy JP, Levinsohn M, Fanaroff A (1975) Familial infantile myasthenia gravis: a cause of sudden death in young children. J Pediatr 87: 428

Crews J, Kaiser KK, Brooke MH (1976) Muscle pathology of myotonia congenita. J Neurol Sci 28: 449

Currie S, Naronha M, Harriman DGF (1974) "Minicore" disease. (abstract). Third International Congress on Muscle Disease. Excerpta Medica, Amsterdam, p 12 (ICS no. 334)

Davidenkow S (1939) Scapulo-peroneal amyotrophy. Arch Neurol 41: 694

Dawkins RL, Mastaglia FL (1973) Cell-mediated cytotoxicity muscle in polymyositis. N Engl J Med 288: 434

Drachman DA (1968) Opthalmoplegia plus: the neurodegenerative disorders associated with progressive external ophthamoplegia. Arch Neurol 18: 654

Drachman DB, Angus CW, Adams RN, Michelson JD, Hoffman GJ (1978) Myasthenic antibodies cross-link acetylcholine receptors to accelerate degradation. N Engl J Med 298: 1116

Drachman DB, Murphy SR, Nigam MP, Hills JR (1967) "Myopathic" changes in chronically denervated muscle. Arch Neurol 16: 14

Dreyfus JS, Shapiro G, Demos J (1960) Etude de la creatinekinase sérique chez les myopathies et leur families. Revue Française d'Etudes Cliniques et Biologiques 5: 384

Dubowitz V (1978) Muscle disorders in childhood. In: Major problems in clinical pediatrics, vol XVI. Saunders, London

Dubowitz V (1985) Muscle biopsy – a practical approach, 2nd edn. Baillìere Tindall, London

Dubowitz V, Brooke MH (1973) Muscle biopsy: a modern approach. Saunders, London

Dubowitz V, Roy S (1970) Central core disease of muscle: clinical histochemical and electron microscopal studies of an affected mother and child. Brain 93: 133

Dunn HG, Lake BD, Dolman CL, Wilson J (1969) The neuropathy of Krabbe's infantile cerebral sclerosis (globoid cell leucodystrophy). Brain 92: 329

Dyck PJ (1966) Histologic measurements and fine structure of biopsied sural nerve: normal and in peroneal muscular atrophy, hypertrophic neuropathy and congenital sensory neuropathy. Mayo Clin Proc 41: 742

Dyck PJ (1975) Pathologic alterations of the peripheral nervous system of man. In: Dyck PJ, Thomas PK, Lambert EH (eds) Peripheral neuropathy. Saunders, Philadelphia, p 296

Dyck PJ, Lambert EH (1968a) Lower motor and primary sensory neuron diseases with peroneal muscular atrophy. I. Neurologic, genetic and electrophysiologic findings in hereditary polyneuropathies. Arch Neurol 18: 603

Dyck PJ, Lambert EH (1968b) Lower motor and primary sensory neuron diseases with peroneal muscular atrophy. II. Neurologic, genetic and electrophysiologic findings in various neuronal degenerations. Arch Neurol 18: 619

Dyck PJ, Lambert EH, Thomas PK (1975) Peripheral neuropathy (2 vols). Saunders, Philadelphia

Edstrom L, Kugelberg E (1968) Histochemical composition, distribution of fibres and fatiguability of single motor units. Anterior tibial muscle of the rat. J Neurol Neurosurg Psychiatry 31: 424

Ellis FR, Kearney NP, Harriman DGF (1973) Histopathological and neuropharmacological aspects of malignant hyperpyrexia. Proc R Soc Med 66: 60

Emery AEH (1980) Duchenne muscular dystrophy: genetic aspects, carrier detection and antenatal diagnosis. Br Med Bull 36: 117

Engel AG (1970a) Acid maltase deficiency in adults: studies in four cases of syndrome which may mimic muscular dystrophy or other myopathies. Brain 93: 599

Engel AG (1970b) Evolution and content of vacuoles in primary hypokalaemic periodic paralysis. Mayo Clin Proc 45: 774

Engel AG, Angelini C, Gomez MR (1972) Finger-print body myopathy. Mayo Clin Proc 47: 377

Engel AG, Gomez MR, Seybold ME, Lambert EH (1973) The spectrum and diagnosis of acid maltase deficiency. Neurology (Minneap) 23: 95

Engel AG, Lindstrom JM, Lambert EH, Lennon VA (1977) Ultrastructural localization of the acetylcholine receptor in myasthenia gravis and its experimental autoimmune model. Neurology (Minneap) 27: 307

Engel WK (1961) Muscle target fibres, a newly recognised sign of denervation. Nature 191: 389

Engel WK (1965) Muscle biopsy. Clin Orthop 39: 80

Engel WK (1970) Selective and non-selective susceptibility of muscle fibre types: a new approach to human neuromuscular disease. Arch Neurol 22: 97

Engel WK (1971) "Ragged-red fibres" in ophthalmoplegia syndromes and their differential diagnosis. In: Abstract. Second International Congress on Muscle Diseases. Excerpta Medica, Amsterdam, p 28 (ICS no. 237)

Engel WK, Brooke MH (1966) Histochemistry of the myotonic disorders. In: Kuhn E (ed) Progressive Muskeldystrophie, Myotonie, Myästhenia. Springer, New York, p 203

Engel WK, McFarlin De (1966) Discussion. Ann NY Acad Sci 135: 68

Engel WK, Resnick JS (1966) Late-onset rod myopathy: a newly recognized, acquired and progressive disease. Neurology (Minneap) 16: 308

Engel WK, Brooke MH, Nelson PG (1966) Histochemical studies of denervated or tenotomized cat muscle, illustrating difficulties in relating experimental animal conditions to human neuromuscular diseases. Ann NY Acad Sci 138: 160

Famborough D, Drachman DB, Satyamart S (1973) Neuromuscular junction in myasthenia gravis: decreased acetylcholine receptors. Science 182: 293

Fardeau M, Harpey J-P, Caille B (1975) Disproportion congénitales des différentes types de fibre musculaire avec petitesse relative des fibres de type 1: documents morphologiques concernant les biopsies musculaires prélevées chez trois membres d'une même famille. Rev Neurol (Paris) 131: 745

Fardeau M, Godet-Guillain J, Tomi FMS et al. (1978) Une nouvelle affection musculaire familiale, définié par l'accumulation intrasarcoplasmique d'un matériel granulo-filamenteux dense en microscopie électronique. Rev Neurol 131: 411

Fenichel GM, Shy GM (1963) Muscle biopsy experience in myasthenia gravis. Arch Neurol 9: 237

Fried K, Emery AEH (1971) Spinal muscular atrophy type II: a separate genetic and clinical entity from type I (Werdnig–Hoffmann disease) and type III (Kugelberg–Welander disease). Clin Genet 2: 203

Gamstorp I (1956) Adynamia episodica hereditaria. Acta Paediatr 108: 1

Gauthier GF (1976) The motor end-plate: structure. In: Landen DN (ed) The peripheral nerve. Chapman & Hall, London, p 464

Gillard E, Otsu K, Fujii J et al. (1992) Polymorphisms and deduced amino acid substitutions in the coding sequence of the ryanodien receptor gene in malignant hyperthermia. Genomics 13: 1247

Goebel HH, Lenard HG, Görke W et al. (1977a) Fibre disproportion in the rigid spine syndrome. Neuropädiatrie 8: 467

Goebel HH, Lenard HG, Kohlschütter A, Pilz H (1977b) The ultrastructure of the sural nerve in Pompe's disease. Ann Neurol 2: 111

Gonatas NK, Shy GM, Godfrey EH (1966) Nemaline myopathy:

the origin of nemaline structures. N Engl J Med 274: 535

Greenbaum D, Richardson PC, Salmon MV, Urich H (1964) Pathological observations in six cases of diabetic neuropathy. Brain 87: 201

Guillain G, Barré JA, Strohl A (1916) Sur un syndrome de radiculo-névrite avec hyperalbuminose du liquide céphalorachidien sans un réaction cellulaire. Remarques sur les caractères cliniques et graphiques des réflexes tendineux. Bulletin Societé Medicale des Hôpitaux de Paris 10: 146

Guiloff RJ, Thomas PK, Contreras M et al. (1982) Evidence for linkage of type 1 sensory and motor neuropathy with the Duffy linkage on chromosome 1. Ann Hum Genet 46: 25

Gutrecht JA, Dyck PJ (1966) Segmental demyelinization in peroneal muscular atrophy nerve fibres teased from sural nerve biopsy specimens. Mayo Clin Proc 41: 775

Haase GR, Shy GM (1960) Pathological changes in muscle biopsies from patients with peroneal muscular atrophy. Brain 83: 631

Hall-Craggs ECB (1972) The significance of longitudinal fibre division in skeletal muscle. J Neurol Sci 15: 27

Hallam PJ, Harding AE, Bercrano J et al. (1992) Duplication of part of chromosome 17 is commonly associated with hereditary motor and sensory neuropathy type 1. Ann Neurol 31: 570

Harley H, Brook J, Rundle S et al. (1992) Expansion of an unstable DNA region and phenotypic variation in myotonic dystrophy. Nature 355: 545

Harper PS (1975) Congenital myotonic dystrophy in Britain. 1. Clinical aspects. 2. Genetic aspects. Arch Dis Child 50: 505

Harriman DGF (1961) Histology of the motor end plate (motor point muscle biopsy). In: Licht S (ed) Electrodiagnosis and electromyography, 2nd edn. Licht, New Haven, p 134

Harriman DGF (1976) Diseases of muscle. In: Blackwood W, Corsellis JAN (eds) Greenfield's neuropathology. Arnold, London, p 849

Hierons R (1957) Changes in the nervous system in acute porphyria. Brain 80: 176

Hiyasaka K, Himuro M, Sato W et al. (1993) Charcot–Marie–Tooth neuropathy type 1B is associated with mutations of the myelin Po gene. Nature Genet 5: 31

Hoffmann EP, Knudson CM, Campbell KP, Kunkel LM (1987) Subcellular fractionation of dystrophin to the triads of skeletal muscle. Nature 330: 754

Hoogendijk JE, Hensels GW, Gabriels-Festen AAWM et al. (1992) De novo mutation in hereditary motor and sensory neuropathy type 1. Lancet 339: 1081

Hopkins IJ, Lindsey JR, Ford FR (1966) Nemaline myopathy: a long-term clinicopathologic study of affected mother and daughter. Brain 89: 299

Howes EL Jr, Price HM, Blumbert JM (1966) Hypokalaemic periodic paralysis: electron microscopic changes in the sarcoplasm. Neurology (Minneap) 16: 242

Illingworth B, Cori GT, Cori CF (1956) Amylo 1,6 glucosidase in muscle tissue in generalized glycogen storage disease. J Biol Chem 218: 123

Isaacs H, Barlow MB (1970) Malignant hyperpyrexia during anaesthesia: possible association with subclinical myopathy. Br Med J i: 295

James NT (1971) The distribution of muscle fibre types in fasciculi and their analysis. J Anat 110: 335

Jerusalem F, Sieb SP (1992) The limb girdle syndromes. In: Vonken PJ, Bruyn GW, Klaurans HL (eds) Myopathies, Handbook of neurology vol. 62. Elsevier, Amsterdam, p 179

Jerusalem F, Rakuska M, Engel AG, MacDonald PD (1974) Morphometric analysis of skeletal muscle capillary ultrastructure in inflammatory myopathies. J Neurol Sci 23: 391

Johnson MA, Polgar J, Weightman D, Appleton D (1973) Data on the distribution of fibre types in thirty six human muscles: an autopsy study. J Neurol Sci 18: 111

Joosten E, Gabreëls F, Bagreëls-Festen A, Vrensen G, Karten J,

Notermans S (1974) Electron microscopic heterogeneity of onion-bulb neuropathies of the Déjerine–Sottas type. Two patients in one family with the variant described by Lyon. Acta Neuropathol (Berl) 27: 105

Kaeser HE (1965) Scapuloperoneal muscular dystrophy. Brain 88: 407

Kamensky E, Philippart M, Cancilla P, Frommes SP (1973) Cultured skin fibroblasts in storage disorders: an analysis of ultrastructural features. Am J Pathol 73: 59

Karch S, Urich H (1975) Infantile polyneuropathy with defective myelination: an autopsy study. Dev Med Child Neurol 17: 504

Karpati G, Carpenter S, Engel AG, Watters G, Allen J, Rothman S, Klassen G, Mamer OA (1975) The syndrome of systemic carnitine deficiency. Neurology (Minneap) 25: 16

Kearns TP, Sayre GP (1958) Retinitis pigmentosa, external ophthalmoplegia and complete heart block. Arch Ophthalmol 60: 280

Keesey J, Lindstrom J, Cokely H, Herrmann C Jr (1977) Antiacetylcholine receptor antibody in neonatal myasthenia gravis. N Engl J Med 296: 55

Kiloh LG, Nevin S (1951) Progressive dystrophy of the external ocular muscles (ocular myopathy). Brain 24: 115

Kissel M, Lynn DJ, Rammohan KW et al. (1993) Mononuclear cell analysis in prednisone and azathioprine-treated Duchenne muscular dystrophy. Neurology 43: 532

Klinkerfuss GH (1967) An electron microscopic study of myotonic dystrophy. Arch Neurol 16: 181

Kocen RS, Thomas PK (1970) Peripheral nerve involvement in Fabry's disease. Arch Neurol 22: 81

Kocen RS, King RHM, Thomas PK, Haas LF (1973) Nerve biopsy findings in two cases of Tangier disease. Acta Neuropathol (Berl) 26: 317

Kunkel LM, Hoffman EP (1989) Duchenne/Becker muscular dystrophy. Br Med Bull 45: 630

Kunkel LM, Hejthnxik JF, Caskey CT (1986) Analysis of deletions in the DNA of patients with Barker and Duchenne muscular dystrophy. Nature 322: 73

Lake BD, Wilson J (1975) Zebra body myopathy: clinical, histochemical and ultrastructural studies. J Neurol Sci 24: 437

Lawrence DG, Locke S (1963) Neuropathy in children with diabetes mellitus. Br Med J ii: 784

Lindstrom JM, Lambert E (1978) Content of acetylcholine receptor and antibodies bound to receptor in myasthenia gravis, experimental autoimmune myasthenia gravis and Eaton–Lambert syndrome. Neurology (Minneap) 28: 130

Lindstrom JM, Seybold ME, Lennon VA, Whittingham S, Duanne DD (1976) Antibody to acetylcholine receptor in myasthenia gravis: prevalence, clinical correlates and diagnostic value. Neurology (Minneap) 26: 1054

Lyon G (1969) Ultrastructure of a nerve biopsy from a case of early infantile chronic neuropathy. Acta Neuropathol (Berl) 13: 131

Mars H, Lewis LA, Robertson AL, Butkus A, Williams GH (1969) Familial hypo β lipoproteinaemia. Am J Med 46: 886

Matsumora K, Naraka I, Campbell KP (1993) Abnormal expression of dystrophin-associated proteins in Fukuyama-type congenital muscular dystrophy. Lancet 341: 521

McArdle B (1951) Myopathy due to a defect in muscle glycogen breakdown. Clin Sci Mol Med 10: 13

McComas AT (1977) Neuromuscular function and disorders. Butterworths, London

McLellan DL, Swash M (1976) Longitudinal sliding of the median nerve during movement. J Neurol Neurosurg Psychiatry 38: 506

Mellick RS, Mahler RF, Hughes BP (1962) McArdle's syndrome: Phosphorylase deficient myopathy. Lancet i: 1045

Milhorat AT, Shafiq SA, Goldstone L (1966) Changes in muscle structure in dystrophic patients, carriers and siblings seen by electron microscopy: correlation with levels of serum creatine phospholeinase. Ann. NY Acad Sci 138: 246

Miranda AF, Nette EG, Hortlage PL, DiMauro S (1979) Phosphorylase isoenzymes in normal and myophosphorylasedeficient human heart. Neurology 29: 1538

Mohire MD, Tandar R, Fries TJ et al. (1988) Early onset benign autosomal dominant limb girdle myopathy with contractures (Bethlem myopathy). Neurology 38: 573

Mokri B, Engel AG (1975) Duchenne dystrophy – electron microscopic findings pointing to a basic or early abnormality in the plasma membrane of the muscle fibre. Neurology (Minneap) 25: 1111

Moosa A, Dubowitz V (1970) Peripheral neuropathy in Cockayne's syndrome. Arch Dis Child 45: 674

Morgan-Hughes JA (1982) Mitochondrial myopathies. In: Mastaglia FC, Walton JN (eds) Skeletal muscle pathology. Churchill Livingstone, Edinburgh, p 309

Morgan-Hughes JA, Daviniza P, Kahn SN, Landon DN, Sherratt RM, Land SM, Clark JB (1978) A mitochondrial myopathy characterized by a deficiency in reducible cytochromes. Brain 100: 617

Morgan-Hughes JA, Hayes DJ, Clark JB, Landon DN, Swash M, Stark R, Rudge P (1982) Mitochondrial myoencephalopathies: biochemical studies in two cases revealing defects in the respiratory chain. Brain 105: 553

Moulds RFW, Denborough MA (1972) Procaine in malignment hyperpyrexia. Br Med J iv: 526

Namba T, Brunner NG, Brown SB, Mugurama M, Grob D (1971) Familial myasthenia gravis. Arch Neurol 25: 49

Namba T, Brunner NG, Grob D (1978) Myasthenia gravis in patients with thymoma with particular reference to onset after thymectomy. Medicine (Baltimore) 57: 411

Neville HE, Brooke MH (1971) Central core fibres: structured and unstructured. (abstract), Excerpta Medica, Amsterdam, p 31 (ICS no. 237)

Neville HE, Brooke MH (1973) Central core fibres: structured and unstructured. In: Kakulas BA (ed) Basic research in myology, part I. Excerpta Medica, Amsterdam, p 497 (ICS no. 294)

Nienhuis AW, Coleman RF, Brown WJ, Munsat TL, Pearson CM (1967) Nemaline myopathy: a histolopathologic and histochemical study. Am J Clin Pathol 48: 1

Ochoa J (1976) The unmyelinated nerve fibre. In: Landon DN (ed) The peripheral nerve. Chapman and Hall, London, p 106

Ochoa J, Mair WG (1969) The normal sural nerve in man. 1. Ultrastructure and numbers of fibres and cells. Acta Neuropathol (Berl) 13: 197

Ochoa J, Danta G, Fowler TJ, Gilliatt RW (1971) Nature of the nerve lesion caused by a pneumatic tourniquet. Nature 233: 265

Olsson Y, Säve-Soderbergh J, Sourander P, Angerwall L (1968) A patho-anatomical study of the central and peripheral nervous system in diabetics of early onset and long duration. Pathol Eur 3: 62

Ontell M (1974) Muscle satellite cells: a validated technique for light microscopic identification and a quantitative study of changes in their population following denervation. Anat Rec 178: 211

Osserman KE (1958) Myasthenia gravis. Grune and Stratton, New York

Othmane KB, Ben Hamida M, Pericak-Vance MA et al. (1992) Linkage of Tunisian autosomal recessive Duchenne-like muscular dystrophy to the pericentromeric region of chromosome 13q. Nature Genet 2: 315

Pearce GW, Pearce JMS, Walton JN (1966) The Duchenne type muscular dystrophy: histopathological studies of the carrier state. Brain 89: 109

Pestronk D, Drachman DB (1978) A new method for demonstrating sprouting at neuromuscular terminals. Muscle Nerve 1: 40

Peter JB, Barnard VR, Edgerton VR, Gillespie CA, Stempel KE (1972) Metabolic profiles of three fibre types of skeletal

muscles in guinea pigs and rabbits. Biochemistry 11: 2627

Petty RKH, Harding AE, Morgan-Hughes JA (1986) The clinical features of mitochondrial myopathy. Brain 109: 915

Pirskanen R (1976) Genetic association between myasthenia gravis and the H-LA system. J Neurol Neurosurg Psychiatry 39: 23

Poewe W, Willeit H, Sluger E et al. (1985) The rigid spine syndrome – a myopathy of uncertain nosological position. J Neurol Neurosurg Psychiatr 48: 887

Polgar J, Johnson MA, Weightman D, Appleton D (1972) Data on fibre size in thirty-six human muscles. J Neurol Sci 19: 307

Prelle A, Moggio M, Comi GP et al. (1992) Congenital myopathy associated with abnormal accumulations of desmin and dystrophin. Neuromusc Disord 2: 169

Price MG, Sanger JW (1982) Intermediate filaments in stricted muscle. In: Dowben RM, Shay JW (eds) Cell and muscle motility, vol. 3. Plenum Press, New York, p 1

Prineas JW (1972) Acute idiopathic polyneuritis: an electron microscopic study. Invest 26: 133

Ptacek LJ, Tarvil R, Griggs RC et al. (1992) Linkage of atypical myotonia congenita to a sodium channel locus. Neurology 42: 431

Ptacek LJ, Johnson KJ, Griggs RC (1993) Genetics and physiology of the myotonic muscle disorders. N Engl J Med 328: 482

Refsum S (1946) Heredopathia atatica polyneuritiformis: a familial syndrome not hitherto described. Acta Psychiatr Scand [Suppl] 381: 303

Reznik N (1973) Current concepts of skeletal muscle regeneration. In: Pearson CM (ed) The striated muscle. Williams and Wilkins, Baltimore, p 185

Reznik M, Engel WK (1970) Ultrastructural and histochemical correlations of experimental muscle regeneration. J Neurol Sci 11: 167

Ridley A (1969) The neuropathy of acute intermittent porphyria. QJ Med 38: 307

Ridley A (1975) Porphyric neuropathy. In: Dyck PJ, Lambert EG, Thomas PK (eds) Peripheral neuropathy, vol 2. Saunders, Philadelphia, p 942

Ringel SP, Bender AN, Engel WK (1976) Extrajunctional acetylcholine receptors: alterations in human and experimental neuromuscular diseases. Arch Neurol 33: 751

Rosman NP, Kakulas BA (1966) Mental deficiency associated with muscular dystrophy: a neuropathological study. Brain 89: 769

Russell DS (1953) Histological changes in the striped muscles in myasthenia gravis. J Pathol Bacteriol 65: 279

Sabin TD, Swift TR (1975) Leprosy. In: Dyck PJ, Thomas PK, Lambert EH (eds) Peripheral neuropathy, vol 2. Saunders, Philadelphia, p 1166

Santa T, Engel AG, Lambert EH (1972) Histometric study of neuromuscular junction. 1. Myasthenia gravis. Neurology (Minneap) 22: 71

Sato T, Walker DL, Peters HA, Reese HH, Chou SM (1971) Chronic polymyositis and myxovirus-like inclusions: electron microscopic and viral studies. Arch Neurol 24: 409

Schaumberg HH, Spencer PS (1979) Toxic neuropathies. Neurology (Minneap) 29: 429

Schmalbruch H (1976) Muscle fibre splitting and regeneration in diseased human muscle. Neuropathol Appl Neurobiol 2: 3

Schmalbruch H (1985) Skeletal muscle. Springer, New York, p 440

Schmid R, Mahler R (1959) Chronic progressive myopathy with myoglobinuria: demonstration of a glycogenolytic defect in the muscle. J Clin Invest 38: 2044

Schotland DL (1977) Duchenne dystrophy – a freeze fracture study. In: Rowland LP (ed) Pathogenesis of human muscular dystrophies. Excerpta Medica, Amsterdam, p 562 (ICS no. 404)

Schubert W, Zimmerman K, Cramer M, Starzinsky-Powitz A (1989) Lymphocyte antigen Leu-19 as a molecular maker of regeneration in human skeletal muscle. Proc Natl Acad Sci

(USA) 86: 307

Schwartz MS, Swash M (1975) Scapulo-peroneal atrophy with sensory involvement: Davidenkow's syndrome. J Neurol Neurosurg Psychiatry 38: 1063

Schwartz MS, Sargeant M, Swash M (1976) Longitudinal fibre splitting in neurogenic muscular disorders: its relation to the pathogenesis of "myopathic" change. Brain 99: 617

Schwartz MS, Moosa A, Dubowitz V (1977a) Correlation of single fibre EMG and muscle histochemistry using an open biopsy recording technique. J Neurol Sci 31: 309

Schwartz MS, Sargeant MK, Swash M (1977b) Neostigmine-induced end-plate proliferation in the rat. Neurology (Minneap) 27: 289

Schwartz MS, Swash M, Gross M (1978) Benign post-infection polymyositis. Br Med J ii: 1256

Seitelberger F, Wanko T, Gavin MA (1961) The muscle fibre in central core disease: histochemical and electron microscopic observations. Acta Neuropathol (Berl)1: 223

Shafiq SA, Dubowitz V, Peterson HdeC, Milhorat AT (1967) Nemaline myopathy: report of a fatal case, with histochemical and electron microscopic studies. Brain 90: 817

Sher JH, Rimalovski AB, Athanassiades TJ, Aronson SM (1967) Familial centronuclear myopathy: a clinical and pathological study. Neurology (Minneap) 17: 727

Sheramata W, Kott S, Cyr DP (1971) The Chediak–Higashi–Steinbrinck syndrome. Arch Neurol 25: 289

Shillito P, Vincent A, Newsom-Davis J (1993) Congenital myasthenic syndromes. Neuromusc Disord 3: 183

Shy GM, Magee KR (1956) A new congenital non-progressive myopathy. Brain 79: 610

Shy GM, Engel WK, Somers JE, Wanko T (1963) Nemaline myopathy: a new congenital myopathy. Brain 86: 793

Sloper JC, Pegrum GD (1967) Regeneration of crushed mamalian skeletal muscle and effects of steroids. J Pathol 93: 47

Sourander P, Olsson Y (1968) Peripheral neuropathy in globoid cell leucodystrophy (Morbus Krabbe). Acta Neuropathol (Berl) 11: 69

Spiro AJ, Shy GM, Gonatas NK (1966) Myotubular myopathy. Arch Neurol 14: 1

Steinberg D, Mize C, Avigan J, Falls HM, Eldjarn L, Try K, Stokke O, Refsum S (1966) On the metabolic error in Refsum's disease. Trans Am Neurol Assoc 91: 168

Stern GM, Hall JM, Robinson DC (1964) Neonatal myasthenia gravis. Br Med J ii: 284

Stevens JC, Lofgren EP, Dyck PJ (1975) Biopsy of peripheral nerves. In: Dyck PJ, Thomas PK, Lambert EH (eds) Peripheral neuropathy. Saunders, Philadelphia, p 410

Sunderland S (1978) Nerves and nerve injuries. Churchill Livingstone, Edinburgh

Suter U, Welcher RA, Snipes GT (1993) Progress in the molecular understanding of hereditary peripheral neuropathies reveals new insights into the biology of the peripheral nervous system. Trends Neurosci 16: 50

Swash M (1979) Guillain–Barré syndrome: clinical aspects. J R Soc Med 12: 670

Swash M (1983) Pathology of the muscle spindle. In: Mastaglia FL, Walten JW (eds) Muscle pathology. Churchill Livingstone, Edinburg, p 508

Swash M, Fox KP (1972) Muscle spindle innervation in man. J Anat 112: 61

Swash M, Fox KP (1974) The pathology of the muscle spindle: effect of denervation. J Neurol Sci 22: 1

Swash M, Fox KP (1975a) Abnormal intrafusal muscle fibres in myotonic dystrophy: a study using serial sections. J Neurol Neurosurg Psychiatry 38: 91

Swash M, Fox KP (1975b) The fine structure of the spindle abnormality in myotonic dystrophy. Neuropathol Appl Neurobiol 1: 171

Swash M, Fox KP (1976) The pathology of the muscle spindle in Duchenne muscular dystrophy. J Neurol Sci 29: 17

Swash M, Schwartz MS (1977) Implications of longitudinal fibre splitting in myopathic and neurogenic disorders. J Neurol Neurosurg Psychiatry 40: 1152

Swash M, Schwartz MS (1981) Familial multicore disease with focal loss of cross striations and ophthalmaplegia. J Neurol Sci 52: 1

Swash M, Schwartz MS (1991) Muscle biopsy pathology, 2nd edn. Chapman and Hall, London

Swash M, Schwartz MS (1996) Neuromuscular diseases: a practical approach to diagnosis and management, 3rd edn. Springer, London

Swash M, van den Noort S, Craig JW (1970) Myopathy associated with diabetes mellitus in two sisters. Neurology (Minneap) 20: 694

Swash M, Sargeant MK, Schwartz MS (1978a) Pathogenesis of longitudinal splitting of muscle fibres in neurogenic disorders and polymyositis. Neuropathol Appl Neurobiol 4: 99

Swash M, Schwartz MS, Sargeant MK (1978b) The significance of ragged-red fibres in neuromuscular disease. J Neurol Sci 36: 347

Swash M, Schwartz MS, Carter ND, Heath R, Leak M, Rogers KLI (1983) Benign X-linked myopathy with acanthocytes (McLeod syndrome) – its relationship to X-linked muscular dystrophy. Brain 106: 717

Swash M, Schwartz MS, Apps MCP (1985) Adult onset acid maltase deficiency: distribution and progression of clinical and pathological abnormality in a family. J Neurol Sci 68: 61

Sweeney VP, Pathak MA, Asbury AK (1970) Acute intermittent porphyria: increased ALA synthetased activity during an acute attack. Brain 83: 369

Tallis R, Staniforth P, Fisher TR (1978) Neurophysiological studies of autogenous sural nerve grafts. J Neurol Neurosurg Psychiatry 41: 677

Tarui S, Oluno G, Ikura Y, Tanaka T, Suda M, Nishikawa M (1965) Phosphofructokinase deficiency in skeletal muscle: a new type of glycogenosis. Biochem Biophys Res Commun 19: 517

Thomas KP, Calne DB, Elliott CF (1972) X-linked scapuloperoneal syndrome. J Neurol Neurosurg Psychiatry 35: 208

Thomas PK, Lascelles RG (1966) The pathology of diabetic neuropathy. QJ Med 35: 489

Thomas PK, Lascelles RG, Hallpike JF, Hewer RC (1969) Recurrent and chronic relapsing Guillain–Barré polyneuritis. Brain 92: 589

Thomas PK, Ochoa J, Berthold C-H et al. (1993) Microscopic anatomy of the peripheral nervous system. In: Thomas PK, Dyck PJ (eds) The peripheral nervous system, 3rd edn. Saunders, Philadelphia, p 28

Thomashefsky AJ, Horwitz SJ, Feingold MH (1972) Acute autonomic neuropathy. Neurology 22: 251

Thornell LE, Edstrom L, Eriksson A, Henriksson KG, Anqvist KA (1980) The distribution of intermediate filament protein (skeletin) in normal and diseased human skeletal muscle. An immono-histochemical and electron-microscopical study. J Neurol Sci 47: 153

Toyka KV, Drachman DB, Griffin DE, Pestronk A, Winkelstein JA, Fischbeck K, Kao I (1977) Myasthenia gravis: a study of humoral immune mechanisms by passive transfer to mice. N Engl J Med 296: 125

Urich H, Wilkinson M (1970) Necrosis of muscle with carcinoma: myositis or myopathy? J Neurol Neurosurg Psychiatry 33: 398

Van Wijngaarden GK, Bethlem J (1971) The facioscapulohumeral syndrome. In: Kakulas BA (ed) Second International Congress on Muscle Diseases. Excerpta Medica, Amsterdam, p 54 (ICS no. 237)

Van Wijngaarden GK, Bethlem J, Dingemans KP, Coers C, Kelerman-Poppet M, Gerard JM (1977) Familial focal loss of cross striations. J Neurol 216: 163

Victor M, Hayes R, Adams RD (1962) Oculopharyngeal muscular dystrophy. A familial disease of late life characterized by dysphagia and progressive ptosis of the eyelids. N Engl J Med 267: 1267

Vincent A, Scadding GK, Thomas HC, Newsom Davis J (1978) In-vitro synthesis of anti-acetylcholine receptor antibody to thymic lymphocytes in myasthenia gravis. Lancet i: 305

Walton JN, Adams RD (1958) Polymyositis. Williams and Wilkins, Baltimore

Walton JN, Rowland LP, McLeod JG (1994) Classification of neuromuscular disorders (for WFN Research Group on Neuromuscular Disorders). J Neurol Sci 124 (Suppl): 109

Webb JN (1977) Cell death in developing skeletal muscle: histiochemistry and ultrastructure. J Pathol 123: 175

Weller RO, McArdle B (1971) Calcification within muscle fibres in the periodic paralyses. Brain 94: 333

Whitaker JN, Engel WK (1972) Vascular deposits of immunoglobulins and complement in idiopathic inflammatory myopathy. N Engl J Med 286: 263

Whitaker JN, Engel WK (1973) Mechanisms of muscle injury in idiopathic inflammatory myopathy. N Engl J Med 288: 434 and 289: 107

Whiteley AM, Schwartz MS, Sachs JA, Swash M (1976) Congenital myasthenia gravis: clinical and HLA studies in two brothers. J Neurol Neurosurg Psychiatry 39: 1145

Wochner RD, Dres G, Stober W, Waldmann TA (1966) Accelerated breakdown of IgG in myotonic dystrophy: a hereditary error of immunoglobulin catabolism. J Clin Invest 45: 321

Young JZ (1942) Functional repair of nervous tissue. Physiol Rev 22: 318

11 · Spleen, Lymph Nodes and Immunoreactive Tissues

Colin L. Berry and J.G. van den Tweel

The varied functions of spleen, lymph nodes and thymus result in their being involved in a widely disparate group of disease processes. A number of these, such as metabolic disease, are dealt with elsewhere in the volume, and this chapter is concerned with certain specific abnormalities, including the pathology of immune deficiency states and of lymphomas.

Embryogenesis and Development

Detailed accounts of the ontogeny of the immune response are available elsewhere (Pabst and Kreth 1980). However, it is worth considering the development of some immune functions as a way of understanding certain abnormalities of this system in childhood, in particular the development of the T lymphocyte series, the B lymphocyte series and the phagocyte series.

The origin of all of these cell types is the fetal yolk sac, which is the source of circulating cells until around the 5th week of gestation, erythropoiesis having begun there at around the 14th day after conception. It is then superseded by the liver; the bone marrow does not assume a dominant role until the 5th month although haemopoiesis can be found there at around 8–10 weeks. There is a differential distribution in skeletal sites: the clavicle, humerus, radius, tibia and ulna are colonized first (8–15 weeks), the vertebrae at the end of this time (15 weeks) and the sternum not until 20 weeks (see pp. 5, 523).

Recent studies suggest that the several populations of cells discussed here may be derived from embryonic stem cells at varying times under appropriate conditions (Wiles and Keller 1991). Although some interactions are clearly necessary in immune system development (thymic epithelium/T lymphocyte), precision in dating a time from which an abnormality will be expressed, based on morphological differentiation in the fetus, may be less sustainable than has been thought in the past.

The brief account of the embryology of the thymus given here is based on the studies of Hammar (1911, 1921) and Kingsbury (1915), together with an examination of human fetal thymuses obtained from Dr H.E.M. Kay.

The primordial thymus develops from the third and probably fourth endodermal pouches during the 6th week of development, approximately 7–10 days after the appearances of these structures (10–12 mm stage). The pouches are simple epithelial cell masses with, initially, a cleft-like lumen. The narrower caudal portion of the third pouch arising from the pharynx forms the corresponding half of the thymus, which at this stage is connected to the pharynx by the ductus pharyngobrachialis III. This later becomes solid, and then breaks (12 mm). Remnants of this duct may become parathyroid or thyroid "rests" or form epithelial cysts.

The walls of the pouch thicken and obliterate the lumen, and the cell mass moves caudally and medially. The parathyroid precursor generally separate from the thymic rudiment at around the 20 mm stage. The thymic precursor thickens caudally and this part is included in the developing thoracic cavity, where it fuses with the similar component of the other side. This fusion is limited to the connective tissue component. With differential growth of the neck and relative descent of the heart and great vessels the thymus is drawn down into the thorax. The cervical portion

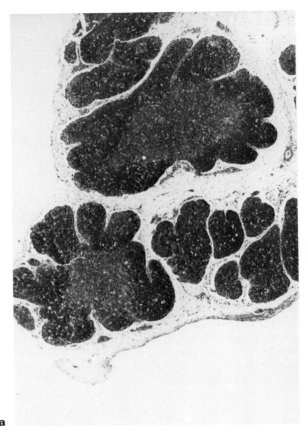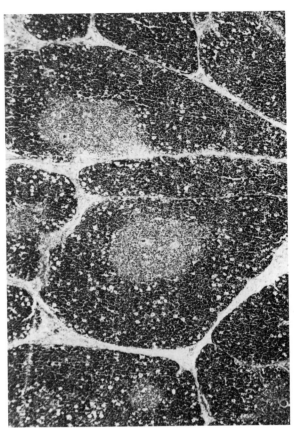

a   b

Fig. 11.1. Thymic appearances in **a** early and **b** late gestation. Initially the lymphocytic component is small and the gland appears to be predominantly epithelial. **a** Thymus at 12 weeks. (H&E, × 40) **b** Thymus at 26 weeks. (H&E, × 160)

becomes elongated and thinned, and extends into the neck in a very variable manner.

At 35–37 mm (approximately 56 days) the dense epithelial mass is surrounded by a mesenchymal condensation, and a lobulated structure develops following vascular invasion of the gland. At around the 40 mm stage the thymic medulla and cortex can be differentiated. Further development of the epithelial component occurs when large cells with eosinophilic cytoplasm appear, collect in small aggregates and become granular and more eosinophilic, and form Hassall's corpuscles. Personal observations suggest that this may occur at around 9–10 weeks after conception, a little earlier than generally suggested. Lymphocytes appear in the gland at the 30–35 mm stage (7–8 weeks) (Gilmour 1941) and are derived from immigrant stem cells of haemopoietic origin.

Ultrastructural studies of the 10–38 mm embryonic thymus have been performed by Pinkel (1968), who described the gland as an epithelial network enclosing lymphocytes and segregating them into groups. A haemo–thymic vascular barrier was described, pre-

venting penetration of antigen into the gland, backed up by a highly phagocytic zone of epithelial cells. Evidence for lymphocyte digestion was found in Hassall's corpuscles, supporting the suggestion of Siegler (1964) that this was an important function of these structures. Essentially similar ultrastructural findings were described by Goldstein et al. (1968), but lymphocytes were seen in passage across the walls of thymic blood vessels in their study.

In Fig. 11.1 the appearances of the gland in early and late pregnancy are shown. An up-to-date account of thymic development with many electromicrographic illustrations of cellular changes is seen in von Gaudecker (1986).

Embryology of Lymph Nodes and Spleen

The spleen first appears as a mesenchymal condensation in embryos of approximately 10 mm, in the dorsal mesogastrium. This development is apparently under the influence of an orphan homeobox gene

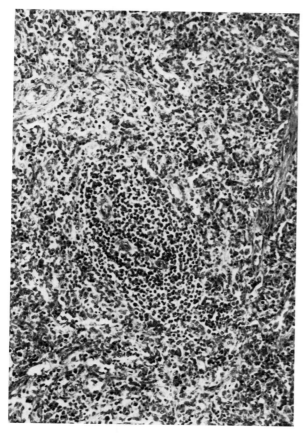

Fig. 11.2. Spleen at 24 weeks, showing early follicular development. (H&E, × 240)

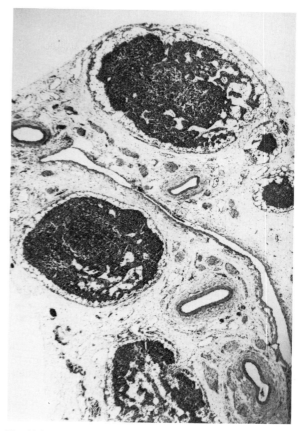

Fig. 11.3. Lymph nodes with well defined lymphocytic populations but a wide subcapsular sinus (26 weeks). (H&E, × 40)

(Hox 11). These unusual genes are not sequentially arranged in a clustered linear array as are most homeoboxes (Berry 1992) and their roles are not understood; however, animals in which this gene is not expressed show absence of the spleen with normal development of other splanchic derivatives (Roberts et al. 1994). The developing spleen is supplied by a branch of the coeliac artery to the greater curve of the stomach which will become the adult splenic artery. At around 30 mm (8–9 weeks) a series of anastomosing trabeculae become visible, in the spaces of which haematopoiesis develops by the 90 mm stage. It is during this stage that splenic sinusoids are formed. Follicular structures are seen by the end of the second trimester (Fig. 11.2).

Accessory masses of splenic tissue often become detached from the main body to form accessory spleens or splenunculi, which are commonly seen at autopsy in childhood.

Lymph nodes can be identified in the neck at the 25 mm stage. During early development erythropoiesis occurs in nodes, but this ceases early in intrauterine life. By 50 mm, when nodes are found in large numbers, the proliferating cells in their stroma are almost entirely lymphoid (Fig. 11.3). Rates of cell division in the fetus are low (Metcalf and Brumby 1966).

Histological Change in the Thymus with Age

Hammar (1926) and Boyd (1932) have discussed in some detail the changes occurring in the thymus gland with age. Boyd also included a quantitative assessment of the numbers of Hassall's corpuscles and their size distribution from prenatal life to the ninth decade.

In general, the initial appearance of closely packed lobules of thymic tissue changes at puberty as a result of enlargement of interlobar septa. At about 15–17 years of age the thymus reaches its maximum weight, and progressive decrease in size then ensues, with more rapid loss of cortex than of medulla. Fat appears in the interlobar septae and eventually the gland remains as a series of epithelial strands separated by fat. A thin rim of cortical lymphocytes is seen. Goldstein and Mackay (1967) have confirmed Boyd's finding that Hassall's corpuscles decrease in number with increasing age – from 12/mm² of medulla at birth to 2/mm² at 70 years of age. A modern study with a detailed account of T-cell changes and changes in immune function in old age is reported by Steinmann (1986).

Development and Function of Immunoreactive Tissues

Some knowledge of the developmental changes of the immunoreactive tissues is essential to a proper understanding of immune deficiency states. The system and its functions are phylogenetically ancient.

In many primitive animals, e.g. the arthropods and protostomes (annelid worms and molluscs), there are specialized phagocytic cells, which engulf injected or foreign particles and fragments of damaged tissue. Specialized lymphocytes first occur in the early vertebrates; both the agnathia and the lampreys and hagfishes have lymphocytes and can reject allografts. Recent work suggests that a self-recognition system, although not very effective, may exist in all animals. It seems likely in view of the importance of complex cell-surface characteristics in a number of processes in development, that a sensitive recognition system developed in association with this type of change, which explains the widespread presence of such systems.

The combination of functions expressed in an immune system capable of recognizing and rejecting allografts, maintaining a memory for previously experienced antigens and producing specifically reactive families of immunoglobulins, is confined to the vertebrates. How is the system formed?

T Lymphocyte Development

At about 8–9 weeks of development, a lymphocyte population appears in the thymic cortex and proliferates there. The origin of these cells is not clear; they may migrate from liver or bone marrow, but some authors support a local origin. The cells migrate to the thymic medulla, where they subsequently proliferate slowly. During this process around 70% of the cells produced will die, and it has been assumed that this extensive cell death represents the elimination of self-reactive clones. A peripheral mechanism may also be involved in this mechanism (Travers 1993).

Thymic inducer hormones act on the cells in the medulla, and the cells acquire most of their specialist reactive capacity there. Certain surface antigens are lost during development (T10); after a transient appearance, others, initally absent in fetal life (T1, T3), appear by term when helper (T1, T3, T4) and suppressor (T1, T3, T5, T8) phenotypes are identifiable.

A mixed leucocyte response to allogenic cells can be demonstrated by 7.5 weeks, but from liver-derived mononuclear cells rather than T cells (Carr et al. 1973). Later studies have shown this to be a non-specific response due to blastogenic substances in the stimulating T cells and involving no antigenic recognition. Response to phytohaemagglutinin (PHA) occurs from about 10 weeks in thymic cells and at 13–15 weeks in spleen cells. Specialist functions (helper, suppressor) are not developed until a little after term, although antiviral mechanisms operate and fetal cells can induce graft-versus-host reactions.

B Lymphocyte Development

B lymphocytes originate in the fetal liver at around 8 weeks' gestation as large pre-B cells, which lack surface antigen receptors and thus are able to develop independently of antigen and T cells. It is at this stage that clonal diversity may develop; in the next stage, at 7–8 weeks, the cells acquire surface immunoglobulin, Fc receptors and antigen receptor sites. They will therefore respond to exposure to antigen, at this stage, by becoming inactive or intolerant. Later (10–12 weeks), mature B cells appear, and by 15–16 weeks differentiation of the series is complete, with expression of surface IgD and IgM and other receptors. There is evidence that several cycles of cell division are necessary before restricted production of a single type of immunoglobulin by individual cells is achieved, but by 10–12 weeks these cells can synthesize IgM in response to antigenic stimulus.

A greater proportion of B cells have surface IgD in the neonate than in the adult, indicating a greater potential repsonsiveness to antigen. However, there is considerable suppression of B-cell function by T cells in the neonate, and in general neonatal B cells are not good responders. Synthesis of immunoglobulin types other than M does not usually begin until well after birth. For a detailed account of these changes see Lawton and Cooper (1980).

Around 75% of circulating lymphocytes are T cells, assessed by their capacity to form rosettes with sheep erythrocytes. Absolute numbers are 1620–4320/mm³ at 1 week of age, and 590–3090/mm³ at 18 months (Fleisher et al. 1975).

Development of the Mononuclear Phagocyte System

Mononuclear phagocytes are derived from a bone marrow precursor and include macrophages in lymph nodes and bone marrow, Kupffer cells, alveolar macrophages and osteoclasts. In general, circulating mononuclear cells replenish this population in adult life. Deficiencies of the system have been well studied in animals, where syndromes of failure of bone resorption mimic osteopetrosis and can be cured by transplantion, as in humans.

Polymorphonuclear Phagocytes

The major acute phagocytic system of polymorphonuclear cells (PMNs) is derived from bone marrow stem cell, which differ from the macrophage stem. However, the mechanisms of phagocytosis and intracellular destruction are comparable in the two lineages. Neonatal PMNs show a number of relative deficiencies of function, which make the diagnosis of abnormal states difficult, but some have been characterized and may depend on associated opsonizing defects.

Fetal Immunoreactivity

There is a considerable body of evidence documenting the immunological competence of the human fetus and its capacity to react to infection. The morphological appearance of the tissues described above is followed by the appearance of lymphocytes in the blood at around the 10th week, at a level of approximately 1000 cells/mm³. At 12 weeks lysozyme (muramidase), a basic protein with a molecular weight of around 15 000 and with pronounced bacteriolytic properties, is produced. Interferon is also found if cells from fetuses older than 18 weeks are exposed to rubella virus (Banatvala et al. 1971). Complement components are the next to appear, at around 15 weeks (C3) and 18 weeks (C4) (Adinolfi 1972). By 20 weeks all components of complement are present.

It used to be argued that the absence of plasma cells in fetal tissues supported the contention that immunoglobulins were not produced in the fetus, despite observations at the turn of the century that plasma cells were seen in congenital syphilis and more recently that they may be found in toxoplasmosis. The relative paucity of plasma cells during gesta-

tion is largely related to lack of stimulus. The timing of antibody production and the sequence in which the various classes appear are clearly under genetic control (Silverstein 1972). In humans, following intrauterine infections, IgM and IgG antibodies may be found in the serum of newborns – for example, in *Toxoplasma gondii*, cytomegalic inclusion disease, and herpes simplex infection. Antibodies to *Listeria monocytogenes* and gram-negative organisms have been found in apparently normal neonates (Cohen and Norins 1968), and the blood group anti-A and anti-B agglutinins of non-maternal origin have been detected in cord sera (Perchalski et al. 1968).

IgG and IgM antibodies are produced in very low concentrations in neonates, and the synthesis of IgD commences after birth. There is some evidence to suggest that IgE may be produced in utero (Adinolfi 1981). Holland and Holland (1966), using what would now be regarded as relatively insensitive techniques, demonstrated antibody production in the 2-month-old child of an aglobulinaemic mother.

A summary of current views of the production of immunoglobulin soon after birth may be given as follows.

IgM

Following stimulation from the gut, IgM production is in progress at the end of the first week of postnatal life, irrespective of maturity. IgM levels rise rapidly for the first 3 weeks of life but do not reach more than 80% of adult levels by the end of the first year. Infection in the perinatal period will act as a powerful stimulus to IgM production, but because of the rapid "normal" rise a significant increment over controls is necessary for diagnosis. An IgM level above 50 mg/dl during the neonatal period is suggestive of systemic infection (Kahn et al. 1969).

IgG

IgG is transferred across the placenta by an active mechanism involving Fc receptors on the trophoblast. This can be demonstrated by the end of the first 8 weeks of pregnancy, but significant transfer occurs only after 32 weeks. Endogenous synthesis does not begin until around 18 weeks. By term, fetal levels usually exceed maternal by a small amount.

IgA

IgA, which like IgM does not cross the placenta, gradually increases in amount in the first year of life, although adult levels are not reached until adolescence. It first appears in the gut at about 1 month of age (Perkkio and Savilahti 1980). IgA is found in tears at 3 weeks after birth.

Immune Deficiency States

Infection may be defined as the entry of self-replicating antigens into the tissues of the host, producing significant injury to the tissues. The establishment of an infection by a virus, fungus or bacterium is dependent on the virulence of the agent concerned, its number, mode of entry and the resistance of the host. Establishment of bacteria in tissues implies a breach of the first line of defence the integrity of mucous membranes or skin with the associated activity of lysozyme, secretory IgA, etc. The bacteria in the tissues are then exposed to a variety of humoral agents with growth-inhibitory or opsonizing effects. Phagocytosis may occur, by granulocytes or mononuclear cells, and intracellular destruction follows, although a number of infective agents may continue to proliferate intracellularly after phagocytosis. The process of intracellular digestion presents antigenic material to responsive cells, and the efferent limb of the immune response (specific antibody production, establishment of delayed hypersensitivity, etc.) is activated.

Immune deficiency states may be considered to affect primarily the "phagocytosis/digestion/antigen recognition" or *afferent* limb of the immune response, or the *efferent* limb, as defined above. However, it will be seen below that such diseases are complex, both in their causation and in the effects of the particular defect considered. The distinction between afferent and efferent limb defects or between cellular or humoral immunity is often not sharply defined, and alterations in one component may indirectly affect another.

T Cell Deficiency States

Patients with T-cell-deficient conditions present with clinical manifestations that include severe or overwhelming infection with ordinarily non-pathogenic bacteria (BCG) or fungi, or with agents that do not normally give rise to serious illness (zoster, varicella, herpes simplex, cytomegalovirus). There may be acute or chronic graft-versus-host disease in those transfused with viable allogenic lymphocytes. Subtle T-cell-deficient states may be manifest in localized

mucosal infections, immunoglobulin deficiency or autoimmunity.

In general, clinical syndromes occur in a way that suggests that all stages of the development of the immunoreactive system may be faulty, with specific effects.

We describe here a number of histopathological entities before making a clinicopathological synthesis. We would emphasize that accurate delineation of these syndromes requires sophisticated laboratory investigation in life, but that in previously unsuspected or uninvestigated causes useful data can be obtained from autopsy and histological examination.

Reticular Dysgenesis

Reticular dysgenesis was described by de Vaal and Seynhaeve (1959) in twins, and few other reports have since been made. The thymus is absent; there is lymphopenia, agranulocytosis and agammaglobulinaemia. Little or no development of peripheral lymphoid tissue is seen, and in a personal case a roll preparation of the entire mesentery revealed no lymph nodes after examination by step sectioning at 100 μm intervals.

The disease is thought to be due to deficiencies of the haemopoietic stem-cell precursor, giving rise to the lymphocytic and granulocytic population. Red cells and platelets are present (Gitlin et al. 1964).

Thymic Agenesis (DiGeorge Syndrome)

In 1968 DiGeorge, in the discussion of a paper, described four cases of thymic agenesis associated with absence of the parathyroid glands. The immunological function of one of these infants was studied and normal immunoglobulin levels were found. Plasma cells were present in lymph node biopsies but there was no demonstrable capacity to develop delayed hypersensitivity reactions. "Runting" was a feature of the clinical syndrome.

In the great majority of reported cases of the syndrome abnormalities of the aortic arch and heart have been present in association with thymic and parathyroid agenesis. Dische (1968) reported an instance of associated tracheo-oesophageal fistula and oesophageal atresia. There is one familial report (Steele et al. 1972), and the disease can occur in either sex.

The expression of the defect of the third and fourth arches is clearly variable: some patients have small thymic masses present, and in only seven of the 19 patients reported by Lischner and Huff (1975) was the thymus completely absent. The fragments present are usually histologically completely normal.

Parathyroid glands can be found in cases with completely absent thymic tissue.

There is a reduction in the thymic-dependent area of the peripheral lymph nodes in most cases, although Huber et al. (1967) have described tonsils, spleen, gut and lymph nodes as all having a normal structure and lymphoid population.

In eight cases of the syndrome that we have encountered, the presenting symptoms have been those of congenital heart disease in five, all dying in the first week of life. One child presented with congenital heart disease and tetany, and a further infant with tetany alone. An intrauterine death was associated with a scaly desquamating skin lesion thought to be a congenital dyskaryosis, but was found to be a disseminated skin infection by *Candida albicans* histologically. The heart lesions present in these cases were truncus arteriosus with right-sided aortic arch (two), transposition of the great arteries, and ventricular septal defect with gross preductal aortic arch hypoplasia and persistent ductus arteriosus. Aortic branching was anomalous in three cases.

Moerman et al. (1987) have emphasized the significance of a right-sided aorta in the syndrome. Four patients with DiGeorge syndrome had a right-sided aorta with a reversed branching pattern and an interruption between the right common carotid and right subclavian artery. In 185 consecutive cases of congenital heart disease, there was no case of an interrupted right aortic arch that was not associated with DiGeorge syndrome. In one further case, from which a thoracic pluck was examined, absence of the thymus was confirmed by serial sectioning (at 20 μm intervals) of the superior mediastinum, and a small nodule of parathyroid tissue was found. Tests with a functional basis had shown severe defects in T-cell activity (failure of sensitization with dinitrochlorobenzene and prolonged survival of allogenic skin grafts). Humoral immune functions are usually well preserved. As the fifth pharyngeal pouch gives rise to the ultimobranchial body, the probable source of C cells in the thyroid C-cell deficiency is present in most cases of DiGeorge syndrome (Burke et al. 1987). In general, the results of such tests suggest that the defect in the DiGeorge syndrome is not at the level of the stem cell giving rise to the T cell population, but is a defect in the thymus anlage, which prevents the proper processing of stem cells to T cells (Waldmann and Broder 1978).

Chisaka and Capecchi (1991) have reported the production of athymic aparathyroid mice with thyroid and submaxillary deficiencies, by the targeted disruption of the mouse homeobox gene Hox-1.5. Defects of the heart and arteries and of the face are also found. The similarity of this phenotype to DiGeorge syndrome is remarkable.

Thymic Dysplasia and Combined Immune Deficiency Syndromes

The term "thymic dysplasia" is used to describe an abnormality of thymic epithelial development resulting in gross reduction in number, or complete absence, of Hassall's corpuscles from the medulla of the gland. This change is accompanied by severe lymphocyte depletion.

A variety of clinical entities may present with this pivotal histopathological finding as a central feature, but we are not convinced that division of the thymic appearances into categories as suggested by Gosseye et al. (1983) is a nosologically significant advance.

If these simple criteria are used to select cases, a number of immune deficiency syndromes may be found when clinical records are examined (Berry 1968; Berry and Thompson 1968). In general, these have the features of the "combined immunity deficiency syndrome" ("Swiss-type" hypogammaglobulinaemia; Glanzmann and Riniker 1950), but cases of the type described by Nezelof et al. (1964), with defective cellular immunity and normal circulating immunoglobulins, are also seen. The Wiskott–Aldrich syndrome (see below and Aldrich et al. 1954) is also associated with thymic dysplasia.

We may regard all of these conditions as examples of the severe combined immunity deficiency syndrome, and should note that the group is variable. Genetically characterized variants are being identified continually, and specific metabolic defects are being found – for example, the T-cell tyrosine kinase deficiency reported by Edler et al. (1994).

Patients with X-linked severe combined immunodeficiency (XSCID) have a number of identifiable deficiencies of immune function, the first of which to be identified was a defect in interleukin 2. A protein that forms part of IL-2 forms part of two other cytokine receptors: IL-4 and IL-7. Each of the three interleukins enhances the growth of T and B cells at different stages of development (see Nowak 1993 for a bibliography).

Pathological Findings

Thymus

The thymus gland is small, weighing less than 2 g in most cases, although weights up to 12 g have been recorded. The abnormal gland tends to be found largely above the innominate vein. Histologically a fetal pattern is preserved, with a simple lobular architecture with conspicuous connective tissue. Corticomedullary demarcation is not marked (Fig. 11.4). The lobules are composed of a mass of mes-

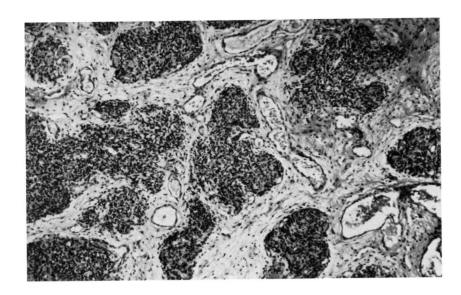

Fig. 11.4. Lobular pattern of the thymus, without corticomedullary demarcation. (H&E, × 40)

enchymal and endothelial cells, with fewer epithelial cells and only occasional lymphocytes, although in some instances variable numbers of these cells are seen. Hassall's corpuscles are absent or grossly reduced in numbers (Fig. 11.5). Reticulin stains confirm the "alveolar" pattern seen at the periphery of the lobules of some glands.

The changes are distinct from those seen in the thymus after involution, in which cortical lymphocyte loss may be extreme, with collapse of the periphery of the gland. Medullary lymphocytes persist and the medulla has a crowded appearance with many Hasall's corpuscles, which may be cystic (Fig. 11.6).

Lymph Nodes

The lymph nodes may be absent, with no trace of such structures despite extensive search by serial section (Berry 1970).

In cases in which nodes are present they may be represented as open-work lattices of supporting tissue, with few sinusoidal histocytes and virtually no lymphocyte population, or as simple masses of ill-organized vessels and connective tissue only recognizable by the distinct subcapsular sinus (Fig. 11.7). Occasionally, follicular collections of lymphocytes are seen, and plasma cells may be present. Varied

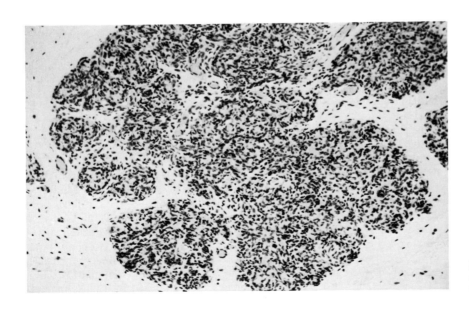

Fig. 11.5. A lobule with no evident development of Hassall's corpuscles. (H&E, × 240)

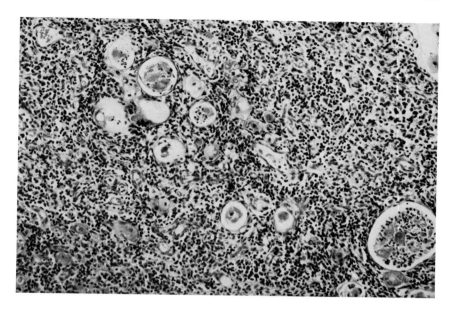

Fig. 11.6. Cystic Hassall's corpuscles with persistence of medullary lymphocytes. The collapsed cortex (*top right*) is lymphocyte-depleted. (H&E, × 240)

appearances may be seen in different nodes in the same case, but follicular structures, if present, are found in most nodes. Haemophagocytosis is not uncommon.

Spleen

In 26 of our autopsy cases the spleen has been present and within the normal weight range for the age. Few lymphocytes may be present in the pulp, but small perivascular lymphocyte cuffs are usually seen about penicillar arteries, although grossly diminished in size compared with age-matched controls (Fig. 11.8).

Gut-associated Lymphoid Tissue

The tonsils, appendix and Peyer's patches, and lymphoid follicles of the gut are here considered as an entity. In our autopsy cases absence of lymphoid

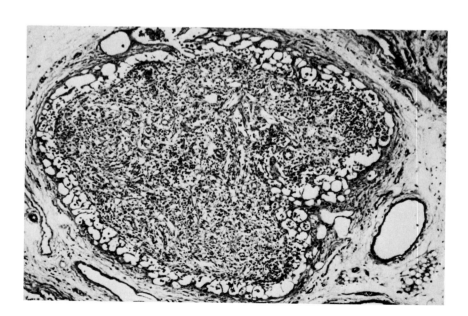

Fig. 11.7. A small lymph node without follicular differentiation or significant lymphocyte population. (H&E, × 40)

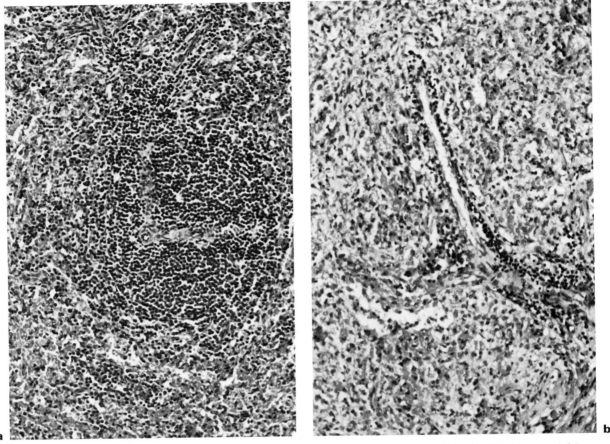

Fig. 11.8. Control spleen. Normal lymphocytes around an artery in a 4-month-old child. (H&E, × 120.) **b** Combined immune deficiency syndrome with small lymphocyte population around a penicillary vessel. (H&E, × 140)

tissue in the tonsillar fossa has invariably been associated with absence of Peyer's patches and appendiceal lymphoid tissue (Fig. 11.9).

The changes found in this group of syndromes are apparently related to an arrest of thymic development at around the 30 mm stage (Blackburn and Gordon 1967) or earlier (Berry 1970), with subsequent changes in the other lymphoid tissues.

Reconstitution therapy has been attempted by grafting of fetal thymus and stem cell transfusion. Graft-versus-host disease may develop in these immunologically incompetent hosts (Robertson et al. 1971) (Fig. 11.10), and this may apparently occur as a result of maternofetal transfusion during pregnancy (Kadowaki et al. 1965).

It must be emphasized that this morphological grouping of cases cuts across clinical syndromes, and is intended to be useful in histopathological diagnosis of the unsuspected case. Nowhere is the value of keeping infant viscera available until after histopathological examination of selected blocks

more clearly seen than in these syndromes, in which accurate diagnosis may have important consequences for genetic counselling. Blocks of the tonsillar bed and appendix are seldom taken for routine histology.

Some views of the pathology of combined immune deficiency syndromes (Heymer et al. 1977) suggest a specificity of association of particular syndromes with morphological findings that in our view is difficult to support.

Thymic Lymphocyte Depletion

In many infants the thymus appears to be grossly depleted of lymphocytes at autopsy. This depletion cannot be confused with the changes seen in immune deficient diseases as the essential structure of the thymus is preserved. Thus, although the cortex is bare, the reticulin structure of this part of the gland persists in a collapsed form, and medullary lymphocytes are present together with many Hassals cor-

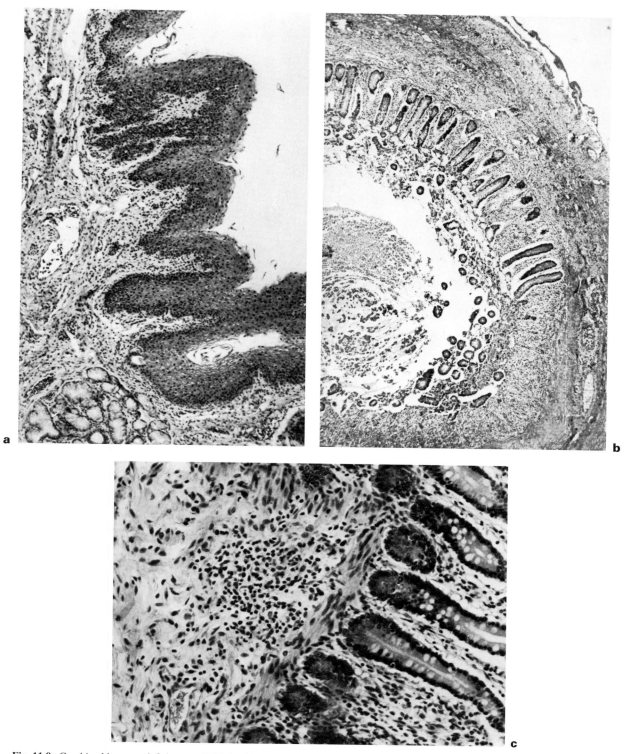

Fig. 11.9. Combined immune deficiency. **a** Folded epithelium from tonsillar fossa, with no lymphocytes. (H&E, × 40) **b** Appendix, with no follicular development. (H&E, × 20) **c** Small lymphoid collection in colon. This is not so large as to interrupt the continuity of the muscularis mucosa, here or in subsequent sections. (H&E, × 140)

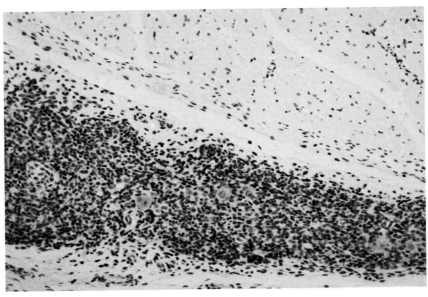

Fig. 11.10. Grafted fetal thymus in the rectus sheath in a case of combined immune deficiency syndrome. Note the presence of Hassall's corpuscles in normal fetal gland. (H&E, × 130)

puscles, which often appear crowded together.

The significance of these changes is far from clear and they do not, in our view, permit any statements to be made about ante-mortem events. In the sequential study referred to above (Berry 1968), lymphocyte loss was evident in 616 cases but was not found in others with a comparable clinical course. We know of no studies relating thymic lymphocyte depletion to ante-mortem cortisol levels or to the ratio of T and B lymphocytes in the circulating blood.

Gurevich et al. (1994) have illustrated a series of changes in immunoreactive tissues in low birth weight infants which they have attributed to antigen exposure. It is not clear that this is the case, and functional studies have not been made – many factors interfere with rapidly dividing cell populations in the middle trimester.

Antibody Deficiency Syndromes

In X-linked infantile agammaglobulinaemia, first described by Bruton (1952), the symptomatology is that of recurrent bacterial infection with pathogenic organisms (pneumococci, streptococci, staphylococci and *Haemophilus influenzae*). These infections, involving the middle ear, lungs, skin or gut, usually occur from 3 months of age. Immunoglobulin is present in very small amounts and blood-group isoagglutinins may be absent. Antibodies are not formed in response to immunization with conventional anti-

gens (e.g. tetanus toxoid). For a useful review see Rosen and Janeway (1966).

The gene for this disease was identified in 1993 (Vetrie et al. 1993). It was mapped to Xq22 by conventional linkage studies, and subsequently the technique of cDNA direct selection was used. In this, yeast artificial chromosomes (YACs) are used to propagate large segments of human DNA in which candidate genes can be identified by various hybridization techniques. The gene encodes a protein which is part of the *src* family of tyrosine kinases, but which is expressed in B cells. Point mutations and deletions in the gene are found in affected patients; these are very varied, and this variation may underlie the different forms of the disease that have been described (late-onset type, isolated light chain anomalies, etc.). There is an apparently close analogy with cystic fibrosis (see p. 227).

Pathological Findings

Lymphoid tissue is greatly reduced in amount, and lymph nodes are difficult to find. The tonsils and adenoids are virtually absent. The thymus is of normal size and form.

Histopathologically there is an absence of reactive two-component follicies in lymphoid tissue. Plasma cells are rarely found in this site. In some cases small follicular structures may be seen and plasma cells discovered; this is presumably the structural expression of the low but detectable immunoglobulin levels present. Lymphoid tissue is found in reduced amounts in the Peyer's patches and appendix. The thymus shows lymphocyte depletion, but the epithelial component is well represented and Hassall's corpuscles are present in normal numbers.

The sequelae of the disease include abscess formation and bronchiectasis, the lesions of which show no specific features, apart from the paucity of plasma cells in the inflammatory exudate.

Selective deficiency of immunoglobulin production also exists. Isolated reduction in the levels of IgM in the serum was reported by Hobbs et al. (1967) and is particularly associated with meningitis. Isolated IgA deficiency is present in about 1 in 1000 adults, but not all of these individuals are symptomatic.

Chronic Granulomatous Disease

Granulomatous disease was first described by Landing and Shirkey (1957). Although it appears as one disease phenotypically, there are two distinct modes of inheritance: X-linked recessive, which is the more common (Windhorst et al. 1968), and autosomal recessive (De Chatelet et al. 1976).

The gene for the sex-linked form is situated on the short arm of the X-chromosome proximal to the muscular dystrophy gene. It codes for a 90 kDa protein which interacts with a smaller (22 kDa) protein to form the functional cytochrome b complex. In the autosomal form the expression of the smaller protein is deficient, but this form of the disease is less well characterized genetically.

When a leucocyte engulfs an organism a phagolysosome is formed by fusion of lysosomes with the phagocytic vacuole. These are of two types, one containing lysozyme, peroxidase and cationic proteins; the other, which is smaller, containing alkaline phosphatase in addition to the other enzymes. Following this fusion there is a rapid increase in metabolic activity with an increase of two to three times in oxygen consumption. Hydrogen peroxide and other superoxides are formed and are bactericidal. Chronic granulomatous disease is a group of conditions in which these processes are defective.

Cell motility, phagocytosis and granule enzyme content and degranulation are essentially normal (see the review by Babior 1978). Staphylococci and the enterobacteriacae are not killed once engulfed, but pneumococci and streptococci are; this difference depends on the fact that the latter organisms themselves produce hydrogen peroxide. This is used by the neutrophil to kill them whereas staphylococci and enterobacteriacae are "protected" by their own catalases.

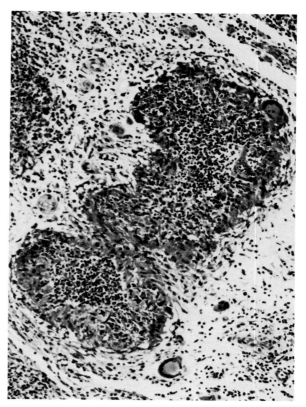

Fig. 11.11. Granuloma in skin from a case of chronic granulomatous disease. *Staphylococcus albus* cultured. (H&E, × 120)

Other immune functions in these individuals are normal; immunoglobulin levels are often high, presumably as a result of chronic infection.

The effect of the persistence of an indestructible agent in phagocytic cells is to induce a granulomatous response in the host. This essential abnormality produces the lesions seen in the disease.

In the skin, discrete tuberculoid granulomas with giant cells are often seen at the site of inflammation (Fig. 11.11), but granulation tissue indistinguishable from that seen around any chronic inflammatory sinus may be seen, with plasma cells present in normal numbers. Regional lymph nodes show reactive changes, and the brown-pigmented histiocytes described by some authors may be present. In our experience of 18 cases, these cells are by no means invariably found, but the pigment is found to be sudanophilic and weakly acid-fast (Fig. 11.12). PAS reactivity is variable. Central necrosis may develop in granulomas in lymph nodes; degenerate polymorphonuclear cells are often seen in the centre of such areas. The spleen is invariably large (Fig. 11.13), and in autopsy material areas of necrosis surrounded by a

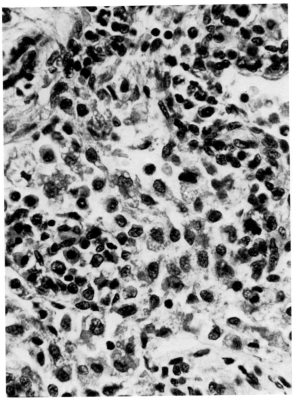

Fig. 11.12. Pigment-containing histiocytes in a lymph node. (H&E, × 240)

granulomatous inflammatory reaction may be seen. The liver shows a variety of changes; discrete focal intraparenchymal granulomas (Fig. 11.14), granulomatous inflammation in the portal tracts, portal fibrosis, and areas of necrosis and repair may all be seen at different stages. A similar range of appearances may be seen in the kidney (Fig. 11.15).

In the lungs the effects of the disease are often masked by superimposed bronchiectatic changes or abscess formation. Granulomatous masses with central necrosis occur and occasional isolated granulomas may be present, but histological material from mildly affected individuals or those in the early stages has not been studied. Symchych et al. (1968) have commented on the frequency with which pigmented histiocytes may be found in the lamina propria of the gut; this is true in our material and in that of Carson et al. (1965). Involvement of bone is not infrequent, and destructive osteomyelitis may ensue (Fig. 11.16).

The organisms involved in these lesions are often "non-pathogenic": from our cases *Aspergillus nidulans* has been isolated from the vertebral bodies, *Serratia marcescens* from the lung, and *Staphylococcus albus* from the renal parenchyma.

Other Granulocyte Defects

A clinical picture closely resembling that of chronic granulomatous disease may occur in glucose-6-phos-

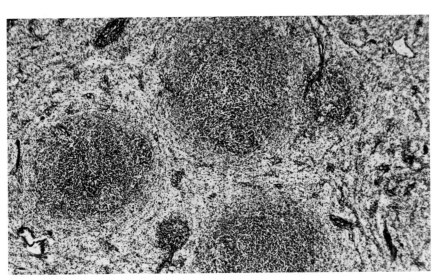

Fig. 11.13. Spleen in chronic granulomatous disease, showing marked sinusoidal hyperplasia. (H&E, × 80)

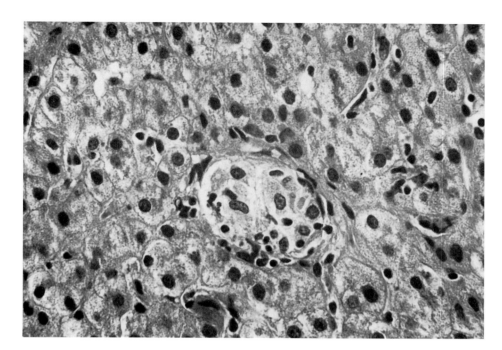

Fig. 11.14. Granuloma in liver parenchyma. (H&E, × 240)

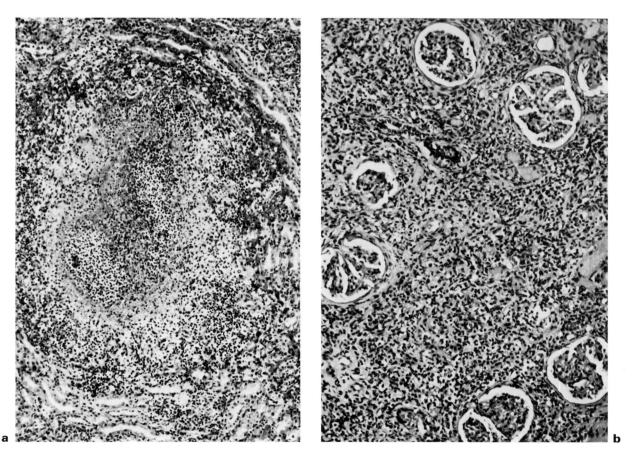

Fig. 11.15. a Intrarenal abscesses. (H&E, × 80) **b** Renal interstitial fibrosis. (H&E, × 120)

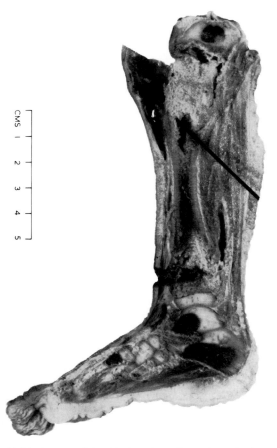

Fig. 11.16. Osteomyelitis with sinus formation and massive bony necrosis in chronic granulomatous disease.

phate dehydrogenase deficiency (see Babior 1978). these patients have similar defects of phagocyte function, but the disease usually presents after the first 5 years of life. In myeloperoxidase deficiency and glutathione deficiency there is no enhancement of susceptibility to infection, but glutathione peroxidase deficiency is associated with the phenotype of chronic granulomatous disease (see Matsuda et al. 1976).

Ataxia Telangiectasia

There are many distinctive features of ataxia telangiectasia. It is inherited as an autosomal recessive characteristic with multisystem effects including cerebellar ataxia, oculocutaneous telangiectasia, recurrent pulmonary infections, and a variable immune deficiency state. There may also be café-au-lait spots, vitiligo and grey hair. Carbohydrate metab-

olism may be abnormal (for a review see McFarlin et al. 1972). The lung infection occurs intermittently but may be progressively destructive, producing pulmonary crippling. A further long-term risk is the development of neoplasia, mainly lymphomatous but including gastric carcinoma, central nervous system malignancy and ovarian tumours (dysgerminoma).

Detailed immunological studies show normal IgG levels, low IgA and IgE, and abnormal IgM (low molecular weight). The low levels of IgA and IgE are due to decreased synthesis (Strober et al. 1968). Immune response to test antigens is poor. Cellular immunity is variable, only 15%–20% of patients responding to common skin test antigens, and there is delayed rejection of skin grafts.

Histopathologically the changes in the lymphoid tissues are those described under thymic dysplasia. Additional lesions include cerebellar atrophy, demyelination of the posterior columns and anterior horn cell loss. The pathology of the cutaneous lesions (e.g. café-au-lait spots) has no special features. Patients with the disease have been shown to have a defect in the repair of DNA and to be extremely sensitive to radiation. Chromosome breaks are common. These changes may explain why large cells with bizarre nuclei are seen in many organs in this condition. α-Fetoprotein levels are high in most cases (Waldmann and McIntire 1972), and this is considered to be an indicator of a widespread failure of gene regulation. Cox et al. (1978) have suggested that the radiosensitivity of cultured skin fibroblasts be used as a diagnostic test in this condition.

Chediak–Higashi Syndrome

A rare familial disorder, Chediak–Higashi syndrome involves partial oculocutaneous albinism (blue eyes, decreased retinal pigmentation associated with photophobia) and severe recurrent infections. Hepatosplenomegaly is common, and the disease causes death in infancy or childhood from infection or neoplasia, the oldest reported survivor being 18 years of age (Kritzler et al. 1964). A history of consanguinity is common, and an autosomal recessive mode of inheritance has been proposed.

Pathologically the classic feature of the disease is the presence of massive intracellular inclusions of lysosomal origin. These are 2–4 μm in diameter, and myeloperoxidase- and lysozyme-positive; they occur in leucocytes, renal tubular epithelial cells, gastric mucosa, pancreas, thyroid, melanocytes and glial cells. The coincidence of enzyme reactivity attributable to more than one type of intracellular inclusion suggests an origin from fused azurophilic and specific granules (Rausch et al. 1978).

Defects of leucocyte function have been described, affecting both their chemotactic response and their bactericidal abilities. The massive inclusions are slow to fuse with phagocytic vacuoles, and this presumably underlies the failure of intracellular bacterial killing (see also p. 613).

Wiskott–Aldrich Syndrome

Wiskott–Aldrich syndrome is inherited as a sex-linked recessive disorder, and is characterized by thrombocytopenic purpura, eczematoid dermatitis and recurrent infections (Cooper et al. 1968). The platelets of affected individuals are small and show a failure to aggregate when exposed to ADP, collagen or epinephrine. Shapiro et al. (1978) have devised a test whereby the carrier state can be detected by assessment of the response of platelets to metabolic stimuli.

Affected individuals may die of infection, haemorrhages or tumours (Table 11.1). The only effective therapeutic measure appears to be bone marrow transplantation (Parkman et al. 1978). Immunoglobulins are present in most cases, but the response to bacterial capsular antigens is poor. Histopathologically there is a varied picture, many cases having relatively normal, although lymphocyte-depleted, thymus and lymph nodes while others are affected by changes resembling those described for thymic dysplasia. The skin lesions are those of a typical eczematous dermatitis (Cooper et al. 1978).

Immune Deficiency States Caused by Protein Loss or Acquired Cellular Defects

Protein-losing enteropathy from any cause is often associated with immunoglobulin deficiency. In intestinal lymphangiectasia, injected labelled immunoglobulin has a short half-life because of excretion via the gut. These patients may have absolute lymphopenia with loss of T cells and failure of cellular immune functions (Strober et al. 1967).

Protein loss in the nephrotic syndrome may lower circulating immunoglobulin levels. Cytotoxic drug therapy may have similar effects, and certainly affects lymphocyte populations.

Enzyme Defects and Immune Deficiency States

There have been a number of descriptions of specific enzyme defects associated with immune deficiency states. Absence of adenosine deaminase gives rise to

Table 11.1. Immune deficiency syndromes and tumours

Disease	Tumours reported
Ataxia telangiectasia	Leukaemia; lymphomas; carcinoma of stomach, skin, parotid Glioma; medulloblastoma; dysgerminoma
Wiskott–Aldrich syndrome	Leukaemia; lymphomas; astrocytoma; leiomyosarcoma
Congenital agammaglobulinaemia (Bruton type)	Leukaemia; lymphomas
Combined immune deficiency syndromes	Leukaemia; lymphoma; carcinoma of stomach, breast, bladder, buccal cavity
Isolated IgA deficiency	Carcinoma of colon, lung, stomach, breast, oesophagus, skin Gliomas
Isolated IgM deficiency	Lymphomas; neuroblastoma

the severe combined immune-deficiency syndrome (probably accounting for half of all cases of the non-X-linked form); purine nucleoside pyrophosphorylase to a cellular immune deficiency syndrome; absence of transcobalamine II to agammaglobulinaemia; and diminished activity of nucleotidase to hypogammaglobulinaemia. The absence of these various enzymes may lead to damage to stem cells or B cells by accumulation of metabolites or, as in the case of transcobalamine II, to failure of transport of vitamin B_{12} into rapidly growing cells. The subject is extensively reviewed by Hirschhorn and Martin (1978).

Tumours and Immune Deficiency States

Enhanced tumour susceptibility occurs in a number of syndromes of immune deficiency. The reasons for this are discussed in detail elsewhere (Berry 1981), and Table 11.1 summarizes reported findings.

Infectious Mononucleosis and Duncan's Disease

Infectious mononucleosis has no specific features in childhood, closely resembling the more usual adolescent disease. Death is rare, and is usually attributable to neurological involvement or to rupture of the spleen (Penman 1971). However, in certain sibships, an anomalous response to the Epstein–Barr virus (EBV) may result in other changes, which were first described in a family called Duncan (see Purtilo et al. 1977 for a review).

In glandular fever EBV infects B lymphocytes. The clinical disease is the manifestation of a "war

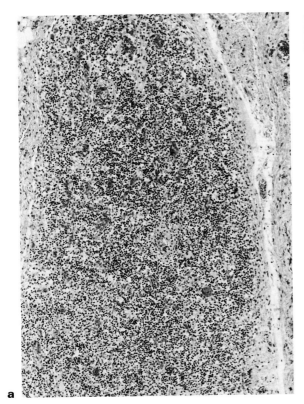

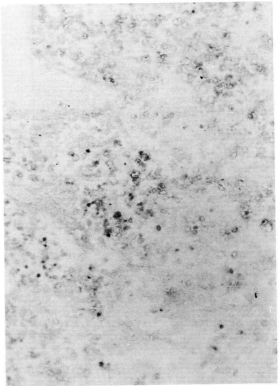

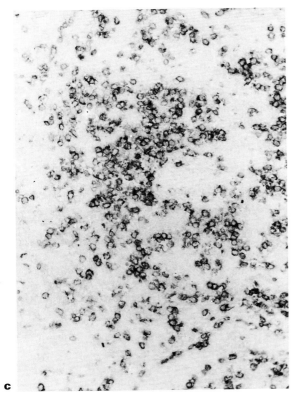

Fig. 11.17. a Post-mortem lymph node from a child dying with AIDS. There is clear lymphocyte depletion and absence of follicular structure. (H&E, × 30) **b** Lymph node section reacted with antibody to T4 cells showing marked depletion. (Immunoperoxidase, × 90) **c** Lymph node section reacted with antibody to T8 cells showing their persistence in normal numbers. (Immunoperoxidase, × 120) (Courtesy of Dr J. Cox, Geneva).

between lymphocytes", with T cells attacking and destroying B cells. In Duncan's disease, an abnormality inherited as an X-linked recessive, this war may result in complete destruction of B cells, producing agammaglobulinaemia. Alternatively, malignant transformation of B cells may occur, with the development of a proliferative state such as Burkitt's lymphoma, plasmacytoma or immunoblastic sarcoma. This change is presumably due to failure of T cells to control the EBV-containing B cells.

Acquired Immune Deficiency Syndrome in Infants

In acquired immune deficiency syndrome (AIDS) the route of infection is commonly maternofetal via the placenta or breast milk, although post-transfusion AIDS has occurred in infants (Nezelof et al. 1986).

About 25% of of HIV-infected children progress to AIDS or death in the first year; by 4 years of age around 40% of infected children have progressed. The spectrum of disease in HIV-infected infants and children differs from that in adults. This reflects differences in the effects of the virus; in congenitally infected infants signs of B-lymphocyte failure generally anticipate those of abnormal T-cell function. Hypergammaglobulinaemia is common, and bacteraemia with common pathogens is an early sign of HIV infection. In the first year of life decrease or reversal of T4 : T8 ratios is not a major characteristic, and where changes occur they are due to decreased numbers of circulating CD8 cells rather than a fall in CD4 numbers.

Lymph node changes include centrofollicular T8 cell hyperplasia, and follicular hyperplasia with loss of the IgD cell mantle in biopsies and cellular depopulation at autopsy. Vascular proliferation was not seen by Nezelof et al. nor in one of our cases, in contrast to the findings of Scott et al. (1984) (Fig. 11.17).

The thymus is small, with a reduced cell population and lack of epithelial differentiation resembling that found in congenital defects of cellular immunity (Berry and Thompson 1968).

Infants rarely develop Kaposi's sarcoma but frequently exhibit lymphocytic interstitial pneumonitis (see p. 825). Children infected in utero have a high incidence of neurological disease.

An extensive report by Schuurman et al. (1989) has confirmed that no specific thymic finding is seen in those affected by AIDS.

Case reports have documented AIDS in children born to high-risk mothers despite delivery by caesarean section or removal at birth to foster families (Cowan et al. 1984; Lapointe et al. 1985).

Other Diseases of the Thymus

Neoplasms

Thymic tumours, which are rare in all age groups, are much commoner in adults than in children. In the assessment of previous reports the designation "malignant thymoma", often the only pathological description, is unhelpful; however, in the three cases aged 15 years or less in the series of 55 cases reported by Friedman (1967), two had benign teratomas and one a malignant teratocarcinoma. In the series of Berg et al. (1968) and Watson et al. (1968), in a total of 59 cases there were three malignant thymomas in individuals less than 15 years of age; these were apparently lymphoepithelial in type. Further confusion with the term "lymphosarcoma" occurs, because of the frequent involvement of the thymus in leukaemia. Examination of the tissues of so-called primary lymphosarcomas of the thymus often reveals evidence of leukaemia, and in a series of 49 autopsy cases of lymphoblastic leukaemia examined by one of us, 43 cases showed evidence of infiltration of the thymus. Of 18 thymic tumours in individuals aged 15 years or less seen by us, seven were teratomas (patients' ages 3, 4, 8 and 9 months and $1\frac{1}{2}$, 8 and 14 years). None of these were malignant, and it is generally true that malignancy in this group of teratomas is manifest in the second decade. Nine cases of benign thymoma or thymic hyperplasia were seen; none of these were associated with myasthenia.

One lymphoepithelial thymoma was removed from a boy of 7 years, who was active and well 6 years after resection. A further example, removed when the patient was 4 years old, proved rapidly fatal. Lynch (1975) has described a lymphoepithelial tumour associated with myasthenia in a 12-year-old (see p. 600 for an account of myasthenia in childhood).

Cases of thymic tumour with acquired immunoglobulin deficiency (Rubin et al. 1964) have not been recorded in children, and of 94 reported cases of thymic tumour and hypoplasia of the bone marrow only one was in a child (aged 5 years) (Talerman and Amigo 1968).

Thymolipoma

Although described as a distinct condition, it seems likely that thymolipoma is a lipoma occurring in the anterior mediastinum. These lesions are rare in infancy, but may be massive in size.

Germinal Follicles

The appearance of germinal follicles in the thymus has been reported in a number of conditions associated with autoimmunity. In infancy and childhood germinal follicles (two cellular component-reactive follicles) are undoubtedly commoner than in adults (Henry 1968), but criteria of what constitutes a follicle and methods of study, e.g. section frequency, have varied widely, accounting for the enormous range described as normal: from 1% (Okabe 1966) to 50% (Middleton 1967).

Cysts

Dyer (1967) has suggested that a number of anterior mediastinal cysts are of thymic origin. If the term is

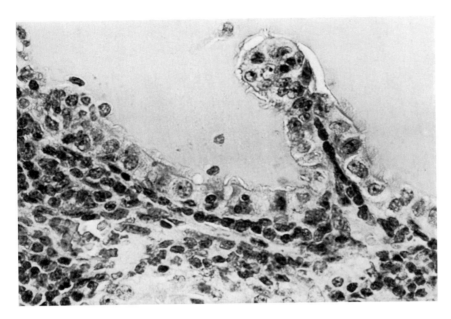

Fig. 11.18. Ciliated epithelium in a thymic cyst, 6 cm in diameter, removed surgically from a 5-year-old boy. (H&E, × 240)

confined to cysts having their origin in the thymus or its analogue, however, they are apparently rare, and are generally regarded as remnants of the ductus phangiobrachialis. They are often lined with a ciliated or columnar epithelium (Fig. 11.18), but other varieties may be seen. For further discussion see Bieger and McAdams (1966) and Indeglia et al. (1967).

Respiratory Obstruction

Sealy et al. (1965) described seven patients in whom the thymus apparently compressed the trachea at the thoracic inlet and caused respiratory obstruction.

It seems from their description that some of these cases may be instances of cartilaginous abnormality of the trachea, which was described as "slit-like" and collapsing in some instances. It is also possible that the compression had affected the viability of the tracheal wall, as has occurred in one of our cases of thymic hyperplasia.

Anatomical Abnormalities of the Spleen

Splenunculi

Splenunculi are often found in neonatal autopsies (in 10%–15%), and in view of an apparently lower inci-

dence in adult life many presumably involute. There is evidence that they may hypertrophy following splenectomy in adult life, e.g. in myelofibrosis and uncommonly in congenital spherocytic anaemia.

Asplenia

Asplenia is an important finding in a neonatal necropsy; it should alert the prosector to the probability of abnormal thoracic situs and abnormalities of the heart. Asplenia is almost always associated with bilateral symmetry of the tracheobronchial tree, with the presence of two eparterial main bronchi and two apparently right (trilobed) lungs. The bronchial findings in turn indicate that two right atria are present and that major cardiac anomalies are probable (see Becker and Anderson 1981).

Associated abnormalities of mesenteric attachment may occur, and renal anomalies are common. The abnormality is commoner in males.

Polysplenia

As with asplenia, polysplenia is a useful indicator of other abnormalities, although these may be less severe than with asplenia. The term should be applied only to cases in which spleens are present on both sides of the mesogastrium; accessory spleens are always on the left of this structure. Both lungs are bilobed and have hyparterial bronchi. In simplistic terms, both are left lungs. Both atria have left-sided characteristics. This syndrome occurs at a similar frequency in both sexes.

Splenomegaly

Splenomegaly is common in many neonatal infections, and in conditions associated with red-cell haemolysis. Detailed pathological findings are available only for conditions in which death is common. The spleen is commonly enlarged in congenital cytomegalovirus infections, and this may be the only abnormality evident at birth. A petechial rash may coexist with splenomegaly. Microscopically, the typical inclusion bodies may be seen in the spleen, and the virus can be isolated from the parenchyma.

Splenomegaly is also common in toxoplasmosis. However, the organism is rarely seen in the tissue, and the only specific finding reported is an eosinophilic infiltrate (Frenkel and Friedlander 1952). The spleen is large in congenital syphilis but shows no distinctive features; the same is true in congenital tuberculosis. In listeriosis, granulomas are commonly seen. Splenomegaly is usual in congenital leukaemia.

Effects of Splenectomy

Splenectomy may be necessary following trauma, or may be indicated in conditions as diverse as congenital spherocytic anaemia, thrombocytopenic purpura, Gaucher's disease and thalassaemia. There has been considerable discussion, over a period of 30 years, of the risks attending splenectomy in the young (see Eraklis and Filler 1972). In general it is agreed that septicaemia is commoner in splenectomized patients and that the commonly associated organisms are *Streptococcus pneumoniae* and other encapsulated bacteria (*Haemophilus influenzae, Neisseria meningitidis*), and less commonly *Escherichia coli*. Classically an overwhelming infection occurs within 2–3 years of the operation and is associated with a mortality rate of up to 80%. Although it has been suggested that post-traumatic splenectomy is less likely to be associated with later infection, a study by Singer (1973) suggests that this is not so. Because of this a conservative approach to the traumatized spleen is now adopted in some centres (Aronzon et al. 1977). There is no evidence that attempts to preserve the spleen in children results in increased surgical morbidity or mortality rate (Buyukunal et al. 1987).

A more recent problem is infection in young patients splenectomized during staging laparotomy for Hodgkin's disease or other lymphoma. A recent report (Chilcote et al. 1976) documented 20 episodes of meningitis and septicaemia in 18 of 200 children after splenectomy during staging. The pneumococci, streptococci, *H. influenzae* and meningococci were the organisms involved in the 75% of cases in which a diagnosis was made (in 25% the causative organism was not identified).

Honigman and Lanzkowsky (1979) have reported a case of overwhelming sepsis in an 8-week-old girl with isolated absence of the spleen diagnosed by computed tomography and by the presence of Howell–Jolly bodies in the blood. Review of the literature reveals only eight children with isolated asplenia, five from one family (see also Kevy et al. 1968).

Cysts, Hamartomas and Heterotopias

Splenic cysts are rare, but McNamara et al. (1968) reported five cases, all in females. They presented between 9 and 15 years of age, with progressive abdominal swelling. Splenectomy revealed pseudocysts (fibrous cavities around areas of presumed necrosis) or epidermoid cysts. The differential diagnosis includes hydatid disease, lymphangioma and haemangioma (see also Qureshi et al. 1964).

It is important that the splenic nodules of hamartomas and heterotopia, which are usually less than 1 cm in diameter, should not be mistaken for more serious lesions. Hamartomas often consist of pancreatic tissue and fat (Butler 1983), but vascular lesions occur. Heterotopia with nodules of normal splenic tissue within the pancreas, adrenal gland or liver may be found in trisomy 13.

Storage Disorders

The diagnosis of storage disorders is described in detail elsewhere (see p. 837). Splenomegaly is a feature of a number of storage disorders, which will be briefly considered here.

Gaucher's Disease

Gaucher's disease is a disease in which glucocerebrosides accumulate in the histiocytes of the entire reticuloendothelial system. The commonest form is

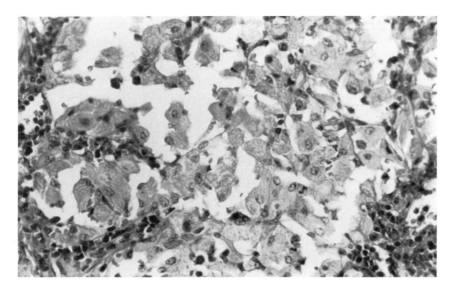

Fig. 11.19. Gaucher cells in the spleen; granular cytoplasm. (H&E, × 240

characterized by hepatosplenomegaly, lymphadenopathy and bone marrow involvement, causing bone pain and various haematological complications, including thrombocytopenia, haemolytic anaemia and neutropenia. The severity of these complications determines the clinical course; the disease is compatible with long life. Macroscopically, tissues involved by Gaucher's disease show an irregular pattern of yellowish-white deposits. These may be confluent in the liver, and the bone marrow appears yellowish-white. Gaucher cells are seen in vast numbers in affected tissues; they are typically massive (up to 120 μm), with granular cytoplasm showing a striated or folded pattern. Figures 11.19 and 11.20 show cells from a 9-year-old boy with the disease who died following a tonsillectomy after haemorrhage associated with thrombocytopenia. The cells are sudanophilic and stain positively with PAS. Electron microscopy shows large inclusions with a single limiting membrane.

Neuropathic Gaucher's disease presents in the first year of life, with failure of neurological development followed by marked regression. Massive hepatosplenomegaly develops and the disease is rapidly fatal.

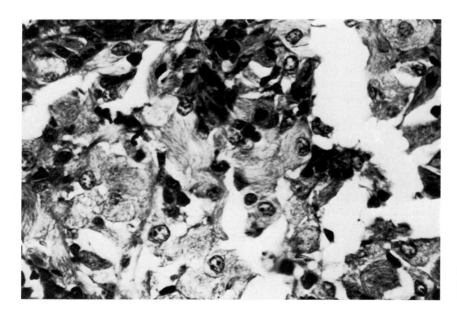

Fig. 11.20. "Folded" cytoplasmic appearance in Gaucher cells. (Azan stain, × 240)

There is no direct cerebral involvement by cerebroside storage; changes in the brain are degenerative and non-specific.

The two forms of the disease appear to be genetically distinct. The non-neuropathic form only is commoner in Jews.

Niemann–Pick Disease

Niemann–Pick disease also occurs in two clinical forms, and involves sphingomyelin accumulation within the reticuloendothelial system and neurons. In the infantile form symptoms are usually evident within the first year of life and include progressive mental and motor retardation, progressive cachexia, and death usually by 2–3 years of age. Massive hepatosplenomegaly occurs, and lymph nodes may enlarge sufficiently to be palpable. In rare cases, neurological involvement is absent and the disease presents later and has a chronic course. An autosomal recessive mode of inheritance seems likely; the infantile form is commoner in Jews.

Macroscopically, the brain appears firm and shrunken; the liver and spleen are hard and uniformly yellowish-white. Reticuloendothelial cell involvement is manifest in the presence of foamy cells up to 80 μm in diameter, with a cytoplasm containing multiple small vacuoles, which are sudanophilic and PAS-positive, and in frozen sections fluoresce under ultraviolet light. Electron microscopy shows multi-amellate inclusions and some amorphous deposits. Similar cytoplasmic deposits are found in neurons and in the dura.

Wolman's Disease

Wolman's disease, often diagnosed clinically by the presence of calcification in the adrenals in a child with hepatosplenomegaly and malabsorption, is characterized by the storage of cholesterol esters. Foamy macrophages can be seen in the marrow, spleen, liver, lymph nodes and lamina propria of the intestine. The central nervous system is not involved (see also pp. 840, 845).

Langerhans' Cell Histiocytosis

Langerhans' cell histiocytosis (LCH) is a group of syndromes characterized by a clonal proliferation of histiocytes (Willman et al. 1994). The majority of cases fall into a group of diseases previously categorized as "histiocytosis X". This occurred in three major forms: Letterer–Siewe disease (now multisystem multifocal LCH), Hand–Schüller–Christian disease (multifocal unisystem LCH) and solitary eosinophilic granuloma (unifocal LCH). Multisystem multifocal disease has been reported in monozygotic twins (Katz et al. 1991).

The review of Sims (1977) described 43 cases of histiocytosis X presenting in children under 12 years of age over a 29-year period. Approximately one-third had died, low age at presentation and soft-tissue involvement being associated with a poor prognosis. Of the survivors, about half had residual disability, including diabetes insipidus, pancytopenia and abnormal lung function tests. Defects of immune function were not found in survivors. Ten of the 29 survivors developed diabetes insipidus, two only temporarily. Histologically, bone lesions often resembled typical eosinophil granuloma (see below), but a "granulomatous" reaction with varying numbers of histiocytes, eosinophils, plasma cells, lymphocytes and polymorphs often led to the diagnosis "compatible with histiocytosis X". Sims' review emphasizes the heterogeneous nature of this disease, and, although pathological findings of typical entities are described below, mixed patterns are commonplace (Avery et al. 1957; Newton and Homoudi 1973).

Reviews by Bokkerink and de Vaan (1980) and Favara et al. (1983) give further details on the the differentiation of histiocytosis X from other disorders, such as familial erythrophagocytic lymphohistiocytosis, combined immunodeficiency and histiocytosis, malignant histiocytosis and virus-associated haemophagocytic syndrome.

Aetiology

Pentalaminar cytoplasmic inclusions have been found in the cytoplasm of histiocytes from all three types of LCH (Basset and Turiaf 1965; Basset et al. 1965, 1972; Shamoto 1970). Although they were initially considered to be possible viral inclusions, identical structures were subsequently found in the Langerhans' cells of the skin. These Langerhans' or Birbeck granules were found in all cases of LCH examined in two series (Nezelof et al. 1979; Mierau et al. 1982), but the numbers of such cells varied in individual cases. The Langerhans' cell has been regarded as a *sine qua non* for the diagnosis of LCH (Favara et al. 1983). Gene rearrangement studies have shown a germ line configuration for the T cell receptor gene (Weiss, 1993). In contrast to macrophages, these cells contain ATPase, lack significant acid phosphatase or esterase,

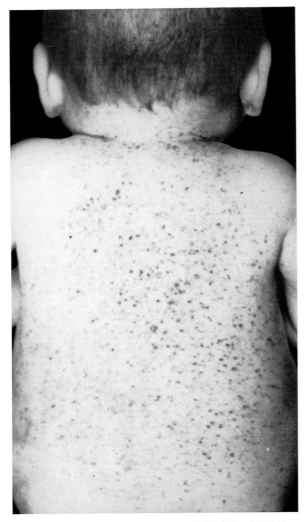

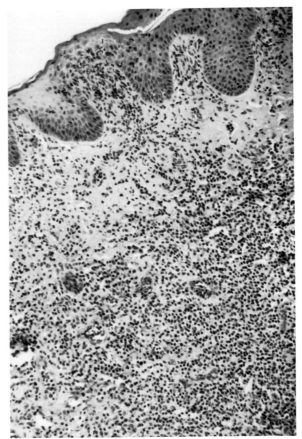

Fig. 11.22. Skin biopsy. The infiltrate is seen in the upper dermis. (H&E, × 120)

Fig. 11.21. Rash in typical distribution of LCH diffuse LCH. Note the abdominal swelling caused by hepatosplenomegaly.

and are S-100 antigen positive by immunohistochemistry. Surface receptors for IgG, the C_3 component of complement, and Ia or Dr molecules are shared with cells of the mononuclear phagocyte system (Thomas et al. 1982; Favara et al. 1983).

The cell is typically negative for CD45 in paraffin sections, but positive for CD1, CD4, CD14 and CD45 in frozen sections. In the majority of cases positive vimentin staining is seen.

Multisystem Multifocal LCH

The disease presents in infancy with generalized symptoms including fever, irritability and anorexia. Lymphadenopathy and hepatosplenomegaly develop, together with a curious scaly papular dermatitis affecting the scalp and trunk, which may be haemorrhagic (Figs. 11.21 and 11.22). At autopsy, liver, spleen and lymph nodes are enlarged and firm, and their cut surfaces appear irregularly speckled with greyish dots. Histologically the structure of the organs is disturbed by a proliferation of well defined histiocytes with ample cytoplasm and typical reniform nuclei and neucleoli. Cellular atypia is uncommon, but cells with two or three nuclei are not. These cells are associated with lymphocytes, other mononuclears and some eosinophils in the cellular infiltrate (Fig. 11.23). A similar cellular infiltration may affect the lung in a very diffuse distribution.

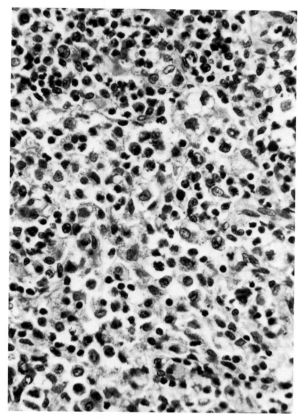

Fig. 11.23. Pleomorphic infiltrate including histiocytes, lymphocytes, occasional polymorphs and eosinophils. Lymph node. (H&E, × 180)

Multifocal Unisystem LCH

This form of the disease is typically characterized by multiple lytic lesions in bone and the syndrome of dwarfism, diabetes insipidus and exophthalmos, a collection of symptoms and signs that is uncommonly seen. Systemic involvement is not uncommon, and mixed cases (multisytem) are seen. They may present with hepatosplenomegaly, lymphadenopathy or honeycomb lung; pancytopenia develops when marrow involvement is severe.

Microscopically, the typical lesion is composed of a granulomatous cellular mass with many histiocytes and eosinophils. Multinucleate forms are common, and lipid accumulates in these cells and in histiocytes. This cellular infiltrate may be found microscopically in many organs, including the skin. Involvement of the ear is common, and in our experience a common presentation is of a non-resolving middle ear infection and an exoriated external audi-tory meatus, associated with temporal bone destruction apparent on radiography (see also p. 558).

Unifocal LCH

These lesions, previously called eosinophil granulomas, typically occur as solitary lesions in bones, usually flat bones, although we have seen examples in the thyroid and lung. The skull, ribs or vertebrae are commonly involved, and lesions are occasionally multiple. Radiological appearances suggest a circumscribed lesion, although a distinct margin may not always be evident. Pathologically the lesions are pinkish-grey or grey, variable in texture, and occasionally gritty due to reactive new bone formation or healing of a fracture. Masses of histiocytes with variable numbers of eosinophils are seen microscopically; giant cells are common. Foam cells and cells containing haemosiderin pigment may also be present (see also p. 558).

Gastrointestinal Involvement

Gastrointestinal tract involvement in Langerhans' cell histiocytosis is not rare and may be manifest as protracted diarrhoea, perforation, malabsorption and protein-losing enteropathy. It is important to entertain this diagnosis in examining gut biopsies; the use of immunocytochemical and other techniques enables a distinction to be made between this and other causes of histiocytic infiltration of the gut (see p. 243).

Malignant Lymphomas

Malignant lymphomas are divided into two groups: Hodgkin's disease (HD) and the non-Hodgkin's lymphomas (NHL). Both groups are relatively rare in children. In a large retrospective Dutch study Coebergh et al. (1991) described an incidence of 0.75 per 100 000 children per year with a male : female ratio of 2 : 5. In about 25% of cases the disease was localized at diagnosis, and in 1% of children an immunodeficiency state preceded the diagnosis. The incidence of HD was 0.3 per 100 000 children per year, with a male : female ratio of 2 : 7. The age-specific incidence rates and the clinical features of NHL and HD correspond to those in other European countries and for white children in the USA. Although there are no types of non-Hodgkin's lym-

Table 11.2. Classification of non-Hodgkin lymphomas

Working formulation	Kiel classification
Low grade	
A. ML small lymphocytic	ML lymphocytic CLL
– CLL type	ML lymphoplasmacytic/lymphoplasmacytoid
– plasmacytoid	
B. ML follicular, predominantly small cleaved cell	ML cb/cc (small) follicular and/or diffuse
C. ML follicular, mixed small cleaved and large cell	ML cb/cc (small) follicular and/or diffuse
Intermediate grade	
D. ML follicular, predominantly large cell	ML cb/cc (large) follicular and/or diffuse
E. ML diffuse, small cleaved cell	ML cc (small)
F. ML diffuse, mixed small and large cell	ML cb/cc (small) diffuse
	ML lymphoplasmocytic/cytoid polymorphic
G. ML diffuse, large cell	ML cb/cc (large), cc (large), cb
High grade	
H. ML large cell immunoblastic	ML immunoblastic
	T-zone lymphoma
	Lymphoepitheloid cell lymphoma
I. ML lymphoblastic	ML lymphoblastic, convoluted type
– Convoluted cell	ML lymphoblastic, unclassified
– Non-convoluted cell	
J. ML small non-cleaved cell	ML lymphoblastic Burkitt (-type) and other B-lymphoblastic
Miscellaneous	

cb, centroblastic; cc, centrocytic; ML, malignant lymphoma.

phoma that occur exclusively in children, there are tumours that show a predominantly paediatric pattern. They will be discussed in more detail in this chapter, as will some features of HD.

Classification

The classification of the NHL is still in a state of flux. Details of the classifications that have been suggested over the past two decades may be found in Rappaport (1966), Lukes and Collins (1974, 1992), Lennert et al. (1975), Nathwani (1979) and Wright and Isaacson (1983). The Working Formulation dating from the early 1980s (National Cancer Institute 1982) is currently widely used in most studies. This classification and the Kiel classification are shown in Table 11.2. The most recent is the REAL classification (Harris et al. 1994).

Many of these types of lymphoma are either not seen in childhood or are extremely rare. More than 98% of childhood lymphomas are of high-grade malignancy (Hvizdala et al. 1991; Ishida et al. 1991), although Lennert (1978) and Bucsky et al. (1990) have described low-grade tumours of both B- and T-cell phenotype that occur very occasionally in childhood.

Modern ideas about the classification of lymphomas centre on the concept of "follicle centre cells" (FCCs). Camera lucida studies were used by Lukes and Collins (1975) to differentiate the types of cell present in lymphomas on the basis of their simi-

larity to the cells present in normal germinal centres. These FCCs are divided into cleaved and non-cleaved types. The former are small to medium-sized, having a notch or indentation in the nucleus, and are referred to as centrocytes by Lennert (1978). The non-cleaved cells are large in size and have round or oval nuclei with several prominent nucleoli, which are usually close to the nuclear membrane. They are called centroblasts by Lennert. Smaller non-cleaved cells with uniform round nuclei and coarse chromatin are involved in Burkitt's type NHL. Non-Hodgkin's lymphomas in childhood are rarely of FCC origin (Frizerra and Murphy 1979; Winberg et al. 1981), and diffuse tumours of lymphocytic type are unusual (Kjeldsberg et al. 1983). Lymphomas in children are virtually limited to three types: Burkitt(-type) lymphomas, lymphoblastic lymphomas and the anaplastic large cell lymphomas (ALCL). The first two groups comprise approximately 75% of malignant lymphomas in children, whereas the ALCLs account for approximately 20%. The rest consist of a diversity of mainly high-grade malignant B-cell lymphomas (centroblastic and immunoblastic). The three main groups distinguish themselves by their clinical presentation, by their specific histological and immunological features and by their cytogenetic profile (Murphy et al. 1989; Link et al. 1990; Table 11.3). A battery of investigative methods is available for the differentiation of these processes, including immuno-

Table 11.3. Correlation between morphology, immunophenotype, cytogenetics and primary presentation in paediatric non-Hodgkin's lymphomas

Histology	Immunophenotype	Cytogenetics	Primary presentation
Small non-cleaved cell	B cell (sIg+)	t(8;14), t(2;8), t(8;22) breaks: 7q, 13q, 14q, 17q, 18q	Jaw, abdomen, digestive tract, Waldeyer's ring
Lymphoblastic	T cell (thymocyte phenotype)	t(11;14), t(8;14), t(10;14) t(1;19), t(2;8)	Mediastinum and upper lymphnodes
	B-cell precursors		Various lymphnodes
Anaplastic large-cell lymphoma	CD30 positive (T, B or null cell)	t(2;5)	Lymphnodes, skin, various places

For an overview of cytogenetic abnormalities in non-Hodgkin's lymphomas, see Mederos et al. (1992).

Table 11.4. Correlation between histology and primary localization of the main groups of paediatric non-Hodgkin's lymphoma

Localization	Total (%)	Histology		
		B-cell (%)	non-B-cell (%)	ALCL
Intra-abdominal	31	1	23	7
Intrathoracal	27	20	1	6
Head and neck	29	7	14	8
Peripheral nodes	6	2	1	3
Others	7	1	2	4
Total	100	31	41	28

After Murphy et al. (1989).

logical, cytochemical, histochemical, immunohisto-chemical and ultrastructural studies.

In the paediatric literature, NHLs are also distinguished as B-cell and non-B-cell NHLs, the latter being mainly T-cell lymphoblastic lymphomas, although also some early precursor B-cell lymphomas are categorized in this group. The ALCLs form a separate entity, even when they are characterized by T-cell markers. The relationships between histology and the primary localization of these tumours is shown in Table 11.4.

Investigation of Lymph Nodes

For optimal diagnosis of malignant lymphomas, biopsies should be received fresh so that imprints and frozen section preparations may be made for cytochemistry, histochemistry and immunohistochemistry. However, most of the currently available monoclonal antibodies against the CD antigens can be applied to paraffin-embedded material, with their better morphology, reducing the need for frozen tissue. Although numerous monoclonal antibodies are available for the differentiation of haematological cell types, only a limited number are required for an adequate diagnosis of paediatric lymphomas. They are summarized as follows.

B-cell NHL

The Burkitt(-like) lymphomas are characterized immunologically by the presence of monotypic surface immunoglobulin with expression of one light chain (there is sometimes cytoplasmic expression and very occasionally complete absence). Positive staining with B-cell-specific monoclonal antibodies such as CD19, CD20 and CD22 also indicates a B-cell origin.

Non-B-cell NHL

A lymphoblastic lymphoma is immunologically defined as an (immature) T-cell process by the presence of TdT or in some cases by CD1, ideally found in combination with two T-cell markers, among which CD3, should be recognized.

The precursor B-cell NHL is characterized by CD19, CD20 and CD22 positivity.

ALCL

This diagnosis is based on histological features. Most ALCLs are positive for the Ki-1 (CD30) antigen. T-cell markers are positive in 60%–70%; the remaining

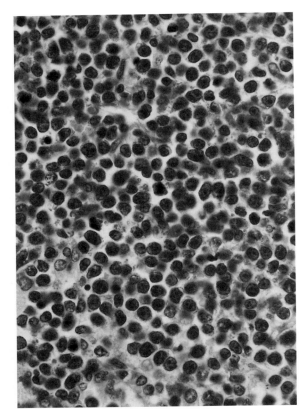

Fig. 11.24. Small non-cleaved cell lymphoma, Burkitt type. The nucleoli are oval to round with small nucleoli.

tumours are positive for B-cell markers or are negative for both T-cell and B-cell markers (null-cell NHL).

B-cell Non-Hodgkin's Lymphomas

Small Non-cleaved Cell Lymphoma

Burkitt's Lymphoma and Burkitt-type Lymphoma. The occurrence of NHL characterized by tumours of the jaw or orbit or by enlargement of abdominal lymph nodes was first described in African children by Burkitt (1958, 1959). Morphological studies of this lymphoma were performed by O'Connor (1961) and Wright (1963). Similar tumours were soon found in many parts of the world – for example, an American variant described by Dorfman (1965). A virus of the herpes group (Epstein–Barr virus, EBV) was identified in cell cultures of Burkitt's lymphoma cells (Epstein et al. 1964). The EBV can be demonstrated in practically all cases of Burkitt's lymphoma in

Africa (Klein 1975; Magrath 1991), whereas only a small percentage of morphologically similar cases from other parts of the world contain EBV. It thus seems likely that although the (immuno) histological and (immuno) cytological appearances of these types of lymphoma are similar, the aetiology may be different in different parts of the world. It is for this reason that the non-African tumour is classified as Burkitt-type lymphoma (or Burkitt-like or non-endemic Burkitt's lymphoma), rather than Burkitt's lymphoma, the latter title being strictly applicable only to EBV-associated (endemic) cases.

Boys are affected two or three times more frequently than girls (Burkitt 1970a; Levine et al. 1975; Lennert 1978). The age distribution shows a peak at 4–7 years in Africa according to Burkitt (1970a), and involvement over the age of 14 years is rare. The data for American and European series show a similar predominance of cases in the first decade, but Burkitt-type lymphoma also occurs in adult life in these parts of the world (Banks et al. 1975; Levine et al. 1975; Lennert 1978).

Tumours of the jaw are present in over half the African cases, but abdominal masses, and kidney, liver and ovarian involvement are also frequent (Burkitt 1970b; Wright 1970). Lymph node involvement was found at autopsy in 69% of affected children in Wright's study, but is rare at the onset of the disease. Coexistent lymphoblastic leukaemia in African Burkitt's lymphoma is rare. Burkitt-type lymphoma occurring in continental Europe involves mainly cervical, rather then abdominal, lymph nodes according to Lennert (1978), whereas abdominal involvement was a prominent feature in the series described by Banks et al. (1975) in the USA. American children with Burkitt-type lymphoma had a higher incidence of lymph node, pulmonary, gastrointestinal and bone marrow involvement, and less tumour replacement in the jaws and gonads than African cases (Magrath and Ziegler 1979).

Cytogenetic analysis shows that a t(8;14) is highly associated with all small non-cleaved cell lymphomas. In a minority of cases also a t(2;8) or a t(8;22) is found. The t(8;14) involves translocation of the *c-myc* oncogene from chromosome 8 to the Ig heavy chain gene locus on chromosome 14.

Burkitt's lymphoma and Burkitt-type lymphoma are small non-cleaved cell NHLs with uniform nuclei showing a coarse chromatin pattern and several prominent nucleoli (Fig. 11.24). Mitoses are frequent. Almost invariably there are macrophages scattered throughout the tumour, with abundant clear cytoplasm, containing cellular debris or intact tumour cells. These give rise to the typical "starry-sky" appearance on low-power microscopy (Fig. 11.25). The appearance of Burkitt(-type) lymphomas in

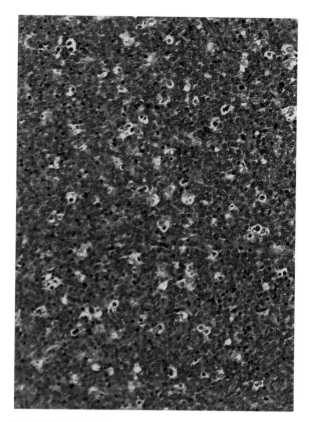

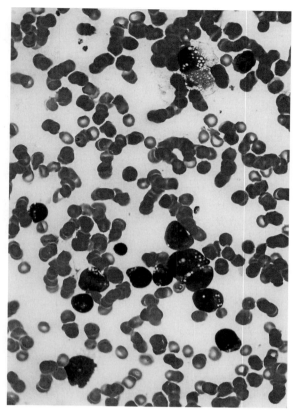

Fig. 11.25. Burkitt's lymphoma (low-power magnification). The starry-sky appearance is evident.

Fig. 11.26. Imprint of small non-cleaved cells with small fat vacuoles in the cytoplasm of the tumour cells.

imprint preparations (Fig. 11.26) and the histochemical and electron microscopic studies are well described by Bernard et al. (1981) and by Lennert (1978). They show L3 blasts in the FAB classification. The tumour cells contain sudanophilic granules, and there are large amounts of neutral fat in the starry sky macrophages. Alkaline phosphatase and non-specific esterase are absent from the tumour cells but present in the macrophages. Immunological studies have shown that the tumour cells have B-cell characteristics (Coccia et al. 1976; Mann et al. 1976; Crist et al. 1981). Common acute lymphoblastic leukaemia antigen (CALLA) is also frequently present (Kjeldsberg et al. 1983). Terminal deoxynucleotidyl transferase (TdT) is negative.

Although bone marrow involvement is usually considered to occur late, Brunning et al. (1977) have described 11 cases with bone marrow replacement at the onset of the disease. All had a rapid clinical course despite chemotherapy. None was frankly leukaemic.

Although differential diagnosis with a number of undifferentiated malignant neoplasms may cause problems, the chief difficulties arise with respect to acute lymphocytic leukaemia (ALL), acute myeloid leukaemia (AML) and lymphoblastic NHLs. For the different features of these neoplasms the reader should consult paediatric haematology textbooks (e.g. Knowles 1992; Nathan and Oski 1993).

Non-Burkitt-type Lymphoma. Although this lymphoma is also considered to be a small non-cleaved cell lymphoma and shows L3 blasts in imprints, there are some morphological features that distinguish it from Burkitt's lymphoma. The nuclei show some variation in shape and size and there may be fewer nucleoli. The starry-sky pattern may be absent.

Clinically, immunologically and cytochemically the two are essentially identical. Treatment for both is the same. Although this tumour usually demonstrates B-cell markers, a non-B-cell non-T-cell variant may be present.

Dayton et al. (1994) compared the features of L3 ALL with those of small non-cleaved cell lymphoma and came to the conclusion that they represent different manifestations of the same disease process.

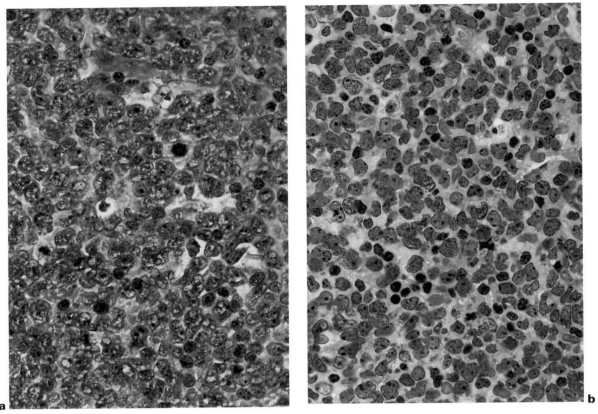

Fig. 11.27. Lymphoblastic lymphoma, morphologically L3-type. **a** Paraffin-embedded section of a lymph node of a 4-year-old girl. **b** Methacrylate-embedded tissue of the same lymph node.

Lymphoblastic (ALL-like) Lymphoma

B-cell lymphoblastic lymphomas form a minority group of paediatric lymphoblastic lymphomas: 4% according to Cossman et al. (1982). Morphologically they are indistinguishable from ALL (Fig. 11.27). They are derived from early B-cell precursors, expressing the antigen profile of early-pre-B or pre-B cells. There is no expression of sIg (Meyers and Hakami 1984; Grumayer et al. 1988). Imprint preparations show L1 or L2 blasts. Wright and Isaacson (1983) suggest the separation of Burkitt's lymphoma from malignant lymphoblastic lymphoma on the basis of cytological and growth pattern differences. TdT is positive in lymphoblastic lymphomas and negative in the Burkitt(-type). PAS stain is occasionally positive in lymphoblastic lymphoma and negative in Burkitt's. For the methyl green pyronine stain, the opposite is true.

Clinically, B-lymphoblastic lymphomas tend to occur in peripheral lymph nodes or as a cutaneous tumour, often in the scalp, in young children.

Large B-cell Lymphomas

Centroblastic lymphoma. This is an usually diffusely growing malignant lymphoma consisting of a proliferation of mainly large non-cleaved FCCs (centroblasts). Centroblastic lymphomas can occur as primary tumours or as secondary lesions after previous evidence of a malignant lymphoma of a lower grade. Childhood centroblastic lymphomas are in general of the primary type; (nodular) low-grade NHLs are extremely rare in this age group. When the diagnosis of a nodular lymphoma in a child is contemplated, the possibility that the lymph node is showing reactive hyperplasia should always be considered seriously. Centroblastic lymphomas are often mixed with varying numbers of immunoblasts. For these cases, the term "polymorphic centroblastic lymphoma" is proposed by Lennert and Feller (1992).

Immunoblastic Lymphoma. B-immunoblastic lymphomas occasionally occur in childhood and adolescence. Males are affected up to three times more

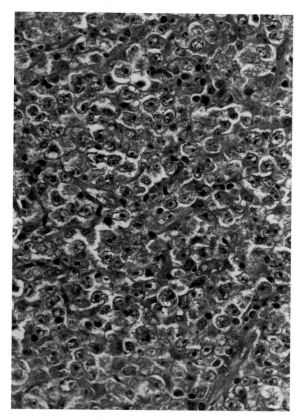

Fig. 11.28. Immunoblastic sarcoma. Note the large, often centrally located, nucleoli in the tumour cells.

often than females. The histological appearance of the tumour comprises diffuse sheets of large cells having oval or round nuclei and one or more prominent, often centrally located, nucleoli (Fig. 11.28). It is sometimes difficult to differentiate this group from polymorphic centroblastic lymphomas. Imprint preparations may be helpful in making the diagnosis.

T-cell Non-Hodgkin's Lymphomas

Lymphoblastic Lymphoma

An ill-defined group of mediastinal tumours with associated leukaemia in children was frequently described in the past as Sternberg sarcoma, following an original description by Sternberg (1908). As an entity it has been recognized by Lukes and Lennert and their colleagues (Barcos and Lukes 1975; Lennert et al. 1975).

T-cell lymphoblastic lymphoma is the commonest

NHL in childhood. Convoluted nuclei are a helpful feature but not present in all cases (Nathwani et al. 1981). The presence of convoluted nuclei is not associated with a particular clinical appearance, prognostic group or specific immunological cell type (Nathwani et al. 1976; Pangalis et al. 1979).

The presence of a large mediastinal mass (in over 80% of patients) is the main clinical feature of this type of lymphoma (Lennert 1978). Males are affected about twice as often as females and the peak incidence is between 10 and 15 years of age (Barcos and Lukes 1975; Lennert 1978). In addition, there may be peripheral lymph node involvement and a leukaemic blood picture. Bone marrow infiltration usually occurs only late in the course of the disease.

The mediastinal mass and replaced lymph nodes comprise a diffuse infiltrate of small to medium-sized lymphoid cells having round or oval nuclei, small nucleoli and a thin rim of basophilic cytoplasm. Intermingled with these cells are other cells, which are large and have large nuclei and prominent nucleoli. The diagnostic convoluted cell of this tumour is present only in small numbers. It is larger than most of the other cells and has an irregularly shaped nucleus, which may have knob-like projections or appear gyrate in outline. Linear subdivisions across the nucleus give a "chickenfoot" appearance (Fig. 11.29), as described by Lukes and Collins (1975). Mitoses are frequent. Imprint preparations show a predominance of small cells, with marked variation of cell size and (usually) the presence of large cells with convoluted nuclei.

Histochemically, a strong focal acid phosphatase activity is present in the paranuclear region of the smaller tumour cells, and this can be demonstrated by electron microscopy to be localized in the Golgi apparatus (Catovsky et al. 1975). The large convoluted cells do not show the presence of acid phosphatase reaction product. The tumour cells are also positive for acid non-specific esterase and ß-glucuronidase, but are negative for other enzymes. Immunologically the vast majority of cases type as immature thymocytes that are TdT positive and nearly always express the early T-cell marker CD7. Most cases also express CD5, CD2 and/or CD3. Others are also positive for CD1, CD4 and/or CD8. The early combination of CD7, CD5 and CD2 is seen in less than one-third of the patients.

Immunological studies have shown that 78% of childhood lymphoblastic lymphomas are of T-cell type (18% are non-B non-T and 4% are pre-B cell in origin). The T cell of lymphoblastic lymphoma is at the "cortical thymocyte" stage of development according to marker studies (Bernard et al. 1981; Cossman et al. 1982). Of T-lymphoblastic lymphomas, 40% express CALLA (Ritz et al. 1981).

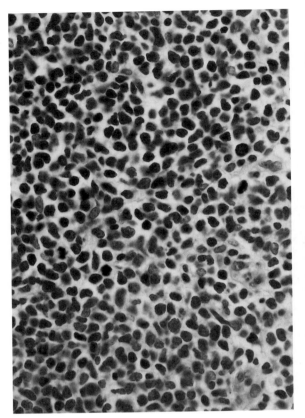

Fig. 11.29. Lymphoblastic lymphoma, convoluted type. The nucleoli show many irregularities in their shape.

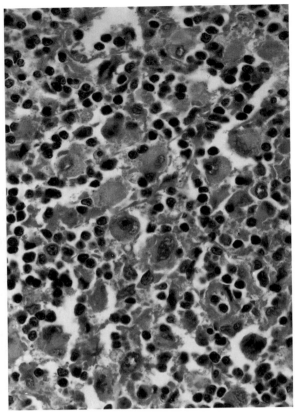

Fig. 11.30. Anaplastic large-cell lymphoma, Ki-1-positive. The tumour cells have abundant cytoplasm and large irregular nuclei with prominent nucleoli. Small lymphocytes are intermingled.

Anaplastic Large-cell Lymphoma

ALCLs can occur at all ages. The average age of the patients is 50 years, with two peaks, one between 10 and 30 years and one over 60 years (Chan et al. 1989; Chott et al. 1990). In the 0–18 year age group, 15–25% of the NHLs are ALCLs. The different aspects of this lymphoma are reviewed by Kinney et al. (1991).

The clinical features are characterized by a (generalized) lymphadenopathy, extranodal localizations (approximately 40%), especially of the skin (25%–30%) and systemic features (50%) such as fever and/or weight loss (Greer et al. 1991; Ebo and Van Hoof 1992). CNS localization is extremely rare in this disease. More than half of the patients already have advanced disease at the time of diagnosis. Vecchi et al. (1993) described 13 cases of ALCL, 85% with T-cell markers, the others with B-cell phenotypes. All patients but one showed more than one involved site, mostly an association of nodal and extranodal sites. One patient was in stage I, seven were in stage II and five in stage III. After 4 years, the survival rate was 100% and the disease-free survival rate 63%. The disease has a good response to salvage therapy and a long duration of second complete remission. This suggests that ALCL is histological a high-grade NHL, but clinically similar to HD. This would confirm the hypothesis that HD and ALCL represent a continuous spectrum of the same disease (Leoncini et al. 1990). The possible correlation is reinforced by the detection of EBV genomes in these tumours (Herbst et al. 1991; Stein et al. 1991; Ross et al. 1992).

Histologically, the tumour comprises large anaplastic cells with vesicular nuclei, prominent nucleoli and varying amounts of cytoplasm. ALCLs often induce capsular thickening and show preferential involvement of the paracortex and sinuses, and focal necrosis. Many mitoses may be found, and various amounts of small lymphocytes may be seen between the tumour cells (Fig. 11.30). Many cases previously diagnosed as true histiocytic lymphomas belong to this group (Ornvold et al. 1992). Chan et al. (1989) divided their cases in two groups. Group I tumours consisted of large polygonal cells with indented, round to oval pleomorphic nuclei and pale cytoplasm. Group II tumours are formed by large cells with basophilic cytoplasm and lobated nuclei, sometimes with perinuclear halos. Frequently multinucleated cells, including Sternberg–Reed-like cells, are present, suggesting a diagnosis of HD. Group II has a slightly better prognosis than group I.

CD30 positivity is, together with morphology, the key characteristic in this NHL. Chott et al. (1990) distinguished two types of CD30+ NHL, a pleomorphic and a monomorphic group, the latter having the poorer prognosis. T-cell markers or T-cell receptor rearrangements are usually positive, although occasional cases of CD30+ lymphomas with B-cell or mixed B-cell/T-cell phenotypes have been described (Kadin 1986; Stein 1988; Vecchi et al. 1993). Some cases of ALCL that express histiocyte-associated antigens have also been reported (Carbone et al. 1990). The CD30+ ALCL often demonstrate the t(2;5)(p23;35) chromosome abnormality (Bitter et al. 1990; Mason et al. 1990; Smith et al. 1993).

Some cases of CD30+ non-ALCL have been described (Bitter et al. 1990); they having poorer outcome than CD30+ LCAL. The differential diagnosis of these tumours versus non-lymphoid malignancies can be complicated because of the not uncommon expression of cytokeratins and vimentin in ALCL (Gustmann et al. 1991).

Hodgkin's Disease

HD occurs in children, although it is not very common. The age range varies from $2\frac{1}{2}$ or 3 years to 16 years in various published series (Pitcock et al. 1959; Norris et al. 1975; McClain et al. 1990; Kung 1991; James et al. 1992). Males are affected twice as frequently as females in most series. However, under the age of 10 years, there is a male predominance of 75%–85% (McMahon 1966; Poppema and Lennert 1980). A bimodal age curve has been shown for HD. In developing countries the first age peak occurs in childhood, whereas in developed countries this first peak is delayed until young adulthood. Armstrong et al. (1993), therefore studied the presence of EBV in a group of 55 paediatric Hodgkin's patients from three different geographical areas. In children under 10 years of age, the disease was particularly likely to be EBV-associated. The difference in EBV association in paediatric and young adult HD was statistically highly significant (P< 0.0001). This is consistent with the hypothesis that paediatric and young adult HD have

different aetiologies, and suggests that EBV is likely to be involved in the pathogenesis of paediatric HD.

Hodgkin's disease is classified according to the Rey classification (Lukes et al. 1966) into lymphocyte predominant, nodular sclerotic, mixed-cellularity and lymphocyte depletion subtypes. (For details on the histological subtypes, see standard pathology textbooks.) The incidence of these particular histological subtypes in childhood varies in different series. Lymphocyte depletion is very rare in this age group. Keller et al. (1968) found mixed-cellularity to be the most common type in the first decade, with nodular sclerosis and lymphocyte predominance occurring in about equal frequency. In the second decade nodular sclerosis is the most frequent type, followed by mixed cellularity and then lymphocyte predominance. In a study of 38 cases of HD in children under 4 years of age, Kung (1992) reports equal frequencies of mixed cellularity and nodular sclerosis. Patients were predominantly male and white, with early-stage disease that responded to therapy with complete remission in more than 90%.

Childhood HD most often presents with cervical or supraclavicular lymphadenopathy. Mediastinal involvement is sometimes found in addition (McClain et al. 1990). The majority of the patients present with stage I or II disease; approximately 40% have stage III or IV disease. McClain et al. (1990) report an overall survival rate of 89% and a disease-free survival rate of 71% after a median follow-up of 10.5 years in 63 children. The disease-free survival rates for patients with stage I–IV disease are 92%, 81%, 78% and 40%, respectively. In an identical study in 169 children, James et al. (1992) describe an overall actuarial survival for the whole group of 81% at 10 years. Of the 169 children, 35 either did not reach a complete remission or relapsed. The estimated actuarial survival from initial relapse or failure of primary treatment was 60% at 5 years and 45% at 10 years. Over half the patients requiring salvage therapy were known within 2 years and only three relapses had occurred more than 3 years after diagnosis. Neither initial histology nor stage affected survival from relapse, although the numbers were small in the study.

Familial Erythrophagocytic Lymphohistiocytosis

The unusual syndrome of familial erythrophagocytic lymphohistiocytosis has been described in over 20 families (Perry et al. 1976). The age of onset is from 2 weeks to 7 years, and the disease mostly affects infants. Neither sex predominates. The clinical onset is non-specific, with failure to thrive, pallor, anorexia and diarrhoea as common features. All affected children have had pyrexia and hepatosplenomegaly at or about the time of onset. Anaemia and progressively deepening jaundice occur, together with bleeding into the skin, gastrointestinal tract and brain. Patients have usually died with bleeding, sepsis or development of a lymphocytic meningitis. The pathological features are a diffuse histiocytic infiltration of the liver, spleen, lymph nodes, bone marrow, lungs, gastrointestinal tract, genitourinary tract and central nervous system. Erythrophagocytosis is often a marked feature, and there are usually lymphocytes intermingled with the histiocytic infiltrate. The disorder has some resemblance to histiocytic medullary reticulosis, but this affects mainly adults and is not familial (apart from one report of an affected father and son by Boake et al. 1965). The histiocytes in familial erythrophagocytic lymphohistiocytosis do not show the marked cellular atypia seen in most cases of malignant histiocytosis (histiocytic medullary reticulosis). Investigations have shown the presence of a primary immunological deficiency in patients with familial erythrophagocytic lymphohistiocytosis (Barth et al. 1972; Ladisch et al. 1978).

Haemophagocytic Syndromes

Excessive phagocytosis of the cellular components of the blood by the cells of the reticuloendothelial system occurs in a wide range of conditions apart from well defined neoplastic conditions. Thus it may be associated with a number of viral infections (cytomegalovirus, varicella, herpes zoster, adenovirus EBV and HIV). It may also occur in gram-negative bacterial, fungal and parasitic infections (leishmaniasis). Ooe (1992) has suggested that activation of histiocytes occurs as a result of the coating of the surface by early products of the coagulation cascade, but as with other hypotheses, involving cyokines for example, supporting data are few and unconvincing.

References

Adinolfi M (1972) Ontogeny of components of complement (C'$_4$ and C'$_3$) in human fetal and new born sera. Dev Med Child Neurol 12: 306

Adinolfi M (1981) Development of lymphoid tissues and immunity. In: Davis JA, Dobbing J (eds) Scientific foundations of paediatrics, 2nd edn. Heinemann, London, p 525

Aldrich RA, Steinberg AG, Campbell DC (1954) Pedigree demonstrating a sex-linked recessive condition characterized by draining ears, eczematoid dermatitis and blood diarrhoea. Pediatrics 13: 133

Armstrong AA, Alexander FE, Paes RP, Morad NA, Gallagher A, Krajewski AS, Jones DB, Angus B, Adams J, Cartwright RA (1993) Association of Epstein–Barr virus with pediatric Hodgkin's disease. Am J Pathol 142: 1683

Aronzon DZ, Arnold WS, Arnold HE, Jerrald MB, Schneider TM (1977) Non-operative management of splenic trauma in children: a report of 6 consecutive cases. Pediatrics 60: 482

Avery ME, McAgee JG, Guild HG (1957) The course and prognosis of reticuloendotheliosis (eosinophilic granuloma, Schüller–Christian disease and Letterer–Siwe disease): a study of forty cases. Am J Med 22: 636

Babior B (1978) Oxygen-dependent microbial killing by phagocytes. N Engl J Med 298: 721

Banatavala JE, Potter JE, Best JM (1971) Interferon response to Sendai and Rubella viruses in human foetal cultures, leucocytes and placenta cultures. J Gen Virol 13: 193

Banks PM, Arsenau JC, Gralnick HR, Canellos GP, DeVita VT, Berard CW (1975) American Burkitt's lymphoma: a clinico-pathologic study of 30 cases. Am J Med 58: 322

Barcos MP, Lukes RJ (1975) Malignant lymphoma of convoluted lymphocytes: a new entity of possible T-cell type. In: Skinks LF, Godden JO (eds) Conflicts in childhood cancer. An evaluation of current management, vol. 4. Liss, New York, p 147

Barth RF, Vergara GG, Khurana SK, Lowman JT, Beckwith JB (1972) Rapidly fatal familial histiocytosis associated with eosinophilia and primary immunological deficiency. Lancet ii: 503

Basset F, Escaig J, Le Crom M (1972) A cytoplasmic membranous complex in histiocytosis X. Cancer 29: 1380

Basset F, Turiaf J (1965) Identification par la microscopie électronique de particules de nature probablement virale dans les liaisons granulomateuses d'une histiocytose "X" pulmonaire. CR Acad Sci (Paris) 261: 3701

Basset F, Nezelof C, Mallet R, Turiaf J (1965) Nouvelle mise en evidence, par la microscopie électronique, de particules d'allure virale dans une seconde forme clinique de l'histiocytose X, le granulome eosinophile de l'os. CR Acad Sci (Paris) 261: 5719

Becker AE, Andeson RH (1981) Pathophysiology of congenital heart disease, Butterworths, London

Berg NP, Rosengren B, Seeman T (1968) Treatment of tumours of the thymus. Scand J Thorac Cardiovasc Surg 2: 65

Bernard A, Boumsell L, Reinherz EL, Nadler LM, Ritz J, Coppin H, Richard Y, Valensi F, Dausset J, Flandrin G, Lemerle J, Schossman SF (1981) Cell surface characterisation of malignant T cells from lymphoblastic lymphoma using monoclonal antibodies: evidence of phenotypic differences between malignant T cells from patients with acute lymphoblastic leukaemia and lymphoblastic lymphoma. Blood 57: 1105

Berry CL (1968) The neonatal thymus and immune paresis. Proc R Soc Med 61(9): 867

Berry CL (1970) Histopathological findings in the combined immunity deficiency syndrome. J Clin Pathol 23: 193

Berry CL (1981) The formation and behaviour of tumours in childhood. In: Davis JA, Dobbing J (eds) Scientific foundations of paediatrics, 2nd edn. Heinemann, London, p 1014.

Berry CL (1992) What's in a homeobox? The development of pattern during embryonal growth. Virchows Archiv A Pathol Anat 420: 291

Berry CL, Thompson EN (1968) Clinico-pathological study of thymic dysplasia. Arch Dis Child 43: 579

Bieger RG, McAdams AJ (1966) Thymic cysts. Arch Pathol 82: 535

Bitter MA, Wilbur AF, Larson RA, McKeithan TW, Rubin CM, Le Beau MM, Stephens JK, Vardiman JW (1990) Non-Hodgkin's lymphoma is correlated with clinical features and the presence of an unique chromosomal abnormality, t(2;5) (p23;q35). Am J Surg Pathol 14: 305

Blackburn WR, Gordon DS (1967) The thymic remnant in thymic alymphoplasia. Arch Pathol 84: 363

Boake WC, Card WH, Kimney JF (1965) Histiocytic medullary reticulosis concurrence in father and son. Arch Intern Med 116: 245

Bokkerink JPM, de Vaan GAM (1980) Histiocytosis X. Eur J Pediatr 135: 129

Boyd E (1932) The weight of the thymus gland in health and in disease. Am J Dis Child 43: 1162

Brunning, RD, McKenna RW, Bloomfield CD, Coccia P, Gajl-Peczalska KJ (1977) Bone marrow involvement in Burkitt's lymphoma. Cancer 40: 1771

Bruton OC (1952) Agammaglobulinemia. Pediatrics 9: 722

Bucsky P, Feller AC, Reiter A, Beck J, Bertram U, Eschenbach C, Gerein V, Lakomek M, Stollman B, Tausch W (1990) Low grade malignant non-Hodgkin's lymphomas and peripheral pleomorphic T-cell lymphomas in childhood – a BFM group report. Klin Pediatr 202: 258

Burke BA, Johnson D, Gilbert EF, Drut RM, Ludwig J, Wicke MR (1987) Thyrocalcitonin-containing cells in the Di George anomaly. Human Pathol 18: 355

Burkitt DP (1958/59) A sarcoma involving the jaws in African children. Br J Surg 46: 218

Burkitt DP (1970a) General features and facial tumours. In: Burkitt DP, Wright DH (eds) Burkitt's lymphoma. Livingstone, Edinburgh, p 6

Burkitt DP (1970b) Lesions outside the jaws. In: Burkitt DP, Wright DH (eds) Burkitt's lymphoma. Livingstone, Edinburgh, p 16

Butler JJ (1983) Pathology of the spleen in benign and malignant conditions. Histopathology 7: 453

Buyukunal C, Danismend N, Yeker D (1987) Spleen saving procedures in paediatric splenic trauma. Br J Surg 74: 350

Carbone A, Gloghini A, De Re V, Tamaro P, Boiocchi M, Volpe R (1990) Histopathologic, immunophenotypic, and genotypic analysis of Ki-1 anaplastic large cell lymphomas that express histiocyte-associated antigens. Cancer 66: 2547

Carr MC, Sites DP, Fudenberg HH (1973) Dissociation of responses to phytohaemagglutinin and adult allogenic lymphocytes in human foetal lymphoid tissues. Nature (New Biol) 241: 279

Carson MH, Chadwick CA, Brubaker RS, Cleland RS, Landing BH (1965) Thirteen boys with progressive septic granulomatosis. Pediatrics 35: 405

Catovsky D, Frisch B, van Noorden S (1975) B, T and "null" cell leukaemias. Electron cytochemistry and surface morphology. Blood Cells 1: 115

Chan JKC, Ng CS, Hui PK, Leung TW, Lo ESF, Lau WH, McGuire LJ (1989) Anaplastic large cell lymphoma. Delineation of two morphological subtypes. Histopathology 15: 11

Chilcote RR, Baehner RL, Hammond D, the Investigators and Special Studies Committee of the Children's Cancer Study Group (1976) Septicemia and meningitis in children splenectomised for Hodgkin's disease. N Engl J Med 295: 798

Chisako O, Capecchi MR (1991) Regionally restricted developmental defects resulting from targeted disruption of the mouse homeobox gene HOX-1.5. Nature 350: 473

Chott A, Kaserer K, Augustine I, Vesely M, Heintz R, Oehlinger W, Hanak H, Radaszkiewicz T (1990) Ki-1 positive large cell lymphoma. A clinicopathological study of 41 cases. Am J Surg Pathol 14: 439

Coccia PF, Kersey JH, Gajl-Peczalska KH, Krivit W, Nesbit ME (1976) Prognostic significance of surface marker analysis in childhood non-Hodgkin's lymphoproliferative malignancies. Am J Hematol 1: 405

Coeberg JW, Van der Does-Van den Berg A, Kamps WA, Rammeloo JA, Valkenburg HA, Van Wering ER (1991) Malignant lymphomas in children in The Netherlands in the period 1973–1985: incidence in relation to leukemia: a report from the Dutch Childhood Leukemia Study Group. Med Pediatr Oncol 19: 169

Cohen IR, Norins LC (1968) Antibodies of IgG, IgM and IgA classes in newborn and adult sera reactive with gram bacteria. J Clin Invest 47: 1053

Cooper MD, Chase HP, Lowman JT, Krivit W, Good RA (1968) Immunologic defects in patients with Wiskott–Aldrich syndrome. Birth Defects 4: 378

Cooper MD, Lawton AR, Preud'homme JL, Seligman M (1978) Primary antibody deficiencies. Springer, New York (Seminars in immunopathology, vol 1), p 265

Cossman J, Jaffe ES, Fisher RI (1982) Diversity of immunologic phenotypes of T-cell lymphoma. Am J Surg Pathol 6: 72 (abstract)

Cowan MJ, Hellman D, Chudwin D et al. (1984) Maternal transmission of acquired immune deficiency syndrome. Pediatrics 73: 382

Cox R, Hosking GP, Wilson J (1978) Ataxia telangiectasia. Arch Dis Child 53: 386

Crist WM, Kelly DR, Ragab AH, Roper MA, Dearth JC, Castleberry RP, Flint A (1981) Predictive ability of Lukes–Collins classification for immunologic phenotypes of childhood non-Hodgkin's lymphoma: an institutional series and review of the literature. Cancer 48: 2070

Dayton VD, Arthur DC, Gajl-Peczalksa KJ, Brunning R (1994) L3 acute lymphoblastic leukemia. Comparison with small non-cleaved cell lymphoma involving the bone marrow. Am J Clin Pathol 101: 130

De Chatelet LR, Shirley PS, McPhail LC (1976) Normal leukocyte glutathione peroxidase activity in patients with chronic granulomatous disease. J Pediatr 89: 598

de Vaal OM, Seynhaeve V (1959) Reticular dysgenesis. Lancet ii: 1123

DiGeorge AM (1968) Congenital absence of the thymus and its immunologic consequences: concurrence with congenital hypoparathyroidism. Birth Defects 4: 116

Dische MR (1968) Lymphoid tissue and associated malformations in thymic agenesis. Arch Pathol 86: 312

Dorfman RF (1965) Childhood lymphosarcoma in St Louis, Missouri, clinically and histologically resembling Burkitt's tumour. Cancer 18: 418

Dyer NH (1967) Cystic thymomas and thymic cysts. Thorax 22: 408

Ebo D, Van Hoof A (1992) Large cell anaplastic lymphoma (Ki-1 lymphoma). Acta Clin Belg 47: 170

Epstein MA, Achong BG, Barr YM (1964) Virus particles in cultured lymphoblasts from Burkitt's lymphoma. Lancet i: 702

Eraklis AJ, Filler RM (1972) Splenectomy in childhood. J Pediatr Surg 7: 382

Favara BE, McCarthy RC, Mierau GW (1983) Histiocytosis X. Hum Pathol 14: 663

Fleisher TA, Luckasen JR, Salad A, Gebrts RC, Kersey JH (1975) T and B lymphocytic sub-populations in children. Pediatrics 55: 162

Frenbel JK, Friedlander S (1952) Toxoplasmosis. Pathology of neonatal disease. Pathogenesis, diagnosis and treatment. Public Health Service Publication No. 141. US Government Printing Office, Washington

Friedman NB (1967) Tumours of the thymus. J Thorac Cardiovasc Surg 53: 163

Frizerra G, Murphy SB (1979) Follicular (nodular) lymphoma in childhood, a rare clinical–pathological entity: report of eight cases from four cancer centres. Cancer 44: 2218

Gilmour JR (1941) Normal haemopoiesis in intra-uterine life. J Pathol Bacteriol 52: 25

Gitlin D, Vawter G, Craig JM (1964) Thymic alymphoplasia and congenital aleukocytosis. Pediatrics 33: 184

Glanzmann E, Riniker P (1950) Essentielle Lymphocytophthise. Ein neues Krankheitsbild aus der Säuglingspathologie. Pediatr Res 175: 1

Goldstein G, Mackay IR (1967) The thymus in systemic lupus erythematosus. A quantitative histopathological analysis and comparison with stress involution. Br Med J ii: 475

Goldstein G, Abbot A, Mackay IR (1968) An electron microscopic study of the human thymus: normal appearances and findings in myasthenia gravis and systemic lupus erythematosus. J Pathol Bacteriol 95: 211

Gosseye S, Diebold N, Griscelli C, Nezelof C (1983) Severe combined immunodeficiency disease: a pathological analysis of 26 cases. Clin Immuno Immunopath 29: 58

Greer JP, Kinney ML, Collins RD, Salhany KJ, Wolff SN, Hainsworth JD, Flexner JM, Stein RS (1991) Clinical features of 31 patients with Ki-1 anaplastic large cell lymphoma. J Clin Oncol 9: 533, 539

Grumayer ER, Ladenstein RL et al. (1988) B-cell differentiation pattern of cutaneous lymphomas in infancy and childhood. Cancer 61: 303

Gurevich P, Czernobilsky B, Ben-Hur H, Nyska A, Zuckerman A, Zusman I (1994) Pathology of lymphoid organs in low-birth-weight human fetuses subjected to antigen-induced influences: a morphological and morphometric study. Pediatrics 14: 679

Gustmann C, Altmannsberger M, Osborn M, Griesser H, Feller AC (1991) Cytokeratin expression and vimentin content in large cell anaplastic lymphomas and other non-Hodgkin's lymphomas. Am J Pathol 138: 1413

Hammar JA (1911) Zür grösseren Morphologie und Morphogenie der Mesenchenthymus. Anatomische Hefte 43: 201

Hammar JA (1921) The new views as to the morphology of the thymus gland and their bearing on the problem of the function of the thymus. Endocrinology 5: 543

Hammar JA (1926) Die Menschenthymus in Gesundheit und Krankheit. I. Das normale Organ. Z Mikrosk Anat Forsch 6: 107

Harris NL et al. (1994) A revised European American classification of lymphoid neoplasms: a proposal from the international lymphoma study group. Blood 84: 1361

Henry K (1968) The thymus in rheumatic heart disease. Clin Exp Immunol 3: 509

Herbst H, Dallenbach F, Hummel M, Niedobitek G, Finn T, Young LS, Rowe M, Muller-Lantzsch N, Stein H (1991) Epstein–Barr virus DNA and latent gene products in Ki-1 (CD30)-positive anaplastic large cell lymphomas. Blood 78: 2666

Heymer B, Niethammer D, Spanel R, Galle J, Kleihauer E, Haferkamp O (1977) Pathomorphology of humoral, cellular and combined primary immunodeficiencies. Virchows Arch A Pathol Anat 374: 87

Hirschhorn R, Martin DW (1978) Enzyme defects in immunodeficiency diseases. Springer, New York (Seminars in immunopathology, vol 1), p 299

Hobbs JR, Milner RDG, Watt PJ (1967) Gamma-M-deficiency predisposing to meningococcal septicaemia. Br Med J iv: 583

Holland NH, Holland P (1966) Immunological maturation in an infant of an agamma-globulinaemic mother. Lancet ii: 1152

Honigman R, Lanzkowsky P (1979) Isolated congenital asplenia: an occult case of overwhelming sepsis. Am J Dis Child 133: 552

Huber J, Cholnoky P, Zoethout HE (1967) Congenital aplasia of the parathyroid glands and thymus. Arch Dis Child 42: 190

Hvizdala EV, Berard C, Callihan T, Falletta J, Sabio H, Shuster JJ, Sullivan M, Wharam MD (1991) Non-lymphoblastic lymphoma in children: histology and stage-related response to therapy: a Pediatric Oncology Group study. J Clin Oncol 9: 1189

Indeglia RA, Shea MA, Grage TB (1967) Congenital cysts of the thymus gland. Arch Surg 94: 149

Ishida Y, Mukai S, Takayama J, Shimoyama M, Konda C, Watanabe S, Ohira M (1991) Non-Hodgkin's lymphoma in patients under twenty years of age. A clinicopathological study. Int J Hematol 54: 241

James ND, Kingston JE, Plowman PM, Meller S, Pinkerton R, Barrett A, Sandland R, McElwain TJ, Malpas JS (1992) Outcome of children with resistant and relapsed Hodgkin's disease. Br J Cancer 66: 1155

Kadin ME, Sako D, Berliner N, Franklin W, Woda B et al. (1986) Childhood Ki-1 lymphoma presenting with skin lesions and peripheral lymphadenopathy. Blood 68: 1042

Kadowaki JI, Zuelzer WW, Brough AJ, Thompson RI, Woolley PV, Gruber D (1965) XX/XY lymphoid chimaerism in congenital immunological deficiency syndrome with thymic alymphoplasia. Lancet ii: 1152

Kahn WN, Ali RV, Werthmann M, Ross S (1969) Immunoglobulin M determinations in neonates and infants as an adjunct to the diagnosis of infection. J Pediatr 75: 1282

Katz AM, Rosenthal D, Jakubovic HR, Pai RK, Qinonez GE, Sauder DN (1991) Langerhans' cell histiocytosis in monozygotic twins. J Am Acad Dermatol 24: 32

Keller AR, Kaplan HS, Lukes RJ, Rappaport H (1968) Correlation of histopathology with other prognostic indicators in Hodgkin's disease. Cancer 22: 487

Kevy SV, Tefft M, Vawter GF (1968) Hereditary splenic hyperplasia. Pediatrics 42: 752

Kingsbury BF (1915) The development of the human pharynx. I. The pharyngeal derivatives. Am J Anat 18: 329

Kinney MC, Greer JP, Glick AD, Salhany KE, Collins RD (1991) Anaplastic large cell Ki-1 malignant lymphomas. Recognition, biological and clinical implications. Pathol Annu 26: 1

Kjeldsberg CR, Wilson JF, Berard CW (1983) Non-Hodgkin's lymphoma in children. Hum Pathol 14: 612

Klein G (1975) The Epstein–Barr virus and neoplasia. N Engl J Med 293: 1353

Knowles D (ed) (1992) Neoplastic hematopathology. Williams and Wilkins, Baltimore

Kritzler RA, Terner JY, Lindenbaum J, Magidson J, Williams R, Preisig R, Phillips GB (1964) Chediak–Higashi syndrome. Cytologic and serum lipid observations in a case and family. Am J Med 36: 583

Kung FH (1991) Hodgkin's disease in children 4 years of age or younger (see comments). J Cancer 67: 1428

Ladisch S, Poplack DG, Holiman B, Blaese RM (1978) Immunodeficiency in familial erythrophagocytic lymphohistiocytosis. Lancet i: 581

Landing BH, Shirkey HS (1957) A syndrome of recurrent infection and infiltration of viscera by pigmented lipid histiocytes. Pediatrics 20: 431

Lapointe N, Michaud JJ, Pekovic D, Chausseau JP, Dupuy JM (1985) Transplacental transmission of HTLV-III virus. New Engl J Med 312: 1325

Lawton AR, Cooper MD (1980) In: Steihm ER, Fulginiti VA (eds) Immunologic disorders in infants and children, 2nd edn. Saunders, Philadelphia, p 36

Lennert K (1978) Malignant lymphomas. Springer, Berlin

Lennert K, Mohri N, Stein H, Kaiserling E (1975) The histopathology of malignant lymphoma. Br J Haematol 31 [Suppl]: 193

Lennert K, Feller AC (1992) High grade malignant lymphomas of B-cell type: centroblastic lymphoma. In: Histopathology of non-Hodgkin's lymphoma. Springer Verlag, Berlin, p 115

Leoncini L, Del Vecchio MT, Kraft R, Megha T, Barbini P, Cevenini G, Poggi S, Pileri S, Tosi P, Cottier H (1990) Hodgkin's disease and CD30-positive anaplastic large cell lymphomas. A continuous spectrum of malignant disorders. A quantitative morphometric and immunohistologic study. Am J Pathol 137: 1047

Levine PH, Cho BR, Connelly RR, Berard CW, O'Conor GT, Dorfman RF, Easton JM, DeVita VT (1975) The American Burkitt Lymphoma Registry: a progress report. Ann Intern Med 83: 31

Link M, Donaldson SS, Berard CW, Shuster JJ, Murphy SB (1990) Results of treatment of childhood localized non-Hodgkin's lymphoma with combination chemotherapy with or without radiotherapy. N Engl J Med 322: 1169

Lischner HW, Huff DS (1975) T cell deficiency in DiGeorge syndrome. In: Bergsama D, Good RA, Finstad J, Paul NW (eds) Immuno-deficiency in man and animals. Sinaver, Sunderland, p 16

Lukes RJ, Collins RD (1974) Immunologic characterization of human malignancy lymphomas. Cancer 34: 1488

Lukes RJ, Collins RD (1975) New approaches to the classification of lymphomata. Br J Cancer 31 [Suppl II]: 1

Lukes RJ, Collins RD (1992) Tumors of the hematopoietic system. Atlas of tumor pathology, second series fascicle 28. Armed Forces Institute of Pathology, Washington DC

Lukes RJ, Craver LF, Hall TC, Rappaport H, Rubin T (1966) Report of the nomenclature committee. Symposium: obstacles to the control of Hodgkin's disease. Cancer Res 26: 1311

Lynch RG (1975) Thymus and immune deficiency. In: Kissane JM (ed) Pathology of infancy and childhood. Mosby, St Louis, p 913

Magrath IT (1991) African Burkitt's lymphoma. History, biology, clinical features and treatment. Am J Pediatr Oncology 13: 222

Magrath IT, Ziegler JL (1979) Bone marrow involvement in Burkitt's lymphoma and its relationship to acute B-cell leukaemia. Leukemia Res 4: 33

Mann RB, Jaffe ES, Braylan RC, Nanba K, Frank MM, Ziegler JL, Berard CW (1976) Non-endemic Burkitt's lymphoma: a B-cell tumor related to germinal centers. N Engl J Med 295: 685

Mason DY, Bastard C, Rimokh R, Dastugue N, Huret JL, Kristofferson U, Magaud JP, Nezelof C et al. (1990) CD30-positive large cell lymphomas (Ki-1 lymphoma) are associated with a chromosomal translocation involving 5q35. Br J Haematol 76: 156

Matsuda I, Oka Y, Taniguchi N (1976) Leukocyte glutathione peroxidase deficiency in a male patient with chronic granulomatous disease. J Pediatr 88: 581

McFarlin DE, Strober W, Waldman TA (1972) Ataxia telangiectasia. Medicine (Baltimore) 51: 281

McClain KL, Heise R, Day DL, Lee CK, Woods WG, Aeppli D (1990) Hodgkin's disease in children: correlation of clinical characteristics, staging procedures, and treatment at the University of Minnesota. Am J Pediatr Hematol Oncol 12: 147

McMahon B (1966) Epidemiology of Hodgkin's disease. Cancer Res 26: 1189

McNamara JJ, Murphy LJ, Griscom NT, Tefft M (1968) Splenic cysts in children. Surgery 64: 487

Meideros LJ, Bagg A, Cossman J (1992) Application of molecular genetics to the diagnosis of hematopoietic neoplasms. In: Knowles DM (ed) Neoplastic hematopathology. Williams and Wilkins, Baltimore, p 263

Metcalf D, Brumby M (1966) The role of the thymus in the ontogeny of the immune system. J Cell Physiol 67: 149

Meyers L, Hakami N (1984) Pre-B cell cutaneous lymphoma in infancy: a unique clinical entity. Med Pediatr Oncol 12: 252

Middleton G (1967) The incidence of follicular structures in the human thymus at autopsy. Aust J Exp Biol Med Sci 45: 189

Mierau GW, Favara BE, Brenman JM (1982) Electron microscopy in histiocytosis X. Ultrastruct Pathol 3: 137

Moerman P, Dumoulin M, Lauweryns J, Van Der Hauwaert LG (1987) Interrupted right aortic arch in DiGeorge syndrome. Br Heart J 58: 274

Murphy SB, Fairclough DL, Hutchison RE, Berard CW (1989) Non Hodgkin's lymphomas of childhood: an analysis of the histology, staging and response to treatment of 338 cases at a single institution. J Clin Oncol 7: 186

Nathan DG, Oski FA (1993) Hematology in infancy and childhood. Saunders, Philadelphia

Nathwani BN (1979) A critical analysis of the classification of non-Hodgkin's lymphoma. Cancer 44: 347

Nathwani BN, Kim H, Rappaport H (1976) Malignant lymphoma, lymphoblastic. Cancer 38: 964

Nathwani BN, Diamond LW, Winberg D, Kim H, Bearman RM, Glick JH, Jones SE, Gams RA, Nissen NI, Rappaport H (1981) Lymphoblastic lymphomas: a clinico-pathologic study of 95 patients. Cancer 48: 2347

National Cancer Institute (1982) NCI sponsored study of classifications of non-Hodgkin's lymphoma. Summary and description of a working formulation for clinical usage. The Non-Hodgkins Lymphoma Pathologic Classification Project. Cancer 49: 2112

Newton WA Jr, Homoudi AB (1973) Histiocytosis: a histologic classification with clinical correlation. In: Rosenberg HS, Bolande RP (eds) Perspectives in pediatric pathology, vol. 1. Year Book Medical Publishers, Chicago, p 251

Nezelof C, Jammet ML, Lortholary P, Labrune B, Lamy M (1964) L'Hypoplasie héréditaire du thymus. Sa place et sa responsabilité dans une observation d'aplasie lymphocytaire normoplasmocytaire et normoglobulinémique du nourisson. Arch Fr Pediatr 25: 897

Nezelof C, Frileux-Herbet F, Cronier-Sachot J (1979) Disseminated histiocytosis X: analysis of prognostic factors based on a retrospective study of 50 cases. Cancer 44: 1824

Nezelof C, Roth A, Blanche S, Barbey S (1986) Le SIDA chez l'enfant. Ann Pathol 6: 300

Norris DG, Burgert EO, Cooper HA, Harrison EG (1975) Hodgkin's disease in childhood. Cancer 36: 2109

Nowak R (1993) Bubble-boy paradox resolved. Science 262: 1818

O'Connor GT (1961) Malignant lymphoma in African children. II. A pathological entity. Cancer 14: 270

Okabe H (1966) Thymic lymph follicles. A histopathological study of 1,356 autopsy cases. Acta Pathol Jpn 16: 109

Ooe K (1992) Pathogenesis and clinical significance of hemophagocytic syndrome: hypothesis. Pediatr Pathol 12: 309

Ornvold K, Carstensen H, Junge J, Gyhrs A, Ralfkiaer E (1992) Tumours classified as "malignant histiocytosis" in children are T-cell neoplasms. APMIS 100: 558

Pabst MF, Kreth HW (1980) Ontogeny of the immune response as a basis of childhood disease. J Pediatr 97: 519

Pangalis GA, Nathwani BN, Rappaport H, Rosen RB (1979) Acute lymphoblastic leukaemia. The significance of nuclear convolutions. Cancer 43: 551

Parkman R, Rappaport J, Geha R, Belli J, Cussaday R, Levey R, Nathan DG, Rosen FS (1978) Complete correction of the Wiskott–Aldrich syndrome by allogeneic bone marrow transplantation. N Engl J Med 298: 921

Penman HG (1971) Fatal infectious mononucleosis: a critical review. J Clin Pathol 23: 765

Perchalski JE, Clem LW, Small PA (1968) 75 Gamma M immunoglobulins in human cord serum. Am J Med Sci 256: 107

Perkkio M, Savilahti E (1980) Time of appearance of immunoglobulin-containing cells in the mucosa of the neonatal intestine. Pediatr Res 14: 953

Perry MC, Harrison EG, Burgert EO, Gilchrist GS (1976) Familial erythrophagocytic lymphohistiocytosis. Cancer 38: 209

Pinkel D (1968) Ultrastructure of human fetal thymus. Am J Dis Child 115: 222

Pitcock JA, Bauer WC, McGaron MH (1959) Hodgkin's disease in children. Cancer 12: 1043

Poppema S, Lennert K (1980) Hodgkin's disease in childhood. Histopathologic classification in relation to age and sex. Cancer 45: 1443

Purtilo DT, De Florio D, Hutt ML, Bhawan J, Yang JPS, Otho R, Edwards W (1977) Variable phenotypic expression of an X-linked recessive lymphoproliferative syndrome. N Engl J Med 297: 1077

Qureshi MA, Hafner DC, Dorchak JR (1964) Non-parasitic cysts of the spleen. Arch Surg 89: 570

Rappaport H (1966) Discussion on: the pathology and nomenclature of Hodgkin's disease. Cancer Res 26: 1082

Rausch PG, Pryswansky KB, Spitznagel JK (1978) Immunocytochemical identification of azurophilic and specific granule markers in the giant granules of the Chediak–Higashi neutrophils. N Engl J Med 298: 693

Ritz J, Nadler LM, Bhan AK, Notis-McConarty J, Pesando JM, Schlossman SF (1981) Expression of common acute lymphoblastic leukaemia antigen (CALLA) by lymphomas of B cell and T cell lineage. Blood 58: 648

Roberts CWM, Shutter JR, Korsmyer SJ (1994) Hox 11 controls the genesis of the spleen. Nature 368: 747

Robertson NRC, Berry CL, Macaulay JC, Southhill JF (1971) Partial immunodeficiency and graft-versus-host disease. Arch Dis Child 46: 571

Rosen FS, Janeway CA (1966) The gamma globulins: III: The antibody deficiency syndromes. N Engl J Med 275: 769

Ross CW, Schlegelmilch JA, Grogan TM, Weiss LM, Schnitzer B, Hanson CA (1992) Detection of Epstein–Barr virus genome in Ki-1 (CD30)-positive, large-cell anaplastic lymphomas using the polymerase chain reaction. Am J Pathol 141: 457

Rubin M, Strauss B, Allen L (1964) Clinical disorders associated with thymic tumours. Arch Intern Med 114: 389

Schuurman H-J, Krone WJA, Broekjuizen R, van Baarlen J, van Veen P, Goldstein AL, Huber J, Goudsmit J (1989) The thymus in acquired immune deficiency syndrome. Am J Pathol 134: 1329

Scott GB, Buck BE, Leterman JG, Blood IL, Parks WP (1984) Acquired immunodeficiency syndrome in infants. N Engl J Med 310: 76

Sealy WC, Weaver WL, Young WG (1965) Severe airway obstruction in infancy due to the thymus gland. Ann Thorac Surg 1: 389

Shamoto M (1970) Langerhans cell granules in Letterer–Siwe disease: an election microscopic study. Cancer 26: 1102

Shapiro RS, Perry GS, Krivit W, Gerrard JM, White JG, Kersey JH (1978) Wiskott–Aldrich syndrome: detection of carrier state by metabolic stress of platelets. Lancet i: 121

Siegler R (1964) The morphology of thymuses and their relation to leukaemia. In: Good RA, Gabrielsen AE (eds) The thymus in immunobiology. Harper and Row, New York, p 623

Silverstein AM (1972) Immunological maturation in the fetus: modulation of the pathogenesis of congenital infectious disease. In: Ontogeny of acquired immunity. Associated Scientific publications, Amsterdam, p 17 (Ciba Foundation Symposium)

Sims DG (1977) Histiocytosis X. Follow up of 43 cases. Arch Dis Child 52: 433

Singer DB (1973) Post-splenectomy sepsis. In: Rosenberg HS, Bolande RP (eds) Perspectives in pediatric pathology. Year Book Medical Publishers, Chicago, p 285

Smith NM, Byard RW, Vasiliou M, Callen DF, Bourne AJ, Leong AS-Y (1993) Pediatric anaplastic large cell (CD30⁺) lymphomas associated with the t(2;5)(p23;q35) chromosomal abnormality. Int J Surg Pathol 1:43

Steele RW, Limas C, Thurman GB, Schulein M, Bauer H, Bellanti JA (1972) Familial thymic aplasia. Attempted reconstitution with fetal thymus in a millipore diffusion chamber. N Engl J Med 87: 787

Stein H (1988) The so-called Ki-1 lymphoma. Proceedings of the European Association for Haematopathology. First Meeting, Geneva, p 13

Steinmann GG (1986) Changes in the human thymus during ageing. In: Muller-Hermelink HK (ed) The human thymus.

Springer, New York, p 43 (Current topics in pathology series, no. 75)

Sternberg C (1908) Über Leukosarkomatose. (Cited by Lennert 1978). Wien Klin Wochenschr 21: 475

Strober W, Wochner AD, Carbone PP, Waldmann TA (1967) Intestinal lymphangiectasia: a protein losing enteropathy with hypogammaglobulinemia, lymphocytopenia and impaired homograft rejection. J Clin Invest 46: 1643

Strober W, Wochner AD, Barlow MH, McFarlin DE, Waldmann TA (1968) Immunoglobulin metabolism in ataxia telangiectasia. J Clin Invest 47: 1905

Symchych PS, Wanstrup J, Anderson V (1968) Chronic granulomatous disease of childhood. Acta Pathol Microbiol Scand 74: 179

Talerman A, Amigo A (1968) Thymoma with aplastic anaemia in a five year old child. Cancer 22: 445

Thomas JA, Janossy G, Chilosi M, Pritchard J, Pincott JR (1982) Combined immunological and histochemical analysis of skin and lymph node lesions in histiocytosis X. J Clin Pathol 35: 327

Travers P (1993) Immunological agnosisa. Nature 363: 117

Vecchi V, Burnelli R, Pileri S, Rosito P, Sabattini E, Civino A, Pericoli R, Paolucci G (1993) Anaplastic large cell lymphoma (Ki-1⁺/CD30⁺) in childhood. Med Pediatr Oncol 21: 402

Vetrie D, Vorechovsky I, Sideras P, Holland J, Davies A, Flinter F, Hammerstrom L, Kinnon C, Levinsky R, Bobrow M, Edvard Smith CI, Bentley DR (1993) The gene involved in X-linked agammaglobulinaemia is a member of the src family of protein–tyrosine kinases. Nature 361; 226–33

von Gaudecker B (1986) The development of the human thymus microenvironment. In: Muller–Hermelink HK (ed) The human thymus. Springer, New York, p 1 (Current topics in pathology series. no. 75)

Waldmann TA, Broder S (1978) T cell disorders in primary immunodeficiency diseases. Springer, New York (Seminars in immunopathology, vol 1), p 239

Waldmann TA, McIntire KR (1972) Serum alpha-fetoprotein levels in patients with ataxia telangiectasia. Lancet ii: 1112

Watson RR, Weisel W, O'Connor TM (1968) Thymic neoplasms. Arch Surg 97: 230

Weiss LM (1993) Histiocyte and dendritic cell proliferation. In: Knowles DM (ed) Neoplastic hematopathology. Williams and Wilkins, Baltimore, p 1474

Wiles MV, Keller G (1991) Multiple haemopoetic lineages develop from embryonic stem cells in culture. Development 111: 259

Willman CL, Busque L, Griffith BB, Favara BE, McClain KL, Duncan MH, Gilliland DG (1994) Langerhans' cell histiocytosis (histiocytosis X). A clonal proliferative disease. N Engl J Med 331: 154

Winberg CD, Nathwani BN, Bearman RM, Rappaport H (1981) Follicular (nodular) lymphoma during the first two decades of life: a clinicopathologic study of 12 patients. Cancer 48: 2223

Windhorst DB, Page AR, Holmes B (1968) The pattern of genetic transmission of the leukocyte defect in fatal granulomatous disease of childhood. J Clin Invest 47: 1026

Wright DH (1963) Cytology and histochemistry of the Burkitt lymphoma. Br J Cancer 17: 50

Wright DH (1970) Gross distribution and haematology: In: Burkitt DP, Wright DH (eds) Burkitt's lymphoma. Livingstone, Edinburgh, p 64

Wright DH, Isaacson P (1983) Biopsy pathology of the lymphoreticular system, Chapman and Hall, London

12 · Bone Marrow

J.G. van den Tweel and W.G.M. Spliet

Development of Haemopoiesis and Bone Marrow

Haemopoiesis starts 14–19 days after conception in the wall of the yolk sac (Bloom and Bartelnew 1940; Gilmour 1941). Primitive blood islands develop into blood vessels, where haemopoietic precursor cells can be found. This intravascular haemopoiesis is almost entirely composed of erthropoiesis in the first 5 weeks. It is magaloblastic, with formation of nucleated red blood cells with a diameter of 10–15 μm. Until the 12th gestational week the red cells mainly contain the embryonic types of haemoglobin Gower I ($\zeta2$, $\epsilon2$), Gower II ($\alpha2$, $\epsilon2$) and to a lesser extent Portland ($\zeta2$, $\gamma2$). There is also some HbF ($\alpha2$, $\gamma2$), which will become the main type of haemoglobin in fetal life. Extra embryonic haemopoiesis continues until the end of the third gestational month.

Haemopoietic stem cells are transported with the blood from extra embryonic to intra embryonic sites (Keleman et al. 1979; Keleman and Calvo 1982). Intra embryonic haemopoiesis starts in the fifth week in the liver. In the second trimester the liver is the main source of blood cells. By this time approximately 50% of the nucleated cells in the liver are erythroid (Fig. 12.1). The erythropoiesis is extravascular and macronormoblastic, with formation of non-nucleated red blood cells that contain mainly HbF, and which are slightly larger than erythrocytes in adults. There is also some granulopoiesis and megakaryopoiesis. Later in gestation, granulopoiesis increases mostly in the portal triads, whereas erythropoiesis is dispersed between the hepatocytes. After gestational weeks 8–12, haemopoietic tissue can also be found in the spleen, thymus and lymph nodes, but normally haemopoiesis at these sites is of short duration and not very extensive. Other organs in which some haemopoiesis can be found are the kidney, adrenal gland, heart, pancreas, gonads and lungs. Extramedullary haemopoiesis decreases at the end of gestation, but in the liver residual haemopoiesis is seen for some weeks after birth.

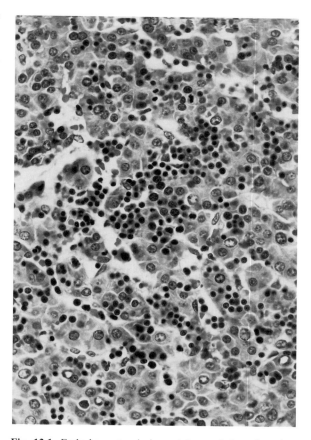

Fig. 12.1. Early haematopoiesis, mainly consisting of erythropoiesis, in a fetal liver of 13 weeks' gestation.

The definitive site of blood cell formation is the bone marrow. Formation of the marrow takes place in two different ways, which relate to the method of formation of the bone. The flat bones of the skull, for example, are formed by desmal or intramembranous ossification from condensations of the neuromesenchyme. This forms thin strands of bone matrix, and primitive mesenchymal cells are transformed into osteoblasts, which form woven bone, which is subsequently replaced by lamellar bone. Two layers of compact bone surrround a layer of spongiosa. All the other bones develop from a cartilaginous primordium by enchondral ossification. (At the periphery of the ossifying cartilage – in the perichondrium – a thin layer of bone is formed by desmal ossification.) The chondrocytes show hypertrophic and regressive changes before dying, and the surrounding matrix, which persists as thin irregular spicula between the cells, becomes calcified. From the surrounding connective tissue, blood vessels penetrate the irregular cavities of the calcified cartilage.

Together with the blood vessels, mesenchymal cells reach the primitive marrow cavities to form a stroma that will, around 2 weeks later, be populated by haemopoietic stem cells from the circulation. Medullary haemopoiesis always develops approximately 2 weeks after formation of an ossification centre. The first medullary haemopoiesis is found in the clavicle at a gestational age of 8 weeks, and subsequently in the humerus, radius, femur, tibia and ribs. At the end of the third month there is blood cell formation in most bones. The appearance of medullary haemopoiesis and decrease of haemopoiesis in the liver are accompanied by a decrease in production of erythropoietin in the liver, and from gestational week 25 the kidney takes over the production of erythropoietin (Clark and Kamen 1987). Medullary erythropoiesis is normoblastic with formation of non-nucleated red blood cells.

Fetal bone marrow is the major site of production of granulocytic and megakaryocytic cells (Fukuda 1974). Megakaryopoiesis is characterized by the formation of microcytic megakaryocytes with two to four nuclear lobes.

From the sixth month of gestation the bone marrow predominates as the site of haemopoiesis (De Waele et al. 1988).

Normal Bone Marrow

Investigation of bone marrow is carried out by aspiration or trephine biopsies. Ideally, both methods are used. Smear preparations of aspirated material give superior cytological detail to histologically examined biopsies. The trephine biopsy allows better evaluation of the bone marrow structure, the cellularity, the amount of connective tissue and the presence of granulomas (Brynes et al. 1978). Bone marrow biopsies can be embedded in plastic or in paraffin; plastic has the advantage that sections can be cut without prior decalcification. Morphological details are usually better appreciated in this material than in the paraffin-embedded tissue; however, immunohistochemical investigation of plastic-embedded samples still raises problems. When sufficient material is available it may be advisable to use both methods.

Both in adults and in children, most trephine biopsies are taken from the posterior part of the iliac crest, where the bone marrow is representative of marrow in general (Harstock et al. 1965). A trephine biopsy should have a length of at least 20 mm and a diameter of 2 mm; biopsies of less than 10 mm must be considered suboptimal. For the investigation of tumour localization, biopsies from both sides of the iliac crest are sometimes recommended (Brunning et al. 1975).

The bone marrow is a dynamic structure, composed of a haemopoietic and stromal compartment. The cellularity of the bone marrow can be assessed semiquantitatively with a scoring system, or by estimating the volume percentage. Normally most non-haematological tissue of the marrow is composed of fat cells, and simple estimation of the ratio of cellular marrow to fatty marrow gives a good indication of percentage cellularity.

After the establishment of haemopoiesis early in fetal life the bone marrow is 100% cellular. By 20 weeks' gestation some fat cells can be found in the bone marrow, but at birth there are few left and the bone marrow has returned to a cellularity of almost 100%. After birth there is a slight increase in the number of fat cells, rising to 20% by the age of 10 (Harstock et al. 1965). These fat cells are located especially at the centre of the diaphyses of long bones, where areas of yellow marrow develop (Custer and Ahlfeld 1932). These areas of yellow marrow slowly extend, and in adults the red haemopoietic marrow is found only in the vertebrae, ribs, sternum, scapula, pelvis, skullbones, and the proximal and distal parts of the long tubular bones. In this red marrow the cellularity is approximately 50%, decreasing slightly with increasing age.

Trilinear haemopoiesis develops from uncommitted stem cells, which cannot be identified morphologically with certainty (Quesenberry 1991). These totipotent stem cells give rise to the myeloid and lymphoid stem cells. From the lymphoid stem cells the precursor cells for the T and B lymphocytes develop (see p. 626). The multipotent myeloid stem cell develops into committed stem cells from which the myeloblasts, erythroblasts, megakaryoblasts and monoblasts develop.

The earliest morphologically recognizable granulocytic cells, the myeloblasts, are arranged along the endost of the bony trabecula and around small arteries. Normally there is a regular maturation, with the mature cells being situated centrally in the intertrabecular spaces. A predominance of immature cells is normal for neonates, but can also be seen during some stages of systemic infection (as the classic left shift). The assessment of a maturation block and the finding of myeloblasts at abnormal sites in the marrow is of diagnostic importance. The eosinophilic and basophilic granulocytes can first be recognized in the promyelocytic stage; however, the basophilic granules cannot normally be seen in biopsies because they are water soluble and disappear during processing.

Erythropoiesis is arranged in small cell groups, the erythrons, in which all maturation stages can be found. These erythrons are situated centrally in the intertrabecular spaces. In the centre of these cell groups histiocytes can be found which normally contain some iron. The earliest recognizable erythroid cell, the erythroblast, has a basophilic cytoplasm and is otherwise hard to distinguish from the myeloblast. During maturation the cytoplasm of the erythroid cell loses its basophilia and becomes acidophilic. At the same time the nucleus becomes pyknotic and is expelled, leaving a reticulocyte. The weakly polychromatic reticulocyte matures in 1–2 days into a mature erythrocyte. In adults the granulocyte: erythrocyte ratio is approximately 3 : 1, but at the end of fetal life and in the first week after birth there is a predominance of erythroid cells, especially immature ones (Kalpaktsoglou and Emery 1965).

Megakaryopoiesis is randomly distributed in the intertrabecular spaces, especially in association with venous sinusoids. In normal individuals megakaryocytes do not form groups, and more than an occasional megakaryocyte along a bony trabeculum should be considered as abnormal; normally, a few megakaryocytes are seen in each high-power field (HPF). Sometimes one can see other cellular elements within the cytoplasm of a megakaryocyte – the phenomenon of emperipolesis. This is seen especially in reactive conditions, but its signficance is not known (Rozman and Vives-Corrons 1981).

Dispersed throughout the bone marrow are monocytic cells and macrophages. These cells regularly show haemophagocytosis, especially in ineffective haemopoiesis and in immune-mediated cell destruction. The same phenomenon can also be seen in leukaemic cells, the cells of rhabdomyosarcoma and medulloblastoma cells, and in other tumour cells.

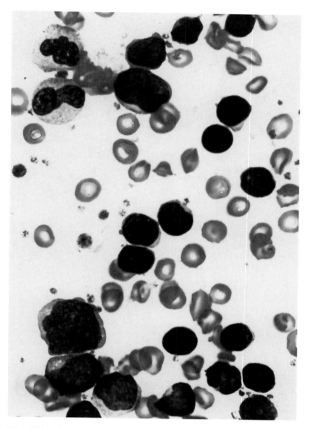

Fig. 12.2. Bone marrow aspirate of a 3-year-old child with neuroblastoma. The centre of the figure shows three haematogones.

In the first years of life, the bone marrow contains many lymphocytes, sometimes comprising up to 50% of the cellularity. Within this group are also gathered the haematogones, described by Longacre et al. (1989). These cells may express CD10, CD19 and terminal deoxynucleotidyltransferase (TdT), and are probably some type of marrow precursor cell (Fig. 12.2). In several benign and malignant disorders these cells may be increased in number (Brunning and McKenna, 1994).

Normally some plasma cells can be seen, especially along capillaries, although in children they are rare. Mast cells will be seen in Giemsa-stained sections.

The haemopoietically active bone marrow contains a very delicate network of small reticulin fibres, especially around bone trabecula and blood vessels. Perls' staining method gives an impression of the iron stores (it is important to realize that decalcification will lead to some loss of iron). A decrease of iron stores can be found with nutritional definciencies and with malabsorption. An increase of iron

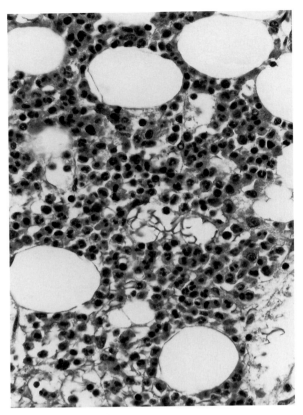

Fig. 12.3. Bone marrow biopsy of a 4-month-old child with Diamond–Blackfan anaemia. The bone marrow shows mainly granulocytic maturation. Erythrocyte precursors are only occasionally seen.

stores is seen in ineffective haemopoiesis and after transfusions of whole blood or packed cells.

Anaemia

Although most anaemias in children share the pathogenesis of anaemias in adults, some cases are seen in the paediatric age group only, and this chapter is restricted to consideration of this group of diseases.

Inherited Anaemias

Pure Red Cell Aplasia

The congenital form of red cell aplasia, also referred to as Diamond-Blackfan anaemia (DBA), usually

manifests itself early in the first year of life. Clinically, the disease is characterized by a severe macrocytic or normocytic anaemic and reticulocytopenia, whereas the leucocyte and platelet counts are normal (Diamond et al. 1976). Although the disease occurs in families in a dominant or recessive pattern, the majority of the cases appear to be sporadic, suggesting new mutations or acquired disease (Freedman 1993). Approximately 30% of children with this disease have congenital abnormalities, among which abnormalities of the thumb are prevalent.

The pathogenesis of the disease is not clear, but many data suggest that the intrinsic defect of the involved erythroid precursor cells is an inability to respond normally to the inducers of erythroid proliferation and/or differentiation (Tsai et al. 1989). Bagnara et al. and colleagues (1991) were able to demonstrate that the CD34+ erythroid progenitor cells in this disease develop normally along the granulocytic and megakaryocytic lines, but in an aberrant way along the erythroid lineage.

Histologically, the bone marrow is normocellular for the age of the child, although there is a selective marked deficiency of red cell precursors. Three patterns of erythroid development can occur. The most common pattern is erythroid hypoplasia or aplasia, which is seen in 90% of patients (Fig. 12.3). In hypoplasia, the erythroid precursors are immature erythroblasts. The second pattern, occurring in 5% of patients, is one of normal numbers and maturation of erythroblasts. The remaining 5% show erythroid hyperplasia with increased numbers of immature cells and maturation arrest. Dyserythropoiesis is occasionally seen. Iron is accumulated after multiple transfusions. Granulopoiesis and megakaryopoiesis are unremarkable. Lymphocytes are often increased. The majority of patients show a good response to steroid therapy. However, a third do not respond, or relapse on this therapy. Most clinicians are cautious about the use of haemological growth-promoting factors because patients with DBA show an increased risk for myelodysplasia and leukaemia.

Sideroblastic Anaemias

This disease is characterized by hypochromic microcytic red blood cells. In childhood it is a rare disease, which is usually X-linked or, very rarely, autosomally recessive (Hines and Grasso 1970).

The bone marrow usually shows erythroid hyperplasia in the presence of many ringed sideroblasts. Iron storage is increased. Longstanding disease may result in systemic haemosiderosis, resulting in dysfunction of the liver, heart and endocrine organs. The acquired form of sideroblastic anaemia has a heterogeneous pathogenesis and is virtually non-existent in children.

Acquired Anaemias

Pure Red Cell Aplasia

Although the majority of patients with acquired pure red cell aplasia (PRCA) belong to the adult age group, some 10% of cases may occur in teenagers. The majority of cases are idiopathic, although thymomas, infections, autoimmune dysfunction and drugs have been implicated as aetiological factors. The pathogenesis of the disease is unclear: cellular and soluble inhibitors of erythropoiesis have been demonstrated in many patients, but others do not show any indication of the origin of the disease (Freedman 1993). Patients present with profound chronic normochromic normocytic anaemia, with decreased or absent number of reticulocytes. Leucocyte and platelet counts are normal. The bone marrow shows absent erythroid precursors but is otherwise normal. Immunosuppressive therapy is the first choice of treatment.

Transient Erythroid Hypoplasia Following Parvovirus Infection

This disorder, considered to be a special form of secondary PRCA, was first described in 1981 by Pattisson et al. in children with sickle cell anaemia in aplastic crisis. The discovery of parvovirus B19 in the serum of these children opened the search for other viruses in patients with a wide range of haemolytic anaemias in aplastic crises. In vitro studies showed that the virus specifically infects and kills the erythroid precursors. Myeloid cells are not affected. The bone marrow cellularity is usually normal. Erythropoiesis often shows giant proerythroblasts (Fig. 12.4), which are presumably the precursors infected by the virus.

Transient Erythroblastopenia of Childhood

This disease develops in previously healthy children and is characterized by a severe normochromic normocytic anaemia with varying reticulocytopenia. Granulopoiesis and platelet formation are unremarkable. The children are usually between 1 and 5 years old and often have a history of recent viral infection or allergic episode. Congenital abnormalities as seen in DBA are not present. In most patients there is

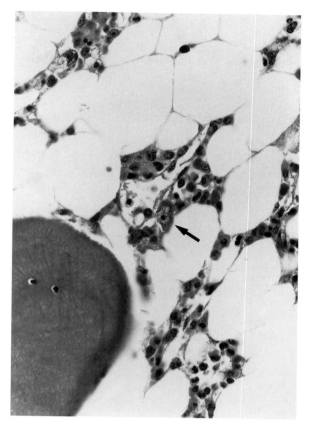

Fig. 12.4. Bone marrow of a 4-year-old child. The centre shows a giant proerythroblast (*arrow*). Hypocellularity is due to treatment for neuroblastoma.

spontaneous complete recovery within a few months of onset. The disease is the result of a transient immunosuppression of erythropoiesis, due to an immunoregulatory abnormality.

The bone marrow is normocellular with erythroid hypoplasia in 60% of patients and aplasia in 10%. The remaining 30% show hypercellular marrow with a recovering erythropoiesis.

Koenig et al. (1979) showed that either whole serum or IgG from patients with this disorder prevented erythroid colony formation from CFU-E in in vitro culture systems; the suppressive activity disappears following recovery.

Imerslund–Grasbeck Syndrome

This disease is a congenital vitamin B_{12} malabsorption, probably due to an abnormality of the ileal receptor for the cobalamin–intrinsic factor complex (Burman et al. 1985). The disorder is the most common inherited cause of paediatric megaloblastic

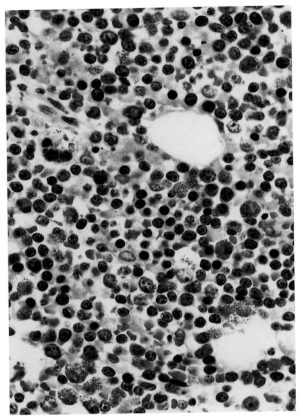

Fig. 12.5. Bone marrow biopsy in a 6-month-old boy with Kostmann's syndrome. Note the absence of normal granulopoiesis. The granuloid cells are eosinophils. Most of the cells that compose the bone marrow are of erythroid origin.

anaemia, occurs between the age of 1 and 15 years, and is autosomally recessive. The bone marrow shows megaloblastic changes as in the adult forms.

Other Causes of (Transient) Red Cell Aplasia

Many other diseases have been described in association with red cell aplasia. Among them are malnutrition, a wide range of drugs and several viral infections.

Granulocytopenia

Granulocytopenia is characterized by an isolated reduction of the number of circulating granulocytes in otherwise normal blood. Isolated neutropenias

usually become manifest by bacterial infections. Two main groups can be distinguished. The first is a consistent neutropenia with a high mortality rate. Kostmann's syndrome is an important representative of this group. Reticular dysgenesis and a form that is associated with X-linked hypogammaglobulinaemia are other examples.

The second group consists of variable neutropenias. The prognosis of these diseases is usually much better than those of the former group. Shwachman's syndrome is a striking example. Other diseases in this group are cartilage hair hypoplasia, dyskeratosis congenita, chronic benign neutropenia and metabolic neutropenia. Kostmann's syndrome and Shwachman's syndrome will be discussed here as the most important representatives of the two groups (Gilman et al. 1970).

Inherited Granulocytopenias

Kostmann's Syndrome

This disease, also called infantile genetic agranulocytosis, is a severe congenital neutropenia, with an autosomal recessive inheritance. It is a rare disease that usually becomes symptomatic within the first 6 month of life. Often the neutrophil counts are nearly normal in the first part of life. Severe pyogenic infections are usually the first symptoms of this disorder and also the main cause of death. Laboratory findings show an average granulocyte count of less then 200 cells/μlitre. However, the total white cell count may be close to normal as a result of increased numbers of monocytes and eosinophils. Kostmann's syndrome is by definition a single-cell cytopenia, and erythrocytes and thrombocytes are therefore present in normal numbers.

The bone marrow usually shows normal cellularity for the age. Myeloid precursors are absent or markedly decreased, but there is usually normal differentiation to the promyelocyte or myelocyte stage. Mature cells are virtually absent (Fig. 12.5). The prognosis of this disease is poor. Most patients die of sepsis or pneumonia within a few years. A few children develop acute leukaemia. The treatment of choice at present is granulocyte colony stimulating factor.

Shwachman's Syndrome

This disease, also called Shwachman–Diamond syndrome, is a rare autosomal recessive trait (Shwachman et al. 1964). A variable neutropenia is accompanied by exocrine pancreatic insufficiency, resulting in malabsorption, steatorrhoea and failure to thrive. The degree of neutropenia varies. Skin infections or pneumonia are usually the first signs of the disease. Although the neutropenia is the most important haematological abnormality, anaemia and thrombocytopenia (or both) occur in more than 20% of cases (Aggett et al. 1980).

The bone marrow is hypocellular in half the cases, most of the others showing a myeloid maturation arrest, but in a few cases normal marrow is found. Erythropoiesis is usually hyperplastic and shows a normal maturation. Megakarryopoiesis is usually normal. The disorder is a premalignant condition with a 5% chance of developing into a form of acute leukaemia. Other patients develop pancytopenia.

Cyclic Neutropenia

This disorder is characterized by cyclic episodes of neutropenia occurring approximately every 3 weeks. During the neutropenic phase (7–10 days long), the patient has serious symptoms that are usually located in and around the mouth (Dale and Hammond 1988).

The bone marrow initially shows hypoplasia of promyelocytes and myelocytes, followed by an increase in more mature cells. The mechanism of the disease is thought to be a defect at stem cell level.

Acquired Granulocytopenias

Most cases of granulocytopenia in childhood are acquired. Among the most important causes are autoimmune diseases, infections and drugs. The autoimmune neutropenias include isoimmune neonatal neutropenia, transient neonatal neutropenia and neutropenia associated with autoimmune disease and thrombocytopenia. However, the most important causes of infectious neutropenias are viruses. Most of the typical paediatric viral infections can result in a transient neutropenia.

Drug-associated neutropenias are usually the result of treatment for malignant disorders.

Thrombocytopenia

Congenital thrombocytopenias can be distinguished into two groups on the basis of bone marrow investigation (Lilleyman 1992). One group, without megakaryocytes, includes amegakaryocytic thrombocytopenia (absent radius syndrome) and Fanconi's anaemia. The other, with megakaryocytes, contains

among others Wiskott–Aldrich syndrome, Montreal syndrome, Grey platelet syndrome and Bernard–Soulier syndrome.

Inherited Thrombocytopenias

Amegakaryocytic Thrombocytopenia

This inherited disease sometimes precedes aplastic anaemia by months or years, and is considered to be an intrinsic haemopoietic stem cell defect (Freedman and Estrov 1990). The thrombocytopenia is usually present at birth. Most children are mentally normal, but some show mental retardation. The disease is sometimes accompanied by hypoplastic or absent radii, resulting in skeletal abnormalities of the forearm (Hall 1987). Other associated congenital abnormalities are heart defects and dysplasia of the jaw and clavicles. The disease may be associated with a Philadelphia chromosome (Xue et al. 1993). Spontaneous bleeding in mucous membranes, the gastrointestinal tract or the skin are usually the first symptoms.

The bone marrow has a normal cellularity, with absent or strongly reduced numbers of megakaryocytes. If megakaryocytes are present they are small. The platelets that are present look normal. The bone marrow often shows a myeloid hyperplasia, sometimes associated with a neonatal leukaemoid blood picture.

Treatment consists of steroids, haemopoietic growth factors (Guinan et al. 1993), antithymocyte globulin (Trimble et al. 1991) and bone marrow transplantation.

Over the years many other cases of amegakaryocytic thrombocytopenia have been described that mimic the thrombocytopenia with absent radius syndrome. One disorder that is highly distinctive has been described by O'Gorman-Hughes (1966). It consists of a congenital amegakaryocytic thrombocytopenia without other abnormalities, which eventually evolves into aplastic anaemia after 3–4 years. Boys are more commonly affected than girls. The bone marrow has a normal cellularity with absent or strongly reduced numbers of megakaryocytes. Survival and platelet morphology are normal.

Thrombocytopenia with Megakaryocytes

There are several situations in which a peripheral thrombocytopenia is observed in the presence of megakaryocytes in the bone marrow. Usually this occurs in combination with other abnormalities as Wiskott–Aldrich syndrome, Bernard–Soulier syn-

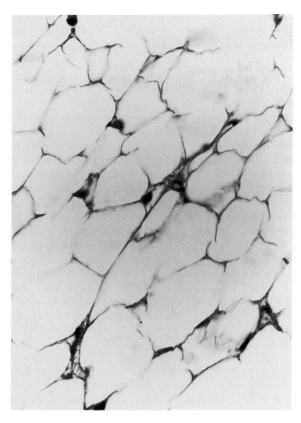

Fig. 12.6. Severely aplastic bone marrow in a 4-year-old child with Fanconi's anaemia. No haemopoiesis is seen.

drome, Grey platelet syndrome or May–Hegglin anomaly.

In the Wiskott–Aldrich syndrome (Wiskott 1937; Aldrich et al. 1954), the basic defect is a cellular and humoral deficiency. The clinical severity of the thrombocytopenia varies from asymptomatic to sometimes extensive purpura. Platelets are approximately half the size of normal platelets, and show ultrastructural abnormalities (Grottum et al. 1969).

Bernard–Soulier syndrome (Bernard and Soulier 1948) is a recessively inherited disorder in which thrombocytopenia is accompanied by abnormal platelet size and shortened survival.

Acquired Thrombocytopenia

Acquired thrombocytopenia is usually the result of aplastic anaemia or myelosuppression by drugs, toxins, irradiation or viral infections (Hoffman 1991). Bone marrow replacement or infiltration by malignant disease (leukaemia, metastatic disease) is an important cause of thrombocytopenia. Megaloblastic

anaemias, as seen in vitamin B_{12} and folic acid deficiency, can cause thrombocytopenia as part of a pancytopenia.

Pancytopenia

Inherited Pancytopenias

Isolated cytopenias are relatively rare diseases. In most diseases, abnormalities of more cell lines present together. The most frequent inherited forms of congenital pancytopenias are Fanconi's anaemia, dyskeratosis congenita and reticular dysgenesis.

Fanconi's Anaemia

This disease was originally described by Fanconi (1927) and represents a pancytopenia associated with multiple congenital abnormalities. The haematological abnormalities may not reveal themselves for some years. Thrombocytopenia is usually the first cytopenia; pancytopenia is usually present by the age of 6–9 years. Some patients develop myelodysplasia or leukaemia.

The congenital abnormalities in Fanconi's anaemia are extensive and include generalized hyperpigmentation of the skin, microsomia, absent or hypoplastic upper limbs, hypogenitalia, and a large number of abnormalities of the skull (microcephaly), eyes and ears. There are renal, gastrointestinal and cardiopulmonary abnormalities.

This disorder is transmitted as an autosomal recessive, although there is a slight excess of males reported in the literature.

The bone marrow is hypocellular, as in aplastic anaemia (Fig. 12.6).

Dyskeratosis Congenita

Dyskeratosis congenita is a very rare X-linked recessive congenital aplasia, associated with hyperpigmentation, dystrophic nails, leukoplakia and mental retardation. This disorder shares many similarities with Fanconi's anaemia. There is an increased incidence of squamous cell carcinoma in these children.

Reticular Dysgenesis

Reticular dysgenesis is characterized by congenital agranulocytosis, lymphopenia and a related cellular

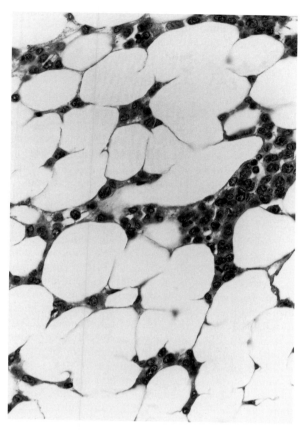

Fig. 12.7. Development of acute myeloid leukaemia in a young patient with acquired aplastic anaemia without known pathogenic mechanism. The leukaemic cells infiltrate between the fat cells.

and humoral immunodeficiency. The disease results from a failure of committed stem cells of the myeloid and lymphoid series. The bone marrow is hypocellular because of the absence of myelopoiesis and lymphocytes, with reduced erythropoiesis. (Findings are described in Chapter 11.)

Bone marrow transplantation is the treatment of choice.

Inherited/Acquired Pancytopenia

Aplastic Anaemia

This somewhat misleading term is applied to a pancytopenia characterized by anaemia, neutropenia and thrombocytopenia. These changes are thought to be the result of failure or suppression of the multipotent myeloid stem cell, resulting in inadequate production or release of the differentiated cell lines. Acquired aplastic anaemia is the most common form of bone marrow failure in both adults and childhood. Drugs

and chemicals are considered to be the most important factors in the aetiology of aplastic anaemia. However, in the majority of the cases, no pathogenic mechanism can be found, and idiopathic cases form the majority of the aplastic anaemias. That they may be caused by immunological course has become apparent as the result of treatment: immunosuppressive drugs can produce recovery of the bone marrow. Treatment with antilymphocyte serum has also been effective.

The bone marrow is hypocellular or aplastic, composed largely of erythroid cells. Scattered foci of lymphocytes and plasma cells may be present. Occasional islands of haemopoietic cells (mainly immature precursors) can be found. As in congenital aplastic anaemia, patients with acquired aplastic anaemia sometimes develop acute leukaemia (Fig. 12.7). This transformation suggests that, at least in a small proportion of cases, aplastic anaemia may represent a preleukemic state. If the anaemia persists after treatment with conventional drugs, bone marrow transplantation is unavoidable.

Differential diagnosis should include hypoplastic acute leukaemia, but this is very uncommon in children.

Myelodysplasia

Primary Myelodysplasia

The myelodysplastic syndromes (MDSs) consist of a heterogeneous group of stem cell disorders, characterized by abnormal maturation of one or more haematological cell lines. MDS is much more common in adults than in childhood, but may occur in the newborn (McMullin et al. 1991). It is estimated that this (premalignant) condition represents less than 3% of haematological malignancies in childhood (Chessels 1991).

The disease usually manifests as a cytopenia of one or more cell lines or as a pancytopenia. Hepatosplenomegaly and granulocytic sarcomas are much more prevalent than in the adult population (Tuncer et al. 1992). The disease may start as refractory anaemia with few other haematological abnormalities in the blood or the bone marrow, but may also present as a preleukaemia as in the elderly.

Myelodysplastic syndrome was originally classified according to the FAB classification (Bennett et al. 1982), as refractory anaemia (RA), refractory anaemia with ringed sideroblasts (RARS), refractory anaemia with excess of blasts (RAEB) and refractory

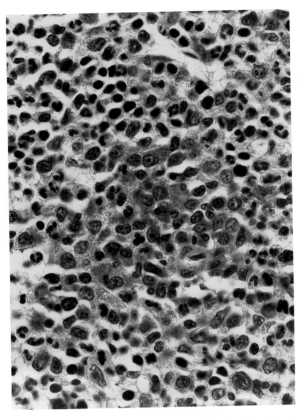

Fig. 12.8. Bone marrow heavily infiltrated by juvenile chronic myeloid leukaemia. Note the dysplastic irregular erythrocyte precursors in a hypercellular marrow, dominated by immature white cells.

anaemia with excess of blasts in transformation (RAEB-t). In the elderly, chronic myelomonocytic leukaemia (CMML) is also included within the myelodysplastic syndrome. This disorder, characterized by an absolute monocytosis in blood and bone marrow, is not seen in children, who suffer instead a chronic leukaemia classified as juvenile chronic myeloid leukaemia (JCML), the paediatric counterpart of CMML. Because of its rarity, the classification of MDS in childhood has been neglected. Recently Brandwein et al. (1990) and Chessels (1991) have tried to classify these disorders.

In MDS, the bone marrow usually shows erythroid hypoplasia, ringed sideroblasts, dyserythropoiesis and megaloblastic (macronormoblastic) maturation. The granulocyte series displays a shift to the left, abnormal maturation and hypogranularity of the cell types beyond promyelocytes. The megakaryocytes are usually small, with one or two small round nuclei. Sometimes there is hardly any cytoplasm, and irregular nuclear forms such as ring nuclei are seen.

In the refractory anaemia group, only the erythroid series shows abnormalities. The number of blasts in the peripheral blood is less than 1%, and in the bone marrow less than 5%. If there are more than 15% ringed sideroblasts in the group of erythroblasts, this disorder is diagnosed as RARS.

If the number of blasts in the peripheral blood varies between 1% and 5% and/or bone marrow blasts are between 5% and 20%, the disease is diagnosed as refractory anaemia with excess of blasts. If the number of blasts in the peripheral blood increases to maximally 29% or is between 20% and 30% in the bone marrow, it is called RAEB in transformation.

Juvenile chronic myeloid leukaemia is a chronic myeloid leukaemia without the Philadelphia chromosome. It is characterized by hepatosplenomegaly and a marked monocytosis in the presence of fetal haemoglobulin. This disease is often associated with neurofibromatosis (Shannon et al. 1992). The peripheral blood shows a moderately raised leucocyte count. The bone marrow shows an increase in monocytes and blast cells, and the other cell lines show dysplastic features (Fig. 12.8). In this respect JCML is truly an MDS. Monocyte-derived haemopoietic growth factors play a role in the regulation of myeloproliferation in JCML (Emanuel et al. 1991).

Many chromosomal changes and gene mutations (Jacobs 1992) are seen in myelodysplasia. Among them are −7, +8 and many deletions and translocations. Because myelodysplasias are a group of chronic disorders rising in a pluripotent or a multipotent stem cell, all daughter cells show the same abnormalities, although there may be variable involvement of the cell lines.

The prognosis of MDS in children is poorer than in adults, the overall mean survival being only 9 years 9 months in one study (Tuncer 1992). Irrespective of the FAB subtype, MDS in childhood seems to run an aggressive clinical course even in the RA group, where a transformation to RAEB-t or AML after an average of 7 months is followed by death in an average of $4\frac{1}{2}$ months. Hasle et al. (1992) reported nine cases with somewhat better survival. Transformation to AML is a frequent complication if the patient survives the complications of the cytopenias. Treatment by bone marrow transplantation is receiving more and more attention. JCML is a disease with a poor prognosis with a median survival of approximately 6 months, usually resulting in bone marrow failure. Transformation of JCML to AML, as seen in the other forms of MDS, is rare. Bone marrow transplantation is again the treatment of choice.

Monosomy 7 related infantile myelodysplastic syndrome is a rare disorder that was first described by Teasdale et al. (1970). It is characterized by monosomy and partial deletion of chromosome 7. The morphological features of monosomy 7 (Fig. 12.9) are those of RA, RAEB or sometimes JCML. Splenomegaly in combination with bone marrow fibrosis is often seen. The disease has been described in families (Paul et al. 1987). Progression to acute myeloid leukaemia is a common feature. Monosomy 7 is a common cytogenetic finding in primary MDS, secondary MDS, de novo AML and secondary AML.

Secondary Myelodysplasia

Myelodysplastic syndromes can also occur as late complications of radiotherapy and/or chemotherapy. Although most of the literature on this subject relates to adults, there are several studies that report on the development of post-therapy myelodysplasia in children (Le Beau 1986; Rubin et al. 1991). Rubin recognizes two subgroups of patients with therapy-related MDS or AML. The first (and largest) includes patients with abnormalities of chromosomes 5 and/or 7, and the second (smaller) patients with abnormalities of chromosome 11 at band q23. Abnormalities at chromosomes 5/7 are usually the result of alkylating agents. The 11q23 abnormalities are seen in patients exposed to the drug epipodyfillotoxin (Pui et al. 1989).

The median interval from initial treatment for the first malignancy to the diagnosis of therapy-related MDS or AML was 46 months in this group. Most of the patients die at a median of 7 months from diagnosis. Morphologically secondary myelodysplasia is indistinguishable from primary myelodysplasia.

Myeloproliferative Disorders

Acute Myeloproliferative Disorders

Acute Non-lymphocytic Leukaemias

Acute non-lymphocytic leukaemias (ANLL) include all leukaemias that are classified M0–M7 in the FAB classification. The majority of the cases, however, are of myeloid origin. Approximately 20% of all acute leukaemias belong to this group.

The clinical features of children with ANLL are usually related to bone marrow failure. Anaemia, pallor, anorexia and headaches are frequent findings. Thrombocytopenia often results in bleeding, especially from the nose or gastrointestinal tract.

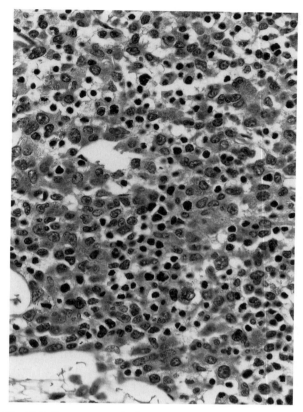

Fig. 12.9. Bone marrow of a 3-year-old child with monosomy 7. Granulopoiesis shows diminished maturation. Erythropoiesis is characterized by many irregular red cell precursors. Both features are characteristic of myelodysplastic syndrome.

The diagnosis of ANLL largely depends on examination of smears of aspirated marrow. The following diagnoses should be considered:

1. *Acute myeloid leukaemia, minimally differentiated* (M0). This designation is sometimes used for cases of acute myeloid leukaemias that are morphologically hard to distinguish from acute lymphoblastic leukaemia. Less than 3% blasts is positive for myeloperoxidase/Sudan black B, whereas more than 20% is positive for myeloid associated antigens. There are no Auer rods present.
2. *Acute myeloid leukaemia with maturation* (M1). This disease consists of myeloblasts that are sometimes very difficult to differentiate from macrolymphoblasts (L2). There are usually no Auer rods, and staining for α-naphthylchloracetate esterase is negative. Sometimes the disease presents as a chloroma in the orbit, cranium or spinal cord.

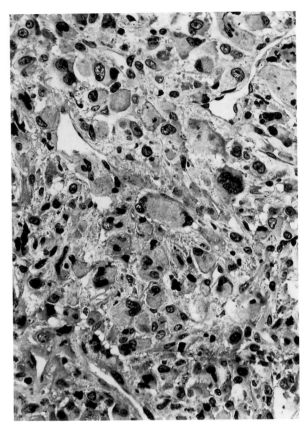

Fig. 12.10. Bone marrow showing large numbers of megakaryoblasts. Reticulin staining (not shown) shows a dense reticulin fibrosis. The biopsy is taken from a 5-year-old girl with Down's syndrome.

3. *AML with maturation* (M2). Although the percentage of myeloblasts is still very high, there is differentiation into more mature forms. Auer rods are present, and the α-naphthylchloracetate esterase reaction is positive.
4. *Acute promyelocytic leukaemia* (M3). Promyelocytes dominate the bone marrow with prominent granulation of the cells and multiple Auer rods.
5. *Acute myelomonocytic leukaemia* (M4). This leukaemia consist of a mixture of myeloblasts, promonocytes and monocytes. The granulocyte series shows differentiation.
6. *Acute monoblastic leukaemia* (M5a) / *Acute monocytic leukaemia* (M5b). In this disease monoblasts or monocytes form more than 80% of the bone marrow cells. Half of the paediatric cases occur before the age of 2 years. Acute monocytic leukaemia (M5b) is quite uncommon in children. Most cases are of the M5a type. The great adhesiveness of the monocytic cells often results in leukostasis.

7. *Erythroleukaemia* (M6). In this disease young forms of erythroblasts and nucleated red cells occur in the blood. In the bone marrow a dominance of megaloblastic erythroblasts is seen. It has been described in a child with monosomy 7 (Shitara et al. 1991).
8. *Acute megakaryocytic leukaemia* (M7). In this disorder the bone marrow shows large numbers of megakaryoblasts, often surrounded by a dense reticulin fibrosis, resulting in a dry tap. This disease is often associated with Down's syndrome (Fig. 12.10).

Chronic Myeloproliferative Disorders

Among the chronic myeloproliferative disorders belong chronic myelocytic leukaemia, essential thrombocytosis (see p. 676), idiopathic myelofibrosis and polycythemia vera (Nix and Fernbach 1981).

Chronic Myeloid Leukaemia

Chronic myeloid leukaemia accounts for only 2% of all leukaemias in children. It is seen in two forms: a juvenile rapidly progressive type with infections, skin lesions, white cell counts below 100 000/mm^3 and absence of Philadelphia chromosomes as main features (at present considered to be a form of myelodysplasia, see p. 669); and a more adult type with gradual onset, high white cell counts and the presence of Philadelphia chromosomes. In the adult form, the bone marrow is hypercellular with many granulocyte precursors, and an increase in the number of megakaryocytes is often accompanied by an increase in reticulin fibrosis. The histological picture is the same as that of adult CML (Fig. 12.11). The disease is often accompanied by splenomegaly due to extramedullary haemopoiesis. Transformation in acute myeloblastic or lymphoblastic leukaemia is frequently seen.

Polycythemia Vera

Polycythemia vera is very rare in children. Symptoms, treatment and prognosis do not differ from those in adults.

Idiopathic Myelofibrosis

Idiopathic myelofibrosis also is a very rare disease in childhood. Most of the cases that were diagnosed as

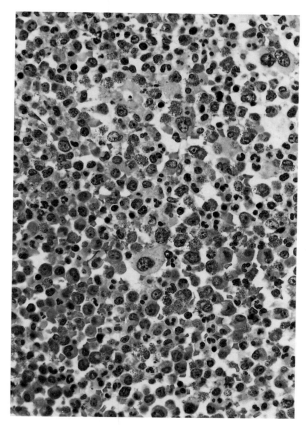

Fig. 12.11. Hypercellular marrow in a young patient with chronic myeloid leukaemia. The bone marrow is hypercellular with a predominance of granulocytic cells in different stages of differentiation.

such in the past appear to be acute megakaryoblastic leukaemias with extensive reticulin fibrosis.

Transient Myeloproliferative Disorder of the Newborn

This disorder is often associated with Down's syndrome. The children develop hepatosplenomegaly and have a leucocytosis with varying numbers of blasts in the blood (Eguchi et al. 1989). The peripheral blood smear may show dysplastic features. It is usually impossible to distinguish this disorder from acute myeloblastic leukaemia. In the first 4 months of life, a "wait and see" policy should be preferred over treatment. In real transient myeloproliferative disorders, many children will show a complete recovery to normal bone marrow (De Alarcon et al. 1987). In others, recovery is only temporarily and eventually an acute myeloproliferative disorder (usually M7 AML) will evolve.

Acute Lymphoblastic Leukaemias

Acute lymphoblastic leukaemia (ALL) is the most common form of neoplastic disease in childhood. It is also the tumour in which progress in treatment is most prominent. The prognosis of ALL in 1960 was still extremely poor, with most patients dying within half a year of the diagnosis; now, over 50% of patients live, with a prospect of complete cure.

Peripheral blood shows white cell counts that are often remarkably raised, although some patients present with counts below 10×10^9/litre. Thrombocytopenia is a frequent finding and often severe. Anaemia is present in variable degrees of severity.

Histopathological findings are similar in many types of leukaemia. In autopsied cases there may be evidence of local (often necrotizing) infections (including stomatitis) and haemorrhage. Moderate hepatosplenomegaly is usual, and lymph node enlargement may be found. The bone marrow is fleshy and pink, and may closely resemble the homogeneous, usually darker red, splenic pulp. It is hypercellular, mainly due to leukaemic blasts, and a dry tap may be the result of aspiration. The liver is uniformly enlarged, but the cut surface may appear normal. Diffuse renal involvement is also common, with often massive enlargement of the kidneys. Focal deposits are sometimes found. Gonadal involvement is common, and the gonads seem to be an important site from which recurrences may begin, as is the central nervous system. Leukaemic masses may be seen in the retina with the ophthalmoscope; meningeal and perivascular intracerebral cuffing with leukaemic cells are commonly found. Changes in an untreated case of ALL in a case of Down's syndrome are seen in Figs. 12.12–12.15.

Therapy produces important modifications of the histopathological findings. Leukaemic cells may almost disappear, the marrow may become hypoplastic, and drug-associated changes may be seen in a number of tissues (Fig. 12.16).

The leukaemic blasts are morphologically classified according to the French–American–British (FAB) classification, which divides ALL into L1 (small microlymphoblastic), L2 (larger more undifferentiated), and L3 (Burkitt type) (Fig. 12.17a, b). It is not always easy to distinguish between the three groups, especially between L1 and L2. Patients with L2 blasts have a somewhat less favourable prognosis then those with L1.

Immunophenotyping of lymphoblastic leukaemias shows several subcategories, among which the common type of ALL is the most frequent (more than 70% of cases over 2 years old). Null cell ALL is seen in approximately 50% of cases in children under 1

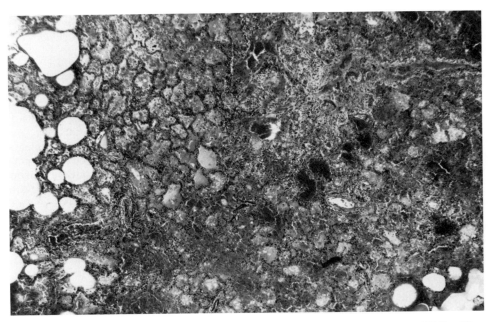

Fig. 12.12. Necrotizing pneumonia from an untreated case of Down's syndrome with ALL. (H&E, × 60)

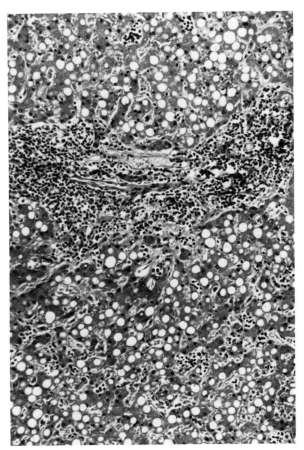

Fig. 12.13. Liver involvement by leukaemic cells in portal tracts (the same case as in Fig. 12.12). (H&E, × 120)

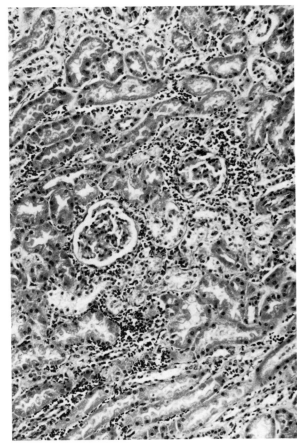

Fig. 12.14. Diffuse renal infiltration in the same case as illustrated in Figs 12.12 and 12.13. (H&E, × 120)

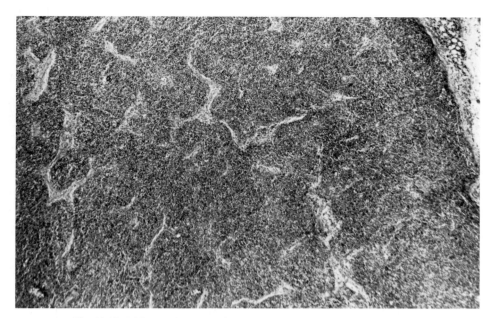

Fig. 12.15. Diffuse replacement of lymph node by leukaemic cells. (H&E, × 60)

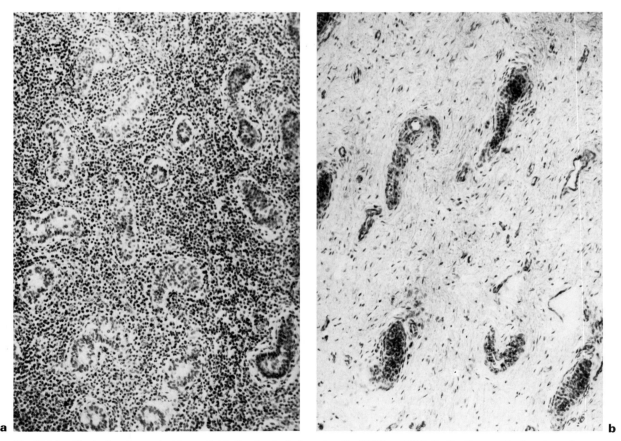

Fig. 12.16. a Testis showing marked interstitial infiltration by leukaemic cells. (H&E, × 120) **b** Testis after combination chemotherapy. The gonads had been diffusely enlarged before treatment. Interstitial fibrosis replaces the cellular infiltrate. (H&E, × 120)

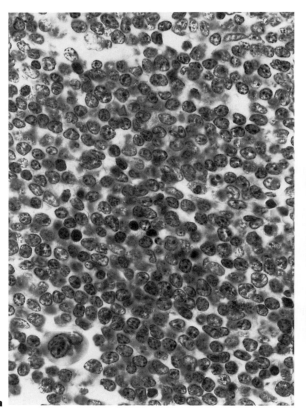
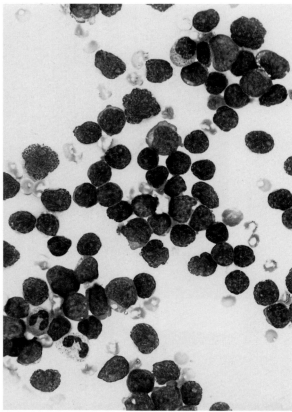

Fig. 12.17. Acute lymphoblastic leukaemia (L1). **a** Hypercellular marrow infiltrated by small lymphoblasts with slightly irregular nuclei with small nucleoli. **b** Bone marrow smear of the same patient. The slight irregularity of the nuclear contours is obvious in this material.

year of age, but only in 2% of children over 2 years of age. A T-cell phenotype is seen in approximately 8% of children over 1 year, whereas B-cell ALL are mainly seen in children under the age of 1 year. There is no clear correlation between the FAB classification of ALL and the immunophenotype, although L3 correlates closely with B-cell ALL (Medical Research Council 1986). Chemotherapy is the treatment of choice in these lesions.

Thrombocytosis

Thrombocytosis of Prematurity

Premature children with low birth weight often have platelet counts ranging from 500 to 900×10^9/litre during the first months of life. There is no other pathology seen in these cases. Bone marrow changes are unremarkable.

Essential Thrombocytaemia

This disorder belongs to the group of the chronic myeloproliferative disorders. It is extremely rare in children, the youngest in the literature being 7 years old (Fernandez–Robles et al. 1990). The clinical features of this disease are the same as are seen in adults, mainly causing thrombosis, headaches and infarctions. The platelet counts are usually over 1000×10^9/litre. Splenomegaly is often part of the disease.

The bone marrow is usually hypercellular and shows an increase of large multilobated megakaryocytes.

Secondary Thrombocytosis

Platelet counts over 500×10^9/litre are often seen in children in a number of diseases (Vora and Lilleyman 1993), especially infection (Thomas and O'Brien 1986; Wolach et al. 1990), idiopathic colitis (Lake et al. 1978) and juvenile rheumatoid arthritis (Calabro et al. 1977).

In many malignant diseases secondary thrombocytosis can be found. Among these are carcinomas, lymphomas and sometimes acute leukaemia (Lascari 1984). Thrombocytosis in hepatoblastomas is probably due to the reduction of thrombopoietin-like substances. These types of thrombocytosis are usually asymptomatic.

Other situations in which a reactive thrombocytosis is seen are iron deficiency, postsplenectomy states, vitamin E deficiency and red cell aplasia.

Benign Familial Thrombocytosis

A few families are described in which an asymptomatic thrombocytosis is seen in different family members (Williams and Shahidi 1991). No sign of other disorders is found.

Histiocytic Disorders

Histiocytic disorders in childhood form a heterogeneous group of diseases. Histiocytes originate in the bone marrow as monocytes and populate the different tissues as macrophages. The interdigitating reticulum cells of the lymph nodes and spleen, and Langerhans' cells, belong to this group. For ease of discussion, childhood histiocytic disorders are classified in this chapter as familial histiocytosis, reactive histiocytosis and Langerhans' cell histiocytosis.

Familial Histiocytosis

Storage Disorders

Most metabolic storage disorders are autosomal recessives, apart from a few (such as Hunter's syndrome and Fabry's disease) that are X-linked recessive. These disorders are discussed elsewhere in this book (see Chapter 16). Scattered or grouped storage cells can be found in bone marrow aspirates and biopsy material.

Familial Erythrophagocytic Lymphohistiocytosis

This autosomal recessive disease was first described by Farquhar and Claireaux (1952). Usually it mani-

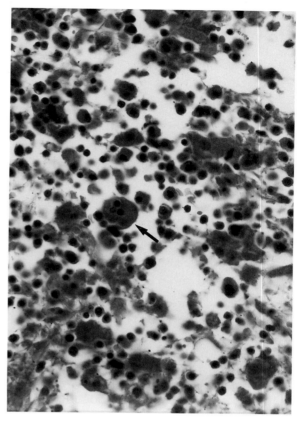

Fig. 12.18. Familial erythrophagic lymphohistiocytes. Extensive erythrophagocytosis is visible (*arrow*).

fests in the first half year of life. Only 10% of cases are seen in children older than 2 years. Diagnostic guidelines are described by Henter and colleagues (Henter and Elinder 1991; Henter et al. 1991).

Patients often present with failure to thrive, pallor, fever, anaemia and hepatosplenomegaly. Lymphadenopathy is seen in approximately 10% of cases. The peripheral blood usually shows a pancytopenia, and the bone marrow is infiltrated to varying degrees with histiocytes, showing erythrophagocytosis (Fig. 12.18) (see also p. 655). Prognosis of this disease is poor. Bone marrow transplantation is the only suggested treatment that may improve prognosis.

Reactive Histiocytosis

Among the group of the reactive histiocytosis are infection-associated haemophagocytic syndromes caused by viruses, such as adenovirus (Reardon et al. 1991), herpes simplex virus, cytomegalovirus and Epstein–Barr virus (Su et al. 1990). Infections by

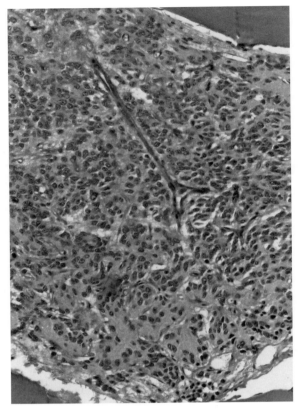

Fig 12.19. Bone marrow involvement by metastatic neuroblastoma merging with haemopoietic tissue.

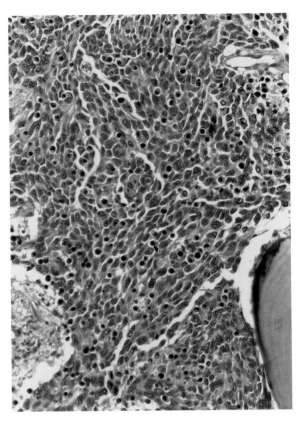

Fig 12.20. Bone marrow infiltration by a rhabdomyosarcoma showing spindle-cell differentiation.

other micro organisms (mycobacteria, cryptococcus, toxoplasma, leishmania, histoplasma and others) are important causes of histiocytic proliferations in the bone marrow. Haemophagocytosis is a frequent feature of these cells. Bone marrow aspirate or biopsy may show reduced erythropoiesis and granulopoiesis, and sometimes fibrosis. The megakaryocytes are usually not affected by the disorder. Sometimes slight dysplastic features may be seen as dyserythropoiesis, megaloblastoid changes and ringed sideroblasts. Clinically, patients usually present with rapidly progressive pancytopenia resulting from the histiocytic haemophagocytosis. Many organs can be involved in the disease. Usually the condition is self-limiting and aggressive treatment is not necessary.

Metastatic Bone Marrow Disease

In children, bone marrow involvement is seen in patients with non-Hodgkin's lymphomas and solid tumours. Solid tumours commonly consist of small round-cell tumours including neuroblastoma (Fig. 12.19), rhabdomyosarcoma (Fig. 12.20) and Ewing's sarcoma (Finkelstein et al. 1970). Neuroblastoma, the most common paediatric solid tumour, has a high frequency of bone marrow involvement. Up to 70% of patients have a positive bone marrow in the course of their disease (Head et al. 1979; Moss et al. 1991). Differential diagnosis on morphological grounds alone may be very difficult. The application of monoclonal antibodies may be very helpful in distinguishing the different entities. Lymphomas are usually positive when stained with leucocyte common antigen and with immature or mature lymphocyte markers. Neuroblastoma is positive for chromogranin, and rhabdomyosarcoma for muscle actin, desmin and vimentin. Ewing's sarcoma also reacts positively with vimentin and is negative with the other markers.

References

Aggett PJ, Cavanagh NP, Matthew DJ (1980) Shwachman's syndrome: a review of 21 cases. Arch Dis Child 55: 331

Aldrich RA, Steinberg AG, Campbell DC (1954) Pedigree demonstrating a sex-linked recessive condition characterized by draining ears, exzematoid dermatitis and bloody diarrhea. Pediatrics 13: 133

Bagnara GP, Zauli G, Vitale L, Rosito V, Vecchi G, Paolucci G, Avanzi GC, Ramenghi U, Timeus F, Gabutti V (1991) In vitro growth and regulation of bone marrow enriched CD34+ hematopoietic progenitors in Diamond–Blackfan anemia. Blood 78: 2203

Bennett JM, Catovsky D, Daniel MT, Flandrin G, Galton DAG, Gralnick HR, Sultan C (1982) Proposals for the classification of the myelodysplastic syndromes. Br J Haematol 51: 189

Bernard J, Soulier JP (1948) Sur une nouvelle variété de dystrophie thrombocytaire hémorrhagipare congenitale. Sem des Hôspitaux, Paris 24: 3217

Bloom W, Bartelnew GW (1940) Hemopoiesis in young human embryos. Am J Anat 67: 21

Brandwein JM, Horsman DE, Eaves AC, Eaves CJ (1990) Childhood myelodysplasia: suggested classification as myelodysplastic syndromes based on laboratory and clinical findings. Am J Pediatr Hematol Oncol 12: 63

Brunning RD, Bloomfield CD, McKenna RW, Peterson L (1975) Bilateral trephine bone marrow biopsies in lymphoma and other neoplastic diseases. Ann Intern Med 82: 365

Brunning RD, McKenna RW (1994) Tumors of the bone marrow. Atlas of tumour pathology, Fascicle 9, third series. Armed Forces Institute of Pathology, Washington DC, p 13

Brynes RK, McKenna RW, Sundberg RD (1978) Bone marrow aspiration and trephine biopsy. An approach to a thorough study. Am J Clin Path 70: 753

Burman JF, Jenkins WJ, Walker-Smith JA, Phillips AD, Sourial NA, Williams CB, Mollin DI (1985) Absent ideal uptake of IF-bound vitamin B_{12} in vivo in the Imerslund Grasbeck syndrome (familial vitamin B_{12} malabsorption with proteinuria). Gut 26: 311

Calabro JJ, Staley HL, Burnstein SL, Leb L (1977) Laboratory findings in juvenile rheumatoid arthritis. Arthritis Rheum 20: 268

Chessels JM (1991) Myelodysplasia. Clin Haematol 4: 459

Christensen RD (1989) Hematopoiesis in the fetus and neonate. Pediatr Res 26: 531

Clark SC, Kamen R (1987) The human hematopoietic colony-stimulating factors. Science 236: 1229

Custer RP, Ahlfeld FE (1932) Studies on the structure and function of bone marrow. II. Variations in cellularity in various bones with advancing years of life and their relative response to stimuli. J Lab Clin Med 17: 960

Dale DC, Hammond WP (1988) Cyclic neutropenia: a clinical review. Blood Rev 2: 178

De Alarcon PA, Patil S, Goldberg J, Allen JB, Shaw S (1987) Infants with Down's syndrome. Use of cytogenetic studies and in vitro colony assays for granulocyte progenitors to distinguish acute non lymphocytic leukaemia from transient myeloproliferative disorder. Cancer 60: 987

De Waele M, Foulon W, Renmans W, Segers E, Smet L, Jochmann K, Van Camp B (1988) Hematologic values and lymphocyte subsets in fetal blood. Am J Clin Pathol 89: 742

Diamond LK, Wang WC, Alter BP (1976) Congenital hypoplastic anemia. Adv Pediatr 22: 349

Eguchi M, Sakakibara H, Suda J, Ozawa T, Hayashi Y, Sato T, Kojima S, Furukawa T (1989) Ultrastructural and ultracytochemical differences between transient myeloproliferative disorder and megakaryoblastic leukaemia in Down's syndrome. Br J Hematol 73: 315

Emanuel PD, Bates LJ, Shu SW, Castleberry RP, Gualtieri RJ, Zuckerman KS (1991) The role of monocyte-derived hemopoietic growth factors in the regulation of myeloproliferation in juvenile chronic myelogenous leukaemia. Exp Hematol 19: 1017

Fanconi G (1927) Familiäre infantile pernizioaartige Anämie. Jahrbuch Kinder 117: 257

Farquhar JW, Claireaux A (1952) Familial haemophagocytic reticulosis. Arch Dis Child 27: 519

Fernandez-Robles E, Vermylen C, Martiat P, Ninane J, Cornu G (1990) Familial essential thrombocytemia. Ped Hematol Oncol 7: 373

Finkelstein JZ, Erkert H, Issacs H Jr, Higgins G (1970) Bone marrow metastasis in children with solid tumours. Am J Dis Child 119: 49

Freedman MH, Estrov Z (1990) Congenital amegakaryocytic thrombocytopenia: an intrinsic hematopoietic stem cell defect. Am J Pediatr Hematol Oncol 12: 225

Freedman MH (1993) Pure red cell aplasia in childhood and adolescence: pathogenesis and approaches to diagnosis. Br J Haematol 85: 246

Fukuda T (1974) Fetal hemopoiesis. II. EM studies on human hepatic hemopoiesis. Virchows Arch B Cell Pathol 16: 249

Gilman PA, Jackson DP et al. (1970) Congenital agranulocytosis: prolonged survival and terminal acute leukaemia. Blood 36: 576

Gilmour JR (1941) Normal haemopoiesis in intrauterine and neonatal life. J Pathol Bacteriol 52: 25

Grottum KA, Hong TH, Holmsen H, Abrahamsen AF, Jeremic H, Seip M (1969) Wiskott–Aldrich syndrome: quantitative platelet defects and short platelet survival. Br J Haematol 17: 373

Guinan EC, Lee YS, Lopez KD, Kohler S, Oette DH, Bruno E, Kozakewich H, Nathan DG, Hoffman R (1993) Effects of interleukin-3 and granulocyte–macrophage colony-stimulating factor on thrombopoiesis in congenital amegakaryocytic thrombocytopenia. Blood 81: 1691

Hall JG (1987) Thrombocytopenia and absent radius syndrome. J Med Genet 24: 79

Harstock RJ, Smith EB, Petty CS (1965) Normal variations with aging of the amount of hematopoietic tissue in bone marrow from the anterior iliac crest. Am J Clin Pathol 43: 326

Hasle H, Brock Jacobson B, Tinggaard Pederson N (1992) Myelodysplastic syndromes in childhood: a population based study of nine cases. Br J Haematol 81: 495

Head DR, Kennedy PS, Goyette RE (1979) Metastatic neuroblastoma in bone marrow aspirate smears. Am J Clin Path 72: 1008

Henter JI, Elinder G (1991) Familial hemophagocytic lymphohistiocytosis. Clinical review based on the findings in seven children. Acta Paediatr Scand 80: 269

Henter JI, Elinder G, Öst A (1991) Diagnostic guidelines for hemophagocytic lymphohistiocytosis. The FHL Study Group of the Histiocyte Society. Semin Oncol 18: 29

Hines JD, Grasso JA (1970) The sideroblastic anemias. Semin Hematol 7: 86

Hoffman R (1991) Acquired pure amegakaryocytic thrombocytopenic purpura. Semin Hematol 28: 303

Jacobs A (1992) Gene mutation in myelodysplastic leukaemia. Res 16: 47

Kalpaktsoglou PK, Emery JL (1965) Human bone marrow during the last three months of intrauterine life. A histological study. Acta Haematol 34: 228

Keleman E, Calvo W (1982) Prenatal hematopoiesis in human bone marrow and its development antecedents. In: Trubowits S, Davids S (eds) The human bone marrow. CRC Press, Boca Raton

Keleman E, Calvo W, Fliedner TM (1979) Atlas of human hemopoietic development. Berlin, Springer Verlag

Koenig H, Lightsey A, Nelson D, Diamond L (1979) Immune suppression of erythropoiesis in transient erythroblastopenia of childhood. Blood 54: 742

Kostmann R (1956) Infantile genetic agranulocytosis. A review with presentation of ten new cases. Acta Paediatr Scand 64: 362

Lake AM, Stauffer JQ, Stuart MJ (1978) Hematostatic alterations in inflammatory bowel disease: response to therapy. Am J Dig Dis 23: 897

Lascari AD (1984) Malignant diseases. In: Lascari AD (ed) Hematologic manifestation of childhood diseases. Thieme-Straton, New York, p 335

le Beau MM, Albain KS, Larson RA (1986) Clinical and cytogenetic correlations in 63 patients with therapy-related myelodysplastic syndromes and acute non-lymphoblastic leukaemia. J Clin Oncol 4: 325

Lilleyman JS (1992) Disorders of platelets. I. Thrombocytopenia and thrombocytosis. In: Lilleyman JS, Hann IM (eds). Paediatric haematology. Churchill Livingstone, Edinburgh, p 148

Lilleymann JS, Hann IM (1992) Paediatric haematology. Churchill Livingstone, London

Longacre TA, Foucar K, Crago S, I-Ming C, Griffith B, Dressler L, McConnell TS, Duncan M, Gribole J (1989) Hematogones: a multiparameter analysis of bone marrow precursor cells. Blood 73: 543

McMullin MF, Chisholm M, Hows JM (1991) Congenital myelodysplasia: a newly described entity? Br J Haematol 79: 653

Medical Research Council (1986) Improvement in outlook for children with lymphoblastic leukaemia in the Britsch Islands. The MRC trial 1972–1985. Lancet i: 408

Moss TJ, Reynolds CP, Sather HN, Romansky SG, Hammond GD, Seeger RC (1991) Prognostic value of immunocytologic detection of bone marrow metastases in neuroblastoma. N Eng J Med 324: 219

Nathan DG, Oski FA (1993) Hematology of infancy and childhood, 4th edn. WB Saunders, Philadelphia

Nix WL, Fernbach DJ (1981) Myeloproliferative diseases in childhood. Am J Pediatr Hematol/Oncol 3: 397

O'Gorman-Hughes DW (1966) The varied pattern of aplastic anaemia in childhood Austr Paediatr J 2: 228

Pattison JR, Jones SE, Hodgson J, Davis LR, White JM, Stroud CE, Murtaza L (1981) Parvovirus infections and hypoplastic crises in sickle-cell anaemia. Lancet i: 644

Paul B, Reid MM, Davison EV, Abela M, Hamilton PJ (1987) Familial myelodysplasia: progressive disease associated with emergence of monosomy 7. Br J Haematol 65: 321

Pui CH, Behm FG, Raimondi SC, Dodge RK, Georgi SL, Rivera GK, Mirro J, Kalvinsky DK, Dahl GY, Murphy SB (1989) Secondary acute myeloid leukaemia in children treated for acute lymphoid leukaemia. N Engl J Med 321: 136

Quesenberry PJ (1991) The blueness of stem cells. Exp Hematol 19: 725

Reardon DA, Roskos R, Hanson CA, Castle V (1991) Virus-associated hemophagocytic syndrome following bone marrow transplantation. Am J Pediatr Hematol Oncol 13: 305

Rozman C, Vives-Corrons JL (1981) On the alleged diagnostic significance of megakaryocytic "phagocytosis" (emperipolesis). Br J Haematol 48: 510

Rubin CM, Arthur DC, Woods WG, Lange BJ, Nowell PC, Rowley JD, Nachman J, Bostrom B, Baum ES, Suarez CR et al. (1991) Therapy-related myelodysplastic syndrome and acute myeloid leukaemia in children: correlation between chromosomal abnormalities and prior therapy. Blood 78: 2982

Shwachman H, Diamond LK, Oski FA, Khaw AT (1964) The syndrome of pancreatic insufficiency and bone marrow dysfunction. J Pediatr 65: 645

Shannon KM, Watterson J, Johnson P, O'Connel P, Lange B, Shah N, Steinherz P, Kan YW (1992) Monosomy 7 myeloproliferative disease in children with neurofibromatosis, type 1: epidemiology and molecular analysis. Blood (US) 79: 1311

Shitara T, Yugami S, Sotomatu M, Oshima Y, Ijima H, Kuroume T (1991) Erythroleukaemia in a child associated with monosomy 7. Cancer 68: 540

Su IJ, Lin DT, Hsieh HC, Lee SH, Chen J, Chen RL, Lee CY, Chen JY (1990) Fatal primary Epstein–Barr virus infection masquerading as histiocytic medullary reticulosis in young children in Taiwan. Hematol Pathol 4: 189

Teasdale JM, Worth AJ, Corey MJ (1970) A missing group C chromosome in the bone marrow cells of three children with myeloproliferative disease. Cancer 25: 1468

Thomas GA, O'Brien RT (1986) Thrombocytosis in children with *Haemophilus influenzae* meningitis. Clin Pediatr 25: 610

Trimble MS, Glynn MF, Brain MC (1991) Amegakaryocytic thrombocytopenia of 4 years duration: successful treatment with antithymocyte globulin. Am J Hematol 37: 126

Tsai PH, Arkin S, Lipton JM (1989) An intrinsic progenitor defect in Diamond–Blackfan anaemia. Br J Haematol 73: 112

Tuncer MA, Pagliuca A, Hicsonmez G, Yetgin S, Ozsoylu S, Mufti GJ (1992) Primary myelodysplastic syndrome in children: the clinical experience in 33 cases. Br J Haematol 82: 347

Vora AJ, Lilleyman JS (1993) Secondary thrombocytosis. Arch Dis Child 68: 88

Williams EC, Shahidi NT (1991) Benign familial thrombocytosis. Am J Hematol 37: 124

Wiskott A (1937) Familiärer, angeborener Morbus Werlhofii? Monatsschr Kinderheilk 68: 212

Wolach B, Morag H, Drucker M, Sadan N (1990) Thrombocytosis after pneumonia with empyema and other bacterial infections in children. Pediatr Infect Dis J 9: 718

Xue Y, Zhang R, Guo Y, Gu J, Lin B (1993) Acquired amegakaryocytic thrombocytopenic purpura with a Philadelphia chromosome. Cancer Genet Cytogenet 69: 51

13 · Endocrine Pathology

Christopher L. Brown

Adrenal Cortex

Development

The cortical tissue of the adrenals arises in the posterior coelomic mesoderm close to the genital ridge and can be identified at the 10 mm stage (6th week). At birth their combined weights average 6.5 g, with the bulk of this relatively large mass comprising a specific fetal cortical zone. This is composed of masses of large eosinophil cells that show ultrastructural characteristics similar to those of the adult adrenal cortex. The definitive cortex forms a sharply contrasting narrow zone of small cortical-type cells beneath the gland capsule. Degenerative involution of the fetal cortex starts at or shortly before birth and is virtually complete within the first few months of postnatal life, although remnants may occasionally be found up to the end of the first year. The definitive cortex shows conspicuous evidence of growth by the 4th day after birth, and the zona glomerulosa and zona faciculata are defined by the 6th week. As a result of involution of the fetal zone the combined weights decrease from birth to an average of 3.5 g at 3 months, after which they increase steadily in size in relation to body weight to reach 6 g at about 12 years of age. The normal development of both the fetal and the definitive cortex is to a large extent dependent on normal hypothalamic and pituitary function because the fetal zone is found to be markedly reduced and the definitive cortex less conspicuously so in cases of anencephaly (Fig. 13.1). Similar failure of development of the rat adrenal can be induced experimentally by destruction of the hypothalamus. The fetal zone is observed to be of increased size in babies born to mothers with diabetes mellitus and in postmaturity.

During intrauterine development the cells of the definitive cortex appear undifferentiated on electron microscopy; those of the fetal zone are large and are active in steroid synthesis. The factors involved in the maintenance and control of the fetal cortex remain uncertain. There is a close functional link between the placenta and the adrenals, the latter producing oestrogen and androgen precursors by removal of a two-carbon side-chain from placental progesterone, a step requiring 17-hydroxylase and desmolase, which the placenta lacks.

Developmental Abnormalities

Absence of one adrenal gland is rare. Failure of both glands to develop probably occurs only in examples of congenital monsters (Benirschke et al. 1956). Occasionally one or both glands are misplaced and are then usually found still related to the urogenital tract. An adrenal has been discovered, well formed, within the skull (Wiener and Dallgaard 1959). Such misplaced glands are usually well organized into the various zones, and the medulla is found separately near the upper renal pole. Ectopic islands of cortical tissue are commonly found adjacent to the main gland, in the retroperitoneal tissues, in the capsule of the liver and kidneys, and in the vicinity of the testes and ovaries. Such islands may become enlarged and prominent in conditions of diffuse hyperplasia of the adrenal cortex, and have been responsible for relapse in some cases of Cushing's disease treated by adrenalectomy.

Congenital hypoplasia is rare but may affect several members in a single family. Two major types are recognized (Kerenyi 1961). In the first the adren-

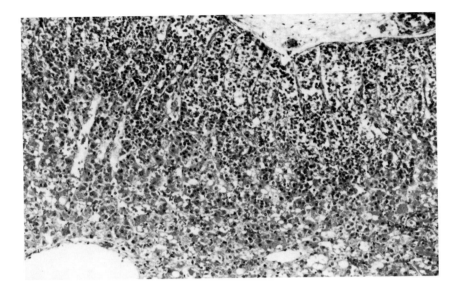

Fig. 13.1. Adrenal from an anencephalic stillborn female. The combined weight of the two glands was 0.2 g. The fetal cortical zone seen in the *lower half* of the picture is greatly reduced, appearing similar in thickness to the definitive cortex. (H&E, × 120)

als are small and similar in detail to those seen in anencephaly (see below). Accompanying abnormalities involving aplasia or hypoplasia of the pituitary and maldevelopment involving the hypothalamus are usually found. In occasional cases of adrenal hypoplasia of anencephalic type the hypothalamus and pituitary appear to be normal, and the small adrenals may reflect their unresponsiveness to trophic hormone. In the second type, with primary congenital adrenocortical hypoplasia, the adrenal cortex is disorganized and consists of clusters of large pleomorphic cells that may reach 100 μm in diameter. Their cytoplasm is eosinophilic and vacuolated and their nuclei are hyperchromatic, some being very large, and often show "inclusions" of invaginated cytoplasm (Fig. 13.2) (Borit and Kosek 1969; Oppenheimer 1970). This "cytomegaly" is accompanied by electron microscopic appearances that suggest cellular activity (Borit and Kosek 1969; Oppenheimer 1970). The pituitary and hypothalamus appear normal. The condition is inherited as an X-linked recessive trait (Weiss and Mellinger 1970). In both types the adrenal medulla is uninvolved, though in some of the cytomegalic cases it may be formed into several islands.

Evidence of adrenal insufficiency is earlier and more severe in the anencephalic type. With better recognition of neonatal "salt-losing" syndromes and

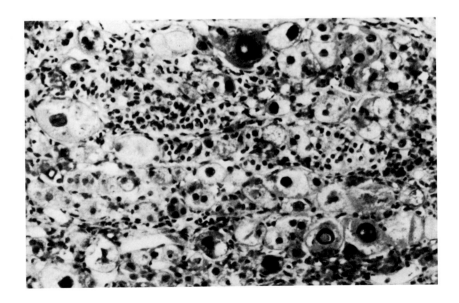

Fig. 13.2. Cytomegaly involving a high proportion of the cells of the fetal adrenal cortex. The enlargement involves both nucleus and cytoplasm, and large infoldings of the nuclear membrane are common, resulting in apparent nuclear inclusions. (H&E, × 240)

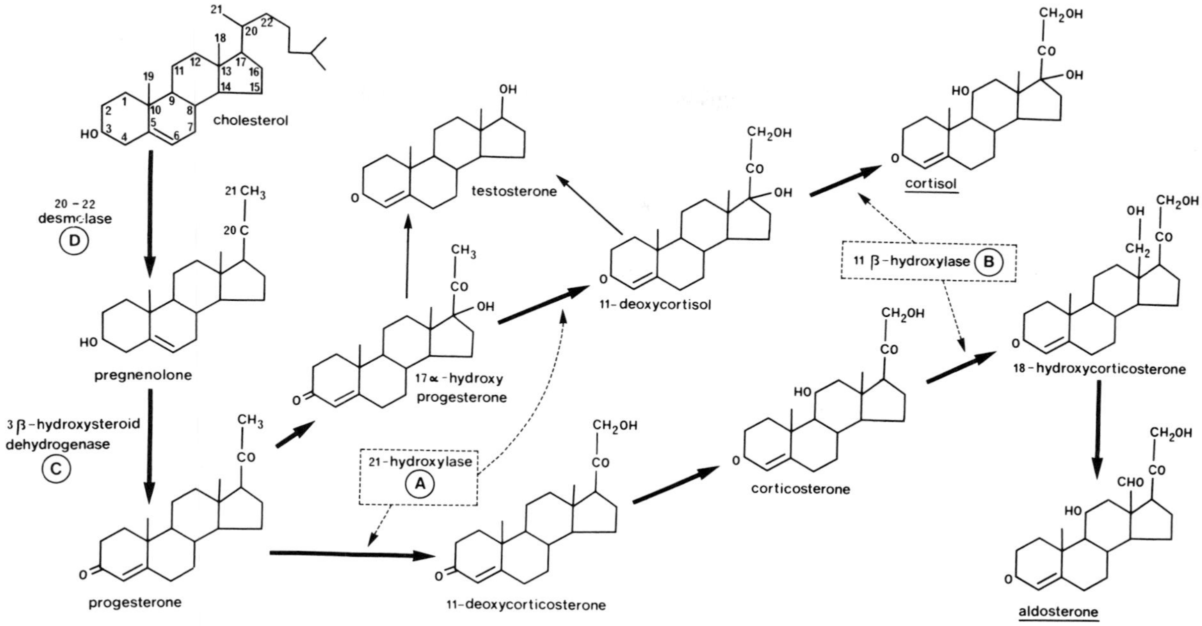

Fig. 13.3. Schematic representation of the major pathways for the synthesis of cortisol and aldosterone. The points at which enzyme defects are most commonly involved in the syndromes of congenital adrenal hyperplasia are indicated (*A, B, C* and *D*).

the possibility of successful treatment, occasional cases of congenital adrenal insufficiency are being recorded in whom associated gonadotrophin deficiency has become apparent (Black et al. 1977; Kelly et al. 1977; Marek 1977). Adrenal cytomegaly is not limited to cases of idiopathic hypoplasia. Similar changes are seen in occasional cells of the fetal zone in normal infants and have been observed in the adrenals in 1% of infants stillborn or dying in the neonatal period (Kohler 1963). Favara et al. (1991) observed adrenal cytomegaly in 0.8% of 2711 paediatric autopsies and found similar changes in cells of the pancreatic islets and acini and in the anterior pituitary. They suggest that the changes are in response to physiological demand. In the Beckwith–Wiedemann syndrome there is extensive cytomegaly in the fetal zone (Wiedemann 1964; Beckwith 1969), and in some cases of autoimmune Addison's disease the surviving cortical cells may appear similar.

In anencephaly adrenal development has been noted to be normal up to the 20th gestational week. The fetal zone then involutes prematurely and the definitive cortex remains smaller than normal, so that at birth the combined weight of the two glands is commonly about 1 g, with the definitive cortex contributing the greater part of the mass. Similar changes were found in the adrenals of five of 25 infants with hydrocephalus (Benirschke et al. 1956).

Congenital Hyperplasia

Lack of specific enzymes involved in the synthesis of steroid hormones (Fig. 13.3) underlies a group of abnormalities inherited as autosomal recessive diseases in which impaired cortisol production is accompanied by enormous adrenal cortical hyperplasia (Fig. 13.4) and formation of large quantities of alternative steroid hormones and their precursors. The resulting clinical picture depends on the severity of the particular enzyme defect, which is consistent in any one pedigree, and its position in the chain of reactions leading to the synthesis of the various hormones. The incidence of these disorders varies greatly in different communities, and for the commonest types has been estimated as 1 in 67 000 births in Maryland (Childs et al. 1956), whereas in an Alaskan Eskimo tribe the incidence is about 1 in 500 (Hirschfield and Fleshman 1969).

21-Hydroxylase Deficiency, 11b-Hydroxylase Deficiency and 3b-Hydroxysteroid Dehydrogenase Deficiency

21-Hydroxylase deficiency accounts for about 90% of cases and occurs as a severe salt-losing form and a less severe virilizing form. In the latter form the

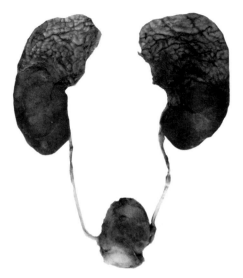

Fig. 13.4. Congenital adrenal hyperplasia. Male aged 14 weeks. Post-mortem specimen showing bilateral extreme diffuse adrenal cortical hyperplasia with characteristic wrinkling of the cortical layers.

increased stimulation of the adrenals results in adequate cortisol output but only at the cost of greatly increased production of the precursor 17α-hydroxyprogesterone, which is converted to testosterone and the excretory product pregnanetriol. There is evidence that the disturbed steroid synthesis is established as early as week 9 of gestation (Kelley et al. 1952), and the consequence of the increased levels of testosterone is virilization of the fetus, resulting in female pseudohermaphrodites and macrogenitosomia praecox in males. Whereas the effects on a female fetus are clinically obvious it appears that a proportion of the less severely affected male infants go unrecognized. If untreated the hormonal imbalance produces somatic changes. Linear growth is accelerated and muscular development increased. Skeletal maturation is even more advanced, however, so that early fusion of the epiphyses results in a reduced final height. Growth of pubic hair may occur as early as 2 years of age, followed by the appearance of axillary, facial and body hair in masculine distribution. Gonadal maturation may be inhibited, the small testes contrasting with the penile development in boys, and breast development and menstruation failing to occur in girls.

The salt-losing form is a little less common than the pure virilizing form, accounting for about one-third of all cases. The more severe defect is accompanied by deficient aldosterone production, but the precise mechanism involved in this further defect is still not understood. The impaired renal salt conservation manifests clinically about the 8th to 10th postnatal day in most cases, but may sometimes be delayed until the end of the 2nd month. The manifestations resemble acute Addisonian crisis, with vomiting, diarrhoea, dehydration and circulatory insufficiency. Without steroid therapy deterioration is rapid and death may occur.

11β-Hydroxylase deficiency is the second commonest cause of congenital adrenal hyperplasia, but even so accounts for only about 5% of cases. There is an increase in 11-deoxy precursors of cortisol, the most important of which is 11-deoxycorticosterone, its strong mineralocorticoid effects resulting in hypertension. There is also excess production of androgens and consequent virilization.

3β-Hydroxysteroid dehydrogenase deficiency affects a very early step in steroid hormone synthesis, affecting cortisol and aldosterone production and allowing formation of only weak androgenic steroids. There is a severe salt-losing syndrome, in most cases without virilization, and many patients die despite full replacement therapy.

In all three, the gross and histological changes in the adrenals are similar. The high levels of pituitary ACTH result in hyperplasia of compact cells, which expand the zona reticularis, with only occasional lipid-containing cells forming the small peripheral zona fasciculata. Large bizarre cortical cells can occur and reflect the high level of cell function. The zona glomerulosa is variously described as increased or decreased in size. The medulla is normal. The weight of each gland averages 15 g, (compared with the normal weight in children of 1.5–3 g). When untreated they are brown in colour; their size continues to increase and they may exceed 30 g in weight. Multiple nodules may develop.

Congenital Lipid Hyperplasia

Congenital lipid hyperplasia is a very rare fourth type of congenital hyperplasia, which produces different appearances in the adrenals. There is a deficiency of 20–22 desmolase, so that conversion of cholesterol to pregnenolone cannot proceed, with consequent impairment of the information of all steroid hormones, including those formed in the gonads. Each gland may exceed 3 g in weight; the enlarged cortex is pale, disorganized and nodular, composed mostly of large lipid filled cells; and there may be deposits of cholesterol. Because virilizing hormones cannot be synthesized, the genital tract in affected male fetuses develops towards the female type (Siebenmann 1957).

Wolman's disease

Wolman's disease is a primary familial xanthomatosis in which the adrenals, among other organs, are involved and appear enlarged with calcification in the inner cortex (Wolman et al. 1961). There is no substantial evidence of functional deficiency (Marshall et al. 1969). (See also pp. 645, 840, 845)

Acquired Adrenocortical Insufficiency

Haemorrhage into the adrenals is seen commonly in newborn infants and is related to prematurity, birth trauma and asphyxia. From their findings at autopsy, de Sa and Nicholls (1972) observed an incidence of 1.7 per 1000 in perinatal deaths. Minor lesions do not cause adrenal insufficiency, but massive haemorrhage may result in acute adrenocortical insufficiency. Calcification is a common secondary change in these lesions. Focal cortical necroses with or without haemorrhage may be found complicating bacterial and viral infections. Haemorrhage into the adrenals sometimes occurs in cases of leukaemia and other bleeding disorders and into metastatic tumour deposits.

Iatrogenic adrenal atrophy is a risk in long-term steroid treatment, and Busuttil (1991) warns of the hazard of subclinical atrophy, having observed its occurrence in two asthmatic children treated since infancy with pulsed steroid inhalers.

Waterhouse–Friderichsen Syndrome

The term "Waterhouse–Friderichsen syndrome" should be reserved for cases that conform to the classic clinical and pathological picture of this well defined condition. The illness is abrupt in onset, with rapid appearance of shock and cyanosis, usually with an accompanying petechial rash (Fig. 13.5). Often, despite prompt treatment, death occurs within 6–24 h. Most cases occur in previously healthy children and young adults as a complication of septicaemia, usually involving *Neisseria meningitidis*. Cases have been described with infection by *Haemophilus influenzae* or pneumococci, and in association with varicella. At autopsy both adrenals are found to be greatly expanded by haemorrhage into the central cortex (Fig. 13.6). The exact causal mechanism of the haemorrhage remains uncertain. Experimentally the lesion can be induced in heparinized animals, suggesting that thrombosis of the vascular sinuses and disseminated intravascular coagulation are not

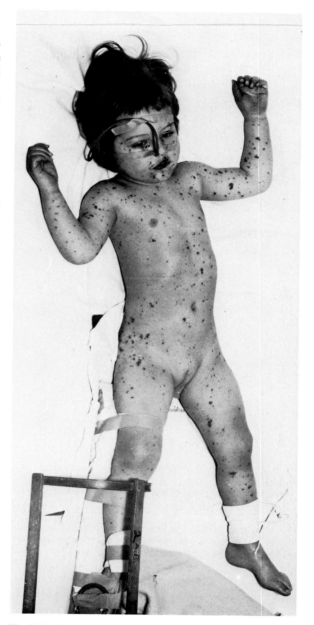

Fig. 13.5. Female aged 3 years. Haemorrhagic rash accompanying meningococcal septicaemia.

primary events. It may be a direct effect of bacterial toxins acting on the stimulated highly vascular gland (Levin and Cluff 1965). Although the syndrome was originally thought to be the result of acute adrenocortical failure, this has not been substantiated. Occasional clinically typical cases have been described in which the adrenals have been normal at autopsy (Hardman

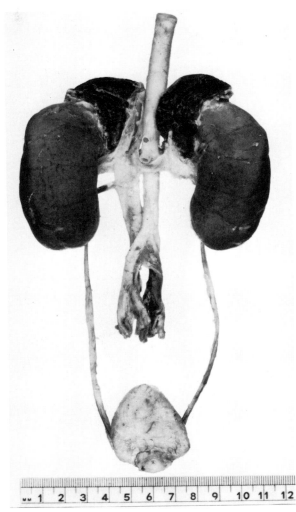

Fig. 13.6. Post-mortem specimen from a girl aged 2 years who died of meningococcal septicaemia with bilateral adrenal haemorrhages (Waterhouse–Friderichsen syndrome).

1968), and in cases that recover adrenal function is usually found to be normal.

Cystic Change in the Definitive Cortex

The appearance of multiple small cysts in the definitive cortex has repeatedly been observed at autopsy in some stillborn fetuses and cases of perinatal death, and has usually been regarded as part of normal development. The studies of Oppenheimer (1969), however, suggest that prematurity and fetal infection are important predisposing factors, and that the changes are the result of focal cortical cell degeneration as a consequence of intrauterine stress.

Addison's Disease

Chronic adrenal insufficiency in childhood is uncommon. In infants it can result from congenital hypoplasia and in some cases follows haemorrhage and calcification in the adrenals. Most other cases are seen in later childhood and adolescence, sometimes from infection by the tubercle bacillus or *Histoplasma capsulatum*, but more often from acquired atrophy. This is usually the result of autoimmune adrenalitis, as originally suggested by Anderson et al. (1957). Not only are circulating antibodies to adrenal cortical cells frequently present, but in some cases there are manifestations of autoimmune diseases involving other endocrine organs, when the total condition is referred to as autoimmune polyendocrinopathy. A history of involvement of other family members with varying combinations of endocrine disturbances is usually found in these cases, and in addition tissues outside the defined endocrine glands may be involved, most notably with resulting pernicious anaemia, areas of cutaneous vitiligo, and sometimes loss of all hair. In cases presenting with these other autoimmune diseases circulating antibodies to adrenal cortex may be present without clinical or laboratory evidence of deficient adrenal function (Blizzard et al. 1962).

In the cases resulting from tuberculous infection the adrenals are almost totally destroyed and enlarged, consisting of central necrotic material and a peripheral inflammatory zone. The infective process does not usually extend beyond the adrenal capsule. There may be extensive calcification in old lesions. In the autoimmune cases the glands are very small and may be misshapen. In some instances no adrenal tissue can be found. Microscopically, there are islands of large eosinophilic compact-type cells surrounded by the collapsed vascular reticulin framework of the original cortex, but no fibrosis. There may be a moderate lymphoid infiltration with some involvement of the medulla, which is otherwise normal.

Cushing's Syndrome

Cushing syndrome is rare in children and more often results from a functioning adrenal adenoma or carcinoma than from pituitary-driven adrenocortical hyperplasia. More than three-quarters of cases occur in females. Clinical manifestations vary largely, according to the underlying cause. In most cases there is some degree of virilization, and if this is marked there is usually associated carcinoma. When andorgenic steroid effects are dominant accelerated muscular and skeletal development are prominent,

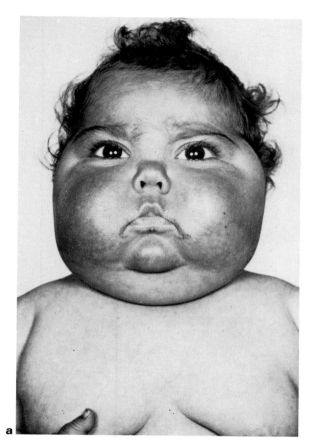 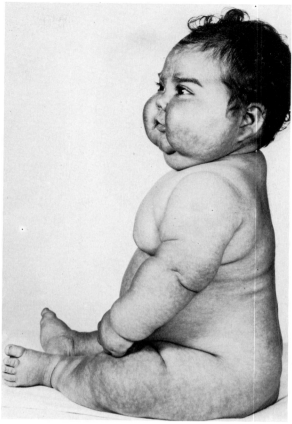

Fig. 13.7. Florid clinical features of Cushing's syndrome due to an adrenal carcinoma in a male infant aged 14 months.

which is in contrast to the findings in cases where cortisol effects dominate. In these more usual cases of Cushing's syndrome obesity with the classic truncal, shoulder and face distribution, impairment of linear growth and osteopenia are the major effects and are regularly associated with acne, hirsutism and a flushed face to produce a highly typical clinical picture (Fig. 13.7). Glucose intolerance is nearly always demonstrable, and there may be symptomatic diabetes. A diastolic blood pressure above 90 mmHg is found in the majority of cases. Adolescent girls usually have amenorrhoea. "Pure" Cushing's syndrome, in which the virilizing effects are not seen, is usually due to an adenoma or primary adrenocortical nodular dysplasia (see below). Occasional tumours, usually carcinomas, are oestrogen-producing and give rise to feminization and abnormal uterine bleeding in young girls; in adolescent boys there may be testicular atrophy and gynaecomastia. Most cases show some acne and growth of sex hair. Aldosterone-producing tumours are particularly rare, and non-functioning carcinomas are also uncommon.

Adrenal cortical tumours associated with Cushing's syndrome occur in all age groups. Adenomas are rounded, encapsulated, firm and pale or brownish, with patches of yellow lipid. They vary in size, usually weighing less than 50 g and rarely exceeding 100 g. Their cells are recognizable as adrenal cortical and are arranged in columns and solid nests separated by a delicate vascular network. The cytoplasm is eosinophilic, like that of the cells of the normal adrenal reticularis, and may contain obvious lipofuscin in pigmented tumours. The nuclei are large, and pleomorphic and bizarre forms are common. These strikingly abnormal nucleated cells may be grouped in well defined areas in the tumour. Clusters of small and large clear cells correspond to the visible lipid-rich patches. Occasional mitoses may be found. There is atrophy of the cortex of both adrenal glands, and the brown zona reticularis is barely visible on the cut surface.

An adrenal cortical carcinoma is the commonest cause of Cushing's syndrome in childhood, being recorded in up to three-quarters of cases, although a lower proportion may be more appropriate (Neville

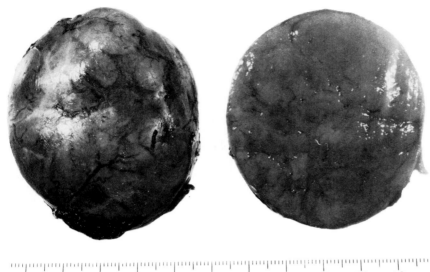

a

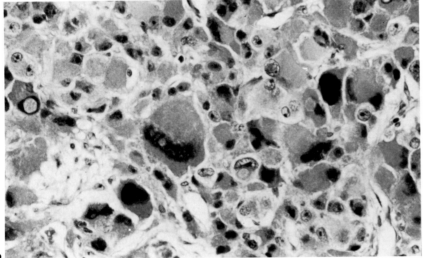

b

Fig. 13.8. a External and cut surfaces of an adrenal tumour weighing 84 g, removed from an 11-year-old girl with mixed Cushing's syndrome. The cut surface is solid and evenly tan coloured with no visible lipid-rich areas. **b** An area of bizarre compact-type adrenal cortical cells from the same tumour. Such cytological changes are not an indication of malignancy. (H&E, × 300)

and Symington 1972). The history in these cases is usually shorter, and features of virilization are more prominent. The tumours (Fig. 13.8a) are soft and lobulated, with a pale or brownish cut surface. Most weigh more than 100 g, occasional cases reaching a very large size. Evidence of malignancy may be obvious from the finding of metastases in local lymph nodes and vascular invasion, but on purely histological grounds their recognition is uncertain more often than not. Apart from the larger size, other findings suggesting malignancy are the presence of areas of necrosis, broad traversing fibrous bands, a diffuse growth pattern, marked disproportionate nuclear enlargement, the presence of monster cells (often with multiple nuclei), numerous mitoses and clinical weight loss (Hough et al. 1979). It is well for the pathologist to bear in mind that metastasizing tumours that appear histologically innocent have been described, and that benign endocrine tumours may show marked nuclear pleomorphism and mitotic activity. All large adrenal cortical tumours should be regarded with suspicion. In carcinomas the cells are mostly of the compact type, with few and scattered lipid-containing cells (Fig. 13.8b).

Occasional cases of pure Cushing's syndrome are described, usually in girls, with onset in later childhood and into early adulthood, in which both adrenals contain numerous pigmented nodules up to 3 mm in diameter throughout a shrunken yellow cortex. The combined weights of the glands have varied from well below to somewhat above normal. The nodules consist of large, pigmented, compact cells with small nuclei, and are sharply demarcated from the rest of the cortex but are not encapsulated. The residual cortex is described as atrophic and composed of clear cells, and in some cases it shows a focal lymphocytic infiltrate. The zoning of the cortex is preserved and the medulla is normal. The condition was identified and described as primary adrenocortical nodular dysplasia by Meador et al. (1967), and was further described by Ruder et al. (1974). Occurrence of the condition in families has also been described (Arce et al. 1978; Donaldson et al. 1981; Schweizer–Cagianut et al. 1982). Corticotrophin is undetectable, and the abnormality appears to be a primary disturbance of the adrenal cortex. It must be distinguished from nodularity in bilateral diffuse adrenal cortical hyperplasia.

Pituitary-driven bilateral adrenocortical hyperplasia accounts for about 35% of childhood Cushing's syndrome, mostly in adolescents and only very rarely before the age of 8 years (Neville and Symington 1972). These authors found that the weights of the adrenal glands usually fell within the normal adult range (4.0–6.0 each). In all cases, however, there is clear histological evidence of hyperplasia (Fig. 13.9). Compact cells of zona reticularis type occupy from one-third to one-half the thickness of the cortex, forming a well defined regular inner band. The zona glomerulosa is conspicuous, with frequent short columns of cells projecting down into the outer zona fasciculata. Microscopic nodules composed of clear cells are found related to the central vein and at the periphery of the cortex. In occasional cases multiple nodules ranging from a few millimetres to 2 cm in diameter may be visible throughout the cortex. The glands in such cases may be much heavier and of markedly unequal size. Histologically the intervening cortex shows diffuse hyperplasia, with the zona reticularis occupying about half the cortical thickness. The nodules usually consist of small compact cells with prominent nuclei.

Almost all cases of Cushing's syndrome in which bilateral adrenal cortical hyperplasia is present are the result of excessive pituitary ACTH secretion (true Cushing's disease), which is characteristically found at a constant concentration in the blood throughout the 24 h rather than at a clearly abnormal elevated level on any single estimation. Recent experience gained from the treatment of cases of Cushing's disease by pituitary microsurgical techniques shows that a pituitary adenoma, often very small, is found in almost every case. The removal of the adenoma is accompanied by cure of the disease and eventual return of normal hypothalamic–pituitary–adrenal

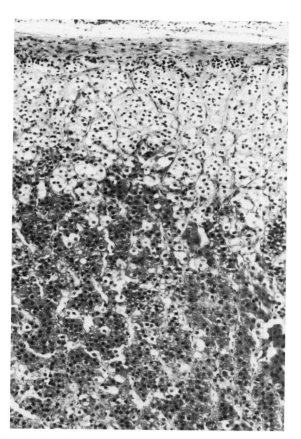

Fig. 13.9. Diffuse adrenal cortical hyperplasia in Cushing's disease. The darkly staining compact cells of the zona reticularis (*below*) have expanded to fill the inner three-quarters of the thickened cortex. The zona glomerulosa forms a distinct narrow band of small clear cells beneath the capsule. The combined weight of the two adrenals was 16.1 g. They were removed from a male aged 15 years who had probably been suffering from Cushing's disease for the preceding 6 years. At the time of treatment clinical features were obvious and severe osteoporosis had resulted in loss of height. (H&E, × 120)

function without loss of other pituitary functions (Salassa et al. 1978; Tyrrell et al. 1978; Fahlbusch et al. 1986). This is the only form of treatment that regularly achieves complete cure, and constitutes strong evidence that the primary abnormality is a pituitary tumour in most cases, rather than a functional hypothalamic disturbance. Radiological evidence of an abnormal pituitary fossa prior to treatment is found in a minority of cases, but following treatment by adrenal ablation Hopwood and Kenny (1977) found increasing pigmentation in 18 and enlargement of the pituitary fossa in eight (Nelson's syndrome) of 31 children treated for Cushing's disease from 1 to $5\frac{1}{2}$ years previously. This is a much higher incidence of this complication than is recorded in adults similarly treated. Very good results can be obtained from the treatment of childhood Cushing's disease with pituitary irradiation, without the risk of occurrence of Nelson's syndrome (Jennings et al. 1977).

The adenomas found in the pituitary in cases of Cushing's syndrome are mostly basophil or chromophobe, and sometimes mixed. Rarely an acidophil tumour is found. In Nelson's syndrome the tumour enlarges progressively and tends to infiltrate surrounding structures. This is sometimes regarded as evidence of malignant change, but although pulmonary metastases have been described the tumours do not usually appear less well differentiated histologically. The corticotrophs in the pituitary gland show Crooke's hyaline change in all cases of active Cushing's syndrome from whatever cause. The cells of a basophil adenoma when present do not show the change.

The rarest form of Cushing's syndrome in children is seen when bilateral adrenal cortical hyperplasia results from ACTH secretion by a non-pituitary tumour. Eleven cases of tumours in children with evidence of ectopic ACTH production are recorded in the review by Omenn (1971). Tumours of neuroblast origin form the largest group and almost all of the remainder are accounted for by tumours of the thymus, pancreatic islets and anaplastic carcinoma of the lung. Medullary carcinoma of the thyroid has also been noted in this context (Williams et al. 1968).

Virilizing Tumours

Virilizing adrenal cortical tumours without features of Cushing's syndrome are more common in children than in adults, and practically all the examples described in males have been in children. More than three-quarters of cases occur in females, and carcinomas account for a similarly large majority. The contralateral adrenal is atrophic in less than 30% of cases, an indication that most of these tumours produce insignificant amounts of cortisol. The anabolic effects of the androgens prevent the growth inhibition and muscle wasting caused by cortisol when present in excess, so that clinically there is precocious growth and muscular development in addition to virilization. Virilizing tumours usually consist exclusively of compact-type cells with eosinophilic granular cytoplasm. Distinction between benign and malignant tumours on histological grounds is often difficult (see p. 688). Virilization in a male child is also seen in late-onset congenital adrenal cortical hyperplasia, interstitial tumours of the testis, true precocious puberty and gonadotrophin-secreting tumours. An androgen-secreting ovarian stromal tumour is a rare cause in females.

Feminizing Tumours

Feminizing adrenal cortical tumours are very rare in children, and although such tumours are in general mostly carcinomas a relatively high proportion in children are adenomas (Gabrilove et al. 1965). Their gross and microscopic features are not specifically different from those of other functioning adrenal tumours. In a girl, distinction from true precocious puberty and from an oestrogen-producing ovarian tumour must be made.

Non-functioning Tumours and Hypoglycaemia

Adrenal cortical carcinomas that show no evidence of hormone production are very rare in children. Occasional large tumours have been associated with episodes of spontaneous hypoglycaemia. In the case involving a girl of 16 recorded by Scholz et al. (1967) immunoreactive insulin was undetectable in the blood during hypoglycaemia, and insulin-like activity could not be detected. The relationship of hypoglycaemia and adrenal carcinoma is complicated because in some cases the tumour has been a part of the Beckwith–Wiedemann syndrome, in which pancreatic islet hyperplasia occurs (Weinstein et al. 1970).

Aldosteronism

Aldosteronism is rare in children. Males are affected more often, and symptoms are typically severe and can usually be traced to infancy (New and Petwood 1966). The commonest change in the adrenals is cortical hyperplasia, often with multiple cortical nodules composed of large clear cells of zona fasciculata type. Grim et al. (1967) discuss nine cases under the age of 18 years, including one case of their own. Seven were in males, the youngest aged 9 years. The adrenals were described as hyperplastic in six cases and nodular in three. In the remaining three the adrenals were thought to be normal. Three reported cases of Conn's adenoma in children aged from 3 to 15 years are quoted by New and Petwood (1966).

Adrenal Medulla and Paraganglia

The adrenal medulla and the extra-adrenal chromaffin tissue differentiate from stem cells (sympathicogonia) of neural crest ectodermal origin. Sympathicogonia migrate laterally in the dorsal wall off the coelom to reach the area of the adrenal mesenchyme by the 6th gestational week. Clusters of these migrant cells penetrate to a central position in the adrenal mesenchyme through the succeeding week, with additional small numbers of cells continuing to arrive through most of the period of gestation. Differentiation of the adrenal medullary sympathicogonia to form chromaffin cells is slow and mostly occurs in early postnatal life, normally being complete by the end of the third year. Groups of primitive cells, sometimes forming rosettes, may be found related to the adrenal vein in neonatal infants. Large collections are not uncommon and have been regarded as localized neuroblastomas (Guin et al. 1969; see also p. 869). Sympathicogonia outside the adrenal differentiate into the paraganglial chromaffin tissue. This matures quickly and is most prominent during intrauterine and early postnatal life, principally in relation to the abdominal aorta. The largest of these masses develops at the end of the second gestational month and forms the para-aortic organ of Zuckerkandle, a paired body found at the level of the origin of the inferior mesenteric artery. The extra-adrenal chromaffin tissue involutes as the adrenal medulla develops and is no longer visible by the time of puberty.

Non-chromaffin paraganglial tissue forming autonomic structures related to vessels, nerves and other tissues is widely distributed. Well defined paraganglia include the carotid bodies, glomus jugulare and aortic (arch) body. The principal cells of these structures have been shown to contain electron-dense granules 100–200 nm in diameter, similar to those found in adrenal phaeochromocytes, and some show formalin-induced cytoplasmic fluorescence, indicating the presence of catecholamine. These features are strong evidence in support of the view that the cells of these structures originate from the neural crest. This has been directly confirmed in the case of the carotid body in the chick (Le Dourain et al. 1972).

The systems of chromaffin and non-chromaffin tissues are clinically important because of the tumours that may develop, often as a part of genetically determined syndromes that also involve hyperplasia in the affected structures.

Conventionally the simple neoplasms are neuroblastoma and its maturing derivatives, phaeochromocytoma and paraganglioma. On the basis of the unifying concept of the neurocristopathies this list can be extended to include carcinoid tumours, medullary carcinoma of the thyroid, at least some tumours of pancreatic islet cells, and anterior pituitary and melanotic progonoma of the jaw. Many of these are described in detail elsewhere.

Phaeochromocytoma

Phaeochromocytomas are rare tumours that occur sporadically and in familial clusters consistent with an autosomal dominant mode of inheritance (Carman and Brashear 1960). Most are found in the adrenal, but they may occur wherever chromaffin tissue is located. Most extra-adrenal tumours are found in the abdomen along the sympathetic chain, but occasional cases have been recorded in the neck, mediastinum and urinary bladder. There is a preponderance in males and in the right adrenal. In children the incidence of bilateral adrenal tumours is higher than the 10% recorded in adults (Hume 1960), at least in part as a consequence of the relatively high proportion of genetically determined cases seen at this age. They are only very rarely malignant. Clinical manifestations are the result of the release from the tumour of large amounts of catecholamines into the blood. Adrenal phaeochromocytomas usually produce both adrenaline and noradrenaline, whereas in extra-adrenal tumours noradrenaline alone is the principal product. In children hypertension is usually sustained rather than paroxysmal, and when severe may produce retinopathy. Noradrenaline-induced cardiomyopathy can occur, producing hypotensive heart failure. Glucose intolerance may produce symptomatic diabetes mellitus, and weight loss with glocysuria may lead to diagnostic confusion. A large number of cases in children have been reviewed by Stackpole et al. (1963).

The tumours are usually well circumscribed and rounded, and they vary greatly in size, from only a few grams to a kilogram. Figure 13.10 shows an adrenal phaeochromocytoma. The cut surface is grey-brown with haemorrhagic areas, and in parts is often cystic. Fixation of fresh tissue in a chromate–bichromate mixture produces a brown reaction product with the contained catecholamines, and is important in confirmation of the diagnosis. Microscopically there is some resemblance to the normal adrenal medulla, with groups of large cells with basophilic granular cytoplasm surrounded by a delicate vascular network. In bichromate-fixed tissue the cytoplasm of many of the tumour cells is coloured brown, and "lakes" of brown pigment are commonly concentrated in the connective tissue around larger vessels. Tumour nuclei are mostly uniform, but scattered large and sometimes bizarre hyperchromatic forms are very typically present. Mitoses are usually difficult to find. Histological recognition of the rare malignant tumour is not possible (Fig. 13.11), and in interpretation of multiple masses of phaeochromocytoma as evidence of malignancy the commoner occurrence of multiple independent tumours must be borne in mind. Good evidence of malignancy is the finding of multiple

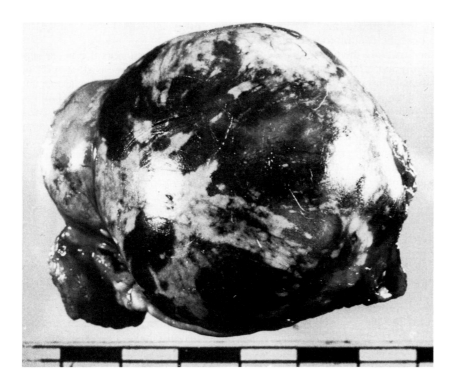

Fig. 13.10. Adrenal phaeochromocytoma weighing 60 g and forming a soft lobulated deep red tumour. The pale areas on the surface represent adrenal cortex. The bulk of the adrenal gland projects from the *lower left* surface of the tumour

deposits in unusual sites for chromaffin tissue. Ultrastructural studies show numerous cytoplasmic electron-dense granules 130–270 nm in size that represent the site of catecholamine storage and correspond to the granules seen on light microscopy. In addition, the electron microscope demonstrates two cells populations, light and dark, but this is apparently unrelated to any functional difference.

The diagnosis of phaeochromocytoma depends on the demonstration of excessive levels of circulating catecholamines in the blood and abnormal amounts of their metabolites in 24 h urine specimens. Ectopic hormone production has been described, including ACTH, erythropoeitin, prostaglandins, and possibly a parathormone-like substance.

Study of the ultrastructure of neuroblastomas, non-chromaffin paragangliomas, and melanotic progonomas shows electron-dense neurosecretory granules in greater or lesser numbers. Catecholamine production occurs in a large proportion of neuroblastomas, with resulting hypertension in up to 10% of cases. Paragangliomas are generally regarded as non-functioning, but occasional cases have been associated with hypertension and increased urinary catecholamine excretion (Weichert 1970). One patient with a melanotic progonoma has been reported, in whom elevated catecholamine excretion was recorded. The characteristics of carcinoid tumours relating to their embryological origins have been set out by Williams and Sandler (1963), and their varied endocrine potential is recorded by Weichert (1970).

Pancreatic Islets

The pancreatic islets are shown to differentiate from cells of pancreatic duct endoderm (Pictet et al. 1976) rather than from migratory cells of the neural crest (Pearse et al. 1973). Cell nests are seen budding from the small ducts in the 3rd month of gestation. The connection with the duct system is subsequently lost. Insulin and glucagon can be demonstrated within the islet cells by the 20th gestational week. Islet tissue forms 1%–2% of the pancreatic mass.

Lymphocytes and lymphoid aggregates are a transitory finding in the exocrine pancreatic tissue of normal fetuses and neonates. They do not involve the islets, which are normal and thus distinct from the infiltrates in diabetics (Jansen et al. 1993).

Hypoglycaemic Disorders

Hypoglycaemia occurring in infants and young children is most commonly a consequence of fasting in an otherwise normal individual (ketotic hypogly-

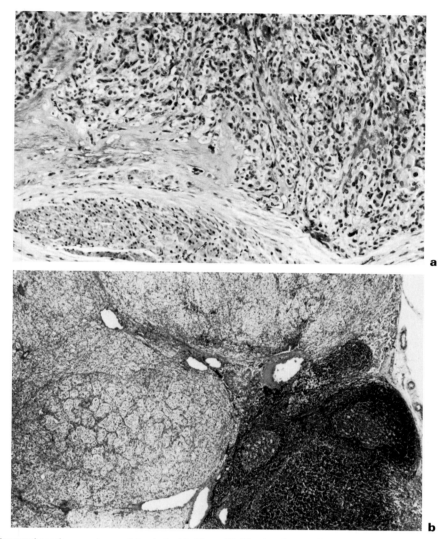

Fig. 13.11. a Malignant phaeochromocytoma arising in the bladder and infiltrating the muscle wall. (H&E, × 120) **b** There are no histological criteria by which malignancy can be recognized in a phaeochromocytoma but in this case a metastasis was present in a local lymph node. (H&E, × 30) (Case 1 of Higgins and Tresidder 1966)

caemia; Chaussain 1973). Liability to hypoglycaemia is particularly great in premature and small-for-gestational age neonatal infants. Less common causes include hepatic enzyme defects, growth hormone and glucocorticoid deficiency, and inappropriate insulin secretion. Most cases of persistent inappropriate insulin secretion occur before the age of 2, and delay in recognition and treatment carries a high risk of permanent neurological and mental damage. The disorder has been attributed to dysfunction of the β-cells without consistent demonstrable histological abnormality (Pagliara et al. 1973) and to agenesis of the glucagon-producing islet A cells (Yakovac et al.

1971) in addition to islet hyperplasia, abnormal β-cell proliferation and β-cell tumour (Misugi et al. 1970; Fischer et al. 1974).

Nesidioblastosis

In nesidioblastosis there is continued uncontrolled proliferation of pancreatic ductular endocrine cells, which replace the normal islets of Langerhans and infiltrate among the acinar tissue. Apparent budding off of endocrine cells from ductular epithelium is seen. Immunohistochemical study has shown near-

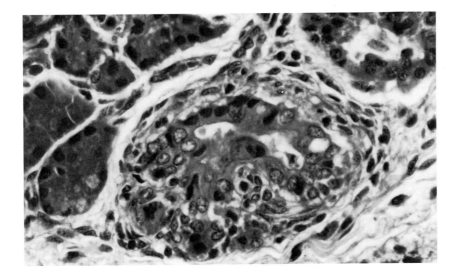

Fig. 13.12. Proliferation of islet cells in a small duct in an infant dying in the postnatal period with nesidioblastosis. (H&E, × 480)

normal proportions of the different islet-cell types (Heitz et al. 1977). Nesidioblastosis has been observed in a proportion of cases of sudden infant death (Fig. 13.12) (Cox et al. 1976; Polak and Wigglesworth 1976) and in cases of hypoglycaemia that have been clinically recognized. In most of the cases described the proliferation of endocrine cells affects the pancreas diffusely, but on occasion only localized ares may be involved, the remaining pancreatic tissue being histologically normal or containing some enlarged islets (Davidson et al. 1974; Gang 1978).

Hyperplasia of the islets of Langerhans is seen as a temporary change in the pancreas of a proportion of infants of diabetic mothers. It is one of the features seen in the Beckwith syndrome and in some cases of erythroblastosis fetalis.

Diabetes Mellitus

Diabetes mellitus is the commonest endocrine disease in childhood, affecting males and females with equal frequency. The prevalence in school-age children is similar in England, Sweden and the USA at about 1.3 per 1000, with a linear increase in incidence from age 5 years to age 16 years (Holmgren et al. 1974; Calnan and Peckham 1977; Kyllo and Nuttall 1978). Most cases are of the insulin-deficiency type with acute onset, although only a minority present with established diabetic ketoacidosis. The major metabolic disturbances are well controlled with insulin, but the later complications that affect small and large vessels and are responsible for retinopathy, nephropathy and large-artery occlusion remain.

Factors relating to the occurrence of insulin-deficiency diabetes have become more clearly defined in recent years, with investigations of genetic make-up, immune responsiveness and virus infections currently providing insight into the hereditary and environmental factors concerned in its aetiology. The major genetic susceptibility is determined by a gene in the HLA regions of the chromosome 6 pair associated with HLA8 and W15 antigens at the B locus and DW3 and DW4 antigens at the D locus. Autoimmune organ-specific diseases show an association with the presence of the HLA8 antigen, and an association has increasingly been detected between insulin-deficiency diabetes and various autoimmune diseases, including Graves' disease, Hashimoto's thyroiditis, pernicious anaemia, Addison's disease and myasthenia gravis (Nabarro et al. 1979). Antibodies that react with pancreatic islet cells are present at the onset of the disease in the serum of a high proportion of cases (Irvine et al. 1977; Lernmark et al. 1978; MacLaren et al. 1975), and abnormalities in the T lymphocytes have been demonstrated (Huang and MacLaren 1976). The anti-islet antibodies bind to the surface of islet cells, those occurring in diabetics being cytotoxic and showing β-cell specificity (Dobersen and Schaff 1982; Van de Winkel et al. 1982). In a study by Gorsuch et al. (1981) of first-degree relatives of patients with insulin-deficiency diabetes, 54 of 582 were found to have anti-islet antibodies. Seven of the antibody-positive relatives became diabetic 3–37 months from entry into the study. None of the antibody-negative relatives developed diabetes or anti-islet antibodies during the period of observation. Pure inheritance and altered immunity are not sufficient in themselves to account for the development of the disease, however, as the concordance rate among pairs of identical twins is only 50%. Whether virus infections are the necessary environmental triggering agent remains open to speculation, but epidemiological observations suggest that diabetes follows Coxsackie virus B4 infections by weeks, mumps infections by months to a few years, and intrauterine exposure to rubella virus by up to 20 years (Gamble et al. 1969; Sultz et al. 1975; Menser et al. 1978). In the acute fatal case described by Yoon et al. (1979) a variant of Coxsackie virus B4 isolated from the pancreas was shown to survive in cell culture and to infect suitable mice with accompanying β-cell damage and hyperglycaemia.

In a small proportion of diabetic children the disease has a different aetiology, usually of obesity-related glucose intolerance, in which case there may be a strong family history of maturity-onset diabetes. A number of rare genetic syndromes account for the remaining occasional cases (Rimoin 1971). In ataxia telangiectasia there is a decrease in the affinity of the insulin receptor probably caused by binding of circulating inhibitors (Bar et al. 1978), whereas in Turner's syndrome there is a reduction in the number of insulin receptors unrelated to obesity (Neufeld et al. 1978).

Changes in the Pancreas

In his study of the pancreas in patients with juvenile diabetes mellitus, Gepts (1965) found abnormalities in the majority of cases both when the disease was clinically of recent onset (less than 6 months) and in those dying after more than 2 years of disease. The weight of the pancreas was found to be normal in the acute group but variably lower than normal in a considerable proportion of chronic cases. Weight deficit, when present, showed no relationship to the severity, duration or age at onset of the disease. Similar observations were made by Doniach and Morgan (1973), who suggest in explanation cessation of normal pancreatic growth from the time of onset of the disease rather than destruction of exocrine tissue.

The most consistent abnormality is seen histologically to involve the islets of Langerhans (Fig. 13.13). Practically all cases show a reduction, usually marked, in the total number of islets and the number of β cells, and depletion of their cytoplasmic granules in aldehyde–fuchsin stained sections that is more marked in cases with longstanding disease. Other changes seen include insular fibrosis, shrinkage of the islet cells, and occurrence of β cells with swollen vacuolated cytoplasm described as hydropic transformation, an appearance resulting from degranulation and accumulation of glycogen. A proportion of the insular cells in some cases contain large irregular nuclei and hyperchromatic nuclei. Gepts (1965) observed an inflammatory infiltrate within and/or around some islets in nearly 70% of his patients with diabetes of recent onset (insulitis). The infiltrating cells were lymphocytes, macrophages and a few polymorphs, but included no plasma cells. None of the cases studied by Doniach and Morgan (1973) showed an inflammatory infiltrate.

In their study of the pancreas in 119 diabetics under 20 years of age, Foulis et al. (1986) observed insulitis in 47 of 60 patients (78%) whose disease was less than 1 year in duration. The inflammatory infiltrate affected 23% of insulin-containing islets. Only rarely were insulin-deficient islets involved, the inflammation apparently subsiding once the β cells in a particular islet have been destroyed. They confirmed that the inflammatory cells were lymphocytes and that occasionally polymorphs were also present but not plasma cells. In many cases it could be seen that the insulitis and loss of β cells involved the pancreas lobule by lobule rather than in a wholesale or random fashion. Focally acute inflammation was seen involving the exocrine pancreas and ducts in six cases and a diffuse lymphocytic infiltrate in nine cases. Acinar cells adjacent to insulin-containing islets were larger and contained more zymogen granules than those in acini surrounding insulin-deficient islets.

Changes in Extrapancreatic Structures

Clinical effects resulting from the changes that take place in the small blood vessels and muscular arteries in diabetes generally become evident only after many years and are therefore rarely seen before the age of 18. Because vascular complications are by far the commonest single cause of major illness and eventual death among diabetics, there is great concern to understand the causal mechanisms and so allow the introduction of logical steps to prevent their development from an early stage in the disease. A central theme common to much contemporary investigation is the suggestion that an abnormally elevated concentration of glucose may of itself lead to the vascular and tissue changes. The tissues principally involved in the late complications of diabetes (blood vessels, nerves, eyes) do not require insulin for glucose uptake. It is possible therefore that the accumulation of by-products from the metabolism of the excessive amounts of glucose by the sorbitol pathway leads to damage in these tissues (Gabbay 1975). The non-enzymatic glycosylation of an increased proportion of long-lived proteins that occurs with an increase in glucose concentration can impair their function.

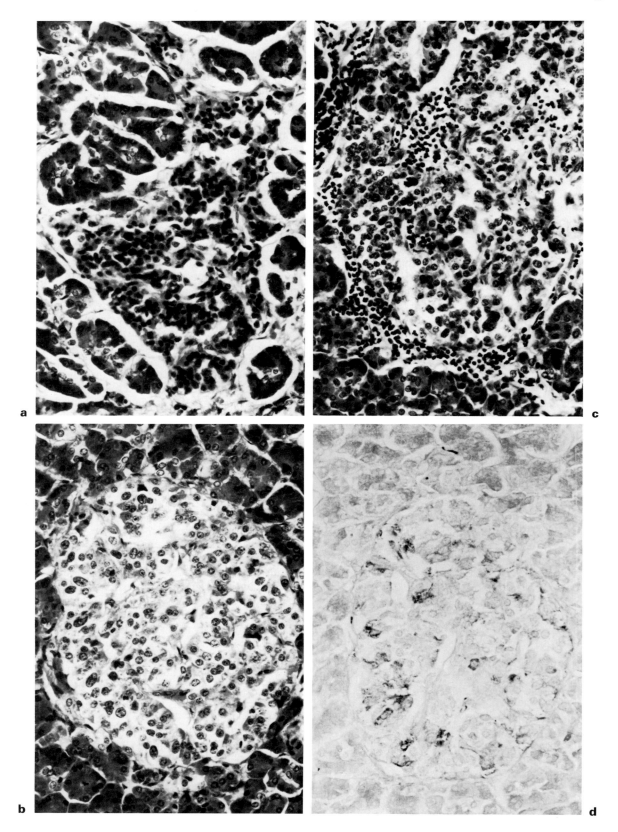

Haemoglobin is markedly affected in this way, with an adverse effect on its affinity for oxygen (Koenig et al. 1976).

Thickening of the basement membrane of small blood vessels is typical in young diabetics. The capillaries are most severely affected and have been found to be abnormal in the glomerulus, retina, muscle, subcutaneous tissue and skin. Thickening of non-vascular basement membrane has also been found in Bowman's capsule, renal tubules, seminiferous tubules, breast, ciliary process of the eye and sweat glands of the skin. Basement membrane change occurs early and has been observed in biopsies taken at the time of presentation and in asymptomatic children with impaired glucose tolerance.

The evolution of the various complications in a large number of juvenile diabetics has been recorded by Knowles et al. (1965) and by the Public Health Service, National Institutes of Health (NIH) of the US Department of Health, Education, and Welfare (1964). Retinopathy and glomerulosclerosis begin to appear after about 10 years of disease and are therefore not seen before the mid to late teens. Knowles et al. recorded retinopathy in as many as 70% of their patients who had had 20 years of disease, and glomerulosclerosis in 30%. Ellis and Pysher (1993) emphasize the importance of overt diabetic nephropathy among adolescent diabetics with proteinuria and/or haematuria, often despite a history of disease as short as 5 years. About 50% of juvenile diabetic patients eventually die of renal disease. Neuropathy is not usually clinically evident before about 10 years of disease, but abnormal electromyographic patterns can be detected much earlier (Eeg-Olofsson and Peterson 1966). The NIH statistics indicate that cataracts are present in at least 5% of diabetic patients under 19 years of age. Accounts of the histological changes in these late diabetic complications are recorded by Williams and Porte (1974) and Bloodworth and Greider (1982).

Fig. 13.13. Histological changes in islets of Langerhans in insulin-dependent diabetes mellitus of recent onset. **a** Ill-defined islet of irregular outline composed of shrunken cells with small uniform darkly staining nuclei. (H&E, × 300) **b** Conspicuous islet smooth in outline composed of large cells forming cords separated by prominent capillaries. The nuclei have a well defined chromatin pattern. There are several unusually large nuclei, and small haematoxyphil bodies can be seen in the cytoplasm of many of the cells. (H&E, × 300) **c** An infiltrate of inflammatory cells (insulitis), pricipally lymphocytes with a few polymorphs, may occasionally be seen within and adjacent to some islets. (H&E, × 300) **d** Marked decrease in number and intensity of staining of beta cells. (Aldehyde Fuchsin, × 300)

Tumours of the Pancreatic Islets

Islet-cell tumours of the pancreas are rare in children. Insulin-secreting tumours are commonest and have been found at all ages, including in a newborn child (Salinas et al. 1968). Children are also recorded in small numbers among cases of gastrin-secreting tumours. Both benign and malignant tumours occur, and they have pathological and behavioural characteristics similar to those of the much commoner adult examples. With better availability of specific antibodies for immunocytochemical use, practice now has moved towards classification of islet-cell tumours according to their secretory product as well as by traditional morphological and staining characteristics (Jones and Dawson 1977; Larsson 1978; Nieuwenhuijzen Kruseman et al. 1978). A proportion of cases of islet-cell tumour show a familial incidence, and many are coincident with abnormalities in other endocrine tissues. This should be considered particularly when more than a single tumour is found in the pancreas and when islets of abnormal appearance are found in the surrounding gland.

Multiple Endocrine Neoplasia Syndromes

The syndromes of multiple endocrine neoplasia (MEN) are familial disorders in which hyperplasia or tumours involve more than one endocrine gland. The pathogenesis of the syndromes is unknown, but both are the clinical manifestation of inheritance of specific autosomal gene defects, the detection of which can be used to screen for carriers in the preclinical phase of the disease. They are disorders principally affecting structures of neuroectodermal origin and their clinical manifestations reflect the local effects and the effects of secretory activity of the particular tumours involved, this usually being the production of the hormone normal for the cell of origin, although sometimes there is ectopic hormone secretion. Evidence of multiple organ involvement may be present at the outset, but in some cases disease of a single organ may be the only apparent abnormality and in others there may be several years' delay in the appearance of disease in the different organs. Although these are uncommon diseases, expression of the abnormality is the rule, so that the identification of a case may bring to light a large number of cases among relatives. In some instances, however, no further cases are found among the family members of a patient with an apparently typical multiple

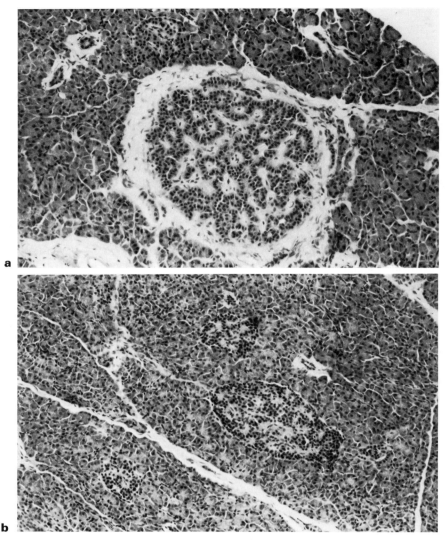

Fig. 13.14. Sections from a partial pancreatectomy specimen from a boy aged 10 years with MEN type 1. Episodes of hypoglycaemia had occurred during the previous year. Several small discrete islet-cell tumours were visible to the naked eye in the resected pancreas. In addition there were several microscopic islet-cell tumours (**a**), and unusually large but otherwise apparently normal islets (**b**). (**a** H&E, × 150; **b** H&E, × 120)

endocrine syndrome, and some of these are undoubtedly examples of mutation.

Type 1 (MEN 1, Wermer's Syndrome)

The anterior pituitary, parathyroids and pancreatic islets are the structures most commonly involved in type 1 as fully documented by Wermer (1974) following his original description in 1954. Adenoma of the pituitary, usually single, is recorded in about half the studied cases. This may be of acidophil, basophil, chromophobe or mixed-cell type, and may interfere with the normal function of the pituitary or produce gigantism and acromegaly or Cushing's disease as a consequence of secretory activity. The parathyroids and pancreas are found to be abnormal in the great majority of cases. Nodular chief-cell hyperplasia involving all four parathyroids is usual, though adenomas have been described. The pancreatic islets (Fig. 13.14) show hyperplasia that may be diffuse and include multiple adenomas and carcinomas. All these changes may be found in the same gland. The tumours may be several centimetres in diameter or may be microscopic, in which case distinction from a large hyperplastic islet can be difficult. They may be found outside the pancreas in the wall of the duodenum and stomach. The histological and ultrastructural appearance of the tumour is similar to that seen in sporadic cases, except that a pronounced ribbon pattern is strongly suggestive of genetic disease (Wermer 1974). The distinction between some of the benign and malignant tumours can be problematic. The most frequent clinical manifestations of islet-cell tumour are the Zollinger–Ellison syndrome and hypoglycaemia. Immunohistochemical studies have also identified tumours that contain glucagon and pancreatic polypeptide.

Benign and malignant tumours in other organs have been recorded in some families with sufficient frequency to allow their inclusion as a part of the syndrome. Most notable among these are carcinoid tumours and adrenal cortical abnormalities. Carcinoids have been described in bronchi, gut, pancreas and thymus. Micronodular and diffuse hyperplasia and adenomas of the adrenal cortex are common and may be accompanied by hyperaldosteronism or Cushing's syndrome. Diffuse adrenocortical hyperplasia with Cushing's disease of pituitary origin also occurs. Cases that have developed lipomas of the subcutaneous tissues and viscera, with adenomas and carcinomas of the large bowel, are also described.

The commonest clinical manifestations in childhood and adolescence are hypoglycaemic attacks, diarrhoea and peptic ulceration from pancreatic tumours, and amenorrhoea associated with a pituitary adenoma. Hypercalcaemia is very frequently the earliest evidence of established disease. Detecting the inheritance of the genetic determinant is likely to be possible in future, allowing identification of those at risk in a kindred, with the benefit of exclusion of normal siblings from repeated biochemical screening (Larsson and Nordenskjold 1994; Thakker 1994).

Type 2 (MEN 2)

The specific association in families of medullary carcinoma of the thyroid with phaeochromocytoma was first recognized by Williams (1965), and the rare further association with mucosal neuromas was described by Williams and Pollock (1966). The parathyroids may also be abnormal, usually showing primary nodular chief-cell hyperplasia. Parathyroid abnormality is sometimes found in cases of sporadic medullary carcinoma of the thyroid but in these cases is not accompanied by elevated levels of serum calcium (Melvin et al. 1972). The simultaneous occurrence of medullary carcinoma of the thyroid, phaeochromocytomas usually in both adrenals and

parathyroid abnormality has been designated MEN type 2 (Steiner et al. 1968) and is usually referred to as MEN 2a to separate these commoner kindreds from those in which neuromas also develop. Rare families showing inheritance of medullary thyroid carcinoma alone also occur (familial MTC). Multiple, and usually bilateral, medullary carcinomas and phaeochromocytomas develop in most cases, although in a small proportion the thyroid or adrenal lesion alone may occur. The adrenal involvement may be very asymmetrical, but if one gland is clinically involved the other will almost certainly be found to be abnormal on microscopic examination. It is suggested, however, that a gland appearing normal at the time of surgery should be conserved (Lairmore et al. 1993). Hyperplasia of the thyroid C cells and the adrenal medulla has been shown to precede the development of tumours (Wolfe et al. 1973; Carney et al. 1976). Hypercalcaemia is found in less than 50% of cases. The incidence of parathyroid hyperplasia and phaeochromocytoma varies considerably in different kindreds, and for phaeochromocytoma may approach 100% (Howe et al. 1993). Keiser et al. (1973) found parathyroid hyperplasia or adenoma in most of their 45 patients. Screening MEN 2a families for evidence of inheritance of the disease determinant using identification of the associated RET proto-oncogene mutation on chromosome 10 is effective (Lipps et al. 1994; Tsai et al. 1994). Carriers of the abnormality can be tested periodically for C-cell hyperplasia by measuring calcitonin release on pentagastrin provocation. In some families pre-emptive thyroidectomy in carriers may be appropriate (Wells et al. 1994). Abnormal calcitonin release on pentagastrin provocation sometimes occurs independent of inheritance of the genetic determinant for medullary carcinoma, and may be a source of confusion in a MEN 2a family (Landsvater et al. 1993). The phaeochromocytomas are mostly benign, but are a significant cause of death unless carefully sought and treated (Evans et al. 1994).

The cases in which mucosal neuromas occur together with medullary carcinoma and phaeochromocytoma have been designated multiple endocrine neoplasia type 2b. This constellation of abnormalities is inherited separately from the other familial medullary carcinoma cases, and is the rarest form seen. The neuromas are most prominent on the eyelids, lips and margin of the tongue, and are accompanied by diffuse enlargement of the lips and sometimes prognathism, producing a characteristic facial appearance (Schimke et al. 1968; Gorlin et al. 1968). Slit-lamp examination reveals abnormal corneal nerves. Ganglioneuromatosis (Fig. 13.15) throughout the gastrointestinal tract is often found, sometimes with accompanying diverticulosis and

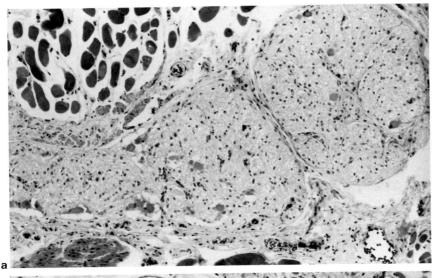

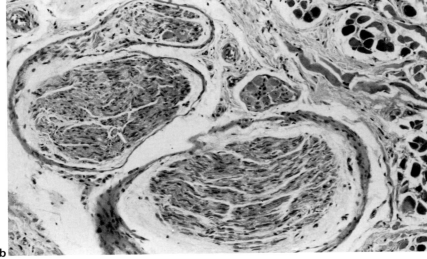

Fig. 13.15. a Ganglioneuromatosis involving the myenteric plexus of the upper oesophagus in a patient with the complete form of familial medullary carcinoma syndrome. (H&E, × 120) **b** Similar neuromas in the tongue produced irregular small projections on the surface. (H&E, × 120)

megacolon. The hereditary nature of this subtype is seen in only a minority of cases, so that most would appear to be the result of mutation. A further factor contributing to the rarity of this group is the much earlier presentation than in other forms of medullary carcinoma syndromes. Many patients with this condition die of thyroid carcinoma while still young (Khairi et al. 1975; Norton et al. 1979).

Parathyroid Glands

The parathyroids appear as solid cellular proliferations of the third and fourth pharyngeal pouch epithe-lium, and can be identified by the 7th gestational week. The solid epithelial masses quickly separate from their pharyngeal pouch, those derived from the fourth arch remaining closely related to the lateral lobes of the thyroid while those from the third arch associate with the migrating thymus and come to lie close to the inferior poles of the thyroid. The cells that make up the parathyroids of infants and children are similar to those of adult glands except that oxyphil cells are not found much before 5 years of age and thereafter occur as occasional single cells until after the age of 10 years, when small clusters begin to appear. Fat is not found incorporated in the infant parathyroid, appearing during early childhood as isolated fat cells and increasing in amount with age, eventually forming small areas of fatty tissue.

Production and release of parathormone are modulated directly by the blood level of ionized calcium. There is little storage of hormone in the normal gland. The present understanding of the synthesis, structure and actions of parathormone are fully discussed by Habener and Potts (1978) and Martin et al. (1979).

Various aspects of parathyroid development, histology and anomalies are dealt with by Gilmour (1937, 1938, 1939, 1941) (see Table 13.1).

Table 13.1 Parathyroid weight

	Mean combined weight of parathyroid glands (mg)	
	Male	Female
Birth to 3 months	6.2	8.8
3 months to 1 year	25.4	15.6
1–5 years	34.9	22.3
6–10 years	49.7	63.3
11–20 years	91.9	95.7

From Gilmour and Martin (1937).

Developmental Abnormalities

One and sometimes more of the parathyroid glands are found in an ectopic site in about 10% of individuals. The inferior pair of glands is most commonly involved and is usually found in association with the superior poles of the thymus in the upper mediastinum. It is common to find a small amount of thymic tissue adjacent to the normally situated inferior parathyroids. Occasionally, a parathyroid is found embedded within the thyroid, and cases of parathyroid adenoma located posterior to the oesophagus have been described.

Apparent failure of development involving a parathyroid appears to be an uncommon event. Gilmour (1938) found only three parathyroids in 6% of his autopsy series and was of the opinion that in most of these cases his dissection had failed to located a gland. Supernumerary concentrations of parathyroid tissue are common, having been detected in three of 14 fetuses (Gilmour 1941) and may be found in an ectopic location. Hypoplasia or agenesis involving all parathyroids is associated with DiGeorge syndrome and also occurs as an accompaniment of congenital malformation in some cases, most conspicuously in those with anomalies involving the head and neck (see p. 628).

Cysts involving the parathyroids are usually found in adults as a secondary change in an adenoma. Developmental cysts are rare and most are probably derived from a pharyngeal pouch remnant, with the parathyroid being involved by association. Microscopical cysts or vesicles are a normal histological feature.

Hypoparathyroidism and Hypocalcaemia

Rapid development of hypocalcaemia involves tetany and convulsions. In more prolonged hypocalcaemia tetany is latent rather than overt and complaints of weakness and pins and needles in the extremities are typical. Chronic hypocalcaemia results in changes in epidermal structures manifesting as scaly coarse skin with patchy hyperpigmentation. There is a liability to chronic cutaneous and mucosal candidiasis. The hair is brittle and there is a tendency for a patchy loss to occur. The nails show deformity with horizontal ridging and become heaped-up when affected by chronic fungous infection. Prolonged hypocalcaemia is likely to be accompanied by soft-tissue calcification, particularly involving the basal ganglia of the brain, retina and subcutaneous tissue. The eyes may also be affected by cataracts. Developing teeth are deformed as a result of irregular hypoplasia of the enamel, producing transverse ridging and a predisposition to caries. Tooth eruption is delayed and radiographs show lack of calcification in the tooth and root and in some cases a thickening of the lamina densa of the adjacent jaw bone.

The different causes of hypocalcaemia fall broadly into those resulting in hypocalcaemia manifesting in infancy and a second group relevant to hypocalcaemia of later onset. Tetany in the neonatal period can be a complication of prematurity and may follow abnormal labour and pregnancy, where it may result from parathyroid injury. A large phosphate load caused by feeding with an unmodified cows' milk formula can result in a sufficient depression of the calcium concentration to produce tetany, typically about the end of the 1st week of life (Tsang et al. 1973). Hypocalcaemia is likely to complicate conditions, primarily producing low blood levels of magnesium. This type has proved more difficult to correct, probably because of the permissive role of magnesium in allowing parathormone to exert its effects (Anast et al. 1972; Suh et al. 1973). A number of instances of neonatal tetany have been described, with onset usually between the 2nd and 20th postnatal days, where the mother has been shown to have primary hyperparathyroidism (Johnstone et al. 1972). On occasion, several offspring have been affected (Hutchin and Kessner 1964). A rare sex-linked recessive form of hypoparathyroidism affects males in the first week or early months of life (Peden 1960).

Hypoparathyroidism occurring in later childhood is seen most commonly between 5 and 15 years of age, although symptoms may be manifest in infancy. It is usually described as idiopathic, but its frequent association with Addison's disease, hypothyroidism, pernicious anaemia, steatorrhoea and diabetes mellitus is well documented, suggesting an autoimmune disorder. Many of the cases have a family history of hypoparathyroidism with or without disturbance involving other endocrine glands (Gorodischer et al. 1970). Circulating antibodies to parathyroid were found in 38% of the patients with idiopathic hypoparathyroidism studied by Blizzard et al. (1966) and in 26% of their patients with Addison's disease without evidence of hypoparathyroidism. Six per cent of their controls also had detectable antibodies. In these autoimmune cases, *Candida albicans* infection of the nails and mouth is particularly common and can spread to become generalized. The infection usually antedates the clinical development of hypoparathyroidism and is not affected by restoring the serum calcium concentration to normal. In cases where hypoparathyroidism and autoimmune disorders involving other endocrines are associated it is usual for the parathyroid disturbance to be the first to develop. Addison's disease is the commonest associated disorder. The pathological changes in the parathyroids in these cases have not been widely studied. In some cases no parathyroid tissue could be found. Almost total replacement by fat and also fibrosis with lymphocytic infiltration have been described (Drake et al. 1939; Chu et al. 1964).

Pseudohypoparathyroidism

The syndrome of unresponsiveness of target organs to parathormone and associated characteristic somatic features, particularly short metacarpals and metatarsals, diminished height and rounded face, was first described by Albright et al. (1942). The disorder appears to be transmitted as an autosomal recessive trait. The hypocalcaemia is the result of failure of 1-hydroxylation of 25-hydroxy vitamin D in the renal tubules through failure of activation of renal cyclic AMP by parathormone (Drezner et al. 1976). The defect in bone growth results from dyschondroplasia with early fusion of epiphyses, and is regarded as an independent genetic trait. Evidence of hyperparathyroid bone disease is found in some cases only, so that the unresponsiveness to parathormone usually also involves the skeleton. It might be expected that the parathyroid glands would be hyperplastic. In the few cases in which the parathyroids have been examined, histological evidence of hyperplasia has been described in some but in others they have been regarded as normal. Raised blood levels of parathormone have been found, with normal suppression on

restoring the blood calcium level to normal (Chase et al. 1969). Cases in which there is evidence of disturbance involving other endocrine glands have been described. These include abnormal thyrotrophin and prolactin secretion and decreased responsiveness of the thyroid to thyrotrophin (Zisman et al. 1969; Marx et al. 1971; Werder et al. 1975; Carlson et al. 1977). The formation of bone in subcutaneous tissue is common, and is probably not directly related to the functional hypoparathyroidism.

Occasional cases involving alternative abnormalities in the synthesis and actions of parathormone have been described and have become entangled incidentally in some of the most confusing nomenclature (summarized by Williams 1978). The distinctive clinical features in pseudohypoparathyroidism and idiopathic hypoparathyroidism are summarized and contrasted by Bronsky et al. (1958).

Hyperparathyroidism

A sustained increase in secretion of parathormone may be primary or, alternatively, a response to a depressed level of plasma calcium. Such responsive hyperparathyroidism may eventually lead to the development of parathyroid tumours and autonomous production of excessive amounts of parathormone with resulting hypercalcaemia (tertiary hyperparathyroidism).

Primary Hyperparathyroidism

Infantile Hyperparathyroidism with Parathyroid Hyperplasia. A few examples of diffuse, nonnodular, chief-cell hyperplasia involving all or several of the parathyroids have been recorded in infants, with evidence of inheritance as an autosomal recessive characteristic in some cases (Hillman et al. 1964; Fretheim and Gardborg 1965; Bradford et al. 1973). Children with this disorder present with hypotonia, dehydration, feeding difficulties, and respiratory distress resulting from impaired development and fractures of the rib cage. There is pronounced osteitis fibrosa and radiological evidence of generalized lack of skeletal mineralization with subperiosteal resorption.

Primary Nodular Hyperplasia. Some cases of primary nodular hyperplasia occur in childhood, mostly in older children and adolescents, though neonatal cases have been recorded (Spiegel et al. 1977). Many are genetically determined and inherited as autosomal dominant disorders. In these cases the parathyroid disorder (Fig. 13.16) may be part of the

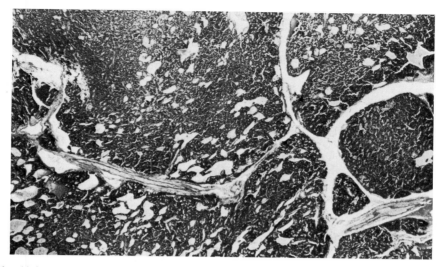

Fig. 13.16. Nodular chief-cell parathyroid hyperplasia in a woman with MEN type 1 manifested in hypecalcaemia, secondary amenorrhoea and an enlarged pituitary fossa. (H&E, × 20)

two syndromes of multiple endocrine neoplasia (MEN 1 and MEN 2), whereas in other cases it is inherited without other endocrine anomalies. Typically, all the parathyroid glands are enlarged and reddish-brown in colour. There may be a marked difference in size among the glands in an individual case, one or more of which may be of normal weight. The normal-sized glands may not be obviously abnormal microscopically. Histologically, the enlarged glands contain multiple nodules composed of chief cells arranged in a variety and mixture of patterns – solid, trabecular and follicular. Occasional nodules may consist predominantly of oxyphil cells. If one nodule dominates, the resulting appearance is difficult to distinguish from that of an adenoma. It has been suggested that the presence of intracellular fat serves to distinguish normal from hyperplastic parathyroid glands (Roth and Gallagher 1976). The intrafollicular material has the characteristics of amyloid in a proportion of cases of primary hyperplasia (Leedham and Pollock 1970).

Secondary Hyperplasia

Some degree of parathyroid hyperplasia occurs in any condition in which the ionized calcium concentration tends to be decreased. Formerly the commonest cause was rickets from dietary vitamin D deficiency, a problem that has re-emerged among the Asian immigrant population in the UK. Disease with accompanying malabsorption and severe hepatic disease have a similar effect. Probably the commonest cause is chronic renal disease, in which phosphate retention is accompanied by a compensatory lowering of calcium levels. This metabolic disturbance is in part the result of an impaired renal excretory capacity, but also reflects reduced hydroxylation of 25-hydroxy vitamin D to form the active 1-25-dihydroxy form, which normally takes place in the renal tubular epithelium. The normal phosphaturic response to parathormone is mediated through the action of the activated vitamin D. A few cases of intrauterine hyperparathyroidism secondary to maternal hypoparathyroidism have been described (Bronsky et al. 1968; Gorodischer et al. 1970; Landing and Kamoshita 1970).

In secondary hyperplasia the parathyroid glands are modestly enlarged and are paler than normal. Microscopically, they are uniformly hypercellular, being composed of normal chief cells. Where the stimulus to hyperplasia has been severe and prolonged, one or more of the parathyroids may develop one or several nodules and will then appear similar to the parathyroids from cases of primary nodular hyperplasia. The clinical history and chemical changes are important in the interpretation of such cases. In chronic renal disease the size of the parathyroids is generally considered to increase in proportion to the duration of the renal failure. However, in children maintained on long-term haemodialysis, parathyroid size has been observed to be related to the amount of calcium loss during dialysis, and was independent of bone disease, which correlated with duration of renal disease (Gruskin et al. 1976). Autonomous hyperparathyroidism supervening on responsive hyperplasia (tertiary hyperparathyroidism) appears to be rare in childhood.

Other Causes of Hypercalcaemia

Tumours

Hypercalcaemia has been recorded with many kinds of tumour, either as a result of extensive bony metastasis or through the action of parathyroid hormone related protein (PTHRP) produced by the tumour. Other bone-mobilizing substances may cause hypercalcaemia, particularly prostaglandins (PGE_2), which stimulates osteoclastic activity. Tumours that have been associated with PTHRP and other hypercalcaemia-inducing products in children include some bone tumours, neuroblastoma, rhabdomyosarcoma and a number of cases of leukaemia and lymphosarcoma (Myers 1960; Stapleton et al. 1976; Joyaraman and David 1977; Hutchinson et al.1978; Ramsay et al. 1979).

Iatrogenic Causes

Both vitamins D and A in excess cause hypercalcaemia and, in vitamin faddism, are likely to be taken together. Thiazide diuretics possibly act through potentiation of the calcaemic effect of parathyroid hormone.

Idiopathic hypercalcaemia of infancy with "elfin facies", mental retardation and supravalvular aortic stenosis appears to be part of the spectrum of Williams' syndrome, in which there is evidence for hypersensitivity to vitamin D. Involvement of more than one member in a family has been observed. Excessive parenteral and dietary intake of vitamin D in infancy has been considered the cause of some cases of supravalvular aortic stenosis and the infantile hypercalcaemia syndrome. Immobilization of an adolescent in the treatment of such problems as fractures and extensive burns can result in a rise in blood calcium level within 4 or 5 days. The rise reaches a peak by the end of 1 week, and, although in most cases the changes are slight, levels as high as 4.5 mmol/litre have occurred. Rarely, temporary hypercalcaemia complicates the uncommon occurrences of subcutaneous fat necrosis in the newborn (Finne et al. 1988; Kruse et al. 1993). Cases occur among neonates suffering birth trauma or asphyxia, and Glover et al. (1991) suggest that hypothermia leading to solidification of the relatively highly saturated fat in neonates is a factor. Hydroxylation of 25-hydroxy vitamin D to the metabolically active 1, 25-dihydroxy form by macrophages in the areas of fat necrosis is implicated. The parathyroid glands in a fatal case were normal (Wilkerson 1964). Hypercalcaemia in sarcoidosis, mediated in a similar manner, has been recorded in a 9-month-old infant (Stamworth et al. 1992).

Benign familial hypercalcaemia is a rare disorder that is apparently inherited as an autosomal dominant trait. The hypercalcaemia is of modest degree and has no apparent ill effect. The underlying disorder is obscure.

Hypercalcaemia is observed in a small proportion of cases of thyrotoxicosis, probably as a direct effect of thyroid hormone excess on bone resorption (Rude et al. 1976). In Addison's disease hypercalcaemia may occur.

Effects of Hypercalcaemia

Hypercalcaemia produces clinical manifestations that include muscular weakness with a combination of irritability, listlessness and lethargy. Examination shows hypotonia and hyperextensible joints, and in young infants there is retardation of all forms of motor development. The bowel is atonic with resulting constipation. Metabolic effects include polyuria as a direct effect of excess calcium on renal tubular water handling. In older children, thirst will tend to compensate for the polyuria unless prevented by nausea, but dehydration is likely to occur in infants and in part may be due to feeding difficulties. Nocturnal enuresis may be the first complaint. A rise in blood urea results from the defective renal tubular function and dehydration. Bradycardia and shortening of the Q–T interval on the ECG may be seen.

Metastatic calcification may occur and can involve the conjunctiva and superficial cornea, joint ligaments, cartilage, blood vessels, lungs and gastric mucosa. In children the kidneys are more often affected by interstitial calcification than stone formation, and their involvement results in impairment of function.

Pituitary

Development

The pituitary develops from two separate ectodermal layers. The *infundibular process* forms from an evagination of the floor of the diencephalon and comes to comprise the *median eminence* at the base of the hypothalamus, a connecting neural stalk or *infundibular stem* and the posterior lobe of the pituitary or *pars nervosa*. Rathke's pouch is a dorsal evagination of the primitive stomatodeum. The devel-

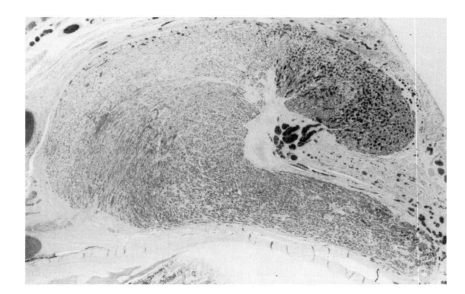

Fig. 13.17. A well organized mass of anterior pituitary tissue from an anencephalic monster. The base of the skull lies below the gland nodule without forming a fossa. There is a convering of disorganized vascular glial tissue. (H&E, × 20)

oping sphenoid bone pinches off the neck of the evagination, leaving a vesicle. The cells of the anterior wall of the vesicle proliferate to form the *adenohypophysis* comprising the *pars distalis* and the *pars tuberalis*. The posterior wall forms the *pars intermedia*, which is vestigial in man, giving rise to the posterior lobe basophils and a group of colloid-filled cysts. The cavity of Rathke's pouch collapses, leaving the hypophyseal cleft, a colloid-filled space between the pars distalis and pars intermedia. Growth hormone has been demonstrated as early as the 9th week of development. A residuum of the neck of Rathke's pouch sometimes persists in the sphenoid bone and is regularly present in the form of clusters of small pituitary-type cells, sometimes including nests of squamous cells in the dorsal pharyngeal wall, and known as the pharyngeal pituitary. It is unlikely that these structures serve any pituitary function.

The blood supply to the pituitary is complex with the superior hypophyseal arteries, one from each internal carotid, supplying the median eminence and upper pituitary stalk by way of numerous special vascular structures, the gomitoli. The capillaries drain into portal sinuses that run down the surface of the stalk to supply the capillary sinuses that ramify between the cells of the anterior lobe. The final venous drainage is to local dural venous sinuses. The posterior lobe and the lower infundibular stem receive blood from a pair of inferior hypophyseal arteries. The effect of this vascular arrangement is to allow releasing and inhibiting hormones, produced in cells of the hypothalamic nuclei and conveyed to their axon terminals in the median eminence, to be transferred in the portal blood to target cells in the anterior pituitary. Axons from neurons of the supraoptic and paraventricular nuclei of the hypothalamus pass into the posterior pituitary where their neurosecretions, antidiuretic hormone and oxytocin, are stored prior to release into the blood stream.

Developmental Abnormalities

Developmental abnormalities of the pituitary are rare and range from harmless separation of the two component parts ("dystopia of the neurohypophysis"; Lennox and Russell 1951) to ectopia (Weber et al. 1977), hypoplasia and aplasia, usually in association with abnormalities of the brain and skull with clinically obvious external defects (Fig. 13.17) (Lundberg and Gemzell 1966; Sadeghi-Nejad et al. 1974). In anencephaly the anterior pituitary is present but small, and being deprived of normal hypothalamic connections is assumed not to function. The constituent cells show electron microscopic evidence of differentiation into the various anterior pituitary cell types. The failure of full development of the fetal zone of the adrenal cortex in this condition is ascribed to lack of pituitary stimulus. There is, however, no notable defect in the development of the thyroid. In holoprosencephaly and septo-optic dysplasia there is failure of pituitary hormone production that often involves growth hormone alone, although sometimes several or all of the interior and posterior pituitary hormones may be deficient.

Failure of normal growth in childhood is found to be related to growth hormone deficiency in 3%–12% of cases. In about a half of these, the defect is the result of a local pituitary lesion and there is then usually additional evidence of deficiency of other pituitary hormones or disturbance to local structures. Pituitary hypoplasia is a rare cause, most cases being related to tumours of the pituitary and adjacent structures or other locally destructive lesions such as eosinophil granuloma, tuberculous infection and autoimmune destruction. Ischaemic necrosis following head injury and birth trauma is rare. In the remaining half no pituitary cause is found and these cases are classed as idiopathic. They are mostly sporadic, but in some instances there is a family history with autosomal recessive inheritance. The growth hormone deficiency may be complete or partial and is usually the sole deficiency in the familial group, whereas in about half the remaining idiopathic cases there is associated deficiency of other pituitary hormones. Thus sexual development may also be impaired and thyroid and adrenal function can be deficient. There are very few post-mortem studies available on the pituitary and hypothalamus in idiopathic cases. The whole pituitary gland tends to be small in dwarfism from any cause, with little evidence of selective depletion in somatotrophs (Russfield and Reiner 1957), although this has been described (Hewer 1944). Evidence thus favours an abnormality involving the hypothalamic nuclei, a suggestion supported by the observation that injection of thyrotrophin-releasing hormone (TRH) provokes normal release of thyrotrophin (TSH) in cases with associated thyrotrophin deficiency. Rare cases have been described in which there is evidence of production of an abnormal growth hormone or failure of induction of peripheral somatomedin generation.

There are several lesions that arise from persisting developmental structures that may destroy the pituitary or interfere with its function and compress surrounding structures. Craniopharyngioma is the commonest tumorous lesion. Most are suprasellar in location, with more than half presenting in childhood and adolescence and rare cases being recorded in the newborn (Iyer 1952; Gass 1956; Tabaddor et al. 1974) (see p. 197). In instances where part of the tumour occupies the sella turcica, greater damage is caused to the pituitary, with resulting hypopituitarism and hypopituitary dwarfism . Suprasellar and dumb-bell cysts are considered to originate from nests of squamous cells commonly found near the junction of the stalk with the pars distalis in adults (Erdheim 1904) and in the newborn (Goldberg and Eshbaugh 1960). Intrasellar cysts are believed to develop from the hypophyseal cleft that represents the remnant of the cavity of Rathke's pouch. Remnants of the compressed pituitary are found in the outer part of the wall of intrasellar cysts and there is usually at least a partial lining of cuboidal ciliated epithelium. The cysts contents are either fluid or inspissated and discoloured from old haemorrhage. Rare tumours include teratomas of typical and "atypical pinealoma" types, and dermoid and epidermoid cysts that must be distinguished from teratomas in the former; the latter should probably be included with the craniopharyngiomas (Russell and Rubinstein 1977, p. 38).

Inflammatory Lesions

Acute hypophysitis can occur as part of a septicaemia or pyaemia and as an extension of infection of the leptomeninges and local air sinuses. The pituitary may be involved diffusely or the inflammation may be localized, most commonly affecting the anterior lobe. Chronic infective disease of the meninges may affect the pituitary either by direct extension of the infection leading to destruction or as a result of inflammatory damage to the pituitary stalk. Causes include tuberculosis, cocidiomycosis and histoplasmosis.

Autoimmune hypophysitis is typically a disease that affects middle-aged and elderly women, but occasionally cases occur in childhood. The process usually involves the anterior lobe only and in most cases giant-cell granulomas are a conspicuous feature, with diffuse lymphocytic and plasma cell infiltration in the intervening pituitary tissue. In some cases there is diffuse lymphocytic infiltrate with a small proportion of plasma cells but no granulomas.

In Hand–Schüller–Christian disease there is usually evidence of disturbance of neurohypophyseal function. The accumulation of cholesterol-containing macrophages in the sphenoid bone and dura and in the basal leptomeninges, pituitary stalk and its posterior lobe produces erosion of the bone and a yellow-grey thickening of the soft structures.

Both the anterior and the posterior lobes of the pituitary are involved in Hunter–Hurler disease.The cytoplasm of the constituent cells, particularly of the acidophils, become distended by the accumulation of mucopolysaccharide (Schochet et al. 1974), but it is unusual for there to be any evidence of functional disturbance.

In fatal head injury, subcapsular haemorrhage and necrosis of both pituitary lobes is a common finding and is often independent of rupture of the stalk. Injury to the hypothalamus may also occur. Similar, though perhaps less severe, lesions in those surviving injury occur, but evidence of anterior pituitary dysfunction is only occasionally documented (Paxson and Brown 1976; Winternitz and Dzur 1976; Fleisher et al.1978; Landon et al. 1978; Miller et al. 1980). The recognition of pituitary disturbance as separate from hypothalamic damage is problematic. Where rupture of the pituitary stalk has occurred, diabetes

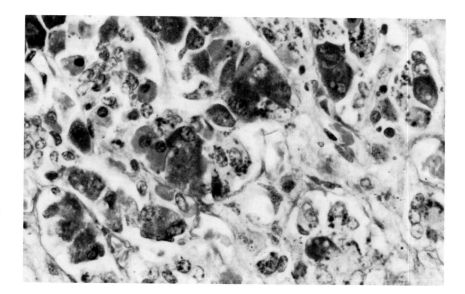

Fig. 13.18. Pituitary from a patient with myxoedema. Several cells with large dark cytoplasmic PAS-positive droplets stand out among the large uniformly dark mucoid basophils and lighter acidophils. (PAS, Orange G, × 480)

insipidus develops either immediately or after a latent period. If the rupture occurs below the median eminence there may be recovery of hormone production.

Adenomas of the Adenohypophysis

Pituitary adenomas are rare before adult life. Traditionally they are classified according to their staining characteristic in histological preparations into chromophobe, acidophil and basophil. With general availability of immunohistochemical methods it is now more appropriate for their classification to be based on the hormones identified in the tumour cells and any associated clinical effects. In contrast to the high proportion of apparently non-functioning chromophobe tumours among adult pituitary adenomas, this type is practically unknown in childhood and adolescence (Russell and Rubinstein 1977 p. 312). Growth hormone-producing tumours and corticotrophin-producing tumours are recorded occasionally and are associated with acromegalic gigantism and Cushing's disease, respectively. Sometimes the tumour cells contain few secretory granules and can then appear chromophobe. In a proportion of cases an acidophil adenoma is present as part of the hereditary syndrome of MEN type 1 and nodular chief-cell hyperplasia of the parathyroids and tumours of the pancreatic islets may be simultaneously present or may develop subsequently. The histological and ultrastructural characteristics of childhood pituitary adenomas are similar to the findings in equivalent adult cases, which are described by Doniach (1977). In a large proportion of

cases of childhood Cushing's disease treated by adrenalectomy there is subsequent enlargement of the pituitary tumour, sometimes with infiltration of the surrounding bone (Hopwood and Kenny 1977), but truly malignant change is extremely rare (Russell and Rubinstein 1977 p. 312). Surgical adenomectomy can produce good results in childhood tumours, but the tendency for persistence of disease in some cases is illustrated in the series reported by Dyer et al. (1994).

Pituitary Changes Reflecting Disease in Target Organs

Impaired function in the various endocrine glands is accompanied by changes in the anterior pituitary consequent to the perturbation of hormone levels or the effects of altered metabolic activity on the pituitary.

In hypothyroidism the pituitary enlarges because of increased size and numbers of thyrotrophs. These can be found in groups within the median wedge and close to the capsule in the anterior and anterolateral areas, and are identified in periodic acid–Schiff (PAS)–stained sections from the presence of PAS–positive droplets and the small number of granules in their cytoplasm (Fig. 13.18). In longstanding untreated hypothyroidism granulated acidophils become less numerous.

Cushing's syndrome is accompanied by characteristic changes in the corticotroph basophils as described by Crooke (1935) (Fig. 13.19a). There is enlargement of the nucleus and cytoplasm, which loses its granules, acquiring a hyaline, slightly refractile appearance. Degranulation occurs first in the

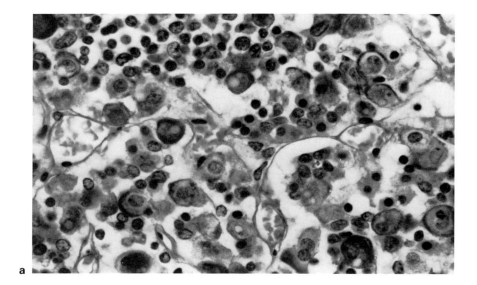

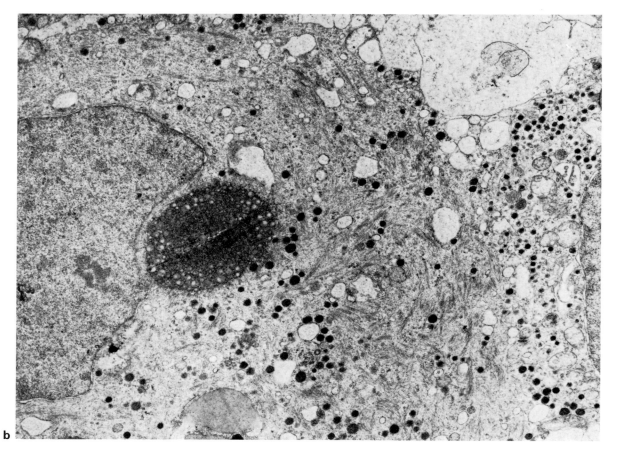

Fig. 13.19. a Crooke cells in the anterior pituitary from a patient with Cushing's syndrome. The hyaline change in the perinuclear cytoplasm and appearance of variable-sized vacuoles is well seen in several of the basophil cells. (PAS, Orange G, × 480) **b** Electron micrograph of an anterior pituitary basophil cell showing Crooke cell change. The cytoplasm contains arrays of fibrils and the secretory granules are reduced in number. (× 14 000)

cytoplasm adjacent to the nucleus and in a band in the mid-zone of the cell body and is accompanied by the appearance of large clear vacuoles. Eventually the cells are totally degranulated. Electron microscopy shows that the hyaline cytoplasm contains a feltwork of fine filaments (Porcile and Racadot 1966) (Fig. 13.19b). Crooke cell change occurs in response to persistently elevated levels of glucocorticoids whether spontaneous or the result of steroid medication. The cells of basophil adenomas in Cushing's disease do not show Crooke cell change but the corticotrophs in the surrounding pituitary do. In untreated Addison's disease the number of partially degranulated basophils is increased and acidophils are reduced in number (Crooke and Russell 1935). Pregnancy and lactation are accompanied by increase in pituitary weight resulting from proliferation of prolactin acidophil cells.

Thyroid

Development

Most, if not the whole, of the human thyroid develops from evagination, proliferation and caudal migration of cells in the midline of the ventral fore-gut epithelium, commencing at the end of the 1st month of gestation. A solid bilobed mass is formed, which is attached by a hollow stalk, the thyroglossal duct, to the pharyngeal floor. At the same time a lateral thyroid mass, the ultimobranchial body, forms from the fourth pharyngeal pouch on each side and fuses with the main median mass. The contribution of the lateral thyroid masses to the developing thyroid remains controversial; they commonly show degenerative changes at an early stage, and in cases of ectopic sublingual thyroid it is unusual for isotope studies to show any cervical uptake of iodine, so that their capacity to form follicular epithelium appears to be insignificant. Studies in animals have shown that the thyroid C cells, or parafollicular cells, which produce calcitonin, are of neural crest origin and migrate to the thyroid via the ultimobranchial bodies (Pearse et al. 1972). It is likely that human thyroid C cells have a similar origin and that the small nests of squamoid and columnar cells commonly found in the lateral thyroid lobes represent remnants of the ultimobranchial body. Further development of the definitive thyroid is by proliferation of its cells in the form of solid cords and later as tubular structures. At about 72 days' gestation an intracytoplasmic vacuole lined

by microvilli forms and is followed by the appearance of demosomes between cell groups, which then extrude their vacuoles to produce an extracellular follicle. Colloid production and the ability to concentrate and bind iodide is established by the 80th gestational day, as has been demonstrated by occasional cases of accidental fetal thyroid ablation resulting from administration of ^{131}I to the mother for therapeutic purposes occurring only when the isotope had been given after the 70th gestational day (Fisher et al. 1963). These early stages in the development of the thyroid are independent of thyrotrophin, but once colloid and thyroid hormone synthesis is established the activity of the thyroid comes under pituitary control. From the 80 mm stage the thyroid weight is established at about 0.046% of the body weight, a proportion that persists into adult life.

Ectopic Thyroid Tissue

Small, and sometimes large, amounts of thyroid tissue are occasionally found outside the normal anatomical site. In most cases the ectopic tissue has been found in the course of the thyroglossal duct as a result of failure of migration early in development. Substantial masses are found most commonly in relation to the posterior part of the tongue (lingual thyroid) and are usually easily visible. Rarely an additional mass separates from the main gland and is found below a lower pole or in the anterior mediastinum with a separate blood supply. It is not very rare to find striated muscle or adipose tissue incorporated in the periphery of a thyroid lobe, and collections of a few thyroid follicles have been demonstrated in cervical lymph nodes in up to 3% of individuals (Meyer and Steinberg 1969). These may represent developmental "tangles" or, in the case of the lymph node foci, benign tissue emboli rather than developmental misplacement.

The importance of misplaced thyroid tissue is, firstly, that it may be misinterpreted as well differentiated carcinoma, especially in the case of inclusions within lymph nodes, and, secondly, that a large ectopic mass may represent the total thyroid tissue. This is commonly the case with a lingual thyroid, so that hypothyroidism is a likely consequence of its excision. Most patients with a lingual thyroid present with a swelling in the throat or mouth, and many are found to have myxoedema. Both problems are easily corrected with oral thyroxine. Carcinoma has been described, and appears to be commoner in lingual thyroids than in normally placed glands (Smithers 1970). It is likely that at least some of the reported cases represent mistaken diagnosis in the presence of a marked hyperplasia accompanying defective thyroid hormone production. Dyshormonogenesis is probably the most frequently associated abnormality accounting for the observed high incidence of hypothyroidism, goitre and development of tumours.

Development of a cyst from remnants of the thyroglossal duct is common and can present in childhood (Brerton and Symonds 1978) or adult life, and even in old age. They occur in the midline between the thyroid and the floor of the mouth, and are often intimately related to the hyoid bone, the mid-portion of which should be resected with the cyst to ensure complete removal. Excised cysts are found to have a lining of respiratory or squamous epithelium or a mixture of both. They have a thick fibrous capsule, which usually includes a variable amount of lymphoid tissue. Apart from size and the disfigurement these cysts may produce, they have a tendency to become infected. Occasionally papillary carcinoma develops in the course of the thyroglossal duct. Such tumours appear to involve no worse a prognosis than their thyroidal counterpart (Page et al. 1974; Saharia 1975).

Goitre

Sporadic

Sporadic or euthyroid simple goitre is not seen in young children but does occur after the age of 6 years, most usually in pubertal and adolescent females. There may be an initial phase of diffuse thyroid enlargement prior to the development of a multinodular goitre similar in morphology to its adult counterpart. Routine tests of thyroid function yield normal results.

Areas of endemic goitre where iodine prophylaxis has not been introduced show a high prevalence of goitre in children of both sexes, with cases occurring at birth and in infancy in the most severely affected districts. It is in these severely goitrous districts that endemic cretinism is found. The level of iodine deficiency alone appears to be only a partial explanation of the incidence of thyroid disease, and severe iodine deficiency has been described without the occurrence of goitre or cretinism (Roche 1959). Even in the most severely goitrous areas there is always a proportion of the population that is spared, although there are no differences in their water supply or diet. The scale of the problem of endemic goitre in world terms is well documented in the detailed survey by Kelly and Snedden (1960). The gross and histological appearances of the thyroid vary according to the severity and duration of the iodine deficiency and also between different goitrous areas. In some

endemic cretins the thyroid appears to atrophy during intrauterine development, leaving only a small fibrotic remnant. The more usual endemic goitre shows an initial phase of parenchymal hyperplasia in response to an elevated blood level of TSH. Later the commonly illustrated and often very large colloid goitre that eventually becomes multinodular supervenes.

Dyshormonogenetic

Dyshormonogenetic goitre comprises a group of uncommon conditions in which there is an inborn defect of thyroid hormone synthesis. The subject has been comprehensively reviewed by Stanbury and Dumont (1983). The capacity of the thyroid to produce hormone is diminished and results in an increased output of TSH from the pituitary, with consequent thyroid hyperplasia. In cases where the block to hormone synthesis is severe, goitre and hypothyroidism are present in infancy. In many instances, however, the disorder is less severe, so that with increased TSH drive the hyperplastic gland maintains sufficient hormone production. The increased demand for thyroid hormone during growth and at puberty often appears to be the time at which a previously compensated defect is revealed by the development of a goitre.

An intrathyroidal metabolic block has been demonstrated to occur on at least five steps in hormone synthesis, resulting in:

1. Failure of iodide trapping
2. Failure of organic binding of intrathyroidal iodide (due to peroxidase deficiency)
3. Failure of iodotyrosine coupling
4. Failure of deiodination of iodotyrosine residues (due to dehalogenase deficiency)
5. Defective thyroglobulin synthesis and production of abnormal iodoproteins

Defect in organification of iodide caused by deficiency in the peroxidase system is by far the commonest of these generally rare inherited disorders and is the defect found in Pendred's syndrome, in which there is associated perceptive deafness. The disturbances of thyroid function among cases of Pendred's syndrome is usually less severe than the apparently similar defect in peroxidase in other cases, so that overt hypothyroidism is uncommon and the size of the goitre is generally modest.

The many cases of Pendred's syndrome that have been described indicate an autosomal recessive mode of inheritance (Nilsson et al. 1965). There appears to be close linkage between the genes determining the thyroidal defect and the deafness, because only very

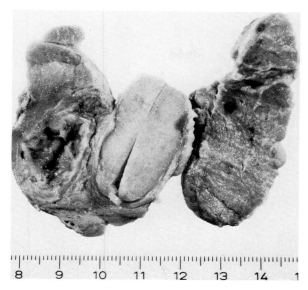

Fig. 13.20. Coronal cut through a dyshormonogenetic goitre weighing 63 g removed from a 17-year-old clinically euthyroid female. The cut surface of the thyroid is paler and more fleshy than normal. An adenoma expands the isthmus and a second partly cystic adenoma occupies the lower pole on the left. In addition, several small nodules are visible scattered in the parenchyma.

demonstrable by cannulation of a salivary gland duct and administration of labelled iodide. Some cases involve the production of abnormal iodoproteins, which may be insoluble in butanol and can be separated by electrophoresis.

The pathological changes in the thyroid are similar in most of the different types of defect and are characteristic. The hyperplastic gland can reach an enormous size, and weights of several hundred grams are not uncommon: occasional cases with a gland weighing in excess of 2 kg have been recorded. The excised thyroid (Fig. 13.20) is firm and fleshy with little visible colloid. Nodules are almost invariably present and in large specimens account for the greater part of the mass. Microscopically, there is intense parenchyma hyperplasia with small, usually empty, follicles lined by columnar epithelium. Pleomorphic nuclei in the thyroid epithelium are usually prominent, including occasional irregular hyperchromatic giant forms (Fig. 13.21a). The nodules vary in size and morphology: most are cellular, comprising solid and empty follicles with only a little vascular stroma. Sometimes the stroma is prominent and oedematous and degenerative changes can occur; the epithelial component can form a wide variety of patterns including papillary structures and large colloid-filled follicles (Fig. 13.21b), and may show extreme nuclear pleomorphism. Individual nodules are usually surrounded by a well defined fibrous compression zone, but their margin may be ill-defined and the nodular tissue may appear to encroach on the adjacent parenchyma and even to invade the walls of blood vessels. The pleomorphism and aggressive appearances can lead to a diagnosis of carcinoma, but caution is needed in assessment and treatment because truly malignant behaviour with metastases is rare (McGirr et al. 1959; Crooks et al. 1963). In a review of reported malignancies in dyshormonogenetic goitre, Vickery (1981) concluded that all the cases in which the diagnosis was acceptable were follicular carcinomas. Occasional papillary carcinomas also occur. In cases in which an abnormal iodoprotein is found the pathological changes may be somewhat different (Kennedy 1969), with a tendency for the goitre to be much larger with a multicystic appearance to the cut surface. The colloid in the large cystic follicles appears pale, fragmented and filamentous on microscopic examination. Multiple nodules are also usually present.

rarely has the thyroidal disorder alone been described among these families. The peroxidase defect may be of variable severity in non-Pendred families, so that although a goitre is invariably present not all cases are hypothyroid. The tendency for the hypothyroid cases to be concentrated mainly within certain families suggests genetic heterogeneity in this disorder. An autosomal recessive mode of inheritance also appears to be operating in the other types of dyshormonogenetic goitre, and clearly is so in the extensively studied large family of tinkers described by Hutchinson and McGirr (1956) and shown to have a defect in deiodinase resulting in goitre, hypothyroidism and, in the majority of their cases, mental retardation.

Identification of the type of defect depends on laboratory investigation. In those with an organification defect, iodide is rapidly concentrated in the thyroid but is largely discharged by the subsequent administration of perchlorate, which blocks the iodide-trapping mechanism. In cases with a deiodinase defect the other tissues show the same defect so that labelled monoiodotyrosine and diiodotyrosine injected intravenously can be recovered unchanged in the urine. The rare cases in which the iodide trap is defective are unable to concentrate iodide tracer or pertechnetate in the thyroid. The salivary gland tissues and gastric mucosa are similarly affected, and the consequent inability to concentrate iodide into the saliva is

Cretinism and Hypothyroidism

The term "cretinism" is liable to some variation in its use, some authors applying it to all cases of congenital hypothyroidism, others only to those in which

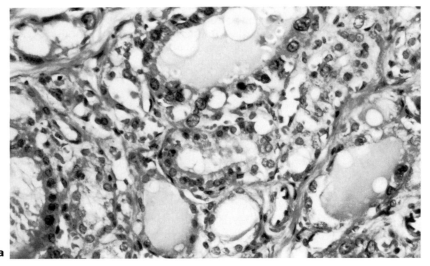

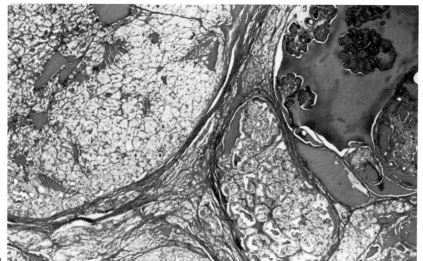

Fig. 13.21. Dyshormonogenetic goitre. **a** Detail from the diffusely hyperplastic parenchyma. The follicles appear empty or contain pale-staining vacuolated colloid. The epithelial cells are cuboid or columnar and in several the nucleus is large and hyperchromatic. (H&E, × 300) **b** There are several nodules with varied histological patterns in the field of view. The parenchyma is diffusely hyperplastic (*bottom left*). (H&E, × 20)

there are associated irreversible mental and neurological sequelae. Congenital hypothyroidism is usually divided into cases associated with severe endemic iodine deficiency and the non-endemic or sporadic form. This latter group includes a variety of entities and can be subdivided into goitrous cases resulting from dyshormonogenesis with a normally placed or ectopic thyroid and non-goitrous cases resulting from thyroidal hypoplasia or agenesis. The reasons for thyroidal hypoplasia and agenesis are not understood, but several specific associations have been observed, including a high incidence of first-cousin marriages among the parents, a high incidence of both thyroid antibodies in the mothers' serum and of hyperthyroidism and hypothyroidism among relatives, and

associations with Down's syndrome and Turner's syndrome. Endemic cretins may be evident at birth and are found in areas with extreme iodine deficiency and a high incidence of goitre, and may account for as much as 8% of the population (Choufoer et al. 1965; Fiero-Benitez et al. 1965), and though usually goitrous some cases occur with a small or impalpable thyroid attributable to associated hypoplasia or agenesis. Sporadic cretins usually appear normal at birth and tend to be large, and in those whose cretinism results from dyshormonogenesis a goitre may be obvious. Reliable early diagnosis is possible by routine assay of serum TSH levels in the neonatal period (Dussault et al. 1975; Hulse et al. 1980; Fisher 1987). Sporadic congenital hypothyroidism is detected with remarkably consistent frequency world-wide, at one case in 3500–4500 births, with twice as many girls as boys. About 90% of cases result from hypoplasia or agenesis of the thyroid, and familial cases are a small minority. The earliest clinical manifestations of hypothyroidism are undue persistence of physiological jaundice, feeding difficulties and constipation with failure to thrive, umbilical hernia, and respiratory problems. Later, thickening, dryness and pallor of the skin, poor hair growth and relative enlargement of the tongue develop, and with time the failure of closure of the fontanelles and retardation of linear growth and mental and motor functions become obvious. The slowing of central nervous development is the most serious effect of fetal and infantile thyroid deficiency because, unlike in the other somatic effects, the delay in growth and maturation of the cerebral cortex and cerebellum is irreparable and results in mental defect and motor disturbances in which ataxia, strabismus, severe spasticity and mild hypotonia are recorded (Smith et al. 1957; Koenig 1968; Hagberg and Westphal 1970; Mäenpää 1972). Skeletal abnormalities in infantile and childhood hypothyroidism are constant findings. The appearance of the ossification centres is delayed, and the absence or small size and fragmentation of the distal femoral epiphysis in a full-term infant is good supporting evidence for hypothyroidism (Dorff 1934; Anderson 1973), having otherwise only been described in babies of diabetic mothers (Pedersen and Osler 1958).

Hypothyroidism developing later in childhood is assumed to be caused by autoimmune thyroid destruction in most cases and affects the sexes with equal frequency (Winter et al. 1966). After the age of 3 years intelligence is not usually irreversibly affected, but slowing of cerebral activity is a common finding, as are the effects on growth and bone maturation.

Autoimmune Thyroid Disease

Both Graves' disease and chronic lymphocytic thyroiditis are recorded at all ages. Some 5% of all graves' disease patients are under 16 years old (Saxena et al. 1964), and more than 40% of childhood non-toxic goitre is attributed to chronic lymphocytic thyroiditis (Saxena and Crawford 1962; Nilsson and Doniach 1964). Girls form the great majority of cases of both disorders. Circulating thyroid antibodies are present, as in the adult disease, and their demonstration is important in diagnosis. A family history of autoimmune thyroid disease is often obtained, and laboratory evidence of thyroid disorder in a parent is very common. The frequent coincidence

of autoimmune thyroid disorders in cases with a chromosomal abnormality, notably Down's syndrome (Hollingsworth et al. 1974) and Tuner's syndrome (Doniach et al. 1968), is recognized.

The changes seen in the thyroid in childhood Graves' disease are similar to those that occur in adults. There is symmetrical smooth, modest, enlargement as a result of diffuse hyperplasia of the parenchyma, with an accompanying depletion of colloid, markedly increased vascularity, and a focal lymphocytic infiltrate of variable amount in most cases. The systemic manifestations are usually of insidious onset, and a rapid pulse rate and accelerated growth rate are often the only changes observed, but enquiry usually draws attention to some falling-off of school performance and an increased appetite. Protuberant exophthalmos from orbital infiltration is rare in children, and sexual maturation is undisturbed in most.

In chronic lymphocytic thyroiditis the gland is enlarged by two to five times, usually symmetrically and with a granular firm consistency and easily palpable outline. The development of a goitre is often the only indication of a thyroid abnormality. Clinical or laboratory evidence of hypothyroidism is found in about one-third of the cases (Saxena and Crawford 1962), and in these the goitre tends to be smaller than in euthyroid cases. The more severely hypothyroid patients show diminished growth and may be myxoedematous (Nilsson and Doniach 1964). Only limited studies of the histological changes in the thyroid are available (Clayton and Johnson 1960; Leboeuf and Bongiovanni 1964). There is an extensive interfollicular infiltrate of lymphocytes and formation of lymphoid follicles with germinal centres. The thyroid epithelium is hyperplastic, the follicles small, and the colloid scanty and inspissated. Fibrosis and oxyphil metaplasia are not usually seen except in longstanding cases.

Other inflammatory disorders affecting the thyroid are rare in children. Rare cases of acute bacterial infection have most often been attributed to β-haemolytic streptococci. De Quervain's subacute giant-cell or granulomatous thyroiditis sometimes occurs in adolescent girls, when it produces the usual symptoms of sore throat and fever followed by painful enlargement of the thyroid, sometimes only one lobe being involved. Symptoms in mild cases resolve in a few days; in others they may last for several months. There is a patchy inflammatory involvement of the thyroid with oedema and an infiltrate of lymphocytes that sometimes extends through the thyroid capsule. Giant cells and granulomas form at the site of destroyed thyroid follicles and here eventual healing is by fibrosis. There is no permanent disturbance of thyroid function.

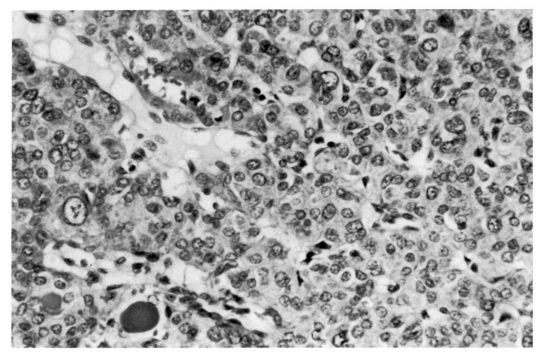

Fig. 13.22. Atypical adenoma. The solid cellular pattern and nuclear pleomorphism are not indications of malignancy. (H&E, × 400)

Tumours

Both benign and malignant tumours of the thyroid are less common in children than in adults. This lowered incidence is greater in benign follicular adenomas and colloid nodules, so that the proportion of solitary thyroid nodules presenting in childhood that are found to be carcinomas is comparatively greater and is probably in excess of 20%. Little is known of naturally occurring factors predisposing to the development of thyroid tumours, but in the hyperplastic dyshormonogenetic gland adenomas, usually multiple, appear sooner or later. Adenomas are also more common in goitrous districts, and follicular and anaplastic carcinomas may be commoner among adults in these areas (Wegelin 1928; Cuello et al. 1969). Papillary carcinoma has a much higher incidence in some countries, notably Japan and Iceland, and it is possible that the high level of dietary iodine may be in part responsible (Williams et al. 1977). Some cases of medullary carcinoma have a familial incidence, with inheritance as a Mendelian autosomal dominant character. There are no data relating to whether chronic lymphocytic thyroiditis has any part to play in the rare cases of childhood thyroid lymphoma. Induction of thyroid tumours in children by irradiation (Saenger et al. 1960; Winship and Rosvoll 1961; Hempelmann et al. 1967) has occurred inad-

vertently on a wide scale as a consequence of the use of X-rays to shrink the thymus in infants to prevent status thymolymphaticus and croup. This was practised particularly in the USA from 1925 to 1955, and the thyroid was inevitably included in the treatment field in these small newborn infants. The use of X-rays as a depilatory agent in the management of tinea capitis and for the treatment of inflammatory and other cutaneous lesions has also contributed cases. Both benign and malignant tumours develop with an increased frequency after a period averaging about 9 years, with the risk persisting throughout life. The accident in 1954 in which radioactive fallout from a hydrogen bomb detonated on Bikini affected islanders on nearby Rongelap was followed by the development in 1969 of one carcinoma and small multinodular goitres in 16 of 19 exposed children (Conard et al. 1970). Thyroid irradiation was principally from radioiodine, with a calculated dose to the gland of up to 14 Gy. An impressive increase in incidence of thyroid carcinomas, the great majority papillary, has been observed in children from the Republic of Belarus following the Chernobyl disaster (Furmanchuk et al. 1992; Nikiforov and Gnepp 1994).

Individual thyroid tumours in children are similar pathologically to their adult counterparts, and are classified accordingly. The following classification is based on the International Histological Classification of Tumours no. 11 (World Health Organization):

1. *Epithelial tumours*
   A. Benign:
      Follicular adenoma
   B. Malignant:
      Papillary carcinoma
      Follicular carcinoma
      Anaplastic carcinoma
      Medullary carcinoma
2. *Non-epithelial tumours*
   Lymphoma
   Teratoma

Adenomas

Adenomas are typically solitary lesions, are encapsulated, and may be subdivided according to whether they are formed from large or small colloid-containing follicles or solid epithelial cords, although no useful purpose is served by this. Adenomas are usually solitary, and mitoses may be easily identified in the more cellular examples. Several sections should be examined to exclude invasion of the capsule and its contained vascular sinuses. This may not be an obvious feature in some of the low-grade follicular carcinomas. Figure 13.22 shows an atypical adenoma.

Carcinoma

The distribution of the different types of carcinoma is a little different when compared with adults. There is greater preponderance of papillary tumours, but anaplastic carcinomas are uncommon.

Papillary. Typically, papillary carcinomas are unencapsulated tumours (Fig. 13.23a), often showing marked central fibrosis and contraction. They are often multifocal. In many cases the primary tumour is less than 2 cm in diameter, and it can be minute. A mixture of neoplastic follicles and papillary structures is usually found (Fig. 13.23b), with a tendency in children for a greater proportion of the tumours to have a predominantly papillary pattern, sometimes with numerous psammoma bodies. Cervical lymph node metastases are present in nearly 90% of cases and may be bilateral in up to 25% of cases (Hayles et al. 1963; Harness et al. 1971). Bulky masses are often formed. The prognosis in most young people is very good, possibly best in cases presenting with local lymph node metastases (Woolner et al. 1961). It does not appear to be influenced greatly by any particular conventional form of treatment (Winship and Rosvoll 1961). Cases in which complete surgical removal of tumour is possible show the best survival figures, but radical surgery may carry high risks of unnecessary damage to recurrent laryngeal nerves and the parathyroids (Richardson et al. 1974). Recorded cases include some that have been observed over several decades, with known metastatic deposits that have shown no evidence of progression.

Follicular. Follicular carcinomas are encapsulated tumours that do not form papillary structures. To the naked eye they usually appear solid and fleshy. They are usually more than 2 cm in diameter and as a group they are larger than the papillary carcinomas but similar in size to the adenomas. The majority cannot be distinguished from the more cellular adenomas on the basis of their gross appearance. Invasion of the tumour capsule with penetration of capsular vascular sinuses and, in the more aggressive tumours, invasion of the surrounding thyroid by pushing rounded tumour masses are the diagnostic features (Fig. 13.24). The invasion of local blood vessels explains the tendency for metastases to involve the lungs and bones. Secondary deposits in cervical lymph nodes are rare. An important source of erroneously diagnosed cases is the inclusion of the often very cellular and sometimes pleomorphic but benign tumours that develop in dyshormonogenetic goitres (see p. 712). Another cause of occasional over diagnosis is the "atypical" adenoma with its solid structure, mitoses and, in some cases, markedly pleomorphic nuclei. Microscopic evidence of invasion through the tumour capsule and into blood vessels is conspicuous in the more aggressive cases, with a correspondingly greater risk of distant metastases and a worse prognosis. The greater proportion of these tumours are, however, indolent in their behaviour and are recognized by less penetrating invasion of their capsule and involvement only of vascular sinuses within the capsule. Evidence of such invasion in some of these cases requires the examination of many tissue blocks taken to include the capsule, and it is recommended that 8–12 such blocks should be taken if possible.

Medullary. Arising from the parafollicular, or C cells, medullary carcinomas have a distinctive morphology and differ in all respects from the papillary and follicular carcinomas that originate from the follicular epithelium. They probably account for between 5% and 10% of thyroid carcinomas, but an accurate figure is difficult to calculate because recorded personal series are small and liable to distortion if a large pedigree of the inherited variety is included.

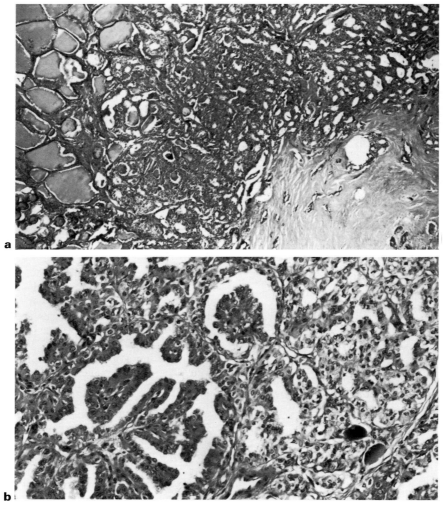

Fig. 13.23. **a** Papillary carcinoma forming an unencapsulated tumour infiltrating between adjacent thyroid follicles. The centre of the tumour is sclerotic. There are several psammoma bodies at the periphery of the tumour. (H&E, × 30) **b** A mixture of papillary structures and neoplastic follicles that is typical of papillary carcinoma as a group. The proportions of the two elements vary, and cases apparently composed exclusively of one or the other can occur. (H&E, × 120)

The genetically determined cases follow an autosomal dominant mode of transmission and can be divided into three subgroups (Williams 1975): one in which thyroid medullary carcinoma alone occurs, a second where medullary carcinoma and phaeochromocytoma are linked, and, least commonly, cases with medullary carcinoma, phaeochromocytoma and multiple mucosal neuromas. In any particular family the subtype is maintained from one generation to the next, with the reservation that in those linked with phaeochromocytoma, which is the commonest form, not all cases will necessarily manifest both thyroid and adrenal tumours. Sometimes the genetic link can be traced in only two generations. This is particularly

so in cases with neuromatous malformations, and suggests a small but definite contribution by mutation. In the familial cases the average age at presentation is lower than in sporadic cases, with the result that more will be seen in children. Another characteristic of the familial type is that in most cases the tumours are multifocal and bilateral, apparently arising in hyperplastic C-cell nests. (See MEN 2, p. 699.)

In about half the cases presenting clinically, local cervical lymph nodes contain metastases. The primary tumour in the thyroid is commonly 2–5 cm in diameter, sharply defined, solid, and often of creamy-yellow colour and gritty when cut. Microscopically,

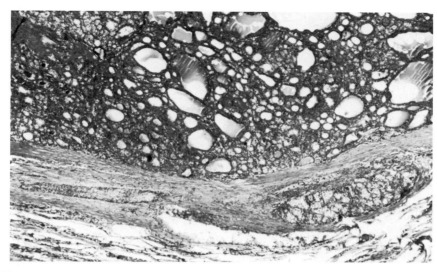

Fig. 13.24. Encapsulated follicular carcinoma identified by tumour invasion into a capsular blood vessel. (H&E, × 30)

the tumour cells are polygonal (Fig. 13.25a) or fusiform and arranged in solid nests and sheets that engulf residual non-neoplastic thyroid follicles. They are broken up by a variable amount of collagenous stroma. Amyloid is usually demonstrable both within the cell masses and in the tumour connective tissue, although on occasions the amount present may be very small. Calcification in amyloid and collagen occurs commonly and can give a characteristic pattern of speckled shadowing on a soft-tissue radiograph. Less common histological patterns occur (Williams et al. 1966), and in these circumstances the almost invariable finding of positive cytoplasmic staining for calcitonin and CEA immunohistochemically is helpful. Electron microscopy with demonstration of electron-dense membrane-bound secretory granules can also be a help in correct identification. The prognosis in individual cases is difficult to predict. The likelihood of tumour dissemination has been correlated with the presence of cervical lymph node metastases (Woolner et al. 1968) and with evidence of more rapid growth assessed by the finding of mitoses and areas of necrosis, features that are more commonly seen with a pronounced spindle-celled pattern (Fig. 13.25b) (Williams et al. 1966). Rapidly fatal cases are uncommon, and even with inoperable or recurrent local disease or distant metastases prolonged survival is more usual.

Calcitonin, the natural product of the C cells, is consistently produced in large quantities by medullary carcinomas. Measurement of levels in the peripheral blood before and after provoked release by alcohol or pentagastrin is a useful test for residual tumour following treatment and for screening of vulnerable members of a family in the genetically determined variants. In some cases additional substances are produced, including ACTH, serotonin, prostaglandins and histaminase. In as many as a quarter of cases a humoral agent that causes severe watery diarrhoea is produced.

Teratoma of the Neck

Teratomas of the neck are rare tumours; they are usually present at birth, occur equally in the two sexes, are associated with hydramnios in 18% of recorded cases, and occasionally cause obstruction during labour. In the younger age group most are benign, only one case of a malignant teratoma having been recorded in infancy. Distinction between teratomas arising within the thyroid (Fig. 13.26) and those arising in extrathyroidal cervical tissues can be difficult (Silberman and Mendelson 1960).

Hormonal Effects of Gonadal Tumours

Testicular

Except for seminoma a substantial proportion of other germ-cell tumours of the testis occur before adulthood, particularly teratomas, in which extraembryonic components (yolk sac and trophoblast) are prominent histologically. Many of the rare stromal

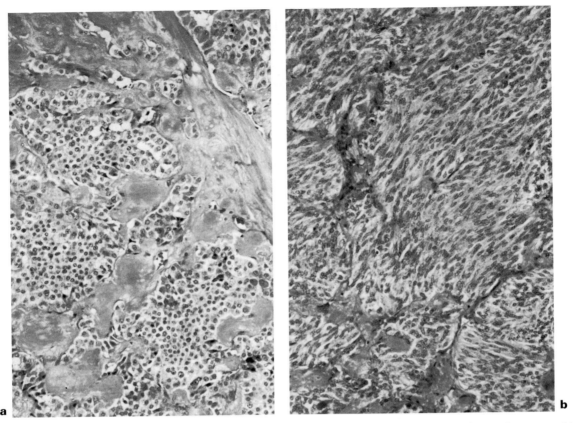

Fig. 13.25. **a** Medullary carcinoma of polygonal cell type. The tumour cells have granular eosinophilic cytoplasm and are arranged in solid nests separated by fibrous tissue and nodular deposits of amyloid. (H&E, × 120) **b** Medullary carcinoma composed of plump spindle cells. Small nodular masses of amyloid are present. (H&E, × 120)

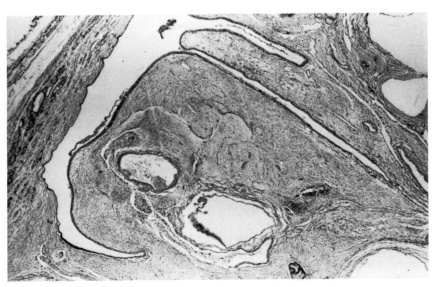

Fig. 13.26. Teratoma within the thyroid removed from a male negro child. The tumour is composed entirely of mature structures of which neuroglia is a prominent solid component. Thyroid follicles are present at the surface of the tumour. (H&E, × 20)

tumours of the testis are seen in childhood. The pathological features and some aspects relating to aetiology and incidence are recorded by Mostofi (1973), and a series of testicular tumours occurring in childhood is recorded by Bormel and Mays (1961).

Germderm Cell Origin

Gynaecomastia occurs in about 30% of all cases of germ cell tumour (Paulsen 1974), particularly among patients with tumours that include histological recognizable trophoblast and measurable levels of chorionic gonadotrophin in their blood and urine. Young children form a prominent group of cases, mostly as a result of the occurrence of tumours that consist predominantly of yolk sac or embryonal carcinoma at this early age (Giebnink and Ruymann 1974). Pure chorion carcinoma and seminoma have virtually never been recorded before puberty.

Testicular Stromal Cell Origin

Tumours of interstitial cell (Leydig cell) origin (Fig. 13.27) are rare. In a review of the literature Gabrilove et al. (1975) quote 23 of 94 recorded cases being in children under 15 years of age. In prepubertal cases the tumour is regularly accompanied by virilization and on occasion gynaecomastia develops in addition. Gabrilove et al. (1975) suggest that gynaecomastia may result from disturbance of the normal ratio of concentration of oestrogen to androgen. Gynaecomastia has also been recorded following administration of methyltestosterone to male eunuchs (McCallagh and Rossmiller 1941). Leydig cell tumours with purely feminizing effects are seen only in adults. Nodules of ectopic hyperplastic adrenal cortical tissue found in relation to the testis in a male infant with congenital adrenal hyperplasia must be distinguished from Lyedig cell tumour.

Sertoli cell tumours are usually benign and are most uncommon. Mostofi et al. (1959) found 23 cases recorded in the AFIP (Armed Forces Institute of Pathology) files, 10 being under 20 years of age. Weitzner and Gropp (1974) found 22 childhood cases recorded in the literature and added one of their own. Sixteen of these cases were less than 1 year old and in two cases there were tumours in both testes. A testicular swelling was the commonest clinical abnormality. Gynaecomastia or sexual precocity occurred in only a few cases. Examination of the pituitary from an adult dying with a malignant Sertoli cell tumour that had been accompanied by gynaecomastia showed changes interpreted as an indication of hyperplasia of the gonadotrophs (Mostofi et al. 1959).

Ovarian

Granulosa theca cell tumours of the ovary are uncommon, with approximately 5% occurring before pubertal age (Lyon et al. 1963) and occasionally even in infancy (Marshall 1965). In most childhood cases the tumours are composed predominantly of granulosa cells. Non-functioning and androgen-secreting tumours occur, but the great majority produce oestrogens, with resultant development of the breasts and genitalia. The appearance of axillary and pubic hair usually follows, but not invariably. The uterus enlarges and endometrial proliferation may be accompanied by irregular bleeding. The contralateral ovary remains infantile.

Other ovarian stromal tumours are even more rare in children. Hilus (Leydig) cell tumours are recorded by Boivin and Richart (1965), and have been reported in association with gonadal dysgenesis (Warren et al. 1964). Sertoli–Leydig cell tumours (androblastomas), though typically occurring in young women, are rare before menarche (Norris and Jensen 1972). Familial occurrence associated with thyroid adenoma has been recorded in adolescents (Jensen et al. 1974). Both tumours usually produce androgens, resulting in pure virilization before puberty and defeminization in postpubertal girls before overtly virilizing effects.

A substantial proportion of germ-cell tumours of the ovary occur in the first two decades. In one series of dysgerminomas (Asadourian and Taylor 1969), 44% were in patients less than 20 years of age. Figure 13.28 shows a dysgerminoma removed from a child. Immature teratoma and embryonal carcinoma are both found predominantly in children and adolescents (Abell et al. 1965). Increased levels of chorionic gonadotrophin in urine and serum suggests that the tumour includes a trophoblastic component and may be accompanied by precocious isosexual development in children, and by menstrual irregularity, amenorrhoea and breast enlargement in postpubertal cases. Occasionally dysgerminoma and gonadoblastoma are associated with virilization (Usizima 1956; Scully 1953).

Details of the clinical and pathological features of ovarian neoplasms occurring in childhood and adolescence are described by Abell (1982).

Ectopic Hormone Syndromes Associated with Tumours

Extensive data have accumulated relating to the production of hormones by tumours of non-endocrine

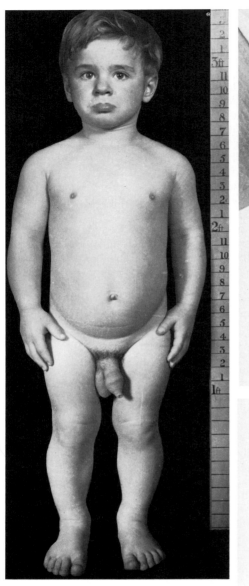

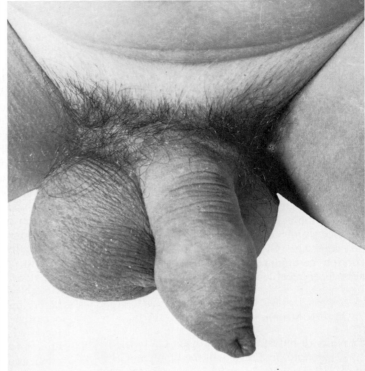

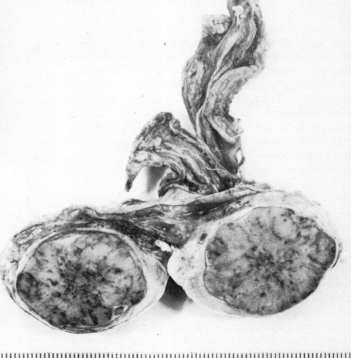

Fig. 13.27. Interstitial cell tumour of the testis in a male aged 2 years 4 months, producing unilateral testicular enlargement, penile development and growth of pubic hair (**a** and **b**). Bisected orchidectomy specimen (**c**) shows the solid sharply circumscribed tumour within the testicular body.

tissues and inappropriate hormones by tumours of endocrine origin in adults (Anderson 1973; Ellison and Neville 1973; Rees and Ratcliffe 1974). Additionally there are examples of hormone-like effects of tumours that it has not been possible to relate to the appropriate hormone (e.g. insulin-like effects). Tumours occurring in children of similar type to those seen in adults have on occasion been reported to produce the same ectopic hormone effects, and additionally there are examples of hormone production by tumours that are more typical of childhood. Many of the reported cases are reviewed by Omenn (1971). Some of the wider implications of paraendocrine and paraneoplastic syndromes are reviewed by Coppes (1993) and Pierce (1993).

Production of ACTH is well documented. Most childhood cases involve tumours now generally regarded as of endocrine cell origin, such as oat cell carcinoma of lung, carcinoid of the thymus, islet-cell tumours, and medullary carcinoma of the thyroid. Of the tumours of childhood those of neuroblast origin are prominent and include phaeochromocytoma. The occurrence of Cushing's syndrome in these circumstances is readily understood. Less obvious is the occasional case in which the tumour produces a corticotrophin-releasing factor that may be CRH itself. Preeyasombat et al. (1992) report such an event in a girl with Ewing's sarcoma of the tibia.

Hypercalcaemia with hypophosphataemia attributed to parathormone-like agents has been recorded with hepatoblastoma and testicular carcinoma among the cases reviewed by Omenn (1971), and in bone sarcoma, neuroblastoma, rhabdomyosarcoma and a number of cases of lymphosarcoma and leukaemia (Myers 1960; Stapleton et al. 1976; Joyaraman and David 1977; Hutchinson et al. 1978; Ramsay et al. 1979). A small-cell ovarian carcinoma occurring in young women and associated with hypercalcaemia has been described by Dickersin et al. (1982). Serum levels of parathormone were normal in the cases in which it was measured, and it is now recognized that several different mechanisms may be involved. In most cases with solid tumours the hypercalcaemia results from production by the tumour of PTHRP. The subjects of calcium homeostasis and mediators of hypercalcaemia in neoplastic disease are reviewed by Gutierre et al. (1990).

Isosexual precocity resulting form gonadotrophin production is recorded in nine males with hepatoblastoma in the review by Omenn (1971). Excluding germ-cell tumours this appears to be the only tumour to produce truly ectopic gonadotrophin. The gonadotrophin is similar in action to pituitary luteinizing hormone (Root et al. 1968; McArthur 1969), a conclusion supported by both the absence of stimulation of the cells of the seminiferous tubules noted in tes-

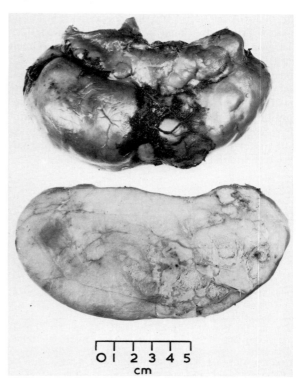

Fig. 13.28. Dysgerminoma removed from a 10-year-old female and apparently restricted to the ovary, though there were some vascular adhesions between the tumour surface and adjacent tissues.

ticular biopsies and the apparent exclusive occurrence of the syndrome in males. The gonadotrophin in the case studied by Braunstein et al. (1972) was similar to chorionic gonadotrophin and distinct from human pituitary luteinizing hormone. The pituitary from the case studied by Behrle et al. (1963) showed a reduced number of acidophils and chromophobes, with increased numbers of basophils and amphophils. Similar pituitary changes were observed in an adult dying with a malignant Sertoli cell tumour of the testis (Mostofi et al. 1959).

Nine childhood cases of hypoglycaemia associated with large non-pancreatic abdominal tumours are collected in the review by Omenn (1971). Four of the tumours were of connective tissue, and included among the remainder were two cases of lymphoma, a large adrenal cortical carcinoma, a Wilms' tumour and a neuroblastoma. The problem of elucidating the cause of the hypoglycaemia associated with tumours of this type, in which low levels of circulating immunoreactive insulin during the hypoglycaemic episode are the usual finding, is discussed by Skrabauek and Powell (1978).

The four tumour-related ectopic hormone and hormone-like conditions so far discussed account for the majority of such syndromes occurring in childhood. Chronic diarrhoea in patients with medullary carcinoma of the thyroid and ganglioneuroma (Green et al. 1959) is mediated by tumour products in much the same way as in some pancreatic islet-cell tumours. In many of the latter cases the gut hormone has been identified and many are not truly ectopic. Similarly, hyperthyroidism provoked by placental thyrotrophin in cases of trophoblastic tumour (Cohen and Utiger 1970) is not strictly the result of production of hormone foreign to the tumour concerned.

References

Abell MR (1982) Ovarian neoplasms of childhood and adolescence. In: Blaustein A (ed) Pathology of the female genital tract, 2nd edn. Springer, New York, p 665

Abell MR, Johnson VJ, Holyz F (1965) Ovarian neoplasms in childhood and adolescence. I. Tumours of germ cell origin. Am J Obstet Gynecol 92: 1059

Albright F, Burnett CH, Smith PH, Parson W (1942) Pseudohypoparathyroidism: an example of "Seabright–Bantom syndrome": report of three cases. Endocrinology 30: 922

Anast CS, Mohs JM, Kaplan SL, Burns TW (1972) Evidence for parathyroid failure in magnesium deficiency. Science 177: 606

Anderson G (1973) Paramalignant syndromes. In: Baron DM, Compston MH, Dawson AM (eds) Recent advances in medicine. Churchill Livingstone, Edinburgh, p 1

Anderson JR, Goudie RB, Gray KG, Timbury GC (1957) Autoantibodies in Addison's disease. Lancet i: 1123

Arce B, Licea M, Hung S, Padron R (1978) Familial Cushing's syndrome. Acta Endocrinol (Copenh) 87: 139

Asadourian LA, Taylor HB (1969) Dysgerminoma. An analysis of 105 cases. Obstet Gynecol 33: 370

Bar RS, Lewis WR, Rechler MM, Harrison LC, Siebert C, Podskalany J, Roth J, Muggeo M (1978) Extreme insulin resistance in ataxia telangiectasia: defect in affinity of insulin receptors. N Engl J Med 298: 1164

Beckwith JB (1969) Macroglossia, omphalocele, adrenal cytomegaly, gigantism, and hyperplastic visceromegaly. Birth Defects 5: 188

Behrle FC, Mantz FA, Olson RL, Trombold JC (1963) Virilization accompanying hepatoblastoma. Pediatrics 32: 265

Benirschke K (1956) Adrenals in anencephaly an hydrocephaly. Obstet Gynecol 8: 412

Benirshke K, Bloch E, Hetig AT (1956) Concerning the function of the fetal zone of the human adrenal gland. Endocrinology 58: 598

Black S, Brook CGD, Cox PJH (1977) Congenital adrenal hypoplasia and gonadotrophin deficiency. Br Med J ii: 996

Blizzard RM, Kyle M, Chandler RW, Hung W (1962) Adrenal antibodies in Addison's disease. Lancet ii: 901

Blizzard RM, Chee D, Davis W (1966) The incidence of parathyroid and other antibodies in the sera of patients with idiopathic hypoparathyroidism. Clin Exp Immunol 1: 119

Bloodworth JMB Jr, Greider M (1982) Endocrine pancreas and diabetes mellitus. In: Bloodworth JMB Jr (ed) Endocrine pathology: general and surgical, 2nd edn. Williams & Wilkins, Baltimore

Boivin Y, Richart RM (1965) Hilus cell tumours of the ovary. A review with a report of three new cases. Cancer 18: 231

Borit A, Kosek J (1969) Cytomegaly of the adrenal cortex, electron microscopy in Beckwith's syndrome. Arch Pathol 88: 58

Bormel P, Mays HB (1961) Testicular tumours of infancy and childhood. J Urol 86: 119

Bradford WD, Wilson JW, Gaode JT (1973) Primary neonatal hyperparathyroidism – an unusual cause of failure to thrive. Am J Clin Pathol 59: 267

Braunstein GD, Bridson WE, Glass A, Hull EW, McIntire KR (1972) In vivo and in vitro production of human chorionic gonadotropin and alpha-fetoprotein by a virilizing hepatoblastoma. J Clin Endocrinol Metab 35: 857

Brerton RJ, Symonds E (1978) Thyroglossal cysts in children. Br J Surg 65: 507

Bronsky D, Kushner DS, Dubin A, Shapper I (1958) Idiopathic hypoparathyroidism and pseudohypoparathyroidism: case reports and review of the literature. Medicine 37: 317

Bronsky D, Kramko RT, Moncada R, Rosenthal IM (1968) Intrauterine hyperparathyroidism secondary to maternal hypoparathyroidism. Pediatrics 42: 606

Busuttil A (1991) Adrenal atrophy at autopsy in two asthmatic children. Am J Forensic Med Pathol 12: 36

Calnan M, Peckham CS (1977) Incidence of insulin dependent diabetes in the first 16 years of life. Lancet i: 589

Carlson HE, Brickman AS, Bottazzo GF (1977) Prolactin deficiency in pseudohypoparathyroidism. N Engl J Med 296: 140

Carman CT, Brashear RE (1960) Phaeochromocytoma as an inherited abnormality. N Engl J Med 263: 419

Carney JA, Sizemore GW, Sheps SG (1976) Adrenal medullary disease in multiple endocrine neoplasia, type 2. Am J Clin Pathol 66: 279

Chase LR, Melson GL, Aurbach GD (1969) Pseudohypoparathyroidism: defective excretion of 3', 5' -AMP in response to parathyroid hormone. J Clin Invest 48: 1832

Chaussain JL (1973) Glycemic response to 24 hour fast in normal children and children with ketotic hypoglycaemia. J Pediatr 82: 438

Childs B, Grumbach MM, Van Wyk JJ (1956) Virilizing adrenal hyperplasia: a genetic and hormonal study. J Clin Invest 35: 213

Choufoer JC, Van Rhijn M, Querido A (1965) Endemic goitre in Western Guinea. II. Clinical picture, incidence and pathogenesis of endemic cretinism. J Clin Endocrinol Metab 25: 385

Chu H-Y, Chang C, Yin W (1964) Idiopathic hypoparathyroidism. Report of 14 cases with one autopsy record. Chin Med J [Eng] 83: 723

Clayton GW, Johnson CM (1960) Struma lymphomatosa in children: report of 12 cases. J Pediatr 57: 410

Cohen JD, Utiger RD (1970) Metastatic choriocarcinoma associated with hyperthyroidism. J Clin Endocrinol Metab 30: 423

Conard RA, Dobyn BM, Sutton WW (1970) Thyroid neoplasm as a late effect of exposure to radioactive iodine in fallout. JAMA 214: 316

Coppes MJ (1993) Serum biological markers and paraneoplastic syndromes in Wilms' tumour. Med Pediatr Oncol 21: 213

Cox JM, Guelpa G, Terrapon M (1976) Islet-cell hyperplasia and sudden infant death. Lancet ii: 739

Craig JM, Schiff LH, Boone JE (1955) Chronic moniliasis associated Addison's disease. Am J Dis Child 89: 669

Crooke AC (1935) A change in the basophil cells of the pituitary gland common to conditions which exhibit the syndrome attributed to basophil adenoma. J Pathol Bacteriol 41: 339

Crooke AC, Russell DS (1935) The pituitary gland in Addison's disease. J Pathol Bacteriol 40: 255

Crooks J, Greig WR, Branwood AW (1963) Dyshormonogenesis and carcinoma of the thyroid gland. Scott Med J 8: 303

Cuello C, Correa P, Eisenberg H (1969) Geographic pathology of thyroid carcinoma. Cancer 23: 230

Davidson DC, Blackwood MJ, Fox EG (1974) Neonatal hypoglycaemia with congenital malformation of pancreatic islets. Arch Dis Child 49: 151

de Sa DJ, Nicholls S (1972) Haemorrhagic necrosis of the adrenal glands in perinatal infants. J Pathol 106: 133

Dickersin GR, Kline IW, Scully RE (1982) Small cell carcinoma of the ovary with hypercalcaemia. Cancer 49: 188

Dobersen MJ, Schaff JE (1982) Preferential lysis of pancreatic B-cells by islet cell surface antibodies. Diabetes 31: 459

Donalson MDC, Grant DB, O'Hare MJ, Shackleton CHL (1981) Familial congenital Cushing's syndrome due to bilateral nodular adrenal hyperplasia. Clin Endocrinol (Oxf) 14: 519

Doniach D, Roitt IM, Polani PE (1968) Thyroid antibodies and sex-chromosome anomalies. Proc R Soc Med 61: 278

Dorniach I (1977) Histopathology of the anterior pituitary. Clin Endocrinol Metabol 6: 21

Doniach I, Morgan AG (1973) Islets of Langerhans in juvenile diabetes mellitus. Clin Endocrinol 2: 233

Dorff GB (1934) Sporadic cretinism in one of twins. Report of cases with roentgen demonstration of osseous changes that occurred in utero. Am J Dis Child 48: 1316

Drake TG, Albright F, Bauer W, Castleman B (1939) Chronic idiopathic hypoparathyroidism: report of six cases with autopsy findings in one. Ann Intern Med 12: 1751

Drezner MK, Neelon FA, Haussler M, McPherson HT, Lebovitz HE (1976) 1,25-dihydroxycholecalciferol deficiency: the probable cause of hypocalcaemia and metabolic bone disease in pseudohypoparathyroidism. J Clin Endocrinol Metab 42: 621

Dussault JH, Coulombe P, Laberge C, Letarte J, Guyda H, Khoury K (1975) Preliminary report on a mass screening program for neonatal hypothyroidism. J Pediatr 86: 670

Dyer EH, Civit T, Visot A, Delalande O, Derome P (1994) Transphenoidal surgery for pituitary adenous in children. Neurosurgery 34: 207

Eeg-Olofsson O, Petersen K (1966) Childhood diabetes neuropathy. A clinical and neurophysiological study. Acta Paediatr Scand 55: 163

Ellis EM, Pysher TJ (1993) Renal disease in adolescents with type 1 diabetes mellitus: a report of the Southwest Pediatr Nephology Study Group. Am J Kidney Dis 22: 783

Ellison ML, Neville Am (1973) Neoplasia and ectopic hormone production. In: Raven RW (ed) Modern trends in oncology. Butterworths, London, p 163

Erdheim J (1904) Uber Hypophysenganggeschwülste und Hirncholesteatome. SB Akad Wiss Wien [3] 113: 537

Evans DB, Lee JE, Merrell RC, Hickey RC (1994) Adrenal medullary disease in multiple endocrine neoplasia type 2. Appropriate management. Endocrinol Metab Clin North Am 23: 67

Fahlbusch R, Buchfelder M, Müller OA (1986) Transsphenoidal surgery for Cushing's disease. J R Soc Med 79: 262

Favara BE, Steele A, Grant JH, Steele P (1991) Adrenal cytomegaly: quantitative assessment by image analysis. Pediatr Pathol ii: 521

Fiero-Benitz R, Alban R, Cordova J, Eguiguren L, Franco R, Moreano M, Malo L, Paltan JD, Paredes M, Rivadeneira I, Sanchez-Jaramillo P, Weilbrauer P (1965) Endemic goitre and endemic cretinism in the Equatorial Andes. VIth Pan American Congress of Endocrinology. Excertpa Medica, Amsterdam (ICS no. 99, Abstract no. 36)

Finne PH, Sanderud J, Aksenes L, Bratlid D, Aarskog D (1988) Hypercalcaemia with increased and unregulated 1, 25-dihydroxyvitamin D production in a neonate with subcutaneous fat necrosis. J Pediat 112: 792

Fisher GW, Vazquez AM, Buist NRM, Campbell JR, McCarty E, Egan ET (1974) Neonatal islet cell adenoma : case report and literature review. Pediatrics 53: 753

Fisher DA (1987) Effectiveness of newborn screening programs for congenital hypothyroidism: prevalence of missed cases.

Pediatr Clin North 34: 881

Fisher WD, Voorhess ML, Gardner LI (1963) Congenital hypothyroidism in infant following maternal I[131] therapy. J Pediatr 62: 132

Fleischer AS, Rudman DR, Payne NS, Tyndall GT (1978) Hypothalamic hypothyroidism and hypogonadism in prolonged traumatic coma. J Neurosurg 49: 650

Foulis AK, Liddle CN, Farquharson MA, Richmond JA, Weir RS (1986) The histopathology of the pancreas in type I (insulin dependent) diabetes mellitus: a 25-year review of deaths in patients under 20 years of age in the United Kingdom. Diabetalogia 29: 267

Fretheim B, Gardborg O (1965) Primary hyperparathyroidism in an infant. Acta Chir Scand 129: 557

Furmachuk AW, Averkin JI, Egloff B, Ruchtic, Abelin T, Schappi W, Korothevich EA (1992) Pathomorphological findings in thyroid cancers of children from the Republic of Belarus; a study of 86 cases occurring between 1986 ("post-chernobyl") and 1991. Histopathology 21: 401

Gabbay KH (1975) Hyperglycemia, polyol metabolism, and complications of diabetes mellitus. Annu Rev Med 26: 521

Gabrilove JL, Sharma DC, Wotiz HH, Dormann R (1965) Feminizing adrenocortical tumours in the male: a review of 52 cases. Medicine (Baltimore) 44: 37

Gabrilove JL, Nicolls GL, MiHy HA, Shoval AR (1975) Feminizing interstitial cell tumour of the testis: personal observations and a review of the literature. Cancer 35: 1184

Gamble DR, Kinsley ML, FitzGerald MG, Bolton R, Taylor KW (1969) Viral antibodies in diabetes mellitus. Br Med iii: 627

Gang DL (1978) Case records of the Masschusetts General Hospital. Case 30. N Engl J Med 299: 241

Gass HH (1956) Large calcified craniopharyngioma and bilateral subdural haematoma present at birth. J Neurosurg 13: 514

Gepts W (1965) Pathologic anatomy of the pancreas in juvenile diabetes mellitus. Diabetes 14: 619

Giebnink GS, Ruymann FB (1974) Testicular tumours in childhood. Am J Dis Child 127: 433

Gilmour JR (1937) The embryology of the parathyroid glands, the thymus and certain associated rudiments. J Pathol 45: 507

Gilmour (1938) The gross anatomy of the parathyroid glands. J Pathol 46: 133

Gilmour JR (1939) The normal histology of the parathyroid glands. J Pathol 48: 187

Gilmour JR (1941) Some developmental abnormalities of the thymus and parathyroids. J Pathol Bacteriol 52: 213

Gilmour JR, Martin WJ (1937) The weight of the parathyroid glands. J Pathol Bacteriol 44: 431

Glover MT, Catterall MD, Atherton DJ (1991) Subcutaneous fat necrosis in two infants following hypothermic cardiac surgery. Paediatr Dermatol 8: 210

Goldberg GM, Eshbaugh DE (1960) Squamous cell nests of the pituitary gland as related to the origin of craniopharyngiomas. A study of their presence in the newborn in infants up to age four. Arch Pathol 70: 293

Gorlin RJ, Sedano HO, Vickers RA (1968) Multiple mucosal neuromas, phaeochromocytoma ad medullary carcinoma of the thyroid – a syndrome. Cancer 22: 293

Gorodischer R, Aceto T Jr, Terplan K (1970) Congenital familial hypoparathyroidism: management of an infant, genetics, pathogenesis of hypoparathyroidism and fetal undermineralization. Am J Dis Child 119: 74

Gorsuch AN, Spencer RM, Lister J, McNally JM, Dean BM, Bottazo FG, Cudworth AG (1981) Evidence for a long prediabetic period in type 1 (insulin dependent) diabetes mellitus. Lancet ii: 1363

Green M, Cooke RE, Lattanzi W (1959) Occurrence of chronic diarrhoea in three patients with ganglioneuroma. Pediatrics 23: 951

Grim CE, McBryde AC, Glenn JF, Gunnells JC (1967) Childhood primary aldosteronism with bilateral adrenocortical hyperplasia: plasma renin activity as an aid to diagnosis. J Pediatr 71: 377

Gruskin AB, Root AW, Duckett GE, Balnarte HJ (1976) Parathyroid function in uremic children during periods of renal insufficiency, haemodialysis and transplantation. J Perdiatr 89: 755

Guin GH, Gilbert EE, Jones B (1969) Incidental neuroblastoma in infants. Am J Clin Pathol 51: 126

Gutierre GE, Poser JW, Katz MS, Yates AJP, Hendry HL, Mundy GR (1990) Mechanisms of hypercalcaemia in malignancy. Baillière's Clin Endocrinol Metab 4: 119

Habener JF, Potts JT Jr (1978) Biosynthesis of parathyroid hormone. N Engl J Med 299: 635

Hagberg B, Westphal O (1970) Ataxic syndrome in congenital hypothyroidism. Acta Paediatr Scand 59: 323

Hardman JM (1968) Fatal meningococcal infections: the changing pathologic picture in the 60's. Milit Med 133: 951

Harness JK, Thompson HW, Nishiyama RH (1971) Childhood thyroid carcinoma. Arch Surg 102: 278

Hayles AB, Johnson LM, Beahrs OH, Woolner LB (1963) Carcinoma of the thyroid in children. Am J Surg 106: 735

Heitz PU, Klöppel G, Häcki WH, Polak JM, Pearse AGE (1977) Nesidioblastosis: the pathologic basis of persistent hyperinsulinemic hypoglycaemia in infants. Diabetes 26: 632

Hempelmann LH, Pifer JW, Burke GJ, Ames WR (1967) Neoplasms in persons treated with X-rays in infancy for thymic enlargement. A report of the third follow-up survey. J Natl Cancer Inst 38: 317

Hewer TF (1944) Ateleiotic dwarfism with normal sexual function: a result of hypopituitarism. J Endocrinol 3: 397

Higgins PM, Tresidder CG (1966) Phaeochromocytoma of the urinary bladder. Br Med J ii: 274

Hillman DA, Scriver CR, Pedvis S, Schragovitch I (1964) Neonatal familial primary hyperparathyroidism. N Engl J Med 270: 483

Hirschfield AJ, Fleshman JK (1969) An unusually high incidence of salt-losing congenital adrenal hyperplasia in the Alaskan Eskimo. J Pediatr 75: 492

Hollingsworth DR, McKeau HE, Roeckel I (1974) Goitre, immunological observations and thyroid function tests in Down syndrome. Am J Dis Child 127: 524

Holmgren G, Samuelson G, Hermansson B (1974) The prevalence of diabetes mellitus: a study of children and their relatives in a northern Swedish county. Clin Genet 5: 465

Hopwood NJ, Kenny FM (1977) Incidence of Nelson's syndrome after adrenalectomy for Cushing's disease in children. Am J Dis Child 131: 1353

Hough AJ, Hollified JW, Page DL, Hartmann WH (1979) Prognostic factors in adrenal cortical tumours. A mathematical analysis of clinical and morphological data. Am J Clin Pathol 72: 390

Howe JR, Norton JA, Wells JA Jr (1993) Prevalence of phaeochromocytoma and hyperparathyroidism in multiple endocrine neoplasia type 2A: results of long-term follow-up. Surgery 114: 1070

Huang SW, MacLaren NK (1976) Insulin dependent diabetes: a disease of autoaggression. Science 192: 64

Hulse JA, Grant DB, Clayton BE, Lilly P, Jackson D, Spracklan A, Edwards RWH, Nurse D (1980) Population screening for congenital hypothyroidism. Br Med J i: 675

Hume DM (1960) Phaeochromocytoma in the adult and in the child. Am J Surg 99: 458

Hutchin P, Kessner DM (1964) Diagnostic lead to hyperparathyroidism in the mother. Ann Intern Med 61: 1109

Hutchinson RJ, Sharpiro SA, Rancy RB (1978) Elevated parathyroid hormone levels in association with rhabdomyosarcoma. J Pediatr 92: 780

Hutchinson JH, McGirr EM (1956) Sporadic non-endemic goitrous cretinism: hereditary transmission. Lancet i: 1035

Irvine WJ, McCallum CJ, Gray RS, Campbell CJ, Duncan LJP, Farquher JW, Vaughan H, Morris PJ (1977) Pancreatic islet-cell antibodies in diabetes mellitus correlated with the duration and type of diabetes, coexistent autoimmune disease and HLA type. Diabetes 26: 138

Iyer CGS (1952) Case report of an adamantinoma present at birth. J Neurosurg 9: 221

Jansen A, Voorbij HA, Jeucken PH, Bruiming GJ, Hooijkass H, Drexhage HA (1993) An immunohistochemical study on organized lymphoid cell infiltrates in fetal and neonatal pancreases. A comparison with similar infiltrates found in the pancreas of a diabetic infant. Autoimmunity 15: 31

Jennings AS, Liddle GW, Orth DM (1977) Results of treating childhood Cushing's disease with pituitary irradiation. N Engl J Med 287: 957

Jensen RD, Norris HJ, Fraumeni JF Jr (1974) Familial arrhenoblastoma and thyroid adenoma, Cancer 33: 218

Johnstone REH, Kreindler T, Johnstone RE (1972) Hyperparathyroidism during pregnancy. Obstet Gynecol 40: 580

Jones RA, Dawson IMP (1977) Morphology and staining patterns of endocrine cell tumours in the gut, pancreas and bronchus and their possible significance. Histopathology 1: 137

Joyaraman J, David R (1977) Hypercalcaemia as a presenting manifestation of leukaemia: evidence of excessive PTH secretion. J Pediatr 90: 609

Keiser HR, Beaven MS, Doppman J, Wells S, Buja LM (1973) Sipple's syndrome: medullary thyroid carcinoma, phaeochromocytoma and parathyroid disease. Ann Intern Med 78: 561

Kelley VC, Ely RS, Raile RB (1952) Metabolic studies in patients with congenital adrenal hyperplasia. Effects of cortisone therapy. J Clin Endocrinol Metab 12: 1140

Kelly FC, Snedden WW (1960) Prevalence and geographical distribution of endemic goiter. In: Endemic goiter. WHO Monogr Ser 44: 27

Kelly WF, Joplin GF, Pearson GW (1977) Gonadotrophin deficiency and adrenocortical insufficiency in children: a new syndrome. Br Med J ii: 98

Kennedy JS (1969) The pathology of dyshormonogenetic goitre. J Pathol 99: 251

Kerenyi N (1961) Congenital adrenal hypoplasia. Report of a case with extreme adrenal hypoplasia and neurohypophyseal aplasia, drawing attention to certain aspects of etiology and classification. Arch Pathol 71: 336

Khairi MR, Dexter RM, Burzynski MJ, Johnston CC (1975) Mucosal neuroma, phaeochromocytoma and medullary carcinoma: multiple endocrine neoplasia type 3. Medicine (Baltimore) 54: 89

Knowles HC Jr, Guest GM, Lampe J, Kessler M, Skillman TG (1965) The course of juvenile diabetes treated with unmeasured diet. Diabetes 14: 239

Koenig MP (1968) Die kongenitale Hypothyreose un der endemische Kretinismus. Springer, Berlin

Koenig RJ, Peterson CM, Jones RL, Saudek C, Lehrman M, Cerami A (1976) Correlation of glucose regulation and haemoglobin ALC in diabetes mellitus. N Engl Med 295: 417

Kohler HG (1963) Karyomegaly of the fetal and adrenal cortex. J Clin Pathol 16: 383

Kruse K, Irle U, Uhlig R (1993) Elevated 1, 25-dihydroxyvitamin D serum concentrations in infants with subcutaneous fat necrosis. J Pediatr 122: 460

Kyllo DF, Nuttall FQ (1978) Prevalence of diabetes mellitus in school-age children in Minnesota. Diabetes 27: 57

Lairmore TC, Ball DW, Baylin SB, Wells SA Jr (1993) Management of phaeochromocytomes in patients with multiple endocrine neoplasia type 2 syndromes. Ann Surg 217: 595

Landing BH, Kamoshita S (1970) Congenital hyperparathyroidism secondary to maternal hypoparathyroidism J Pediatr 77: 842

Landon H, Adin I, Spitz IM (1978) Pituitary insufficiency following head injury. Isr J Med Sci 14: 785

Landsvater RM, Rombouts AG, TE Meermai GJ, Schillhorn-van-Veeh (1993) The clinical implications of a positive calcitonin test for C-cell hyperplasia in genetically unaffected members of an MEN 2A kindred. Am J Hum Genet 52: 335

Larsson L-I (1978) Endocrine pancreatic tumours. Hum Pathol 9: 401

Larsson C, Mordenskjold M (1994) Family screening in multiple endocrine neoplasia type I (MEN 1). Ann Med 26: 191

Leboeuf G, Bongiovanni AM (1964) Thyroiditis in childhood. Adv Pediatr 13: 183

Le Dourain N, Le Lièvre C, Containe J (1972) Recherches expérimentales sur l'origine embryologique du corps carotidien chez les oiseaux. C R Acad Sci [D] (Paris) 275: 583

Leedham PW, Pollocak DJ (1970) Intrafollicular armyloid in primary hyperparathyroidism. J Clin Pathol 23: 811

Lennox B, Russell DS (1951) Dystopia of the neurohypophysis: two cases. J Pathol 63: 485

Lernmark A, Freedman ZR, Hofmann C, Rubenstein AH, Steiner DF, Jackson RL, Winter RJ, Traisman HS (1978) Islet-cell-surface antibody in juvenile diabetes mellitus. N Engl J Med 299: 375

Levin J, Cluff LE (1965) Endotoxemia and adrenal haemorrhage. A mechanism for the Waterhouse–Friderichsen syndrome. J Exp Med 121: 247

Lipps CJ, Landsvater RM, Hoppener JW, Geerdink RA et al. (1994) Clinical screening as compared with DNA analysis in families with multiple endocrine neoplasia type 2A. N Engl J Med 331: 828

Lundberg PO, Gemzell C (1966) Dysplasia of sella turcica. Acta Endocrinol (Kbh) 52: 478

Lyon Fa, Sinykin MB, McKelvey JL (1963) Granulosa-cell tumours of the ovary, review of 23 cases. Obstet Gynecol 21: 67

MacLaren NK, Huang SW, Fogh J (1975) Antibody to cultured human insulinoma cells in insulin-dependent diabetes. Lancet i: 997

Mäenää J (1972) Congenital hypothyroidism; etiological and clinical aspects. Arch Dis Child 47: 914

Marek J (1977) Gonadotrophin deficiency and adrenocortical insufficiency in children. Br Med J ii: 828

Marshall JR (1965) Ovarian enlargement in the first year of life: review of 45 cases. Ann Surg 161: 373

Marshal WC, Ockenden BG, Fosbrook AS, Cummings JN (1969) Wolman's disease. A rare lipidosis with adrenal calcification. Arch Dis child 44: 331

Martin KJ, Kruska KA, Freitag JJ, Klahr S, Slatoposky E (1979) The peripheral metabolism of parathyroidism. N Engl J Med 301: 1092

Marx SJ, Hershaman JM, Aurbach GD (1971) Thyroid dysfunction in pseudohypoparathyroidism. J Clin Endocrinol Metab 33: 822

McArthur JW (1969) Discussion. Recent Prog Horm Res 25: 306

McCallagh EP, Rossmiller HR (1941) Methyltestosterone. I. Androgenic effects and production of gynaecomastia and oligospermia. J Clin Endocrinol Metab 1: 496

McGirr Em, Clement WE, Currie ARE, Kennedy JS (1959) Impaired dehalogenase activity as a cause of goitre with malignant change. Scott Med J 4: 232

Meador CK, Bowdoin B, Own WC, Farmer TA (1967) Primary adrenocortical nodular dysplasia: a rare cause of Cushing's disease. J Clin Endocrinol Metab 27: 1255

Melvin KEW, Tashjian AH Jr, Miller HH (1972) Studies in familial (medullary) thyroid carcinoma. Recent Prog Horm Res 28: 399

Menser MA, Forrest JM, Bransby RD (1978) Rubella infection and diabetes mellitus. Lancet i: 57

Meyer JS, Steinberg LS (1969) Microscopically benign thyroid follicles in cervical lymph nodes. Cancer 24: 302

Miller WL, Kaplan SL, Grumbach MM (1980) Child abuse as a cause of post-traumatic hypopituitarism. N Engl J Med 302: 724

Misugi K, Misugi N, Sotas J, Smith B (1970) The pancreatic islets of infants with severe hypoglycaemia. Arch Pathol 89: 208

Mostofi FK, (1973) Testicular tumours. Epidemiologic, etiologic and pathologic features. Cancer 32: 1186

Mostifi FK, Theiss EA, Ashley DJB (1959) Tumours of specialized gonadal stroma in human male patients. Cancer 12: 944

Myers WPL (1960) Hypercalcemia in neoplastic disease. Arch Surg 80: 308

Nabarro JD, Mustaffa BE, Morris DV, Walport MJ, Kuntz AB (1979) Insulin deficient diabetes: contrasts with other endocrine deficiencies. Diabetologia 16: 5

Neufeld ND, Lippe BM, Sperling M, Kaplan SA (1978) Insulin resistance with reduction in monocyte insulin binding in gonadal dysgenesis. Clin Res 26: 190A

Neville AM, Symington T (1972) Bilateral adrenocortical hyperplasia in children with Cushing's syndrome. J Pathol 107: 95

New MI, Petwoon RE (1966) Disorders of aldosterone secretion in childhood. Pediatr Clin North Am 13: 43

Niewenhuijzen Kruseman AC, Knijnenburg G, Burtel de la Rivière G, Bossman FT (1978) Morphology and immunohistochemically-defined endocrine function of pancreatic islet cell tumours. Histopathology 2: 389

Nikiforov Y, Gnepp DR (1994) Paediatric thyroid cancer after the Chernobyl disaster. Pathomorphologic study of 84 cases (1991–1992) from the Republic of Belarus. Cancer 74: 748

Nilsson LR, Doniach D (1964) Autoimmune thyroiditis in children and adolescents: 1. Clinical studies. Acta Pediatr Scand 53: 255

Nilsson LR, Bogfors M, Gamstorp I, Holst H-E, Liden G (1964) Non-endemic goitre and deafness. Acta Paediatr Scand 53: 255

Norris HJ, Jensen RD (1972) Relative frequency of ovarian neoplasms in children and adolescents. Cancer 30: 713

Norton JA, Frooke LC, Farrell RE, Wells SA (1979) Multiple endocrine neoplasia type IIb. the most aggressive form medullary thyroid carcinoma. Surg Clin North Am 59: 109

Omenn GS (1971) Ectopic hormone syndromes associated with tumours in childhood. Pediatrics 47: 613

Oppenheimer EH (1969) Cyst formation in the outer adrenal cortex; studies in the human fetus and newborn. Arch Pathol 87: 653

Oppenheimer EH (1970) Adrenal cytomegaly: studies by light and electron microscopy. Arch Pathol 90: 57

Page CP, Kemmerer WT, Haff RC, Mazzaferri EL (1974) Thyroid carcinomas arising in thyroglossal ducts. Ann Surg 180: 799

Pagliara AS, Karl IE, Haymond M, Kipnis DM (1973a) Hypoglycaemia in infancy and childhood, I. J Pediatr 82: 363

Pagliara AS, Karl IE, Haymond M, Kipnis DM (1973b) Hypoglycaemia in infancy and childhood, II. J Pediatr 82: 558

Paulsen CA (1974) The testis. In: Williams RH (ed) Textbook of endocrinology, 5th edn. Saunders, Philadelphia, p 362

Paxson CL Jr, Brown DR (1976) Post-traumatic anterior hypopituitarism. Pediatrics 57: 893

Pearse AGE, Polak JM, van Nooreden S (1972) The neural crest origin of the C cells and their comparative cytochemistry and ultrastructure in the ultimobranchial gland. In: Talmag RV, Munson PL (eds) Calcium, parathyroid hormone and calcitonins. Excerpta Medica, Amsterdam, p 29

Pearse AGE, Polak JM, Heath CM (1973) Development, differentiation and derivation of the endocrine polypeptide cells of the mouse pancreas. (Immunofluorescence, cytochemical and ultrastructural studies). Diabetalogia 9: 120

Peden VH (1960) True idiopathic hypoparathyroidism as a sex-linked recessive trait. Am J Hum Genet 12: 323

Pedersèn J, Osler M (1958) Development of ossification centres in infants of diabetic mothers. Acta Endocrinol (Kbh) 29: 467

Pictet RL, Rall LB, Phelps P, Rutter WJ (1976) The neural crest and the origin of the insulin producing and other gastrointestinal hormone producing cells. Science 191: 191

Pierce ST (1993) Paraendocrine syndromes. Curr Opin Oncol 5: 639

Polak JM, Wigglesworth JS (1976) Islet-cell hyperplasia and sudden infant death. Lancet ii: 570

Porcile E, Racadot J (1966) Ultrastructure des cellules de Croke observées dans l'hypophyse humaine au cours de la maladie de Cushing. C R Acad Sci [D] (Paris) 263: 948

Preeyasombat C, Sirikulchayamonta V, Mahachokelerwattana P, Sriphrapradang A, Boompuckmavig S (1992) Cushing's syndrome caused by Ewing's sarcoma secreting carticotrophin releasing factor-like peptide. Am J Dis Child 146: 1103

Ramsay NKC, Brown DM, Nesbit ME, Coccia PF, Krivit W, Krutzik S (1979) Autonomous production of parathyroid hormone by lymphoblastic leukaemia cells in culture. J Pediatr 94: 623

Rees LH, Ratcliffe JG (1974) Ectopic hormone production by non-endocrine tumours. Clin Endocrinol (Oxf) 3: 263

Richardson JE, Beaugie JM, Doniach I, Brown CL (1974) Thyroid cancer in young patients in Great Britain. Br J Surg 61: 85

Rimoin DL (1971) Inheritance of diabetes mellitus. Med Clin North Am 55: 807

Roche M (1959) Elevated thyroidal I^{131} uptake in the absence of goitre in isolated Venezuelan Indians. J Clin Endocrinol Metab 19: 1440

Root AW, Bongiovanni AM, Eberlein WR (1968) A testicular intersitial cell-stimulating gonadotrophin in a child with hepatoblastoma and sexual precocity. J Clin Endocrinol Metab 28: 1317

Roth SI, Gallagher MJ (1976) The rapid identification of "normal" parathyroid glands by the presence of intracellular fat. Am J Pathol 84: 521

Rude RK, Oldham SB, Singer FR, Nicoloff JT (1976) Treatment of thyrotoxic hypercalcaemia with popranolol. N Engl J Med 294: 431

Ruder HJ, Loriaux DL, Lipsett MB (1974) Severe osteopenia in young adults associated with Cushing's syndrome due to micronodular adrenal disease. J Clin Endocrinol Metab 39: 1138

Russell DS, Rubinstein LJ (1977b) Pathology of tumours of the nervous system, 4th edn. Arnold, London, p 312

Russfield AB, Reiner L (1957) The hypophysis in human growth failure: report of three dwarfs. Lab Invest 6: 334

Sadeghi-Nejad A, Seniar B (1974) Familial syndrome of isolated aplasia of the anterior pituitary. J Pediatr 84: 79

Saenger EL, Silverman FN, Sterling TD, Tuner ME (1960) Neoplasia following therapeutic irradiation for benign conditions in childhood. Radiology 74: 889

Saharia PC (1975) Carcinoma arising in thyroglossal duct remnant: case reports and review of the literature. Br J Surg 62: 689

Salassa RM, Laws ER Jr, Carpenter PC, Northcutt RC (1978) Trans-sphenoidal removal of pituitary microadenoma in Cushing's disease. Mayo Clin Proc 53: 24

Salinas ED Jr, Mangurten HH, Roberts SS, Simon WH, Cornblath M (1968) Functioning islet cell adenoma in the newborn. Pediatrics 41: 646

Saxena KM, Crawford JD (1962) Juvenile lymphocytic thyroiditis. Pediatrics 30: 917

Saxena KM, Crawford JD, Talbot NB (1964) Childhood thyrotoxicosis: a long-term perspective. Br Med J ii: 1153

Schimke RN, Hartmann WH, Prout TE, Rimoin DLL (1968) Syndrome of bilateral pheochromocytoma, medullary thyroid carcinoma and multiple neuromas. N Engl J Med 279: 1

Schochet SS, McCormick WF, Halmi NS (1974) Pituitary gland in patients with Hurlers syndrome. Arch Pathol 97: 96

Scholz DA, Horton ES, Lebowitz HE, Ferris DO (1967) Spontaneous hypoglycaemia associated with an adrenocortical carcinoma. J Clin Endocrinol Metab 27: 991

Schweizer-Cagianut M, Solomon F, Hedinger CHR E (1982) Primary adrenocortical nodular dysplasia with Cushing's syndrome and cardiac myxomas. A peculiar familial disease. Virchows Arch A Pathol Anat 397: 183

Scully RE (1953) Gonadoblastoma. A gonadal tumour related to the dysgerminoma (seminoma) and capable of sex hormone production. Cancer 6: 445

Siebenmann RE (1957) Die kongenitale Lipoidhyperplasie der Nebennierenrinde bei Nebennierenrindeninsuffizienz. Schweiz Z Pathol 20: 77

Silberman R, Mendelson IR (1960) Teratomas of the neck: report of 2 cases and review of the literature. Arch Dis Child 35: 159

Skrabuck P, Powell D (1978) Ectopic insulin and Occam's razor: reappraisal of the riddle of tumour hypoglycaemia. Clin Endocrinol (Oxf) 9: 141

Smith DW, Blizzard RM, Wilkins L (1957) The mental prognosis in hypothyroidism of infancy and childhood: review of 128 cases. Pediatrics 19: 1011

Smithers DW (1970) Tumours of the thyroid gland. In: Monographs on neoplastic disease. Livingstone, Edinburgh, p 155

Spiegel AM, Harrison HE, Marx SJ, Brown EM, Aurbac GD (1977) Neonatal primary hyperparathyroidism with autosomal dominant inheritance. J Pediatr 90: 269

Stackpole RH, Melicow M, Uson AC (1963) Pheochromocytoma in children. Report of 9 cases and review of the first 100 published cases with follow-up studies. J Pediatr 63: 315

Stanbury JB, Dumont JE (1983) Familial goitre and related disorders. In: Stanbury JB, Wyngaarden JB, Fredrickson DS, Goldstein JL, Brown MD (eds) The metabolic basis of inherited disease, 5th edn. McGraw-Hill, New York, p 231

Stanworth SJ, Kennedy CTC, Chetcuti PAJ, Carswell F (1992) Hypercalcaemia and sarcoidosis in infancy. R Soc Med 85: 177

Stapleton FB, Lukert BP, Linshaw MP (1976) Treatment of hypercalcaemia associated with osseous metastases. J Pediatr 89: 1029

Steiner AC, Goodman AD, Powers SR (1968) Study of a kindred with pheochromocytoma, medullary thyroid carcinoma, hyperparathyroidism and Cushing's disease: multiple endocrine neoplasia, type 2. Medicine (Baltimore) 47: 371

Suh SM, Tashjian AH Jr, Matsuo M, Parkinson DK, Fraser D (1973) Pathogenesis of hypocalcaemia in primary hypomagnesaemia: normal end-organ responsiveness to parathormone. Impaired parathyroid gland function. J Clin Invest 52: 153

Sultz HA, Hart BA, Zielezny M, Schlesinger ER (1975) Is mumps virus an etiologic factor in juvenile diabetes mellitus? J Pediatr 86: 654

Tabaddor K, Shulman K, Dal Canto MC (1974) Neonatal craniopharyngioma. Am J Dis Chid 128: 381

Thakker RV (1994) The role of molecular genetics in screening for multiple endocrine neoplasia type 1. Endocrine Metab Clin North Am 23: 117

Tsai MS, Ledger GA, Khosla S, Gharib H, Thibodeau SN (1994) Identification of multiple endocrine neoplasia type 2 gene carriers using linkage analysis and analysis of the RET proto-encogene. J Clin Endocrinol Metab 78: 1261

Tsang RC, Light IJ, Sutherland JM, Kleinman LI (1973) Possible pathogenetic factors in neonatal hypocalcemia of prematurity. J Pediatr 82: 423

Tyrrell JB, Brooks RM, Fitzgerald PA, Cofoid PB, Forsham PH, Wilson PB (1978) Cushing's disease: selective transsphenoidal resection of pituitary microadenomas. N Engl J Med 198: 753

US Department of Health, Education and Welfare (1964) PHS Publication number 1168. HEW, Washington DC

Usizima H (1956) Ovarian dysgerminoma associated with masculinization. Report of a case. Cancer 9: 736

Van de Winkel M, Smets G, Gepts W, Pipeleers D (1982) Islet cell surface antibodies from insulin-dependent diabetics bind specifically to pancreatic B cells. J Clin Invest 70: 41

Vickery AL (1981) The diagnosis of malignancy in dyshormonogenetic goitre Clin Endocrinol Metab 10: 317

Warren JC, Erkman B, Cheatum S (1964) Hilus-cell adenoma in a dysgenetic gonad with XX/XO mosaicism. Lancet i: 141

Weber FT, Donnelly WH, Bejar RL (1977) Hypopopituitarism following extirpation of a pharyngeal pituitary. Am J Dis Child 131: 525

Wegelin C (1928) Malignant disease of the thyroid gland and its relations to goitre in man and animals. Cancer Treat Rev 3: 297

Weichert RF(1970) III. The neural ectodermal origin of peptidesecreting endocrine glands. Am J Med 49: 232

Weinstein RL, Kliman B, Neeman J, Cohen RB (1970) Deficient 17-hydroxylation in a corticosterone producing adrenal tumour from an infant with hemihypertrophy and visceromegaly. J Clin Endocrinol Metab 30: 456

Weiss L, Mellinger RC (1970) Congenital adrenal hypoplasia an X-linked disease. J Med Genet 7: 27

Weitzner S, Gropp A (1974) Sertoli cell tumour of testis in childhood. Am J Dis Child 128: 541

Wells SA Jr Chi DD, Toshima K, Denmer LP, Coffin CM et al. (>10 an's) (1994) Predictive DNA testing and prophylactic thyroidectomy in patients at risk for multiple endocrine neoplasia type 2A. Ann Surg 220: 237

Werder EA, Illig R, Bernasconi S, Kind H, Prader A, Fischer JA, Fanconi A (1975) Excessive thyrotropin response to thyrotropin-releasing hormone in pseudohypoparathyroidism. Pediatr Res 9: 12

Wermer P (1974) Multiple endocrine adenomatosis; multiple hormone-producing tumours, a familial syndrome. Clin Gastroenterol 3: 671

Wiedemann HR (1964) Complex malformatif familial avec hernie ombilicale et macroglossie – un "syndrome nouveau"? J Genet Hum 13: 223

Wiener MF, Dallgaard SA (1959) Intracranial adrenal gland. A case report. Arch Pathol 67: 228

Wilkerson JA (1964) Idiopathic infantile hypercalcaemia with subcutaneous fat necrosis. Am J Clin Pathol 41: 390

Williams ED (1965) A review of 17 cases of carcinoma of the thyroid and phaeochronocytoma. J Clin Pathol 18: 288

Williams ED (1975) Medullary carcinoma of the thyroid. In: Harrison CV, Weinbred K (eds) Recent advances in pathology, vol 9. Churchill Livingstone, Edinburgh, p 156

Williams ED (1978) The parathyroid glands. In: Symmers W St C (ed) Systemic pathology, vol 4. Churchill Livingstone, Edinburgh, p 2045

Williams ED, Pollock DJ (1966) Multiple mucosal neuromata with endocrine tumours: a syndrome allied to von Recklinghausen's disease. J Pathol Bacteriol 91: 71

Williams ED, Sandler M (1963) The classification of carcinoid tumours. Lancet i: 238

Williams ED, Brown CL, Doniach I (1966) Pathological and clinical finding in a series of 67 cases of medullary carcinoma of the thyroid. J Clin Pathol 19: 103

Williams ED, Morales AM, Horn R (1968) Thyroid carcinoma and Cushing's syndrome. J Clin Pathol 21: 129

Williams ED, Doniach I, Bjarnason O, Michie W (1977) Thyroid cancer in an idodide rich area. Cancer 39: 215

Williams RH, Porte D Jr (1974) The pancreas. In: Williams RH (ed) Textbook of endocrinology, 5th edn. Saunders, Philadelphia, p 566

Winship T, Rosvoll RV (1961) A study of thyroid cancer in children. Am J Surg 102: 747

Winter J, Eberlein WR, Bongiovanni AM (1966) The relationship of juvenile hypothyroidism to chronic lymphocytic thyroiditis. J Pediatr 69: 709

Winternitz WW, Dzur JA (1976) Pituitary failure secondary to head trauma: case report. J Neurosurg 44: 504

Wolfe HJ, Melvin KEW, Cervi-Skinner SJ et al. (1973) C-cell hyperplasia preceding medullary thyroid carcinoma. M Eng J Med 289: 437

Wolman M, Sterk VV, Gatt SL, Frenkel M (1961) Primary familial xanthomatosis with involvement and calcification of the adrenals. Report of two more cases in siblings of a previously described infant. Pediatrics 28: 742

Woolner LB, Beahrs OH, Black BM, McConahey WM, Keating FR Jr (1961) Classification and prognosis of thyroid carcinoma: a study of 885 observed cases in a thirty year period. Am J Surg 102: 354

Woolner LB, Beahrs OH, Black BM, McConahey WM, Keating Fr Jr (1968) Thyroid carcinoma: general considerations and follow-up data on 1181 cases. In: Young S, Inman DR (eds) Thyroid neoplasia. Academic Press, London, p 51

Yakovac WC, Baker L, Hummeler K (1971) Beta cell nesidioblastosis in idiopathic hypoglycaemia of infancy. J Pediatr 79: 226

Yoon JW, Austin M, Onodera T, Notkins AL (1979) Isolation of a virus from the pancreas of a child with diabetic ketoacidosis. N Engl J Med 300: 1173

Zisman E, Lotz M, Jenkins ME, Bartter FC (1969) Studies in pseudohypoparathyroidism: two cases with a probable selective deficiency of thyrotropin. Am J Med 46: 464

14 · Infectious Diseases

Ronald O.C. Kaschula

Infections in Newborn Infants and Fetuses

Role of the Placenta

The fetus may be infected by the maternal systemic route and by organisms gaining access via the birth canal. Partial protection of the fetus is provided by the placenta in rubella, malaria and tuberculosis. The placenta is not known to have any specific immunological defence against infection but produces interferon, which seems to be a factor limiting transplacental spread of viral infections (Banatvala et al. 1971). Hofbauer cells (tissue macrophages of placental villi) were thought by Wood (1980) to have a role in limiting transplacental spread of infection.

Haematogenous infections affecting the fetus usually first produce an inflammatory response in chorionic villi. Such villitis is most often focal rather than diffuse and may be unrecognized if limited microscopic examination of placental tissue is undertaken. Altshuler and Russell (1975) have classified villitis into the following histological types:

1. Proliferative villitis: an infiltration by inflammatory cells with tissue necrosis
2. Necrotizing villitis: inflammatory cell infiltration accompanied by necrosis of villous tissue
3. Reparative villitis: resolution of inflammation with the formation of granulation tissue and proliferation of fibroblasts
4. Stromal fibrosis: fibrous scarring of villi without evidence of active inflammation

It is recognized that stromal fibrosis with endothelial vascular proliferation, occurring in the absence of evidence of active inflammation, also has causes other than maternal infection (Fox 1981).

Placental villitis is associated with intrauterine fetal growth retardation (Altshuler et al. 1975; Russell 1979). It seems that retarded fetal growth is a consequence of inflammatory damage to villi, occurring as a consequence of the infection as well as being due to infection of the fetus (Fox 1981).

Perinatal and Neonatal Pneumonia

The age of the infant at the time that the disease is manifested is not always helpful in distinguishing between perinatal and neonatal pneumonia. Some infections such as group B β-haemolytic streptococci (B-βHS), staphylococci, *Escherichia coli* and *Klebsiella* can pursue a very rapidly progressive course, whereas *Chlamydia* and *Mycoplasma* infections may only be slowly progressive.

Following rupture of the membranes, organisms including aerobic and anaerobic bacteria, *Chlamydia*, *Mycoplasma*, fungi and viruses may have access to the amniotic fluid and fetus. Pathogens that are commonly encountered during the neonatal period include B-βHS, *Streptococci fetalis*, *Listeria monocytogenes*, *E. coli*, *Klebsiella*, *Staphylococcus aureus* and *Staph. epidermidis*, *Pseudomonas aeruginosa*, *Mycoplasma* and *Chlamydia*. Where there has been prolonged rupture of the membranes prior to birth (in excess of 24 h) the amniotic fluid is frequently infected and there is an inflammatory response from both fetus and mother. Occasionally, amniotic fluid may become infected when membranes are intact, either by organisms that have ascended through the cervical canal or by those that have come via the maternal blood stream. Viruses such as cytomegalovirus, rubella, parvovirus and herpes tend to reach the amniotic fluid by haematogenous spread. Inflammatory exudate and bacterial organisms in amniotic fluid infection can be inhaled into the lungs in fetal life and, should hypoxia occur before birth, respiratory movements are accentuated and more vigorous inhalation occurs. Meconium discharged in hypoxic episodes may initiate a chemical pneumonitis.

Large numbers of inflammatory cells together with epithelial squames can be present in the lungs without active infection. In contrast, virulent organisms such as B-βHS and *Haemophilus influenzae* may cause death within 24 h and yet be associated with a minimal inflammatory response (Naeye et al. 1971; Blanc 1981).

The pathological features will vary according to the causative organism. Most often the lungs are congested and airless, having a macroscopic resemblance to hyaline membrane disease. *H. influenzae* produces features similar to those described for B-β HS infection, with emphasis on a low-protein fluid exudate. Staphylococcal infections are generally associated with septicaemia, generalized disease such as bullis impetigo, toxic epidermal necrolysis, furunculosis, purulent conjunctivitis, breast abscess and osteomyelitis. *E. coli* and *Klebsiella* spp. tend to be associated with neonatal meningitis and urinary tract infections in addition to the confluent haemorrhagic bronchopneumonia, with a tendency to necrosis of tissue, cavitation, abscess formation, purulent pleurisy and pyopneumothorax, which occurs with these two organisms and staphylococci. *P. aeruginosa* infections are also associated with extensive necrosis, with large numbers of organisms particularly concentrated around blood vessels.

Chlamydia trachomatis is a common cause of neonatal and perinatal pneumonia, which is associated with ophthalmia neonatorum. The pneumonia has an insidious onset and pursues a slowly progressive course (March 1982).

Mycoplasma and *Ureaplasma* infections of the lungs have been encountered in stillbirths, abortions and preterm infants, where they are associated with chorionamnionitis, pneumonia and meningitis (Tafari et al. 1976; Waites et al. 1990).

Viral pneumonia occurring in the first month after birth is generally considered to be postnatally acquired. Respiratory syncytial virus accounts for most, but Enterovirus, Rhinovirus, Adenovirus, Parainfluenza and Herpes simplex virus are also implicated. Adenovirus is the most virulent (Abzug et al. 1990).

Group B β-Haemolytic Streptococcal Infection

Neonatal infection by group B β-haemolytic streptococci (B-βHS), manifesting as pneumonia and meningitis, has become increasingly frequent. There has been a tendency for epidemic infections to occur in various localities (Hood et al. 1961). Early infections are considered to be acquired from the mother's birth canal, whereas late infections probably come from other maternal sites or by cross-infection from other babies or from nursing attendants. During pregnancy and in parturient women, the incidence of colonization by B-βHS is significantly increased (Craig 1981). The risk factors for infant infection are preterm labour, prolonged rupture of membranes, chorioamnionitis, multiple gestation, a previous history of maternal B-βHS infection and prolonged stay in hospital. Over the past two decades the mortality rate has fallen from 30%–50% to 5%–15% (Wessels and Kasper 1993).

Clinical Features

Early-onset streptococcal pneumonia manifests very shortly after birth and may be difficult to distinguish from hyaline membrane disease. Affected infants rapidly develop shock, a bleeding tendency due to prolonged coagulation time, and neutropenia. Mortality rates may exceed 90% among infants whose birth weight is less than a kilogram.

In late-onset disease symptoms develop 10 days to 3 months after birth. Infection is almost invariably due to the serotype III strain of organism (Baker et al. 1973; Baker and Barrett 1974). In 15% of cases the organisms may be cultured from peripheral blood (Baker et al. 1978). The infants are less severely clinically ill than those with early-onset disease, but they tend to have meningitis and disseminated suppurative lesions in many sites.

Pathology

Acute villitis of the placenta occurs as a consequence of haematogenous spread, and is usually associated with meningitis, but it is thought that pneumonia is usually due to organisms reaching amniotic fluid as a consequence of spread through the birth canal. Although the inflammatory response in the lungs is fairly intense in almost half the autopsy cases studied, about a third have only minimal infiltration by neutrophils (Fig. 14.1). These cases simulate and may be misdiagnosed as pulmonary oedema. Patients who have survived for a day or more, particularly when assisted ventilation has been provided, often have deposits of hyaline fibrin in peripheral alveoli, which is not associated with atelectasis. Interstitial pulmonary haemorrhages are seen in about a quarter of cases. Involution of the thymus and inflammatory

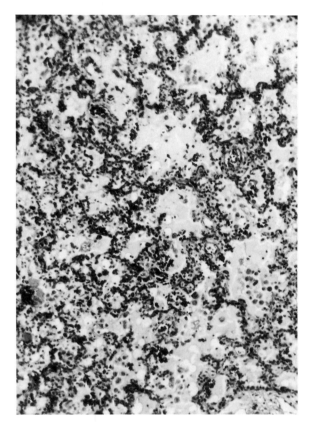

Fig. 14.1. B-βHS pneumonia. Mild intra-alveolar oedema with interstitial infiltration by neutrophils.

reactive changes with follicular hyperplasia are generally found in the spleens of patients who have survived for more than a week or two.

Congenital Syphilis

In syphilis the fetus becomes infected by haematogenous spread through the placenta during episodes of maternal spirochetaemia. Within hours of venereal exposure, and long before serological tests for syphilis become positive or a primary lesion has appeared, the fetus is in danger. Women who contract syphilis before becoming pregnant usually have immunological defences that prevent or restrict spirochetaemia, although intermittent episodes of spirochetaemia tend to occur for the succeeding 2–3 years in the absence of appropriate antibiotic therapy.

The fetus is susceptible to infection by *Treponema pallidum* throughout gestation. However, infection occurring during the first trimester, before the fetus has fully acquired inflammatory responsiveness and

immunological reactivity, produces no destructive lesions (Stowens 1966; Harter and Benirschke 1976).

Live-born infants are likely to be premature and have overt features of congenital syphilis. Maternal infection late in pregnancy may be associated with negative serology, and signs of disease may only become evident weeks or months after birth (Dorfman and Glaser 1990).

Clinical Features

Clinical recognition of the condition depends very much on familiarity with the disease. The varied manifestations range from macerated stillbirth or early neonatal death with gross signs, to an apparently normal infant in whom infection is proved only because investigation has been initiated by a positive maternal serological test result.

Radiological lesions of bone are the most frequent manifestation of congenital syphilis, affecting more than 80% of cases (Malan 1985). The long bones, particularly the femur, tibia and humerus, are most often affected. Involvement is almost always multiple and bilateral without being symmetrical, and the lesions are thus considered to be a consequence of disturbed endochondral and periosteal bone formation rather than being due to direct infection. In preterm infants one usually sees porosis or rarefaction in the distal metaphysis. Sometimes the parotic zone may be associated with bands of enhanced provisional calcification. In infants born at or near term the lesions are more florid, with the zone of porosis becoming irregular and associated with variable destruction of bone giving a sawtooth appearance. Wimberger's sign, which refers to destruction of proximal medial metaphysis, is not infrequently encountered (Cremin and Fisher 1970). Pseudoparesis of a limb, apparently due to painful bony lesions, occurs in about 20% of cases with radiological lesions of bone. Subperiosteal layering of new bone along the diaphysis is an infrequent early lesion but is the most common anomaly seen in infants older than 2 months. The lesion becomes more conspicuous as the infant gets older. There is the radiographic appearance of a double contour along the shaft of the bones, which does not reach the termination of the metaphysis (Fig. 14.2). The simultaneous presence of typical diaphyseal and metaphyseal lesions in areas having a high incidence of disease is regarded as highly suggestive of syphilis (Malan 1985).

Premature birth occurs in more than 80% of cases in developing countries; about 40% of patients are growth retarded. Enlargement of the placenta relative to the size of the fetus is encountered in about 50% of

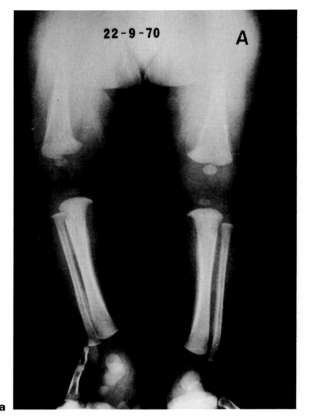

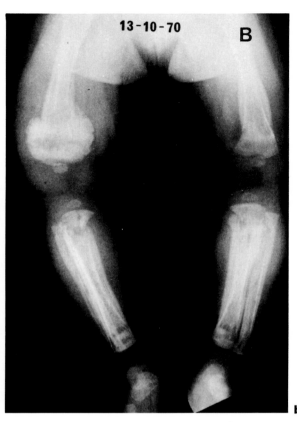

a   b

Fig. 14.2. a Radiograph of the lower limbs of a newborn infant with congenital syphilis. There is subperiosteal layering of new bone of the right femur with early destruction of the distal medial metaphysis. **b** The same infant after 21 days of therapy. There is gross bilateral layering of new bone formation along all long bones, with porotic destruction of the medial metaphyses of both tibias, gross reactive calcification of the distal metaphysis of the right femur, and rarefaction of the left femur.

cases. This increase in placental–fetal weight ratio tends to be associated with fetal growth retardation but is often not clinically recognized.

Hepatosplenomegaly occurs in more than 75% of cases, and splenomegaly without liver enlargement is encountered in approximately 15%. Thirty per cent of cases have conjugated hyperbilirubinaemia, raised liver enzyme levels and disturbance of liver function tests indicative of hepatitis with obstructive jaundice. Disturbance of liver function may persist for a year before becoming normal.

Skin lesions are found in almost 50% of cases and occur in a number of forms. Excessive fissuring and deep desquamation particularly occurs on the palms and soles. Maculopapular lesions may be prominent in lightly pigmented individuals, and seem to precede desquamation. Bullous eruptions containing large numbers of organisms break down to leave a weeping denuded area, which may become pustular. Very infrequently one may see annular or circinate skin lesions and "blueberry muffin" lesions (due to

haemopoiesis in the skin). Mucocutaneous lesions are occasionally encountered in the form of nasal or mouth ulcers, punched-out ulcers of the tongue (Fig. 14.3), rhinitis with a highly infectious nasal discharge (snuffles), and condylomata of genitoanal region.

Purpura and bleeding occur to a variable extent and generally take the form of spots or large ecchymoses on the chest and abdomen. Bleeding is attributed to thrombocytopenia, deficiency of clotting factors because of liver involvement, and disseminated intravascular coagulation. Haemolytic anaemia with associated reticulocytosis is seen in 25%–50% of cases. Generalized oedema is seen in about 25% of cases and is associated with severe hypoalbuminaemia and often with ascites as well. These changes may be so severe that the term "hydrops fetalis" is applicable. A small number of newborn infants suffer a nephritic type of nephrotic syndrome, due to preformed immune complexes, with proteinuria and haematuria (Kaschula et al. 1974) (Fig. 14.4).

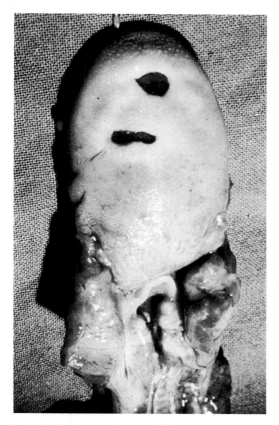

Fig. 14.3. Bland punched-out syphilitic ulcers of the tongue.

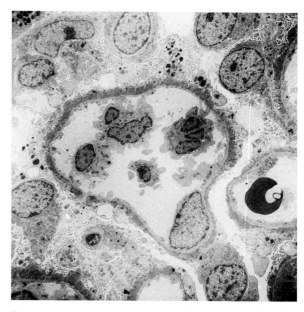

Fig. 14.4. Electron micrograph of a glomerular capillary with numerous subepithelial immune complex deposits on the epithelial surface of the basement membrane of a newborn infant with a nephritic type of nephrotic syndrome caused by congenital syphilis. (× 1424)

Respiratory difficulties because of pneumonitis are encountered in about 40% of cases with radiological features of diffuse pulmonary infiltration which is not specific for syphilis.

Pathology

Although *Treponema* are present in the blood stream in large numbers and become widely distributed, certain viscera are more frequently affected. These are the pancreas, liver, bone, lung, nasal mucosa and gastrointestinal tract. The morphological features vary according to the stage of fetal development at the time of infection, the number of organisms transmitted, the duration of survival of the fetus after infection and the effectiveness of any therapy that may have been given. Late-gestation infection, where the fetus has effective immune responsiveness, stimulates lymphoid follicle development and plasma cell proliferation. In addition to the clinical observation of infants being small for their gestational period, the developmental maturation of many organs is retarded. Glomerular development in kidneys is impaired and retarded. The lungs and pancreas contain excessive amounts of mesenchymal tissue for their stage of development, and the air spaces of lungs retain a fetal glandular configuration. During the postnatal period, there is prolonged persistence of the fetal adrenal cortex. Haemolytic anaemia with intense and widespread extramedullary haemopoiesis occurs.

Miliary granulomas or microgummata occur diffusely in some cases and mainly affect liver and pituitary. Healing occurs by fibrous replacement.

Small muscular arteries and arterioles sometimes develop an accumulation of mononuclear inflammatory cells, including plasma cells, in the outer layers of the vessel wall and surrounding tissues. These lesions also seem to heal by fibrosis, often producing a typical "onion skin" pattern.

Acute abscess-like lesions occur rarely in thymus, spleen, lymph nodes and other organs, where there is a central area of necrosis and an intense infiltration by neutrophils.

The liver generally shows varying degrees of bile staining, but the classic picture of pericellular cirrhosis is now rarely encountered and is usually a late

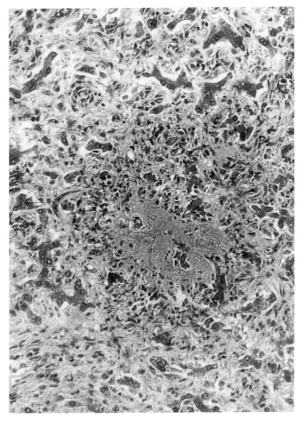

Fig. 14.5. Liver with fragmentation of parenchymal cell plates, diffuse fibrosis and a microgumma. Congenital syphilis.

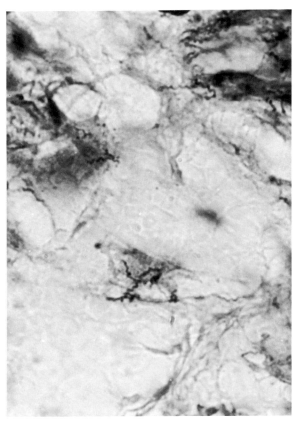

Fig. 14.6. *Treponema pallidum* spirochaetes occurring in small clusters and individually in the pancreas of a patient with congenital syphilis. (Warthin–Starry stain)

manifestation of untreated infection in infants who were born at term. In this condition there is disruption of the normal architecture, with diffuse fibrosis occurring in all areas of the lobule. The parenchymal cell plates become fragmented so that individual hepatic cells are surrounded by connective tissue fibres (Fig. 14.5). Excessive extramedullary haemopoiesis is a frequent finding, which occurs in portal areas and diffusely or focally within sinusoids. Miliary granulomas may accompany either cirrhosis or haemopoiesis, and very rarely one may encounter parenchymal giant cell formation. In untreated cases spirochaetes are usually widely scattered in large numbers but predominate in Disse's space. In cases in which the patient dies within a few hours of a single dose of penicillin, small clusters of agglutinated organisms may be found (Fig. 14.6).

The pancreas is more often affected than the liver. There is haemopoiesis and diffuse pancreatitis which undergoes healing by fibrosis. Initially acini, ductules and islets become separated by oedema and

inflammatory cells, but, as fibrosis develops, compression atrophy of parenchymal tissue occurs (Fig. 14.7). Dilatation of acini and ducts are not features of syphilitic infection. Occasionally, large granulomas with extensive areas of necrosis may be seen and, when these heal, large focal scars of fibrous tissue are found.

The lungs are most often macroscopically normal, but may be pale, voluminous and heavy with extensive pneumonia alba (see below). Microscopically, they appear very immature for their gestational age. There is persistence of extramedullary haemopoiesis, with retention of mesenchymal connective tissue and a glandular rather than an alveolar pattern to the airspaces. The thickened alveolar walls initially contain plasma cells with lymphocytes and macrophages in addition to haemopoietic foci. Spirochaetes may be present in large numbers, and, as the pneumonia heals, fibrosis with thickening of the walls of the airspaces occurs. "Pneumonia alba" refers to sharply outlined zones or sheets of fibrosis with tiny airless

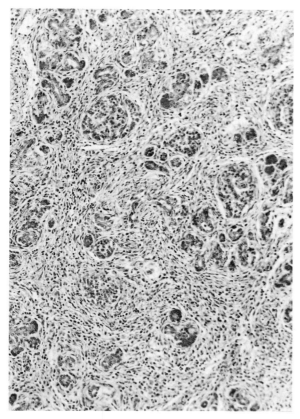

Fig. 14.7. Pancreas in congenital syphilis. There is separation of acini by loose fibrous tissue and a mild mixed inflammatory cell infiltration.

alveolar structures (Oppenheimer and Dahms 1981). The rudimentary alveoli may contain entrapped inflammatory cells as well as shed epithelial cells.

The long bones of the limbs are almost always affected, and symmetrical radiological changes are almost invariably present at birth. Most often the periosteum along the shaft and at the epiphyses is thickened by granulation tissue and plasma cell infiltration with subperiosteal new bone formation. At the epiphyses of the long bones, there is osteochondritis with granulation tissue formation and fibrosis. This is associated with irregular vascular penetration and absorption of cartilage (Fig. 14.8). The symmetrical nature of the lesions in long bones, and the fact that similar radiological changes are encountered in conditions such as congenital rubella, prematurity, erythroblastosis, congenital cytomegalovirus infection and rickets, strongly suggests a dystrophic process. The progression of the lesions demonstrated in Fig. 14.2, which occurred while the patient was receiving therapy, supports this hypothesis (Cremin and Fisher 1970).

The gastrointestinal tract is affected fairly frequently. Most often there is focal infiltration of the intestinal wall by mononuclear inflammatory cells, but diffuse infiltration of such inflammatory cells may widen the mucosa and submucosa. Perivascular inflammatory cell infiltration may be conspicuous and compress vessel lumina. Healing occurs by fibrosis, which may cause stenosis, and rarely discontinuity of the intestinal lumen, manifested as intestinal atresia (Siplovich et al. 1988). Acute focal lesions

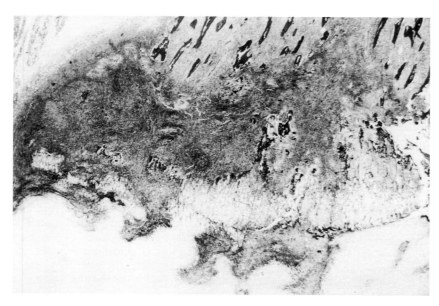

Fig. 14.8. Destruction of epiphyseal cartilage with inflammatory granulation tissue formation and fibrosis of the metaphysis in the proximal tibia of a patient with congenital syphilis.

in the muscular wall can be responsible for intestinal rupture and consequent meconium peritonitis (Oppenheimer and Dahms 1981).

In the kidneys in neonates extramedullary haemopoiesis may be prominent, with an associated mixed lymphocytic and plasma cell infiltration in interstitial areas. This picture is not generally associated with symptoms of renal disease. Features that conform with those of immune glomerulopathy are seen in association with clinical features of the nephrotic syndrome or glomerulonephritis in infants who are older than 1 month (Kaschula et al. 1974) (Fig. 14.4).

The skin rashes that occur are associated with focal accumulation of lymphocytes and plasma cells around adnexal structures and small vessels. Mucous membranes are thickened by mononuclear inflammatory infiltrates and granulation tissue proliferation. Punched-out ulcers, without surrounding hyperaemia, are occasionally seen in the nose, mouth and tongue (Fig. 14.3).

The placenta is usually enlarged without being hydropic. Microscopic examination may show spirochaetes and other non-specific features of intrauterine infection. Most often there is extreme immaturity of chorionic villi with some concentric perivascular fibrous tissue around the blood vessels of terminal and stem villi. Very occasionally there may be intimal thickening of fetal vessels with narrowing of the lumina. Focal villitis with infiltration by lymphocytes and plasma cells is another non-specific feature.

A variety of other organs may also be affected. The pituitary may undergo extensive necrosis with large abscess-like granulomas. The adrenals may contain large numbers of spirochaetes without granulomas, and intense inflammation followed by fibrosis may occur in the testes. The spleen and lymph nodes may have focal lesions with hyperplastic lymphoid aggregates and extramedullary haemopoiesis. In the central nervous system, including the spinal cord, focal mononuclear infiltrates and extramedullary haemopoiesis may be seen in pia-arachnoid. Granulomas tend to be sited in choroid plexus, medulla, spinal cord and eye. In the heart, mononuclear inflammatory infiltrations may be seen in pericardium and endocardium in association with granulomas of the myocardium or non-specific degeneration of myocardial fibres with inflammatory cell infiltration.

Neonatal Tetanus

Neonatal tetanus is usually caused by the introduction of the spores of *Clostridium tetani* to the umbilical stump. Vegetative organisms multiply at this site without evoking an inflammatory response, but liberate exotoxins. Neurotoxins have both local and central effects (Malan 1985). In the brain, tetanospasmin is bound to gangliocides and, once fixed, cannot be neutralized by antitoxin.

In some societies various mixtures, which often include animal manure, are placed on the umbilical stump. In such societies mothers are not generally immunized and there is a high incidence of the disease. A survey in Bangladesh revealed that 27% of all infant deaths are due to tetanus (Stoll 1979). It is estimated that 700 000 children die of this illness each year in the world (EPI Newsletter 1992).

Without treatment the mortality rate in neonatal tetanus is approximately 90%, with most deaths occurring during the second week of life. The mechanism of death has not been fully determined. Inconsistent neuronal degeneration of the dorsal vagal nuclei of the 4th ventricle, with surrounding oedema and some round-cell infiltration, have been reported (Montgomery 1961). Most often no satisfactory pathological changes that can explain death are demonstrated. In cases treated in special centres, septicaemia or hypostatic pneumonia may be the immediate cause of death. Attacks of respiratory failure often occur without convulsions and point to medullary intoxication. Hyperpyrexia, tachycardia with hypotension, bulbar palsy and cardiac arrest are frequent features in fatal cases. Myocardial damage with electrocardiographic changes as well as myolysis of striated muscle have been encountered.

Perinatal Listeriosis

Listeria monocytogenes causes perinatal disease with early-onset and late-onset forms. Infection is generally acquired by transplacental haematogenous spread, by inhalation of infected amniotic fluid or by direct contact and aspiration at the time of vaginal delivery. The organism may be responsible for mid-trimester abortions, premature onset of labour, intrauterine distress, amniotic fluid infection syndrome, neonatal pneumonia, septicaemia and meningitis. It produces transient infections of intestines and female genitourinary tract as well as being pathogenic to many animals. Without being implicated as the causative agent, genital listerial infection is frequently associated with repeated abortion. Severe infection of conceptuses may occur with little or no overt clinical evidence of infection in the mother's genital tract. Gastroenteritis and non-specific septicaemic symptoms in the mother or other family members often herald premature birth of an infant with listerial septicaemia. The mortality rate is almost 50% (Bortolussi 1985).

Infection occurs more often in the infants of diabetic mothers, and it is thought that maternal physical and hormonal changes during pregnancy may facilitate listerial infections. Iron and adrenocorticosteroids are known to promote listerial infection (Buchner and Schneirson 1968). Epidemics have been attributed to sheep manure used in cabbage fields prior to the preparation of coleslaw (Schlech et al. 1983) and to cheese prepared from unpasteurized milk (Klatt et al. 1986).

Pathology

Placentae that have been infected as a consequence of haematogenous spread are often enlarged. Often there is inflammation of membranes and umbilical cord (Evans et al. 1985). Within the villous parenchyma one may find scattered yellowish-white lesions. They may resemble tubercles but range from 0.5 to 10.0 mm in diameter and consist of areas of necrosis with an infiltration by neutrophils and a peripheral pallisade of histiocytes. Fibrin thrombi containing entrapped inflammatory cells may be present in the adjoining intervillous space, and a non-specific focal villitis may occur (Driscoll 1962). When infection is the result of ascending spread through the cervix, there is extensive acute inflammation of the membranes and small abscesses may be seen within the decidua (Vawter 1981).

Specific inflammatory granulomas, called "listerioma" by Vawter (1981), occur in many organs including placental villi, adrenals, liver, lung, spleen, bone marrow, meninges and arteries. They range from a microscopic size of 0.1 mm to 10 mm, are yellowish-white in colour and solid without liquefactive necrosis. Early lesions have a macroscopic resemblance to miliary tubercles, having a central area of necrosis with preservation of reticulin framework. The central zone initially contains gram-positive bacilli with necrotic cells and fibrin. Peripherally there are bacteria, acute inflammatory cells and macrophages. As the lesion matures the central zone is found to contain fewer organisms, cellular debris becomes sparse, and the lesion collapses and is repaired by regeneration fibrosis leading to an inconspicuous scar.

Other lesions encountered include a generalized bleeding tendency from small blood vessels. Purpuric rashes with petechiae, pulmonary haemorrhages, intraventricular haemorrhages, subarachnoid haemorrhages and blood-stained pleural and pericardial effusions with laboratory features of a consumptive coagulopathy occur. In addition, the brain may show paraventricular leucomalacia or massive necrosis, and focal meningitis may occur in infants who have survived for 2 days. Newborn infants usually become jaundiced because of haemolysis and prematurity. There is also an increased frequency of cholangitis and of extrahepatic biliary atresia. In addition to focal miliary inflammatory lesions the liver may show sinusoidal congestion, a consequence of circulatory compromise, together with central necrosis and microvesicular fatty change. Thymus, spleen and lymph nodes contain reduced numbers of lymphocytes in association with features of immunological stimulation.

Congenital Rubella (see also Chapter 2)

Clinical Features

Approximately two-thirds of infected infants are asymptomatic at birth and during the neonatal period. However, most of the infants with silent infection develop long-term sequelae during the ensuing 5–10 years. Overt manifestation of infection at birth is subtle and non-specific.

The risk of fetal damage from congenital rubella is very high when infection occurs early in pregnancy. The chances have been estimated at 90% before 11 weeks' gestation, when multiple defects are common. Thereafter about 34% will have neurosensory hearing loss alone, but this figure falls to 17% at 13–16 weeks and becomes zero after 18 weeks (Miller et al. 1982). Infection occurring during the first 11 weeks often leads to premature birth, intrauterine growth retardation, thrombocytopenia and purpura, and neonatal hepatitis with hepatomegaly. In addition, congenital heart disease, interstitial pneumonia, blotchy retinopathy, cataracts, bone changes manifesting as radiolucency in the metaphysis of long bones, and encephalopathy manifesting as lethargy, irritability and seizures may occur. Isolation of rubella virus is most often obtained from vitreous, cerebrospinal fluid, lung and liver. The presence of elevated levels of specific IgM antibody in a single serum specimen from a young infant is regarded as diagnostic, although this is found only in about 50% of confirmed cases (Hanshaw and Dudgeon 1978).

Pathology

Infection of the conceptus occurs about a week before the onset of the rash in the mother (Rosenberg et al. 1981b). Fetal infection seems to result from immobilization of portions of necrotic placental vascular endothelium which has been infected with rubella during the first trimester (Menser and Reye 1974), when abortion may occur. Therapeutically aborted infected fetuses usually demonstrate scattered foci of cell necrosis without inflammatory infiltration. There seems to be tropism for endothelial and myocardial cells (Tondury and Smith 1966).

Infants who are infected during the early gestational period tend to have fewer mitoses during early growth and development and are small for gestational age at birth with allometric inhibition of growth of all organs and tissues. They eventually become small adults. When infection occurs later in the gestational period (after 14 weeks) the small for gestational age infant has asymmetrical inhibition of growth with sparing of brain development at the expense of skeletal tissues and internal organs. The ratio of brain weight to liver weight may increase from 3 : 1 to 6 : 1. These infants are able to grow into normal-sized adults. All rubella-infected infants with low birth weight usually have radiographic changes in long bones, which are attributed to inhibition of growth at the metaphyseal plate. In males the incisor, canine and second mandibular molar teeth are smaller than normal (Cohen 1974).

There is a high risk of congenital heart disease during the first 16 weeks' gestation. Way (1967) has estimated the rates as 50% during the first 4 weeks, 25% during the second 4 weeks, 17% during the third 4 weeks, 11% during the fourth 4 weeks, and 0% thereafter.

In different series the incidence of cardiovascular anomalies varies from 30% to 90% (Singer et al. 1967; Esterly and Oppenheimer 1969; Fortuin et al. 1971; Tang et al. 1971).

The sites that are most susceptible to damage are the ductus arteriosus, great vessels, cardiac septa and valves. Persistent patency of the ductus arteriosus is most often encountered. Other frequently occurring anomalies are pulmonary artery stenosis, atrial and ventricular septal defects, stenosis of pulmonary and aortic valves, tetralogy of Fallot, transposition of the great arteries and coarctation of the aorta (Way 1967; Rosenberg et al. 1981b). A characteristic microscopic feature of the aorta and large arteries is fibrovascular intimal proliferation without significant damage to internal elastic lamina and media. Focal myocardial necrosis with or without an inflammatory response, myocardial scarring without calcification, and valvular sclerosis are also seen fairly frequently (Campbell 1965). In the ductus arteriosus there is collagenous replacement of elastica and muscle. Stenosis of renal arteries may cause systemic hypertension, whereas it has been suggested among long-term survivors vascular lesions are potential causes of coronary, cerebral and peripheral vascular disease in adults (Forrest et al. 1969).

There is a high incidence of interstitial pneumonitis with patchy collapse among newborn infants with congenital rubella syndrome. The respiratory distress that the infants suffer is mainly due to congestion attributed to congestive heart failure. On microscopic examination one generally sees mild infiltration of interstitial tissue by mononuclear inflammatory cells, vascular congestion and intra-alveolar oedema with some hyaline membrane formation.

Jaundice and hepatomegaly are commonly found in the neonatal period and are due to hepatitis. Microscopically, the parenchymal hepatic cells become swollen and hyalinized. There is extramedullary haemopoiesis with giant cell transformation and cholestasis. In some cases bile duct proliferation suggestive of extrahepatic biliary obstruction is seen, and biliary atresia is known to occur (Esterly and Oppenheimer 1973; Rosenberg et al. 1981a, b).

Newborn infants with congenital rubella syndrome often have transient splenomegaly, thrombocytopenia, purpura and anaemia. The anaemia is due to haemolysis and is associated with extramedullary haemopoiesis in liver, gastrointestinal tract, pancreas, adrenals and kidneys. Initially there is precocious development of lymphoid aggregates with prominent germinal centres in spleen and lymph nodes. Persistence of infection in older infants and children causes the lymphoid aggregates to decrease in size progressively, whereas the thymus is usually small and relatively lymphopenic from birth. In young infants lymph nodes have atrophic T-dependent paracortical zones with proliferation of vessels and B-dependent cells (Singer et al. 1969). A number of disorders of cellular immune reactivity have been observed in congenital rubella syndrome and these are thought to account for the persistence of virus excretion despite antibody production during the early years after birth (South et al. 1975).

In the pancreas, focal mixed inflammatory cell infiltration between acini occurs. Active or latent diabetes mellitus develops in about 20% of survivors who, at autopsy, have been shown to have an apparent decrease in number of islets and stainable β cells (Menser et al. 1978; Rosenberg et al. 1981b).

There are reports of late-onset thyrotoxicosis and hypothyroidism among survivors of congenital rubella syndrome. Such cases have demonstrated lymphocytic infiltrates in the thyroid, sometimes with germinal centres and destruction of thyroid acini. Acinar cells tend to be enlarged and eosinophilic, and reduced amounts of colloid are found (Rosenberg et al. 1981b).

Addison's disease has been encountered in a 10-year-old child who had congenital rubella syndrome (Ziring et al. 1977).

Transitory and symmetrical radiological changes are encountered in the very young. Radiolucencies in the metaphysis of long bones (considered to resemble a celery stalk) correlate with osteoporotic zones, containing increased osteoblasts, ground substance and myxoid tissue. There is irregularity of the line of provisional calcification at the epiphyses with irregular resorption of cartilage. Newly formed bony trabeculae retain a central zone of cartilage which is surrounded by a thin layer of osteoid (Rosenberg et al. 1981b). The pattern of inhibited bone growth has, like that of congenital syphilis, been attributed to a generalized retardation of cell division.

Cataracts are frequent but generally become evident after the neonatal period, whereas microphthalmus, iridocyclitis and retinitis (focal degeneration and proliferation of pigment epithelium) may be seen at any early age.

In the ear, Esterly and Oppenheimer (1973) consider that deafness is due to inflammation, cystic degeneration and atrophy of the stria vascularis lining the periphery of the cochlear duct. Reissner's membrane is often collapsed and adherent to the stria, and the tectorial membrane is rolled up and displaced into the inner sulcus.

In the central nervous system, microcephaly may be a manifestation of generalized inhibition of growth. Other lesions include malformation, cerebral vasculitis, meningitis, focal necrosis and subarachnoid haemorrhage. Necrosis occurs in parenchymal areas, around vessels and in periventricular embryonic matrix (Desmond et al. 1969). The necrotic foci are attributed to vascular disease in cases which have deposits of calcium and acid mucopolysaccharide in the walls of arteries (Rosenberg et al. 1981b). Focal destruction of vessel walls with disruption of internal elastic lamina, pericapillary collections of granular material, endothelial proliferation and ischaemic necrosis of adjacent brain are also seen (Rorke 1973). The malformations that are encountered include meningomyelocele and Dandy–Walker syndrome. Progressive rubella panencephalitis is a late manifestation (second decade) in cases that seem to have persistent latent infection. There is diffuse mononuclear inflammation of meninges and perivascular areas of white matter in the hippocampus and brain stem. This is associated with focal and nodular areas of gliosis.

The placenta is generally reduced in size, apparently due to generalized inhibition of growth and mitotic activity. There are not other destructive gross changes apart from foci of haemorrhage and necrosis of decidua. Microscopically, the most striking feature is disseminated acute necrosis with mixed inflammatory cell infiltration and rare intracytoplasmic eosinophilic inclusion bodies occurring in decidua and chorionic villi (Driscoll 1969). Among the chorionic villi there is massive hypoplasia with arrested development of terminal branches, whereas stem villi become broad with reduced vascularity. There is necrosis of the endothelium of villous capillaries as well as fragmentation of intraluminal blood vessels and small haemorrhages.

Congenital Cytomegalovirus Infection

Congenital cytomegalovirus (CMV) infection is a very frequent cause of perinatal viral infection. It is estimated to involve 3 in 1000 births in the UK (Peckham et al. 1983) and 8 in 1000 in the USA, where it causes brain damage in 1 per 1000 births (Rosenberg et al. 1981a). Congenital CMV infection is most frequently symptomless and without sequelae. It is estimated that approximately 80%–90% of cases are not recognized. In addition, infection can occur during the perinatal period and is then indistinguishable from latent prenatal infection. The incubation period has been found to vary between 30 and 60 days (Reynolds et al. 1973). Severely affected infants usually have evidence of symmetrical intrauterine growth retardation. Other features include hepatosplenomegaly, jaundice, thrombocytopenic purpura, haemolytic anaemia, chorioretinitis, pneumonitis, and central nervous system disease which includes microcephaly, hydrocephaly and intracranial calcification (McCracken et al. 1969). Some infants may have a large placenta and be hydropic. Although virus infection persists after birth, there is little evidence for continued tissue destruction, as occurs with rubella infection. Symptomatic infants often have long-term problems such as cerebral palsy, epilepsy, mental retardation and sensorineural deafness.

In developing countries and in the low socioeconomic group of developed countries, there is a relatively high rate of maternal immunity and a high incidence of latent fetal infection. These infections are mainly due to reactivation of latent maternal infection. Overt neonatal disease with serious sequelae occurs most often when the mother is exposed to the virus for the first time during pregnancy (Becroft 1981).

Pathology

The most striking morphological feature of CMV infection is the presence of characteristic enlarged cells having intranuclear and intracytoplasmic inclusions (Figs. 14.9 and 14.10). In the early stages the CMV-infected cell may be difficult to distinguish from cells with herpes group inclusions. At this stage a distinguishing feature is the presence and persistence of the nucleolus in the infected cell (Strano 1976). With development, the cell enlarges and the

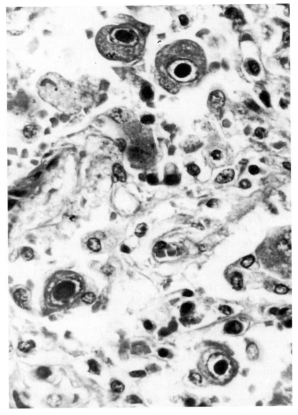

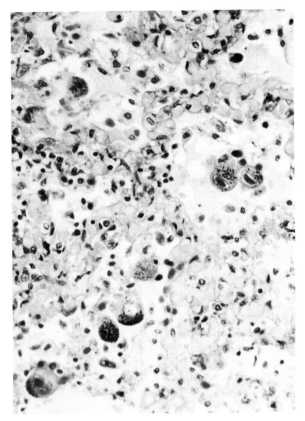

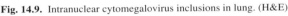

Fig. 14.9. Intranuclear cytomegalovirus inclusions in lung. (H&E)

Fig. 14.10. Intranuclear and intracytoplasmic cytomegalovirus inclusions. (PAS)

nucleus becomes very prominent. The centrally sited inclusion material may be eosinophilic or basophilic, and sometimes has a round clear object in the centre which, together with a peripheral halo, resembles a target or an "owl's eye". The intracytoplasmic inclusions do not have a halo, consistently stain with methenamine silver and are periodic acid–Schiff (PAS)-positive (Gorelkin et al. 1986). The basic features are preserved in autolysed tissues of severely macerated fetuses when differential staining is lost. The ultrastructural features of individual virus particles cannot be distinguished from other viruses in the herpes group.

Fetal growth retardation is a feature of both symptomatic and asymptomatic infection (Berge et al. 1990). The placenta and central nervous system are the most frequently involved sites of infection. In the placenta, specific lesions containing characteristic inclusion-bearing cells tend to be sited near or at the endothelium of fetal capillaries and in Hofbauer or stromal cells of chorionic villi (Blanc 1978). The lesions are more often less specific, and, in the early stages, foci of necrosis in the stroma or vessels of ter-

minal and stem villi occur. Later there is intense invasion by lymphocytes, plasma cells, histiocytes and fibroblasts. The stroma of stem villi may contain haemosiderin deposits, and calcification may occur within villi or their basement membranes. Non-specific changes include focal or diffuse oedema of villi (which can produce a hydropic placenta weighing more than a kilogram), chorioamnionitis, and intervillitis (which may be due to concurrent infection by a bacterial agent).

Central nervous system involvement is responsible for the most important clinical effects of congenital CMV infection. Almost all descriptions of the pathology of CNS infection are from infants or children who were severely affected at birth. Acute lesions tend to be localized to the periventricular regions and comprise small necrotic foci with swollen eosinophilic microglial cells (Becroft 1981). Some lesions may contain cells with CMV inclusions but the majority resemble a non-specific acute viral encephalitis. Acute lesions are indicative of continuing active infection and may be encountered in cases of chronic disease. Inclusion may occur in neurons, glia, ependyma, choroid plexus, meninges and vascular endothelium. Inclusion-bearing cells have been reported in cerebrospinal fluid (Arey 1954). Nonspecific lesions that may be encountered include haemorrhages and leucomalacia.

Chronic lesions are recognized as foci of necrosis, usually associated with glial proliferation and haemosiderin- or lipid-containing macrophages. Calcification is common and the lesions tend to localize in periventricular regions. Sometimes glial proliferation may occur without necrosis in juxtaependymal regions. These proliferations extend into the ventricular cavities as empendymal buds and are considered to be responsible for hydrocephalus. Abnormalities of cellular migration from germinal matrix and disorganized gyration are particularly seen in microencephalic brains. Small brains are encountered in severe infection, subclinical infection and growth-retarded cases.

Ear involvement is manifested as sensorineural deafness and is estimated to occur in almost 20% of cases with subclinical infection (Stagno et al. 1977). Inclusion-bearing epithelial cells may be seen in the lining of the semicircular canals, sacules and utricles, in the maculae, in the cristae, in the vestibular (Reissner's) membranes and on the striae vascularis of the cochleae.

Eye abnormalities due to severe CMV infection are chorioretinitis, optic neuritis and atrophy, cataract, nystagmus, strabismus, microphthalmia and colobomata (Blattner 1974; Stagno et al. 1977). The incidence of chorioretinitis has been reported to be 25% of symptomatic infants (Blattner 1974).

The lungs are a frequent site for the identification of inclusion-bearing cells in macerated stillborn infants. In newborn infants these organs most frequently show inclusions, which may be seen as early as 20 weeks' gestation (Rosenstein and Navarette-Reyna 1964). An inflammatory reaction is seldom seen, although small numbers of lymphocytes and plasma cells are sometimes present. However, pneumonitis is a common manifestation of infection occurring after the neonatal period and also occurs in acquired postnatal infections (Hanshaw 1979). (See also p. 371.)

Renal involvement is slightly less frequent than are pulmonary manifestations. Inclusions occur in distal convoluted tubules, collecting ducts and the proximal nephron. There is interstitial infiltration by lymphocytes and plasma cells in severe infection, and proliferative glomerulonephritis has been reported (Beneck et al. 1986).

Hepatic lesions are as frequent, but significant liver disease is not common. Hepatomegaly and icterus tend to develop after the neonatal period and persist for some months. Hyperbilirubinaemia is due to both hepatocellular dysfunction and haemolysis. CMV inclusions tend to occur in the lining cells of small bile ducts in variable numbers. Extramedullary haemopoiesis is usually prominent, with intracellular and intralobular cholestasis, necrosis of parenchymal cells, giant cell transformation and some bile duct proliferation.

The salivary glands are frequently involved in both congenital and acquired infection, but tissue necrosis and inflammatory response are inconspicuous. Similar involvement of the pancreas, thyroid and pituitary gland occurs, but the adrenals are rarely affected in congenital infection (Becroft 1981).

The spleen is moderately enlarged (usually twice normal weight) in cases of congenital CMV infection. Extramedullary haemopoiesis and congestion account for this, as the lymphoid follicles are usually reduced in size.

The thymus is reduced in size as a response to the stress of ongoing intrauterine infection.

Congenital and Neonatal Herpes Simplex Infection

There are two basic types of inclusion in herpesvirus infection. Type A inclusions have a clear halo separating the inclusion material from the nuclear membrane. Type B inclusions are amphophilic, homogeneous or glassy, and push nuclear chromatin against the nuclear membrane (Fig. 14.11). Type A inclusions are not infectious, whereas type B are (Singer 1981). The source of most neonatal infections due to *Herpesvirus hominis* (HSV) is maternal genital infection, which in more than two-thirds of cases is HSV type 2 (Kalmyak 1977; Sharon 1977). Latent intrauterine infection may be associated with intrauterine death, fetal growth retardation, cystic brain degeneration, hydrops, interstitial pneumonitis, hepatitis, myocarditis, encephalitis and renal failure (Robb et al. 1986). Neonatal infection with HSV type 1 is more often due to postnatal contact with parents with *Herpes labialis*. There are no perceptible differences in the expression of the infections produced by the two strains of virus, and prognosis for the neonate is uniformly poor.

Pathology

The organs that are most consistently affected by HSV infection in the neonate are liver, adrenal, oesophagus, skin, eye and brain. The characteristic lesion begins as a focus of inclusion-bearing parenchymal cells, which undergoes coagulative necrosis to which there is a subsequent inflammatory response with peripheral dilation of vessels and mild

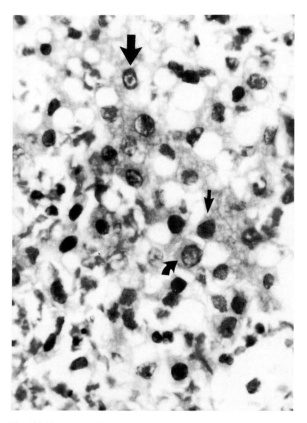

Fig. 14.11. Herpesvirus inclusions in liver. *Thick arrow*, Cowdry type A inclusion (a clear halo between the inclusion material and the nuclear membrane). *Curved arrow*, Cowdry type B inclusion (glassy inclusion material pushing chromatin against the nuclear membrane). *Thin arrow*, Cowdry type B inclusion (dense amphophilic homogenous inclusion material fills the nucleus).

inflammatory cell infiltration. Lysis of the nuclear membrane of affected cells leads to coagulative necrosis of the cell without detectable virus particles being liberated.

In the liver, affected parenchymal cells have enlarged nuclei prior to the appearance of inclusions. The pattern of necrosis sometimes tends to radiate from blood vessels in which fibrin thrombi are found. Disseminated intravascular coagulopathy is frequently associated with this type of lesion (Miller et al. 1970; Whitaker and Hardison 1978). In other radiating lesions it seems that the virus produces a cellular toxin which diffuses out from the infected focus (Darlington and Granoff 1973). Portal tissues and bile ducts are not affected.

The adrenal glands are usually simultaneously affected with liver lesions. Here the lesions are smaller and less numerous. They are confined to the definitive cortex.

The incidence of placental involvement is not known, but placental infection is considered to be a cause of spontaneous abortion (Nahmias et al. 1983). Necrosis of individual or groups of chorionic villi occurs without any significant inflammatory response (Witzleben and Driscoll 1965). Herpetic inclusions may also occur in syncytial trophoblasts, amnion and the chorionic plate and around fetal blood vessels of the umbilical cord. All cases of placental infection are associated with fetal or neonatal lesions.

Involvement of the brain in cases of intrauterine infection varies from devastating destruction to mild meningoencephalitis. There may be extensive necrosis in cerebral grey matter, basal ganglia, superficial white matter periventricular regions and cerebellar folia (Singer 1981). The necrotic lesions tend to be centred around small blood vessels, with intranuclear inclusions occurring in the nuclei of oligodendroglia and neuronal cells. Necrotic foci may undergo calcification. Meningeal lesions consist of an infiltration by lymphocytes and macrophages. Children who survive severe neonatal infection may develop porencephaly, hydranencephaly and multiple brain cysts.

Little is know about the frequency with which eyes are involved in autopsy cases. Abnormalities of vision occur in cases that survive neonatal infection. Lesions encountered are conjunctivitis, corneal opacification, iritis, uveitis, retinitis and cataracts.

Vesicular lesions of the skin particularly occur at sites that have prolonged exposure to the mother's birth canal during vaginal delivery: the scalp in cephalic presentations and buttocks in breech presentations (Nahmias et al. 1983). Recurrent eruptions of vesicles may occur for a number of years after birth.

In the lungs, focal necrotic lesions usually with intranuclear inclusions and associated with fibrin exudation into alveolar spaces, may occur in the parenchymal areas. They evidently reflect haematogenous dissemination of the virus.

In the gastrointestinal tract, the lips, tongue, pharynx and oesophagus may be affected by direct contact with swallowed infected amniotic fluid. Following the initial formation of vesicles, which are rarely seen, there may be extensive and deep ulceration of mucosa. Lesions with intact epithelium may contain inclusion-bearing cells, and occasional multinuclear giant cells may be seen. Acanthosis of squamous epithelium with acantholysis and a mild inflammatory cell infiltration into epithelium and subepithelial tissues are occasionally encountered. Lesions of the stomach and intestines are rare. Focal superficial lesions may be found in the stomach and intestinal mucosa of cases with gastroenteritis.

At the height of infection there is fairly widespread depletion of thymic-dependent lymphocytes in the lymphoreticular system. The periarteriolar sheaths of the spleen and paracortical zones of lymph nodes are most strikingly affected in infants who die within 2 weeks of birth. Repopulation of these zones and stimulation of areas attributed to B lymphocytes occurs with healing (Sterzl and Silverstein 1967). There is advanced involution of the thymus in almost all fatal cases of disseminated infection, with loss of cortical lymphocytes and an abundance of Hassall's corpuscles.

In severe disseminated disease, additional organs such as kidneys, bladder mucosa, ovaries, testes, pancreas and striated muscle may have focal necrotic lesions with surrounding haemorrhage.

Congenital Parvovirus Infection

Parvoviruses are among the smallest DNA-containing viruses known, and generally cause illnesses in small mammals. Human infection causes erythema infectiosum, erythrocyte aplasia, arthropathy, purpura and intrauterine fetal infection. Intrauterine infection was first recognized and associated with non-immunogenic hydrops fetalis by Brown et al. (1984) and with stillbirth by Knot et al. (1984). It is now recognized as a cause of intrauterine anaemia, thrombocytopenia and congestive heart failure leading to spontaneous abortion mainly occurring between 18 and 28 weeks' gestation. At autopsy, the frequently hydropic stillborn fetuses may have large oedematous placentas, and there is diffuse extramedullary haemopoiesis. Infected erythroblasts develop expanded nuclei with eosinophilic, slightly marginal inclusions (lantern cells). These viral inclusions occur in the sinusoids and capillaries of liver, spleen, bone marrow and placenta (Anand et al. 1987) and stain with phloxine-tartrazine (Burton 1986). The virus is also effectively demonstrated by in situ hybridization techniques (Schwarz et al. 1991).

Coxsackie and Other Enterovirus Infections

Coxsackie and echovirus infections are common during the neonatal period and frequently lead to significant mortality rates. An incidence of 50 per 100 000 live births has been estimated compared with 12 per 100 000 live births for Herpes simplex (Kaplan et al. 1983). Most infections are due to Coxsackie B2–5 viruses with Coxsackie B1 and A9 occurring less often (Wong et al. 1989).

Neonatal enterovirus infection occurs twice as frequently in males as in females. The incubation period is about 5–8 days. Infections mainly occur during national or local epidemics, and may be congenital (during the latter stages of pregnancy), natal or postnatal. In congenital infection the mother has symp-toms before the onset of labour, but with natal and perinatal infection the mother is usually infected before the onset of symptoms in her infant. Virus has been isolated from the placenta in cases with congenital infection (Brightman et al. 1966). When the onset of symptoms occurs in the infant 5–10 days after birth, infection is considered to have been acquired during the natal period; when symptoms appear after 10 days, infection is probably postnatal. Infants with congenital Coxsackievirus infection usually have problems with control of body temperature. They develop anorexia with lethargy and vomiting. When severe infection occurs during the postnatal period, there is usually a biphasic course to the disease: an initial mild pyrexial illness is followed by meningitis or myocarditis after an interval of 7–10 days.

Pathology

Transplacental transmission of the virus probably occurs during maternal viraemia. In the fetus there is tropism for the central nervous system and the endothelial cells of vessels in the heart, liver, lungs, kidneys and adrenals. Coxsackievirus B frequently affects myocardial muscle, the liver and the lungs, and is often fatal. Coxsackievirus B4 and B5 infections also produce inflammation of the islets of Langerhans. Echovirus affects the liver, adrenals, kidneys, central nervous system and lungs. Focal myocardial necrosis or massive hepatic necrosis occurs with a number of enterovirus infections. With Coxsackievirus, disseminated intravascular coagulopathy and massive adrenal and pulmonary haemorrhages with necrosis may occur (Gear and Measroch 1973; Krous et al. 1973). In fatal cases of Coxsackievirus infection the heart is usually pale and dilated, and has petechial haemorrhages. Microscopic changes are variable, ranging from patchy necrosis, which varies in intensity, progressing from minimal inflammatory cell infiltration or nuclear pyknosis to obvious karyorrhexis and karyolysis. Muscle necrosis can be extensive and after 8–10 days calcification occurs. The inflammatory cell infiltration comprises histiocytes and polymorphs in the early stages with Anitschkow myocytes, lymphocytes and plasma cells becoming more numerous in the later stages. Fibrinous pericarditis and vasculitis are not features of Coxsackievirus infection. The liver is often congested, with focal fatty metamorphosis. Focal necrotic lesions with polymorph infiltration and fibrinous exudation on the surface of the liver are occasionally encountered. There is usually excessive extramedullary haemopoiesis. The lungs tend to be congested, with oedema of the pleura and fibrous septae. Microscopic features of meningoencephalitis

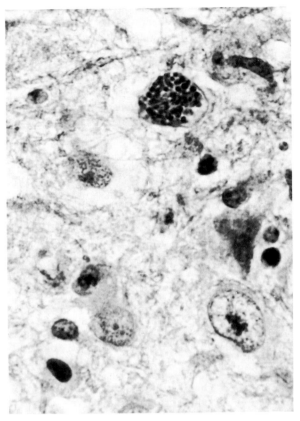

Fig. 14.12. *Toxoplasma* cyst with neighbouring pseudocysts in brain.

take the form of macrophage and lymphocyte infiltration into focal areas, with dilatation and congestion of meningeal vessels and some perivascular cuffing with oedema of cerebral vessels (Simenhoff and Uys 1958).

Congenital Toxoplasmosis

Toxoplasmosis has a worldwide distribution and is caused by infection with *Toxoplasma gondii*, an obligate intracellular parasite. Felines, particularly the domestic cat, are the definitive hosts. Humans and other animals, particularly mice, become infected from oocysts, which the cat excretes within 3 or 4 days of becoming infected. Mice are the chief consumers of shed oocysts. The process of carnivorism together with transplacental infection is important in maintaining the life-cycle of the organism. Non-feline animals do not excrete oocysts but may develop toxoplasmosis, whereas congenital

toxoplasmosis is a disease which is recognized only in humans and sheep. The organism is lunate or banana-shaped, 4–7 μm in length and 2–4 μm in width. The actively multiplying tachyzoites destroy infected cells, probably as a result of their competition with vital cell processes (Frenkel 1973). Varying numbers of tachyzoites may enter host cells, where they have been referred to as pseudocysts. After multiplication within the host cell, they are liberated and enter new cells and so resume multiplication. Bradyzoites are slowly multiplying forms of the organism which accumulate PAS-positive material and become surrounded by an argyrophilic membrane. These structures are referred to as cysts (Fig. 14.12). They persist for months or years and so maintain a chronic form of infection.

In the USA approximately 6 in 1000 women acquire toxoplasmosis during pregnancy, but only one infant in 1000 newborns is infected (Alford et al. 1974). In another survey (Couvreur 1971) it has been shown that 60% of infants born to mothers who become infected during pregnancy are unaffected; 30% have subclinical infection and 10% are aborted. When infection takes place early in pregnancy, there is a higher chance of the fetus having severe infection, although the fetus is affected more frequently when infection takes place late.

Animal studies indicate that the brain and eye are protected sites for infection, as organisms survive in these sites for longer periods than in other viscera and the bloodstream (Frenkel 1973). It is also known that proliferation of organisms begins in the central nervous system when chronically infected individuals are immunosuppressed. Necrosis of uninfected cells that follows rupture of cysts during chronic infection is considered to be due to delayed hypersensitivity.

Tachyzoites cause necrosis of tissues, particularly brain, eye and muscle, during acute infection. These destructive lesions tend to be associated with an inflammatory cell infiltration consisting of macrophages and lymphocytes with a few polymorphs and sometimes occasional plasma cells. A microglial response is found in the brain. Occasionally, small blood vessels become involved in the infective and destructive process, leading to thrombosis and infarction which, in the brain, eventually undergoes calcification. Large numbers of organisms may get into the cerebrospinal fluid of the ventricles of the brain and infect the ependymal lining cells. This results in an inflammatory process affecting the ependymal and subependymal tissues, causing ulceration. The shedding of tissue debris may in turn obstruct the aqueduct of Sylvius (Fig. 14.13). Infection of the ependyma usually results in extensive

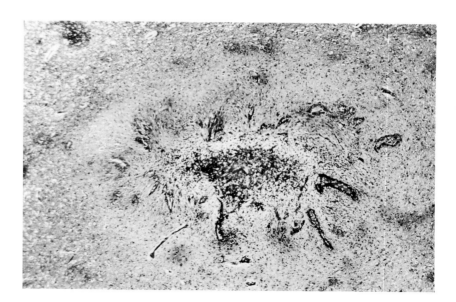

Fig. 14.13. Congenital toxoplasmosis causing ulceration and subependymal oedema of the aqueduct of Sylvius. The aqueduct is obstructed by inflammatory exudate and shed necrotic debris.

necrosis of cerebral tissue, although the total number of recognizable organisms may be small.

Laboratory Diagnosis

Direct microscopic examination of tissues has little application during life. The organisms are rarely seen in infected lymph glands, but are frequently encountered in the brain and eye of necropsy cases. The toxoplasmin skin test for cell-mediated immunity and hypersensitivity has a role in population surveys. Among the available serological tests the methylene blue dye test, IgM indirect fluorescent antibody test and Double–Sandwich IgM ELISA test are most widely used. The latter is considered to be the most sensitive and specific.

Pathology

Most infants with congenital toxoplasmosis have subclinical infection, and a significant proportion of these cases become mentally retarded or have subnormal intelligence. Cases of this type often have placentitis with inflammatory cell infiltration into chorionic villi and focal necrosis of individual villi. Occasionally, organisms may be found.

The central nervous system is most frequently and extensively involved in cases of overt infection. The affected brain may show hydrocephalus and hydranencephaly with focal polymicrogyri and microcephaly. When infection occurs before the 6th month of gestation, there are usually extensive areas of necrosis with cyst formation. Infections occurring late in pregnancy tend to be associated with granulomas and foci of reactive gliosis. Although necrotic lesions are randomly placed in the central nervous system, the cerebellum and spinal cord are less frequently affected. The lesions are often superficial, well defined, yellowish and may contain calcific granules or chalky material. Congestion of the meningeal vessels and subarachnoid haemorrhages, which can be extensive, are concomitant lesions. Hydrocephalus is caused both by loss of cerebral substance from necrosis and by obstruction of the aqueduct by necrotic debris. The ependymal lining of the ventricular system undergoes inflammation, and the adjoining cerebral tissue becomes necrotic, usually containing focal chalky calcification.

Microscopic examination reveals many lesions in different stages of evolution. Near the surface of the brain, focal chronic areas of meningoencephalitis are encountered, but more deeply liquefactive necrosis with calcification or focal areas of oedema associated with inflammatory cell infiltration may be seen. The inflammatory infiltrate is variable but usually consists of macrophages, polymorphonuclear leucocytes, lymphocytes with pleoplasma cells and variable numbers of eosinophils. Perivascular cuffing of inflammatory cells around neighbouring blood vessels is frequently encountered. In these areas there may be large numbers of organisms that have been released from cysts. The ventricular lining is frequently involved. The choroid plexus, although not itself extensively involved, is often surrounded and covered by necrotic debris. The ependyma may be totally destroyed or may be the site of nodular ependymitis. The adjoining surviving cerebral tissues have granulation tissue capillaries and show reactive gliosis with astrocytic proliferation. Throughout the brain there may be scattered encysted organisms. As healing occurs, the inflammatory cell infiltration becomes gradually reduced and cysts become fewer, but glial scars with calcification are retained.

Ocular lesions occur in 60%–80% of cases with generalized disease. Sometimes the eye is the only organ involved in overt disease and is often microphthalmic or becomes microphthalmic. Involvement is usually manifested as chorioretinitis affecting the macular region and is most often bilateral (O'Connor 1974). In the acute phase of the disease, the vitreous becomes turbid and there is accumulation of yellowish exudate over the posterior pole. As organisms are released from the retina, hypersensitivity develops which progresses to iridocyclitis with corneal opacification, cataracts, posterior synechia, glaucoma and occasionally retinal detachment. Microscopic examination shows diffuse inflammation of all layers of the retina associated with varying degrees of necrosis, infarction and calcification. The endothelial cells of small capillaries tend to become parasitized. There may be considerable disorganization of the layers of the retina with intense inflammatory cell infiltration and calcification. Choroidal lesions are sited adjacent to the retinal lesions, and secondary atrophy of the optic nerve may result. As healing occurs there is proliferation of granulation tissue capillaries, which penetrate the posterior portion of the vitreous and may masquerade as a neoplasm (Pettapiece et al. 1976).

The ears may be involved with otitis media and mastoiditis. Microscopic examination shows many free-lying organisms in areas of inflammation, with necrosis and calcification (Callahan et al. 1946).

Involvement of the cardiovascular system is frequent because of the apparent tropism of the organisms for endothelial cells of small blood vessels of the myocardium. When tachyzoites are released from endothelial cells, they produce necrosis of the vessel wall with inflammation as well as thrombosis, resulting in small infarcts of tissues. Parenchymal involvement of cardiac muscle as well as striated muscle is frequent. When the heart is involved it is generally a dilated and flabby organ with focal haemorrhages. Microscopic examination reveals interstitial necrosis with inflammatory cell infiltration, occasional inflammatory granulomas or nodular aggregates of mixed inflammatory cells. Interstitial oedema separates muscle fibres. The fibres become fragmented necrotic and occasionally hyalinized. Free and encysted organisms tend to occur near such cardiac lesions.

Involvement of the placenta is usually not well documented in overt neonatal infection. Organisms reach the placenta through the maternal circulation and become localized in chorionic villi and fetal vessels. When infection has occurred early in pregnancy and placental involvement is in the chronic stage, encysted parasites occur in avascular areas such as Wharton's jelly and the chorionic plate. Organisms may get into the amniotic fluid, but do not seem to infect the lungs or the gastrointestinal tract. The severity of fetal disease is usually not reflected by the degree of placental involvement. Macroscopically, the placenta is usually enlarged, pale and oedematous.

Microscopic examination shows inflammation and necrosis of chorionic villi with free tachyzoites and occasional cysts. Necrotic lesions, sited superficially in chorionic villi, often involve syncytiotrophoblasts and are associated with inflammation and necrosis of fetal vessels. Granulomas may be seen in some villi. As the disease progresses, the inflammatory infiltrate contains fewer polymorphs with a greater proportion of lymphocytes and plasma cells; free organisms disappear and are replaced by occasional cysts (Elliott 1970; Dische and Gooch 1981).

When the kidneys are involved, petechial haemorrhages with some bile staining may be seen macroscopically. Microscopic examination, in addition, shows interstitial oedema, inflammatory cell infiltration, variable degrees of extramedullary haemopoiesis and bile casts in tubules. Very rarely, focal necrotizing glomerular nephritis may occur with organisms in affected glomeruli (Zeulzer 1944). Acute nephritis and acute nephrotic syndrome due to immune complexes have been described, and these patients make a full clinical recovery (Shahin et al. 1974).

Pathological changes in the liver are mild and inconspicuous, in spite of the fact that clinical involvement may be severe. The liver is slightly enlarged with varying degrees of bile staining and congestion. Microscopic examination shows extramedullary haemopoiesis, which may be very prominent, with icterus and mild periportal fibrosis. Focal and diffuse hepatitis occurs in some cases and giant cell transformation has been reported (Zeulzer 1944). Organisms are very rarely found in vascular endothelial cells, areas of necrosis and Kupffer cells. Changes in the lung consist of mild interstitial pneumonitis with septal oedema and inflammatory cell infiltration.

The endocrine organs that may be affected include the adrenals, pancreas and thyroid. Involvement of the adrenal is partly attributed to stress reaction with reduced cortical lipid, but areas of necrosis of variable size with free tachyzoites, inflammatory cell infiltration and calcification may also be encountered. Lesions with organisms occur more often in the testes than they do in the ovaries. In the testes there is a tendency for encysted organisms to be found inside seminiferous tubules (Dische and Gooch 1981).

Infections in Malnourished Children

Children with severe protein–energy malnutrition are immunologically compromised. They suffer from opportunistic infections and have a severe course in common diseases. Depression of immunocompetence is indicated by lowered levels of almost all complement factors, depressed T-lymphocyte function and defective intracellular bacterial killing by leucocytes. There is impaired chemotaxis by polymorphs. Hypergammaglobulinaemia is attributed to frequent and continued infections starting before the onset of malnutrition. However, chronic and/or repeated infections may also lead to malnutrition by affecting a wide range of metabolic functions including food intake, intestinal function, haemoglobin and cell protein synthesis. Normal non-specific immune functions and repair mechanisms may also be affected.

Among malnourished children extremely high morbidity and mortality rates have been attributed to septicaemia and bacteraemia (Smythe and Campbell 1959), to supervening pneumonia or diarrhoea, and to measles. Studies in West Africa and South Africa have shown that although the mortality rate for measles is high (10%–25%) among children less than 3 years of age, protein–energy malnutrition has little influence on the rate (Aaby et al. 1983, 1984; Beckford et al. 1985). The high measles mortality rate that occurs in areas where protein–energy malnutrition is prevalent is now attributed to associated vitamin A (retinol) deficiency (Hussey and Klein 1990). Other factors that increase the mortality rate of measles are high doses of infection, overcrowding, large family size, poor hygiene and early age of exposure (Aaby et al. 1983, 1984, 1986).

Interaction of Nutrition with Specific Infections

Measles (see also pp. 771–776)

There is a widely held view that undernourished children whose weights fall below the 10th centile for age experience a particularly severe and lethal form of measles. However, as indicated above, substantive evidence for this view is not strong. It is recognized that there is a high mortality and morbidity rate following measles in impoverished communities where malnutrition is prevalent. Often death occurs some weeks after recovery from measles infection. The causes of such deaths are predominantly pneumonia, but also include gastroenteritis, myocarditis and

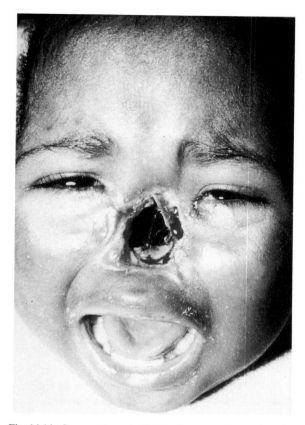

Fig. 14.14. Cancrum (noma) affecting the nose and occurring after measles in an oedematous infant with features of kwashiorkor.

meningitis (Beckford et al. 1985). These infections are attributed to lowered immune responses in the postmeasles state and the general deleterious effect of measles on nutritional status, particularly the demand on vitamin A reserves. There is evidence that measles virus activity persists longer in malnourished than in well nourished children. Virus secretion could be at a higher level and continue for a longer time than in controls (Scheifele and Forbes 1972). In poor and non-industrialized countries children are particularly susceptible to supervening herpesvirus and adenovirus infection during the 4–6 weeks following the onset of the measles rash (Kipps and Kaschula 1976).

Cancrum oris or noma is closely associated with malnutrition and measles. The condition usually occurs shortly after a malnourished child has had measles. It is characterized by rapid spread of a gangrenous process involving all tissues related to the oral or nasal cavity (Fig. 14.14). The organisms that are cultured from the lesion have been anaerobic spirochaetes and fusiform bacilli, as well as commensal organisms of the mouth. These organisms have been considered to develop invasive properties during the

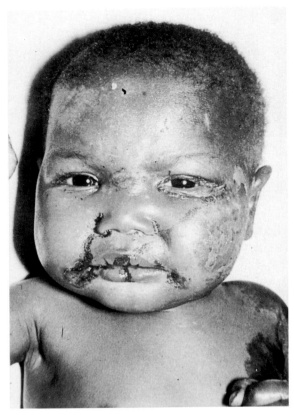

Fig. 14.15. Infant with overt kwashiorkor (facial oedema, sparse depigmented hair and hypopigmentation and hyperpigmentation of skin) with extending ulcerative herpes stomatitis.

anergy that follows measles in a malnourished child. However, a number of clinical observers have drawn attention to the fact that herpes stomatitis may have initiated the process. Such progressive tissue destruction by herpesvirus infection is seen in the lungs and liver and seems to be a more acceptable explanation for this condition (Morley 1983).

In Africa the most frequent cause of blindness among rural black children has been considered to be measles. These children suffer a fulminating necrotizing keratitis, which rapidly leads to corneal perforation and finally to corneal staphyloma or leukoma. Infection with a supervening organism has been considered to be responsible for the sequence of events (Sutter 1973). It has been surmised that the supervening infecting agent is most frequently herpesvirus.

Herpesvirus

Herpes simplex is a life-threatening disease among children with overt protein–energy malnutrition and

in children with active or recent measles. More than 95% of non-neonatal cases of fatal disseminated herpesvirus infection occur in children aged 2–25 months (Kipps et al. 1967). In this condition the child develops a primary herpetic lesion on the lips, tongue, oesophagus or the external genitalia. The vesicles enlarge, become confluent and eventually produce superficial ulcers (Fig. 14.15). There is a fibrinous exudate over the floor of the ulcers, and the adjoining epithelium may contain giant cells. The giant cells, together with other adjoining epithelial cells, may contain varying numbers of typical intranuclear inclusions (Fig. 14.11). The nuclei of affected squamous epithelial cells become enlarged with fragmentation of the chromatin network. The chromatin and nucleolus become marginated, followed by the appearance of eosinophilic intranuclear inclusion material. Occasionally, there may be more than one such inclusion within a nucleus. The inclusion bodies increase in size and, when multiple, seem to coalesce eventually to fill the nucleus. Similar lesions are encountered on the lips, in the oesophagus and on the genitalia. The ulcers of the tongue and oesophagus often coalesce and become serpiginous (Fig. 14.16). Accumulations of fibrinous exudate and epithelial cells in the floors of the ulcers may masquerade as nodules in the oesophagus (McKenzie et al. 1959). The most striking lesions are encountered in the liver, which is yellowish because of fatty change, often due to kwashiorkor. Superimposed on this are variable numbers (usually very numerous) of focal areas of necrosis having a deep white centre and surrounded by a hyperaemic border, giving a target-like appearance (Fig. 14.17). Microscopically, the lesions resemble ischaemic infarcts, having a haphazard distribution. The central necrotic area may contain small numbers of red blood cells, but there is an abrupt change to surviving liver parenchyma (Fig. 14.18). The adjoining parenchyma shows no evidence of inflammatory cell reaction, although liver sinusoids tend to be dilated and congested with blood. The neighbouring liver cells contain variable numbers of intranuclear inclusion bodies. The sequence of changes encountered in affected liver cells begins with swelling of the nucleus and loss of staining density followed by fragmentation and stippling of the chromatin. Chromatin becomes marginated to resemble an irregularly staining basophilic lining to the nuclear membrane. The rest of the nucleus becomes very uniformly eosinophilic and homogeneous. As the lesions mature, the nucleus becomes irregularly chromated, and under high magnification the inclusions have a honeycomb appearance of small round eosinophilic bodies set in a bluish coloured matrix, the whole filling the entire nucleus (McKenzie et al. 1959). Macroscopic lesions

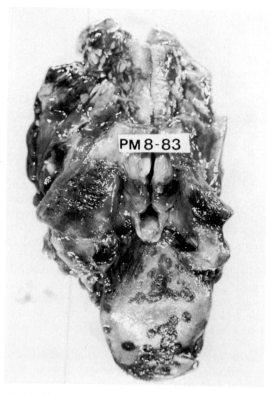

Fig. 14.16. Herpes ulcers on tongue. The ulcers have coalesced to give a serpiginous pattern.

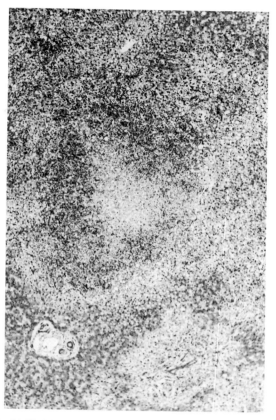

Fig. 14.18. Disseminated herpesvirus infection in liver. There is a central pale area of advanced necrosis surrounded by a haemorrhagic and congested zone where extension of infection, with many inclusion-bearing cells, is found, and an abrupt change to unaffected liver parenchyma.

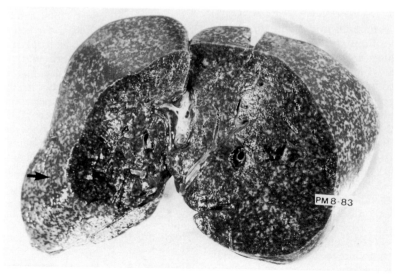

Fig. 14.17. Post-mortem specimen from a child with kwashiorkor and disseminated herpesvirus infection involving the liver. A fatty liver with haemorrhagic and congested zones surrounding necrotic foci. A target-like lesion is arrowed.

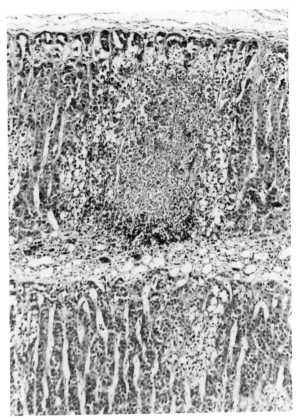

Fig. 14.19. Disseminated herpesvirus infection in an adrenal gland. A small focal area of necrosis in the cortex is surrounded by oedematous degenerating haemorrhagic adrenal tissue where viral inclusions occur.

inclusions have been encountered in the spleen and heart.

Gastroenteritis

Malnourished children are prone to have repeated and prolonged episodes of acute diarrhoeal disease, during which time they develop progressive intestinal villous atrophy and thymic atrophy (Berkowitz 1992). Many of these children die from dehydration, electrolyte imbalance or other complications.

In most cases of infantile gastroenteritis no causative organism is isolated even in well equipped laboratories. The more frequently encountered causative organisms include *Campylobacter*, *Escherichia coli*, rotavirus, *Shigella*, *Salmonella* and *Giardia lamblia*. Malnourished children who experience repeated attacks of acute diarrhoeal disease are prone to develop disaccharidase deficiency. Such enzyme deficiency perpetuates chronic diarrhoea (Barbezat et al. 1967). In addition to lactase deficiency these children also have reduced acid phosphatase activity in the intestinal mucosa (Kaschula et al. 1979).

Pathological changes in the small intestine in cases of non-specific enteritis are minimal even in severe infection. Intestinal villi become oedematous and swollen with reduced replacement of shed epithelial lining cells. There is initially infiltration by a small number of polymorphonuclear leucocytes, but after repeated infections plasma cells and lymphocytes accumulate in large numbers. As the disease progresses, villi become increasingly atrophic, and regenerative epithelium is flattened and lacks the normal complement of goblet cells (Fig. 14.20). The submucosa is generally oedematous, and the blood vessels are usually congested during the acute phase. Lymphoid aggregates become depleted of lymphocytes.

Gastroenteritis is particularly prevalent among populations where faecal contamination of drinking water is high and the mother needs to work, foregoes breastfeeding and places her infant in the care of a foster mother in poor hygienic circumstances. Children coming from this background and who have survived repeated attacks of acute gastroenteritis are prone to develop Mediterranean lymphoma during the second and third decades of life (Dutz et al. 1976).

Bacterial Infections

Children with protein–energy malnutrition have increased susceptibility to infections with organisms encountered predominantly during the neonatal

are occasionally encountered in the adrenal glands. These are similar to those seen in the liver but are very much less frequent and also have a congested or haemorrhagic border (Fig. 14.19). Microscopically, the lesions are found to occur in both the cortex and the medulla. They closely resemble those encountered in the liver and have the same type of inclusion bodies. Disseminated lesions may also be found in the lungs. In addition, a lesion which is attributed to inhalation of virus from primary lesions in the mouth or pharynx produces necrosis of the epithelium of bronchi, trachea and bronchioles, with inclusions being encountered in surviving respiratory epithelial cells. The destructive process in bronchioles can be extensive enough to destroy the elastica and muscle, and large numbers of inclusion body-containing cells can be found in the adjoining parenchyma (Kaschula et al. 1983). Brain is usually congested and oedematous and only very rarely are inclusions found. Necrotic infarct-like lesions unassociated with virus

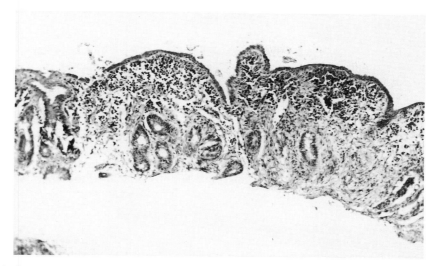

Fig. 14.20. Jejunal microscopy in protein–energy malnutrition with repeated episodes of acute gastroenteritis. There is advanced villous atrophy (flattened mucosa), focal shedding of epithelial cells and a superficial mild infiltration of neutrophils, plasma cells and lymphocytes.

period. These organisms include *Escherichia coli*, *Pseudomonas aeruginosa*, *Klebsiella* and *Candida albicans*. The jejunal microflora of malnourished children contains vastly increased numbers of *E. coli*, *Bacteroides* and *Streptococcus faecalis*. Such abnormal colonization may cause diarrhoea or variable degrees of malabsorption, which may further lead to deterioration in the nutritional status. In developing countries bacteraemia and septicaemia are highly prevalent among malnourished children. In many areas *Salmonella* is the predominant organism (Berkowitz 1992).

Malnourished children do not seem to have increased susceptibility to *Bordetella pertussis* infection. However, the combined effects of anorexia, exhaustive coughing, persistent vomiting and malaise which are associated with pertussis can quickly convert a relatively well nourished state into marasmus. Children who have borderline nutrition at the onset of whooping cough and who are deprived of food can very quickly become malnourished and die.

Malnourished children are known to have increased susceptibility to tuberculosis and the infection is associated with poor localization of the organisms.

Pneumonia. In developing countries pneumonia is very prevalent among young children. It is more frequent and more severe in malnourished than in well nourished children (Spooner et al. 1989). The causative organisms are mainly *Streptococcus pneumoniae*, *Haemophilus influenzae* and *Staphylococcus aureus*. However, among severely malnourished children "opportunistic" organisms make up a significant

proportion of the total (Mimica et al. 1971) and enteric bacilli are encountered more often.

Fungal Infections

Depressed cellular immune reactivity in the malnourished child permits a number of opportunistic fungal infections to occur. Fungi that are frequently responsible for such infection include *Candida*, *Aspergillus*, *Crytococcus* and *Zygomycetes* (*Mucor*).

Candidiasis. Candida commonly colonize the mouth, the oesophagus and the lower gastrointestinal tract as well as the vagina in malnourished children. Severely malnourished children may have extensive lesions in the mouth and oesophagus associated with candida pneumonia, gastritis or colitis. Rarely, there may be systemic spread to other organs, particularly the liver, brain, spleen, skin and kidneys. Such lesions may be associated with fungal endocarditis. The lesions have a chalky white necrotic centre in which budding yeasts and mycelia may be found. The inflammatory infiltrate consists predominantly of lymphocytes and histiocytes, with fewer polymorphonuclear leucocytes and plasma cells. On epithelial surfaces there is a heaped-up appearance producing a pseudomembrane (Fig. 14.58).

Aspergillosis. Aspergillus infection occurs by inhalation of spores. In malnourished children invasive proliferation of the organism takes place in the lungs, after which there may be haematogenous spread to the central nervous system, liver, kidneys and skin (Fig. 14.60). Bone marrow invasion also occurs occasionally, producing osteomyelitis. Children with aspergillosis have intermittent fever, and radiographs usually show pulmonary infiltrates. Macroscopically, the lesions in the lung appear as reddish, dark-bluish or purple nodular zones of consolidation with surrounding congestion and haemorrhage. The central zone undergoes necrosis with cavitation and abscess formation. Microscopically, septate mycelia are found to proliferate in the lesion and within blood vessels. Blood vessel involvement leads to thrombosis with subsequent pulmonary infarction and haemorrhage.

Cryptococcus. This infection is relatively uncommon in childhood, but it occurs in malnourished children (mainly boys) and in immunosuppressed children. Malnourished children often have overt pulmonary infection with diffuse infiltrative pneumonia and regional lymphadenopathy. Involvement of the central nervous system draws attention to the infection, where it affects both the substance of the brain and the meninges.

Zygomycosis. It has been reported that zygomycosis is mainly a hospital-acquired infection in children being treated for leukaemia or organ transplantation (Medoff and Kobayashi 1981). However, in my experience pulmonary and disseminated infections are also often encountered in children with kwashiorkor and marasmus.

Pneumocystis. This organism is now included with the fungi following studies of ribosomal RNA sequences (Edman et al. 1988). *Pneumocystis carinii* causes severe endemic interstitial plasma cell pneumonia in institutionalized infants with marasmus (Dutz et al. 1974). An incidence of 10% of kwashiorkor fatalities has been reported (Hughes et al. 1974). Bottle feeding is associated with a high incidence of chronic and persistent diarrhoea leading to marasmus with low levels of serum immunoglobulins. When the serum IgG level falls to below 2 g/litre before the 4th month of life, there is a marked propensity for such infection. Infants who recover from Pneumocystis infection develop protective immunity to the organism.

Protozoal Infections

Amoebiasis. This condition, caused by *Entamoeba histolytica*, is one in which the nutritional status of the host clearly determines the clinical pattern of the disease. The pathogenicity of the organism seems to be influenced by the nutritional status of the host and the bacterial environment in the colon. Among malnourished children, saprophytic organisms confined to the lumen of the bowel more readily become invasive, producing colitis and amoebic liver abscess. Maternal infection of infants may occur at the time of birth. Liver abscesses in children most frequently occur in endemic areas in a background of low socio-economic status, poor hygiene and malnutrition and have been recorded in children as young as 1 month (Rode et al. 1978). Proliferating fungating lesions may be encountered in the perianal and perineal regions.

Cryptosporidium. This protozoa causes a diarrhoea that is severe and protracted in malnourished children (MacFarlane and Horner-Bryce 1987).

Plasmodium. Malaria is prevalent in tropical and subtropical areas of Africa, Asia and Central America. *Plasmodium falciparum* has tropism for the placenta as a favourite site for erythrocytic schizogony. Transplacental transmission of malaria occurs. *P. malariae* infection tends to be chronic. Although chronic malaria has an adverse effect on nutrition in endemic areas (MacGregor 1971), malnourished children seem to have fewer and less severe attacks of acute malaria than their well nourished counterparts. Children with kwashiorkor in endemic areas have lower parasite rates, and attacks of severe malaria, such as cerebral involvement with convulsions and coma, occur more frequently in better than in poorly nourished children.

Splenomegaly and hepatomegaly occur, and enlargement of the spleen may be so great that it may rupture. The enlarged liver has a chocolate-greyish-red colour because of accumulation of malaria pigment. Microscopically, there is mononuclear inflammatory cell infiltration in the portal triads and adjoining parenchyma. When the brain is affected malarial pigment accumulates around blood vessels, which become congested, and there is cerebral oedema with petechial haemorrhages. Parasitized red blood cells may be seen in the vessels of the brain in association with fibrin thrombi. The kidneys may be subject to acute tubular necrosis, or immune complex membranoproliferative glomerulonephritis may particularly occur with *P. falciparum* and *P. malariae* infections. In chronic malaria due to *P. malariae* infection serum levels of IgM become significantly raised. In endemic areas children who have undergone splenectomy have an increased risk of severe and fatal malaria.

Parasitic Disease

It is commonly assumed that, because intestinal parasites consume host fluids or compete with the host for nutrients, they predispose to, or enhance, pre-existing malnutrition. Apart from hookworm, considerable numbers of parasites such as *Ascaris*, *Strongyloides* and *Trichuris* are required to produce any real impact on nutrition. The social and environmental factors that predispose to malnutrition also do so for many parasitic infestations. Heavy infestation with *Ascaris* and hookworm is highly prevalent in developing countries. Hyperinfection with *Strongyloides* occurs in immune-suppressed malnourished children, and then accentuates their state of malnutrition.

Deficiency of Specific Nutrients

A number of specific nutritional deficiency states are associated with increased susceptibility to infection.

Iron Deficiency

Children with iron deficiency have a diminished capacity to synthesize DNA and have hypochromic microcytic anaemia associated with a decreased capacity to transform lymphocytes (Hershko et al. 1970; Chandra 1975). The cytotoxic effect of leucocytes on phagocytosed staphylococci is reduced. However, the administration of therapeutic free iron often enhances the growth of pathogenic organisms such as *Pseudomonas*, *Salmonella*, *Streptococcus*, *Klebsiella* and *Listeria*. Iron is thought to facilitate the growth of bacteria by negating the bacteriostatic effects of iron-binding proteins such as transferrin and lactoferrin (Stockman 1981). The administration of iron to children with kwashiorkor results in increased mortality rates, which is attributed to elevated levels of unbound serum iron, causing an acute imbalance between oxidants and scavengers of free radicals (McFarlane et al. 1970; Sive et al. 1993).

Trace Elements and Vitamins

Zinc, copper, chromium, selenium, folic acid, vitamin A, pyridoxine and ascorbic acid are all required in order to mount a normal and effective inflammatory response to infection. When these factors are deficient, the inflammatory process tends to be inhibited or may be inappropriate. Under such circumstances, otherwise mild infection may become severe or chronic. In megaloblastic anaemia due to folic acid deficiency, depressed cell-mediated immunity has been demonstrated (Gross et al. 1975).

Mycobacterial Infections

Tuberculosis

With measles, tuberculosis ranks as the most prevalent cause of death and chronic ill-health in poor countries. The prevalence of tuberculosis increases very rapidly when rural people become urbanized in substandard housing with unemployment and malnutrition as aggravating factors. Most deaths occur before the age of 5 years, but complications of tuberculosis most often become manifest some 20 years later (Hinman et al. 1976). The incidence of childhood infection is highest during winter months, when children are crowded indoors. Children generally become infected by adults in the immediate household in which they live. The incubation period for the disease is said to vary between 19 and 56 days (Smith and Marquis 1981). The causative organism is most often *Mycobacterium tuberculosis*; however, *Mycobacterium bovis* is particularly prevalent in the rural parts of Africa, where inhabitants are infected by consuming contaminated milk and beef. In industrialized countries childhood tuberculosis is most frequently encountered among recently arrived immigrants from non-industrialized countries.

Primarily immunodeficient children develop severe systemic tuberculosis or disseminated BCG infection. Children with secondary severe T-cell immunodeficiency due to either immunosuppressive drugs, AIDS, malnutrition or malignancy are predisposed to a more severe form of disease. In addition, during active tuberculosis, a number of suppressor mechanisms have been recognized. These include proliferation of suppressor macrophages, suppressor T cells and inhibitors of chemotaxis, and lymphopenia has frequently been recorded in the advanced stages of tuberculosis. The predominance of these suppressor mechanisms may in part explain the anergy that occurs in severe tuberculosis.

Pathology

The basic lesion is an inflammatory granuloma with caseous necrosis. Primary infection usually occurs in early childhood, most often by inhalation. The primary focus produced in the lung is usually sited subpleurally at the base of an upper lobe or the apex

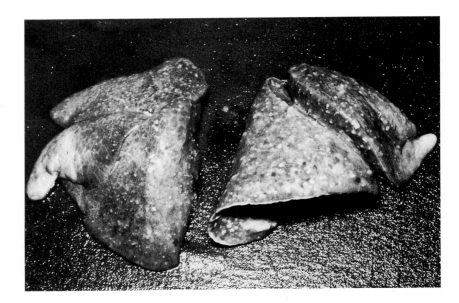

Fig. 14.21. Miliary tuberculosis of the lungs in a 3-month-old boy.

of a lower lobe. In most instances there is healing of both the primary pulmonary focus and the associated lymph node lesions. In some children there is local spread from the primary pulmonary focus; bronchogenic spread produces pyramidal lesions with a base on the pleura, and when a larger bronchus is involved in this way there is wider dissemination with multiple foci of caseous necrosis throughout the lung. The cut surface of such an involved lung shows many small foci of caseation, which have an irregular (clover-leaf) pattern. This is referred to as "tuberculous bronchopneumonia" and is usually fatal.

Haematogenous dissemination occurs when host resistance is low (malnutrition) and caseous infected material enters a vessel. Alternatively, infected macrophages and infected caseous necrotic material can pass from caseous lymph nodes through the lymph vessels into the thoracic duct and so into the circulation. When large numbers of organisms suddenly flood the bloodstream, miliary tuberculosis results. Smaller numbers of organisms produce subacute haematogenous tuberculosis, whereas very small numbers of organisms produce localized organ tuberculosis.

Miliary Tuberculosis

"Miliary tuberculosis" is a term which is derived from the size and shape of the tubercles scattered throughout the involved organ, reminding one of millet seeds (Fig. 14.21). When large numbers of organisms enter a pulmonary vein, the resulting miliary tubercles are found mainly in the spleen, the liver and kidneys. In severe disease there may also be involvement of the adrenals, the gonads and the peritoneum. Tuberculous meningitis is often associated with miliary tuberculosis in children.

When large numbers of organisms enter the superior vena cava from the thoracic duct or enter a pulmonary artery, miliary tuberculosis is found in the lungs. When a pulmonary artery is a site of such entry, only one lung is involved.

Subacute Tuberculosis. This term refers to a milder form of miliary spread. The tubercles are fewer in number, larger and caseous, measuring up to 5 mm in diameter. Both miliary and subacute tuberculosis may be fatal.

Organ Tuberculosis

"Organ tuberculosis" is a term referring to chronic tuberculous involvement of an organ as a result of haematogenous dissemination. Usually only one organ or an organ system is involved, and the primary site of tuberculosis may no longer be conspicuous. In children the organs most frequently involved are the meninges (with the brain), bones (with joints), kidneys and epididymis. The heart is rarely a site for such lesions (Fig. 14.22).

Post-primary Tuberculosis

Post-primary tuberculosis is due to either reinfection or reactivation of a previously quiescent primary

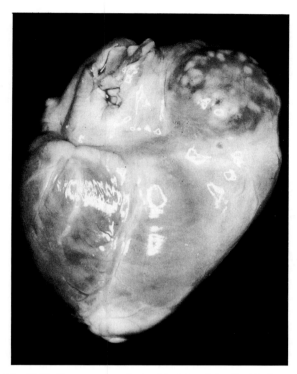

Fig. 14.22. Caseous tuberculosis of the left atrial wall of the heart.

tuberculosis process. Because there is some impairment of cellular immunity or overwhelming infection with highly virulent organisms, there is reactivation of the disease process. Lesions are characterized by extensive caseation, which is attributed to a prominent hypersensitive reaction, and fibrosis, which is due to the immune responsiveness of the individual. There is little or no lymph node involvement.

Gastrointestinal Tuberculosis

Gastrointestinal tuberculosis may be caused by swallowing of infected material from the lungs or of foods, particularly dairy products, which have been contaminated with *Mycobacterium bovis*. The former route of infection produces a postprimary response, whereas the latter occurs in the absence of previous exposure and leads to a primary type of response. The terminal ileum is most commonly involved. Lesions are initially localized to Peyer's patches, where caseation occurs, producing ulcers which slough off infected material. The ulcers become secondarily infected with bacterial organisms and progressively enlarge. They often have a circumferential configuration with edges that are ragged, nodular and undermined. Small tubercles may be seen on the

serosal surface of the affected ileum. Microscopically, the base of the ulcer shows a non-specific chronic inflammatory process due to superimposed infection. Deeper in the wall one finds typical tuberculous granulomas.

Massive caseation of mesenteric lymph nodes occurs with primary infection. Occasionally, a hyperplastic type of intestinal lesion occurs, in which there is a prominent fibrous and granulomatous response, giving a localized mass and/or intestinal obstruction. Infection may occur in the crypts of Morgagni of the rectum, from which extension through the bowel wall into the surrounding tissues may occur. In the terminal rectum it is possible for such lesions to rupture into the ischiorectal fossa to produce a tuberculous fistula-in-ano.

A primary tuberculous complex may also be sited in the pharynx and mouth, involving the tonsils and lymph glands of the neck. There is then massive cervical lymphadenitis. Secondary tuberculosis of the tongue, mouth and pharynx occasionally occurs from sputum from a pulmonary cavity.

Tuberculosis Affecting Pleura, Pericardium and Peritoneum

The pleura, pericardium and peritoneum may all be involved in tuberculous infection. The massive caseous mesenteric lymph nodes of primary intestinal tuberculosis may rupture into the peritoneal cavity. This produces diffusely scattered acute caseating granulomas of the peritoneum.

Tuberculous Meningitis

Tuberculosis meningitis is a frequent cause of death among children who have tuberculous infection. There is blood-borne infection, usually from a primary complex, which reaches the meninges from multiple foci sited in the brain, most often adjacent to the ventricular system, the choroid plexus or just deep to the pia arachnoid. As this focus (Rich focus) undergoes caseation, it discharges organisms into the cerebrospinal fluid. The meningitis that is produced is sited predominantly at the base of the brain. The exudate is scanty, grey-white in colour and cheesy in consistency. Microscopically, there are small tubercles close to small arteries within the meninges. Initially there is prominent exudation of lymphocytes with mononuclear cells, much fibrin and very few giant cells. This exudate in time undergoes necrosis, the lesions extend along the course of blood vessels, and vasculitis is found. The cerebrospinal fluid contains increased amounts of protein and lymphocytes, with decreased levels of chloride and sugar. A "spider-web" clot forms when such cerebrospinal fluid is left to stand for half an hour. Tuberculous encephalitis occurs as a result of multiple small tubercles sited in the brain substance. Sometimes only a small number of tubercles is found. These may enlarge and become caseous, and are referred to as tuberculomas; they have the effect of a space-occupying lesion within the cranial cavity.

Tuberculous Infection of Bones and Joints

Bones and joints are affected from blood-borne spread. The lesions begin in cancellous bone, usually near the ends of long bones, and from there extend into joint cavities to cause destruction of cartilage. The hips and knees are frequently affected. Young boys are particularly prone to have vertebral involvement, in which the vertebral bodies may collapse and produce angular deformity (Pott's disease). When the lumber vertebral bodies are affected, extension into the psoas muscle may occur, and the whole psoas muscle may be replaced by caseous material, which can extend to below the inguinal ligament.

Renal Tuberculosis

Tubercles occur in the cortex, but extension is along tubules to the pyramids. From there extension to the pelvis, ureter and bladder may occur.

Genital Tuberculosis

Genital tuberculosis in children is more frequent in boys than in girls; the epididymis is occasionally the site of a granulomatous process. Involvement of the female genital tract is very rare in pre-adolescent children.

Congenital Tuberculosis

Congenital tuberculosis is rarely diagnosed and occurs in the infants of women who have pulmonary or uterine tuberculosis. Infants with congenital infection are often born prematurely and usually develop clinical manifestations of disease within 3 weeks of birth (Horley 1952; Hudson 1956). The primary focus is usually in the placenta, rarely in the liver, but is not always demonstrable. The lymph node component is sited in the porta hepatis at the junction of the cystic and common hepatic ducts. Rarely, tubercle

bacilli can get into amniotic fluid without having produced lesions in the body of the placenta. Such organisms may be inhaled or swallowed, and so a primary lesion may be established in the lungs or in the gut. Infants who have congenital tuberculosis may have progressive primary lesions. The liver is extensively involved and may be the source of miliary spread. When the primary focus is sited in the lung, it usually progresses to tuberculous pneumonia. Tuberculous meningitis and miliary spread are frequent consequences of congenital infection (Le Roux et al. 1978; Hageman et al. 1980). Neonatal tuberculosis may be a consequence of the infant being infected as it passes through the birth canal and swallows infected material.

Childhood Leprosy

Because of the social stigma associated with the words "leprosy" and "leper", Hansen's disease is now the more acceptable term for chronic infection by *Mycobacterium leprae*. The bacillus seems preferentially to affect cooler parts of the body such as skin, upper respiratory tract (especially nasal mucosa), eyes, testes and superficial nerves. Infection is considered to be from one person to another, although armadilloes and chimpanzees may act as an animal reservoir, with undetermined insect vectors. There is still a high incidence of the disease in Africa, the northern coast of South America, India and South East Asia. Children have increased susceptibility to infection and comprise between 20% and 30% of diagnosed cases (Noussitou 1976). In children early lesions occur singly and have been identified in infants less than 6 months of age. Such cases may be due to transplacental infection or from breast milk from an infected mother (Pedley 1967). Large numbers of organisms occur in the lepromatous form of the disease and it seems that, when such lesions break down and ulcerate, infectivity is highest. Disease prevalence does not seem to be associated with protein–energy malnutrition, but the possible role of subclinical hypovitaminosis A still needs to be evaluated. Aerosolized spread from nasal lesions and direct skin-to-skin contact under conditions of poor housing and living conditions are considered to be highly important in facilitating dissemination of the disease (Meyers 1992).

The bacillus is able to survive and multiply in macrophages. Survival of the organisms and expression of the disease depend on the host's immune response. There is a continuous decrease in sensitivity to lymphocytes in patients from tuberculoid leprosy to lepromatous leprosy. The incubation period for the disease is variable, being shorter in children than in adults, and generally varies between 2 and 5 years. The classification of the disease proposed by Ridley and Jopling (1966) is still widely used.

Intermediate leprosy represents the earliest manifestation. It may heal, remain static or progress. There are a few skin macules without nerve involvement. Diagnosis is made by the histological demonstration of small numbers of weakly acid-fast bacilli. They may be found in superficial nerves or arrectores pilorum muscles.

Tuberculoid leprosy manifests as single or multiple asymmetric anaesthetic macules, papules or plaques of sharply demarcated hypopigmented skin. Cutaneous peripheral nerves are commonly involved and then become clinically palpable. There is an active cellular immune response with the formation of generally non-caseating granulomas with lymphocytes, epithelioid cells and Langhans' giant cells in the superficial dermis and subcutaneous nerves. Bacilli are found only in small numbers, but destructive fibrosis and Schwann cell proliferation may be prominent in affected nerves and nerve trunks.

Lepromatous leprosy manifests as a disseminated infection with numerous freely multiplying bacilli. It was particularly prevalent among the institutionalized children of parents with Hansen's disease (Muir 1936). In this juvenile form, skin changes are initially inconspicuous with vague indistinct macules without changes in sensation or sweating. Untreated, the macules coalesce and progress to form large hypopigmented areas of skin. The organisms are readily found in skin smears or biopsy specimens. There is loss of hair from affected parts, and nerves become involved with extensive sensory loss. There is a gradual accumulation of macrophages around vessels, nerves and skin appendages. Initially the bacilli are sparse, but in advanced disease large numbers of bacilli occur in each cell virtually to take up all the cytoplasmic space (globi). A variable plasma cell response may be associated. Distant organs that are often affected include larynx, upper respiratory tract, liver, testes (mainly in adults), sclera and lymph nodes.

Borderline leprosy has features of both tuberculoid and lepromatous leprosy and tends to evolve slowly towards either tuberculoid or lepromatous forms of disease. Intermediate steps in this evolutionary process have been recognized as borderline tuberculoid leprosy and borderline lepromatous leprosy. In the former there are more numerous lesions that are less well defined than occurs in typical tuberculoid leprosy. A broad spectrum of intermediate histopathological changes are encountered. Nerves are less damaged and more easily recognized as such than in tuberculoid leprosy. Bacilli are also more often identified and may be seen within Schwann cells. The subepidermal area of skin is generally free of infiltrating cells. In borderline lepromatous leprosy the granulomas are composed of macrophages with small numbers of lymphocytes. Nerves are not destroyed and contain many bacilli. BCG vaccine has a role in preventing the disease, and dapsone is very useful in treating patients and interrupting transmission (Crawford 1992).

Atypical Mycobacterial Infections

Many non-tuberculous mycobacteria cause disease in humans. In children the most frequently found types are *M. fortuitum*, *M. scrofulaceum* and *M. avium-intercellulare*. Infections due to *M. chelonei*, *M. marinum*, *M. ulcerans* and *M. kansasii* also occur. Children with acquired immune deficiency syndrome (AIDS) not infrequently have pulmonary or disseminated infection with *M. avium-intercellulare*. It seems that BCG vaccination carries some protection from these infections, but the response to antituberculous drugs is generally poor.

Cervical Lymphadenopathy

Cervical lymphadenopathy is a frequent manifestation of mycobacterial infection in children, but ulcerating lesions of the skin, and bone and joint disease also occur. In the USA non-tuberculous mycobacterial lymphadenopathy of the neck is six times more frequent than cervical lymphadenopathy caused by *Mycobacterium tuberulosis* (Margileth et al. 1984). These mycobacterial organisms are commonly found in soil, dust, water and food such as eggs, milk and vegetables.

The classical cervical form of infection is usually unilateral, occurring in urbanized children younger than 5 years (Joshi et al. 1989), whereas tuberculous lymphadenitis in the USA mainly occurs after the age of 12 (Lai et al. 1984). The involved lymph glands are sited close to the mandible. They are firm, rubbery and non-tender, but are confluent or matted together. There may be some erythema of the overlying skin. As the lesions progress there is softening, and eventually the overlying skin breaks, forming a discharging sinus. In time, fibrosis and calcification take place, but there are no significant systemic symptoms. Microscopic examination of biopsied lymph nodes shows stellate zones of caseous necrosis. Giant cells are infrequent and resemble foreign-body-type rather than Langhans-type giant cells (Jones and Campbell 1960).

Superficial Skin Lesions

Superficial skin lesions occur particularly with *M. scrofulaceum* and *M. marinum*, which causes swimming pool granuloma in children. Skin lesions are usually associated with abrasion from barnacles, shrimp or fish and repeated exposure to fresh or seawater. An inflamed nodule with a wart-like excrescence usually develops, but sometimes abscesses or deep ulcers occur. Treatment usually requires extensive surgical excision, although most lesions will heal slowly by fibrosis over a period of several months or years.

Mycobacterium ulcerans

Mycobacterium ulcerans produces a special form of ulceration in children who have daily contact with tropical or subtropical rain forests and river or lake water. There are specific localities in Australia, Papua New Guinea and Africa, where there is a high incidence of infection (MacCullum et al. 1948; Hutt 1966; Hayman 1993). The disease usually begins as a skin papule, a subcutaneous nodule or an area of localized oedema because of necrotizing panniculitis. The initial lesion is painless but enlarges and ulcerates. Ulcers may be very extensive, and generally occur on limbs but also on the face and trunk in children. Healing occurs with fibrosis and contractures, but calcification may also be seen. Sometimes there is disseminated or deep infection with bone involvement. Smaller satellite ulcers may occur. Pathological examination shows extensive coagulative necrosis of subcutaneous fat. The fat develops a firm consistency and has a grey-white colour. The necrotic fat forms lipid lacunae and amorphous gelatinous collections. Large numbers of acid-fast bacilli occur as extracellular globular clusters in the lacunae. Only small numbers of organisms are found in necrotic dermis, fibrous septae and areas where the lesion is enlarging. After secondary bacterial infection has occurred, polymorphonuclear leucocytes, histiocytes containing phagocytosed lipids, plasma cells and lymphocytes appear in increasing numbers. Langhans' giant cells are occasionally encountered. The undermined edge of the ulcer undergoes epithelialization.

Bacterial Infections

Staphylococcus

Factors that predispose towards staphylococcal infection are the presence of foreign material (in skin abrasions and surgical procedures), viral infections such as measles, granulocytopenia, abnormalities of chemotaxis and certain immune-deficiency syndromes. Examples are Job and Chediak–Higashi syndromes, hypogammaglobulinaemia and agammaglobulinaemia, and chronic granulomatous disease. Staphylococcal infection remains a problem in nurseries of maternity hospitals.

Skin Suppuration

Impetigo is a common form of staphylococcal skin infection, which is manifested as tender erythematous papules or patches at the site of previous injury or insect bites. There is a transient vesicular stage, which becomes encrusted and hyperaemic. Satellite lesions from autoinfection often develop. Furuncles or boils are more common in children than in adults. Cellulitis also occurs very frequently in situations of poverty. The cause is not limited to staphylococci, as streptococci and *Haemophilus influenzae* may occur individually or mixed with *Staphylococcus aureus*.

Scalded Skin Syndrome

Scalded skin syndrome (also called Ritter's disease or pemphigus neonatorum) is due to particular strains of *Staph. aureus* that produce an epidermolytic toxin (Margileth 1975). Mild erythroderma of the skin is followed by sudden acute bullous desquamation of large areas. The bullae are intraepidermal; the denuded area becomes moist and red but later becomes dry and is followed by secondary scaly desquamation. If there is no supervening bacterial infection, healing with complete regeneration of squamous epithelium takes place over 2 weeks.

Abscesses

Infantile breast abscess is usually unilateral, and constitutional signs are minimal. Abscess formation is preceded by marked induration and erythema of the tissues of the breast. Surgical drainage is required to limit the progress of the disease. Septic myositis and/or deep abscess usually follow a bacteraemia from a skin infection, whereas liver abscess is often a consequence of umbilical cord infection in the newborn or of ascariasis of the common bile duct in older children. Staphylococcal conjunctivitis is fairly common in infants, but stye is encountered in older children.

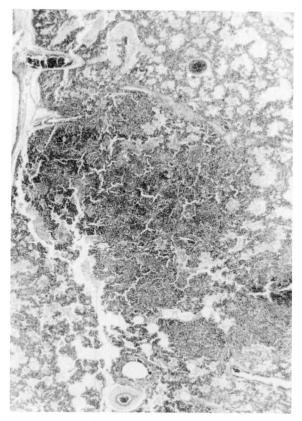

Fig. 14.23. Haemorrhagic bronchopneumonia caused by *Staphylococcus aureus* in a child who had a preceding upper respiratory tract viral infection.

Acute Suppurative Lymphadenitis

Acute suppurative lymphadenitis may be due to *Staphylococcus* or mixed infection with *Staphylococcus* and *Streptococcus*. The condition is frequently preceded by a minor throat or mouth infection.

Pneumonia

Pneumonia due to *Staph. aureus* is prevalent among infants less than a year of age. There is usually pre-existing skin infection or viral pneumonia caused by measles, influenza or certain strains of adenovirus. There is also an association with cystic fibrosis and leukaemia. The pneumonia takes the form of a haemorrhagic bronchopneumonia (Fig. 14.23) and has a propensity to develop lung abscesses, pneumatoceles, pneumothorax (particularly tension pneumothorax), empyema and bronchial wall necrosis. This necrosis

may progress to bronchiectasis (Kaschula et al. 1983).

Bacteraemia and Septicaemia

Bacteraemia and septicaemia are often not recognized until satellite lesions such as osteomyelitis, arthritis and pericarditis have become established, by which time there may be severe toxaemia with constitutional symptoms. Blood cultures, if taken, are frequently positive, and acute bacterial endocarditis may develop.

Toxic Shock Syndrome

A syndrome of fever, profound hypotension and diffuse macular erythroderma followed by skin desquamation after 1–2 weeks has been attributed to the liberation of toxins by *Staphylococcus aureus*. Other organisms such as group A streptococci, *Streptococcus pneumoniae* and *Pseudomonas aeruginosa* have also been implicated. There is massive capillary vasodilatation with intravascular fluid loss, causing oedema and multisystem organ damage (Todd 1988). Many cases have been associated with tampon usage in menstruating girls, but staphylococcal enteritis, skin burns, focal infections and osteomyelitis are also responsible.

Osteomyelitis

In areas where there is a high incidence of acute osteomyelitis, almost all cases occurring in children older than 2 years are due to *Staphylococcus aureus*. In younger children (1 month to 2 years) *Haemophilus influenzae* is the predominant organism (Hoffman et al. 1990; Faden and Grossi 1991). In western countries other organisms such as streptococci and gram-negative bacteria have a role. Before 1 year of age, there is a tendency for the infection to spread across the growth plate of long bones along transphyseal vessels to cause arthritis. Lesions are often multiple and poorly localized. The most common site is the diaphysis of the long bones, but small cancellous bones of the hands and feet may also be involved.

The condition has an abrupt onset, with toxaemia, pyrexia and pain. Pseudoparalysis often occurs in the very young, and toxic shock syndrome is a feature in some older children.

The lesions are localized to the metaphysis adjacent to the epiphyseal plate as organisms become

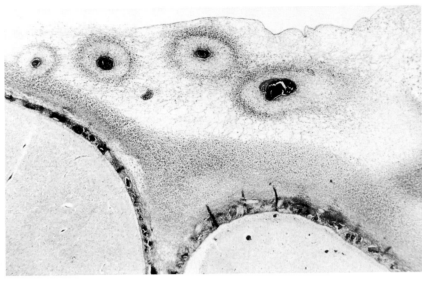

Fig. 14.24. Acute purulent meningitis caused by *Streptococcus pneumoniae* in a 15-month-old boy. Note the perivascular cuffing of meningeal vessels by neutrophils.

localized in venous lakes at this site. There is rapid production of pus, which extends along the length of the medullary cavity. Symptoms are rapidly relieved by surgical decompression. Occasionally, osteomyelitis may be due to trauma as occurs with infected compound fractures. Adolescent boys may have vertebral osteomyelitis due to gram-negative organisms or streptococci (Walbogel et al. 1970).

During the early acute stage of infection, radiological changes are usually not apparent, although isotope bone scans are helpful in arriving at a diagnosis. When adequate drainage of pus is not established, cortical bone may undergo necrosis to leave a sequestrum. This is usually followed by chronic infection and a discharging sinus. The prognosis is influenced by the state of overall nutrition, immobilization of the affected limb and the status of the nutrient artery of the affected bone.

Arthritis

Arthritis may also be due to *Haemophilus influenzae* type B, *Pneumococcus, Neisseria* and *Streptococcus* in children less than 2 years of age. After the age of 2 the cause is usually staphylococcal or tuberculous. In young infants there is often more than one joint affected. When synovium is biopsied it shows the features of an acute inflammatory reaction on a serous surface. There is exudation of pus and fibrin with a granulation tissue response.

Group A Streptococcus

Group A streptococcal infections are common in childhood. They are due to β-haemolytic streptococci of Lancefield group A, most often spread by droplets. The clinical manifestations of infection include tonsillitis and pharyngitis, scarlet fever, impetigo, erysipelas, rheumatic fever and acute glomerulonephritis. Streptococcal pharyngitis and tonsillitis are said to be subclinical in 30%–50% of cases (Kaplan 1992). Severe infection, with toxaemia, pyrexia, nausea, vomiting and shock, occurs in 10% of cases. As the organism is highly sensitive to penicillin and/or erythromycin, infection is no longer the formidable disease that it was in the preantibiotic era. Scarlet fever is rarely encountered even in developing countries. However, impetigo, rheumatic fever and acute glomerulonephritis due to streptococcal infection remain common.

Pneumococcus

Streptococcus pneumoniae is an important cause of morbidity and mortality in children. It usually causes acute otitis media, bronchopneumonia, meningitis (Fig. 14.24), osteomyelitis and primary peritonitis in young girls. Fulminating septicaemia occurs particularly in children who have undergone splenectomy (see p. 643). Infections are more common during the winter and spring months and the 6- to 24-month age group is most prone to infection (Teele 1981). Infection occurs more often in black children; those with sickle cell disease are more susceptible (Fraser et al. 1973). The organism is often a commensal in the pharynx, and ear infection is thought to be via the Eustachian tube. It is suggested that pneumonia follows aspiration of pharyngeal organisms after a viral infection, where there has been increased production of mucin and inhibition of the epithelial ciliary activity.

Neisseria gonorrhoeae

The true incidence of gonorrhoeal infections in children is not known, as the studies that have been carried out have been based on symptomatic cases. The incidence of childhood infections has been increasing since 1958. It is high in the 15–19 year age group, and in the 10–14 year group, where girls have symptomatic infection more frequently than boys (Wilfert and Gutman 1981).

Ophthalmia neonatorum due to *Neisseria gonorrhoeae* occurs most often in the lower social classes. A mother may or may not be symptomatic. The infant develops a conjunctival discharge between 2 and 21 days after birth. Initially the discharge is watery, but it becomes thick, mucopurulent and blood-stained. Infection is usually bilateral. There is oedema of the lids and conjunctiva. Without appropriate treatment the cornea may become involved and undergo ulceration and perforation. Infection may also spread to other parts of the body to produce arthritis and septicaemia.

Children aged 1 month to 9 years may become infected by fomites from infected adults usually by way of bath towels or bed clothing. There may also be involuntary sexual contact. Vaginitis is the commonest form of infection in pre-adolescent children. It is, however, a mild disease with infection restricted to the superficial mucosa. There is purulent discharge with itching and dysuria, and occasionally urethritis, proctitis and peritonitis may occur (Benson and Weinstock 1940). Infected prepubertal boys develop urethritis, which is less common than vaginitis in girls. Disseminated disease with septicaemia, polyarthritis and osteomyelitis occasionally occurs.

Neisseria meningitidis

There is a uniformly high prevalence of the disease in children less than 2 years of age when bactericidal antibody activity against the organism is low. Twenty per cent of children are found to harbour *Neisseria*

meningitidis in the nasopharynx, but most isolated organisms are not pathogenic (Goldschneider et al. 1969). Some immunity is acquired by exposure to other organisms that have a common antigen with *N. meningitidis* (Gotschlich et al. 1977). Communities have periodic epidemics as immunity wanes, and in 1972 Sao Paolo had a major epidemic affecting thousands of children. The genitourinary tract is another site where the organism may be harboured without causing overt disease.

The primary site of infection by virulent organisms is usually the pharynx, but may also be the conjunctiva in young children. The organisms disseminate through the bloodstream from the site of primary infection to produce a mild bacteraemia or an explosive and fulminating disease, often resulting in death within hours. Boys are affected at an earlier age and more often than girls. The clinical manifestations usually show evidence of upper respiratory tract infection with pyrexia, headache, vomiting and occasionally muscle and joint pains. In severe infection, petechial haemorrhages of the skin, ecchymoses and purpura occur in 50%–60% of cases. In Cape Town, where the disease is continuously prevalent, most cases present with septicaemia. Acute circulatory collapse is seen in 16% and pure meningitis in only 15% (Ryder et al. 1987). Approximately 70%–80% of fatalities have meningococcaemia, and less than 30% have meningitis without septicaemia (Neveling and Kaschula 1993). It is notable that, in communities with a high incidence of malnutrition, the fatalities tend to occur in the better nourished individuals. Most cases die within 72 h of onset of the disease, and approximately 30% have myocarditis. When the heart is affected one finds collections of inflammatory cells in the myocardial interstitium associated with focal myolysis (Fig. 14.25). There is some extravasation of red blood cells with acute vasculitis, and occasionally the atrioventricular node may be involved. Focal pericarditis occurs rarely, in less than 5% of cases, who also have meningococcaemia. These children develop a pericardial effusion which requires aspiration. The skin lesions appear early, are often extensive and massive, with large ecchymoses and purpura. These lesions are due to underlying acute vasculitis associated with fibrin thrombi. Major vessels are occasionally involved, and amputations of digits and limbs may be necessary (Fig. 14.26). Involvement of the central nervous system takes the form of acute suppurative meningitis affecting the leptomeninges with vasculitis and perivascular cuffing of the vessels of the superficial cortex (Fig. 14.27).

Adrenal haemorrhages occur in about 60% of fatalities (Neveling and Kaschula 1993). Microscopic examination does not reveal any inflammatory lesion,

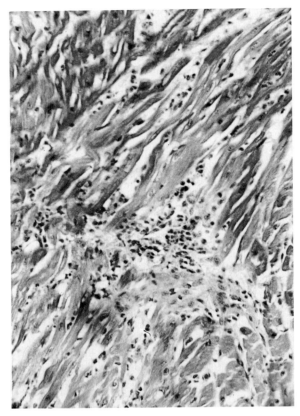

Fig. 14.25. Focal cardiomyolysis and acute myocarditis in meningococcaemia.

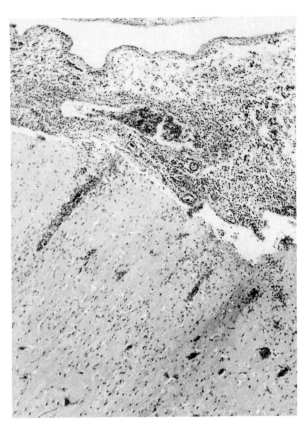

Fig. 14.27. Microscopy of meningoencephalitis caused by *Neisseria meningiditis*. A purulent exudate occurs into the subarachnoid space and around the blood vessels of the superficial cortex.

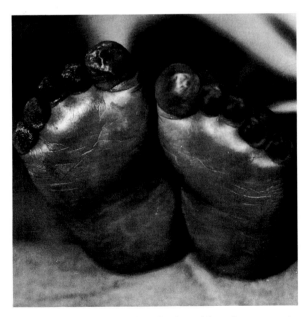

Fig. 14.26. Acute gangrene of toes in a boy with meningococcaemia.

but fibrin thrombi may be encountered in small vessels. The typical Waterhouse–Friderichsen syndrome (purpura and circulatory collapse) is not always associated with adrenal haemorrhage and is probably due to endotoxic shock (Hardman 1968). It seems that endotoxin also activates the coagulation system to produce disseminated intravascular coagulopathy, which is frequently associated with meningococcaemia (Rodriquez-Erdmann 1965).

Gastrointestinal Infections

Cholera

In pandemic areas where children form a large sector of the population, they are often affected; they are especially prone to infection after the first year of life. The mortality rate in certain Third World countries varies between 15% and 20%. However, when an epidemic occurs in a new area, the disease affects adult males predominantly (Cohen et al. 1971). A carrier state is present before overt disease and/or during convalescence.

Large doses of *Vibrio cholerae* need to be ingested to produce infection. The organisms adhere to the intestinal epithelium on the brush border and proliferate at this site to produce an enterotoxin. The enterotoxin causes a number of biochemical derangements, which cause water to be transported from the extracellular space into the lumen of the intestine. This causes severe dehydration with diarrhoea, circulatory collapse, acidosis and hypokalaemia (Cassel and Pfeuffer 1978). The clinical onset of the disease is variable: it may be insidious or abrupt. There is diarrhoea, which initially includes faecal material but soon becomes watery (isotonic) with flecks of mucus but no blood. There is progressive dehydration and children become pyrexial. They often develop seizures and this may go on to coma. Acute renal failure may develop because of circulatory collapse, and cardiac arrythmias may occur because of the hypokalaemia. Treatment is directed at rehydration and giving attention to acid–base and electrolyte balance.

Escherichia coli

The pathogenicity of particular serotypes of enteropathic *Escherichia coli* in neonatal and infantile diarrhoeal disease was first demonstrated in the late 1940s (Bray and Beavan 1948). At least five pathogenetic mechanisms are now known to be operative (Hart et al. 1993). Enterotoxogenic *E. coli* (ETEC) produce two enterotoxins, one heat-stable and the other heat-labile that closely resembles and acts like cholera toxin. Both cause enterocytes to secrete fluids. They are the main cause of diarrhoea in the tropics (Sack 1975) and among international travellers (Steffen 1986). They also produce fimbrial adhesions that facilitate colonization in the small intestine (Gracey 1993).

Enteropathogenic *E. coli* (EPEC), like ETEC, produces a non-inflammatory diarrhoea that is particularly prevalent during the summer in developing countries. The organism has an attaching and effacement capacity on the brush borders of enterocytes. Enteroinvasive *E. coli* (EIEC), enterohaemorrhagic *E. coli* (EHEC) and enteroaggregative *E. coli* (EAggEC) produce inflammatory diarrhoea. The EIEC biotypes mainly affect infants and causes a disease which is very similar to *Shigella* infection and often requires intravenous rehydration (Hart et al. 1993). The EHEC biotypes are normal commensals in the intestines of cattle and pigs. The main mode of infection is considered to be from undercooked contaminated meat or from manure. Infection causes haemorrhagic colitis and haemolytic uraemic syndrome. Verocytotoxin 1 or 2 is released and causes necrosis of enterocytes in the terminal ileum and colon, where an attaching and effacement phenomenon occurs. Affected patients experience abdominal cramps and watery diarrhoea that becomes haemorrhagic as surface ulceration ensues. When bacilli enter the bloodstream, they damage endothelial cells and precipitate haemolytic uraemic syndrome (Hart et al. 1993). The EAggEC group has recently been defined among previously untypable O serotypes. The group is an important cause of acute and persistent diarrhoea in rural India (Bhan et al. 1989). The organisms adhere and aggregate on colonic mucosa and in Peyer's patches.

E. coli are important causes of diarrhoea, and in developing countries cause much morbidity and mortality. Transferable plasmids have a role in conferring virulence (Sack et al. 1971). Specific diagnosis requires sophisticated laboratory facilities and expensive reagents, and is time-consuming. The necessary facilities are consequently usually not available where they are most needed.

Salmonella

Salmonella infection is a frequent cause of gastroenteritis in areas of poor sanitation, and infection is usually by way of contaminated food and drink. The virulence of salmonella organisms depends upon the serotype and phagetype. Typhoid and paratyphoid fevers are the most severe forms of salmonella infection, but gastroenteritis due to *S. enteritidis* now has worldwide prevalence as a consequence of mass production of chickens and eggs. Children with sickle cell disease are particularly prone to develop salmonella osteomyelitis of the small bones of the hands and feet; young children are also prone to develop salmonella meningitis.

In the lymphoid aggregates of the small intestine, the organisms proliferate without attracting polymorphonuclear leucocytes. Lymphoid aggregates become swollen as a result of accumulation of fibrin and small haemorrhages with an infiltration of lymphocytes, macrophages and plasma cells. During the later stages of infection macrophages become increasingly prominent and phagocytose cellular debris. In severe infection inflammation may extend to the muscularis propria. Lymphoid aggregates and Peyer's patches ulcerate late in the bacteraemic phase of typhoid fever (Fig. 14.28). Extensive haemorrhage and perforation may occur, and perforation with subsequent peritonitis is often fatal. Mesenteric lymph glands become enlarged and softened. They develop focal

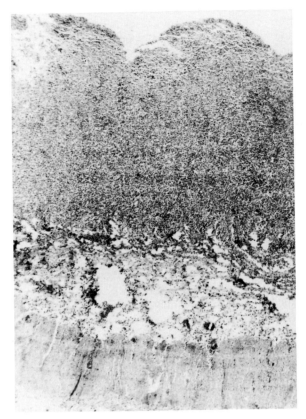

Fig. 14.28. Typhoid ulceration of small intestine. The lymphoid tissue of a Peyer's patch is swollen because of proliferation of lymphocytes, macrophages and plasma cells. Note the local haemorrhage at the *upper right*.

Fig. 14.29. A mesenteric lymph node in typhoid fever. There is an accumulation of macrophages, lymphocytes and plasma cells with many areas of focal necrosis.

areas of necrosis with oedema and have an inflammatory infiltration similar to that which occurs in the lymphoid aggregates of the intestine (Fig. 14.29). The spleen becomes considerably enlarged with a tense capsule, but the parenchyma is soft. There is marked sinusoidal hyperplasia, with focal areas of necrosis and haemorrhage. The liver also undergoes enlargement due to hyperplasia of the Kupffer cells and swelling of liver parenchymal cells. Parenchymatous degeneration and focal necrosis may occur. Release of endotoxin is responsible for pyrexia and the focal necrosis that is seen in heart and striated muscle. Endotoxin is also considered to be responsible for depression of bone marrow and leucopenia. Children often have an accompanying laryngitis, pharyngitis and pneumonia. Complications due to distant localization of organisms include meningitis, endocarditis, arthritis and perichondritis. Persistent infection of the gall bladder is considered to be the cause of the carrier state.

Shigella

Infection is by the anal/oral sequence from symptomatic and non-symptomatic carriers. Epidemics from contaminated water or food occur, and in areas of poor sanitation flies have a role in the spread of disease. The maximal age incidence is 1–4 years. Only a small number of organisms is required to produce infection (ten organisms have been found to be sufficient) (DuPont et al. 1969). Organisms invade the colonic epithelium, where cell necrosis and an intense inflammatory response occurs. A toxin that binds to villous enterocytes but not to crypt cells is produced. Necrosis is most intense along the tips of mucosal folds. Goblet cells quickly disappear. There is extravasation of fibrin, and gland crypts become obstructed with the formation of crypt abscesses (Takeuchi et al. 1968). Endotoxin causes the epithelial cells to lose rather than absorb water, and this is

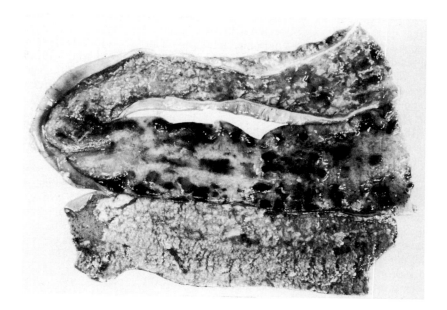

Fig. 14.30. Colon in bacillary dysentery caused by *Shigella dysenteriae*. There is congestion of the mucosa with ulceration and the formation of an inflammatory pseudomembrane.

mainly responsible for the watery diarrhoea. The organisms do not normally enter the bloodstream.

The clinical manifestations and pathology are to some extent dependent on the strain of infecting organism. All cases have watery diarrhoea with blood and mucus. Tenesmus is often prominent, but toxic megacolon, hypoglycaemia, haemolytic uraemia syndrome and pneumonia may complicate infection (Bennish 1991). The incubation period for *Shigella sonnei* and *S. flexneri* is 1–3 days, whereas that for *S. dysenteriae* is 3–7 days. *S. sonnei* infection is more common in the UK and *S. flexneri* in Continental Europe. *S. dysenteriae* mainly occurs in developing and tropical countries. *S. dysenteriae* type 1 (Shiga's bacillus), which causes a severe form of disease, mainly occurs in the Far East. Infection becomes manifest clinically as acute malaise with pyrexia, abdominal cramps, diarrhoea and tenesmus. Blood and mucus appear in the stools, which become increasingly copious and watery, leading to dehydration. Febrile convulsions may be encountered in children, particularly when they have *S. dysenteriae* or *S. flexneri* infection.

There is intense hyperaemia of the mucosal surface with congestion of the blood vessels in all forms of infection. Many small bleeding ulcers occur and are more frequent in *S. flexneri* and *S. dysenteriae* infections (Fig. 14.30). Crypt abscesses with diffuse infiltration of polymorphonuclear leucocytes into the lamina propria occur in all forms of infection. In *S. flexneri* infection there is prominent loss of surface epithelium, which commences over the mucosal folds. In *S. sonnei* infection a thick, purulent mucous

exudate tends to cover the surface of the affected areas, whereas in *S. dysenteriae* infection there is extensive necrosis of the lamina propria to produce a pseudomembrane in which fibrin, mucus and necrotic cells are mixed together and replace the surface mucosa. Children with chronic infection may develop rectal prolapse, although this is rare.

Yersinia

There are three species of *Yersinia* that are pathogenic to humans. These include *Y. pestis*, which causes plague with adenitis, septicaemia, pneumonia and meningitis; *Y. enterocolitica*, a common cause of gastroenteritis; and *Y. pseudotuberculosis*, which causes mesenteric adenitis, erythema nodosa, polyarthritis and septicaemia, but is not common in humans. There is a large reservoir of *Y. enterocolitica* infection in animals, and the organism survives for a long time in water. They seem to require a hot–cold cycle (such as in and out of refrigeration) to facilitate the production of virulence factors (Gracey 1993). Infection probably occurs more often than is recognized, as special culture facilities are needed for organism identification.

Disease occurs more frequently during winter months in temperate zones. Children less than 5 years of age develop acute diarrhoeal disease with vomiting and pyrexia. The stools are watery and usually without blood and mucus, but may contain large numbers of pus cells. Children usually recover after 7–21 days, but some may develop chronic infection with periodic attacks of acute diarrhoea. Older children (more than 5 years) infected with serotypes 0 : 3 and 0 : 9 may develop a syndrome simulating acute appendicitis or mesenteric adenitis. The disease is increasingly being reported in neonates and infants up to 3 months of age who are prone to develop septicaemia (Challapalli and Cunningham 1993; Naqvi et al. 1993).

Initial sites of infection are the lymphoid aggregates of the terminal small intestine and appendix. The draining mesenteric lymph nodes are also quickly involved. After about 5 days microabscesses appear in Peyer's patches and in the lymph nodes. Superficial ulcers develop in the mucosa of the terminal ileum. In cases of severe infection, small abscesses may also be found in distal lymph nodes, the spleen and liver. A suppurative pneumonia which contains microabscesses has been described (Bradford et al. 1974). The severity of the disease seems to depend on the size of the inoculum. A number of older children undergo surgery as possible cases of appendicitis or mesenteric adenitis. Mesenteric lymph nodes are found to be enlarged and matted, producing a retroperitoneal mass. The appendix is not significantly inflamed but may contain microabscesses. Acute septicaemic illness resembling typhoid, which may be fatal, has been reported in children (Spira and Kabins 1976). As a consequence of septicaemia, localization to distant organs such as joints, eyes, meninges, liver and soft tissues of the perineum have been reported (Rabson et al. 1975).

Campylobacter and Helicobacter

During the past two decades *Campylobacter* infection has become recognized as one of the most important causes of acute diarrhoea in both developed and developing countries. *C. jejuni* accounts for 96% of such infections in a developing population (Lastovica et al. 1986), where it is responsible for 18% of acute diarrhoeal illness in infants (Househam et al. 1988), whereas in industrialized countries it seems to account for between 5% and 10% of cases (Ruiz-Palacios and Pickering 1992). Among urban slum dwellers in Liberia, campylobacters account for 45% of diarrhoeas in children younger than 5 years (Molbak et al. 1988). The incubation period from infection to the onset of symptoms varies from 1 to 7 days. *C. jejuni* and *C. coli* have a capacity to adhere to cells and produce a cholera-like enterotoxin that induces intraluminal accumulation of fluid. Campylobacters may also invade the mucosa to cause cell damage and inflammation, or they may cause bacteraemia with disseminated lesions such as

meningitis, endocarditis, cholecystitis, adenitis and urinary tract infections. *C. fetus* is particularly prone to cause bacteraemia with a systemic illness similar to typhoid (Guerrant et al. 1978; Schewitz and Le Roux 1978). The disease may also manifest as intrauterine infection associated with stillbirths and abortion, when there is usually placental infarction, haemorrhage and necrosis. There is a tendency for neonatal meningitis (Rettig 1979) and Guillain–Barré syndrome to occur in older children (Kuroki et al. 1991).

The most frequent clinical manifestation is of an acute diarrhoeal disease resembling viral gastroenteritis and lasting from 1 and 7 days. Symptoms of secretory diarrhoea are predominant in developing countries, whereas in developed countries inflammatory diarrhoea is more common (Ruiz-Palacios and Pickering 1992). Occasionally, there may be relapsing colitis simulating ulcerative colitis or Crohn's disease. The most predominant symptoms are diarrhoea and abdominal pain, but malaise, fever, nausea and vomiting also occur. Blood is often present in the stools and true rigors occur occasionally. Prolonged severe infection occurs in about 20% of cases (Blaser and Reller 1981). Pathological examination of the gut reveals an oedematous exudative enteritis with congestion and haemorrhage. Biopsies of the colon have shown non-specific colitis with infiltration of polymorphonuclear leucocytes, mononuclear inflammatory cells and eosinophils. There is degeneration and atrophy of surface epithelium, loss of mucus, crypt abscesses and ulceration of the epithelium (Lambert et al. 1979). The gram-negative bacilli are curved and stain with Giemsa and silver.

Complications of the disease include toxic megacolon, pseudomembranous colitis, massive lower gastrointestinal tract haemorrhage, mesenteric adenitis, appendicitis, meningitis, arthritis, cholecystitis, urinary tract infection, bacterial endocarditis, pericarditis, peritonitis and lung abscess (Blaser and Reller 1981).

Helicobacter has recently been separated as a genus distinct from *Campylobacter*. The organism is associated with chronic antral type B gastritis and peptic ulceration in adults and children (Czinn et al. 1986; Hazell et al. 1986). There is active inflammation with mucosal infiltration by neutrophils and plasma cells, hyperplasia of lymphoid aggregates and epithelial cells, and mucus depletion. *H. pylori* occurs in the mucus layer covering the mucosa immediately adjacent to surface gastric epithelial cells. Young children with such infection have been reported to have acute protein-losing enteropathy with organisms adherent to epithelial cell junctions (Fig. 14.31). Recovery from protein-losing enteropathy is accompanied by resolution of the gastritis and disappearance of the organisms (Hill et al. 1987).

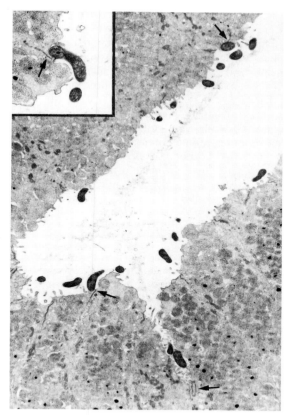

Fig. 14.31. Electron micrograph of the superficial portion of a gastric gland from helicobacter gastritis. Numerous *H. pylori* organisms are concentrated at cell junctions (*arrows*). (× 2250) *Inset*, *H. pylori* attached to a gastric epithelial cell at an intercellular tight junction (*arrow*). (× 20 000) (Courtesy of Dr C.C. Sinclair-Smith, University of Cape Town)

Diphtheria

Diphtheria is an acute infectious disease caused by *Corynebacterium diphtheriae*. There are three biotypes, all of which may be toxigenic or non-toxigenic, depending on the presence of bacteriophages having genes for toxin production. Non-toxigenic strains of organism commonly infect the ear, nasopharynx and vagina. During the past 30 years the virulence of the organism seems to have been declining. Eighty per cent of infections occur in children less than 15 years of age who have not been immunized. The incidence of infection is highest among poor people living in overcrowded housing conditions. Respiratory infections are acquired by inhalation of organisms; skin infection is usually by contact with fomites.

The primary site of infection is usually the nasopharynx and larynx, but can also be the nose, mouth and skin. Local tissue necrosis occurs, with an associated acute inflammatory response. As the lesions enlarge a fibrinopurulent exudate is discharged. The lesion becomes deeper and wider as increasing amounts of toxin are produced. The fibrinous exudate now becomes adherent due to encrustation, and contains altered blood. Microscopically, the membrane is composed of necrotic epithelial cells, inflammatory cells, red blood cells, fibrin and organisms (Fig. 14.32). Deep to the membrane there is proliferation of granulation tissue capillaries, and hence attempts at removing the membrane produces bleeding. The membrane, together with oedema of the underlying soft tissue, narrows the lumen to the airways. Very high levels of toxin are

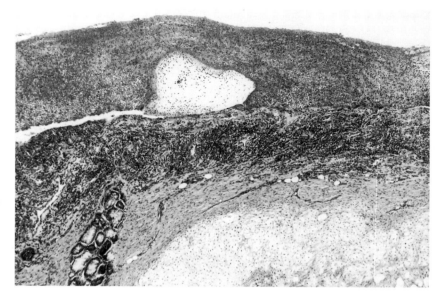

Fig. 14.32. Microscopic appearance of diphtheritic membrane, which is composed of necrotic epithelial cells, inflammatory exudate, fibrin, red blood cells and organisms. Deep to the membrane is a zone of vascular granulation tissue and oedematous loose connective tissue.

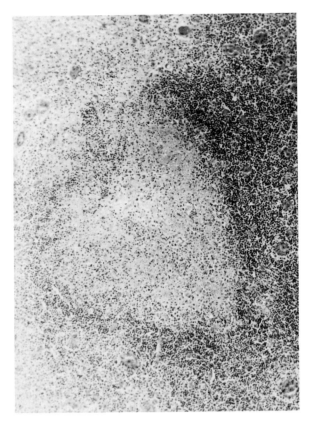

Fig. 14.33. A cervical lymph node with hyperplastic follicle caused by diphtheria.

discharged into the bloodstream when vascular areas such as the pharynx and tonsils are the site of infection. The regional lymph glands undergo prominent hyperplasia with marked enlargement of follicles (Fig. 14.33). Enlargement of the follicles of the spleen and distant lymph nodes may also occur, and the centres of hyperplastic follicles may become necrotic. The skin may be a site of primary infection when the organisms gain access to pre-existing wounds. Ulcers having sharp edges and a membranous base are formed.

Myocarditis generally occurs 10–14 days after onset of symptoms. Myocardial involvement may cause acute heart failure and circulatory collapse. Cardiac arrhythmia may cause sudden death. Initially the myocardial fibres are oedematous; they then develop cloudy swelling and progressively acquire fine granules of lipid. Infiltration of polymorphs and lymphocytes is associated with congestion of small vessels. Hyaline degeneration of myocardial fibres and cardiomyolysis follow. Necrotic muscle is replaced by fibrosis and, when this is extensive, congestive cardiac failure may result.

Peripheral nerves become involved 3–7 weeks after onset of the disease. The nerves most commonly affected are those that supply the area of infection. There is degeneration and destruction of myelin sheaths and swelling of axon cylinders. Cranial nerve paralysis may lead to aspiration pneumonia.

The liver may be enlarged owing to cloudy swelling of hepatocytes, and focal necrosis may be found. The kidneys may be the site of non-specific non-suppurative interstitial nephritis and acute tubular necrosis. Adrenal haemorrhages occur rarely. Occasionally there are haemorrhages from multiple sites, associated with prolonged bleeding time (Havaldar et al. 1989).

Haemophilus influenzae

Haemophilus influenzae is a gram-negative coccobacillus. There are six antigenic capsular types, designated a–f; capsule type b confers invasive properties on the organism and accounts for over 95% of *Haemophilus* infections in children. Between 60% and 90% of children harbour *H. influenzae* in the upper respiratory tract, but only 5% have encapsulated type b organisms. The attack rate of invasive disease is 0.01 that of the carrier rate (Michaels et al. 1976). *H. influenzae* b is now considered to be responsible for most life-threatening infections in children aged 1 month to 5 years in the USA. Infection is most prevalent among poor urban dwellers, but is also particularly high among Eskimoes and Navajo indians. Siblings of infected children have a 6% chance of contracting the disease.

Meningitis is the most frequent form of clinical disease, with a peak incidence from 7 to 12 months, with 66% of cases occurring before the age of 18 months. The disease seems to be a consequence of bacteraemia, with organisms reaching the cerebrospinal fluid through the choroid plexus. Fatal cases of meningitis usually have extensive and diffuse bilateral exudation of pus cells and fibrin into the subarachnoid space. Complications include 8th nerve deafness and obstructive hydrocephalus.

Intense acute epiglottitis occurs almost exclusively in Caucasians. The disease occurs most frequently after the age of 2 years. There is generally no associated bacteraemic phase, and hence additional foci of infection are rare. However, aspiration of organisms may cause pneumonia. There is considerable oedema of the larynx, associated with acute inflammatory cell infiltration and exudation of fibrin, but no significant epithelial ulceration.

Pneumonia due to *H. influenzae* varies in its clinical manifestation. It mainly occurs before the age of 2 years and has a low mortality rate. Some cases have an insidious onset of mild focal pneumonia, whereas others may have severe bilateral pneumonia progressing to empyema with a high fatality rate.

Septic arthritis occurs predominantly in children less than 2 years old who also have meningitis. It tends to affect large joints and is frequently associated with osteomyelitis. Black children are more frequently affected than Caucasians.

Cellulitis occurs in young children usually less than a year of age, often those who are bottle-fed. The face, head and neck, but particularly the retro-orbital region, are the favoured sites. There is acute onset, with erythematous discolouration of the skin later changing to a bluish-purple colour. Blood cultures are frequently positive.

Other complications from infection include pericarditis, osteomyelitis, epididymitis, urinary tract infection and soft tissue abscesses. Neonatal sepsis due to non-typable *H. influenzae* is increasingly being reported. It is associated with premature birth and has a high mortality rate (Takala et al. 1991). Children treated with chloramphenicol remain infective for a variable duration after being clinically cured.

Pertussis

In developing countries there is still a high prevalence of infection with high mortality rates. Most clinical cases are due to *Bordetella pertussis*, but *B. parapertussis* and *B. bronchiseptica* and adenovirus types 1,2,3 and 5 can produce an identical illness (Connor 1970). Pertussis is a highly communicable disease with a high mortality rate among infants less than 12 months of age (Brooks and Buchanan 1970). *B. pertussis* is an obligate human parasite that normally proliferates only in the presence of ciliated respiratory epithelium. The incubation period for infection varies between 6 and 20 days but is most often about 7 days. Immunity prevents adherence of the organism to epithelial cells (Aftandalians and Connor 1973). There is usually diffuse involvement of the respiratory epithelium of the larynx, trachea, bronchi and bronchioles. Following infection there is infiltration of the mucosa by lymphocytes and polymorphonuclear leucocytes, with congestion. Inflammatory cells become discharged into the lumina of bronchi and bronchioles, and peribronchiolar lymphoid aggregates undergo hyperplasia. Bronchial and bronchiolar epithelium undergoes necrosis and is shed into the lumen. Interstitial bronchopneumonia develops, with shedding of inflammatory cells and mucus into the lumina of bronchioles, resulting in atelectasis and air trapping. Frequently there is additional infection by other organisms. The most frequent complications are bronchiectasis and an encephalopathy with features of cerebral hypoxia.

Pseudomonas

Children with burns or cystic fibrosis, or those receiving immunosuppressive therapy or having an immune-deficiency disease are most prone to infection. *Pseudomonas* is a gram-negative bacillus that normally occurs in soil and water, but *P. aeruginosa* is also a commensual of the gastrointestinal tract of between 5% and 30% of individuals. The organism is often resistant to antibiotics, and infection is frequently acquired within hospitals. Colonization of skin burns is common, and active infection impairs attempts at skin grafting. Extensive infection in large burns is a frequent cause of death from septicaemia. Children with cystic fibrosis often acquire chronic pseudomonas infection of the tracheobronchial passages, and a necrotizing haemorrhagic bronchopneumonia sometimes occurs.

Children with malignancy (especially leukaemia) or those on immunosuppressive therapy are highly susceptible to infection, which is likely to become generalized. One of the hallmarks of pseudomonas infection is an acute vasculitis, where vessel walls are infiltrated by large numbers of organisms (Fig. 14.34). These organisms and the tissue necrosis that is produced give the vessels a bluish hue on haemotoxylin and eosin (H&E)-stained sections. As a consequence of the vasculitis, haemorrhages and thromboses occur. Gangrenous areas of skin are often seen in cases of septicaemic disease.

Other conditions that predispose to infection are prolonged usage of indwelling catheters or intravenous lines, prolonged usage of assisted ventilatory apparatus, and myelomeningocele. Infection may also occur before and after open heart surgery.

Nocardiosis

Nocardia asteroides is the main cause of systemic disease, whereas *N. madurae, N. brasiliensis* and *N. kaecaviae* tend to cause localized chronic disease. The normal habitat of the organism is the soil. Infection often occurs in immunosuppressed individuals. Children become infected by inhaling the organisms, and the lungs are the usual site of primary infection (Law and Marks 1982), which causes necrotizing lobular pneumonia and abscesses. Boys are affected more often than girls. Metastatic lesions in the brain, kidney, spleen, liver, skin, pericardium, myocardium, adrenals and bone may occur. The branching organisms are not seen on H&E stains, but are readily revealed on Gram and methenamine silver stains. *N. brasiliensis* and *N. madurae* cause mycetomas of the skin in tropical areas, particularly in South and Central America, and in Africa.

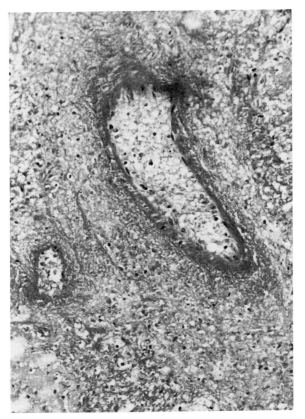

Fig. 14.34. Acute necrotizing vasculitis caused by infection with *Pseudomonas*. The deep staining of the necrotic vessel wall is caused by proliferation of large numbers of bacilli.

Anaerobic Infections

Anaerobic infections less frequently affect children than adults. The process is most often peritonitis resulting from appendicitis, gastric perforation or sigmoid volvulus. In newborn infants necrotizing enterocolitis due to anaerobic bacteria may also occur. The organisms responsible are usually a mixture of *Bacteroides*, *Clostridium* and *Fusobacterium*, together with *Escherichia coli*. Often there is an underlying immune deficiency, particularly in leukaemia or lymphoma, and in such circumstances the child is predisposed to developing septicaemia from the anaerobe. Another initiating site for anaerobic infection is the paranasal sinuses, where chronic infection may lead to a local abscess; this can progress to osteomyelitis. When *Clostridium perfringens* contributes to the anaerobic infection, gas formation will be seen in the involved tissues. Toxins produced by anaerobic organisms lead to significant systemic symptoms. These include circulatory collapse, haemolysis and jaundice, and toxic diarrhoea.

Complications are brain abscess, deep abscesses of the retroperitoneum and perinephric sites, and acute tubular necrosis.

Cat Scratch Disease

Cat scratch disease is a subacute relatively benign, regional lymphadenitis that follows cutaneous inoculation with a pleomorphic gram-negative bacillus (Wear et al. 1983). A candidate organism (*Afipia feles*) was cultured by English et al. (1988) in 10 of 19 patients with the disease. Since then further culture (Dolan et al. 1993) and serologic (Zangwill et al. 1993) studies indicate a very close association with *Rochalimaea henselae*.

In temperate zones there is a higher incidence during the autumn and winter. The highest age incidence seems to be between 2 and 14 years. A small erythematous papule or pustule forms at the site of inoculation, and persists for several weeks. Subsequently the draining lymph nodes become enlarged and tender. The microscopic features of the primary lesion and lymph nodes are similar. In the skin there are small areas of dermal necrosis surrounded by a larger zone of acellular necrobiosis, around which there is a palisade of epithelioid histiocytes and giant cells with a mantle of small lymphocytes. Polymorphonuclear leucocytes and plasma cells are found in perivascular areas, and a diffuse mild infiltration of eosinophils may occur (Winship 1953; Najii et al. 1962).

The lymph node lesions have been classified into three evolutionary stages. Initially there is enlargement caused by expansion of the cortex and hyperplasia of germinal centres (Fig. 14.35). Epithelioid granulomas, often with Langhans' giant cells, are scattered throughout the gland. During the next stage increasing numbers of enlarging granulomas fuse with each other and become infiltrated by polymorphonuclear leucocytes (Fig. 14.36). There is central necrosis of the granulomas with progressive suppuration and sinus formation. During the final stage there are many pus-filled sinuses, and pus may rupture through the capsule of the node into surrounding tissue. The resulting inflammatory response and fibrosis binds adjoining glands together and to adjacent tissues. The early lesions need to be differentiated from lymphoma, sarcoid and infectious mononucleosis. Later lesions resemble those of mycobacterial infections, lymphogranuloma venerium, brucellosis and tularemia. The pathological evolution of the lesions has been described by Winship (1953), Najii et al. (1962) and Campbell (1977).

Patients may develop an encephalopathy with cranial or peripheral nerve involvement and convulsions

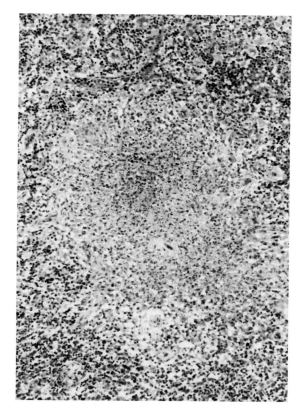

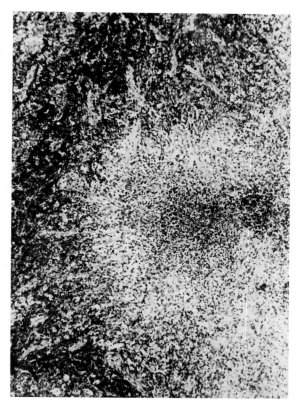

Fig. 14.35. Lymph node with an early epithelioid granuloma caused by cat scratch disease.

Fig. 14.36. Lymph node with an enlarging granuloma containing pus cells caused by cat scratch disease. (Courtesy of Dr J.A.H. Campbell, University of Cape Town)

(Carithers and Margileth 1991). Additional complications that have been reported are hepatic abscesses, osteolytic lesions, erythema nodosum, haemolytic anaemia, thrombocytopenia and pneumonia.

Lyme Disease

Lyme disease is a tick-borne multisystem infection caused by the spirochaete *Borrelia burgdorferi*. It is transmitted through the bite of *Ixodes* ticks and probably occurs worldwide but is endemic in particular localities of North America (Anonymous 1993). After a variable incubation period (3–32 days, but mainly 7–20 days), skin lesions appear. The initial lesion is centred around the site of the tick bite and takes the form of a raised erythematous plaque (erythema chronicum migrans). Secondary lesions appear a few days later and resolve after about 3 weeks. Systemic symptoms include asymmetrical arthralgia/arthritis, flu-like symptoms, facial nerve palsy, aseptic meningitis and neurological disturbances (Williams et al. 1990). The neurological disturbances

tend to occur a month or two after the tick bite and take the form of meningitis, meningoencephalitis, chorea, cranial neuritis, ataxia and myelitis. Rarely the heart (myocarditis and pericarditis), liver (hepatitis and jaundice) and lymph nodes (eosinophilic lymphadenitis) may be involved. Maternofetal transmission has been reported (Schlesinger et al. 1985). At present there is no reliable laboratory test for diagnosis. False-positive serologic tests occur at a rate of 5%–10%.

Viral Infections

Measles

Some aspects of measles virus (Rubeola) infection are discussed in the section dealing with malnutrition and infection (see p. 747). It is a formidable infection in developing countries, where death rates of 30%–40% have been reported (Cantrelle et al. 1960).

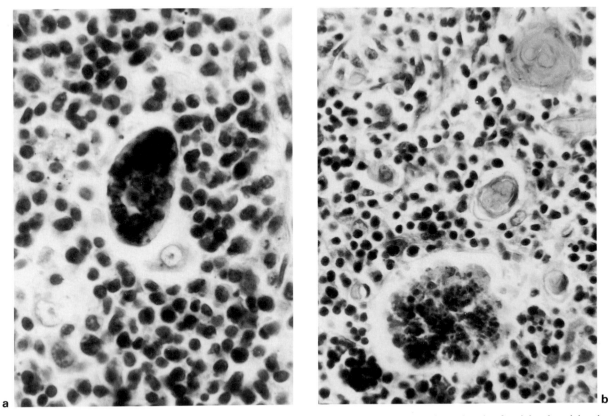

Fig. 14.37. Warthin–Finkeldey giant cells in acute measles infection. **a** A splenic follicle showing pyknosis of peripheral nuclei and inclusions in central nuclei. **b** Medulla of thymus showing a large number of pyknotic nuclei and paler cytoplasmic inclusions.

Nosocomial bacteraemias occur six times more often than in general paediatric patients, and significantly contribute to morbidity (Hussey and Simpson 1990). Measles vaccine has greatly reduced the incidence of infection, which is now rare in the USA but remains common in the UK and France, where vaccination of children is not compulsory. The severity of infection has been related to the initial infective dose (Aaby et al. 1986), but deficient reserves of vitamin A (retinol) are now considered to be the main factor (Hussey and Klein 1990; Butler et al. 1993). In industrialized countries the incidence is maximal beyond 5 years, whereas in impoverished non-industrialized areas the maximum age incidences very between 7 months and 2 years (Morley 1962; Hayden 1974). Transmission of infection is mainly by aerosolized droplets of respiratory infections from symptomatic cases. Infectivity is greatest during the prodrome.

The port of entry for the virus is usually the nasopharynx or conjunctiva. Virus replication occurs in inoculated epithelial cells and draining lymph nodes. Viraemia follows after 2–3 days, with more extensive infection of respiratory, conjunctival and salivary epithelial cells. The lymphoreticular system also becomes diffusely involved. A week after initial infection there is secondary viraemia with pyrexia and toxaemia. Natural killer cells and cytotoxic T cells limit spread while B cells are primed to produce antibodies. The measles rash appears between days 11 and 15 and signifies the onset of effective immune responsiveness with the appearance of antibodies (Graves et al. 1984). Lymphocytes infiltrate areas of virus replication, where they facilitate the clearance of the organisms. Anergy occurs at this time, with suppression of delayed hypersensitivity and reduced lymphocyte proliferation and lymphokine production. Serum interleukin-2 levels rise during the week before the appearance of the rash and remain increased for at least another 4 weeks (Anonymous 1989; Griffin et al. 1989).

Pathology

A characteristic of measles infection is widespread occurrence of two similar types of multinucleate

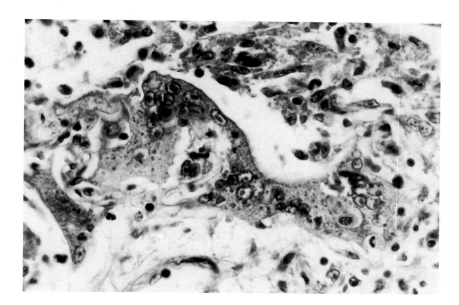

Fig. 14.38. Epithelial measles giant cells derived from alveolar lining cells (type 2 pneumocytes) containing both intranuclear and intracytoplasmic inclusions.

giant cells. Warthin–Finkeldey giant cells occur mainly in lymphoid aggregates, whereas epithelial measles giant cells develop from type 2 pneumocytes, respiratory epithelium, salivary gland epithelium and other epithelial tissues. Warthin–Finkeldey giant cells may contain more than 50 or 100 nuclei, usually much fewer, and may have very few or many intracytoplasmic and intranuclear inclusions. They are mostly encountered in the tonsils, adenoids, Peyer's patches, appendix, spleen, thymus and lungs (Fig. 14.37). When few or no inclusions are present, as often occurs in lymphoid tissues, the nuclei become clumped and are pyknotic.

Epithelial measles giant cells are often encountered during the prodrome of the illness, when large numbers may be sloughed off and can be identified on buccal smears. They generally have fewer nuclei than do Warthin–Finkeldey giant cells but, like them, have intranuclear and intracytoplasmic inclusions. Initially these giant cells are adherent to the basement membrane of the epithelium from which they are derived (Fig. 14.38).

Epithelial giant cells are frequent in Koplik spots, lesions which are seen in the mouth before the onset of the measles rash. There is oedema of subepithelial tissues as well as intracellular oedema of adjoining epithelium. A non-specific and relatively inconspicuous inflammatory infiltration occurs.

In the measles exanthem epithelial giant cells with up to 30 nuclei are found with parakeratosis, dyskeratosis, spongiosis and intracellular oedema. Underlying dermal blood vessels are congested, and there is a mild perivascular lymphocytic infiltration (Suringa et al. 1970).

Detailed studies of the respiratory system have been made only in fatal cases, most of which have pharyngitis, tracheitis, bronchitis, bronchiolitis and pulmonary parenchymal involvement. Draining lymphatics and lymph nodes often contain Warthin–Finkeldey giant cells. The epithelium of the trachea and main bronchi becomes heaped up and may undergo squamous metaplasia. Epithelial giant cells may be present among surface epithelial cells as well as mucous glands. Involvement of the lungs is seen as interstitial pneumonia with epithelial measles giant cells adherent to or in airspaces with an infiltration of polymorphonuclear leucocytes, macrophages and smaller numbers of lymphocytes and eosinophils (Fig. 14.39). Late in the disease large Warthin–Finkeldey-like giant cells may be seen inside airspaces. Alveoli are often oedematous and may be lined by hyaline membranes.

The bronchioles are often lined by hyperplastic epithelium, which may have surface epithelial giant cells (Fig. 14.40). In many children there is metaplasia of bronchial and bronchiolar epithelium. The epithelial cells may become hydropic and swollen (Fig. 14.41), or squamoid, infiltrating (apparently through pre-existing pores) adjoining alveoli and resembling a squamous carcinoma (Becroft and Osborne 1980) (Fig. 14.42). This proliferative response is sometimes associated with a peripheral fibrous inflammatory response, producing a fibroepithelial nodule, and the squamous metaplasia may be an index of vitamin A deficiency.

During the anergic period lasting 4–6 weeks after the onset of clinical measles, young children in developing countries are prone to supervening infection with herpesvirus, adenovirus, *Staphylococcus* and

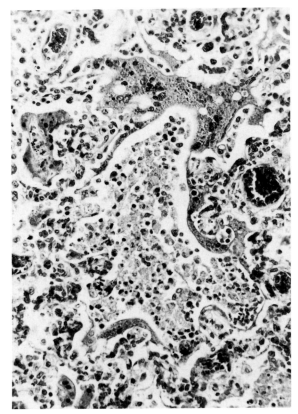

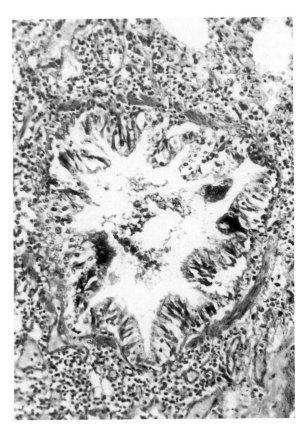

Fig. 14.39. Measles pneumonia: epithelial measles giant cells adherent to the alveolar wall and pleomorphic inflammatory cell infiltration into interstitium and airspaces.

Fig. 14.40. Bronchiole in measles pneumonia showing heaped-up epithelium with small bizarre surface-epithelial measles giant cells.

other organisms (Orren et al. 1981; Kaschula et al. 1983; Beckford et al. 1985). Fatal measles virus pneumonia may also be encountered without the clinical evidence of a skin rash (Enders et al. 1959). Severe laryngotracheobronchitis due to supervening bacterial infection (mainly *Staph. aureus*) may occur during or shortly after measles in children less than 2 years of age in western countries (Fortenberry et al. 1992).

Modified measles occurs in partially immune individuals in whom a milder form of disease develops after a shorter prodrome. Atypical measles occurs in some previously immunized individuals, but mainly those who received vaccine containing killed viruses. The clinical manifestations of infection are similar to those of typical measles except that Koplik spots are rarely seen and there is a rapid and considerable increase in serum antibody levels. The rash begins at the tips of the extremities and spreads in a cephalad direction. Almost all cases have lobular or segmental pneumonia with hilar lymphadenopathy. Often there is an associated hepatosplenomegaly with hyperaes-

thesia. Radiographic evidence of persistence of the nodular pneumonia may be found for up to 1–2 years after onset of the infection.

Clinically evident acute measles encephalitis occasionally follows secondary viraemia in non-industrialized countries and in immune-suppressed children (Hughes et al. 1993). However, most children, the world over, have electroencephalographic disturbances during acute measles and/or shortly thereafter. In the brain there is a mild to moderate inflammatory response with inclusion bodies and perivenous demyelination, as occurs in other viral encephalitides. Measles virus may be cultured from the cerebrospinal fluid and from brain tissue.

Acute allergic measles encephalitis is a postinfectious encephalitis occurring after viraemia. It may also occur in the wake of varicella, vaccinia and rubella. There is demyelination, necrosis and haemorrhage (Fig. 14.43). Measles virus cannot be isolated from the cerebrospinal fluid or from brain tissue.

Subacute sclerosing panencephalitis (SSPE) occurs on a basis of genetic predisposition. It is almost

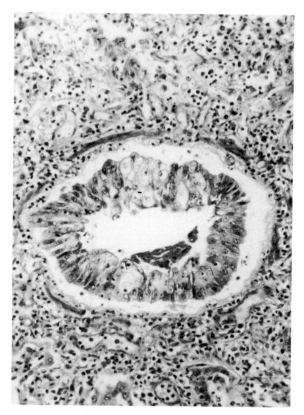

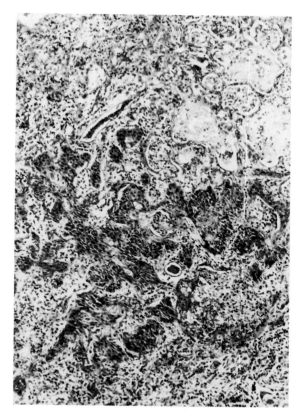

Fig. 14.41. Hyperplastic bronchiolar mucosa in measles pneumonia. Some epithelial cells are hydropic and distended.

Fig. 14.42. Measles pneumonia: squamoid metaplasia of bronchiolar epithelium extending diffusely into alveoli to simulate a carcinoma.

always fatal and symptoms begin about 6–7 years after having natural measles at an early age; it rarely follows vaccination. There are behavioural changes with ataxia and seizures with mental and motor deterioration. High levels of measles antibody are present in cerebrospinal fluid. Incomplete virus particles replicate in the central nervous system and are able to spread from cell to cell while the immune system is unable to overcome the infection (Sever 1983). Pathological lesions may be widespread in the central nervous system and comprise proliferation of microglial cells and astrocytes, with an infiltration of lymphocytes and plasma cells around small blood vessels as well as into the meninges (Fig. 14.44). In longstanding disease focal demyelination occurs. Intranuclear and intracytoplasmic inclusions which stain for measles antigen are found in affected areas (Fig. 14.45). Ultrastructural examination reveals nucleocapsids of paramyxoviruses but no complete measles virus. Infectious measles virus may be recovered after long-term cocultivation and/or fusion with susceptible cells (Kipps et al. 1983).

Another form of encephalitis with measles inclusion bodies occurs in children who are immune-suppressed when becoming infected with measles. The encephalitis develops 1–6 months after the onset of, or exposure to, measles. Pathological lesions comprise focal necrosis with glial proliferation, usually associated with perivascular cuffing. Demyelination is conspicuous, but intranuclear and intracytoplasmic inclusions are frequent and ultrastructural study reveals tubular structures resembling paramyxovirus nucleocapsids (Kipps et al. 1983).

Adenovirus

Adenoviruses produce a variety of illnesses in children. Children less than 5 years of age are particularly susceptible to infection. This is enhanced in day-care centres, orphanages and nursery schools. Respiratory infections are most frequent, but gastrointestinal, cardiac, neurological, lymphatic, cutaneous and urinary manifestations also occur. As with

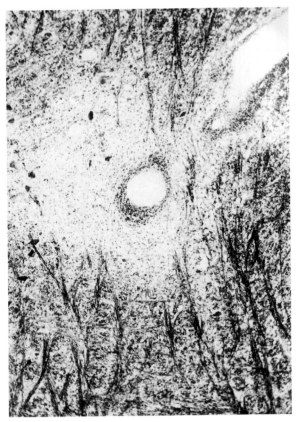

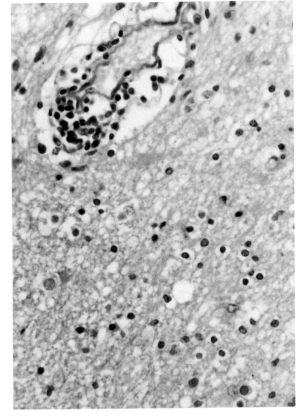

Fig. 14.43. Acute allergic postinfectious encephalitis: demyelination and necrosis around haemorrhagic blood vessels. (Luxol fast blue cresyl violet)

Fig. 14.44. Subacute sclerosing panencephalitis: perivascular cuffing of a small blood vessel by lymphocytes and plasma cells. Microglial proliferation and cells with intranuclear inclusions are present.

herpesvirus, adenovirus infection may be persistent with long periods of latency. The virus has a DNA genome and there are at least 47 antigenic types that affect humans. Adenovirus accounts for a significant proportion of aetiologically identifiable respiratory infections in children. Epidemics of infection occur from time to time in children's hospitals. More frequent and severe disease occurs in the wake of measles and in conditions of poverty, poor housing and malnutrition. Transmission of infection is by aerosolized droplets reaching the nose, throat and conjunctiva, or by the faecal–oral route. The nature of infection depends on the serotype of the virus and the immune status of the host. Cytopathic changes are generally seen 4–5 days after infection in epithelial cells. Infected cells develop intranuclear inclusions and initially respiratory epithelial cells retain their cilia, but after cell death has occurred regenerative epithelial cells lack cilia and are cuboidal. Goblet cells are absent or sparse, but in time there is reconstitution to a normal epithelial structure. In severe

infection there is a necrotizing bronchitis, bronchiolitis and pneumonia. Marked exudation occurs from ulcerated surfaces, with hyaline membrane formation and exudation of cellular debris. Muscle and elastica may be partly or completely destroyed (Becroft 1967; Kaschula et al. 1983) (Fig. 14.46). In bronchi and larger bronchioles a subepithelial infiltration of lymphocytes, plasma cells, macrophages and occasional polymorphonuclear leucocytes occurs. In the lungs there may be extensive necrosis of interstitial walls, with accumulation of much nuclear debris and inclusion-bearing cells in a fibrin-rich inflammatory exudate. At the periphery of such areas, vessels are congested, interstitial walls are oedematous and dilated lymphatics are found. Two types of inclusion are often encountered simultaneously, in large numbers. The first has diffuse accumulation of homogeneous amphophilic or basophilic inclusion material, which fills the nucleus, having pushed the nuclear chromatin to the nuclear membrane. In the second there is discrete basophilic or eosinophilic inclusion material

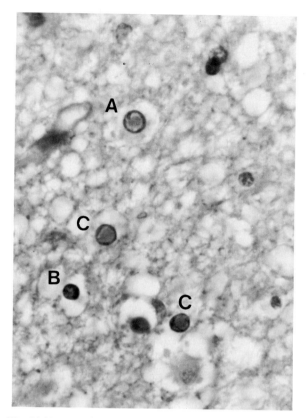

Fig. 14.45. Cowdry type A (*A*), type B (*B*) and intermediate (*C*) intranuclear inclusions in subacute sclerosing panencephalitis.

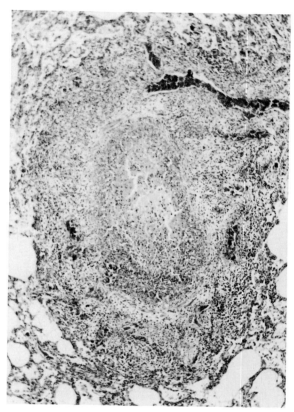

Fig. 14.46. Microscopy of necrotizing bronchiolitis caused by adenovirus type 7a infection, occurring in the wake of measles.

surrounded by a relatively clear zone or halo in the nuclear chromatin. Narrow strands of stainable material seem to link the inclusion to the nuclear membrane. These inclusions have a similarity to those of cytomegalovirus but they are smaller and do not have stainable granules in their cytoplasm (Fig. 14.47). Rarely, one may encounter giant cells with two or three nuclei, all of which may contain similar inclusions. In cells with multiple nuclei the intranuclear inclusions may overlap and give a smudgy appearance. In addition, the nuclear membrane in dying cells may be lost and the inclusion material will have an indistinct smudgy border (Nahmias et al. 1967).

There is much evidence to suggest that post-measles adenovirus infection is an important cause of follicular bronchiectasis, which often develops shortly after measles (Kaschula et al. 1983). In follicular bronchiectasis there is destruction and ectasia of bronchioles and bronchi, abscess formation, parenchymal cysts and a prominent accumulation of lymphoid aggregates around bronchi and bronchioles and in the lung parenchyma.

Other organs that may be involved and have similar inclusions are the liver, lymph nodes, spleen and tonsils. When large numbers of inclusions are present in these organs, there may be focal necrosis. Electron microscopic study of such infected tissues will reveal icosahedral viral particles (60–90 nm in diameter) consisting of a central core and an outer coat. These particles are arranged in a lattice-like pattern or crystalline array within the nucleus (Schonland et al. 1976). In meningoencephalitis there will be oedema and congestion of the brain, often with perivascular cuffing by lymphocytes, and, occasionally, intranuclear inclusions may be found within neurons. Epidemic conjunctivitis has been caused by adenovirus type 8, which affects blood vessels of the conjunctiva, forming small aneurysms and producing oedema, congestion and haemorrhages (Vass 1964). Adenovirus types 7 and 21 have been known to cause bronchiolitis obliterans, a chronic illness that follows severe necrotizing bronchiolitis, which heals by fibrous obliteration of small airways (Becroft 1971; Wohl and Chernick 1978). In recent years adenovirus has been found to be a significant cause of gastroen-

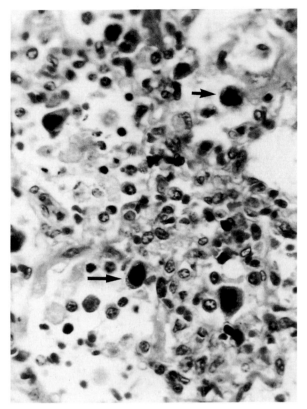

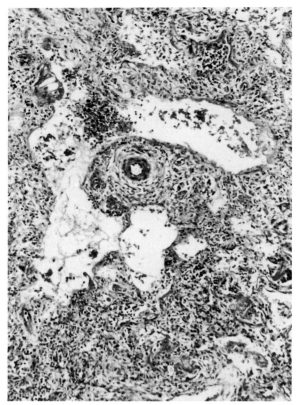

Fig. 14.47. Adenovirus inclusions occurring in pulmonary airspaces, with smudgy edges where the nuclear membranes have been lost (*short arrow*) and a partial halo effect caused by inclusion material not reaching the nuclear membrane (*long arrow*).

Fig. 14.48. Influenza infection causing epithelial necrosis of a terminal bronchiole, local oedema and pleomorphic inflammatory cell infiltration.

teritis in children younger than 4 years (Krajden et al. 1990). The virus is also implicated in young children with intussusception (Porter et al. 1993), where typical inclusions are demonstrable in mucosal epithelial cells.

Influenza Virus

The influenza virus remains an important cause of mortality and morbidity among children with asthma, congenital heart disease and malignancy. In children less than 5 years of age, there is pyrexia, cough, pharyngitis and upper respiratory tract infection. Febrile convulsions are common and patients may have severe abdominal pain with gastrointestinal symptoms, simulating an acute surgical emergency. Pneumonia occurs in most hospitalized cases, and croup, bronchitis and bronchiolitis may be prominent.

In older children and adolescents pyrexia is less intense but there is a sudden onset of severe toxaemia, headache and cough. Abdominal pain, nausea, vomiting and cervical lymphadenopathy are relatively prominent features.

Primary viral pneumonia is characterized by bronchiolar epithelial necrosis, peribronchial lymphocytic infiltration extending into parenchymal interstitium with intra-alveolar haemorrhages, necrosis of alveolar lining cells and hyaline membrane formation (Fig. 14.48). During the recovery phase regenerative alveolar epithelium may be temporarily represented by a monolayer of cuboidal cells.

Other organs that are affected by influenza are the heart, lymph nodes, brain, liver, gastrointestinal tract and striated muscle. The affected heart may be pale and flabby, with scattered petechial haemorrhages being present in the myocardium. Microscopic examination reveals focal interstitial inflammatory infiltration with cardiomyolysis and interstitial oedema. Tracheobronchial lymph glands may become reac-

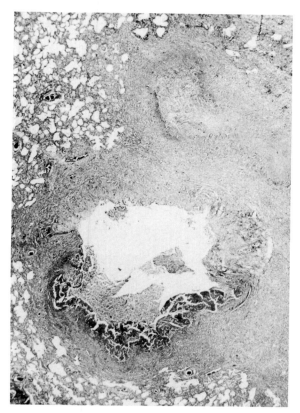

Fig. 14.49. Acute necrotizing bronchiolitis caused by parainfluenza viral infection. There is necrosis of epithelium and muscle with oedema of adjoining tissue.

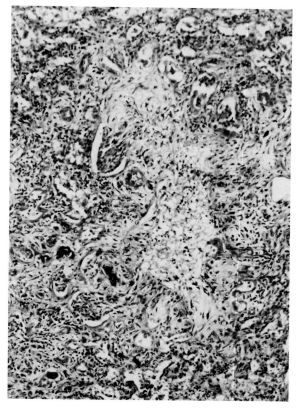

Fig. 14.50. Interstitial pneumonia caused by parainfluenza virus with necrosis of the lining cells of terminal bronchioles, alveolar ducts and alveoli. There is oedema and inflammatory infiltration of interstitial walls with multinucleate giant cells varying in shape and size.

tive, with hyperplasia of sinusoids and follicles. There is oedema, congestion and haemorrhages. Necrosis of germinal centres is often encountered (Oseasohn et al. 1959). The brain is usually oedematous and congested with occasional parenchymal petechial haemorrhages. The liver may be the site of diffuse microgranular fatty change in cases with associated Reye's syndrome (see p. 296). In cases with abdominal pain and diarrhoea, there is necrosis of enterocytes and epithelial cells of pancreatic ducts. This may be associated with a mixed inflammatory cell infiltration into the pancreas. Striated muscle will show rhabdomyolysis with a mild mixed mononuclear inflammatory cell infiltration.

Parainfluenza Virus

Parainfluenza is a frequent cause of lower respiratory tract infection in infants and young children, causing acute laryngotracheobronchitis (croup). Infection is mainly by droplets from other people or animals (serotypes 1–3). Type 3 infection occurs mainly in children aged 6–12 months, whereas types 1, 2 and 4 occur mainly in preschool children. Infection of the respiratory epithelium does not always destroy the cell, which may become hyperplastic and extrude virus. Infection spreads from cell to cell as well as by the bloodstream. In severe infection there is extensive necrosis of epithelium, with prominent inflammatory cell infiltration into subepithelial tissues (Channock et al. 1961; Zinserling 1972). The lumen of infected airways, particularly in the subglottic area, becomes narrowed as a result of inflammatory congestion and oedema, which is responsible for severe respiratory distress and hypoxia. Prominent oedema of subepithelial tissues also occurs in association with acute necrotizing bronchiolitis (Figs. 14.49 and 14.50). Interstitial pneumonia with necrosis of alveolar lining cells, the formation of hyaline membranes and

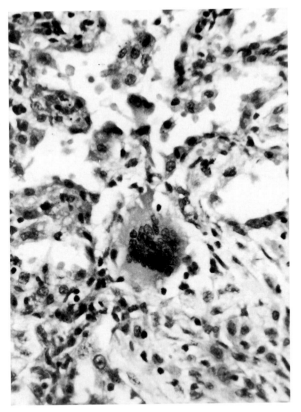

Fig. 14.51. An intra-alveolar giant cell in parainfluenza viral infection. There are no cytoplasmic or nuclear viral inclusions.

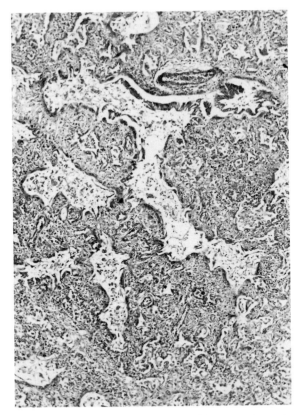

Fig. 14.52. Respiratory syncytial virus (RSV) pneumonia causing necrosis of bronchiolar and alveolar epithelium. Lumina contain copious mucin and cellular debris causing atelectasis. A mild lymphocytic infiltration involves interstitial walls near the bronchiole.

oedema of alveolar walls with occasional multinucleated giant cell formation may be seen in the lungs (Fig. 14.51).

Respiratory Syncytial Virus

Respiratory syncytial virus (RSV) is an important pathogen in infancy and early childhood. The most severe form of disease occurs before 6 months of age while the infant still has maternal antibodies, or after 12 months (Groothuis et al. 1990). Children are frequently reinfected each year. Annual outbreaks of infection occur in most urban communities and most often this is during the winter or spring (Gardner 1977). RSV is the main cause of pneumonia and bronchiolitis in early infancy. More severe forms of infection occur among boys, children who are immunosuppressed and children living in poor housing conditions (Hall et al. 1986). Infection seems to be by direct contact with secretions or large

droplets. The incubation period is between 2 and 8 days. Primary infection occurs on the respiratory epithelium of the nose or conjunctiva. There is cell-to-cell transfer of virus.

In fatal cases, the most significant changes are found in the bronchioles and lungs. There is necrosis of the epithelium of the airways associated with oedema of the walls of the bronchioles. The lumina of the terminal airways become plugged by sloughed epithelium, inflammatory cells and copious mucin (Fig. 14.52). There is a peribronchiolar mononuclear inflammatory cell infiltration consisting predominantly of lymphocytes. Atelectasis and areas of hyperinflation from air trapping may be prominent (Aherne et al. 1970; Ferris et al. 1973). Healing begins within a few days, but may take weeks for full restoration. The regenerative epithelium may have multiple nuclei and is without cilia for about 2 weeks. The mucosal glands of the bronchi and bronchioles may enlarge, and increased numbers of goblet cells are formed. Muscular hypertrophy may persist for a long time (Reid 1977). Pneumonia due to RSV is characterized by interstitial infiltration by lymphocytes and histiocytes, which extends to involve bronchiolar walls. Alveolar walls are expanded by oedema and areas of necrosis in which exudation of fibrin and inflammatory cells into airspaces occurs. Multinucleate giant cells containing intranuclear inclusions may be seen (Fig. 14.53). RSV has been implicated as a cause of sudden infant death syndrome (SIDS) (Downham et al. 1975).

Reovirus

Although most reovirus infections are trivial, they are a noted cause of respiratory and enteric infections in children. In Boston about 50% of schoolchildren have antibodies to Reovirus type 2 (Lerner et al. 1962). Human infection is thought to be mainly by the faecal–oral route, but also occasionally by inhalation. Infected children may have exanthem with rhinorrhoea, pharyngitis, mild fever and diarrhoea (Rosen et al. 1960). In cases of fatal infection there may be an interstitial pneumonia associated with myocarditis, hepatitis and encephalitis (Joske et al. 1964; Tillotson and Lerner 1967).

On the basis of serologic studies Reovirus type 3 has been implicated as a cause of extrahepatic biliary atresia and neonatal hepatitis (Glaser et al. 1984; Brown et al. 1988), but contrary evidence has also been presented (Dussaix et al. 1984).

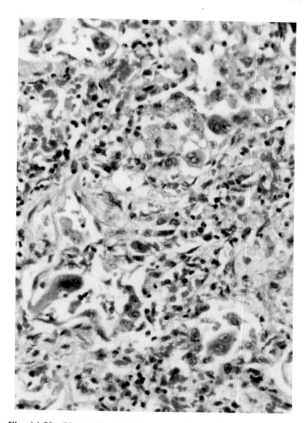

Fig. 14.53. Giant cells in RSV pneumonia at high magnification. One giant cell has indistinct intranuclear inclusion material.

Non-polio Enteroviruses: Coxsackievirus and Echovirus

These viruses frequently cause mild non-specific febrile illness, but some types are associated with a severe and fatal course. The enteroviruses have been classified into three sub-categories: poliovirus, Coxsackievirus and echovirus. However, as some strains have been reclassified into other genuses or categories, it is becoming convenient to call them all enterovirus followed by a specific type number. The more recently identified types are Enterovirus 68–72. There are some minor cross-reactions between strains of Coxsackievirus and echovirus, but there are no common antigens that would be of diagnostic value. Humans are the natural hosts for these viruses, although many animals, birds and molluscs may be infected. Transmission is mainly by the faecal–oral and oral–oral routes.

There is much variation in clinical expression of infection. This largely depends on the tropism of the virus, its type, the age and HLA blood group of the patient, and the dose of infection. Expression of

infection may include the common cold, pharyngitis, herpangina, parotitis, croup, bronchitis, bronchiolitis, pneumonia, pleurodynia, acute diarrhoeal disease, constipation, vomiting, mesenteric adenitis, pancreatitis, juvenile-onset diabetes, hepatitis, acute haemorrhagic conjunctivitis, photophobia, myocarditis, pericarditis, epididymitis, orchitis, nephritis, acute arthritis, myositis, various xanthomatous reactions, aseptic meningitis, encephalitis, Guillain–Barré syndrome, SIDS, congenital anomalies, abortion, prematurity and stillbirth.

Primary infection is usually in the pharynx and lower alimentary tract, with involvement of draining lymph nodes. After 3 days there is minor viraemia leading to disseminated infection and the onset of symptoms. This is followed by major viraemia and dissemination of the disease. Neonatal infections are more severe than infections in older infants and children.

Coxsackievirus A usually causes mild illness, but has been isolated from the brain of SIDS cases without demonstrable lesions being seen (Gold et al. 1961). Coxsackievirus B commonly causes severe myocarditis, meningoencephalitis and lesions of adrenal glands, pancreas, liver, lungs and striated muscle.

Echovirus occasionally causes fatal disease in infants and children. There is usually enlargement and congestion of the liver with hepatic necrosis (Philip and Larson 1973). Echovirus 11 has been reported to be associated with cot deaths as well as an acute shock-like illness with diffuse haemorrhages attributed to disseminated intravascular coagulation in infants (Berry and Nagington 1982). The kidneys, adrenal medulla, gastrointestinal tract and central nervous system are most often affected in severe echoviral infections.

Poliomyelitis

In common with other enteroviruses, poliovirus has a single-stranded RNA genome. Epidemics of infection occurred regularly until the introduction of vaccines in the late 1950s and early 1960s. During epidemics more than 90% of paralytic cases were children aged less than 5 years, but inapparent non-paralytic infections far outnumbered clinically apparent disease. Transmission is evidently by the faecal–oral route. The incubation period is 7–10 days.

Infection of the central nervous system may occur via the bloodstream or peripheral nerves. Affected neurons become swollen and then shrink. As they undergo necrosis, there is chromolysis and neuronophagia. Involvement is associated with congestion and inflammatory cell infiltration of the meninges. There may be intense inflammatory cell infiltration, initially including polymorphonuclear leucocytes but followed by lymphocytes, plasma cells and macrophages. Satellitosis around degenerating neuronal cells is seen. Only a proportion of the neuronal cells in an affected area undergo necrosis. Loss of neuronal cell bodies is followed by degeneration of axons and neurogenic atrophy of muscle. Healed lesions are seen as foci of neuronal cell loss, with some astrocytic gliosis and collapse of supporting tissue. The anterior horn cells of the lumbar and cervical regions and sensory neurons are most often affected. In the brain the main sites are the vestibular nuclei, reticular formation of the pons and medulla, cerebellar vermis and basal ganglia.

Infectious Mononucleosis (Epstein–Barr Virus Infection)

Epstein–Barr virus (EBV) has structural similarities to herpesvirus with a DNA genome. It is fragile and easily inactivated. Transmission is by close interpersonal contact, mainly through saliva. Young children often experience a subclinical or mild non-specific illness. Most infections manifest pyrexia, malaise, fatigue, tonsillitis, pharyngitis and lymphadenopathy. Splenomegaly and hepatomegaly with or without cholestasis may follow. Infection is followed by prolonged shedding of virus in oropharyngeal secretions (Niederman et al. 1976). There is a long incubation period ranging from 30 to 50 days. Various types of immune deficiency predispose persons infected with EBV to potentially fatal lymphoproliferative diseases, B-cell lymphomas (including Burkitt's lymphoma) and severe atypical infection. In the X-linked lymphoproliferative syndrome, there is selective vulnerability to EBV, terminating in agammaglobulinaemia, fatal infectious mononucleosis or lymphoma (Purtilo et al. 1985) (see also p. 600). Infection with EBV is also associated with nasopharyngeal carcinoma in children.

Following infection there is intense stimulation of the lymphoreticular tissues by EBV, which has tropism for B lymphocytes. A brisk immune response with increased production of cytotoxic-suppressor (T8) lymphocytes and prominent natural killer cell activity follows (Schooley et al. 1984). In infectious mononucleosis atypical lymphocytes (inactivated T lymphocytes) are found in the peripheral blood. The EBV genome is not carried in the atypical cells but in B lymphocytes (Pagano 1975). The genome exists in a state of latency in B lymphocytes, and there is a lifelong potential for reactivation (Sheldon et al. 1973). There is, however, continuous shedding of the virus from the parotid gland (Morgan et al. 1979). Circulating cytotoxic T killer cells capable of lysing EBV genome are always present (Svedmyr and Jondal 1975).

Atypical lymphocytes are slightly enlarged and have a pale blue vacuolated cytoplasm with a scalloped border. The oval or indented nucleus has a coarse network of chromatin. The cells have a heterogeneous appearance relative to the monomorphic appearance encountered in Burkitt's lymphoma. These atypical lymphocytes may be sufficiently bizarre to resemble lymphoblasts of acute leukaemia (Fig. 14.54). In affected enlarged lymph nodes there may be some effacement of architecture with enlargement of the paracortex and some follicular hyperplasia (Fig. 14.55). Atypical lymphocytes are present in the sinusoids, and there may be focal necrosis. Occasionally, cells resembling Reed–Sternberg cells may be found. Splenic enlargement is due to infiltration by atypical lymphocytes into the red pulp, which is not associated with follicular hyperplasia. The atypical cells also infiltrate into the capsule, the trabeculae and the walls of blood vessels. Rupture of

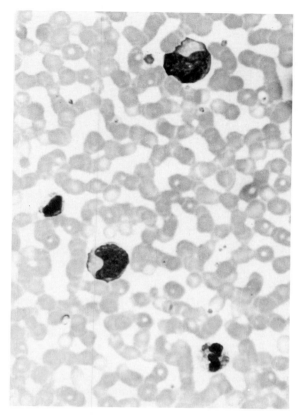

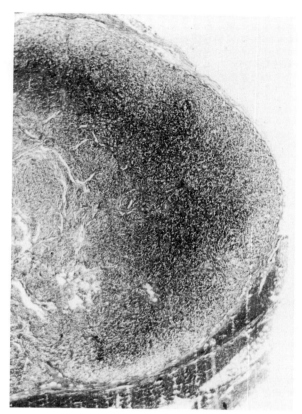

Fig. 14.54. Atypical lymphocytes on a blood smear from a patient with infectious mononucleosis. The two atypical lymphocytes are enlarged and have scalloped borders, indented nuclei with coarse chromatin and pale vacuolated cytoplasm.

Fig. 14.55. Lymph node in infectious mononucleosis showing effacement of architecture with widening of the paracortex and a hyperplastic follicle.

the spleen may occur following minor trauma. In the liver there is infiltration of mononuclear cells into the sinusoids and the portal tracts. Focal non-epithelioid granulomatous necrosis may occur. Mononuclear infiltration of heart, pancreas, brain and lung has also been encountered (Seemayer et al. 1981).

Acquired Herpes Simplex Virus Infections
(see also p. 678)

The herpes group of viruses (herpes simplex virus, EBV, cytomegalovirus, varicella–zoster virus and human herpesvirus 6) are relatively large, with double-standard DNA genomes. There are two serological subtypes of herpes simplex virus (HSV). Infection is through close interpersonal contact by direct apposition with infected tissue, saliva or mucus. There is a danger of extended primary infection in abraded skin, especially in burn patients, patients with eczema and infants with nappy rash.

Neonatal HSV infection is mainly due to type 2 virus from the maternal birth canal. The virus has tropism for epithelial cells of ectodermal origin, especially skin and mucous membranes. Infected cells swell and degenerate, but a small number of multinucleate giant cells may form. The infected cells usually develop intranuclear inclusions with marginated nuclear chromatin (Cowdry type A inclusion). There is thus a narrow halo separating inclusion material from the nuclear membrane with the aggregated chromatin. At the site of infection much intercellular oedema develops, which leads to the formation of a vesicle. The surrounding tissues become erythematous and have congested blood vessels. Rupture of the vesicle generally leads to secondary bacterial infection, the formation of a pustule and encrustation. The lesions are superficial and there is no scarring (Fig. 14.56). Infection of the eye may involve the conjunctiva and cornea, and may be mild and localized or extend to produce significant ulceration and scarring with visual impairment. In a small number

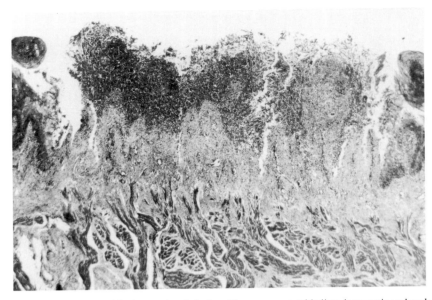

Fig. 14.56. Ulceration of the tongue caused by herpesvirus infection. The squamous epithelium is necrotic and replaced by an irregular floor of granular necrotic debris with a mild vascular response but no scarring.

of cases encephalitis follows primary infection. The orbital region of the frontal lobes and the bases of the temporal lobes are then most often affected. Focal lesions consisting of necrosis with local oedema, but sometimes progressing to extensive diffuse oedema, giving signs of raised intracranial pressure, may be encountered. Focal lesions are usually associated with small haemorrhages. Latent infection seems to be in sensory neural ganglia innervating tissues originally involved by the primary infection. When reactivation occurs it is in the region of the primary infection.

Varicella–Zoster

Varicella–zoster is a member of the herpes group of viruses with a DNA genome. It may be isolated from vesicle fluid, and electron microscopic examination of such fluid was useful in its differentiation from vaccinia and smallpox. The virus is labile and hence is only transmitted by direct person-to-person contact. On rare occasions transplacental infection of the fetus occurs during the first trimester of pregnancy (Siegel 1973).

The chickenpox exanthem usually starts on the scalp or trunk and spreads to other sites. Mucous membranes and conjunctiva may also be involved. The vesicles are in the superficial squamous epithelium and may be preceded by small erythematous macular lesions before becoming vesicular. Later the vesicles encrust and may become infected by bacteria. Microscopically, the lesions are indistinguishable from those of herpesvirus. As with herpesvirus, there may be dissemination of infection to the lungs, liver and adrenals in children with a compromised cellular immune system. Meningoencephalitis, thrombocytopenia, myocarditis, arthritis, Guillain–Barré syndrome, nephritis and Reye's syndrome are uncommon complications that may occur.

Acquired Cytomegalovirus Infections

Cytomegalovirus is a member of the herpes group of viruses, having a DNA genome, a state of latency and persistent shedding of virus. The virus is labile, and hence transmission is mainly by direct person-to-person contact. Severe infections have followed organ transplantation or blood transfusion from carrier donors. The organism is shed into saliva, breast milk, urine, semen, uterine cervix, the gastrointestinal tract and blood. Most children become infected before reaching adulthood. Some primary infections may be associated with mild interstitial pneumonitis or mild anicteric hepatitis. Sometimes primary infection is manifested as pyrexia of unknown origin with or without lymphadenopathy. Reactivation of latent infection with wide dissemination may occur when children are therapeutically immune suppressed, are malnourished or have AIDS. All organ systems are susceptible to infection, but the salivary gland ducts, proximal renal tubules, pulmonary pneumocytes and phagocytic cells of the brain are prone to harbour the virus. There is a slow cycle of replication, with minimal and focal evidence of tissue necrosis.

Mumps

Mumps virus produces a highly contagious generalized infection characterized by fever and parotitis. In some young children the infection is subclinical whereas adolescents are usually severely ill with systemic symptoms. The virus belongs to the paromyxoviruses and has a single-stranded RNA genome. Transmission is mainly by inhalation, and the organism may be isolated from throat swabs from 2 days before until 7 days after the onset of parotid swelling (Deinhardt and Shramek 1970). The incubation period for infection is usually 16–18 days.

Before the introduction of a vaccine, about 50% of children were infected before 5 years, the peak age of onset being between 3 and 4 years. Mumps produces a generalized infection, although emphasis is most often focused on the parotid glands. Parotitis is usually bilateral, but may be unilateral, and occasionally there is involvement of other salivary glands. The infected salivary glands become swollen and oedematous and there may be small capsular haemorrhages. Microscopically, there are degenerative changes in duct epithelium with infiltration by lymphocytes and macrophages around the ducts. Acinar cells are usually not affected, but some pressure atrophy may occur.

Meningoencephalitis due to mumps is uncommon. When it occurs early in the disease, it is considered to represent replication of the virus within neurons and is associated with neuronophagia, satellitosis by inflammatory cells and perivascular cuffing. Late-onset encephalitis is considered to be an allergic post infectious demyelinating process (Taylor and Torenson 1963). Deafness may occur after acute mumps and is not necessarily associated with encephalitis; it is considered to be due to labyrinthitis and retrograde demyelination. The deafness is usually unilateral. Pancreatitis is considered to be a common cause for abdominal pain and to contribute to hyperamylasaemia. Inflammation is usually self-limiting, although haemorrhagic pancreatitis with pseudocyst formation does occur (Feldstein et al. 1974). Diabetes sometimes develops after mumps infection but is not related to the severity of pancreatitis.

Nephritis with haematuria and polyuria has been reported as a cause of death (Hughes et al. 1966). Orchitis with focal haemorrhage, necrosis and poly-

morphonuclear leucocyte infiltration occurs mainly in adults and adolescent boys.

Inclusion body myositis, which mainly occurs during the second and third decades of life, has recently been linked to persistent infection with mumps. There is progressive weakness of distal and proximal muscles with both neurogenic and myopathic features. Microscopically, there are features of polymyositis with rimmed vacuoles having basophilic granules within the sarcoplasm of affected fibres (Chou 1986).

Acquired Parvovirus Infection

This disease (erythema infectiosum) has recently been attributed to Parvovirus B19 (Anderson et al. 1983). It causes a minor acute illness with malar erythema (slapped cheeks), a generalized reticular or lace-like maculopapular eruption mainly on the limbs, and mild constitutional symptoms (arthralgia in adults). Outbreaks of infection occur in schools and institutions, mainly during the winter and spring in temperate climates. The incubation period is 4–14 days (Cherry 1992). Parvovirus are among the smallest viruses (20–25 nm) having a DNA genome, and mimic the particles of hepatitis B virus surface antigen (HBsAg). B19 is the only serotype.

Infection is by the respiratory tract, and following viraemia there seems to be tropism for early erythrocytic precursor cells. There is severe reticulocytopenia with some neutropenia, lymphopenia and thrombocytopenia. Skin biopsies taken during the exanthematous stage have not shown specific features. Dilatation of blood vessels with lymphocytic and occasional plasma cell perivascular infiltration have been reported (Grimmer and Joseph 1959). Infection has been found to cause aplastic crisis in sickle cell disease (Pattison et al. 1981) and in hereditary erythrocytic multinuclearity associated with a positive acidified (Hams) test (HEMPAS) (West et al. 1986). It is considered that parvovirus infection may be the cause of transient haemolytic anaemia (Mortimer 1986) and that it may have a role in idiopathic aplastic anaemia (Bentley 1986). Immunocompromised children, particularly those with acute lymphocytic leukaemia, may develop persistent anaemia as a consequence of B19 infection.

Viral Gastrointestinal Infections

Rotavirus

Rotavirus was first regarded as a cause of infantile gastroenteritis in 1973 by Bishop et al. As the name implies, the virus resembles a wheel measuring approximately 70 nm in diameter and has a double-stranded RNA genome. There are several serotypes. Transmission is by the faecal–oral route, and the organism is highly contagious, with frequent nosocomial infections in hospitals. The incubation period is less than 48 h. In temperate regions infection occurs mainly during the winter months. The peak age incidence is between 6 months and 3 years. High infant mortality rates in developing countries are partly attributed to this virus (Househam et al. 1988).

Duodenal biopsies in rotavirus gastroenteritis reveal shortened blunted villi with increased lymphocytes and plasma cells in the lamina propria. Surface enterocytes become cuboidal and lose their brush border. Often there are reduced disaccharidase levels within the cells. Morphology may be restored to normal within 48 h of the onset of infection (Mebus et al. 1977). Symptoms last between 2 and 14 days, but most often the duration is 5 or 6 days. Complications of the disease include intussusception, Reye's syndrome, encephalitis, haemolytic uraemic syndrome and disseminated intravascular coagulopathy.

Norwalk Agent

"Norwalk agent infection" refers to infection with a virus-like particle measuring 27 nm in diameter and first seen by Kapikian et al. in 1972. The agent has not been cultivated in vitro, but volunteers have been infected (Dolin et al. 1971). The agent is highly contagious and transmission seems to be from faeces and/or vomitus (Greenberg et al. 1979). The incubation period for infection is 1–2 days, and infection usually lasts for less than 48 h (Blacklow et al. 1972).

Biopsies of small intestines of cases show villous shortening with crypt hypertrophy and increased cellularity of the lamina propria, including infiltration by neutrophils. Surface enterocytes become disorganized, increased mitoses appear in the crypts and brush border enzyme activity is depressed (Schreiber et al. 1973).

Other Virus Infections

Other viruses that primarily infect the gastrointestinal tract and may cause diarrhoeal disease are enteroviruses and adenoviruses. Caliciviruses and astrovirus are small round virus particles similar to Norwalk agent, known to cause diarrhoea in animals, and are occasionally identified in humans without yet having been shown to be human pathogens.

Post-infection Diarrhoea

Persistent diarrhoea that follows viral infection of the gastrointestinal tract seems to be brought about by a number of mechanisms. These include:

1. Reduction of the absorptive surface by decrease of the villous surface : crypt ratio and loss of microvilli
2. Replacement of specialized absorptive villous tip cells by secretory crypt cells
3. Inflammatory exudation with inflammatory cells secreted into the intestinal contents and stimulation of adenyl cyclase
4. Loss of brush border lactase with consequent passage of unhydrolysed lactose in the large bowel and subsequent oxygenation by intestinal bacteria to lactic acid, which is an irritant

Mycoplasma and Ureaplasma Infections

Mycoplasmas and ureaplasmas are the smallest free-living organisms known to survive outside host cells. There are more than 100 recognized species, 13 of which infect humans. *Mycoplasma pneumoniae, M. hominis* and *Ureaplasma urealyticum* are aetiologically related to disease. *M. pneumoniae* is the most prevalent and most important. All members of these species lack a cell wall, are pleomorphic and do not stain well with the usual bacteriological dyes. Their size varies from that of myxoviruses (120–150 nm) to that of small bacteria. They are able to multiply in cell-free media by binary fission, and their growth is inhibited by specific antibody (Broughton 1986).

Mycoplasma

Mycoplasma has a worldwide distribution, but infections are more frequently diagnosed in temperate zones. Infection is most prevalent in the 5–9 and 10–14 years age groups. Pneumonia due to *M. pneumoniae* is very uncommon in infants less than 6 months of age. This may be because of protection from maternally derived antibodies. The incubation period for infection varies between 1 and 3 weeks, but is usually 11–14 days (Biberfeld and Sterner 1969). Within families the disease is highly communicable, although slow to spread: approximately 65% of family members become infected from an index case. In schools the communicability rate is slightly lower. Individuals may suffer recurrent infections.

Infection is acquired by the respiratory route from small particle aerosols and large droplets of secretion.

M. pneumoniae has an attachment factor which reacts with receptors on host cells to enable the organism to become attached to sensitive epithelial cells. Once attached, the organism remains extracellular but causes cell damage. Cell injury is associated with defective ciliary action of respiratory epithelium. Although infection in young children is frequent, symptomatic disease occurs most often in older children and young adults. Immunodeficient animals experience a less severe form of disease than immunocompetent controls (Clyde 1979).

Pathological changes are seen in the epithelium of bronchi, bronchioles and alveoli. Changes are less conspicuous in the trachea and upper respiratory tract, where ciliated epithelium may become degenerate. In the distal air passages there is shedding of epithelial cells with exudation of fibrin and mononuclear inflammatory cells into the lumina. The walls of bronchi and bronchioles become oedematous and there is peribronchial infiltration by lymphocytes, macrophages and plasma cells. Alveolar walls become thickened because of congested blood vessels and an infiltration of lymphocytes and macrophages. Focal interstitial haemorrhages may be seen. Pneumonia and bronchiolitis may be associated with pharyngitis (present in 32% of infected children), otitis media (present in 27% of patients with pneumonia) (Stevens et al. 1978), sinusitus and croup.

An erythematous maculopapular rash involving the trunk and back often occurs (Foy et al. 1970). Its distribution is variable and may also be associated with conjunctivitis. Microscopy of affected skin shows mild acanthosis with marked intracellular oedema. A mixed polymorphonuclear and mononuclear inflammatory cell infiltration into the upper dermis occurs, which may be associated with haemorrhagic foci. Blisters form, which contain plasma and polymorphonuclear leucocytes. Other complications of infection include haemolytic anaemia, gastroenteritis (which may be associated with mesenteric adenitis), anicteric hepatitis (in which focal necrosis of the liver may be seen), pancreatitis, splenomegaly with follicular hyperplasia, a flitting polyarthritis, acute myocarditis, haemorrhagic encephalitis and acute transverse myelitis.

M. hominis and *M. fermentans* have caused persistent infection in blood, bones, joints and kidneys in immunodeficient patients (Bauer et al. 1991).

Ureaplasma

Ureaplasma is distinguished from *Mycoplasma* in that it has the ability to hydrolyse urea. There is one species, *U. urealyticum,* with 8–11 serotypes. The reservoir for human infection is the genital tract of adult men and women. Infants become infected in utero from chorioamnionitis or as they pass through the birth canal during childbirth. The organism may be recovered from infected infants for up to 2 years after birth, and thereafter infection is rare until after adolescence, when sexual activity begins. Infants that have been infected or exposed to the organisms in utero are often of low birth weight and fail to thrive. Cases of neonatal pneumonia with persistent pulmonary hypertension and meningitis with hydrocephalus have been reported (Waites et al. 1989; 1990).

Fungal Infections

Compared with other infectious agents, fungi rarely cause overt disease in children. Fungal infections are, however, of special interest as they tend to cause protracted illness, often difficult to diagnose, and have high morbidity and mortality rates. Subclinical infections with some fungi, especially *Candida albicans* and *Histoplasma capsulatum*, are common in children. Systemic infection by fungi tends to be associated with the administration of cytotoxic immunosuppressive agents, steroids, prolonged use of antibiotics and malnutrition.

Fungal organisms that cause superficial skin infections (dermatomycoses) lead a predominantly saprophytic existence and only rarely penetrate into the dermis. The incidence of infection is highest in tropical humid climates, and boys are affected more often than girls. Ringworm of the scalp (tinea capitis), caused by species of the genera *Microsporum* and *Trichophyton*, is extremely common in children aged 5–10 years. More than 40% of children in certain South African institutions and orphanages have been found to be infected, whereas in the USA rates of 4.5% and 8.2% have been reported (Terreni 1961; Bocobo et al. 1965). Tinea pedis (athletes foot) and tinea cruris (dhobie itch) occur mainly in adolescents and young adults. However, tinea unguium (a nail plate fungal infection) mainly occurs in older children who also have a scalp ringworm (Padhye 1973).

Candida

Candida albicans is the most common species of the fungus causing disease in humans, but other species of *Candida* are becoming increasingly responsible for infections. Many factors are known to increase susceptibility to infection. These include all causes of depressed cellular immunity, various endocrine dis-

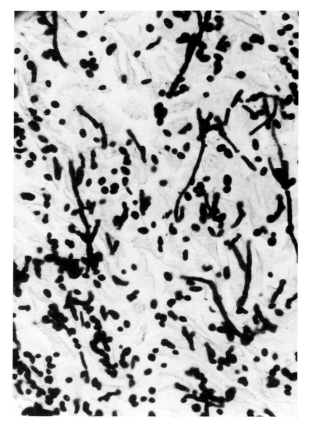

Fig. 14.57. Smear from the oral membrane in thrush, stained with Gomori methenamine silver. Budding yeasts occur together with hyphae and pseudohyphae (constricted at the cell junctions).

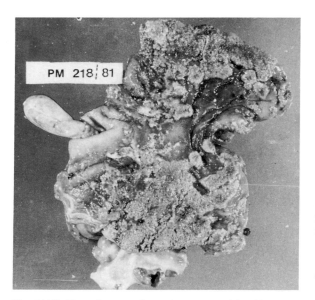

Fig. 14.58. Heaped-up pseudomembranous gastritis with ulceration caused by *Candida* infection.

orders (especially diabetes), anaemia, malignancy, prolonged antibiotic usage, indwelling catheters, hypovitaminosis A, burns and prematurity.

Thrush

Oral thrush due to invasion of the mucosa of the mouth occurs in many newborn infants, in whom pneumonia due to *Candida* is uncommon. Infection is often acquired from the genital tract of the mother, and the infant is usually bottle-fed. The focal lesions in the mouth have a creamy white pseudomembrane consisting of budding yeast with septate hyphae (Fig. 14.57). Removal of the membrane leaves a bleeding surface. Often the angles of the mouth become involved, where cracks and fissures covered by a creamy membrane appear.

Nappy Rash

Nappy rash is an eczematous and erosive dermatitis that develops in the moist area of a nappy in infants with diarrhoeal disease and candida infection of the gastrointestinal tract. The peak age incidence is 1–4 months. Initially macules and papules form, which progress to weeping and ulceration. The ulcers have a red base with scalloped overhanging borders.

Congenital Systemic Infection

Congenital systemic infection is usually a consequence of amniotic fluid infection or blood spread to the fetus across the placenta. When amniotic fluid infection syndrome is the underlying cause, the lungs and the gastrointestinal tract are most prominently involved. Lesions may also occur in the kidneys, liver, spleen and brain. Meningitis is increasingly becoming a life-threatening complication (Buchs 1985).

Gastroenteritis

Gastroenteritis is caused by invasive growth of the organism on the mucosa of the stomach and intestines (Fig. 14.58). Invasive growth on the mucosa of the stomach has been associated with neonatal gastric perforation.

Systemic Candidiasis

Systemic candidiasis occurs in children who are immunocompromised from leukaemia, steroid

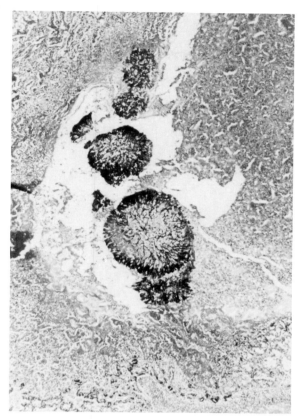

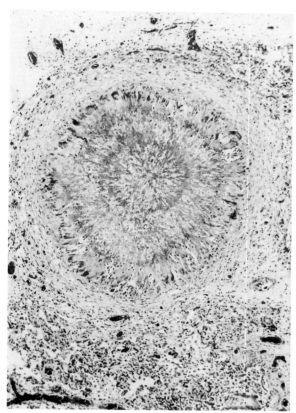

Fig. 14.59. Low-magnification microscopy of an aspergilloma occurring in a pulmonary tuberculous cavity of an 11-month-old girl with kwashiorkor.

Fig. 14.60. Invasive pulmonary infection by *Aspergillus* in a marasmic child, producing a progressively expanding, well defined, rounded lesion with central necrosis, peripheral invasion, chronic inflammation and fibrosis.

therapy, major surgery during the neonatal period, peritoneal dialysis or parenteral nutrition, and produces disseminated low-grade inflammatory lesions. The children may have endocarditis with vegetations occurring on normal heart valves, particularly when indwelling catheters are present in the venous system or after prophylactic antibiotic therapy for major surgery. Meningitis due to *C. albicans* occurs as a consequence of systemic infection in both newborn infants and older children. Affected children often develop a maculopapular rash, endophthalmitis and lymphadenitis.

Aspergillus

Aspergillus is a rare cause of infection in paediatric practice. Children with defective phagocytic activity, as occurs in chronic granulomatous disease (Dean et al. 1993), leukaemia and other primary haematological malignancies, are prone to infection by both

Candida and *Aspergillus* (Levine et al. 1974). Sites that are usually affected are the external ear, nasal sinuses, lungs, eyes, genitourinary tract and heart, as well as skin, bone and brain from traumatic inoculation. Immunocompromised children are more likely to suffer invasive spread from paranasal sinuses to adjoining tissues, aspergilloma in a pre-existing pulmonary cavity (Fig. 14.59), invasive lung disease (Figs. 14.60 and 14.61) and disseminated blood-borne infection.

Zygomycosis

Infection with Zygomycetes has often been referred to as mucormycosis or phycomycosis. The fungi in this group are normally found in soil and on fruit and vegetables. They lead to rapidly fatal infections in hospitalized immunosuppressed children. Newborn, diabetic and malnourished children are also particularly prone to infection (Kahn 1963). The distinctive

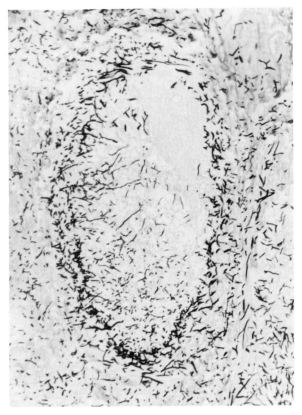

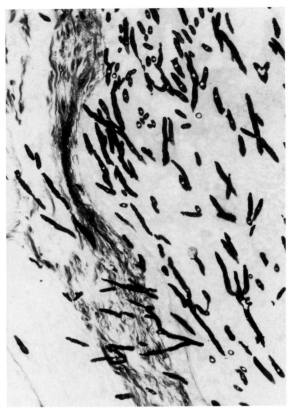

Fig. 14.61. Invasion of a thrombosed pulmonary vein by *Aspergillus*, having small septate hyphae and exhibiting dichotomous branching. (Gomori methenamine silver stain)

Fig. 14.62. An 8-year-old girl with acute leukaemia and fata disseminated fungal infection. Sparsely septate haphazardly branched hyphae of *Mucor* transversing the wall of a vein. (Gomori methenamine silver)

capacity of the organism to penetrate blood vessel walls is shown in Figs. 14.62 and 14.63. Following such penetration there is usually widespread haematogenous dissemination, but in children there is a tendency for the infection to affect stomach and intestines, where perforation and massive haemorrhages occur as complications. In newborn infants, infection may be associated with circulatory collapse and features of necrotizing enterocolitis (Woodward et al. 1992).

Cryptococcosis

Cryptococcosis, also known as torulosis, is caused by *Cryptococcus neoformans* and mainly affects pigeon fanciers and persons who have become immunosuppressed. Disseminated infection often occurs in older boys (Figs. 14.64–14.66) and adults. Primary pul-

monary lesions occur as a consequence of inhalation of organisms, but involvement of the brain and meninges as a result of haematogenous spread is more frequently clinically diagnosed (Fig. 14.67). The tissue response to infection varies between a mucous cavity with many macrophages to a granuloma with many lymphocytes, giant cells and fibroblasts. Large numbers of organisms are found in the lesions.

Histoplasmosis

Histoplasma capsulatum var. *duboisii* has a worldwide distribution, often occurring in the soil of chicken runs and caves frequented by bats. Primary infection usually occurs at an early age in lungs and draining lymph nodes, where the lesions undergo fibrosis and may calcify. The clinical and pathological manifestations

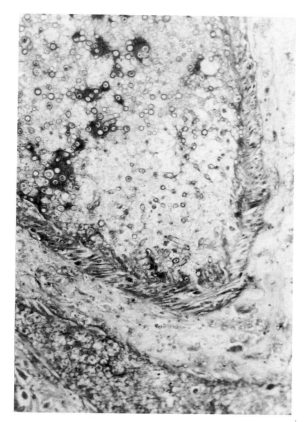

Fig. 14.63. Cross-sections of broad empty hyphae of *Mucor* proliferating within the lumen of a blood vessel and resembling *Coccidioides*. Leukaemic child with pulmonary infection. (H&E)

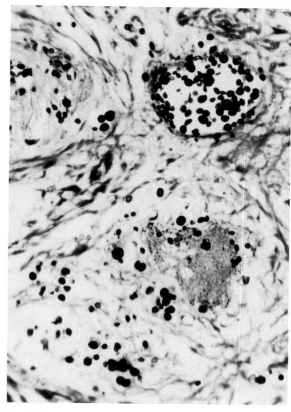

Fig. 14.64. Free-lying and phagocytosed *Cryptococcus neoformans* showing the narrow base of budding yeasts. A 7-year-old boy with Hodgkin's lymphoma and infected abdominal lymph nodes. (Gomori methenamine silver)

are similar to tuberculosis. Cellular immune responses are depressed early in infection, while antibody titres rise. There is a tendency for children to have disseminated infection involving spleen, liver, lymph nodes, pancreas, adrenals, eyes, central nervous system and bone marrow. Primary gastrointestinal infection has been reported in children (Soper et al. 1970). In a South American study of 19 fatal cases, 63% occurred in prepubertal children (36% before the first birthday), boys being affected twice as often as girls (Salfelder et al. 1970).

Histoplasma capsulatum var. *duboisii* occurs together with *H. capsulatum* in middle Africa between the Sahara and the Limpopo river. Infection is most prevalent in boys and young men. The organism has tropism for skin and bones, where numerous yeasts may be found. Draining lymph nodes are frequently involved and, unlike in infection by *H. capsulatum*, the lesions rarely calcify. The yeasts are relatively resistant to

digestion after being phagocytosed by macrophages and giant cells (Fig. 14.68).

Coccidioidomycosis

Coccidioidomycosis is due to infection by *Coccidiodes immitis*, which occurs in semi-arid regions of the western hemisphere, the former USSR and Australia. Primary infection is mostly in the lungs as a consequence of inhaling the fungus, but skin puncture by contaminated objects may also initiate the disease. Disseminated infection is more frequent in immunosuppressed persons living in endemic areas. Young infants have increased susceptibility to disseminated disease. Primary lesions are characterized by granulomas containing giant cells, macrophages and acute inflammatory cells. There is localization of the organisms to lungs and regional

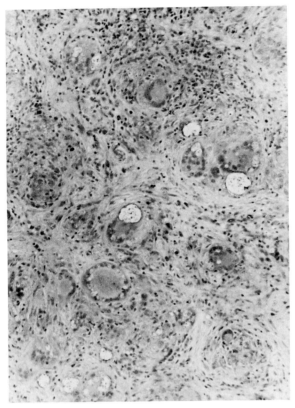

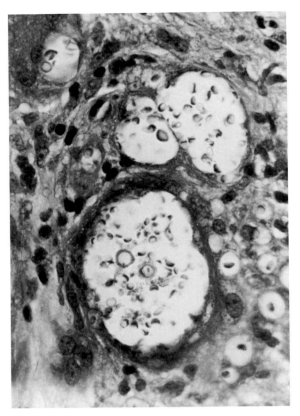

Fig. 14.65. Fibromucinous lymphadenitis caused by *Cryptococcus neoformans* with numerous phagocytosed yeasts in multinucleate giant cells. (Same case as Fig. 14.64.)

Fig. 14.66. Cryptococcal lymphadenitis showing encapsulated and non-encapsulated yeasts, free lying and phagocytosed by giant cells at high magnification. (Same case as in Figs. 14.64 and 14.65.)

lymph nodes in most infections (Pappagianis 1972). Disseminated lesions occur in bone, lymph nodes, soft tissues and meninges (Kafka and Catanzaro 1981).

Sporotrichosis

Primary infection by *Sporothrix schenckii* is a subacute or chronic epithelioid granulomatous process of skin, mucous membranes or lungs. There is a worldwide distribution with greater prevalence in warm temperate regions. Cutaneous infection usually follows scratches from thorns, grasses, wooden splinters or tree bark, whereas pulmonary infection occurs by inhalation of spores. Childhood infection has been reported following exposure to hay, junk and domestic animals (Singer and Muncie 1952). Pulmonary lesions are often misdiagnosed as tuberculosis because of the development of cavities or fibrocaseous lesions with lymph node involvement. Multiple bone and joint lesions often occur which

resemble typical osteomyelitis or arthritis with hypertrophic synovium and degeneration of articular cartilage. Following inoculation into skin there is hyperkeratosis, parakeratosis, pseudoepitheliomatous hyperplasia and the formation of intradermal microabscesses (Lurie and Still 1969). The classic lesion is of a chronic granuloma with an asteroid body in the centre. The asteroid body is derived from antigen–antibody complexes and inflammatory cell debris (Williams et al. 1969).

Rhinosporidiosis

Rhinosporidium seeberi causes slowly enlarging polypoid or papilliferous tumours with a vegetative wart-like appearance that most often occur on the conjunctiva or nose. Most infections occur in childhood and manifest as relatively asymptomatic growths. The peak age of definitive diagnosis is 20–40 years. As the lesions enlarge, they cause irritation, after which autoinfection of other sites may

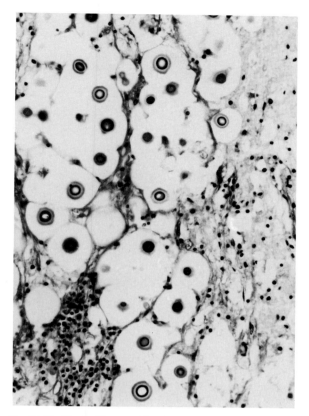

Fig. 14.67. Meningitis caused by *Cryptococcus neoformans* seen as dispersed yeast-like organisms having a refractile PAS-positive mucopolysaccharide capsule. The 6-year-old daughter of a pigeon fancier. (PAS)

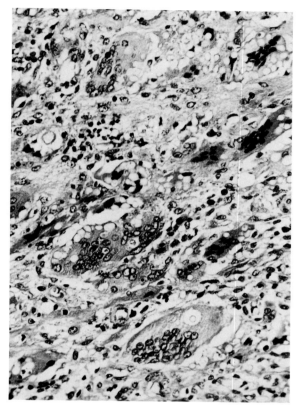

Fig. 14.68. African histoplasmosis of the subcutis in a 12-year-old cattle herder. Numerous surviving yeasts have been phagocytosed by macrophages and multinucleate giant cells.

occur from scratching. Initially nasal lesions resemble benign nasal polyps without mucinous cysts. Pedunculated lesions may also occur on the palpebral conjunctiva, anus, vagina and penis (Kutty and Unni 1969).

Microscopic examination of early lesions shows invagination of epithelium in which typical rounded flask-shaped cysts containing spores, inflammatory cells and free spores are found (Figs. 14.69 and 14.70). Surgical excision is the only effective treatment that avoids disfiguring destruction of tissues.

Protozoal Infections

Amoebiasis due to *Entamoeba histolytica*

Amoebiasis has a worldwide distribution but is a particular problem in the tropics. It is estimated that only about 10% of individuals who harbour the organism develop invasive disease (Ravdin 1989). There is much speculation about the organism's change from a commensual to a virulent pathogen. Diet and intestinal flora seem to influence these events. In a Nigerian necropsy study 26% of cases with invasive disease occurred in children aged 1 month to 14 years, with an equal sex incidence (Abioye and Edington 1972). The causative organism (*Entamoeba histolytica*) is a protozoan with trophozoite and cyst forms. Non-invasive trophozoites are 10–20 μm in diameter with a single nucleus 3–5 μm in diameter and a slightly eccentric karyosome. Spherical cysts (10–20 μm in diameter) with one to four nuclei are found in the stools of those who are colonized (Fig. 14.71). Such individuals do not have invasive disease but may pass loose stools.

Infection is transmitted by cysts by the faecal–oral route. The carrier state of non-invasive trophozoites varies considerably in different communities. It is highest in the age group 0–9 years, but lowest among children aged 15–19 years (Hart et al. 1984).

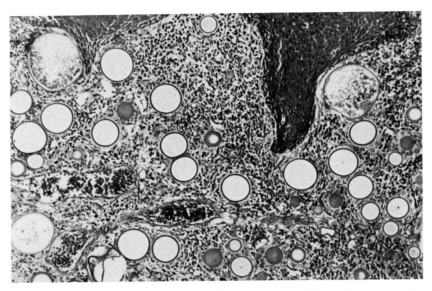

Fig. 14.69. Subconjunctival rhinosporidiosis in a 6-year-old boy. There are many rounded cysts having refractile walls and sometimes containing spores. An intense infiltration of mixed inflammatory cells is among the cysts.

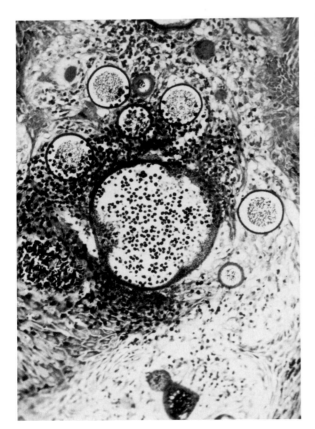

Fig. 14.70. Mature spores being released from a spherule. Adjoining spherules contain immature spores. (Same case as in Fig. 14.69.) (Gomori methenamine silver)

Trophozoites colonize the caecum and ascending colon preferentially. Invasive disease may occur after a variable delay. Then there is epithelial microulceration, with an initial mild inflammatory response by neutrophils and mononuclear cells. Thereafter the amoebae penetrate the damaged epithelial basement membrane to form flask-shaped ulcers, which extend to and through the muscularis mucosa. Surviving surrounding mucosa becomes oedematous and there is a hyperaemic border to the ulcers (Figs. 14.72 and 14.73). In areas of necrosis, cellular outlines are progressively lost. The cytoplasm and nuclei of necrotic cells become deeply eosinophilic and finely granular. The presence of this destructive necrotic material often alerts the experienced pathologist to search for amoebae when examining a rectal biopsy. Amoebae stain PAS-positive in necrotic and viable tissue (Fig. 14.74). The trophozoites of virulent amoebae produce proteolytic enzymes, which digest host tissues and seem to facilitate spread of the organism.

The ulcers enlarge to penetrate through the muscularis mucosae. Granulation tissue capillaries without significant fibrosis forms the bed of such large ulcers. Supervening bacterial infection produces a mixed inflammatory response.

At times there is extensive ulceration with diffuse oedema of the whole colon. The mucosa resembles gelatinous velvet, and the gut wall becomes extremely friable and often perforates. Children rarely recover from this condition (Lami and Moore 1989). Recent studies in South Africa indicate that amoebae tend to invade the walls of the blood vessels that

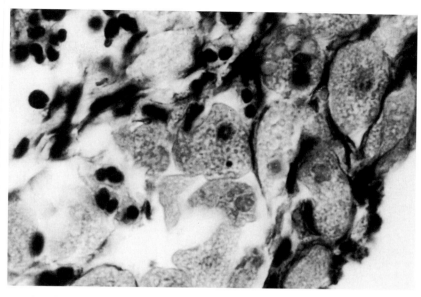

Fig. 14.71. Numerous trophozoites and cysts of *Entamoeba histolytica* showing nuclear characteristics and including red cells. (Courtesy of Dr J. Cox, Geneva) (H&E, × 400)

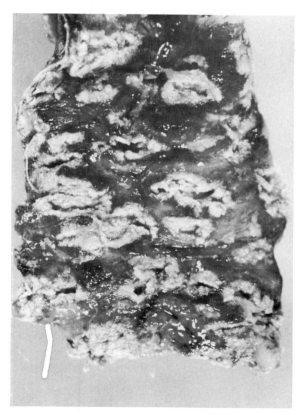

Fig. 14.72. Gross appearance of ulcerative amoebic colitis occurring in a young girl. The ulcers have raised oedematous edges with necrotic debris in the floor.

supply the affected areas of colon. This invasion is often the blood vessels that supply the affected areas of colon. This invasion is often associated with thrombosis, subsequent infarction and perforation of the colon (Luvuno et al. 1985). The veins draining areas of amoebic ulcers may become oedematous (apparently because of partial enzymatic digestion), with narrowing of the lumina (Fig. 14.75).

An amoeboma is found more frequently in children than in adults. The lesion is most often seen in or near the caecum, as a polypoid mass almost filling the lumen (Connor et al. 1976a).

Rectal amoebiasis can extend to involve the anus and perianal skin, producing multiple small ulcers which are associated with pseudoepitheliomatous hyperplasia. This may simulate squamous carcinoma macroscopically. The phenomenon is particularly seen in homosexual boys and young men. In the vagina, vulva and penis, similar cauliflower-like lesions may develop in areas where amoebiasis is sexually transmitted (Mylins and Ten Seldam 1962). Microscopically, these lesions show papillary acanthosis of epithelium and a hyperaemic dermis, infiltrated by lymphocytes, plasma cells and smaller numbers of eosinophils. Amoebae are found near the areas of ulceration (Connor et al. 1976a).

Amoebic liver abscesses occur as a consequence of haematogenous spread from colonic infection, and have been found in the first month of life. They are initially free of bacterial organisms and contain few pus cells. The contents are usually opaque yellow-

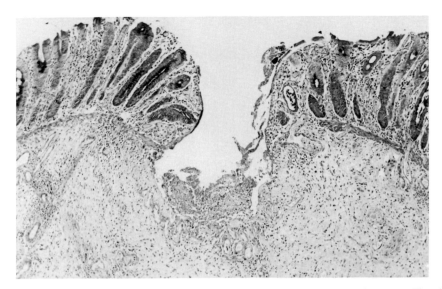

Fig. 14.73. Microscopy of a flask-shaped amoebic ulcer of the colon extending through the muscularis mucosa. The adjoining mucosa is oedematous without any significant inflammatory cell response. The floor of the ulcer contains digested debris, and trophozoites may be seen in the undermined edges.

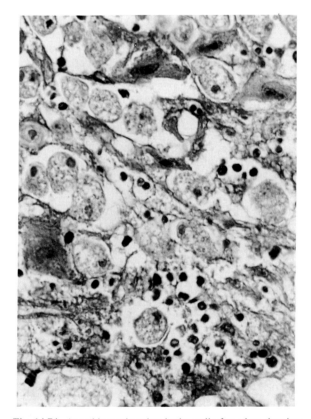

Fig. 14.74. Amoebic trophozoites in the wall of an ulcer showing cytoplasmic vacuoles with phagocytosed cellular debris.

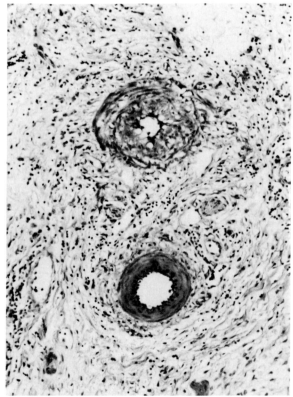

Fig. 14.75. Small artery and vein in the sigmoid mesentery in a case of diffuse colonic amoebiasis. The vein wall is oedematous with leiomyolysis and narrowing of the lumen.

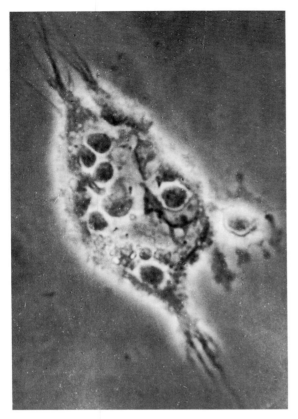

Fig. 14.76. Flagellate form of *Naegleria* showing bipolar flagellae and phagocytosed cells. (Courtesy of Dr A.J. Lastovica, University of Cape Town)

green or grey-brown, having the classic resemblance to anchovy paste. The material is acidic with a pH ranging from 5.2 to 6.7 (Ramachandran et al. 1976). Children often have multiple small abscesses, which may rarely perforate. However, when this occurs, perforation is into the right pleural cavity or right lung, into the pericardial cavity or into the peritoneum. Haematogenous dissemination to distant organs is rare.

Meningoencephalitis due to *Limax* Amoebae

Two genera of slug-like free-living amoebae have been found to cause meningoencephalitis in humans since Derrick's report in 1948. The possibility of "limax amoebas" being pathogenic in acidic fluid had already been reported in 1896 by Von Leyden and Schaudinn. Initially reported cases were the result of swimming in particular lakes, rivers and swimming pools, but suppressed immunity is now an increasingly important predisposing factor. *Naegleria* are

biphasic amoeboflagellates (Fig. 14.76), whereas *Acanthamoeba* have no flagellate form.

Naegleria fowleri

Naegleria fowleri produces an acute meningoencephalitis with suppurative inflammation of the brain and meninges. In an Australian series 75% of cases were in children of 15 years or younger (Dorsch et al. 1983). Boys are affected almost twice as often as girls. Infection is through the nasal passages and becomes clinically manifest 5–15 days after swimming in infected freshwater lakes, rivers or swimming pools. Although many people are exposed to the organisms, invasive disease is rare (Seidel 1985). Acute amoebic rhinitis followed by rapid spread to the meninges and brain through the cribriform plate occurs in invasive disease, leading to death within 5–16 days of exposure (Culbertson 1976).

There is severe infection of the meningeal space, producing a rapidly spreading purulent meningitis, which extends to involve the brain tissue, producing necrosis with an acute inflammatory response. Amoebae are present within the inflammatory exudate, and the base of the brain, cerebellum and spinal cord are often heavily involved. The amoebae are readily recognized in tissue sections on routine H & E stains (Fig. 14.77). The trophozoites are small (8–15 μm in diameter) with sharply defined nuclear membranes and small slightly eccentric nucleoli. They resemble macrophages and often occur in closely packed clusters (Carter 1972). The amoebae often invade vessel walls, grow within the vessels and produce thrombosis and haemorrhage. They seem to ingest portions of erythrocytes rather than whole cells, leading to haemolytic anaemia and haemosiderin deposits in their cytoplasm. The organisms may be cultured from cerebrospinal fluid and brain tissue.

Acanthamoeba

Acanthamoeba tends to produce chronic meningoencephalitis. Infection occurs mainly in patients who have reduced resistance to infection because of pre-existing chronic ill-health or immunosuppression. Trophozoites have clear cytoplasm with a denser nucleus, a well defined nuclear membrane and a dense nucleolus. The cysts are slightly smaller than a rounded trophozoite (12–15 μm) but larger than a *Naegleria fowleri* trophozite (4–6 μm) (Allen and Culbertson 1992). The organism has been isolated from children and young adults with purulent otitis media, keratitis, skin infections and acute and chronic

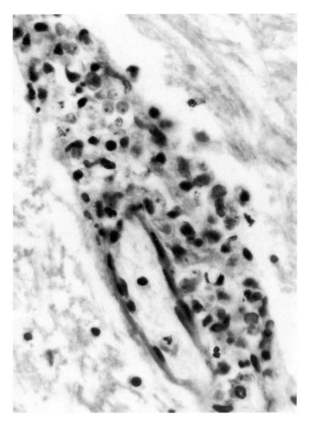

Fig. 14.77. Intracerebral perivascular accumulation of *Naegleria fowleri* amoebae with a mononuclear inflammatory cell infiltration. The amoebae resemble macrophages but have small eccentric nuclei.

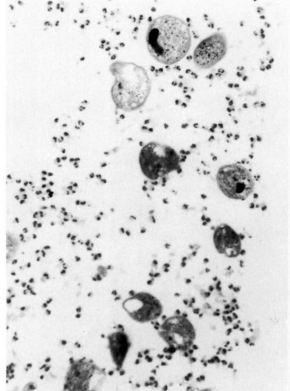

Fig. 14.78. Oval and rounded *Balantidium coli* organisms with prominent macronuclei, vacuolated cytoplasm and thin cell membranes. One organism has a pointed anterior end. Many have phagocytosed material in their cytoplasm. The host was a 14-year-old tribal African boy.

lung infections (Seidel 1985). The lesions in the brain resemble those of *Naegleria* but are more focal, patchy and granulomatous. Thrombosed vessels and infarction also occur. Trophozoites as well as cysts may be seen (Callicott 1968; Jager and Stamm 1972).

Balantidiasis

The protozoan *Balantidium coli* is an uncommon cause of intermittent diarrhoea and constipation in humans. Infection mainly occurs in tropical and subtropical regions. Institutions for mentally retarded children occasionally have outbreaks in temperate climates. Pigs, rats and primates harbour the organism, and many outbreaks in adults and children have followed the consumption of inadequately cooked or raw pork at festive occasions. The oval trophozoite is the largest of the protozoa that parasitize humans (Marcial and Marcial-Rojas 1985) (Fig. 14.78).

Infection varies from an asymptomatic carrier state to severe fulminating dysentery with abdominal pain, pyrexia, anorexia, nausea, headache, cachexia and loss of weight (Neafie 1976). Invasion of colonic mucosa produces flask-shaped ulcers with undermined edges, as occurs in amoebiasis. The ulcers may perforate or cause severe haemorrhage. Distant spread of infection to liver, vagina, bladder and ureter rarely occur (Neafie 1976).

Giardiasis

Giardiasis is an intestinal infestation caused by *Giardia lamblia*, a protozoan with worldwide distribution. It commonly occurs in malnourished children with diarrhoea (Sullivan et al. 1990). Infestation is frequent in areas that lack adequate water and sewage provision. Person-to-person infection may occur by the faecal–oral route and via shared toys. Ingested

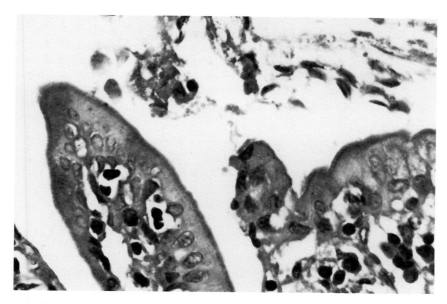

Fig. 14.79. Intestinal giardiasis with trophozoites at the tips of jejunal villi with accumulation of intraepithelial and subepithelial lymphocytes. (H&E, × 400)

cysts are excysted in the stomach, and the emerging trophozoites colonize the duodenum, upper jejunum and common bile duct. Trophozoites adhere to surface epithelium and rarely penetrate into tissues. Infestation is associated with varying degrees of villous atrophy, increased shedding of enterocytes and accumulation of intraepithelial lymphocytes (Fig. 14.79). In previously healthy individuals plasma cells in the lamina propria may increase, but in malnourished or hypogammaglobulinaemic children they are reduced and local production of secretory IgA becomes impaired.

Children with giardiasis usually have upper abdominal pain and diarrhoea or steatorrhoea. Very young preschool children often have symptomless infection (Ish-Horowicz et al. 1989), whereas in adolescents infection may mimic chronic inflammatory bowel disease (Gunasekaran and Hassall 1992). Protuberance of the abdomen, peripheral oedema, hypochromic microcytic anaemia and weight loss may also occur.

Malaria

Malaria is a major infectious disease in a large segment of the population in developing countries. Almost a third of the world's population is at risk of infection. Several million persons contract the disease each year, and in children the mortality rate is almost 10%. Human disease is caused by infection by four species of a protozoan of the genus *Plasmodium*, transmitted by female anopheline mosquitoes. Asexual reproduction of the plasmodia within erythrocytes causes fever and other symptoms. The four species commonly causing malaria in humans are *P. falciparum*, *P. vivax*, *P. malariae* and *P. ovale*. *P. knowlesi* normally affects non-human primates but has also naturally affected humans (Chin et al. 1965). There is a small but real risk that non-human primates may serve as a reservoir for infection.

The mode of transmission and life cycles of the plasmodia have been recorded by many authors (Connor et al. 1976b; Markell and Voge 1981; Randall and Seidel 1985).

P. falciparum and *P. vivax* account for 95% of infections in humans, although *P. vivax* is exceptionally rare in Africa south of the Sahara (Thomas 1986). *P. falciparum* causes the most virulent form of disease, often with very heavy invasion of erythrocytes, so that 10% of the cells may be parasitized. *P. vivax* is characterized by long persistence of tissue forms, which can cause recurrence of clinical malaria after intervals of 7–10 years after leaving malarial areas.

Malaria may be transmitted accidentally with blood transfusion and across the placenta. In endemic areas the fetus may be infected, and neonatal presentation with symptoms of fever, irritability, jaundice and hepatosplenomegaly 3–5 weeks after birth may occur (Quinn et al. 1982). Severe anaemia, which is preventable by chemoprophylaxis, may occur between 24 and 39 weeks' gestation. Heavy malarial infestation may be a cause of premature labour. The placenta is a privileged site for erythrocyte schizogony by *P. falciparum*, which may be a cause of intrauterine growth retardation.

Anaemia

Anaemia may be out of proportion to the degree of parasitaemia. Immune reaction contributes to the destruction of red blood cells, but the role is considered to be relatively small (Anonymous 1975).

Cerebral Malaria

Cerebral malaria is a dreaded emergency in nonimmune individuals who have severe infection with *P. falciparum*. It is reported to occur in 5% of children with malaria in India (Gautam et al. 1980). In Europe and North America it is the most common form of fatal malaria encountered among recent arrivals from endemic areas. In tropical countries it is considered to be a significant cause of neurological handicap (Brewster et al. 1990). Patients become confused and disorientated, convulse and go into coma. The brain may have a grey colour from malarial pigment, and becomes oedematous and congested. The cut surface reveals petechial haemorrhages in white matter. Microscopic examination shows congestion of small vessels and capillaries by parasitized erythrocytes. Some vessels become obstructed and surrounded by necrotic parenchyma with small "ring" haemorrhages.

Liver

The liver enlarges during acute attacks of haemolysis. Kupffer cells proliferate and accumulate pigment, merozoites and parasitized erythrocytes. Malarial pigment is eventually concentrated in portal areas, where increased lymphocytes and macrophages are found in repeated acute or chronic infection. The liver becomes deeply pigmented (chocolate-red, grey or black).

Spleen

The spleen becomes considerably enlarged early in acute infections of children, and may rupture while being palpated. It tends to be soft or rubbery and diffusely pigmented. In chronic malaria or after repeated acute attacks, the spleen may reach a kilogram in weight. Microscopic examination indicates intense engorgement of parasitized cells in the sinusoids during acute attacks, with the sinusoidal lining cells phagocytosing malarial pigment, merozoites and parasitized and unparasitized red blood cells. Infarcts and haemorrhage may result from vessels being occluded by sequestered parasitized erythrocytes. In chronic malaria, fibrosis and mineralization may be noted.

Kidneys

The kidneys are the site of a variety of lesions. They are usually slightly enlarged. Acute renal failure with haemoglobin casts in the tubules may occur as a consequence of interference with the microcirculation of the kidneys. The glomeruli often contain grains of pigment, which is birefringent. Immune complex membranoproliferative glomerulonephritis with nephrotic syndrome sometimes occurs with falciparum malaria (Boonpucknavig and Sitprija 1979).

Blackwater Fever

Blackwater Fever is a complication of severe falciparum malaria that occurs mainly in adults and teenagers. Symptoms comprise high fever, chills, rigours, jaundice, vomiting, rapidly progressive anaemia and the passing of red or black urine. There has been a high frequency of cases among individuals receiving quinine therapy, or who have undergone excessive exertion. In addition, persons with various underlying illness, adults following excessive alcohol intake, and non-immune persons (who temporarily stop taking antimalarial drugs while in an endemic area) are prone to the condition. There is a haemolytic crisis with massive destruction of erythrocytes, which leads to haemoglobinaemia, haemoglobinuria, intense icterus and acute renal failure leading to anuria and death.

Lungs

The lungs are often oedematous and congested, with mononuclear inflammatory cells in the alveolar walls.

Heart

The heart may be dilated and flabby with haemorrhagic petechiae. Capillaries may be occluded by parasitized erythrocytes, and interstitial oedema may be noted.

Bone Marrow and Lymph Nodes

Bone marrow and lymph nodes undergo reactive changes with accumulation of phagocytosed pigment and merozoites. Haemopoieties cells undergo hyperplasia in response to haemolysis and infection.

Diagnosis

Examination of thick and thin blood films for the parasites gives a definitive diagnosis. However, in tissue sections, the recognition of malarial pigment (haemozoin) examined for birefringence on sections stained with Wright's stain has been reported (Lawrence and Olson 1986).

Tropical Splenomegaly

Tropical splenomegaly is a syndrome in which there is massive enlargement of the spleen, repeated low-grade fever and anaemia; it occurs in postpubertal residents of the tropics, and has been attributed to repeated plasmodial infection. The spleen is usually in excess of a kilogram in weight and has a thickened capsule, which may be calcified. The cut surface is dark and fleshy with occasional small infarcts. The splenic cords are filled with lymphocytes and fewer plasma cells. Malarial pigment is not a feature, but phagocytosed haemosiderin is present. In the liver sinusoids there is a prominent infiltration of lymphocytes and macrophages (Fig. 14.80). Kupffer cells undergo reactive hyperplasia and accumulate haemosiderin without malaria pigment. Cirrhosis is not a feature of this condition. Serum levels of IgM and IgG are very high, with high titres of malarial antibodies to *P. malariae* (Hutt 1966, Crane 1977, Hoffman et al. 1984). Many patients also develop a nephrotic syndrome with progressive renal failure, due to deposition of soluble antigen–antibody complexes. Circulating suppressor T lymphocytes are reduced (Hoffman et al. 1984).

Babesiosis

Babesiosis is an underdiagnosed condition that occurs worldwide and simulates malaria (Krause et al. 1992). It is caused by an intraerythrocytic zoonotic protozoan, usually *Babesia microti*. It is transmitted by *Ixodes* ticks from rodents and other animals. Infection causes fever, haemolytic anaemia, jaundice, haemoglobinaemia, haemoglobinuria and acute renal failure. As in malaria, parasitized erythrocytes may obstruct blood vessels, causing ischaemia and necrosis. Hepatosplenomegaly and cerebral dis-

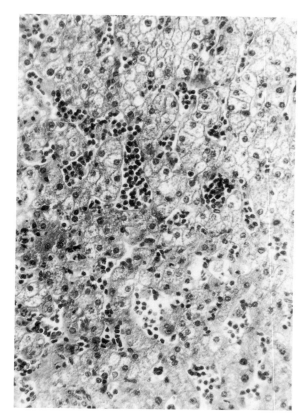

Fig. 14.80. Microscopy of liver in tropical splenomegaly caused by repeated plasmoidae infection with *Plasmodium malariae*. The sinusoids are infiltrated by lymphocytes and macrophages, and there is some reactive hyperplasia of Kupffer cells.

turbances may follow. The condition is diagnosed by identifying the organisms on blood smears stained by Giemsa or Wright stains. Several serological tests are available to identify antibodies.

Pneumocystis carinii

Pneumocystis carinii causes pneumonia as an opportunistic infection in neonates and children with immunological and neoplastic disease. Studies of DNA sequences now suggest that *Pneumocystis* is a fungus; it has common staining reactions with other fungi (PAS and Silver) (Edman et al. 1988). It is, however, insensitive to antifungal drugs, although drugs used to treat protozoal infections are generally effective. The organism occurs in three forms. Cysts may be seen in lungs and respiratory secretions. They are rounded structures approximately 5 μm in diameter containing up to eight oval "sporozoites" (1–2 μm in diameter). The sporozoites are released from the

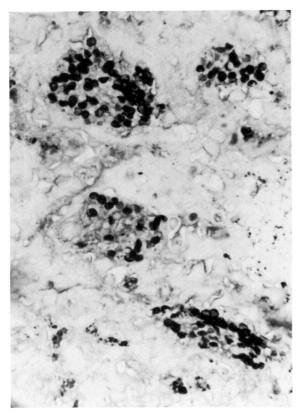

Fig. 14.81. Microscopy of *Pneumocystis carinii* infection of the lung. There are rounded hemispherical and sickle-shaped trophozoites in the alveoli. (Gomori methenamine silver)

cysts and quickly mature into "trophozoites". Trophozoites are sickle-shaped and 2–5 μm in diameter (Fig. 14.81). They have short pseudopodial extensions, which attach to host tissue cells without penetration, although they may be phagocytosed. They undergo morphological changes and encyst (Pifer et al. 1977).

Transmission of infection seems to be from one human to another, with epidemics occurring in orphanages and children's cancer clinics (Dutz 1970). An animal reservoir is possible as the organisms are widespread as saphrophytes in a variety of animals. Many children have clinically inapparent infections (Perera et al. 1970). The severity of illness is based on host susceptibility, and predisposing conditions include lymphocytic leukaemia and other generalized lymphoproliferative malignancies, protein–energy malnutrition and primary and acquired immune deficiency syndromes. Dutz et al. (1974) have reported a high incidence of infection in an orphanage among infants less than 5 months old with marasmus and having IgG levels below 2 g/litre.

Infection with *P. carinii* is almost always limited to the lungs. Disseminated infection to multiple organs is very rare (Telzak et al. 1990). Two basic forms of disease have been recognized by Dutz (1970): interstitial plasma cell pneumonia and hypoimmune hypoergic pneumocystosis.

Interstitial Plasma Cell Pneumonia

Interstitial plasma cell pneumonia occurs in debilitated, malnourished, institutionalized, prematurely born infants, often receiving artificial nutrition, between the ages of 3 and 6 months. Organisms rapidly proliferate on the surface of alveolar lining cells and apparently produce a powerful antigenic stimulus. The alveolar walls become distended with fluid, plasma cells and lymphocytes. There may be a five- to ten-fold thickening of alveolar wall and pulmonary septae. High levels of IgM immunoglobulin are produced.

The children may die within 2 or 3 days or become chronically ill for weeks and months. At autopsy the lungs are voluminous with liver-like consistency, and the infiltration by plasma cells and lymphocytes persists long after treatment has eliminated the organisms.

A less severe focal form of infection occurs more frequently and tends to involve subpleural portions of lung. There is an early plasma cell response but the *Pneumocystis* organisms proliferate slowly.

Hypoimmune Hypoergic Pneumocystosis

Hypoimmune hypoergic pneumocystosis occurs in infants, children and adults who are immunosuppressed (mostly due to AIDS or immunosuppressive therapy). *Pneumocystis* infection is commonly concurrent with fungal and/or viral infections (particularly cytomegalovirus). Alveolar air spaces accumulate large numbers of organisms in vacuolated cellular debris which interferes with gaseous exchange. There is no significant inflammatory cell response (Fig. 14.82). Alveolar lining cells may proliferate, desquamate and may form giant cells. This response may be initiated by a concurrent viral infection. There is exudation of fibrin, which tends to become organized, and carnification of the lung may occur as macrophage phagocytic activity is impaired. Relatively small numbers of organisms are encountered and they tend to be sited in vacuolated cellular debris in airspaces (Price and Hughes 1974).

Congenital infection is a rare occurrence (Pavlica 1962). When disseminated disease occurs, infected necrotic lesions may appear in liver, hilar lymph

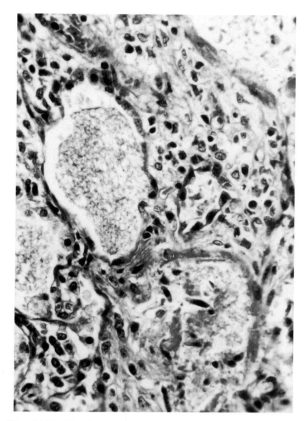

Fig. 14.82. Hypoimmune hypoergic pneumocystosis of lung. Alveolar spaces are filled with fibrin, vacuolated cellular debris and organisms which are not seen on haematoxylin and eosin stains. The inflammatory response is mild and insignificant.

nodes, spleen, retina, bone marrow, adrenals, gastrointestinal tract, pancreas and heart with or without organisms in peripheral blood (Telzak et al. 1990).

Diagnosis. Diagnosis of the condition is best achieved by microscopic examination of sputum, bronchial aspirates or material from bronchoalveolar lavage. The organisms stain with Papanicolaou, methenamine silver, toluidine blue and May–Grünwald–Giemsa. The Papanicolaou stain has recently been found to be highly satisfactory (Young et al. 1986).

Acquired Toxoplasmosis

Toxoplasmosis is a common, often asymptomatic, protozoal infection which rarely causes illness beyond the neonatal period (see p. 744).

Transmission of infection is by ingestion of cysts in infected meat, ingestion or inhalation of sporulated oocysts from cat faeces, inoculation, blood transfu-

sion or organ transplantation. Trophozoites reach the bloodstream and are carried throughout the body within leucocytes. Although infection usually produces no clinical illness, some children and young adults may develop tender non-suppurative cervical lymphadenitis. Rarely, there is accompanying fever, myocarditis, maculopapular rash, myalgia and pneumonia.

Involved lymph nodes have specific changes where parasites are only occasionally seen. The nodes undergo a striking degree of follicular hyperplasia with large germinal centres containing many macrophages (Fig. 14.83). In the interfollicular areas large epithelioid cells are focally distributed and are less frequently encountered in germinal centres (Fig. 14.84). There is usually no giant cell response, but there may be focal distention of sinusoids by immature histiocytes. Plasma cells and immunoblasts may be found in medullary cords (Dorfman and Remington 1973).

Other organs such as heart, lungs, spleen, voluntary muscles and liver may have necrotic lesions (Kass et al. 1952). Disseminated disease is often found in patients with AIDS. The calcific lesions of the central nervous system that are encountered in congenital infection are not seen in acquired disease. However, retinal lesions may become reactivated, particularly during early adolescence.

Leishmaniasis

Leishmaniasis is a group of diseases caused by protozoal haemoflagellates of the genus *Leishmania,* which are transmitted by various species of phlebotomous flies from animal reservoirs. *L. donovani* invades cells of the reticular endothelial system of viscera, producing enlargement of liver and spleen with severe anaemia and is usually fatal if not treated. *L. tropica* invades the reticular endothelial cells of the skin and is usually a self-limited disease. *L. braziliensis* and *L. mexicana mexicana* produce cutaneous lesions in the western hemisphere. Infection with *L. mexicana mexicana* tends to be self-limiting, whereas infection with *L. braziliensis* tends to metastasize to mucous membranes of the nose, mouth and pharynx, where much disfigurement is caused. The *Leishmania* organisms are obligate intracellular parasites of vertebrates. They stain readily with Giemsa and Wright's stains to show a red nucleus and pale blue cytoplasm (Figs. 14.85 and 14.86).

Visceral Leishmaniasis due to L. donovani

L. donovani causes a visceral form of leishmaniasis, which is also known as kala-azar or ponos. There is

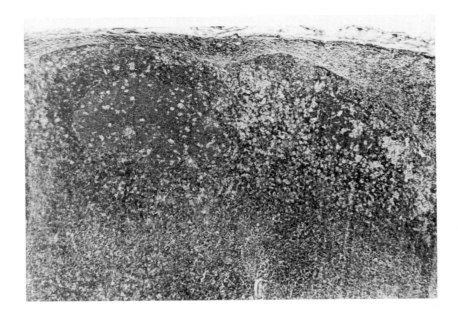

Fig. 14.83. Microscopy of toxoplasmosis in a 10-year-old girl. There is follicular hyperplasia, with macrophages in the germinal centres of a biopsied cervical lymph gland.

diffuse lymphadenopathy with considerable enlargement of the spleen and liver. Sinusoidal lining cells and Kupffer cells are hyperplastic and accumulate phagocytosed organisms. In the intestine macrophages containing phagocytosed organisms may be seen in the mucosa and submucosa of the duodenum and jejunum. Villi may become oedematous and distended. Erythrophagocytosis by macrophages, leucopenia and anaemia are additional early features of infection. In chronic disease the liver may undergo centrilobular fatty infiltration or necrosis and become cirrhotic. Infarcts appear in the spleen, and the marrow may be largely replaced by parasitized histiocytes (Manson-Bahr 1971).

Old World Cutaneous Leishmaniasis due to L. tropica, L. major and L. aethiopica

These organisms are the cause of Old World cutaneous leishmaniasis, also referred to as oriental sore (Delhi boil, Aleppo button). At the site of inoculation

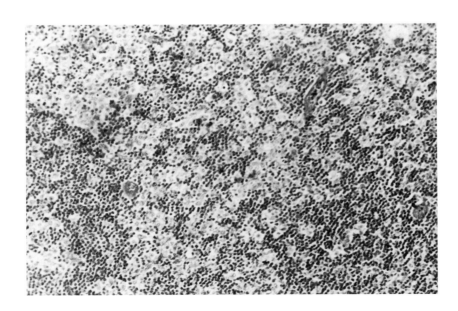

Fig. 14.84. Interfollicular area of lymph node in toxoplasmosis. Large numbers of epithelioid macrophages are present.

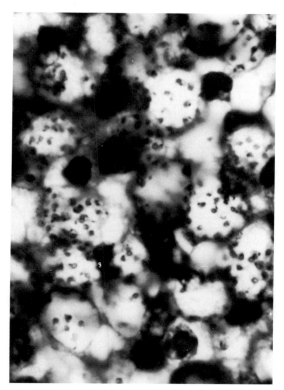

Fig. 14.85. Giemsa stain of phagocytosed *Leishmania tropica* in a skin biopsy from a teenage girl.

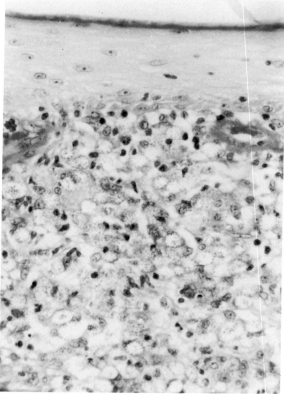

Fig. 14.86. Microscopy of cutaneous leishmaniasis. (Same case as in Fig. 14.85). The finely granular organisms are phagocytosed by histiocytes, and there is an associated mild infiltration of lymphocytes and plasma cells.

histiocytes engulf the organisms, but they multiply and destroy the phagocytes. There is infiltration by increasing numbers of histiocytes, lymphocytes and plasma cells. Granulomas with epithelioid and giant cells form. Capillary obstruction leads to necrosis and ulceration. A depressed ulcer with a raised indurated border and a base of granulation tissue forms. Healing is protracted with infections by *L. tropica*. Florid infection may lead to satellite lesions developing so that a mistaken diagnosis of malignancy may be made (Turk and Bryceson 1971).

American Leishmaniasis

American leishmaniasis is caused by several species of *Leishmania* and has a variety of clinical forms. They produce skin lesions with a variety of characteristics. Outbreaks of the disease are centred around forested areas where the particular vectors are found (Lainson 1983).

Trypanosomiasis

African Trypanosomiasis

African trypanosomiasis or sleeping sickness is due to the protozoal haemoflagellates *Trypanosoma brucei gambiense* and *Trypanosoma brucei rhodesiense*. The Rhodesian form of disease is more acute and usually kills the host within weeks or months, whereas the Gambian form evolves over years. The protozoal organisms may be seen on Giemsa-stained blood smears (Fig. 14.87). *T. b. gambiense* does not have an important animal reservoir; however, whereas game animals serve as a reservoir for *T. b. rhodesiense*, the tsetse fly is the vector for both organisms, which are not morphologically distinguishable. Males older than 30 years are most commonly affected, but there is a significant incidence among teenaged children in endemic areas (Davies 1982).

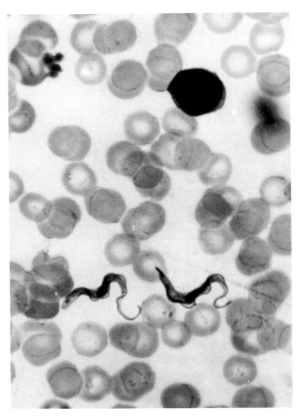

Fig. 14.87. Giemsa-stained blood smear of *Trypanosoma brucei rhodesiense* showing the typical flagellum and undulating membrane.

The organisms are inoculated into the skin, where they multiply to produce a painful chancre. After 10 days slender forms of haemoflagellates are found in the bloodstream. This is followed by waves of parasitaemia as new antigenic strains of organisms develop. There is a brisk outpouring of IgM immunoglobulins with lesser amounts of IgG from a prominent plasma cell response. Immune complex glomerular disease may supervene.

Cervical and mesenteric lymph nodes become hyperplastic with diffuse proliferation of lymphocytes and plasma cells. Initially they may be haemorrhagic and contain large numbers of organisms. When the central nervous system is invaded by the protozoal organisms, progressive leptomeningitis develops. The brain becomes oedematous, with gliosis and perivascular cuffing by lymphocytes and plasma cells (Goodwin 1971).

American Trypanosomiasis

American trypanosomiasis, also referred to as Chagas' disease, is caused by the haemoflagellate *Trypanosoma cruzi*. The disease is transmitted by reduviid bugs in South and Central America, where infection is prevalent, affecting between 7 and 10 million. There is a reservoir of infection among wild and semi-domestic animals. *T. cruzi* has been shown to cause abortion, placentitis and congenital infection (Bittencourt 1976).

After being inoculated into the skin, the organisms become phagocytosed and divide within macrophages. A nodular swelling (chagoma) develops at the site of entry. There is infiltration by lymphocytes, macrophages, eosinophils and polymorphs. Spread to regional lymph glands, which undergo reactive hyperplasia, follows. After local proliferation of the organism has occurred, parasitaemia with dissemination to multiple sites follows. The host responds with leucocytosis and prominent plasma cell proliferation. The organs that are most sensitive to disseminated disease are cardiac muscle, skeletal muscle, the reticuloendothelial system and neuroglial cells.

The heart is frequently involved. Myocardial cells swell and become necrotic. There is a mixed inflammatory cell reaction. Some organisms may develop into pseudocysts (amastigote form of the organism) in various parts of the body including the heart (Fig. 14.88). Pseudocysts are large and frequent during the acute phase of infection, when there is diffuse necrosis of myocardial fibres and an intense mononuclear inflammatory cell response (Fig. 14.89). In fatal cases the heart is found to be dilated and diffusely fibrosed. Often cardiac aneurysms develop, which may rupture or be associated with mural thrombi and embolic phenomena. The ganglion cells of the parasympathetic nervous system are particularly sensitive to infection. More than 90% of the ganglion cells of myenteric plexus of the oesophagus and colon may be destroyed. Such destruction leads to megaoesophagus and megacolon, with features of chronic intestinal pseudo-obstruction (de Rezende and Moreira 1988).

Rickettsial Diseases

Rickettsia are bacteria which (like viruses) are obligate intracellular parasites. They appear as coccobacilli measuring 0.3–0.5 μm in diameter and often occur in short chains. *Rickettsia* remain viable in blood at 4 °C for several days. They produce acute infections with high fever, often with a rash and headache. With the exception of Rocky Mountain spotted fever, these infections tend to occur in poor socioeconomic conditions with overcrowding. The majority of infections thus occur in children, who

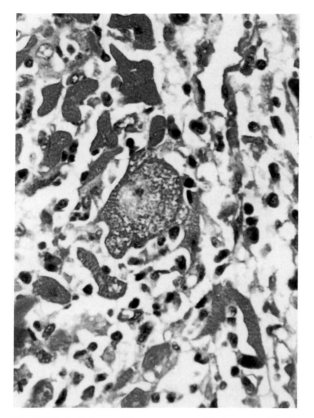

Fig. 14.88. Amistigote of *Trypanosoma cruzi* in the myocardium in Chagas' disease. Myocardial fibres show hyalinization, vacuolation and lysis.

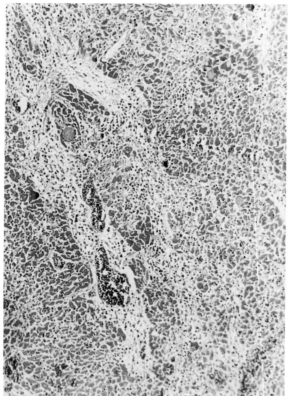

Fig. 14.89. Diffuse acute myocarditis in Chagas' disease, with degeneration and necrosis of myocardial fibres, mixed inflammatory cell infiltration and the presence of pseudocysts.

form the bulk of the population exposed to the organisms and their vectors. The basic lesion is either a vasculitis or pneumonia, and almost all infections are transmitted through an arthropod vector. In all infections agglutinins are produced to OX19, OX2, or OXK strains of *Proteus vulgaris* (Weil–Felix reaction). The organisms may be demonstrated by immunofluorescent techniques or the Gimenez stain, which stains them bright red (Murray 1981).

Epidemic Typhus

Epidemic louse-borne typhus is caused by *Rickettsia prowazekii*. The disease occurs mainly in children, although all ages are affected. Infection is from louse faeces, which may be inhaled or contaminate punctured skin. After an incubation period of 10–14 days an acute shock-like systemic illness with rash, sparing the face, arms and soles, develops. Patients often become stuporose and go into coma; diffuse purpura may occur. They usually die from encephali-

tis, myocarditis, pneumonia or acute renal failure (Meheus et al. 1974).

The organisms disseminate through the bloodstream without producing a local lesion. Generalized vasculitis with fibrin thrombi in very small blood vessels develops. Rickettsia have a tropism for endothelial cells, where they multiply preferentially. Sometimes large vessels are occluded by thrombi, when tissue necrosis develops. Microscopic collections of mononuclear inflammatory cells may be found in various organs around small blood vessels. Mild interstitial pneumonia, myocarditis, meningoencephalitis, gangrene, parotitis, pancreatitis, otitis media, effusions and focal interstitial nephritis may occur (Diab et al. 1989).

Brill–Zinsser Disease

Brill–Zinsser disease is a recrudescent form of typhus acquired several years earlier. The clinical symptoms are similar to but milder than those of acute epidemic typhus. This condition indicates persistence of the organism in humans (Gaon and Murray 1966).

Endemic Typhus

Endemic murine typhus is caused by the organism *Rickettsia mooseri*. Humans acquire the disease from rat fleas, and rats and other rodents serve as an animal reservoir. The clinical symptoms are similar to those of epidemic typhus but milder. In untreated cases the mortality rate is less than 5%. The pathology of endemic typhus closely resembles that of louse-borne epidemic typhus, and acute interstitial myocarditis, interstitial orchitis and meningoencephalitis occur (Binford and Ecker 1947).

Rocky Mountain Spotted Fever

Rocky Mountain spotted fever is caused by *Rickettsia rickettsia*. Humans acquire the disease from tick bites, and western hemisphere rodents (rats) together with ticks serve as a reservoir for the disease. This disease is an increasing clinical problem in the USA because of the growing popularity of hiking in mountainous or scrub areas (Walker and Bradford 1981). Nearly two-thirds of patients are less than 15 years of age and there is a 5%–7% mortality rate, mainly due to delays in diagnosis (Murray 1981). The clinical features are similar to those of endemic murine typhus, except that the rash begins at the wrists and ankles, spreads to the whole body and also involves the face, palms and soles. Cutaneous gangrene, severe hyponatraemia and peripheral circulatory collapse occur more often than in typhus.

To inoculate the organisms, ticks must feed long enough to engorge (about 10 h). In common with other rickettsial illnesses, there is infection of endothelial cells of small vessels, with extensive vasculitis and increased capillary permeability. This leads to severe oedema and peripheral circulatory collapse. The rickettsia have their long axis aligned with the length of blood vessels and are thus not easily seen on transverse sections. Infected endothelial cells become swollen, and there is infiltration of macrophages, lymphocytes and plasma cells around the affected arterioles, venules and capillaries.

The brain may be congested and oedematous, with many punctuate haemorrhages (Lillie 1941). Micro-infarcts occur in white matter, but typhus nodules (focal intense collections of mononuclear inflammatory cells around vessels) are small and less conspicuous than in epidemic typhus.

The heart is affected in almost all fatal cases. There is slight increase in weight, and haemorrhagic petechiae are scattered in the myocardium. A diffuse interstitial mononuclear inflammatory cell infiltration occurs with interstitial oedema.

The lungs become congested and oedematous with focal haemorrhages. They are often the site of intercurrent bacterial bronchopneumonia, but also have interstitial pneumonia (Walker et al. 1980). The alveolar walls are thickened by oedema fluid, mononuclear inflammatory cells, fibrin and haemorrhages. Pulmonary oedema can be massive and is often a serious iatrogenic problem.

The kidneys are usually unaffected, but may have parenchymal haemorrhages and be oedematous. Occasionally, acute tubular necrosis or multifocal interstitial nephritis occurs.

Tick Typhus Fever

A number of other typhus-like fevers caused by different rickettsial organisms are transmitted by ticks that occur in Asia, Africa and Australia. In these infections there is a milder form of clinical disease, but indurated lesions develop at the site of the tick bite. The lesion becomes necrotic, ulcerates and becomes encrusted. Regional lymph nodes become enlarged. Children experience a milder form of disease than adults.

Tsutsugamushi Fever

Tsutsugamushi fever (scrub typhus) is caused by *Rickettsia tsutsugamushi,* which has antigenic heterogeneity, with variable severity of clinical disease. The vectors are certain trombiculid mites (chiggers), and infection occurs in south-east Asia and the Pacific islands. Latent infection occurs in small rodents, and humans are infected by the bite of the larval form of the mites.

A small necrotic ulcer develops at the site of infection, leading to an eschar with regional lymphadenopathy. A sudden headache with fever and myalgia occurs, followed a week later by a macular or maculopapular rash without haemorrhagic features. Patients may suffer from interstitial pneumonia, meningitis, myocarditis and peripheral circulatory collapse (Silpapojakul et al. 1991). The basic vasculitic lesion of other rickettsial illnesses is found (Ognibene et al. 1971).

Q Fever

This acute rickettsial infection is underdiagnosed in children (Richardus et al. 1985). It is primarily a disease of animals that is transmitted to humans by

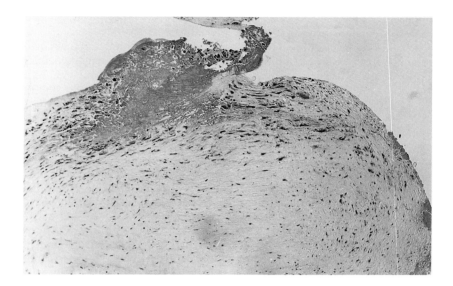

Fig. 14.90. A fibrin-rich vegetation is attached to a valve leaflet removed from a chronically ill child with serologic evidence of Q fever. (H&E, × 50)

inhalation. The organism, *Coxiella burnetti*, is resistant to heat and desiccation. It occurs worldwide, but is particularly prevalent in rural Australia (Wisniewski and Krumbiegel 1970). Q fever usually manifests as sudden fever, severe headache, malaise, myalgia, arthralgia, abdominal pain and vomiting. Hepatosplenomegaly, radiological pneumonitis, haemolytic anaemia, leucopenia and menigitis may follow (Ruiz-Contreras et al. 1993). Biopsies of liver or bone marrow trephines demonstrate granulomas with lipid vacuoles and dense fibrin deposits. Endocarditis with fibrin-rich vegetations may be found on heart valves (Fig. 14.90). The diagnosis may be made by a number of serological tests, but it is notable that there is no cross-reaction with *Proteus* agglutinins.

Parasitic disease

Parasitic infestations are prevalent in the tropics, particularly in areas where standards of housing, sewage, education and personal hygiene are low. Some, such as *Ascaris, Strongylcoides* and hookworm, accentuate pre-existing malnutrition, and the severity of infestation is enhanced by malnutrition and its associated immune suppression.

Ascariasis

Infestation with *Ascaris lumbricoides* is highly prevalent and probably affects between 600 and 1000 million people throughout the world (Stoll 1947; Katz 1992). During 1970s, in rural communities in the southern USA, between 20% and 67% of children were affected (Blumenthal and Shultz 1975). Some individuals seem to have increased susceptibility to heavy and repeated infection (Hall et al. 1992). Infection is acquired by the ingestion of ova, from which larvae hatch in the upper intestine. The larvae penetrate blood vessels, are carried through the bloodstream to the heart and lungs, and from there down the oesophagus to the upper intestinal tract where they mature into adult worms. During their migratory cycle, tissue responses are initiated in the lungs and eosinophilia results. IgG antibodies are produced, but they do not confer significant immunity. Symptoms and signs produced include abdominal pain and tenderness, abdominal mass due to worm bolus, and vomiting of worms because of intestinal obstruction. Complications include volvulus, bowel gangrene, biliary obstruction, liver abscess, liver granulomas, acute pancreatitis (Rode et al. 1990), intestinal perforation and mesenteric adenitis. In the small intestines the worms produce antienzymes, which seem to be responsible for malabsorption. This accentuates any malnutrition that may be present. Extra-abdominal complications include pulmonary worm embolism (Daya et al. 1982), bronchial obstruction (Ramchander et al. 1991), otitis media and septicaemia associated with liver abscess.

Hookworm

Infestation with hookworm probably affects approximately a billion people, most of whom are free of symptoms; however, hookworm is an important cause of anaemia (Hotez 1989). Heavy infestation contributes to malnutrition through loss of blood and serum. Two species of hookworm affect humans. These are *Ancylostoma duodenale* and *Necator americanus*. A single adult *A. duodenale* is responsible for the loss of approximately 0.25 ml blood per day. Infection follows exposure of the skin to moist soil infested with the larvae, which penetrate the skin, reach the bloodstream and are carried to the gastrointestinal tract. There they mature into adult worms, which become attached to the intestinal wall. Transmission of larvae through colostrum, breast milk and across the placenta are additional modes of infestation (Hotez 1989). An IgA antibody response provides partial protection to further infection by damaging worms, which are subsequently expelled (Katz 1992). Infection causes eosinophilia and iron-deficiency anaemia. Pre-existing malnutrition is exacerbated, and intellectual retardation is more frequent in heavily infected children.

Pinworm

Pinworm infection, caused by *Enterobius vermicularis*, is highly prevalent, occurs worldwide and affects children of all social classes. Ova are picked up from perianal skin, towels, bedclothes, underwear and the air. Larvae emerge in the duodenum, and mature worms normally inhabit the caecum and colon. Gravid female worms deposit their ova on perianal skin, where larvae can hatch within a few hours and migrate into the rectum. Infected humans experience anal pruritus, and mature worms are often found in the appendix. Females may suffer vulval itching and vaginal discharge from worms entering the vagina.

Whipworm

Infection with the whipworm *Trichuris trichiura* is almost as prevalent as ascariasis and enterobiasis. Most infections are light and asymptomatic. When heavy infestation occurs, there may be a dysentery syndrome with diarrhoea, blood and mucus in the stools (MacDonald et al. 1991). Ova are picked up from contaminated soil and are ingested. Larvae hatch in the jejunum, where they penetrate the intestinal villi and migrate to the caecum and colon after maturing. The worms become attached to the mucosal wall, from which nutrients are derived without affecting the host unless there is heavy infestation.

Strongyloidosis

Infection with *Strongyloides stercoralis* is much less frequent than infections with *Ascaris*, *Enterobius* and *Trichuris*. As with hookworm, infection occurs through the skin by exposure to infective larvae in moist soil. After the larvae have reached the intestines, through the bloodstream, maturation to adult worms occurs. Mature worms reside between mucosal folds without attaching to mucosa and do not consume blood. Ova are passed out with faeces for larvae to emerge in moist soil. Sometimes larvae hatch from intestinal ova, penetrate the mucosa and enter the bloodstream to cause hyperinfection. Because of the autoinfection life-cycle, strongyloidiasis sometimes occurs in mental hospitals and homes for retarded children (Katz 1992). Infection is associated with eosinophilia and eosinophilic infiltration into the intestinal wall. Malnourished and immune-suppressed children have a greater tendency to auto-infection. Infection is mostly symptomless, but diarrhoea and constipation occur with massive infection. In addition, larvae may be caught up in tissues such as the central nervous system. The condition is diagnosed by identifying ova or larvae in the stools.

Schistosomiasis

Schistosomiasis is due to infection by a trematode (fluke). There are many species, of which five affect humans. The three most commonly encountered members are *Schistosoma haematobium*, which occurs in Africa and parts of south-west Asia including India, *S. mansoni,* which occurs in South and Central America and much of Africa, and *S. japonicum*, which occurs in south-east Asia. The disease affects more than 200 million people, and infection mainly occurs in childhood. Infected persons pass ova in faeces and/or urine. In fresh water, miracidia emerge from the ova and must gain access to particular species of snail. Infected snails discharge cercariae, which are able to pass through intact human skin to reach the lymphatics and blood circulation. Mature adult worms reside as copulating pairs in the venules of the intestines and spinal cord (*S. mansoni* and *S. japonicum*) or urinary system (*S. haematobium*), where large numbers of ova are deposited into the tissues. An intense immune response occurs, with eosinophilia and accumulation of autofluorescent immune complexes on the surface of worms and dead ova. Inflammatory granulomas, with a foreign body giant cell response and calcification of dead ova follow. The ova of *S. mansoni* and *S. japonicum* have lateral spines and are acid-fast when stained by the

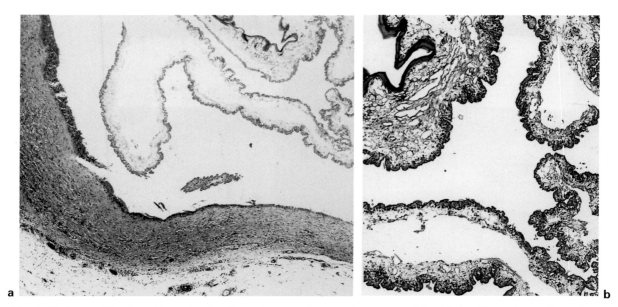

Fig. 14.91. Larva of *Taenia multiceps* showing fibrous tissue reaction around a narrow peripheral lining. Within the cyst is a delicate membrane from which multiple scolices may arise. (**a** H&E, × 20; **b** H&E, × 50)

modified Ziehl–Nielsen stain; those of *S. haematobium* are negative and have terminal spines.

Cercarial penetration of human skin causes a mild pruritus, with the appearance of macules within minutes of invasion in unsensitized persons. Subsequent exposure to cercariae causes a more intense reaction that may take the form or urticaria. Katayama fever is an explosive delayed reaction occurring 2–8 weeks after penetration by the cercariae of *S. japonicum* or large numbers of *S. mansoni* in an initial exposure. There is fever, colic, weakness, lassitude, diarrhoea, anorexia, nausea, myalgia, sweating and headache. These symptoms are often misdiagnosed as malaria. There is also hepatosplenomegaly, some lymph adenopathy, purpura, urticaria and eosinophilia. The reaction is initiated by the deposition of ova. Liver biopsy may demonstrate granulomas centred around ova with large numbers of eosinophils.

Genitourinary lesions are mainly due to *S. haematobium* and are manifested as subepithelial granulomas. There may be polypoid lesions with ulcers that cause haematuria and later lead to fibrosis, calcification, squamous metaplasia and eventually neoplasia.

In the intestines, ova that are not extruded into the lumen cause an inflammatory granuloma with infiltration by eosinophils, as occurs in the urinary system. Papillomas and fibrosis may occur but involvement is generally symptomless.

In the spinal cord, focal granulomas may cause tranverse myelitis. Occasionally *S. japonicum* causes diffuse encephalitis with or without granulomas (Kaufmann 1969).

Hepatic lesions occur as a result of adult worms or schistosoma egg embolism. A granulomatous inflammatory response with much fibrosis occurs around thrombosed portal veins. The fibrosis does not obstruct the bile ducts or hepatic arteries and veins, and is referred to as pipestem or Symmers fibrosis (Ramos et al. 1964). There is presinusoidal portal hypertension with hepatosplenomegaly. Haematin, indistinguishable from malarial pigment by light microscopy, often accumulates in portal areas and in Kupffer cells.

Embolization of ova to the lungs produces granulomas that rarely progress to vascular bed obstruction with pulmonary hypertension.

Cestode Infestations

The flatworms or tapeworms that tend to affect children are *Taenia solium* (pork tapeworm) and *Echinococcus* species. *T. saginata* (beef tapeworm), *Diphyllobothrium latum* (fish tapeworm), *T. multiceps* (bladder worm), *Hymenolepis nana* (dwarf tapeworm) and *Dipylidium caninum* (dog tapeworm) also occur, but are of less clinical importance. The larvae of *T. multiceps,* like those of *T. solium,* have a tendency to become located in the central nervous system but form multiple scolices (Fig. 14.91). *D.*

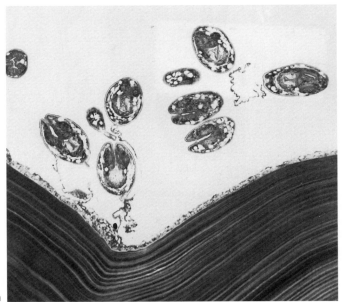
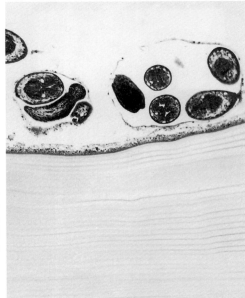

a   b

Fig. 14.92. a Part of a hydatid cyst showing a laminated acellular ectocyst with a narrow germinal layer and several immature invaginated head segments of potential future adult worms. (PAS, × 63) **b** Portion of a hydatid cyst illustrating the very thin and delicate brood capsule containing invaginated head segments of the parasite. (H&E, × 50)

latum is sometimes associated with megaloblastic anaemia. Heavy infestation with *H. nana* is said to be associated with vague non-specific irritability, diarrhoea, abdominal pain, anal and nasal pruritus, and lethargy.

Cysticercosis

Cysticercosis due to *T. solium* is generally acquired from undercooked infected pork. A scolex evaginates from the cysticercus to form an intestinal tapeworm. As well as being the usual definitive host, humans may become the intermediate host by ingesting ova from infected human faeces. Larvae emerge from the ova in the stomach and enter the circulation. Encysted larvae then appear in various organs. The brain is the most common and devastating site for such infection. Occasionally skeletal muscle, heart, liver and lungs are also involved. When the larvae die, there is an inflammatory reaction with calcification. Within the cranium the encysted larvae act as expanding space-occupying lesions that may produce hydrocephalus or seizures. Eye lesions may cause blindness and glaucoma.

Hydatid Disease

Hydatid disease, due to *Echinococcus* species, mainly *E. granulosus,* occurs when humans ingest ova that

have been passed in the faeces of an infected dog. Sheep are the usual intermediate host. Embryos that emerge from ingested ova penetrate the intestinal wall and enter the portal circulation. Most are filtered out in the liver and lungs, but some reach the capillary bed of the systemic circulation. Surviving embryos develop into hydatid cysts (cystic larvae), which contain many protoscoleces of suckers and hooklets. The cyst wall is composed of an outer laminated, acellular, elastic membrane with an inner narrow, cellular, germinal layer. The spherical brood capsules grow out from the inner layer and contain the hooklets and suckers. They become infective daughter cysts (Fig. 14.92). About 70% of hydatid cysts occur in the liver, and symptoms due to a slowly enlarging mass occur after a long interval. There is profound eosinophilia if hydatid fluid slowly enters the circulation. When much fluid rapidly enters the circulation there is an allergic reaction with urticaria and angioneurotic oedema. When hydatid cysts occur in confined spaces, such as long bones, they produce large numbers of daughter cysts.

References

Aaby P, Bukh J, Lisse IM, Smits AJ (1983) Measles mortality, state of nutrition and family structure: a community study from

Guinea Bissau. J Infect Dis 147: 693

Aaby P, Bukh J, Lisse IM, Smits AJ (1984) Overcrowding and intensive exposure as determinants of measles mortality. Am J Epidemiol 120: 49

Aaby P, Bukh J, Hoff G et al. (1986) High measles mortality in infancy related to intensity of exposure. J Pediatr 109: 40

Abioye AA, Edington GM (1972) Prevalence of amoebiasis at autopsy in Ibadan. Trans R Soc Trop Med Hyg 66: 754

Abzug MJ, Beam AC, Gyorkos EA, Levin MJ (1990) Viral pneumonia in the first month of life. Pediatr Inf Dis J 9: 881

Aftandalians R, Connor JD (1973) Bacteriacidal antibody in serum during infection with *Bordetella pertussis*. J Infect Dis 128: 555

Aherne WA, Bird T, Court SDM et al. (1970) Pathological changes in virus infections of the lower respiratory tract in children. J Clin Pathol 23: 7

Alford CA Jr, Stagno S, Reynolds DW (1974) Congenital toxoplasmosis: clinical laboratory and therapeutic considerations with special reference to subclinical disease. Bull NY Acad Med 50: 160

Allen SD, Culbertson CG (1992) *Naegleria* and *Acanthamoeba*. In: Feigin RD, Cherry JD (eds) Textbook of pediatric infectious disease, 3rd edn. Saunders, Philadelphia, p 2020

Altshuler G, Russell P (1975) The human placental villitudes: a review of chronic intrauterine infection. Curr Top Pathol 60: 64

Altshuler G, Russel P, Ermocilla R (1975) The placental pathology of small-for-gestational-age infants. Am J Obstet Gynecol 121: 351

Anand A, Gray ES, Brown T, Clewley JP, Cohen BJ (1987) Human parvovirus infection in pregnancy and hydrops fetalis. N Engl J Med 316: 183

Anderson MJ, Jones SE, Fisher-Hock SP et al. (1983) Human parvovirus, the cause of erythema infectiosum (fifth disease). Lancet i: 1378

Anonymous (1975) WHO Report. World Health Organization, Geneva

Anonymous (1989) Editorial: Immunology of measles. Lancet ii: 780

Anonymous (1993) Lyme disease – United States 1991–1992. Morbidity Mortality Weekly Report 42: 345

Arey JB (1954) Cytomegalic inclusion disease in infancy. Am J Dis Child 88: 525

Baker CJ, Barrett FF, Gordon RC, Yow MD (1973) Suppurative meningitis due to Streptococci of Lancefield group B – a study of 33 infants. J Pediatr 82: 724

Baker CJ, Barrett FF (1974) Group B streptococcal infections in infants. JAMA 230: 1158

Baker JP, Chalhub LB, Shackelford PG (1978) Ventriculitis in group B streptococcal meningitis. Pediatr Res 12: 549

Banatvala JE, Potter JE, Best JM (1971) Inteferon response to Sendai and rubella viruses in human fetal cultures. J Gen Virol 13: 193

Barbezat GO, Bowie MD, Kaschula ROC, Hansen JDL (1967) Studies on the small intestinal mucosa of children with protein–calorie malnutrition. S Afr Med J 41: 1031

Bauer FA, Wear DJ, Angritt P, Lo S-C (1991) *Mycoplasma fermintans* (incognitus strain) infection in kidneys of patients with AIDS and associated nephropathy. Hum Pathol 22: 63

Beckford AP, Kaschula ROC, Stephen C (1985) Factors associated with fatal cases of measles. A retrospective autopsy study. S Afr Med J 68: 858

Becroft DMO (1967) Histopathology of fatal adenovirus infection of the respiratory tract in young children. J Clin Pathol 20: 561

Becroft DMO (1971) Bronchiolitis obliterans, bronchitis and other sequelae of adenovirus type 21 infection in young children. J Clin Pathol 24: 72

Becroft DMO (1981) Prenatal cytomegalovirus infection: epidemiology, pathology and pathogenesis. Perspect Pediatr Pathol 6: 203

Becroft DMO, Osborne DRS (1980) The lungs in fatal measles

infection in childhood: pathological, radiological and immunological correlations. Histopathology 4: 401

Beneck D, Greco MA, Feiner HD (1986) Glomerulonephritis in congenital cytomegalic inclusion disease. Hum Pathol 17: 1054

Bennish ML (1991) Potentially lethal complication of shigellosis. Rev Infect Dis 13 (suppl 4) : 319

Benson RA, Weinstock E (1940) Gonorrhoeal vaginitis in children. A review of the literature. Am J Dis Child 59: 1083

Bentley DP (1986) Hyperplastic anaemia and parvovirus infection. Br Med J 293: 836

Berge P, Stagno S, Federer W et al. (1990) Impact of asymptomatic congenital cytomegalovirus infection on size at birth and gestational duration. Pediatr Infect Dis J 9: 170

Berkowitz FE (1992) Infections in children with severe protein–energy malnutrition. Pediatr Infect Dis J 11: 750

Berry PJ, Nagington J (1982) Fatal infection with Echovirus 11. Arch Dis Child 57: 22

Bhan MK, Raj R, Levine MM et al. (1989) Enteroaggregative *Escherichia coli* associated with persistent diarrhoea in a cohort of rural children in India. J Infect Dis 159: 1061

Biberfeld G, Sterner GA (1969) A study of *Mycoplasma pneumoniae* infections in families. Scand J Infect Dis 1: 39

Binford CH, Ecker HD (1947) Endemic (murine) typhus. Am J Clin Pathol 17: 797

Bishop RF, Davidson GP, Holmes IH et al. (1973) Virus particles in epithelial cells of duodenal mucosa from children with acute gastroenteritis. Lancet ii: 1281

Bittencourt AL (1976) Congenital Chagas' disease. Am J Dis Child 130: 97

Blacklow NR, Dolin R, Fedson DS et al. (1972) Acute infectious non-bacterial gastroenteritis. Etiology and pathogenesis. Ann Intern Med 76: 993

Blanc WA (1978) Pathology of the placenta and cord in some viral infections. In: Hanshaw JB, Dudgeon JA (eds) Viral Diseases of the Fetus and Newborn. Saunders, Philadelphia, Chap 17: p. 237

Blanc WA (1981) Pathology of the placenta, membranes and umbilical cord in bacterial, fungal and viral infections in man: In: Naeye RL, Cassane JN, Kaufman N (eds) Perinatal diseases. Williams and Wilkins, Baltimore, p 67

Blaser MJ, Reller LB (1981) Campylobacter enteritis. N Engl J Med 305: 1444

Blattner RJ (1974) The role of viruses in congenital defects. Am J Dis Child 128: 781

Blumenthal DS, Shultz MG (1975) Incidence of intestinal obstruction in children affected with *Ascaris lumbricoides*. Am J Trop Med Hyg 24: 801

Bocobo FC, Eadie GA, Miedler LJ (1965) Epidemiologic study of tinea capitis caused by *T. tonsurans* and *M. audouinii*. Public Health Rep 80: 891

Boonpucknavig V, Sitprija V (1979) Renal disease in acute *Plasmodium falciparum* infection in man. Kidney Int 16: 44

Bortolussi R (1985) Neonatal listeriosis. Where do we do go from here? Pediatr Infect Dis J 4: 228

Bradford WD, Noce PS, Gutman LT (1974) Pathologic features of enteric infection with *Yersinia enterocolitica*. Arch Pathol 98: 17

Bray J, Beavan TED (1948) Slide agglutination of *Bact. coli neopolitanum* in summer diarrhoea. J Pathol 60: 395

Brewster DR, Kwiatkowski D, White NJ (1990) Neurological sequelae of cerebral malaria in children. Lancet 336: 1039

Brightman BJ, Scott TFM, Westphal M et al (1966) An outbreak of Coxsackie B5 virus infection in a newborn nursery. J Pediatr 69: 179

Brooks GF, Buchanan TM (1970) Pertussis in the United States. J Infect Dis 122: 123

Broughton RA (1986) Infections due to *Mycoplasma pneumoniae* in childhood. Pediatr Infect Dis J 5: 71

Brown T, Anand A, Ritchie LD, Clewley JP, Reid TMS (1984) Intrauterine parvovirus infection associated with hydrops fetalis.

Lancet ii: 1033

Brown WR, Skol RJ, Levin MJ et al. (1988) Lack of correlation between infection with reovirus 3 and extrahepatic biliary atresia or neonatal hepatitis. J Pediatr 113: 670

Buchner LH, Schneirson SS (1968) Clinical and laboratory aspects of *Listeria monocytogenes* infection. Am J Med 45: 904

Buchs S (1985) Candida meningitis: a growing threat to premature and full term infants. Pediatr Infect Dis J 4: 122

Burton P (1986) Intranuclear inclusions in marrow of hydropic fetus due to parvovirus. Lancet ii: 1155

Butler JC, Havens PL, Sowell AL et al. (1993) Measles severity and serum retinol (vitamin A) concentration among children in the United States. Pediatr 91: 1176

Callahan WP Jr, Russell WO, Smith MG (1946) Human toxoplasmosis. Medicine 25: 343

Callicott JH Jr (1968) Amebic meningo-encephalitis due to free-living amebas of the *Hartmanella- (Acanthameba) Naegleria* group. Am J Clin Pathol 49: 84

Campbell JAH (1977) Cat scratch disease. In: Sommers SC, Rosen PP (eds) Path Ann 12(1). Appleton-Century-Crofts, New York, p 277

Campbell PE (1965) Vascular abnormalities following maternal rubella. Br Heart J 27: 134

Cantrelle PA, Etifier J, Masse N (1960) Mortalité et morbidité de l'enfant N. Afrique. Journées Africaines de Pädiatrie. Centre Internationale de l'Enfant, Paris, p 66

Carithers HA, Margileth AM (1991) Cat-scratch disease: acute encaphalopathy and other neurologic manifestations Am J Dis Child 145: 98

Carter RF (1972) Primary amoebic meningo-encephalitis – an appraisal of present knowledge. Trans R Soc Trop Med Hyg 66: 193

Cassel D, Pfeuffer T (1978) Mechanism of cholera toxin action: covalent modification of the guanyl nucleotide binding protein of the adenylate cyclase system. Proc Natl Acad Sci USA 75: 2669

Chandra RK (1975) Impaired immunocompetence associated with iron deficiency. J Pediatr 86: 899

Channock RN, Bell JA, Parrott RH (1961) Natural history of parainfluenza infection. Perspect Virol 2: 126

Challapalli M, Cunningham DG (1993) *Yersinia entercolitica* septicaemia in infants younger than three months of age. Pediatr Infect Dis J 12: 168

Cherry JD (1992) Parvoviruses. In: Feigin RD, Cherry JD (eds) Textbook of pediatric infectious diseases, 3rd edn. Saunders, Philadephlia, p 1626

Chin W, Contacos PG, Coatney GR et al. (1965) A naturally acquired quotididian-type malaria in man transferrable to monkeys. Science 149: 865

Chou SM (1986) Inclusion body myositis: a chronic persistent mumps myositis? Hum Pathol 17: 765

Clyde WA (1979) *Mycoplasma pneumoniae* infections of man. In: Tully JT, Whitcomb RF (eds) The mycoplasmas, vol 2. Academic Press, New York, p 275

Cohen J, Schwartz T, Kalsmer R et al. (1971) Epidemiological aspects of cholera El Tor outbreak in a non-endemic area. Lancet ii: 86

Cohen MM Sr (1974) The effect of maternal rubella on dental development. Birth Defects 10: 25

Connor DH, Neafie RC, Meyers WM (1976a) Amebiasis. In: Binford CH, Connor DH (eds) Pathology of tropical and extraordinary diseases, vol 1. AFIP, Washington DC, p 308

Connor DH, Neafie RC, Hockmeyer WT (1976b) Malaria. In: Binford CH, Connor DH (eds) Pathology of tropical and extraordinary diseases, vol 1. AFIP, Washington DC, p 273

Connor JD (1970) Evidence for an aetiological role of adenoviral infection in pertussis syndrome. N Engl J Med 283: 390

Costa J, Rabson AS (1985) Viral diseases. In: Kissane JM, Anderson WAD (eds) Anderson's pathology. Mosby, St Louis, p 345

Couvreur J (1971) Prospective study of acquired toxoplasmosis in pregnant women with a special reference to the outcome of the foetus. In: Hentsch D (ed) Toxoplasmosis. Huber, Bern, p 119

Craig JM (1981) Group B beta hemolytic streptococcal sepsis in the newborn. Perspect Pediatr Pathol 6: 139

Crane GG (1977) The pathogenesis of tropical splenomegaly syndrome: the role of immune complexes. Papua New Guinea Med J 20: 6

Crawford CL (1992) Controlling leprosy. Br Med J 305: 774

Cremin BJ, Fisher RM (1970) The lesions of congenital syphilis. Br J Radiol 43: 333

Culbertson CG (1976) Amoebic encephalitides. In: Binford CH, Connor DH (eds) Pathology of tropical and extraordinary diseases, vol 1. AFIP, Washington DC, p 317

Czinn SJ, Dahms BB, Jacobs GH, Kaplan B, Rothstein RC (1986) *Campylobacter*-like organisms in association with symptomatic gastritis in children. J Pediatr 109: 80

Darlington RW, Granoff A (1973) Replication-biological aspects. In: Kaplan AS (ed) The herpesviruses. Academic Press, New York, p 94

Davies JE (1982) Sleeping sickness and the factors affecting it in Botswana. J Trop Med Hyg 85: 63

Daya H, Allie A, McCarthy R (1982) Disseminated ascariasis: a case report. S Afr Med J 62: 820

Dean AF, Janota I, Thrasher A, Robertson I, Mieli-Vergani G (1993) Cerebral aspergilloma in a child with autosomal recessive chronic granulomatous disease. Arch Dis Child 68: 412

Deinhardt FW, Shramek GJ (1970) Mumps virus. In: Blair JE, Lennette EH, Truant JP (eds) Manual of clinical microbiology. Williams and Wilkins, Baltimore, p 515

de Rezende JM, Moreira H (1988) Chagasic megaesophagus and megacolon: historical review and present concepts. Arq Gastroenterol 25: 32

Derrick EH (1948) A fatal case of generalised amoebiasis to a protozoon closely resembling, if not identical with, *Iodamoeba butschlii*. Trans R Soc Trop Med Hyg 42: 191

Desmond MM, Montgomery JR, Melnick JC, Cochran, GG, Verniaud W (1969) Congenital rubella encephalitis. Am J Dis Child 118: 30

Diab SM, Araj GF, French FF (1989) Cardiovascular and pulmonary complications of epidemic typhus. Trop Geogr Med 41: 76

Dische MR, Gooch WM (1981) Congenital toxoplasmosis. Perspect Pediatr Pathol 6: 83

Dolan MJ, Wong MT, Regnery RL et al. (1993) Syndrome of *Rochalimaea henselae* adenitis suggesting cat scratch disease. Ann Intern Med 118: 331

Dolin R, Blacklow NR, DuPont H et al. (1971) Transmission of acute infectious non-bacterial gastroenteritis to volunteers by oral administration of stool filtrates. J Infect Dis 123: 307

Dorfman RF, Remington JS (1973) The value of lymph node biopsy in the diagnosis of acute acquired toxoplasmosis. N Engl J Med 289: 878

Dorfman DH, Glaser JH (1990) Congenital syphilis presenting in infants after the newborn period. N Engl J Med 323: 1299

Dorsch MM, Cameron AS, Robinson BS (1983) The epidemiology and control of primary amoebic meningoencephalitis with particular reference to South Australia. Trans R Soc Trop Med Hyg 77: 372

Downham MAPS, Gardner PS, McQuillin J, Ferris JAJ (1975) Role of respiratory viruses in childhood mortality. Br Med J i: 235

Driscoll SG (1962) Congenital listeriosis: diagnosis from placental studies. Obstet Gynecol 20: 216

Driscoll SG (1969) Histopathology of gestational rubella. Am J Dis Child 118: 49

DuPont HL, Hornick RB, Dawkins AT et al. (1969) The response of man to virulent *Shigella flexneri* 2a. J Infect Dis 119: 296

Dussaix E, Hadchouel M, Tardieu M et al. (1984) Biliary atresia and reovirus type 3 infection. N Engl J Med 310: 658

Dutz W (1970) *Pneumocystis carinii* pneumonia. In: Sommers SC (ed) Pathol Annu. Butterworths, London, 5: 309

Dutz W, Jennings-Khodadad E, Post C, Kohout E, Nazarian I, Esmaili H (1974) Marasmus and *Pneumocystis carinii* pneumonia in institutionalized infants. Z Kinderheilk 117: 241

Dutz W, Kohout E, Rossipal E, Vessal K (1976) Infantile stress, immune modulation and disease patterns. In: Sommers SC (ed) Pathol Annu 11. Appleton-Century-Crofts, New York, p 415

EPI Newsletter (1992) First ladies' support elimination of neonatal tetanus. In: Expanded program on immunization, maternal and child health program. Pan American Health Organization, Washington DC, 14(6): 8

Edman JC, Kovacs JA, Masur H, Santi DV, Elwood HJ, Sogin ML (1988) Ribosomal RNA sequence shows *Pneumocystis carinii* to be a member of the Fungi. Nature 334: 519

Elliott WG (1970) Placental toxoplasmosis. A report of a case. Am J Clin Pathol 53: 413

Enders JF, McCarthy K, Mitus A, Cheatham WJ (1959) Isolation of measles virus at autopsy in cases of giant cell pneumonia without rash. N Engl J Med 261: 875

English CK, Wear DJ, Margileth AM, Lissner CR, Walsh GP (1988) Cat-scratch disease: isolation and culture of the bacterial agent. JAMA 259: 1347

Esterly JR, Oppenheimer EH (1969) Pathological lesions due to congenital rubella. Arch Pathol 87: 380

Esterly JR, Oppenheimer EH (1973) Intrauterine rubella infection. Perspect Pediatr Pathol 1: 313

Evans JR, Allen AC, Stinson DA, Bortolussi R, Peddle LJ (1985) Perinatal listeriosis: report of an outbreak. Pediatr Infect Dis J 4: 237

Faden H, Grossi M (1991) Acute osteomyelitis in children. Am J Dis Child 145: 65

Feldstein JD, Johnson FK, Kallick CA et al. (1974) Acute haemorrhagic pancreatitis and pseudocyst due to mumps. Ann Surg 180: 85

Ferris JAJ, Aherne WA, Locke WS, McQuillan J, Gardner PS (1973) Sudden unexpected death in infants. Histology and virology. Br Med J ii: 439

Forrest JM, Menser MA, Reye RDK (1969) Obstructive arterial lesions in rubella. Lancet i: 1263

Fortenberry JD, Mariscalco M, Louis PT, Stein F, Jones JK, Jefferson LS (1992) Severe laryngiotracheobronchitis complicating measles. Am J Dis Child 146: 1040

Fortuin NJ, Morrow AG, Roberts WC (1971) Late vascular manifestations of the rubella syndrome. Am J Med 51: 134

Fox H (1981) Placental involvement in maternal systemic infection. Perspect Pediatr Pathol 6: 63

Foy HN, Kenny GE, McMahan R et al. (1970) *Mycoplasma pneumoniae* in the community. Am J Epidemiol 93: 55

Fraser DW, Darby CP, Koehler RE et al. (1973) Risk factors in bacterial meningitis: Charleston County, South Carolina. J Infect Dis 127: 271

Frenkel JK (1973) Pathology and pathogenesis of congenital toxoplasmosis. Bull NY Acad Med 50: 182

Gaon JA, Murray ES (1966) The natural history of recrudescent typhus (Brill–Zinsser disease) in Bosnia. Bull WHO 35: 133

Gardner PS (1977) How etiologic, pathologic and clinical diagnoses can be made in a correlated fashion. Pediatr Res 11: 254

Gautam OP, Thawrani YP, Mathur PS (1980) Pattern of malaria in children and its therapeutic evaluation. Indian Pediatr 17: 511

Gear JHS, Measroch V (1973) Coxsackie virus infection of the newborn. Prog Med Virol 15: 42

Glaser JH, Balistrevi WF, Morecki R (1984) Role of reovirus type 3 in persistent infantile cholestasis. J Pediatr 105: 912

Gold E, Carver DH, Heinberg H et al. (1961) Viral infection: a possible cause of sudden unexpected death in infants. N Engl J Med 264: 53

Goldschneider I, Gotschlich EC, Artenstein MS (1969) Human immunity to the meningococcus. II. Development of natural immunity. J Exp Med 129: 1327

Goodwin LG (1971) The pathology of African trypanosomiasis. Trans R Soc Trop Med Hyg 64: 797

Gorelkin L, Chandler FW, Ewing EP (1986) Staining qualities of cytomegalovirus inclusions in the lungs of patients with the acquired immunodeficiency syndrome: a potential source of diagnostic misinterpretation. Hum Pathol 17: 926

Gotschlich EC, Goldschneider I, Lepow ML et al. (1977) The immune response to bacterial polysaccharides in man. In: Haber E, Krause RM (eds) Antibodies in human diagnosis and therapy. Ravan Press, New York, p 391

Gracey M (1993) Bacterial diarrhoea. Ann Trop Paediatr 13: 107

Graves M, Griffiths DE, Johnson RT et al. (1984) Development of antibody to measles virus polypeptides during complicated and uncomplicated measles virus infections. J Virol 49: 409

Greenberg B, Wyatt RG, Kapikian AZ (1979) Norwalk virus in vomitus. Lancet i: 55

Griffin DE, Ward BJ, Jauregui E, Johnson RT, Vaisberg A (1989) Immune activation in measles. N Engl J Med 320: 1667

Grimmer H, Joseph A (1959) An epidemic of infectious erythema in Germany. Arch Dermatol 80: 283

Groothuis JR, Slabenblatt CK, Laver BA (1990) Severe respiratory syncytial virus infection in older children. Am J Dis Child 144: 346

Gross RL, Reid JVO, Newberne PM, Burgess B, Marston R, Hift W (1975) Depressed cell-mediated immunity in megaloblastic anaemia due to folic acid deficiency. Am J Clin Nutr 28: 225

Guerrant RL, Lahaita RG, Winn WC Jr, Roberts R (1978) Campylobacteriosis in man: pathogenic mechanisms and review of 91 blood stream infections. Am J Med 65: 584

Gunasekaran TS, Hassall E (1992) Giardiasis mimicking inflammatory bowel disease. J Pediatr 120: 424

Hageman J, Schulman S, Schreiber M, Luck S, Yogev R (1980) Congenital tuberculosis: critical reappraisal of clinical findings and diagnostic procedures. Pediatr 66: 980

Hall CB, Powell KR, MacDonald NE et al. (1986) Respiratory syncytial virus infection in children with compromised immune function. N Engl J Med 315: 77

Hall A, Awar KS, Tomkins AM (1992) Intensity of reinfection with *Ascaris lumbricoides* and its implications for parasite control. Lancet 339: 1253

Hanshaw JB (1979) A new cytomegalovirus syndrome? Am J Dis Child 133: 475

Hanshaw JB, Dudgeon JA (1978) Viral diseases of the fetus and newborn. Saunders, Philadelphia, p 17

Hardman JM (1968) Fatal meningococcal infections: the changing pathologic picture in the sixties. Mil Med 133: 951

Hart CA, Batt RM, Saunders JR (1993) Diarrhoea caused by *Escherichia coli*. Ann Trop Paediatr 13: 121

Hart J, Spirman U, Shattach J (1984) An outbreak of amoebic infection in a kibbutz population. Trans R Soc Trop Med Hyg 78: 346

Harter CA, Benirschke K (1976) Fetal syphilis in the first trimester. Am J Obstet Gynecol 124: 705

Havaldar PV, Patil VD, Siddibhavi BM (1989) Haemorrhagic diphtheria. Ann Trop Paediatr 3: 178

Hayden RJ (1974) The epidemiology and nature of measles in Nairobi before the impact of measles immunization. East Afr Med J 51: 199

Hayman J (1993) Out of Africa: observations on the histopathology of *Mycobacterium ulcerans* infection. J Clin Pathol 46: 5

Hazell SL, Lee A, Brady L, Hennessy W (1986) *Campylobacter pyloridis* and gastritis. Association with intercellular spaces and adaption to an environment of mucus as important factors in colonization of gastric epithelium. J Infect Dis 153: 685

Hershko C, Karsai A, Eylon L et al. (1970) The effect of chronic iron deficiency on some biochemical functions of human haemopoietic tissue. Blood 36: 321

Hill IJ, Sinclair-Smith CC, Lastovica AJ, Bowie MD, Emms M (1987) Transient protein losing enteropathy associated with acute gastritis and *Campylobacter pylori*. Arch Dis Child 62: 1215

Hinman AR, Judd JM, Kolnik JP et al. (1976) Changing risks in tuberculosis. Am J Epidemol 103: 486

Hoffman SL, Piesseus WF, Ratiwayanto et al. (1984) Reduction of suppressor T lymphocytes in the tropical splenomegaly syndrome. New Engl J Med 310: 337

Hoffmann EB, Knudsen CJ, Paterson MP (1990) Acute osteomyelitis and septic arthritis in children: a spectrum of disease. Pediatr Surg Int 5: 382

Hood M, Jannery A, Dameron G (1961) β Hemolytic streptococci, group B associated with the perinatal period. Am J Obstet Gynecol 82: 809

Horley JF (1952) Congenital tuberculosis. Arch Dis Child 27: 167

Hotez PJ (1989) Hookworm disease in children. Paediatr Infect Dis J 8: 516

Househam KC, Mann MD, Bowie MD (1988) Enteropathogens associated with acute infantile diarrhoea in Cape Town. S Afr Med J 73: 83

Hudson FP (1956) Clinical aspects of congenital tuberculosis. Arch Dis Child 31: 136

Hughes WT, Price RA, Sisko F et al. (1974) Protein–calorie malnutrition : a host determined for *Pneumocystis carinii* infection. Am J Dis Child 128: 44

Hughes I, Jenny MEM, Newton RW, Morris DJ, Klapper PE (1993) Measles encephalitis during immunosuppressive treatment for acute lymphoblastic leukaemia. Arch Dis Child 68: 775

Hughes WT, Steigman AJ, Delong HF (1966) Some implications of fatal nephritis associated with mumps. Am J Dis Child 111: 297

Hussey G, Simpson J (1990) Nosocomial bacteremias in measles. Pediatr Infect Dis J 9: 715

Hussey GD, Klein M (1990) A randomized controlled trial of vitamin A in children with severe measles. N Engl J Med 323: 160

Hutt MSR (1966) Buruli ulcer, subcutaneous phycomycosis, and idiopathic tropical splenomegaly: 3 recent aspects of pathology in Africa. Sommers SC (ed) Path Annu 1. Appleton-Century-Crofts, New York, p 241

Ish-Horowicz M, Korman SH, Shapiro M et al. (1989) Asymptomatic giardiasis in children. Pediatr Infect Dis J 8: 773

Jager BV, Stamm WP (1972) Brain abscesses caused by free-living amoeba probably of the genus *Hartmanella* in a patient with Hodgkin's disease. Lancet ii: 1343

Jones PG, Campbell PE (1960) Tuberculous lymphadenitis in childhood. The significance of anonymous mycobacteria. Br J Surg 50: 302

Joshi W, Davidson PM, Jones PG, Campbell PE, Roberton DM (1989) Non-tuberculous mycobacterial lymphadenitis in children. Eur J Pediatr 148: 751

Joske RA, Keall ED, Leak PJ et al. (1964) Hepatitis encephalitis in humans with reovirus infection. Arch Intern Med 113: 811

Kafka JA, Catanzaro AT (1981) Disseminated coccidio-idiomycosis in children. J Pediatr 98: 355

Kahn LB (1963) Gastric mucormycosis: report of a case with a review of the literature. S Afr Med J 37: 1265

Kalmyak JE (1977) Incidence and distribution of Herpes simplex virus types 1 and 2 from genital lesions in college women. J Med Virol 1: 175

Kapikian AZ, Wyatt RG, Dolin R et al. (1972) Visualization by immune electron microscopy of a 27 nm particle associated with acute infectious non-bacterial gastroenteritis. J Virol 10: 1075

Kaplan EL (1992) Group A streptococcal infections. In: Feigin RD, Cherry JD (eds) Textbook of pediatr infectious diseases, 3rd edn. Saunders, Philadelphia, p 1296

Kaplan MH, Klein SW, McPhee J, Harper RG (1983) Group B coxsackievirus infections in infants younger than three months of age: a serious childhood illness. Rev Infect Dis 5: 1019

Kaschula ROC, Uys CJ, Kuijten RH, Dale JRP, Wiggelinkhuizen J (1974) Nephrotic syndrome of congenital syphilis. Arch Pathol 97: 289

Kaschula ROC, Gajjar PD, Mann M, Bowie MD et al. (1979) Infantile jejunal mucosa in infection and malnutrition. Isr J Med Sci 15: 356

Kaschula ROC, Druker J, Kipps A (1983) Late morphological consequences of measles: a lethal and debilitating lung disease among the poor. Rev Infect Dis 5: 395

Kass EH, Andrus SB, Adams RD et al. (1952) Toxoplasmosis in the human adult. Arch Intern Med 89: 759

Katz M (1992) Nemathelminthes. In: Feigin RD, Cherry JD (eds) Textbook of pediatric infectious diseases. Saunders, Philadelphia, 3rd edn, p. 2078

Kaufmann JCE (1969) Bilharziasis with particular reference to South Africa: the pathology of bilharzia of the central nervous system. Med Proc 15: 355

Kipps A, Becker W, Wainwright J, McKenzie D (1967) Fatal disseminated primary herpesvirus infection in children: epidemiology based on 93 non-neonatal cases. S Afr Med J 41: 647

Kipps A, Kaschula ROC (1976) Virus pneumonia following measles. A virological and histological study of autopsy material. S Afr Med J 50: 1083

Kipps A, Dick G, Moody JW (1983) Measles and the central nervous system. Lancet ii: 1406

Klatt EC, Pavlova Z, Teberg AJ, Yonekura ML (1986) Epidemic perinatal listeriosis at autopsy. Hum Pathol 17: 1278

Knot PD, Welply GAC, Anderson MJ (1984) Serologically proved intrauterine infection with parvovirus. Br Med J 289: 1660

Krajden M, Brown M, Petrasek A, Middleton P (1990) Clinical features of adenovirus enteritis: a review of 127 cases. Pediatr Infect Dis J 9: 636

Krause PJ, Telford SR, Pollack RJ et al. (1992) Babesiosis: an underdiagnosed disease of children. Pediatrics 89: 1045

Krous HF, Dietzman D, Ray CG (1973) Fatal infections with echovirus type 6 and 11 in early infancy. Am J Dis Child 126: 842

Kuroki S, Haruta T, Yoshioka M, Kobayashi Y, Nukina M, Nakanishi H (1991) Guillain–Barré syndrome associated with campylobacter infection. Pediatr Infect Dis J 10: 149

Kutty MK, Unni PN (1969) Rhinosporidiosis of the urethra. A case report. Trop Geogr Med 21: 338

Lai KK, Stottmeier KD, Shermann IH et al. (1984) Mycobacterial cervical lymphadenopathy: relation of etiologic agents to age. JAMA 251: 1286

Lainson R (1983) The American leishmaniasis: some observations on their ecology and epidemiology. Trans R Soc Trop Med Hyg 77: 569

Lambert ME, Scofield PF, Ironside AG, Mandal BK (1979) *Campylobacter* colitis. Br Med J i: 857

Lami JL, Moore TC (1989) Colectomy for necrotizing amebic pancolitis in early childhood with survival. J Pediatr Surg 24: 1174

Lastovica AJ, Le Roux E, Congi RV, Penner JL (1986) Distribution of sero-biotypes of *Campylobacter jejuni* and *C. coli* isolated from paediatric patients. J Med Microbiol 21: 1

Law BJ, Marks MI (1982) Pediatric nocardiosis. Pediatr 70: 560

Lawrence C, Olson JA (1986) Birefrigent haemozoin identifies malaria. Am J Clin Pathol 86: 360

Lerner AM, Cherry JD, Klein JO et al. (1962) Infections with reovirus. N Engl J Med 267: 947

Le Roux FB, Schwersenski J, Greeff MJ (1978) Congenital tuberculosis. A report of a probable case. S Afr Med J 53: 946

Levine AS, Schimpff SC, Graw RG et al. (1974) Haematologic malignancies and other marrow failure states: progress in the management of complicating infections. Semin Hematol 11: 141

Lillie RD (1941) The pathology of Rocky Mountain spotted fever. Natl Inst Health Bull 177: 1

Lurie HI, Still WJS (1969) The "capsule" of *Sporotrichium schenckii* and the evolution of the asteroid body: a light and electron microscopic study. Sabouraudia 7: 64

Luvuno FM, Mtshali Z, Baker LW (1985) Vascular occlusion in the pathogenesis of complicated amoebic colitis. Br J Surg 72: 123

MacCallum P, Tolhurst JC, Buckle G, Sissons HA (1948) New mycobacterial infection in man. Clinical aspects. J Pathol Bacteriol 60: 93

MacDonald TT, Choy M-Y, Spencer J et al. (1991) Histopathology and immunohistochemistry of the caecum with *Trichuris* dysentery syndrome. J Clin Pathol 44: 194

MacFarlane DE, Horner-Bryce J (1987) Cryptosporidiosis in well nourished and malnourished children. Acta Paediatr Scand 76: 474

MacGregor IA (1971) Immunity of plasmodial infection: consideration of factors relevant to malaria in man. Int Rev Proc Med 4: 1

Malan AF (1985) Syphilis tetanos tuberculose. In: Vert P, Stern L (eds) Medicine neonatale. Masson, Paris, p 619

Manson-Bahr PE (1971) Leishmaniasis. Int Rev Trop Med 4: 123

March DH (1982) Prematurity and perinatal mortality in pregnancies complicated by maternal *Chlamydia trachomonas* infections. JAMA 247: 1585

Marcial MA, Marcial-Rojas RA (1985) Protozoal and helminthic disease. In: Kissane JM, Anderson WAD (eds) Anderson's pathology. Mosby, St Louis, p 401

Margileth AM (1975) Scalded skin syndrome: diagnosis, differential diagnosis and management of 42 children. South Med J 68: 447

Margileth AM, Chandra R, Altman RP (1984) Chronic lymphadenopathy due to mycobacterial infection. Clinical feature, diagnosis, histopathology and management. Am J Dis Child 138: 917

Markell EK, Voge M (1981) Medical parasitology, 5th edn. Saunders, Philadelphia

McCracken GH, Shinefield HR, Cobb K, Rausen AR, Disch ER, Eichenwald HF (1969) Congenital cytomegalic inclusion disease. A longitudinal study of 20 patients. Am J Dis Child 117: 522

McFarlane H, Reddy S, Adcock KJ, Adeshina H, Cooke AR, Akene J (1970) Immunity, transferrin and survival in kwashiorkor. Br Med J iv: 268

McKenzie D, Hansen JDL, Becker W (1959) Herpes simplex virus infection: dissemination in association with malnutrition. Arch Dis Child 34: 250

Mebus CA, Wyatt RG, Kapikian AZ (1977) Pathology of diarrhoea in gnotobiotic calves induced by the human reovirus-like agent of infantile gastroenteritis. Vet Pathol 14: 273

Medoff G, Kobayashi GS (1981) Zygomycosis. In: Feigin RD, Cherry JD (eds) Textbook of pediatric infectious diseases. Saunders, Philadelphia, p 1510

Meheus AZ, Mubiligi V, Rugamra A (1974) A louse-borne typhus epidemic in the prefecture of Butare, Rwanda. East Afr Med J 5: 675

Menser MA, Reye RDK (1974) The pathology of congenital rubella – a review. Pathology 6: 215

Menser MA, Forrest JM, Bransby RD (1978) Rubella infection and diabetes mellitus. Lancet i: 57

Meyers WM (1992) Leprosy. In: Feigin RD, Cherry JD (eds) Textbook of pediatric infectious diseases, 3rd edn. Saunders, Philadelphia, p 1149

Michaels RH, Poxiviak CS, Stonebraker FE et al. (1976) Factors affecting pharyngeal *Haemophilus influenzae* type b colonization rates in children. J Clin Microbiol 4: 413

Miller DR, Hanshaw JB, O'Leary DS, Hnilica JV (1970) Fatal disseminated Herpes simplex virus infection and hemorrhage in the neonate. J Pediatr 76: 409

Miller E, Cradock-Watson JE, Pollock TM (1982) Consequences of confirmed maternal rubella at successive stages of pregnancy. Lancet ii: 781

Mimica I, Donoso E, Howard JE, Lederman GW (1971) Lung puncture in the etiological diagnosis of pneumonia: a study of 543 infants and children. Am J Dis Child 122: 278

Molbak K, Hojlyng N, Gaarslev K (1988) High prevalence of campylobacter excretors among Liberian children related to environmental conditions. Epidemiol Infect 100: 227

Montgomery RD (1961) The cause of death in tetanus. West Indian Med J 10: 84

Moortey B, Mehta S, Mitra SK et al. (1977) Amoebic liver abscess in a 4 month old infant. Aust Paediatr J 13: 53

Morgan DG, Niederman JC, Miller G, Smith HW, Dowaliby JM (1979) Site of Epstein–Barr virus replication in the oropharynx. Lancet ii: 1154

Morley DC (1962) Measles in Nigeria. Am J Dis Child 103: 230

Morley D (1983) Severe measles: some unanswered questions. Rev Infect Dis 5: 460

Mortimer PP (1986) The eighty years of fifth disease. Br Med J 289: 338

Muir E (1936) Juvenile leprosy. Int J Leprosy 4: 45

Murray ES (1981) Rickettsial diseases. In: Feigin RD, Cherry JD (eds) Textbook of pediatric infectious diseases. Saunders, Philadelphia, p 1437

Mylins RE, Ten Seldam REJ (1962) Venereal infection by *Entamoeba histolytica* in a New Guinea native couple. Trop Geogr Med 14: 20

Naeye RL, Dellinger WS, Blanc WA (1971) Fetal and maternal features of antenatal bacterial infections. J Pediatr 79: 733

Nahmias AJ, Griffith D, Snitzer J (1967) Fatal pneumonia associated with adenovirus type 7. Am J Dis Child 114: 36

Nahmias AJ, Keyserling HL, Kerrick GM (1983) Herpes simplex. In: Remington JS, Klein JD (eds) Infectious diseases of the fetus and newborn. Saunders, Philadelphia, p 636

Najii AF, Carbonell F, Barker HJ (1962) Cat scratch disease. Am J Clin Pathol 38: 513

Naqvi SH, Swierkosz EM, Gerard J, Mills JR (1993) Presentation of *Yersinia enterocolitica* enteritis in children. Pediatr Infect Dis J 12: 386

Neafie RC (1976) Balantidiasis. In: Binford CH, Connor DH (eds) Pathology of tropical and extraordinary diseases. AFIP, Washington DC, p 325

Neveling U, Kaschula ROC (1993) Fatal meningococcal disease in childhood: an autopsy study of 86 cases. Ann Trop Paediatr 13: 147

Niederman JC, Miller G, Pearson HA et al. (1976) Infectious mononucleosis: Epstein–Barr virus shedding in saliva and in oropharynx. N Engl J Med 294: 1355

Noussitou FM (1976) Leprosy in children. World Health Organization, Geneva O'Connor GR (1974) Manifestations and management of ocular toxoplasmosis. Bull NY Acad Med 50: 192

Ognibene AJ, O'Leary DS, Czarnecki SW et al. (1971) Myocarditis and disseminated intravascular coagulation in scrub typhus. Am J Med Sci 261: 233

Oppenheimer EH, Dahms BB (1981) Congenital syphilis in the fetus and neonate. Perspect Pediatr Pathol 6: 115

Orren A, Kipps A, Moodie JW, Beaty DW, Dowdle EB, MacIntyre JP (1981) Increased susceptibility to herpes simplex virus infections in children with acute measles. Infect Immun 31: 1

Oseasohn R, Adelson L, Kaji M (1959) Clinico-pathological study of 33 cases of Asian flu. N Engl J Med 260: 509

Padhye AA (1973) *Microsporum persiolor* infection in the United States. Arch Dermatol 108: 561

Pagano JS (1975) Diseases and mechanisms of persistent DNA virus infection: latency and cellular transformation. J Infect Dis 132: 209

Pappagianis E (1972) Coccidioidomycosis. In: Hoeprich PD (ed) Infectious diseases. Harper and Row, Hagerstown, p 405

Pattison JR, Jones SE, Hodgson J et al. (1981) Parvovirus infections and hypoplastic crisis in sickle-cell anaemia. Lancet i: 664

Pavlica F (1962) The first observation of congenital pneumocystis in a fully developed stillborn child. Ann Pediatr (Basel) 198: 177

Peckham C, Coleman J, Hurley R, Chin K, Henderson K (1983) Cytomegalovirus infection in pregnancy: preliminary finding from a prospective study. Lancet i: 1352

Pedley JC (1967) The presence of *M. leprae* in human milk. Leprosy Rev 38: 239

Perera DR, Western KA, Johnson HD et al. (1970) *Pneumocystis carinii* in pneumonia in a hospital for children. Epidemiologic aspects. JAMA 214: 1074

Pettapiece MC, Hiles DA, Johnson BL (1976) Massive congenital ocular toxoplasmosis. J Pediatr Ophthalmol 13: 259

Philip AGS, Larson EJ (1973) Overwhelming neonatal infection with echo 19 virus. J Pediatr 82: 391

Pifer LL, Hughes WT, Murphy MJ (1977) Propagation of *Pneumocystis carinii* in vitro. Pediatr Res 11: 305

Porter HJ, Padfield CJH, Peres LC, Hirschowitz L, Berry PJ (1993) Adenovirus and intranuclear inclusions in appendices in intussusception. J Clin Pathol 46: 154

Price RA, Hughes WT (1974) Histopathology of *Pneumocystis carinii* infestation and infection in malignant disease in childhood. Hum Pathol 5: 737

Purtilo DT, Tatsumi E, Manolov G et al. (1985) Epstein–Barr virus as an etiologic agent in the pathogenesis of lymphoproliferative and aproliferative diseases in immune deficient patients. Int Rev Exp Pathol 27: 112

Quinn TC, Jacobs RF, Murtz GJ, Hook EW, Locksley RM (1982) Congenital malaria: a report of 4 cases and review. J Pediatr 101: 229

Rabson AR, Hallot AF, Koornhof HJ (1975) Generalised *Yersinia enterocolitica* infection. J Infect Dis 131: 447

Ramchander V, Ramcharan J, Muralidhara K (1991) Fatal respiratory obstruction due to *Ascaris lumbricoides* – a case report. Ann Trop Paediatr 11: 293

Ramachandran S, Induruwa PAC, Pereira MVF (1976) pH of amoebic liver pus. Trans R Soc Trop Med Hyg 70: 159

Ramos O, Saad F, Lesser WP (1964) Portal haemodynamics and liver cell function in hepatic schistosomiasis. Gastroenterology 47: 241

Randall G, Seidel JS (1985) Malaria. Pediatr Clin North Am 32: 893

Ravdin JI (1989) *Entamoeba histolytica:* from adherence to enteropathy. J Infect Dis 159: 420

Reid L (1977) Influence of the pattern of structural growth of lungs on susceptibility to specific infectious diseases in infants and children. Pediatr Res 11: 210

Rettig PJ (1979) Medical progress: campylobacter infections in human beings. J Pediatr 94: 855

Reynolds DW, Stagno S, Hosty TS, Tiller M, Alford CA (1973) Maternal cytomegalovirus excretion and perinatal infection. N Engl J Med 289: 1

Richardus JH, Dumas AM, Huisman J, Schaap GJP (1985) Q fever in infancy: a review of 18 cases. Pediatr Infect Dis J 4: 369

Ridley DS, Jopling WH (1966) Classification of leprosy according to immunity. A five group system. Int J Leprosy 34: 255

Robb JA, Benirschke K, Mannino F, Voland J (1986) Intrauterine latent herpes simplex virus infection: II. Latent neonatal infection. Hum Pathol 17: 1210

Rode H, Davies MRQ, Cywes S (1978) Amoebic liver abscesses in infancy and childhood. S Afr J Surg 16: 131

Rode H, Cullis S, Millar A, Cremin B, Cywes S (1990) Abdominal complications of *Ascaris lumbricoides* in children. Pediatr Surg Int 5: 397

Rodriquez-Erdmann F (1965) Intravascular activation of the clotting system with phospholipids. Blood 26: 541

Rorke LB (1973) Nervous system lesions in the congenital rubella syndrome. Arch Otolaryngol 98: 249

Rosen L, Hovis JF, Mastrota FM et al. (1960) An outbreak of infection with a type I reovirus among children in an institution. Am J Hyg 71: 266

Rosenberg HS, Kohl S, Vogler C (1981a) Viral infections of the fetus and the neonate. In: Naeye RL, Kissane JM, Kaufman N (eds) Perinatal diseases. Williams and Wilkins, Baltimore, p 133

Rosenberg HS, Oppenheimer EH, Esterly JR (1981b) Congenital rubella syndrome: the late effects and their relation to early lesions. Perspect Pediatr Pathol 6: 183

Rosenstein DL, Navarette-Reyna A (1964) Cytomegalic inclusion disease. Am J Obstet Gynecol 89: 220

Ruiz-Contreras J, Montero RG, Amador JTR, Corradi EG, Vera AS (1993) Q Fever in children. Am J Dis Child 147: 300

Ruiz-Palacios G, Pickering LK (1992) Campylobacter and helicobacter infections. In: Feigin RD, Cherry JD (eds) Textbook of pediatr infectious diseases, 3rd edn. Saunders, Philadelphia, p 1072

Russell P (1979) Inflammatory lesions of the human placenta. II. Villitis of unknown etiology in perspective. Am J Diagn Gynecol Obstet 1: 339

Ryder CS, Beatty DW, Heese HdV (1987) Group B meningococcal infection in children during an epidemic in Cape Town, South Africa. Ann Trop Paediatr 7: 47

Sack RB (1975) Human diarrhoeal disease caused by enterotoxogenic *Escherichia coli*. Annu Rev Microbiol 29: 333

Sack RB, Gorbach SL, Banwell JG et al. (1971) Enterotoxic enterogenic *Escherichia coli* isolated from patients with severe cholera-like disease. J Infect Dis 123: 378

Salfelder K, Brass K, Doehnert G, Doehnert R, Sauerteig E (1970) Fatal disseminated histoplasmosis – anatomic study of autopsy cases. Virchows Arch A Pathol Anat 350: 303

Scheifele DW, Forbes CE (1972) Prolonged giant cell excretion in severe African measles. Pediatr 50: 867

Schewitz IA, Le Roux E (1978) Campylobacter infections: first reports from Red Cross War Memorial Children's Hospital, Cape Town. S Afr Med J 54: 385

Schlech WF, Levigne PM, Bortolussi RA et al. (1983) Epidemic listeriosis. Evidence for transmission by food. N Engl J Med 308: 203

Schlesinger PA, Duray PH, Durk BA et al. (1985) Maternal–fetal transmission of the Lyme disease spirochaete, *Borrelia burgdorferi*. Ann Intern Med 103: 67

Schonland M, Strong ML, Wesley A (1976) Fatal adenovirus pneumonia: clinical and pathological features. S Afr Med J 50: 1748

Schooley RT, Arbit DI, Henle W et al. (1984) T lymphocyte subset interactions in the cell mediated immune response to Epstein–Barr virus. Cell Immunol 86: 402

Schreiber DS, Blacklow NR, Trier JS (1973) The mucosal lesion of the proximal small intestine in acute infectious nonbacterial gastroenteritis. N Engl J Med 288: 1318

Schwartz TF, Nerlich A, Hottentrüger B et al. (1991) Parvovirus B 19 infection of the fetus: histology and in situ hybridization. Am J Clin Pathol 96: 121

Seemayer TA, Olgny LL, Gartner JG (1981) The Epstein–Barr virus: historical, biologic, pathologic and oncologic considerations. Perspect Pediatr Pathol 6: 1

Seidel JS (1985) Primary amebic meningoencephalitis. Pediatr Clin North Am 32: 881

Sever JL (1983) Persistent measles infection of the central nervous system: subacute sclerosing panencephalitis. Rev Infect Dis 5: 467

Shahin B, Papadopoulou ZL, Jenis EH (1974) Congenital nephrotic syndrome associated with congenital toxoplasmosis. J Pediatr 85: 366

Sharon N (1977) The prevalence of Herpesvirus hominis in genital lesions with suggestive chancre morphology. Am J Clin Pathol 68: 628

Sheldon PJ, Hemsted EH, Holborow EJ et al. (1973) Thymic origin of atypical lymphocytes in infectious mononucleosis. Lancet ii: 1153

Siegel M (1973) Congenital malformations following chickenpox, measles, mumps and hepatitis. JAMA 226: 1521

Silpapojakul K, Chupuppakarn S, Yuthasompob S et al. (1991) Scrub and murine typhus in children with obscure fever in the tropics. Pediatr Infect Dis J 10: 200

Simenhoff ML, Uys CJ (1958) Coxsackie virus myocarditis of the newborn: a pathological study of 4 cases. Med Proc 4: 389

Singer DB (1981) Pathology of neonatal herpes simplex virus infection. Perspect Pediatr Pathol 6: 243

Singer DB, Rudolph AJ, Rosenberg HS, Rawls WE, Bonink M (1967) Pathology of the congenital rubella syndrome. J Pediatr 71: 665

Singer DB, South MA, Montgomery JR, Rawls WE (1969) Congenital rubella syndrome. Am J Dis Child 118: 54

Singer JI, Munci JE (1952) Sporotrichosis: etiologic considerations and report of additional cases from New York. N Y State J Med 52: 2147

Siplovich L, Davies MRQ, Kaschula ROC (1988) Intestinal obstruction in the newborn with congenital syphylis. J Pediatr Surg 23: 810

Sive AA, Subotzky EF, Malan H, Dempster WS, Heese H de V (1993) Red blood cell antioxidant enzyme concentrations in kwashiorkor and marasmus. Ann Trop Paediatr 13: 33

Smith MHD, Marquis JR (1981) Tuberculosis and other mycobacterial infections. In: Feigin RD, Cherry JD (eds) Textbook of pediatric infectious diseases. Saunders, Philadelphia, p 1016

Smythe PM, Campbell JAH (1959) The significance of bacteraemia of kwashiorkor. S Afr Med J 33: 777

Soper RT, Silber DL, Holcomb GW (1970) Gastrointestinal histoplasmosis in children. J Pediatr Surg 5: 32

South MA, Montgomery JR, Rawls WE (1975) Immune deficiency in the congenital rubella and other viral infections. Birth Defects 11: 234

Spira TJ, Kabins SA (1976) Yersinia enterocolitica septicaemia with septic arthritis. Arch Intern Med 136: 1305

Spooner V, Barker J, Tulloch S et al. (1989) Clinical signs and risk factors associated with pneumonia in children admitted to Goroka Hospital, Papua New Guinea. J Trop Pediatr 35: 295

Stagno S, Reynolds DW, Amos CS et al. (1977) Auditory and visual defects resulting from symptomatic and subclinical congenital cytomegaloviral and toxoplasma infections. Pediatr 59: 669

Steffen R (1986) Epidemiologic studies of traveller's diarrhoea, severe gastrointestinal infections and cholera. Rev Infect Dis 8: S122

Sterzl J, Silverstein AM (1967) Developmental aspects of immunity. Adv Immunol 6: 337

Stevens D, Swift PGF, Johnston PGB et al. (1978) Mycoplasma pneumoniae infections in children. Arch Dis Child 53: 38

Stockman JA (1981) Infections and iron. Too much of a good thing. Am J Dis Child 135: 18

Stoll BJ (1979) Tetanus. Pediatr Clin North Am 26: 415

Stoll NR (1947) This wormy world. J Parasitol 33: 1

Stowens D (1966) Pediatric Pathology, 2nd ed. Williams and Wilkins, Baltimore, p 249

Strano AJ (1976) Light microscopy of selected viral diseases – morphology of viral inclusion bodies. Pathol Annu 11: 53

Sullivan PB, Marsh MN, Phillips MB et al. (1990) Prevalence and treatment of giardiasis in chronic diarrhoea and malnutrition. Arch Dis Child 65: 304

Suringa DWR, Bank LB, Ackerman AB (1970) Role of measles virus in skin lesions and Koplik's spots. N Engl J Med 283: 1139

Sutter EE (1973) Blindness among South African negroes. S Afr Arch Ophthalmol 1: 105

Svedmyr E, Jondal M (1975) Cytotoxic effector cells specific for B cell lines transformed by Epstein–Barr virus are present in patients with infectious mononucleosis. Proc Natl Acad Sci USA 72: 1622

Tafari N, Ross S, Naeye RL, Judge DM, Marboe C (1976) Mycoplasma T strains and perinatal death. Lancet i: 108

Takala AK, Pekkanen E, Eskola J (1991) Neonatal Haemophilus influenzae infections. Arch Dis Child 66: 437

Takeuchi A, Formal SB, Sprinz H (1968) Experimental acute colitis in the Rhesus monkey following per oral infection with Shigella flexneri. Am J Pathol 52: 503

Tang JS, Kauffman SL, Lynfield J (1971) Hypoplasia of the pulmonary arteries in infants with congenital rubella. Am J Cardiol 27: 491

Taylor EB, Torenson WE (1963) Primary mumps meningeal encephalitis. Arch Intern Med 112: 216

Teele DW (1981) The pneumococcus: its role in infectious disease. In: Feigin RD, Cherry JD (eds) Textbook of pediatric infectious diseases. Saunders, Philadelphia, p 940

Telzak EE, Cote RJ, Goed IWM et al. (1990) Extrapulmonary Pneumocystis carinii infections. Rev Infect Dis 12: 380

Terreni AA (1961) Tinea capitus survey in Charleston SC. Arch Dermatol 83: 88

Thomas JET (1986) Malaria. S Afr J Cont Med Education 1: 31

Tillotson JR, Lerner AM (1967) Reovirus type 3 associated with fatal pneumonia. N Engl J Med 275: 1060

Todd JK (1988) Toxic shock syndrome. Clin Microbiol Rev 1: 432

Tondury G, Smith DW (1966) Fetal rubella pathology. J Pediatr 68: 867

Turk JL, Bryceson AD (1971) Immunological phenomenon in leprosy and related diseases. Adv Immunol 13: 209

Vass Z (1964) Histological findings in epidemic keratoconjunctivitis. Acta Ophthalmol 42: 119

Vawter GF (1981) Perinatal listeriosis. Perspect Pediatr Pathol 6: 153

Von Leyden E, Schaudinn F (1896) Leydenia gemmipara Schaudinn, ein neuer, in der ascites-Flussigkeit des lebenden menschen gefunder amoebenüchnlicher Rhizotode. Sitzunsber Berl Akad Wiss 29: 951

Waites KB, Crouse DT, Phillips JB III et al. (1989) Ureaplasmal pneumonia and sepsis associated with persistent pulmonary hypertension of the newborn. Pediatr 83: 79

Waites KB, Crouse DT, Cassell GH (1990) Ureaplasma and mycoplasma CNS infections in newborn babies. Lancet i: 658

Walbogel FA, Medoff G, Swartz MV (1970) Osteomyelitis: a review of clinical features, therapeutic consideration and unusual aspects. N Engl J Med 282: 206, 260, 316

Walker DH, Bradford WD (1981) Rocky Mountains spotted fever in childhood. Perspect Pediatr Pathol 6: 35

Walker DH, Crawford CG, Cain BG (1980) Rickettsial infection of the pulmonary microcirculation: the basis for interstitial pneumonitis in Rocky Mountain spotted fever. Hum Pathol 11: 263

Way RC (1967) Cardiovascular defects and the rubella syndrome. Can Med Assoc J 97: 1329

Wear DJ, Margilith AM, Hadfield TL et al. (1983) Cat scratch disease: a bacterial infection. Science 221: 1403

Wessels MR, Kasper DL (1993) The changing spectrum of group B streptococcal disease. N Engl J Med 328: 1843

West NC, Meight RE, Mackie M, Anderson MJ (1986) Parvovirus infection associated with aplastic crisis in a patient with HEMPAS. J Clin Pathol 39: 1019

Whitaker JA, Hardison JE (1978) Severe thrombocytopenia after generalized herpes simplex virus (HSV-2) infection. South Med J 71: 864

Wilfert C, Gutman L (1981) Venereal disease. In: Feigin RD, Cherry JD (eds) Textbook of pediatric infectious diseases. Saunders, Philadelphia, p 376

Williams AO, Lichtenberg F, Smith JH et al. (1969) Ultrastructure of phycomycosis. Arch Pathol 87:459

Williams CL, Strobino B, Lee A et al. (1990) Lyme disease in childhood: clinical and epidemiologic features of ninety cases. Pediatr Infect Dis J 9: 10

Winship T (1953) Pathological changes in so-called cat scratch fever. Am J Clin Pathol 23: 1012

Wisniewski HJ, Krumbiegel ER (1970) Epidemiological studies of Q fever in humans. Arch Environ Health 21: 66

Wittner M (1992) Trypanosomiasis. In: Feigin RD, Cherry JD (eds) Textbook of pediatric infectious diseases. 3rd edn. Saunders, Philadelphia, p 2070

Witzleben CL, Driscoll SG (1965) Possible transplacental trans-mission of herpes simplex infection. Pediatr 36: 192

Wohl MEB, Chernick V (1978) Bronchiolitis. Am Rev Respir Dis 118: 759

Wong SN, Tam AYC, Ng THK, Ng WF, Tong CY, Tang TS (1989) Fatal coxsackie B1 virus infection in neonates. Pediatr Infect Dis J 8: 638

Wood GW (1980) Mononuclear phagocytes in the human placenta. Placenta 1: 113

Woodward A, McTigue C, Hogg G, Watkins A, Tan H (1992) Mucormycosis of the gut: a "new" disease or a variant of necro-tizing enterocolitis. J Pediatr Surg 27: 737

Young JA, Stone JW, McGonigle RJS, Adu D, Michael J (1986) Diagnosing *Pneumocystis carinii* pneumonia by cytological examination of bronchoalveolar lavage fluid: report of 15 cases. J Clin Pathol 39: 945

Zangwill KM, Hamilton DH, Perkins BA et al. (1993) Cat scratch disease in Connecticut: epidemiology, risk factors and evalua-tion of a new diagnostic test. N Engl J Med 329: 8

Zeulzer WW (1944) Infantile toxoplasmosis. Arch Pathol 38: 1

Zinserling A (1972) Peculiarities of lesions in viral and mycoplasma infections of the respiratory tract. Virchows Arch A Pathol Anat 356: 259

Ziring PR, Gallo G, Finegold M, Buimovici-Klein E, Orga P (1977) Chronic lymphocytic thyroiditis: identification of rubella virus antigen in the thyroid of a child with congenital rubella. J Pediatr 90: 419

15 · AIDS

Ronald O.C. Kaschula

Acquired immune deficiency syndrome (AIDS) is a severe immune deficiency caused by infection with human immunodeficiency virus (HIV). This is an RNA retrovirus of the subfamily *Lentivirnae*, members of which typically have a slow progression from infection to overt disease. In addition to a propensity to opportunistic infection, the disease is often also associated with central nervous system degeneration, lymphadenopathy and anaemia. Initially it was thought that the virus had tropism for T cells with the CD4 receptor, mainly helper T lymphocytes, where it replicates and becomes part of the host cell's genetic material. It is now known that the virus may infect a variety of tissues such as brain, gastrointestinal tract, kidney, lung and possibly heart (Levy 1990). Although the virus core is composed of a single strand of RNA reverse transcriptase, it enables transcribed double-stranded DNA to become permanently imprinted into infected cells. Fully expressed AIDS usually occurs after replication has caused progressive destruction of the body's cellular immune system. In 1981 the Centres for Disease Control in the USA first drew attention to a new syndrome, predominantly affecting homosexual men, and causing Kaposi sarcoma, *Pneumocystis carinii* pneumonia and other opportunistic infections (Anonymous 1981a, b). Since then, seropositive testing of a specimen taken from a patient in Zaire in 1959 has indicated that the disease had long existed at a low level of prevalence and awareness (Nahmias et al. 1986). Shortly thereafter an additional virus was identified and reported to cause a similar syndrome in West Africa (Clavel et al. 1987). The viruses are now distinguished as types 1 and 2. HIV-2 still has a restricted geographic distribution, but is reported to occur on continents other than Africa.

Childhood AIDS was first reported in 1983 (Oleske et al. 1983; Rubinstein et al. 1983). Paediatric AIDS initially constituted a small proportion (1%–2%) of all cases. However, the incidence in children is now rapidly increasing. Initially most childhood cases were attributed to transfusion of infected blood and/or blood products or to drug abuse, but mother-to-fetus and mother-to-infant infection are now much more prevalent (Italian Multicentre Study 1988). It seems that about one-third of infants born to HIV-positive mothers contract prenatal AIDS. In addition, there is increasing evidence that postnatal transmission of infection in colostrum and breast milk is a factor, in Central Africa, among women who seroconvert after delivery (Hira et al. 1990; Van de Perre et al. 1992). In a European study a significantly higher rate of HIV-1 transmission has been strongly associated with duration of breast feeding (de Martino et al. 1992).

Diagnosis of HIV Infection in Infants

Tests demonstrating the presence of antibody to HIV infection are the mainstay of laboratory diagnosis in adults and children older than 18 months. Almost 100% of infants born to HIV-positive mothers test positive at birth. Uninfected infants lose maternal antibody over the succeeding 6–12 months. It is important to identify truly infected infants as soon as possible after birth. High levels of IgG antibodies block the binding of IgM antibodies to test reagents.

Consequently, alternative tests have had to be devised to make early diagnosis in newborn infants. HIV culture has limited use because it is slow and expensive and strict biosafety precautions are required. At present, the most effective reliable tests for infants are the polymerase chain reaction and Elispot tests (Rogers et al. 1991; Nesheim et al. 1992). HIV-specific IgA and p24 antigen assays detect only a small proportion of cases, and in vitro antibody production assays are not reliable during the first 2 months of life (Rogers et al. 1991). There is a tendency for clinicians to accept two or more positive results on sequentially collected samples.

Clinical Features

A dysmorphic syndrome exhibiting growth retardation, microcephaly and abnormal facies has been attributed to maternal HIV infection (Marion et al. 1986), but not confirmed in another study (Qazi et al. 1988). It is not clear how much additional factors, such as drug and alcohol abuse and smoking, contribute to the features seen in the first study. Most often, affected infants fail to thrive, and develop frequent fevers, generalized lymphadenopathy, respiratory symptoms and signs, and neurological abnormalities. Most cases manifest symptoms before 18 months of age, but presentation in older children is now increasingly being reported. Recurrent infections with commonly occurring organisms as well as with opportunistic organisms are also increasingly being reported. Immunological investigation reveals a state of anergy with reduced T helper cell counts for age and a polyclonal hypergammaglobulinaemia (Connor et al. 1988). Lymphocyte subsets in healthy young children and HIV-infected children at various ages have been determined and are considered to be of diagnostic value (Rogers et al. 1991; McKinney and Wilfert 1992). A classification system for the disease in adolescents and young adults, in whom the disease is mostly acquired either sexually or parenterally, has been set by the American Centres for Disease Control and has recently been updated (Anonymous 1992). The classification is mainly used in public health surveillance in North America, and is based on the occurrence of a number of clinical conditions that are frequently associated with AIDS, as well as reduced absolute values of CD4 + T lymphocytes (helper cells). In developing counties where AIDS is more prevalent and laboratory resources are considerably more restricted, adaptations have had to be made. Conditions included in the 1993 surveillance case definition are: candidiasis of bronchi, trachea, lungs or oesophagus; invasive cervical cancer; extrapulmonary coccidioidomycosis; extrapulmonary cryptococcosis; prolonged intestinal cryptosporidiosis (lasting more than a month); cytomegalovirus infection other than of liver, spleen and lymph nodes; HIV-related encephalopathy; prolonged herpes simplex or herpes bronchitis, pneumonia or oesophagitis; extrapulmonary histoplasmosis; chronic intestinal isosporiasis; Kaposi sarcoma; lymphoma (Burkitt, immunoblastic or primary of the brain); mycobacterial infections (including tuberculosis, *Mycobacterium kansasii*, avium complex and other species); *Pneumocystis carinii* pneumonia; recurrent pneumonia; progressive multifocal leucoencephalopathy; recurrent salmonella septicaemia; cerebral toxoplasmosis and HIV-related wasting syndrome. In developing countries such as Zambia a more simplified, yet accurate, set of criteria for case definition has greater relevance (Chintu and Zumla 1993). In the Zambian system of paediatric clinical case definition, at least two of the following three major criteria must be present:

1. Recurrent fever of at least 1 month's duration
2. Recurrent oropharyngeal candidiasis
3. Recurrent respiratory infections

together with at least two of the following seven minor criteria:

1. Chronic diarrhoea of at least 1 month's duration
2. Weight loss or abnormally slow growth
3. Generalized lymphadenopathy
4. Persistent cough of at least 1 month's duration
5. Extrapulmonary tuberculosis
6. *Pneumocystis carinii* pneumonia
7. Confirmed maternal HIV-1 infection

These criteria apply only in the absence of known causes of immunodeficiency (Chintu et al. 1993).

Although long-term follow-up of children categorized into clinical severity groups has indicated prognostic significance, the clinical onset of symptomatic AIDS before the age of 6 months is uniformly bad (Turner et al. 1993).

Systematic Pathology

The whole spectrum of lesions that occurs in the various organs of adults with AIDS is also found in children, but often with a different frequency. In children there is greater emphasis and more frequent

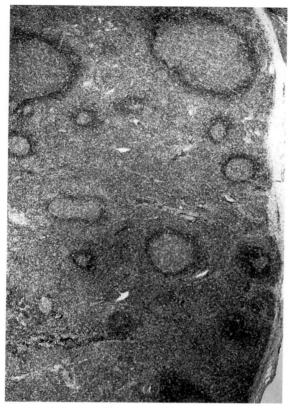

Fig. 15.1. AIDS lymphadenopathy in the hyperplastic phase, with increased follicles of variable size and shape extending into the medullary region. (H&E, × 16)

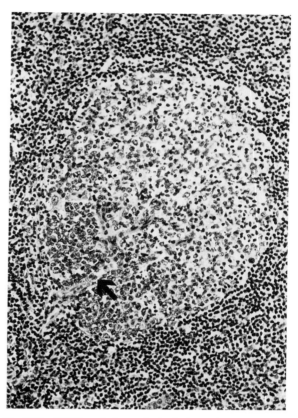

Fig. 15.2. AIDS lymphadenopathy in the hyperplastic phase, with a thin-walled blood vessel penetrating a reactive germinal centre. (H&E, × 50)

involvement of the lymphoreticular system (including the thymus) and the development of pulmonary lymphoid lesions and of fibrocalcific arterial lesions (Joshi 1990). In addition, the morphology of encephalopathic lesions in children differs from that seen in adults.

Persistent Generalized Lymphadenopathy

"Persistent generalized lymphadenopathy" (PGL) refers to a spectrum of histopathological changes that occur in HIV-positive individuals. The phenomenon is often the first indication that infection is progressing to clinical AIDS. Although the morphological changes are characteristic, they are not diagnostically specific (Stanley and Frizzera 1986), but mononuclear cell proliferation in cortical or medullary sinuses, in close proximity to reactive follicles during the hyperplastic phase, is characteristic and suggestive of HIV infection (Butler and Osborne 1988). Most often the cervi-

cal and axillary lymph nodes are affected, and biopsies reveal significant changes in the follicles (Baroni and Uccini 1993). In the initial reaction there is follicular hyperplasia with increase in size and numbers of follicles, so that they occur throughout the node (Fig. 15.1). Often the germinal centres have an irregular outline and contain numerous mitoses and macrophages with tingible bodies. Small blood vessels with flat endothelium may be seen within the germinal centres and may be associated with clusters of small lymphocytes (Fig. 15.2). In the interfollicular and paracortical zones, small lymphocytes with immunoblasts, neutrophils and macrophages are found with arborizing vessels having thickened endothelium (Baroni and Uccini 1993). As this stage of hyperplasia (early regression or fragmentation), haemorrhages appear within the germinal centres, and the mantle zones of small lymphocytes become reduced (Fig. 15.3). As regression progresses, increasing foci of necrosis, often associated with lymphocytic infiltration, appear in the germinal

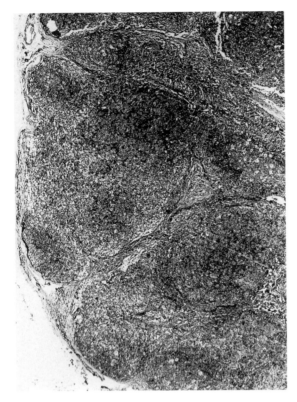

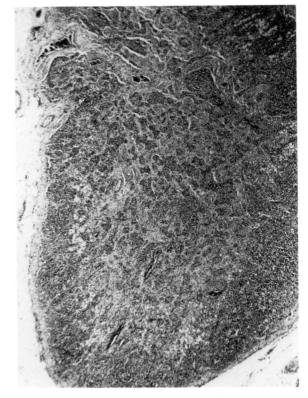

Fig. 15.3. AIDS lymphadenopathy in the early regressive phase, with attenuation of previously hyperplastic germinal centres with small haemorrhages. (H&E, × 25)

Fig. 15.4. AIDS lymphadenopathy in the late regressive phase, with loss of cortical follicles and hyperplastic medullary sinuses in which lymphocytes and neutrophils accumulate. (H&E, × 20)

centres. Eventually, the germinal centres virtually disappear and the medullary sinuses become hyperplastic and dilated with lymphocytes and neutrophils (Fig. 15.4).

As involution progresses the follicles become smaller but hypervascular, with the vessels assuming features similar to those seen in the hyaline vascular form of Castleman's disease. Increased vascularity of the interfollicular and paracortical areas occurs in association with increasing depletion of lymphocytes. Eventually, as clinical AIDS develops, there is obliteration of architecture by diffuse fibrosis isolating small numbers of lymphocytes and plasma cells.

Immunocytochemical studies have shown reduction in CD4+T lymphocytes (helper cells) with increased CD8+T lymphocytes (killer cells) during follicular fragmentation. During the early hyperplastic phase, stains for Ki67 (monoclonal antibody that stains for proliferating cells in G1–G2 phases) is strongly positive in germinal centres when most cells also stain for CD19+ B lymphocytes, and small numbers of mature T lymphocytes (CD2+) are present (Baroni and Uccini 1993). Changes in the

subsets of T lymphocytes in the paracortical areas parallels those in the germinal centres.

Thymic Pathology

Progressive alterations in thymic morphology have been recorded from biopsy and autopsy studies (Joshi and Oleske 1985; Joshi et al. 1986). On the basis of these studies and subsequent experience with the disease, the following categories of reaction have been suggested (Joshi 1990; Joshi et al. 1990).

Precocious Involution

Here the normal age-related involutionary changes occur earlier and in greater intensity than would be expected for the degree of stress. There is marked shrinkage of the gland with depletion of cortical lymphocytes, loss of corticomedullary differentiation and microcystic dilatation of Hassall's corpuscles. Some hyalinization of cortex and medulla may be seen.

Dysinvolution

Here the features are similar to those of precocious involution, with the exception that Hassall's corpuscles are mostly inconspicuous or absent (Fig. 15.5). The features are reminiscent of those seen in some congenital immune deficiency syndromes; however, when multiple levels of tissue are examined, small Hassall's corpuscles are found.

Thymitis

There is an added inflammatory process indicated by the presence of any of: lymph follicles with germinal centres; local or diffuse accumulations of macrophages; plasma cell infiltration with disruption of architecture; or the presence of multinucleated giant cells in the medulla.

Biopsy studies followed by autopsy in individual patients indicate that thymitis tends to be followed by precocious involution or dysinvolution at autopsy. However, a case with biopsy features of precocious involution has been reported to have reconstituted its thymic architecture at subsequent autopsy (Joshi 1990). It seems that thymic injury accentuates the immune suppression that results from derangements to CD4+ and CD8+ T lymphocytes in HIV infection and AIDS.

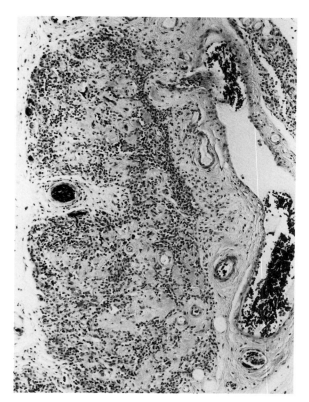

Fig. 15.5. Shrunken thymic lobule with depletion of cortical lymphocytes, absent Hassall's corpuscles and sclerotic medulla representative of thymic disinvolution. (H&E, × 40)

Splenic Changes

Massive enlargement of the spleen is frequently seen in children with active AIDS. This is due to hyperplasia of splenic cords and sinusoids. In autopsy cases there is obliteration of white pulp with loss of T lymphocytes and their replacement by plasmacytoid cells. Giant cells, haemorrhagic infarcts, fibrosis and Gamna–Gandy bodies have been described (Anderson 1992).

Pulmonary Lymphoid Lesions

Bronchioalveolar lavage, transbronchial biopsy and open lung biopsy have provided invaluable information in resolving the nature of various radio-opaque lesions that are encountered in the lung fields of children with HIV infection. Although infections by bacterial and opportunistic organisms are common, pulmonary lymphoid lesions are much more frequent in children than in adults (Joshi 1990). Open lung biopsy is generally necessary to diagnose pulmonary lymphoid hyperplasia and lymphoid interstitial pneu-

monitis complex (PLH/LIP) (Joshi et al. 1985; Joshi and Oleske 1986).

In pulmonary lymphoid hyperplasia there are many, often large, peribronchiolar lymphoid nodules that normally have germinal centres and may include a few plasma cells. Lymphoid interstitial pneumonitis manifests as a diffuse infiltration of alveolar walls by mature and immature lymphoid cells and plasma cells with Russell bodies. There may be some focal nodular aggregates of lymphoid cells, and less frequently collections of mononuclear cells with or without giant cells may resemble granulomas (Joshi 1990). Viral inclusions, fungi, acid-fast bacilli and *Pneumocystis carinii* are not a feature. However, Epstein–Barr virus (EBV) genome has been demonstrated in living tissue of children with PLH/LIP (Andiman et al. 1985). The infiltrative lymphocytes in both forms of pulmonary involvement are polyclonal, and often there are overlapping features with the cellular infiltrates involving alveolar septae as well as occurring as peribronchial nodules. Pulmonary fibrosis is not a recognized feature of this condition, but occasionally there may be progression to generalized systemic lymphoproliferative disorder. Intra-alveolar accumulations of mononuclear macrophages containing diastase-resistant periodic acid–Schiff (PAS)-positive granules associated with cuboidal change of alveolar lining cells occurs occasionally. In such cases, a mild lymphoplasmacytic infiltration into alveolar walls is seen. As HIV and EBV genomes are found in the lungs of patients with these types of lymphoplasmacytic infiltration, it seems reasonable to assume that they have a synergistic effect in producing the pulmonary lesions (Joshi 1990). The lower incidence of such lesions in adults may be because of previous exposure and thus development of immunity to EBV.

Lymphocytic infiltration into the lungs is usually a prominent feature of a systemic lymphoproliferative disorder that involves lymph nodes and such extranodal sites as liver, spleen, kidneys, skin, salivary glands and muscle but not the brain (Joshi et al. 1987a). Para-aortic lymph nodes are particularly enlarged. As pertains to pulmonary lymphoid lesions associated with EBV infection, there is a polymorphic infiltration that includes polyclonal B lymphocytes and plasma cells in all grades of maturation.

Hepatic Lesions

In children with hepatomegaly and increased serum levels of aniline and aspartate aminotransferase, percutaneous liver biopsies have demonstrated features consistent with chronic active hepatitis (Duffy et al. 1986). There is prominent hyperplasia of sinusoidal lining cells, with increased numbers of T lymphoytes (particularly the CD8+ subset) occurring in a patchy or diffuse distribution. Apoptosis of a small number of hepatocytes occurs, together with increased accumulation of nuclear glycogen. Piecemeal necrosis occurs in portal areas that are infiltrated by lymphocytes, plasma cells and histiocytes. Bile ducts are often damaged, with degeneration and disruption of epithelium. In addition, protal fibrosis with bridging and endothelialitis with adherence of lymphocytes to the endothelium of portal veins have been described.

Arteriopathy

Small and medium-sized muscular arteries of several organs (e.g. heart, lungs, kidneys, spleen, intestines and brain) are prone to intimal fibrosis with fragmentation of elastica and fibrosis in the media as well as calcification of internal elastic lamina and media. These changes are associated with variable degrees of luminal narrowing, aneurysm formation and

thrombosis (Joshi 1990). Coronary arteries are consistently affected, but cerebral arteries are relatively spared. It seems that the process may be a consequence of a circulating noxious agent (possibly from an opportunistic infection) that damages the elastica of the arteries. As a consequence of luminal narrowing, ischaemic changes including infarcts occur in affected organs.

Heart

In children myocardial infarction occurs as a consequence of coronary artery arteriopathy, where there is generally medial calcification, disruption of elastic lamina and intimal fibrosis (Joshi et al. 1987b). In addition, heart failure due to dilated cardiomyopathy mainly affecting the right atrium and ventricle with pericardial effusion has been described (Joshi et al. 1988). Tricuspid valve thickening and nodularity has been reported in children (Steinherz et al. 1986). Electrocardiographic abnormalities that indicate right or left ventricular hypertrophy and various abnormalities of the conduction system are reported (Bharati and Lev 1990). In these cases there is constant involvement of small and medium-sized vessels in the conduction system and adjoining myocardium. Sometimes there is thrombosis and/or calcification of the arteries with perivascular inflammatory cell infiltration, fibrosis of adventitia and intimal proliferation. Within the myocardium there may be degeneration of myocardial fibres, fatty infiltration, focal calcification and myocarditis. The SA and AV nodes as well as the bundle of His and the bundle branches are also subject to alteration in the form of vascular changes, fibrosis, fatty infiltration, inflammatory cell infiltration and focal calcification. The pathogenesis of these changes in unclear. All affected cases had HIV in the myocardium, but it is possible that the abnormalities were a consequence of harmful substances released from various opportunistic infections to which the heart may be sensitive.

Central Nervous System

HIV has tropism for neural tissue, and invasion of the CNS probably occurs very early in infection, as HIV-1 specific antibody synthesis is demonstrable within the blood–brain barier before the onset of symptoms (Epstein et al. 1986). Affected children usually have progressive encephalopathy, delayed milestones, retarded intellect and microcephaly. Pathological lesions most often occur in subcortical white matter, the pons and basal ganglia. Vascular and juxtavascular calcification is the most constant finding, occur-

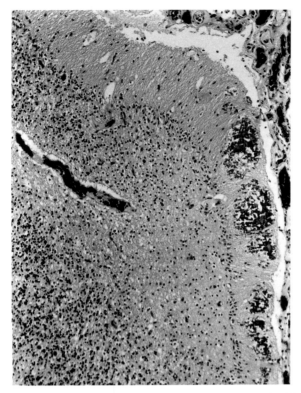

Fig. 15.6. Calcification of cerebellar cortex in infantile AIDS with cytomegalovirus infection. (H&E, × 63)

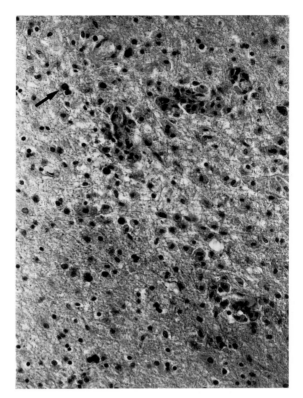

Fig. 15.7. AIDS-associated focal inflammatory gliosis with intranuclear inclusions (*arrowed*). (H&E, × 128)

ring in more than 90% of autopsy cases (Sharer et al. 1986). The basal ganglia (especially the putamen) and white matter are particularly prone, but other sites such as the cerebellum are not resistant (Fig. 15.6). Fibrinoid necrosis of small vessels occurs occasionally. Inflammatory gliosis takes the form of focal perivascular or diffuse accumulation of glial cells, lymphocytes, macrophages and sometimes plasma cells (Fig. 15.7). Necrosis sometimes occurs in association with microglial nodules. Multinucleate giant cells resembling Langhans' or Touton giant cells, as well as closely packed nuclei without visible cytoplasm, resembling giant cells, are all associated with inflammatory infiltrates in AIDS encephalopathies (Budka 1986). The giant cells as well as intravascular macrophages may contain HIV particles (Navia et al. 1986; Gartner et al. 1986). Alterations in white matter are influenced by the age of the child in relation to the process of myelination. At autopsy the total amount of white matter tends to be diminished and myelination is often impaired, but where there is demyelination as a consequence of inflammatory gliosis the bare axons tend to be preserved (Fig. 15.8). It has recently been shown that multifocal necrotizing leucoencephalopathic lesions with a predilection for involvement of the pons is not specific for AIDS (due to HIV infection), but may occur in a variety of immunosuppressed persons (Anders et al. 1993). Opportunistic infections in the central nervous system of childhood AIDS patients are less frequent than in adults, but lymphomas may be more frequent. Peripheral neuropathy is less common in children than in adults, but subclinical abnormalities are probably as prevalent as in adults.

Gastrointestinal Involvement

In addition to many opportunisitic infections, children with AIDS are liable to have non-specific persistent diarrhoea that is attributed to AIDS enteropathy. There is malabsorption with or without an identifiable organism, although HIV-infected cells have been found in the rectum of adults with a similar syndrome (Gelb and Miller 1986; Nelson et al. 1988). In the jejunal mucosa there is partial villous atrophy, crypt hypoplasia and increased numbers of intraepithelial lymphocytes.

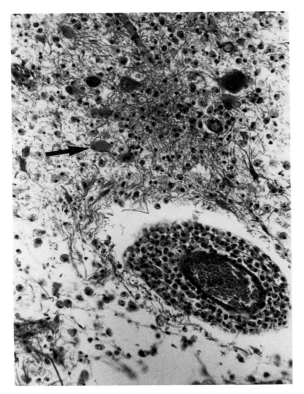

Fig. 15.8. Inflammatory gliosis in AIDS, with preservation of bare axons and presence of intranuclear homogeneous inclusions (*arrows*). (H&E, × 160)

Renal Involvement

Nephropathy manifesting as proteinuria, oedema and uraemia occurs in almost 10% of children with AIDS (Scott et al. 1989), who have a wide range of pathological lesions. These include mesangial proliferation, focal glomerulosclerosis, segmental necrotizing glomerulonephritis, minimal change disease and tubuloreticular accumulations within glomerular endothelial cells (Strauss et al. 1989).

Perinatal and Placental Changes

Infants of HIV-positive mothers are often small for gestational age and have been shown to be associated with preterm birth, fetal death (Gichangi et al. 1993) and a higher death rate during the first 2 years of life (Lallemant et al. 1989). In addition, placentas of HIV-positive mothers are larger and heavier than expected and have a higher incidence of placental inflammation. The fetoplacental weight ratio is

significantly reduced. Haemorrhagic endovasculitis attributed to viral infection has been reported in a placenta (Sander 1980). Villi are found to be coarse, cellular and hypovascular with increased calcification and fibrin deposition (Jauniaux et al. 1988). Although a dysmorphic HIV embryopathy comprising growth retardation, microcephaly and abnormal facies has been reported, it has not gained general acceptance as a specific syndrome (Marion et al. 1986; Qazi et al. 1988).

Opportunistic Infections

Prospective studies have shown that asymptomatic HIV-1 infected children contract infections at much the same rate as uninfected children, whereas symptomatic HIV-1 infected children have significantly more frequent infections (Principi et al. 1991). Pneumonia-bronchitis, candidiasis, diarrhoea, urinary tract infections, sepsis, non-tuberculous mycobacterial infection, otitis media and cytomegalovirus infection are the most frequent severe infections encountered.

Disseminated Non-tuberculous Mycobacterial Infection

This is a common systemic pathogen in AIDS and has been reported in 5.7% of over 3000 children with AIDS aged less than 13 years in the USA over a 10 year period. More than 85% had *Mycobacterium avium* complex, and there is increased propensity to affect older children who have haemophilia or transfusion-associated HIV-1 infection. Before the recognition of the infection the CD4+ T lymphocyte count drops to less than 50 cells/mm^3 in 70% of cases (Horsburgh et al. 1993). Infected children usually fail to gain weight, develop anorexia with abdominal pain or tenderness, and become anaemic (Hoyt et al. 1992). The organisms accumulate in very large numbers within histiocytic-type cells in lymph nodes, liver, spleen, intestinal lamina propria and bone marrow. Unlike in immunocompetent individuals, necrosis and granuloma formation is rarely seen and pulmonary involvement is uncommon.

Tuberculosis

Persons previously infected with *Mycobacterium tuberculosis* tend to experience reactivation of the original infection. This often occurs simultaneously with a state of anergy, and hence active tuberculosis may not be clinically diagnosed, so that spread of the organism through the community is increased. The morphological appearance of AIDS-associated tuberculosis depends on the degree of immunodeficiency at the time that reactivation occurs. Caseation and necrosis become less conspicuous with increasing immunodeficiency (Fig. 15.9), but lymph nodes are the most frequent extrapulmonary site to be affected (Sunderam and Reichman 1988).

Opportunistic Pulmonary Infections

The majority of HIV-infected children develop pulmonary infection at some stage in the disease. *Pneumocystis carinii* pneumonia is the most frequent opportunistic infection seen in HIV-infected children. It tends to manifest acute symptoms of fever, tachypnoea, cough and progressive hypoxia over a short period. In the early acute phase chest radiographs may be normal, but they soon show diffuse bilateral alveolar and interstitial obliteration. The diagnosis is made by demonstrating the organisms in sputum, bronchioalveolar lavage fluid or open lung biopsy specimens. Extrapulmonary lesions due to *Pneumocystis carinii* may occur in any of many organs. In childhood AIDS, pulmonary and extrapulmonary lesions usually show focal necrosis, foamy eosinophilic exudation and numerous organisms. Children with AIDS often contract bacterial pneumonia, and most often this is due to encapsulated organisms such as the Enterobacteriaceae and *Pseudomonas aeruginosa*. Cytomegalovirus (CMV), respiratory syncytial virus (RSV), varicella and measles are among the more common supervening viral infections that affect the lungs. Pulmonary CMV is particularly common and often occurs simultaneously with pneumocystis infection. Infection with CMV may involve the gastrointestinal tract mucosa as well as the enteric nervous system (Anderson et al. 1990), heart, brain, liver, adrenals, kidney and haemopoietic system. Pulmonary infection with RSV tends to occur at an early age, has a high (15%–40%) mortality rate (Chandwani et al. 1990) and is associated with prolonged shedding of virus. A very high proportion of HIV-infected children who contract measles develop fatal measles pneumonia. Prior immunization produces a poor antibody response, so that measles is a recognized formidable supervening infection (Palumbo et al. 1992; Nadel et al. 1991).

Enteric Opportunistic Infections

In developing countries, persistent life-threatening diarrhoea associated with fever and dehydration

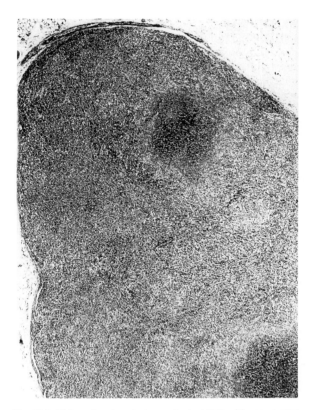

Fig. 15.9. Tuberculous lymphadenopathy in AIDS, with non-caseous necrosis in a node that lacks lymph follicles. (H&E, × 50)

occurs more often in HIV-infected infants. It is often associated with malnutrition and a symptomatic mother. The causative organism is most often an enteroadherant *Escherichia coli* (Pavia et al. 1992). In industrialized countries, novel enteric viruses such as *Astrovirus* and *Picobirnavirus* have an important role as aetiological agents of diarrhoea in HIV-infected patients (Grohmann et al. 1993). Rotaviruses, enteric adenovirus and Norwalk agent are not considered to be significant aetiological agents. Enteric protozoa are now recognized as having an important role in causing diarrhoeal disease in HIV-infected children.

Cryptosporidium

In Africa, *Cryptosporidium* is a highly prevalent cause of diarrhoea in persons with symptomatic AIDS, and it accounts for up to 10% of cases in the UK and the USA (Curry et al. 1991). The organism has a complicated life-cycle, with asexual, sexual and sporogenous phases. Organisms invade the gastrointestinal tract from the oesophagus to the rectum, including the biliary system. The organism occupies an extracytoplasmic location within an intracellular parasitophagous vacuole. Laboratory diagnosis is achieved by staining oocysts in faecal smears with modified Ziehl–Nielsen or auramine stains (Casemore et al. 1985) or by demonstrating the parasite in duodenal or rectal biopsy specimens. There seems to be no effective treatment, and relapses are common.

Isospora

Infections with *Isospora belli* have mainly occurred among American Hispanics and Haitians and in Africa (Curry et al. 1991). It produces a chronic watery diarrhoea, and the organisms infect enterocytes of the small intestine where they take up an intracytoplasmic location and cause symptoms after a variable latent period (Sorvillo et al. 1990). In the intestine there is mild mucosal inflammation, with eosinophilia and crypt hyperplastic atrophy. Rarely, the organisms may spread to draining lymph nodes. Laboratory diagnosis is based on faecal examination for oocysts or biopsy of small intestine. The organism has a close morphological resemblance to *Sarcocystis* and to *Toxoplasma*.

Sarcocystis

Infections with *Sarcocystis hominis* and *S. suihominis* are rare even in patients with AIDS, and occur from eating poorly cooked infected meat. In humans the organisms infect small intestinal enterocytes and cause diarrhoea. The organisms are smaller and more spherical than those of *Isospora*.

Microsporidiosis

The microsporidia are a group of obligate intracellular protozoans that have a coiled filament within their small spores which facilitates penetration of host cells in the process of infection (Canning and Lom 1986). *Enterocytozoan bieneusi* and *Encephalitozoan cuniculi* are the commonest human microsporidia that have been associated with malabsorption and diarrhoea in symptomatic AIDS (Lucas et al. 1989; Curry et al. 1991). Routine histological sections demonstrate the organisms within enterocytes of duodenal or jejunal biopsies, but ultrastructural examination is required for definitive verification (Peacock et al. 1991).

Giardiasis

Most often, enteric infection with *Giardia lamblia* is asymptomatic. It is not significantly more frequent in patients with AIDS than in those without.

Amoebiasis

Invasive amoebiasis due to *Entamoeba histolytica* is not a feature of AIDS, and there may be a significant negative association.

Infections with Opportunistic Non-enteric Protozoa

Toxoplasmosis

Previously exposed persons, mainly adults, often develop reactivation of previously dormant infection as immunity wanes following HIV infection. The brain and eyes are usually targeted for tissue destruction, but pulmonary, enteric and peritoneal infection may also occur.

Acanthamoeba

Disseminated infection with *Acanthomoeba* has been reported in an 8-year-old child with symptomatic HIV infection who had multiple previous opportunistic infection as well as inflammatory demyelinating polyneuropathy (Friedland et al. 1992). Dissemination was mainly to skin, but motor weakness with spasticity occurred during the terminal phase of the illness.

Leishmaniasis

Visceral leishmaniasis due to *L. infantum* occurs as a supervening infection in Mediterranean countries (Cook 1990). The typical features of kala-azar, with hepatosplenomegaly, skin lesions and fever, occur. Abundant organisms may be seen in spleen or marrow aspirates and in liver biopsies.

Trypanosomiasis

Both American and African forms of infection have occurred in patients with AIDS, but do not seem to be more prevalent in HIV-infected persons than in the normal population.

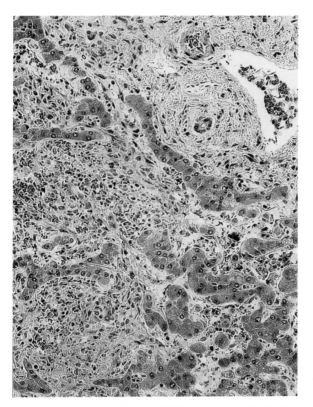

Fig. 15.10. Pseudoneoplastic angiofibromatous nodules in liver due to bacterial infection in AIDS. (H&E, × 100)

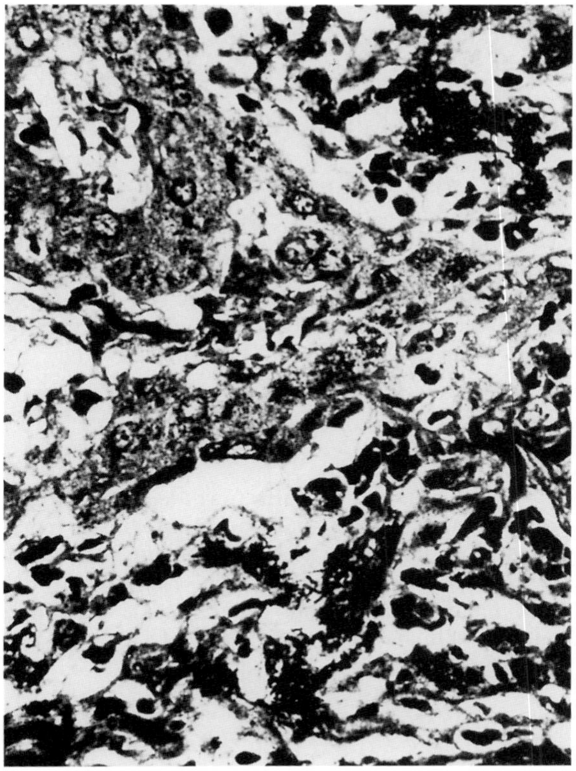

Fig. 15.11. Clumps of bacilli that occur in pseudoneoplastic angiofibromatous nodules in AIDS. (Wharthin–Starry stain, × 400)

Malaria and Babesiosis

The clinical manifestations of these infections do not seem to be different from those in the HIV-negative population.

Bacillary Angiomatosis

A newly recognized infectious disease that affects immunocompromised persons, especially adults with AIDS, manifests as a pseudoneoplastic vascular proliferation containing bacteria (Fig. 15.10). The condition presents as erythematous papules and nodules on the skin or within the liver, where they have been likened to peliosis hepatis. Involvement of spleen and bone has also been reported (Koehler et al. 1992). The clinical and histological features resemble Kaposi's sarcoma. The responsible organisms have been identified as being closely related to those associated with cat scratch disease, and many patients manifesting bacillary angiomatosis have been associated with cats. The offending organisms are considered to be *Rochalimaea quintana* and *R. henselae*

and are demonstrable as colonies within the vascular lesions by means of silver stains. Haematoxylin and eosin (H&E) stains show peliotic spaces in a fibromyxoid stroma containing mixed inflammatory cells, dilated capillaries and clumps of purple-staining material that can be shown to be clumps of bacilli (Perkocha et al. 1990) (Fig. 15.11). The organisms may be cultured from homogenized tissue on agar or on eukaryotic tissue-culture monolayers (Koehler et al. 1992).

Opportunistic Viral Infections

In addition to CMV, EBV, RSV, measles and the enteric viruses already discussed, children with AIDS are extremely prone to reactivation of localized Herpes simplex (Ewing 1990) and possibly also of Parvovirus B19 (Nigro et al. 1992). In AIDS, reactivated Herpes simplex of the skin and mucosa causes large chronic painful ulcers that may reach 20 cm in diameter. The lesions are generally sited on the face, mouth, genital or anal areas and within the oesophagus. Disseminated infection, as occurs in malnourished children, has not been reported, but is a rare complication of varicella–zoster virus infection.

Opportunistic Fungal Infections

Candidiasis

Recurrent oral thrush is one of the earliest symptomatic features of AIDS in children (Principi et al. 1991). Infection often spreads to the lower oesophagus and stomach. In addition, intravascular infection occurs when indwelling catheters are used.

Torulosis

Supervening infection with *Cryptococcus neoformans* is fairly common and serious. It seems to represent primary exposure to the organism rather than reactivation of an earlier infection. The lungs (interstitial pneumonia without granulomas), meninges, brain and skin are most often involved.

Histoplasmosis

On the basis that the condition occurs in non-endemic areas, it is deduced that supervening infection with *Histoplasma capsulatum* var. *capsulatum* in patients with AIDS represents reactivation of previous infection in at least a proportion of cases (Salzman et al. 1988). Dissemina-tion to multiple organs is common, and the encapsulated yeasts tend to be found in histiocytes. Lungs and draining lymph nodes are most often affected and the lesions may be caseating granulomas, non-caseating granulomas or non-granulomatous.

Coccidioidomycosis

The fungus *Coccidioides immitis* occurs in arid parts of the Americas and seems to occur both as a primary infection and as reactivation of previous infection (Bronnimann et al. 1987). In AIDS this fungus manifests multiple small nodules, usually granulomas or suppurative lesions in the lungs. Dissemination is not uncommon.

AIDS-associated Neoplasms

In contrast to adults with AIDS, malignancies are rarely encountered among HIV-infected children.

However, as supportive therapy extends to the period that HIV-infected children survive, it is anticipated that more malignancies may be reported. At present there is no evidence to suggest that HIV infection influences the biological behaviour and outcome of malignant neoplasms. Most HIV-infected children who develop neoplasms die from causes other than the neoplasm. Tumours that have occurred in children with AIDS include leiomyomatous tumours, rhabdomyosarcomas, Kaposi's sarcoma, Burkitt's lymphoma, and B-cell leukaemia and lymphoma of the central nervous system.

Myogenic Tumours

Nine children with AIDS, aged between 3 and 9 years, have been reported to develop myogenic tumours. All either had vertically acquired infection or were given transfusions very shortly after birth. Leiomyosarcoma is extremely rare in non-HIV-infected children, occurring at a rate of less than 1.6 per 10 million. The association of benign and malignant visceral leiomyomatous tumours with HIV infection suggests that HIV infection has a direct role in their causation (Chadwick et al. 1990). Smooth muscle tumours are not known to have a particular association with other causes of immunodeficiency. Girls are affected twice as often as boys, and the usual age range is 3–9 years (Van Hoeven et al. 1993). In addition, the lesions tend to occur in unusual sites such as lungs, liver and gastrointestinal tract, and some have been associated with high titres of EBV nuclear antigen (Van Hoeven et al. 1993).

Kaposi's Sarcoma

In Uganda, Kaposi's sarcoma is becoming increasingly prevalent among children with AIDS (Coulter 1993). Cutaneous lesions are most common (Fig. 15.12), but the lymphadenopathic form has been reported to occur in young American HIV-infected infants. The neoplastic lesions are small, with the affected lymph nodes often not discernibly enlarged (Buck et al. 1983). The spleen and thymus may also be involved by the tumour. Microscopic examination of affected lymph nodes shows Kaposi's sarcoma tumour nodules, generally peripherally sited, with some effacement of architecture and intermixed with plasma cells and immunoblasts.

Lymphoma and Leukaemia

The lymphomas and leukaemias reported to occur in HIV-infected children are almost entirely of B-cell

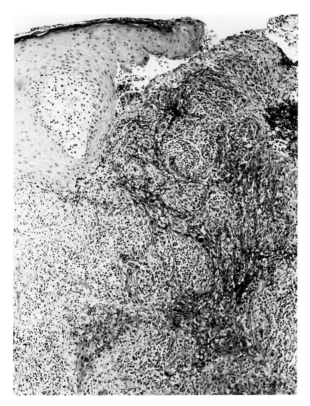

Fig. 15.12. Ulcerated cutaneous Kaposi sarcoma in a child with AIDS. (H&E, × 50)

origin or Hodgkin's disease. In addition, there is a strong association with EBV infection. Primary B-cell lymphoma is the most frequent cause of a focal mass in the central nervous system of HIV-infected children (Epstein et al. 1988). This tumour is otherwise very rare in children. Sporadic Burkitt's lymphoma associated with EBV infection is reported in USA (Kamani et al. 1988), but no relationship of endemic Burkitt's lymphoma with HIV infection has been demonstrated (Mbidde et al. 1990). Sometimes the diagnosis of lymphoma is the first symptom of AIDS in an HIV-infected child who has been symptom free for a long time (Montalvo et al. 1990).

AIDS in African Children

AIDS has become a devastating disease in parts of Africa, where many cases are unrecorded or not diagnosed. A Zairian study in 1986 revealed that 11% of children aged 2–14 years admitted to hospital and 1% of healthy siblings had HIV antibody (Mann et al.

1986). All cases of AIDS occurring in Central, East and Southern Africa have been caused by HIV-1 infection, whereas in West Africa both HIV-1 and HIV-2 infections occur, with HIV-2 more prevalent in some countries, such as Senegal (Coulter 1993). It seems that pure HIV-2 infection leads to a longer incubation period and a less severe form of the disease (Boccon-Gibod 1990). The great majority of African cases are caused by perinatally acquired infection, and most manifest symptoms before 6 months of age (Friedland and McIntyre 1992); many die during their first hospital admission. The infant mortality rate is three to five times that of infants born to HIV-negative mothers.

The clinical diagnosis of AIDS in young children in Africa is not always easy to distinguish from marasmus and marasmic kwashiorkor (Schuerman et al. 1988). In addition, among African children there is a high background incidence of non-specific infection and intestinal parasitic infestation. Nevertheless, generalized lymphadenopathy attributed to AIDS seems to occur more often in African children. The main presenting features of clinical AIDS are lymphadenopathy, failure to thrive, hepatomegaly, splenomegaly, oral thrush, diarrhoea and respiratory distress, and these occur in more than 50% of cases (Friedland and McIntyre 1992). HIV-infected African children seem to contract pneumonia more often than their European counterparts, and the pneumonia is usually caused by bacterial organisms or measles rather than *Pneumocystis carinii* (Boccon-Gibod 1990). The gastrointestinal infections more commonly found are *E. coli*, *Cryptosporidium*, *Isospora belli* and candidiasis. Lymphoid interstitial pneumonitis is probably more common in African children with AIDS than is diagnosed because most die without undergoing sophisticated investigation and never come to autopsy. Kaposi's sarcoma is increasingly being recognized as an expression of AIDS in HIV-infected children in Uganda (Katongole-Mbidde et al. 1991).

References

Anders KH, Becker S, Holden JK et al. (1993) Multifocal necrotizing leukoencephalopathy with pontine predilection in immunosuppressed patients: a clinicopathologic review of 16 cases. Hum Pathol 24: 897

Anderson VM (1992) Acquired immunodeficiency syndrome (AIDS). In Stocker JT, Dehner LP (eds) Pediatric Pathology. Lippincott, Philadelphia, p 376

Anderson VM, Greco MA, Recalde AL, Chandwani S, Church JA, Krasinski K (1990) Intestinal cytomegalovirus ganglioneuronitis in children with human immunodeficiency virus infection

Pediatr Pathol 10: 167

Andiman WA, Eastman R, Martin K et al. (1985) Opportunistic lymphoproliferations associated with Epstein–Barr viral DNA in infants and children with AIDS. Lancet ii: 1390

Anonymous (1981a) Kaposi's sarcoma and pneumocystis pneumonia among homosexual men – New York City and California. MMWR Morb Mortal Wkly Rep 30: 305

Anonymous (1981b) Follow-up on Kaposi sarcoma and pneumocystis pneumonia. MMWR Morb Mortal Wkly Rep 30: 409

Anonymous (1992) 1993 revised classification system for HIV infection and expanded surveillance case definition for AIDS among adolescents and adults. MMWR Morb Mortal Wkly Rep 41: 1

Baroni CD, Uccini S (1993) The lymphadenopathy of HIV infection. Am J Clin Pathol 99: 397

Bharati S, Lev M (1990) Conduction system in children with AIDS. In: Joshi VV (ed) Pathology of AIDS and other manifestations of HIV infection. Igaku-Shoin, New York, p 187

Boccon-Gibod L (1990) Pathology of AIDS in African patients. In: Joshi VV (ed) Pathology of AIDS and other manifestations of HIV infection. Igaku-Shoin, New York, p 329

Bronnimann DA, Adam RD, Galgiani JN et al. (1987) Coccidioidomycosis in the acquired immunodeficiency syndrome. Ann Intern Med 106: 372

Buck BE, Scott GB, Valdes-Dapena M, Parks WP (1983) Kaposi sarcoma in two infants with acquired immunodeficiency syndrome. J Pediatr 103: 911

Budka H (1986) Multinucleate giant cells in brain: a hallmark of the acquired immune deficiency syndrome (AIDS). Acta Neuropathol Berl 69: 253

Butler JJ, Osborne BM (1988) Lymph node enlargement in patients with unsuspected human immunodeficiency virus infections. Hum Pathol 19: 849

Canning EU, Lom J (1986) The microsporidia of vertebrates. Academic Press, London

Casemore DP, Armstrong M, Sands RL (1985) Laboratory diagnosis of cryptosporidiosis. J Clin Pathol 38: 1337

Chadwick EG, Connor EJ, Hanson CG et al. (1990) Tumours of smooth-muscle origin in HIV infected children. JAMA 263: 3182

Chandwani S, Barkowsky W, Kransinski K, Lawrence R, Welliver R (1990) Respiratory syncytial virus infection in human immunodeficiency virus infected children. J Pediatr 117: 251

Chintu C, Zumla A (1993) AIDS case definitions in developing countries. Lancet 342: 1054 (letter)

Chintu C, Malek A, Nyumbu M et al. (1993) Case definitions for paediatric AIDS: the Zambian experience. Int J STD AIDS 4: 83

Clavel F, Mansinho K, Chamaret S et al. (1987) Human immunodeficiency virus type 2 infection associated with AIDS in West Africa. N Engl J Med 316: 1180

Connor EM, Minnefor AB, Oleske JM (1988) Human immunodeficiency virus infection in infants and children. Curr Top AIDS 1: 185

Cook GC (1990) "Exotic" parasitic infections: recent progress in diagnosis and management. J Infect 20: 95

Coulter JBS (1993) HIV infection in African children. Ann Trop Paediatr 13: 205

Curry A, Turner AJ, Lucas SB (1991) Opportunistic protozoan infections in human immunodeficiency virus disease: review highlighting diagnostic and therapeutic aspects. J Clin Pathol 44: 182

de Martino M, Tovo P-A, Tozzi AE et al. (1992) HIV-I transmission through breast-milk: appraisal of risk according to duration of feeding. AIDS 6: 991

Duffy LF, Daum F, Kahn E et al. (1986) Hepatitis in children with acquired immune deficiency syndrome: histopathologic and immunocytologic features. Gastroenterology 90: 173

Epstein LG, Sharer LR, Oleske JM et al. (1986) Neurologic manifestations of human immunodeficiency virus in children. Pediatrics 78: 678

Epstein LG, Boucher CAB, Morrison SH et al. (1988) Persistent human immunodeficiency virus type 1 antigenemia in children correlates with disease progression. Pediatrics 82: 919

Ewing EP (1990) Systemic opportunistic and other infections with special reference to pulmonary involvement. In: Joshi VV (ed) Pathology of AIDS. Igaku-Shoin, New York, p 65

Friedland IR, McIntyre JA (1992) AIDS – the baragwanath experience: part II, HIV-infection in pregnancy and childhood. S Afr Med J 82: 90

Friedland LR, Raphael SA, Deutsch ES et al. (1992) Disseminated *Acanthamoeba* infection in a child with symptomatic human immunodeficiency virus infection. Pediatr Infect Dis J 11: 404

Gartner S, Markovitz P, Markovitz DM et al. (1986) The role of mononuclear phagocytes in HTLV-III/LAV infection. Science 233: 215

Gelb A, Miller S (1986) AIDS and gastroenterology. Am J Gastroenterol 81: 619

Gichangi PB, Nyongo AO, Timmerman M (1993) Pregnancy outcome and placental weights: their relationship to HIV-I infection. E Afr Med J 70: 85

Grohmann GS, Glass RI, Pereira HG (1993) Enteric viruses and diarrhoea in HIV-infected patients. N Engl J Med 329: 14

Hira SK, Mangrola UG, Mwale C et al. (1990) Apparent vertical transmission of human immunodeficiency virus type 1 by breast-feeding in Zambia. J Pediatr 117: 421

Horsburgh CR, Caldwell MB, Simonds RJ (1993) Epidemiology of disseminated non-tuberculous mycobacterial disease in children with acquired immunodeficiency syndrome. Pediatr Infect Dis J 12: 219

Hoyt L, Oleske J, Holland B, Connor E (1992) Nontuberculous mycobacteria in children with acquired immunodeficiency syndrome. Peidatr Infect Dis J 11: 354

Italian Multicentre Study (1988) Epidemiology, clinical features and prognostic factors of paediatric HIV infection. Lancet ii: 1043

Jauniaux E, Nessmann C, Imbert MC, Meuris S, Poissant F, Hustin J (1988) Morphologic aspects of placenta in HIV pregnancies. Placenta 9: 633

Joshi VV (1990) Pathology of acquired immunodeficiency syndrome (AIDS) in children. In: Joshi VV (ed) Pathology of AIDS and other manifestations of HIV infection. Igaku-Shoin, New York, p 239

Joshi VV, Oleske JM (1985) Pathologic appraisal of the thymus gland in acquired immunodeficiency syndrome in children. A study of four cases and a review of the literature. Arch Pathol Lab Med 109: 142

Joshi VV, Oleske JM (1986) Pulmonary lesions in children with the acquired immunodeficiency syndrome: a reappraisal based on data in additional cases and follow-up study of previously reported cases. Hum Pathol 17: 641

Joshi VV, Oleske JM, Minnefor A et al. (1985) Pathologic pulmonary findings in children with acquired immunodeficiency syndrome: a study of ten cases. Hum Pathol 16: 241

Joshi VV, Oleske JM, Saad S et al. (1986) Thymus biopsy in children with acquired immunodeficiency syndrome. Arch Pathol Lab Med 110: 837

Joshi VV, Kauffman S, Oleske JM et al. (1987a) Polyclonal polymorphic B-cell lymphoproliferative disorder with prominent involvement in children with acquired immune deficiency syndrome. Cancer 59: 1455

Joshi VV, Pawel B, Connor E et al. (1987b) Arteriopathy in children with acquired immune deficiency syndrome. Pediatr Pathol 7: 261

Joshi VV, Gadol C, Connor E et al (1988) Dilated cardiomyopathy in children with acquired immunodeficiency syndrome: a pathologic study of five cases. Hum Pathol 19: 69

Joshi VV, Oleske JM, Connor EM (1990) Morphologic findings in children with acquired immune deficiency syndrome: pathogenesis and clinical implications. Pediatr Pathol 10: 155

Kamani N, Kennedy J, Brandsma J (1988) Burkitt lymphoma in a child with human immunodeficiency virus infection. J Pediatr 112: 241

Katongole-Mbidde E, Kazura JW, Banura C et al. (1991) Latency period to the development of childhood AIDS-associated Kaposi sarcoma in African children. VII International Conference on AIDS, Florence 1991 (abstract MC 3185)

Koehler JE, Quinn FD, Berger TG, Le Boit PE, Tappero JW (1992) Isolation of *Rochalimaea* species from cutaneous and osseous lesions of bacillary angiomatosis. N Engl J Med 327: 1625

Lallemant M, Lallemant-le-Coeur S, Cheynier D et al. (1989) Mother–child transmission of HIV-I and infant survival in Brazzaville, Congo. AIDS 3: 643

Levy JA (1990) Changing concepts in HIV infection: challenges for the 1990s. AIDS 4: 1051 (editorial)

Lucas SB, Papadaki L, Conlon C, Sewankambo N, Goodgame R, Serwadda D (1989) Diagnosis of intestinal microsporidiosis in patients with AIDS. J Clin Pathol 42: 885

Mann JM, Francis H, Davachi F et al. (1986) Human immunodeficiency virus seropositivity in pediatric patients 2 to 14 years of age at Mama Yemo Hospital, Kinshasa, Zaire. Pediatrics 78: 673

Marion RW, Wizna AA, Hutcheon G et al. (1986) Human T-cell lymphotropic virus type III (HTLV-III) embryopathy. A new dysmorphic syndrome associated with intra-uterine HTLV-III infection. Am J Dis Child 140: 638

Mbidde EK, Banura C, Desmond-Hellman SD, Kizito A, Kazura J, Hellman NS (1990) African Burkitt's lymphoma and HIV infection. VI International Conference on AIDS, San Francisco. Abstract SB 26

McKinney RE, Wilfert CM (1992) Lymphocyte subsets in children younger than two years old: normal values in a population at risk for human immunodeficiency virus infection and diagnostic and prognostic application to infected children. Pediatr Infect Dis J 11: 639

Montalvo FW, Casanova R, Clavell LA (1990) Treatment outcome in children with malignancies associated with human immunodeficiency virus infection. J Pediatr 116: 735

Nadel S, Rutstein R, Chatten J (1991) Measles giant cell pneumonia in a child with human immunodeficiency virus infection. Pediatr Infect Dis J 10: 542

Nahmias AJ, Weiss J, Yao X et al. (1986) Evidence for human infection with HTLV-III/LAV-like virus in Central Africa, 1959. Lancet i: 1279

Navia BA, Cho E-S, Petito CK et al. (1986) The AIDS dementia complex: II. Neuropathology. Ann Neurol 19: 525

Nelson JA, Wiley CA, Reynolds-Kohler C et al. (1988) Human immunodeficiency virus detected in bowel epithelium from patients with gastrointestinal symptoms. Lancet i: 259

Nesheim S, Lee F, Sawyer M et al. (1992) Diagnosis of human immunodeficiency virus infection by enzyme-linked immunospot assays in prospectively followed cohort of infants of human immunodeficiency virus positive women. Pediatr Infect Dis J 11: 635

Nigro G, Luzi G, Fridell E et al. (1992) Parvovirus infection in children with AIDS: high prevalence of B19 specific immunoglobulin M and G antibodies. AIDS 6: 679

Oleske, J, Minnefor A, Cooper R Jr et al. (1983) Immune deficiency syndrome in children. JAMA 249: 2345

Palumbo P, Hoyt L, Demasio K, Oleske J, Connor E (1992) Population-based study of measles and measles immunization in human immunodeficiency virus-infected children. Pediatr Infect Dis J 11: 1008

Pavia AT, Long EG, Ryder RW et al. (1992) Diarrhoea among African children born to human immunodeficiency virus I-infected mothers: clinical, microbiologic and epidemiologic features. Pediatr Infect Dis J 11: 996

Peacock CS, Blanshard C, Tovey DG, Ellis DS, Gazzard BG (1991) Histological diagnosis of intestinal microsporidiosis in patients with AIDS. J Clin Pathol 44: 558

Perkocha LA, Geaghan SM, Yen TSB et al. (1990) Clinical and pathological features of bacillary peliosis hepatis in association with human immunodeficiency virus infection. N Engl J Med 323: 1581

Principi N, Marchisio P, Toruaghi R et al. (1991) Occurrence of infections in children infected with human immunodeficiency virus. Pediatr Infect Dis J 10: 190

Qazi QH, Sheikh TM, Fikrig S et al. (1988) Lack of evidence for craniofacial dysmorphism in perinatal human immunodeficiency virus infection. J Pediatr 112: 7

Rogers MF, Ou C-Y, Kilbourne B, Schochetman G (1991) Advances and problems in the diagnosis of human immunodeficiency virus infection in infants. Pediatr Infect Dis J 10: 523

Rubinstein A, Sreklick M, Gypta A et al. (1983) Acquired immunodeficiency with reversed T4/T8 ratios in infants born to promiscuous and drug addicted mothers. JAMA 249: 2350

Salzman STT, Smith RL, Aranda CP (1988) Histoplasmosis in patients at risk for acquired immunodeficiency syndrome in a nonendemic setting. Chest 93: 916

Sander CH (1980) Hemorrhagic endovasculitis and hemorrhagic villitis of the placenta. Arch Pathol Lab Med 104: 371

Schuerman L, Seynhaeve V, Bachschmidt I et al. (1988) Severe malnutrition and paediatric AIDS: a diagnostic problem in rural Africa. AIDS 2: 232

Scott GB, Hutto C, Makuch RW et al. (1989) Survival in children with perinatally acquired human immunodeficiency virus type I infection. N Engl J Med 321: 1791

Sharer LR, Epstein LG, Cho E-S et al. (1986) Pathologic features of AIDS encephalopathy in children: evidence for LAV/HTLV-III infection of brain. Hum Pathol 17: 271

Sorvillo F, Lieb L, Iwakoshi K, Waterman SH (1990) *Isospora belli* and the acquired immunodeficiency syndrome. N Engl J Med 322: 131

Stanley MW, Frizzera G (1986) Diagnostic specificity of histologic features in lymph node biopsy specimens from patients at risk for acquired immunodeficiency syndrome. Hum Pathol 17: 1231

Steinherz LJ, Brochstein JA, Robins J (1986) Cardiac involvement in congenital acquired immunodeficiency syndrome. Am J Dis Child 140: 1241

Strauss J, Abitol C, Zilleruelo G et al. (1989) Renal disease in children with acquired immunodeficiency syndrome. N Engl J Med 321: 625

Sunderam G, Reichman LB (1988) Tuberculosis and human immunodeficiency virus infection. Semin Resp Med 9: 481

Turner BJ, Denison M, Eppes SC, Houcheus R, Fanning T, Markson LE (1993) Survival experience of 789 children with the acquired immunodeficiency syndrome. Pediatr Infect Dis J 12: 310

Van de Perre P, Simonon A, Msellati P et al. (1992) Postnatal transmission of human immunodeficiency virus type 1 from mother to infant – a prospective cohort study in Kigali, Rwanda. N Engl J Med 325: 593

Van Hoeven KH, Factor SM, Kress Y, Woodruff JM (1993) Visceral myogenic tumours: a manifestation of HIV infection in children. Am J Surg Pathol 17: 1176

16 · Metabolic Disorders: a Simplified Approach to their Diagnosis

Brian D. Lake

In many laboratories the mention of the possibility of a biopsy or sample for the evaluation of a metabolic problem causes consternation and questions of what to do. This chapter outlines an approach to diagnosis and the examination of various samples for a range of metabolic disorders.

The spectrum of metabolic disorders presenting to the histopathologist is constantly changing as biochemical and molecular diagnostic tests are refined and become more specific and capable of being performed on smaller samples. The role of the histopathologist in the diagnosis of metabolic disease will vary from hospital to hospital, and will depend on the degree of enthusiasm of the clinical staff for metabolic disease and on the diagnostic facilities available. The most useful role is in initial screening, using simple microscopic tests which can point to a precise diagnosis or the most likely group of disorders, confirm a suspicion or exclude a variety of disorders.

In the following pages the usefulness of examination of blood and bone marrow films, urinary sediment, hair, and liver, rectal, conjunctival and skin biopsies will be evaluated in relation to a range of metabolic disorders. Electron microscopy, often regarded as of vital importance in metabolic disorders, is needed only occasionally. Further details of the clinical features and biochemistry of these disorders and others can be found in Scriver et al. (1995).

It must be remembered that metabolic disorders affect only a very small proportion of children; thus each disorder is rare and few paediatricians will be familiar with the whole range. It may be better to refer the patient to a specialist centre rather than to attempt a diagnosis with limited experience and expertise. However, some tests that can confirm or exclude the presence of metabolic disease can be performed in most laboratories.

The simplest possible approach to the problem will often lead to a diagnosis in the shortest time with least discomfort to the patient and minimal involvement of the laboratory. As in all branches of medicine, there is no substitute for a well informed clinical appraisal, and it is most important to establish a dialogue between paediatrician and pathologist to ensure adequate investigation. Any surgeon to be involved should also be aware of the reasons for the biopsy and, more importantly, of what should and should not be done to it.

Occasionally a biopsy will arrive in the laboratory without prior warning or consultation, even in the best-regulated centres. Under these circumstances, provided the specimen has arrived fresh and without undue delay, part should be fixed in formalin for routine histopathology, part should be frozen by the most rapid means available for histochemistry and biochemistry, and part should be fixed for electron microscopy. The two best methods for freezing tissue are:

1. Freezing in isopentane cooled to $-160°C$ in liquid nitrogen
2. Freezing in hexane cooled to $-79°C$ in an acetone/solid carbon dioxide bath

An adequate but less desirable method is freezing directly in liquid nitrogen, although if the tissue is well dusted with starch powder (Biosorb glove powder) perfect freezing can be obtained even in inexperienced hands. If these methods are not practicable, freezing on solid carbon dioxide, or in the last resort by placing in a deep freeze, will preserve the tissue

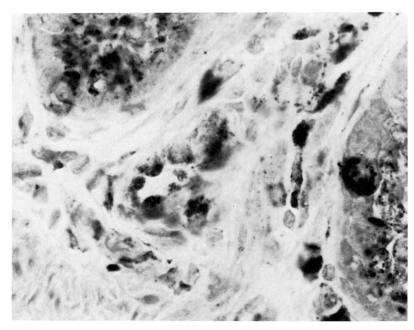

Fig. 16.1. Acid phosphatase activity can be used as a marker to demonstrate an abnormal reaction in an otherwise normal-looking cell. The endothelial cells normally show no acid phosphatase activity, but in this figure their involvement is clearly shown in a suction rectal biopsy from a patient with Niemann–Pick disease type A. Similar involvement may be demonstrated in Batten's disease and G_{M1}-gangliosidosis. ($\times$ 1000)

for biochemical analysis but may leave it in a state unsuitable for sectioning. Whichever freezing technique is used, the frozen tissue should be carefully wrapped in aluminium cooking foil or parafilm to prevent drying, and stored in a precooled small bottle at –20 °C or below. It is a useful principle to "fix some, freeze some, and take some for electron microscopy" from most biopsies, whether or not they are from patients suspected of having a metabolic disorder.

The sections below set out the principal tests that can be performed in the majority of hospital laboratories. The number of special stains required is not large. Considerable information can be derived from:

1. A periodic acid–Schiff (PAS) reaction to detect glycogen and compounds containing 1 : 2 glycol groups (e. g. oligosaccharides, gangliosides).
2. Sudan black for lipids. Some indication of the presence of neutral fat or complex lipids can be inferred from the colour of the stained section.
3. A reaction to show acid phosphatase activity. A change in the intensity of the reaction, or of its distribution within the cell, indicates altered cellular function.

Other methods will be necessary from time to time, but these three and a haematoxylin and eosin (H&E)

preparation will allow the general nature of the disorder to be appreciated. Figure 16.1 shows a rectal suction biopsy stained to reveal acid phosphatase activity.

The enzyme defects and substances stored in various types of lysosomal storage disease are shown in Table 16.1.

Blood Film Examination

It is often thought that examination of blood films for evidence of metabolic disease is a difficult procedure only to be undertaken in specialist centres. The contrary is true. The examination of standard blood films – as performed every day by all routine haematology laboratories using a May–Grünwald–Giemsa or similar stain – can be very informative and will support a diagnosis, exclude a diagnosis or point in a particular direction for further tests. The test requires simple observation of the morphology of lymphocytes, particularly in the tail and trails of the film. This area of the film is one usually avoided by the haematologist because of the vagaries of cell spreading. However, the abnormal morphology of cells is

Table 16.1. Lysosomal storage disease: stored substance and enzyme defect

Disorder	Enzyme defect	Stored substance
Pompe (glycogen storage disease II)	Acid maltase (α-1 : 4 - glucosidase)	Glycogen
Niemann–Pick type A and B	Sphingomyelinase	Sphingomyelin (and cholesterol)
Niemann–Pick type C	Abnormality of cholesterol esterification	No major substance identified
Gaucher (all forms)	Glucocerebrosidase (β-glucosidase)	Glucocerebroside
Wolman	Acid esterase	Cholesteryl esters and triglycerides
Fabry	α-Galactosidase	Ceramide trihexoside
Cystinosis	Transport defect	Cystine
Tay–Sachs	Hexosaminidase A	G_{M2}-Ganglioside
Sandhoff	Hexosaminidases A and B	G_{M2}-Ganglioside
Generalized gangliosidosis	β-Galactosidase	G_{M1}-Ganglioside
Batten's	Unknown	Subunit c of mitochondrial ATP synthase in late infantile and juvenile forms
Farber	Ceramidase	Ceramides
Mannosidosis	α-Mannosidase	Oligosaccharides with terminal α-mannose
Cherry-red spot – myoclonus syndrome	Sialidase (2 types)	Oligosaccharides with sialic residues, and gangliosides
Metachromatic leucodystrophy	Arylsulphatase A	Cerebroside sulphates
Krabbe's leucodystrophy	Galactocerebrosidase	Galactocerebroside
Mucopolysaccharidoses	Various (see Table 16.4)	Water-soluble acid mucopolysaccharides and ganglioside

rarely seen in the well spread areas because the vacuolated cells tend to congregate in the tail owing to their size or density. It is also thought that vacuolation is non-specific. However, given an adequate clinical history, the presence or absence of lymphocytic vacuolation can be a valuable diagnostic pointer. Abnormal granulation of neutrophils and eosinophils can also be assessed in the film, but not necessarily in the trails. Preparation of a buffy coat for electron microscopy is not needed except in special circumstances where no abnormality can be or is expected to be seen by light microscopy.

In many instances a confident diagnosis can be made and confirmed by a specific enzyme assay. In this way valuable time and expensive reagents – some of which have to be prepared and radiolabelled in the laboratory – can be saved. In contrast with this is the blunderbus approach, where the patient is investigated for every condition for which there is an enzyme assay on leucocytes. More often than not, no inborn error is detected under these circumstances. Screening by light microscopy can avoid many of these tests and the costs involved. Vacuolation, particularly in lymphocytes, is found in the conditions shown in Table 16.2. The change may be marked, with numerous well defined large vacuoles in many cells, or minor, with small vacuoles in few cells. Occasionally, all lymphocytes contain vacuoles. It should be noted that the vacuolation induced in monocytes by an anticoagulant is coarse, irregular, and without well defined margins to the vacuoles. Even with prolonged immersion in anticoagulant, similar induced vacuolation is not apparent in neutrophils or lymphocytes.

Table 16.2. Conditions in which vacuolated lymphocytes are found

Small vacuoles (1–6 per cell)	Larger vacuoles (often numerous)
Niemann–Pick type A	G_{M1}-Gangliosidosis type 1
Wolman's disease	Mannosidosis
Pompe's disease the juvenile and and adult forms of glycogen storage disease	Fucosidosis
	I-cell disease (mucolipidosis II)
	Mucolipidosis I and III
	Aspartylglucosaminuria
	Juvenile Batten's disease
	Salla disease and sialic acid storage disease

Pompe's Disease

In Pompe's disease, the infantile glycogen storage disease type II (see p. 853), each lymphocyte contains one or more small discrete vacuoles in which glycogen can be demonstrated. The demonstration of glycogen is best accomplished by the PAS reaction after a thin protective film of celloidin has been applied to the slide by dipping it in dilute (0.25%) celloidin in ethanol, shaking and air-drying. A nuclear counterstain is added to define the cell type. Although B lymphocytes contain glycogen deposits, these deposits are usually all round the periphery of the cell; they do not show vacuolation and their proportion of the lymphocyte population is small. The glycogen deposits in Pompe's disease coincide with acid phosphatase activity, showing the lysosomal connection with the storage material, and by electron microscopy the glycogen deposits are shown to be membrane bound (Trend et al. 1985). The vacuolation and glycogen deposition is also detectable in fetal blood samples.

The milder forms of this disorder, affecting juveniles and adults, also show glycogen deposits within lymphocyte vacuoles, but fewer lymphocytes appear to be affected. Confirmation of the diagnosis is by assay of acid maltase (α-1 : 4-glucosidase) activity in leucocytes or cultured fibroblasts.

Niemann–Pick Disease Types A and B

The lymphocytic vacuoles in Niemann–Pick disease type A are also small and discrete, but they do not affect every lymphocyte. The deposited sphingomyelin cannot be demonstrated because the staining reactions for small amounts are not sufficiently intense. The diagnosis can be confirmed by assay of sphingomyelinase activity in leucocytes or cultured fibroblasts, by examination of bone marrow (see p. 844), or by suction rectal biopsy (see p. 849). Lymphocytes in Niemann–Pick disease type B (juvenile/adult without neurological involvement) show no significant vacuolation.

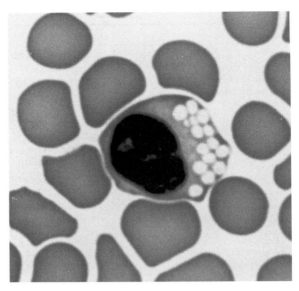

Fig. 16.2. Vacuolated lymphocyte in the blood film. Coarse vacuolation similar to this occurs in G_{M1}-gangliosidosis, juvenile Batten's disease, sialic acid storage disease and mannosidosis. (May–Grünwald–Giemsa, $\times 2800$)

Niemann–Pick Disease Type C (see p. 845)

Small discrete vacuoles may occur in some patients, affecting a small but significant proportion of lymphocytes (Hagberg et al. 1978).

Wolman's Disease and Cholesteryl Ester Storage Disease

Wolman's disease and cholesteryl ester storage disease show lymphocytic vacuoles similar to those in Pompe's disease and type A Niemann–Pick disease. In this instance the vacuoles contain neutral fat (triglyceride and cholesteryl esters), which is readily stained with Oil Red O or Scharlach R. Deficiency of acid esterase activity can be reliably shown by a histochemical method in which 1-naphthyl acetate is used as substrate (Lake 1971). Large foam cells similar to those in marrow are rarely found in blood films, but have occasionally been seen in the acute infantile form.

G_{M1}-Gangliosidosis

Numerous larger, well defined, vacuoles occur in the majority of lymphocytes in infantile G_{M1}-gangliosidosis (type 1), but in the late infantile form (type 2)

vacuolation is sparse or absent. No storage substance can be shown within the vacuoles. The deficiency of β-galactosidase activity in neutrophils and lymphocytes from patients with types 1 and 2 disease can be shown histochemically by means of a substituted indoxyl substrate (Lake 1974). Similar prominent lymphocytic vacuolation is also seen in infantile sialic acid storage disease.

Mannosidosis

Similar coarse vacuolation, but affecting a smaller percentage of lymphocytes, is found in mannosidosis. In this instance the condition clinically resembles one of the mucopolysaccharidoses, but coarse lymphocytic vacuolation is not a feature of that group of conditions. In mannosidosis (Fig. 16.2) the stored substances are water-soluble oligosaccharides, which can be demonstrated by the PAS method for glycogen (see p. 839) in the affected lymphocytes in the thicker regions of the blood film. Even though the vacuoles are prominent in the tail of the film the stored substance cannot be demonstrated, probably because in this thinly spread region the cells have ruptured and their contents are thus freely soluble. Occasional lymphocytes with numerous small vacuoles occupying almost all the cytoplasm may also be present.

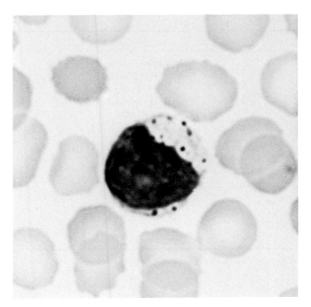

Fig. 16.3. Gasser cell in blood film. Mucopolysaccharidosis. These cells can occur in most mucopolysaccharidoses, and are not specific for any particular type. (May–Grünwald–Giemsa, × 2800)

Batten's Disease

In Batten's disease (which may also be known as neuronal ceroid-lipofuscinosis), the most common group of neurodegenerative disorders seen in children, the type of lymphocyte abnormality varies with the subgroup of the disease. The juvenile type of Batten's disease (also known as Spielmeyer–Vogt or Sjögren disease), shows prominent coarse vacuoles in about 10%–30% of lymphocytes, particularly in the tail of the blood film (Fig. 16.2). Electron microscopy shows mainly membrane-bound vacuoles, which are mostly empty, but occasional small fingerprint bodies may be found within a small proportion of vacuoles. Electron microscopy of blood for juvenile Batten's disease is unnecessary because the vacuoles are well seen by light microscopy. Rectal biopsy is the investigation of choice for confirmation of this condition. In contrast, late-infantile Batten's disease (or Bielschowsky–Jansky disease) is readily identifiable by the presence of curvilinear bodies in many lymphocytes at electron microscopy. No light microscopical abnormality is noted, and in particular no vacuoles are seen. Similarly, in the infantile form (or Santavuori or Hagberg type) no vacuoles are present, but electron microscopy of the lymphocytes shows membrane-bound granular osmiophilic deposits (GROD) measuring 0.5–1 μm in diameter, with one or two of these present in about 50% of lymphocytes. In the early juvenile form, also known as the variant late infantile form by Finnish workers, no abnormality is found in lymphocytes by light or electron microscopy.

The Mucopolysaccharidoses and Mucolipidoses

Occasional vacuolation is seen in the lymphocytes from patients with mucopolysaccharidosis, and in some of the vacuoles small densely staining inclusions may be present. The cells correspond to those initially described by Gasser (1950) in a patient with presumed Hurler's disease (MPS I-H), and can be present in any of the mucopolysaccharidoses (Fig. 16.3). Lymphocytic vacuolation is prominent in the mucolipidoses, but in this group of disorders there is no mucopolysaccharide deposition and the metachromasia characteristic of the mucopolysaccharidoses is absent.

The degree of metachromasia is helpful in predicting the type of mucopolysaccharidosis, and following the staining procedure described by Muir et al. (1963) 100 lymphocytes are examined under an oil-immersion objective and the percentage of those with metachromatic inclusions is recorded. Table 16.3 is a general guide to the conclusions that can be drawn from the percentage of lymphocytes with metachromatic inclusions.

Table 16.3. Mucopolysaccharidosis: metachromatic inclusions in lymphocytes

Percentages of lymphocytes containing metachromatic inclusions	Significance
20% or more	Sanfilippo (MPS III) is the first choice; some patients with Hunter (MPS II) may also have high counts
5%–20%	Hurler (MPS I-H) or Hunter (MPS II)
Less than 5%	Hurler–Sheie (MPS I-H/S) or Scheie (MPS I-S)

Patients with Morquio's syndrome (MPS IV) (Table 16.4) show no metachromasia, but basophilic inclusions of doubtful significance and specificity are sometimes present in neutrophils (Hansen 1972).

Although lymphocyte metachromasia is present in patients with Maroteaux–Lamy syndrome (MPS VI), the much more striking and specific Alder granulation is the better diagnostic pointer. All neutrophils show what appears to be marked toxic granulation in routine Giemsa stains. The Alder granulation,

Table 16.4. The mucopolysaccharidoses

Type[a]	Eponym	Enzyme defect	Urinary glycosaminoglycan
I-H	Hurler	α-L-Iduronidase	Dermatan sulphate
I-S	Scheie		Heparan sulphate
I-H/S	Hurler/Scheie		
II	Hunter	Sulphoiduronate sulphatase	Dermatan sulphate
			Heparan sulphate
III A	Sanfilippo	Heparan sulphate-N-sulphatase	Heparan sulphate
B	Sanfilippo	N-acetyl-α-D-glucosaminidase	
C	Sanfilippo	Acetyl CoA: α-glucosaminide N-acetyltransferase	
D	Sanfilippo	N-acetylglucosamine-6-sulphate sulphatase	
IV	Morquio	Chondroitin sulphate N-acetylhexosamine sulphate 6-sulphatase	Keratan sulphate
VI	Maroteaux–Lamy	Chondroitin sulphate-N-acetylgalactosamine sulphate-4-sulphatase (aryl sulphatase B)	Dermatan sulphate
VII	Sly	β-Glucuronidase	Dermatan sulphate

[a] Type V is vacant: Scheie syndrome (originally type V) was transferred to type I on recognition of its enzyme defect.

however, is coarser than toxic granulation and stains with a reddish lilac hue. Alder granulation (Fig. 16.4) is not metachromatic with the standard toluidine blue method (neither are toxic granules), but in the more sensitive toluidine blue staining method of Haust and Landing (1961) Alder granulation is basophilic while toxic granulation remains unstained. It is interesting to note that the first description of the Maroteaux–Lamy syndrome must be ascribed to Alder (1939), who clearly described two patients with the mild form of Maroteaux–Lamy syndrome (MPS VI B), each of whom had the neutrophil granules. Alder granulation

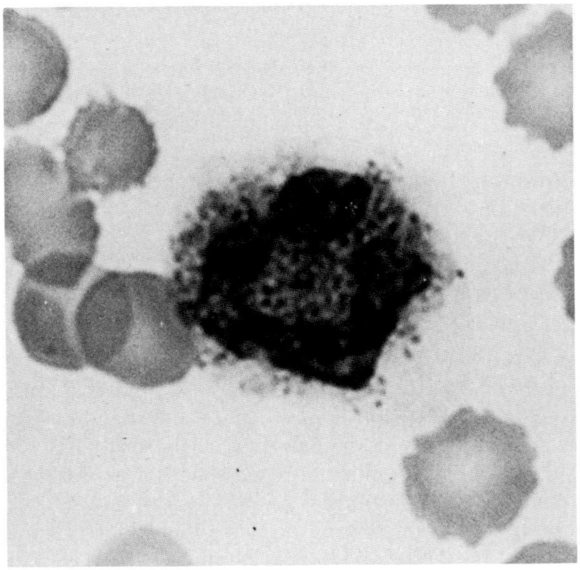

Fig. 16.4. Alder granulation in neutrophil in a blood film from a patient with Maroteaux–Lamy syndrome (MPS VI). (× 2800)

is present in cases of mucosulphatidosis (Rampini et al. 1970) and of β-glucuronidase deficiency (Pfeiffer et al. 1977), where it may be quite coarse.

Other Conditions

Lymphocytic vacuolation occurs in a number of other, much rarer, conditions. Aspartylglucosaminuria, which was first described in England (Jenner and Pollitt 1967) and later found to be relatively common in Finland (Haltia et al. 1975), may show very marked coarse vacuolation similar to that seen in juvenile Batten's disease, type 1 G_{M1}-gangliosidosis, Salla disease (Aula et al. 1979) and sialic acid storage diseases.

Some patients with fucosidosis and some with the cherry red spot–myoclonus syndrome, also known as sialidosis (Rapin et al. 1978), show a small number of vacuolated lymphocytes which may be missed without extensive searching.

Neutrophil Vacuolation (Jordans Anomaly)

This phenomenon, which should not be confused with the less conspicuous neutrophil vacuolation sometimes seen in acute infections, was described by Jordans (1953) in two brothers, who, in retrospect, may have had carnitine deficiency. However, not all patients with carnitine deficiency have neutrophil vacuolation. Jordans anomaly, in which neutral lipid can be demonstrated in the vacuoles, is an important diagnostic finding in neutral lipid storage disease where patients with ichthyosis have systemic involvement and deposition of triglyceride in many cell types (Judge et al. 1994). No lymphocytic vacuolation is found in neutral lipid storage disease.

Eosinophil Abnormalities

Irregular eosinophil granulation with grey and/or larger than normal granules (not to be confused with the giant eosinophil granules of the Chediak–Higashi syndrome or some of the preleukaemic states) is present in G_{M1}-gangliosidosis (Gitzelmann et al. 1984) and in sialic acid storage disease (Lake 1990). In mucosulphatidosis eosinophils have been reported absent, but may fall into the above category.

Bone Marrow Examination

The judicious use of bone marrow sampling can be of great help in deciding whether a patient with hepatosplenomegaly has a storage disease or whether the hepatosplenomegaly is caused by malignancy, infection or some other process. Most histopathologists are unused to looking at marrow films and prefer their samples fixed, embedded and sectioned. If this practice is followed it will not be possible to draw any conclusions about storage disorders. For the diagnosis of this group of conditions, several films should be made from the aspirate, either directly from the needle or preferably from an anticoagulated sample. A standard haematological stain will show storage cells, which are usually numerous, although on rare occasions only a few may be found in an otherwise adequate sample. There is no need to fix the other films, and as long as they remain dry their cytochemical reactions will be preserved for many weeks and can if necessary be sent by post for further study.

It is important that purely histochemical methods are used, so that appropriate conclusions can be made. For example, the Sudan black method commonly used by haematologists does not demonstrate fat but peroxidatic activity characteristic of the granulocytic series of cells. The methods that give the most useful information are Sudan black for lipids, PAS for carbohydrates and an acid phosphatase reaction for lysosomal activity. Normal bone marrow cells do not show much acid phosphatase activity after short incubation (30 min in a Gomori medium), and the strong activity of histiocytes or macrophages is easily visible under a lower-power objective. These methods are also useful for the detection of haemophagocytosis. Evidence of ingestion of red blood cells or white cells is more readily found in a PAS or

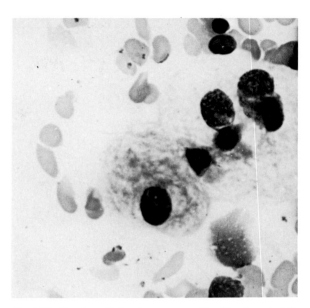

Fig. 16.5. Gaucher cells in a bone marrow film. The characteristic stripy appearance is not always easily seen. (May–Grünwald–Giemsa, × 1000)

acid phosphatase preparation than in a routine. May–Grünwald-Giemsa (MGG) stain. Other staining methods may occasionally be necessary for specific disorders.

Gaucher's Disease

Two main types of storage cell occur in bone marrow, and to the inexperienced eye they can cause problems of identification. The Gaucher cell is large, is sometimes multinucleate, and has a cytoplasm which stains a bluish-grey with Giemsa or similar stains (Figs. 16.5 and 16.6). In addition, the cytoplasm is often described as having the appearance of crumpled tissue paper. Many of the cells have this stripy look, in complete contrast to the foamy vacuolated appearances of the storage cells in Niemann–Pick disease and most other lipid storage diseases. Gaucher cells stain only weakly with Sudan black, and moderately with PAS, these two reactions being in keeping with the staining properties of glucocerebroside. Gaucher cells, like all storage cells and histiocytes with activated lysosomal systems, show strong acid phosphatase activity, which in Gaucher's disease is tartrate stable. The deficiency of the glucocerebrosidase as a β-glucosidase cannot be shown by histochemical methods.

The number of Gaucher cells is variable, but in general terms the infantile cases show numerous pos-

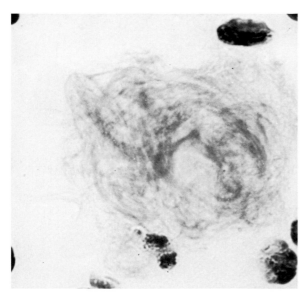

Fig. 16.6. A Gaucher cell in a bone marrow film. The fibrillar stripy nature of the cytoplasm is clearly visible. (Sudan black, × 1800)

itive cells in a marrow aspirate, while the juvenile and adult forms tend to have fewer Gaucher cells. Cells similar to those in Gaucher's disease have been reported in chronic myeloid leukaemia and thalassaemia. In G_{M1}-gangliosidosis type 2 (*late infantile*), Gaucher-like cells are present, but the cytoplasm is less fibrillar, more closely packed, and stains a more intense blue than that of Gaucher cells in a Giemsa preparation. In these cases the deficiency of β-galactosidase activity can be detected in the marrow sample or in blood films (see p. 840).

Niemann–Pick Disease Type A

Large foamy vacuolated histiocytes occur in most storage disorders, and differentiation of one from another rests on subtle morphological changes and correlation of the appearances of foamy cells with other cellular changes and their histochemical staining properties.

In Niemann–Pick disease type A (infantile) (Fig. 16.7), the foamy marrow storage cells stain weakly with Sudan black, and when the Sudan black preparations are examined in polarized light a reddish birefringence can be seen in the storage cells in most cases. The vacuoles of the storage cell are mostly small and uniform in size, and only rarely are ingested white cells or nuclear debris present. The PAS reaction is variably positive. Acid phosphatase activity is strong and mainly confined to the periphery of the vacuoles. Niemann–Pick type A cells will be stained blue with the ferric haematoxylin stain after alkaline hydrolysis. Lymphocytic vacuolation should also be present.

Adult Niemann–Pick Disease Type B and Sea-blue Histiocytes

In the juvenile non-neurological form of Niemann–Pick disease type B, marrow cells similar to those in the infantile form are found but the lymphocytic vacuolation is usually absent. Adult Niemann–Pick disease (the distinction between the adult and juvenile forms may be spurious) shows *numerous* unmistakable sea-blue histiocytes. These cells are so striking that "they should alert even the most casual of haematopathologists" (Reynolds 1973). To be of significance these cells should be numerous and easily seen in all parts of the film. Cells with one or two blue granules should never be regarded as sea-blue histiocytes. The cytoplasm of the cells is packed with granules, stains deep blue with Giemsa or Wright stains, is PAS- and Sudan black-positive, and shows strong autofluorescence. This material has the staining characteristics

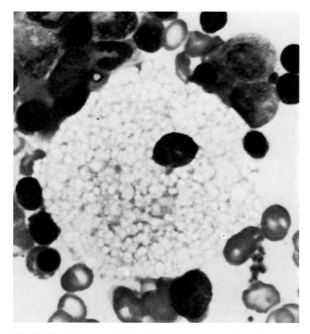

Fig. 16.7. A Niemann–Pick cell in a bone marrow film. The fairly uniform vacuolation in the cytoplasm and the absence of other features are characteristic. (May–Grünwald–Giemsa × 1000)

and ultrastructure to suggest a type of lipofuscin. Older patients have more of these cells, to such an extent that the vacuolated Niemann–Pick cells containing sphingomyelin may be overlooked.

Confirmation of the diagnosis of Niemann–Pick disease can be made by assay of sphingomyelinase activity in white blood cells or in cultured fibroblasts.

Cells similar to sea-blue histiocytes are found in lecithin–cholesterol–acyltransferase deficiency, but in much smaller numbers. Small numbers of cells of this type are occasionally present in older patients with Niemann–Pick disease type C.

Niemann–Pick Disease Type C

Some confusion may be caused by the classification of Niemann–Pick diseases and the similarity of the storage cells in the various types. In types A (infantile with neurological involvement) and B (juvenile/adult without neurological involvement), accumulation of sphingomyelin and deficiency of sphingomyelinase is well documented. In the other types (C and D) there is no such deficiency, although marked sphingomyelin accumulation is found in the spleen. These types (C and D), often referred to as "atypical Niemann–Pick disease", are now regarded as part of the spectrum of Niemann–Pick disease type C. The classification of the various types of Niemann–Pick disease has become less cumbersome and more easily understood since the 1982 international meeting in Prague (Elleder and Jirásec 1983). Cases are now defined on the basis of the presence or absence of sphingomyelinase activity as:

Group 1: Deficient sphingomyelinase activity
  I Type A with neuronal storage
  II Type B without neuronal storage
Group 2: No deficiency of sphingomyelinase activity
  III Type C with neuronal storage (includes type D)
  IV A form without neuronal storage has yet to be positively identified

This is a convenient classification for the moment, but it will undoubtedly be revised when the group 2 disorder is better understood. For a review of the historical background to the classification see Lake (1992). A defect in cholesterol esterification has been detected (Vanier et al. 1988) and this is sufficiently reliable for successful prenatal diagnosis (Vanier et al. 1989). The foam cells found in the marrow (Fig. 16.8) resemble those of Niemann–Pick disease type A, but the vacuoles are of widely varying sizes and densely staining inclusions are frequently present in Giemsa preparations. The cells contain no demonstrable fat, show PAS positivity, and have strong acid

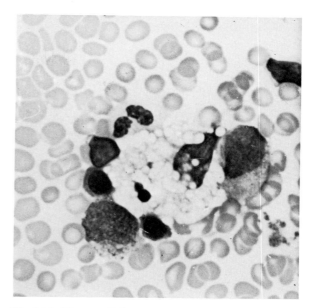

Fig. 16.8. Niemann–Pick disease type C. Foamy cell in a bone marrow film. Variable vacuole size and darkly stained inclusions differentiate these cells from other foamy storage cells. (May–Grünwald–Giemsa, 1000)

phosphatase activity. The course is long, with over 50% of patients presenting with neonatal hepatitis (Kelly et al. 1993), and neurological symptoms are slow to appear; thus it is important to be certain of the diagnosis, and to confirm the neuronal storage by rectal biopsy (see p. 849). Note that heterozygotes may have storage cells in marrow (and other tissues, but have no neuronal storage), but the number of cells is less than the homozygote state. Care in testing younger siblings is thus important.

Gangliosidosis

The large foamy histiocytes found in G_{M1}-gangliosidosis type 1 have no characteristic staining reactions. Diagnosis rests on the presence of coarsely vacuolated lymphocytes and the absence of β-galactosidase activity, which can be shown by a histochemical method (Lake 1974) or by quantitative biochemical assay. No histiocytes can be found in the marrow in cases of G_{M2}-gangliosidosis (Tay–Sachs disease).

Wolman's Disease

Histiocytes that contain much neutral fat (cholesterol, cholesteryl esters, triglycerides) and stain strongly with Sudan black or Oil Red O are present in

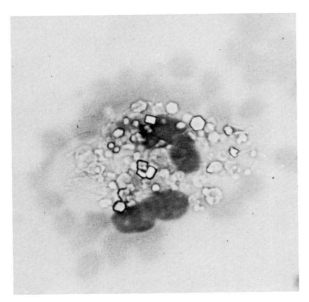

Fig. 16.9. Bone marrow film. Cystinosis. Cystine crystals in typical hexagonal and brick shapes within a macrophage are readily visible in partially polarized light. Some fine needle-shaped crystals are also visible. The film has been lightly stained with alcoholic basic fuchsin to show nuclei. (× 1100)

system in conditions such as chronic myeloid leukaemia and thalassaemia. In Langerhans' cell histiocytosis large foamy marrow cells may be encountered, particularly in advanced cases, but these cells, although striking in Giemsa preparations, have no demonstrable storage substance. Their acid phosphatase reaction is very strong and sharply localized, in contrast with the strong but diffuse reaction of genuine storage cells. Where screening for systemic involvement in Langerhans' cells histiocytosis is necessary, films may be stained for α-mannosidase activity. Unfixed films are incubated in a medium that contains 5% polyethylene glycol 6000 to prevent diffusion of the very soluble enzyme (Filipe and Lake 1990). Normal marrow shows very little α-mannosidase activity apart from a pale blush in some cells. Where abnormal cells are present in Langerhans' cell histiocytosis, intense α-mannosidase activity is found in the abnormal cells. The reaction is so strong that a single abnormal cell can be detected in a marrow film scanned at low power. Conditions leading to lipid overload, particularly disorders involving lipid metabolism (hyperlipoproteinaemias, hyperlipidaemia and Tangier disease) may show prominent lipid-laden macrophages, which can be mistaken for Niemann–Pick cells (type A).

Wolman's disease (infantile and juvenile forms), and these stain a distinctive purple colour with Nile blue. Vacuolated lymphocytes containing neutral fat and the absence of acid esterase activity are necessary for the diagnosis. The storage cells of cholesteryl ester storage disease are less prominent in the marrow.

Mucopolysaccharidosis

The foamy cells are readily seen in May–Grünwald–Giemsa preparations. Within the vacuoles basophilic granules are present which are strongly metachromatic with toluidine blue. The cells are particularly prominent in or around the marrow fragments. Although storage cells are found in the bone marrow from patients with mucopolysaccharidosis (Hansen 1972), bone marrow biopsy should never be necessary except for haematological reasons. There are simpler and more reliable methods available for the diagnosis of mucopolysaccharidosis (see Tables 16.3 and 16.4 and p. 841).

Acquired Storage Cells

Acquired storage cells occur occasionally and can be related to an overload of the reticuloendothelial

Cystinosis

It is not always appreciated that cystine crystals, although relatively insoluble, have sufficient solubility to disappear almost completely from routinely stained films. For the diagnosis of cystinosis a slightly different approach is needed. Films should be made with great care, because the act of making the films can easily rupture the histiocytes in which the crystals are situated, in which case the crystals of cystine are much more likely to be lost. The films are air-dried, fixed in absolute alcohol, and stained with 1% basic fuchsin in 70% alcohol for 10 min, followed by rinsing in alcohol, clearing and mounting. The small amount of water in the stain is insufficient to dissolve any cystine present but allows a reasonable degree of nuclear staining. The slides are then examined between partly crossed polarizers for cystine crystals, which are birefringent in their longitudinal plane. This means that the characteristic brick-shaped crystal is easily seen under these conditions, but the hexagonal end of the crystal is not so readily visible (Fig. 16.9). Most marrow samples contain a large preponderance of the brick-shaped crystals, but occasionally the less visible hexagonal shape may predominate.

A wet preparation is also invaluable for the diagnosis of cystinosis. This is made by placing one drop of the anticoagulant-treated marrow sample on a slide and covering with a large cover slip. The gently made thin preparation is ideal for searching for the intact histiocytes containing cystine crystals, and individual cystine crystals from histiocytes ruptured by the action of aspirating the marrow are also readily visible. Dirt, dust and glass fragments (from diamond marking of the slides) are birefringent but have an irregular outline.

Bone Marrow Biopsy as an Exclusion Test

The absence of storage-type cells from an appropriately stained adequate sample almost certainly means that a storage disease can be excluded, often a useful exclusion test in a child with unexplained hepatosplenomegaly.

It is a general principle that, if storage cells are seen in a bone marrow sample and their precise identity is not known, all that should be reported is that storage cells are present. In many cases a diagnostic label has been attached to a finding and has subsequently (sometimes many years later) been proved wrong. The course of the disease may be different from that diagnosed, and in some instances prenatal diagnosis has been attempted on the basis of wrong information. In all storage diseases, enzyme assay is an essential part of the diagnosis. The histopathologist's task is to point the enzymologists in the right direction and to eliminate cases in which no storage disease is present.

Urine Examination

The study of urinary sediment by light microscopy is of help only in metachromatic leucodystrophy and in Fabry's disease.

Chemical study of urinary deposit or supernatant by thin-layer chromatography can be extremely helpful in the diagnosis of the mucopolysaccharidoses, Fabry's disease and the rarer mannosidosis, fucosidosis and sialidoses.

Metachromatic Leucodystrophy

The presence in the urinary sediment of intracellular deposits of a substance staining golden yellow-brown after staining with the toluidine blue method as described by Bodian and Lake (1963) is pathognomonic for metachromatic leucodystrophy, although in a different clinical setting patients with mucosulphatidosis also show these deposits. The demonstration of intracellular deposits is vital to the diagnosis, but a high index of suspicion should be maintained if extracellular material is seen in the form of tubular casts. The intracellular and extracellular deposits show a greenish birefringence when examined in polarized light.

The appearance of the metachromatically stained deposits is identical in both metachromatic leucodystrophy and mucosulphatidosis. These two conditions can be differentiated in the laboratory by examination of routinely stained blood films, where Alder granulation (see p. 842) is present in mucosulphatidosis but absent in metachromatic leucodystrophy.

The substance inducing metachromasia in the exfoliated renal epithelial cells is a mixture of sulphatides (cerebroside sulphates), similar to the sulphatide found in the brain in metachromatic leucodystrophy. The presence of sulphatide can be confirmed by thin-layer chromatography of a lipid extract of the urinary sediment. It has become apparent in recent years that there is a pseudodeficiency of arylsulphatase A that gives low arylsulphatase A activity on biochemical testing, yet the patients under investigation do not have metachromatic leucodystrophy. The pseudodeficiency is more common than metachromatic leucodystrophy and may well be found on general screening in a neurological setting. No metachromatic material is found in the urinary sediment in the pseudodeficiency.

Fabry's Disease

Large tubular casts and mulberry-like cells staining intensely with PAS are found in the urinary sediment from patients with Fabry's disease. The cells do not exhibit metachromasia but do show a silvery birefringence. It is not always easy to see these cells and deposits, because normal urine often contains cells that stain with PAS, albeit to a lesser extent. It is possible to extract the deposit with chloroform/methanol (2 : 1 v/v) and after washing and drying the extract to perform thin-layer chromatography (TLC) (Lake and Goodwin 1976) to show the large excesses of both ceramide di- and trihexosides (Fabry's disease is X-lined); the normal individual rarely shows both di- and trihexoside, although either substance can be present separately.

Mucopolysaccharidoses

The excess urinary glycosaminoglycan (GAG) excretion in the mucopolysaccharidoses cannot be detected by light microscopy and is best demonstrated by one of the several precipitation methods available (Pennock 1976). The Alcian blue precipitation method described by Whiteman (1973) is sensitive and allows quantification, and is in routine screening use at the Hospital for Sick Children, Great Ormond Street, London. Further characterization of the GAG is made by two-way chromatography and electrophoresis, followed by staining by Alcian blue. The pattern of GAG excretion is of particular importance in pointing to the appropriate enzyme assay.

Oligosaccharidoses

Water-soluble oligosaccharides can be detected by TLC in the supernatant of centrifuged urine from patients with sialidosis, mannosidosis, fucosidosis and aspartylglucosaminuria.

Neuronal Storage Disease: Diagnosis by Rectal Biopsy

General Considerations on Rectal Biopsy

Rectal biopsy gives a positive indication of neuronal storage in all the neuronal storage diseases, and with the use of appropriate staining methods and electron microscopy the precise diagnosis should be possible in all cases. However, whether rectal biopsy is justifiable depends on the biochemical facilities available and the expertise of the surgeon.

Since the inception of rectal biopsy for neurological diagnosis biochemical advances have been enormous, and in the majority of cases the diagnosis can be made by enzyme assay in white blood cells, serum or cultured fibroblasts. There are a few conditions (Batten's disease, Niemann–Pick type C) in which neuronal involvement must be demonstrated before the diagnosis, with its grave prognosis, can be made. Confirmation of neuronal storage in the rare cases of Tay–Sachs disease with normal hexosaminidase activity is necessary before embarking on the search for activator protein deficiency.

Suction rectal biopsy of the type taken for the diagnosis of Hirschsprung's disease is usually adequate, and because it can be taken without anaesthetic is now preferred to a full-thickness biopsy. It has the advantage that several biopsies may be taken and repeated if necessary.

Examination of appendix is preferred in some centres; electron microscopy of skin or conjunctiva is preferred by others.

Staining Methods

The diagnostic appearances in rectal biopsies will be given for the whole range of neuronal storage diseases to provide an overall picture. Routinely prepared sections of formalin-fixed, paraffin wax-embedded tissue are of no help in differential diagnosis, because the lipids are dissolved during processing and their characteristic staining reactions are lost. Cryostat sections of fresh-frozen tissue are therefore essential and these should be stained by the following methods:

1. Haematoxylin and eosin
2. PAS (after 10 min fixation in 4% formaldehyde)
3. PAS celloidin (the slide is dipped in 0.25% celloidin in ethanol and dried; retains water-soluble compounds)
4. Luxol fast blue, neutral red
5. Sudan black (no fixation required)
6. An acid phosphatase reaction
7. An unstained, unfixed, mounted section for examination for autofluorescence (excitation 365 nm, barrier 410 nm; dark ground or epi-illumination conditions)

All these methods should be used. To ensure that sufficient neurons are found for each staining method, several serial sections should be cut. A single section on a slide is inadequate.

Gangliosidoses, Sialidoses and Farber's Disease

In the gangliosidoses the neurons are markedly enlarged and foamy, and stain strongly with both PAS methods. Confirmation of the presence of sialic acid can be obtained by the sodium metaperiodate–Schiff reaction (Roberts 1977). Weak staining is found with Sudan black and luxol fast blue. There is almost no autofluorescence. Tay–Sachs disease (of all types) can be differentiated from G_{M1}-gangliosidosis by the presence of PAS-positive histiocytes in the lamina propria and vacuolation of endothelial cells in G_{M1}-gangliosidosis and by the presence of β-galactosidase activity in Tay–Sachs disease. The histochemical method for detecting hexosaminidase activity cannot demonstrate the deficiency of the A component of this enzyme in Tay–Sachs disease (Lake and Ellis 1976), but can be used to show the total deficiency of hexosaminidase activity in Sandhoff's disease.

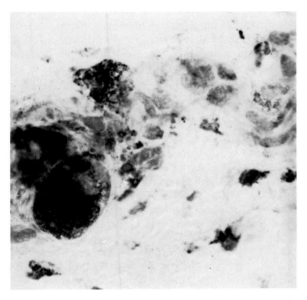

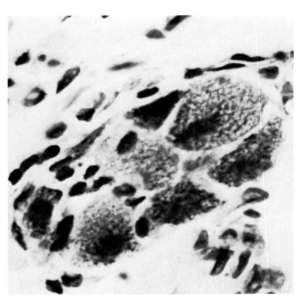

Fig. 16.10. Niemann–Pick disease type A. Cryostat section of a suction rectal biopsy stained to show acid phosphatase activity. Three neurons showing strong activity can be seen with their nerve supply. Macrophages in the loose connective tissue also show strong activity. (× 700)

Fig. 16.11. Rectal biopsy; Niemann–Pick disease type A. The neurons in Meissner's plexus have a distended foamy cytoplasm, an appearance also seen in the gangliosidoses. (× 950)

The sialidoses (cherry red spot–myoclonus syndrome) (Rapin et al. 1978) have very similar staining reactions, and differentiation from the gangliosidoses may not be possible by rectal biopsy.

In Farber's disease (Toppet et al. 1978), neuronal changes similar to those in the gangliosidoses may cause some confusion. Although ceramidase deficiency causes accumulation of ceramides, there is also an increase of a ganglioside-like substance giving rise to PAS positivity. However, in this condition a silvery birefringence in polarized light is seen in the neurons after staining with Sudan black. This is in contrast with the red birefringence in Niemann–Pick disease type A and Fabry's disease.

Niemann–Pick Disease

Some patients with Niemann–Pick disease of the infantile type (type A) are late in showing neurological involvement, and despite proof of the disease (enzyme assay in leucocytes, liver biopsy, bone marrow) there may be some doubt as to the neuronopathic nature of the disease. Suction rectal biopsy will provide the necessary evidence.

The neurons of Meissner's plexus are large and have a foamy ground-glass cytoplasm. They are very similar in appearance to the classic neuronal storage pictures of Tay–Sachs disease (Figs. 16.10 and

16.11). The cytoplasm stains with Sudan black (with reddish birefringence in polarized light) and has a honeycomb-like appearance in the acid phosphatase reaction. It is not always easy to be sure that the cells are neurons, but they often occur in small clusters of two or three with the tell-tale nerves leading to them.

The lamina propria is filled with histiocytes, which stain positively with Sudan black (Fig. 16.12) and show reddish birefringence in polarized light, are variably PAS-positive, and exhibit strong acid phosphatase activity. Endothelial cells are involved and this is best shown in the acid phosphatase preparation. Smooth-muscle cells contain sudanophilic deposits, and numerous histiocytes are present throughout the submucosa. The deposited sphingomyelin can be specifically stained by the ferric haematoxylin method after alkaline hydrolysis (Elleder and Lojda 1973). In type B Niemann–Pick disease there is no neuronal storage, but otherwise the changes are identical to those of type A.

Niemann–Pick Disease Type C

Patients with Niemann–Pick disease type C (Neville et al. 1973; Lake 1977, 1992; Vanier et al. 1988) may present with hepatosplenomegaly or spleno-megaly alone in mid-childhood, but more than 50% have severe prolonged jaundice in the neonatal period

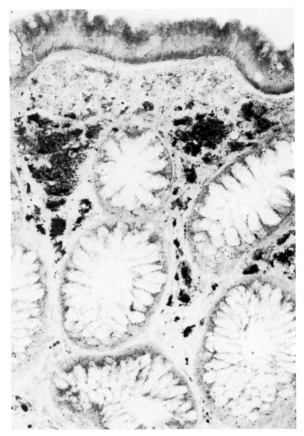

Fig. 16.12. Niemann–Pick disease type A. Cryostat section of suction rectal biopsy stained with Sudan black, showing numerous sudanophilic macrophages in the lamina propria. (× 280)

and are often regarded as having neonatal hepatitis (Kelly et al. 1993). Some patients are followed undiagnosed, as posthepatitic fibrosis problems and the significance of the numerous PAS-positive Kupffer cells and histiocytes in the liver biopsy may be overlooked. The neurological symptoms, regardless of the initial presentation, begin around 5–6 years, but can be delayed to the early teens. In others the neurological symptoms may occur much earlier or much later

(Vanier et al. 1988). The diagnosis, initially made by examination of bone marrow films, needs confirmation by demonstration of neuronal involvement. Neuronal storage is present at an early age and can be found at 32 weeks' gestation (Adam et al. 1988) and earlier. Demonstration of this deposition is essential before the diagnosis, with its attendant grave prognosis, can be made.

The substance(s) accumulating in the neurons is water-soluble and best demonstrated by the protected PAS reaction (PAS cell) (Fig. 16.13). The intensity of the PAS reaction is diminished by prior aqueous fixation and in some instances may be negative under these conditions. Apart from an intense acid phosphatase reaction the neurons display no other staining reactions. The presence of histiocytes in the lamina propria is a non-specific and not uncommon finding, but in this condition they are also present in the submucosa. Electron microscopy of the neurons is essential because the degree of storage may be minimal at an early age.

Batten's Disease

Neuronal storage in Batten's disease (also known as *ceroid lipofuscinosis*) is accompanied by smooth muscle and endothelial cell storage. The combination of these and their staining characteristics makes the differential diagnosis from other neuronal storage conditions comparatively easy (Lake 1976). Table 16.5 shows the differences in the neuronal staining patterns of the different subgroups and other major storage disorders. Smooth muscle and endothelial cell storage is best seen in Sudan black and acid phosphatase preparations and by autofluorescence (Fig. 16.14). It should be noted that the neuronal storage may be subtle and not easily seen, and that evaluation of the other cell types is an important part of the investigation. In addition to the smooth muscle and endothelial cell storage there are acid phosphatase-positive histiocytes among the smooth muscle cells of the muscularis mucosae (and muscularis propria) in the juvenile forms. The rectal biopsy appearances

Table 16.5. Neuronal staining reactions in the more common storage disorders

Disorder	PAS	Sudan black	Luxol fast blue	Autofluorescence
Batten's disease				
Infantile	++	++	−	++
Late infantile	+/−	+	+/− +	+
Juvenile and early juvenile	++	++	++	++
Gangliosidosis	+++	+	++	−
Niemann–Pick disease				
Type A	+/−	+	−	−
Type C	+	−	−	−

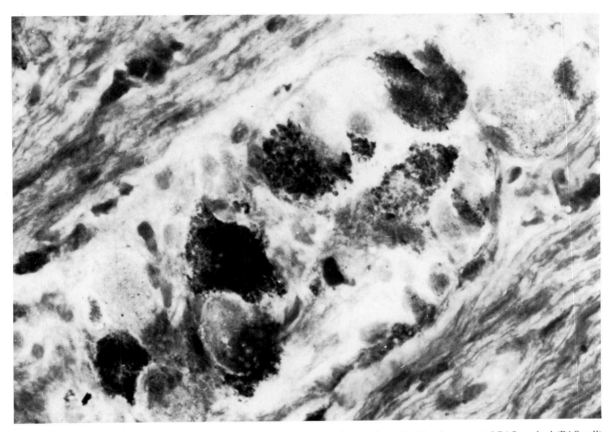

Fig. 16.13. Niemann–Pick disease type C. Neurons in a cryostat section of appendix stained by the protected PAS method (PAS cell) show storage of a substance that is removed by aqueous fixatives. (× 800)

of the early juvenile form are identical to those of the juvenile form (even to the ultrastructure), but the two may be differentiated by the presence of vacuolated lymphocytes in the juvenile but not the early juvenile form. The vacuolation of lymphocytes is apparent from soon after birth (and probably before), long before any clinical symptoms occur, and the test may be used to screen younger siblings – if the parents want to know. As with all neuronal storage disorders, the neuronal storage is present long before the neurological symptoms occur. The rectal approach can be used in a positive way to diagnose affected patients, and in a negative way to exclude the possibility of

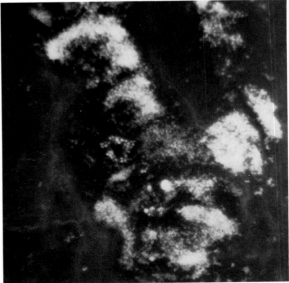

Fig. 16.14. Juvenile Batten's disease. Neurons in a cryostat section of a rectal biopsy, showing autofluorescence in an unstained unfixed section. Excitation with UG5 or BG3 filter. (× 800)

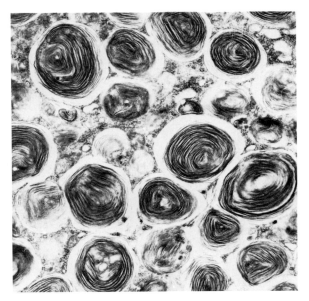

Fig. 16.15. Electron micrograph. Membranous cytoplasmic bodies in a neuron from the appendix of a patient with generalized gangliosidosis. The same appearance is also found in Tay–Sachs disease and in sialidosis. (× 18 000)

younger siblings being affected. Examination of blood buffy coat preparations by electron microscopy are also useful for the infantile and late infantile forms. It should be noted that DNA probes are available for most families with the infantile form (on chromosome 1, Jarvela et al. 1992) and for the juvenile form (on chromosome 16, Gardiner 1992), and biopsy approaches for sibling screening may be best carried out by this route.

Paraffin sections may be used for the diagnosis of Batten's disease if frozen tissue is not available, because the stored protein in the late infantile and juvenile forms and the substance in the infantile form are not extracted by fixation or processing. It retains not only the sudanophilia (grey-black) and autofluorescence, but also the immunoantigenicity to antibodies prepared to the stored protein (subunit c of ATP synthase, Hall et al. 1991) in the late infantile and juvenile forms.

Electron Microscopy

Ultrastructural studies of the neuronal deposits in storage diseases reveal membranous cytoplasmic bodies (MCBs) in the gangliosidoses and sialidoses (Fig. 16.15), zebra-like bodies in Farber's disease and mucopolysaccharidoses, and pleomorphic lipid bodies in Niemann–Pick disease type C (Fig. 16.16). Axonal swellings with granular and lamellar debris are

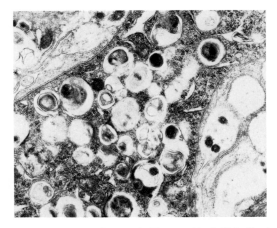

Fig. 16.16. Electron micrograph. Pleomorphic lipid bodies in a neuron from a rectal biopsy from a patient with Niemann–Pick disease type C. (× 18 000)

evident in many of the storage disorders and are non-diagnostic.

In infantile Batten's disease, GRODs (finely granular osmiophilic deposits) are present in most cell types (Fig. 16.17). In late infantile Batten's disease all the affected cell types (see Lake 1992) contain curvilinear profiles exclusively (Fig. 16.18). In the juvenile and early juvenile forms of Batten's disease, neurons of the gastrointestinal tract contain fingerprint profiles (Fig. 16.19), in contrast to the brain in which mixtures of curvilinear and fingerprint profiles may be found. Mixed curvilinear and fingerprint

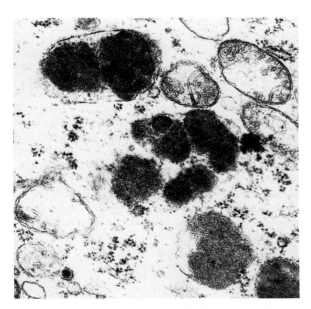

Fig. 16.17. Electron micrograph. Infantile Batten's disease. GRODs in a neuron. (× 45 000)

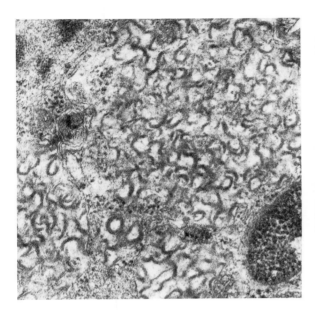

Fig. 16.18. Electron micrograph. Late infantile Batten's disease. Curvilinear bodies in a smooth muscle cell. Similar deposits are also found in neuron and lymphocytes. (× 68 000)

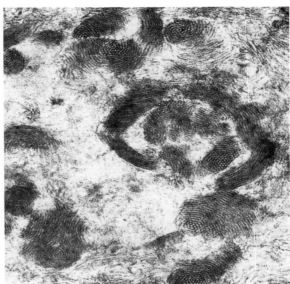

Fig. 16.19. Electron micrograph. Juvenile Batten's disease. Fingerprint bodies are present in the neuronal cytoplasm in a rectal biopsy. (× 110 000)

profiles are present in other cell types, and skeletal muscle may have squashed or tightly packed curvilinear bodies in the juvenile forms.

A tissue diagnosis of the late infantile Batten's disease has been made prenatally (Chow et al. 1993).

Glycogen Storage Disease

Glycogen storage disease (GSD) in its various forms is an important cause of failure to thrive associated with hepatomegaly. Biochemical screening (fasting blood sugar levels, glucagon stimulation after fasting, lactate and urate levels) will often give some indication of the type of GSD (Spencer-Peet et al. 1971), and confirmation can sometimes be obtained by assay of the appropriate enzyme in red blood cells or leucocytes. Table 16.6 shows the various types of GSD encountered. Types I, III and IX are most frequent. Other much rarer types (e.g. phosphorylase b kinase deficiency of heart) also exist. Type IX was formerly known as type VIB. True liver phosphorylase deficiency is extremely rare and may not exist. Figure 16.20 shows the pathways of glycogen and glucose metabolism, and in Figure 16.20b the glucose-6-phosphatase system with the phosphate and glucose channels is shown in diagrammatic form.

If a liver biopsy is necessary, this should only be performed after discussion between pathologist,

surgeon and clinician. The division of material is best directed by the metabolic physician in charge of the case, who will know, from clinical impression and biochemical tests, what emphasis is needed for each investigation. An open liver biopsy provides most material, but two cores with the Trucut needle will give adequate tissue for biochemistry and histochemistry with a small amount for routine histology. Open biopsies (now rare) are divided similarly, with the piece for histology having a large surface area but little depth. The biopsies should be collected from the operating theatre and either taken directly to the laboratory or dealt with on the spot, because delay in freezing can affect the enzyme activities. If an open biopsy is taken, it is also good practice to take a small piece of muscle (rectus abdominis or internal oblique) from the edge of the incision for freezing, so that it can be studied to determine whether there is muscle involvement. Where facilities permit, a small piece of skin can also be put into culture medium to establish a fibroblast line on which enzyme and metabolic studies can be made.

Routine histology in GSD gives only minimal information except for showing the degree of enlargement of the hepatocytes, the extent of fibrosis and the presence and extent of nuclear glycogenation. This latter feature is different from the normal nuclear glycogen usually seen as vacuolation of nuclei in periportal regions in haematoxylin and eosin preparations. In particular, the glycogen content

Table 16.6. Glycogen storage disorders

Type	Enzyme defect	Signs and symptoms	Liver pathology
O	Glycogen synthetase	Hypoglycaemia Fits	Fatty Very low glycogen content
IA	Glucose-6-phosphatase	Hepatomegaly Hypoglycaemia Lactic acidosis Hyperuricaemia	Very fatty Absent glucose-6-phosphatase Normal glycogen content Nuclear glycogenation becomes prominent in older patients

IB	Glucose-6-phosphate
	  translocase
		As above plus
		  neutropenia
			As IA
			Fibrosis increases with age

IC	Phosphate transport defect	As IA	As IA
ID	Glucose transport defect	As IA Neutropenia	As IA Fibrosis increases with age
IIA	Acid maltase (infantile)	Hypotonia Cardiomegaly No hypoglycaemia Hepatosplenomegaly	Glycogen increased in hepatocytes and Kupffer cells Strong acid phosphatase activity
IIB	Acid maltase (juvenile and adult)	Affects skeletal muscle only	
III	Debranching enzyme	Mildly hypoglycaemic Hepatomegaly Raised LFTs	Very high but very soluble glycogen content Portal fibrosis Usually no fat Nuclear glycogenation prominent in older patients
IV	Branching enzyme	Hepatomegaly Jaundice Rarely hypoglycaemic	Cirrhosis Bile stasis Indigestible glycogen
V	Myophosphorylase	Affects skeletal muscle only	
VII	Phosphofructokinase	Affects skeletal muscle only	
IX	Phosphorylase kinase	Hepatomegaly (asymptomatic)	Very high glycogen Mild to moderate fat No fibrosis

cannot be related to the colour density of specific stains, because the glycogens in these storage diseases have differing solubilities and much may be lost in the fixation and processing. This is especially true in type III GSD, where the stored limit dextrin is very soluble and almost none remains after fixation. Cryostat sections are essential to show glycogen and enzymes, and can also give perfectly adequate histological results if the freezing and sectioning are carefully controlled. It should be noted that an increased glycogen content can be found in liver and muscle in patients who have been receiving intravenous dextrose for hypoglycaemia, and this should be considered before making a diagnosis of GSD of unknown type. A high liver glycogen content may also be found in some organic acidaemias.

In some types of GSD, hepatocellular adenomas may occur asymptomatically, only being discovered incidentally. They are of no clinical significance and rarely or never have malignant potential. Hepatocellular adenomas have been described in type I, type III and recently type IV GSD (Alshak et al. 1994).

Type 0

Very few patients with glycogen synthetase deficiency have been described (Aynsley-Green 1981).

Liver biopsies contain increased fat and very little glycogen, and there is no evidence of necrosis or fibrosis. Skeletal muscle is entirely normal. The diagnosis must be made by biochemical assay of liver because leucocytes and erythrocytes have normal glycogen synthetase activity in this condition. Care should be taken to exclude Reye's syndrome and disorders of fatty acid oxidation where a similar lack of glycogen and increased fat are found (Howat et al. 1984).

Type I

In type IA GSD the liver shows marked panlobular fatty change without excessive glycogen deposition (Fig. 16.21). Nuclear glycogen is present and becomes more prominent with age. No glucose-6-phosphatase activity can be detected with the standard Gomori lead capture method, but a control liver section (rat, mouse or human) is essential to show that the method is working. The activity must be entirely absent – not just lowered – because the other types of GSD may show subnormal activity of this enzyme with the activity confined to the periphery of the hepatocyte. The absence of glucose 6-phosphatase activity can also be demonstrated in jejunal mucosa, but very low levels are also seen in the

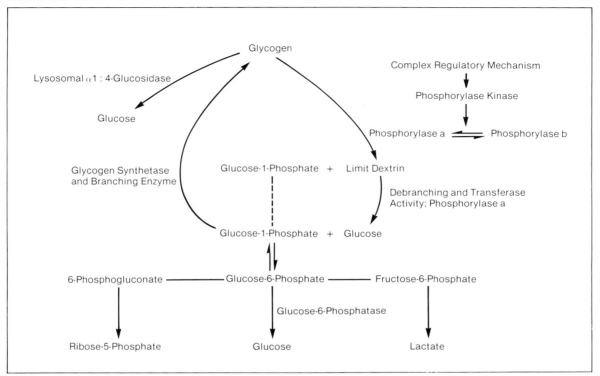

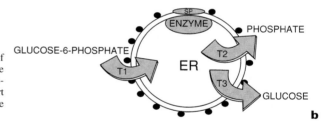

Fig. 16.20. Glycogen and glucose metabolism. **a** Pathways of glycogen breakdown and synthesis. **b** The glucose-6-phosphatase system, the endoplasmic reticulum (*ER*) with the glucose-6-phosphate translocase (*T1*), phosphate (*T2*) and glucose (*T3*) transport systems. Hydrolysis takes place within the lumen. *SP* is a putative stabilizing protein.

jejunal mucosa in coeliac disease and in fructose intolerance. Glucose-6-phosphatase activity is present mainly in the perinuclear and supranuclear regions of the enterocytes, and should not be confused with the intense brush border alkaline phosphatase activity which also hydrolyses glucose 6-phosphate. There is massive glycogen accumulation throughout the renal proximal tubular epithelium, where absence of glucose-6-phosphatase can also be demonstrated.

There are other forms of type I GSD (Burchell and Waddell 1990; Waddell and Burchell 1993), each very similar in morphological terms although the degree of fibrosis may vary (see Table 16.6). The regulation of glucose 6-phosphate transport through the endoplasmic reticulum to the lumen where hydrolysis by glucose-6-phosphatase takes place, and the need to transport the released glucose and phosphate from

the lumen of the endoplasmic reticulum each require specific translocating mechanisms. Defects in each of these are known. Thus what appeared initially as a simple defect of failure to hydrolyse glucose 6-phosphate has grown to encompass four different defects, each giving the same symptoms as the originally described glucose-6-phosphatase deficiency. Biochemical assay of the system is necessary for the complete evaluation of type I GSD once it has been shown that glucose-6-phosphatase activity is deficient. Fresh tissue (unfrozen) is required.

Type II

Biopsy of liver or muscle should not be necessary in Pompe's disease, because examination of the blood

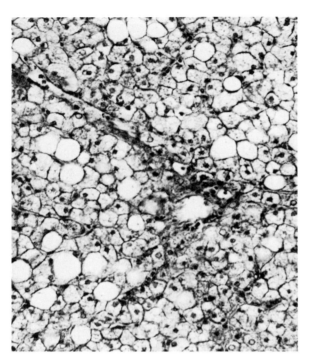

Fig. 16.21. Glycogen storage disease type I. Routine section of liver showing fatty change. Margination of nuclei and occasional nuclear vacuolation (glycogen). (H&E, × 200)

by light microscopy and enzyme assay on blood or cultured fibroblasts secures the diagnosis. Extensive vacuolation of the heart muscle and skeletal muscle fibres with a gross excess of glycogen and striking acid phosphatase activity are the main pathological features. Increased glycogen in smooth muscle cells and in neurons of the gastrointestinal tract are also seen.

Type III

In type III GSD the liver shows marked glycogen accumulation without fat deposition. The liver cells are enlarged and the nucleus is often off-centre, the general appearance resembling that of a plant cell. Nuclear glycogen is a prominent feature, particularly in older patients. There is often portal fibrosis. Glucose-6-phosphatase activity is lowered and confined to the periphery of the hepatocytes. Histochemical methods for the demonstration of phosphorylase activity in liver give falsely low results and cannot be relied on to differentiate debranching enzyme deficiency from phosphorylase or phosphorylase kinase deficiencies.

Type IX

Phosphorylase kinase deficiency (type IX GSD storage disease) is becoming a relatively commonly recognized condition, often found incidentally as asymptomatic hepatomegaly. The liver shows marked glycogen storage, with swollen hepatocytes and mild to moderate fat deposition. No fibrosis is found and nuclear glycogen is not a feature. These findings serve to differentiate this type of glycogen storage disease from debranching enzyme deficiency.

Type IV

The rare type IV GSD shows hepatic cirrhosis with bile stasis and can confidently be diagnosed by the total resistance of the glycogen present to digestion by diastase or saliva. The glycogen (long-chain-length amylopectin) shows a lasting brown-lilac colour with Gram's iodine, whereas all other glycogens give only a yellow or fleeting yellow-brown colour.

Other Types Including Those with Muscle Involvement

Other forms of GSD may be encountered which do not fit into any particular category. Frozen tissue should be kept from each biopsy so that at some future time the tissue can be assayed when newer enzyme defects are recognized.

Glycogen storage in skeletal muscle is found in GSD types II and III and in type V (myophosphorylase deficiency; McArdle's disease) and type VII (phosphofructokinase deficiency; Tarui's disease). The two latter disorders may not always show a gross excess of glycogen, but the enzyme deficiency in each is reliably demonstrated by histochemical techniques.

Normal neonates also have relatively high muscle glycogen levels, and the diagnosis of a GSD on a muscle biopsy from a neonate should be resisted unless there are overwhelming reasons for doing so. Intravenous dextrose given to a sick neonate may also induce a high glycogen content.

Disorders of Fructose Metabolism

Two disorders of fructose metabolism can be confused with GSD. Fructose-1: 6-diphosphatase deficiency can present in a manner resembling glucose-6-phosphatase deficiency, and in a fatty liver with glucose-6-phosphatase activity this possibility must be considered.

Children with fructose intolerance (fructose-1-phosphatase aldolase deficiency) who have not presented in early life with neonatal hepatitis present later with mild hepatomegaly and failure to thrive. On close questioning the information that the child has always avoided eating foods containing fructose often emerges. The similarity to the milder forms of glucose-6-phosphatase deficiency is striking, except that the glucagon stimulation test is positive. The histochemical method for the demonstration of fructose 1-phosphate aldolase activity is not very sensitive, and not all cases show the elevation of glucose-6-phosphatase reported earlier. The glycogen content may appear raised in stained sections. There is marked fatty change and this may be found even when the child is apparently well and seems to avoid food containing fructose (Fig. 16.22).

Other Tissues and Techniques

Brain

In neuronal storage diseases brain biopsy has been superseded by examination of intestinal neurons, and in most instances this technique has in turn been superseded by enzyme assay of white blood cells or cultured fibroblasts. In a few conditions, which can be considered to be metabolic diseases, brain biopsy is the only means of diagnosis. Alexander's leucodystrophy and spongiform leucodystrophy with abnormal astrocytic mitochondria (Adachi et al. 1973) are two such examples, although the latter (Canavan's disease) can now be diagnosed by demonstration of N-acetyl aspartate in urine or by the deficiency of aspartoacylase in white blood cells or cultured fibroblasts (Matalon et al. 1989).

Neuroaxonal dystrophy is a difficult diagnosis to make in a brain biopsy by light microscopy alone. The axonal spheroids, although fairly common in the brain stem at autopsy, are inconspicuous in the frontal cortex on biopsy stained by haematoxylin and eosin. Dense staining of the spheroids can be obtained with the non-specific esterase method (Fig. 16.23). Although the neuronal cell bodies also show esterase activity, their intensity is less. The spheroids have characteristic ultrastructural changes and may be found on electron microscopy without too much searching. Most centres now, however, will prefer electron microscopic examination of the myelinated and unmyelinated nerves in a skin or conjunctival biopsy (Arsénio-Nunes and Goutières 1978) (Fig. 16.24).

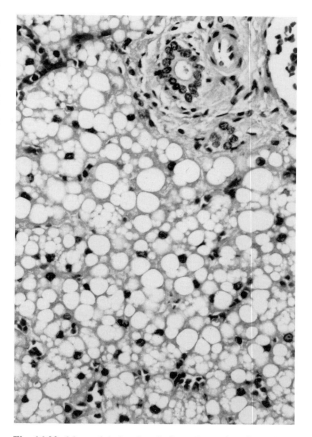

Fig. 16.22. Macroglobular chronic fatty change in a liver biopsy. This appearance may be seen in several metabolic disorders, including fructose intolerance and medium-chain acyl-CoA dehydrogenase deficiency, and may be present without any clinical symptoms.

Hair

In Menkes' disease there is a deficiency of copper transport. This affects all enzymes which have copper as an essential component of the enzyme. In skin biopsies from patients with Menkes' disease a lower staining intensity than normal can be shown for DOPA oxidase and presumably also for cytochrome oxidase in other organs. A simpler test is to examine hair. Scanning electron microscopy will give more dramatic pictures, but simple light microscopy of a few hairs on a microscope slide, held down by the weight of a cover slip, allows more hairs to be examined, is quicker, and is adequate for most purposes. Polarizing microscopy of the hair sample also gives insight into the structural organization of the hair, and will show the alternate banding found in trichothiodystrophy. The macroscopic appearance of the short, frizzy, brittle, white hair is almost diagnostic,

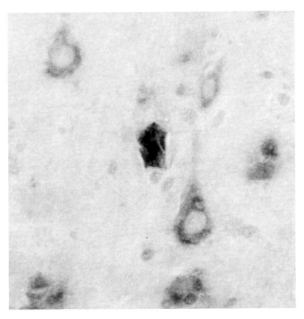

Fig. 16.23. Infantile neuroaxonal dystrophy. Cryostat section of cortex of a brain biopsy stained by the non-specific esterase method. An axonal spheroid is strongly stained and the characteristic clefts are shown. The neurons are much weaker. (× 640)

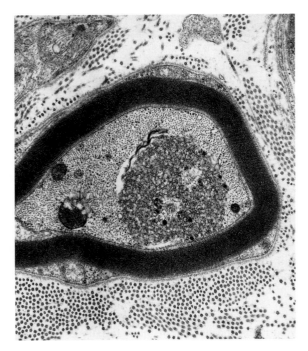

Fig. 16.24. Infantile neuroaxonal dystrophy. Electron micrograph of a nerve in a conjunctival biopsy, showing the axonal "spheroid" characteristic of the disorder. Similar bodies are found in unmyelinated nerve fibres. (× 17 400)

and microscopy with a dissecting microscope is sufficient to confirm the clinical diagnosis in a classic case of Menkes' disease. The hair shows pili torti (Figs. 16.25 and 16.26) and occasional thickenings with breakage (trichorrhexis nodosum), although the latter are always present. Not all hairs show pili torti, so a careful search is necessary. In older patients, the hair may appear relatively normal and samples from different areas of the scalp may be necessary. Samples from obligate carriers may show an occasional pili torti but this is rare. Fragile hair with trichorrhexis nodosum can also be found in about 50% of patients with argininosuccinic aciduria. In Netherton's syndrome the hair shows occasional "bamboo nodes" and other foci of tight twisting of the hair shaft giving an incipient bamboo node appearance (Figs. 16.27 and 16.28).

Skin and Conjunctiva

Electron microscopy of a skin or conjunctival biopsy allows examination of many different cell types (e.g. fibroblasts, endothelial cells, epithelial cells, smooth muscle cells, Schwann cells and macrophages), and it is tempting to succumb to a screening programme using these tissues for confirmation of a clinical suspicion. More often than not such biopsy material is used as a general screen to see whether a diagnosis can be found, and under these circumstances chances of success are slender.

The mucopolysaccharidoses, oligosaccharidoses, mucolipidosis IV, Fabry's disease, each form of Batten's disease and adrenoleucodystrophy have each been shown to have characteristic ultrastructure (Ceuterick and Martin 1984), although it would be difficult to differentiate between any of the mucopolysaccharidoses and the oligosaccharidoses. In the latter disorders the endothelial cells and fibroblasts (and possibly the epithelial cells in a conjunctival biopsy) contain membrane-bound vacuoles that are essentially empty. The changes in a conjunctival biopsy in mucolipidosis IV are more characteristic, with membranous cytoplasmic bodies present not only in endothelial cells (as in Fabry's disease) but also in the basal epithelial cells (Fig. 16.29). The outermost epithelial cells are grossly vacuolated, with a few loose lipid lamellae present (Fig. 16.30). The disorder may be mild and present later than expected (Casteels et al. 1992). Membranous cytoplasmic bodies are also found in cultured fibroblasts from mucolipidosis IV, but care is needed because the antibiotic added to the culture medium may also induce similar changes. The ultrastructural appearances of cultured fibroblasts in mucolipidosis IV are sufficiently distinctive to be of value in the prenatal

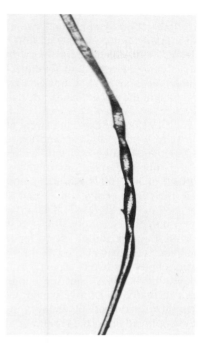

Fig. 16.25. Menkes' kinky hair disease. A single hair showing pili torti over a short length. This feature is not present over the whole length and is not found in every hair. (× 75)

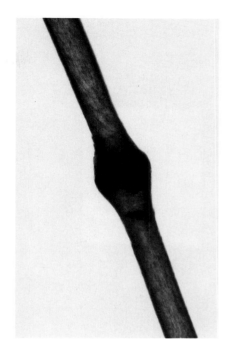

Fig. 16.27. Netherton's syndrome. Hair showing a bamboo node.

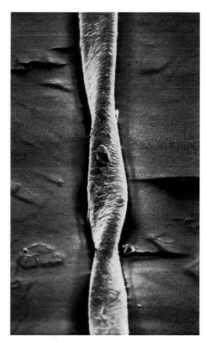

Fig. 16.26. Menkes' kinky hair disease. Scanning electron micrograph of a single hair, clearly showing pili torti. (× 200)

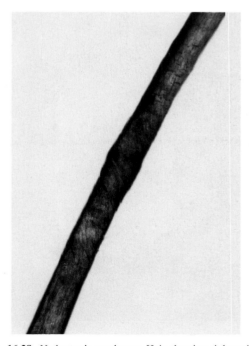

Fig. 16.28. Netherton's syndrome. Hair showing tight twisting, which is found more frequently than the bamboo nodes.

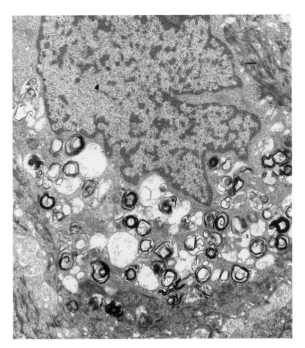

Fig. 16.29. Mucolipidosis IV. Electron micrograph of a conjunctival biopsy showing the membranous cytoplasmic bodies present in the basal epithelial cells. (× 8700)

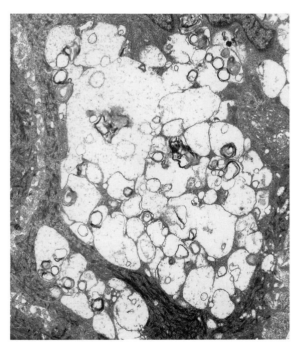

Fig. 16.30. Mucolipidosis IV. Electron micrograph of a conjunctival biopsy showing the loose lamellar arrangement of the storage material in the more superficial epithelial cells. (× 6600)

diagnosis on cultured amniotic fluid cells (Kohn et al. 1982). Curvilinear bodies are found in endothelial cells in late infantile Batten's disease, GROD in the infantile form, and mixed curvilinear/fingerprint profiles in the early juvenile and juvenile forms in both conjunctival and skin biopsies at electron microscopy. In skin the sweat glands are also a prime site for storage in Batten's disease of all types (Berkovic et al. 1986). The apocrine sweat glands are involved in Lafora body disease, and characteristic large PAS-positive diastase-resistant inclusions are present in the subnuclear regions of the cell (Fig. 16.31) (Busard et al. 1987). These inclusions are stained dark blue by Lugol's iodine and stand out against the yellow background. The glycoprotein secretions, which are strongly PAS-positive, are unstained with Lugol's iodine. It is reported that eccrine gland duct cells can also be used for the diagnosis of Lafora body disease (Carpenter and Karpati 1981; Berkovic et al. 1986), but the inclusions are less frequent in that site. Unmyelinated and myelinated nerves show characteristic changes in the neuroaxonal dystrophies (Fig. 16.24), and conjunctival biopsy is the method of choice (Arséunio-Nunes and Goutières 1978), although skin biopsy may also be used (Berkovic et al. 1986; Kimura 1991). Conjunctival biopsy has also been used for the diagnosis of adrenoleucodystrophy, but the angulate lysosomes characteristic of the liver and brain in infantile Refsum's disease, Zellweger syndrome and adrenoleucodystrophy may occur in *normal* conjunctiva (Fig. 16.32), and false-positive diagnoses would be possible (Dingemans et al. 1983). Skin biopsy has also been reported in Niemann–Pick disease type C (Boustany et al. 1990), and the characteristic inclusions were noted particularly in macrophages. It should be noted, however, that in Niemann–Pick type C "pathognomonic" inclusions may also be found in heterozygotes for the disease (see also p. 845).

Disorders of the Peroxisome

In recent years the metabolic pathways relating to peroxisomes have become recognized, and it is now clear that the peroxisome is involved in a wide range of metabolic processes, including catabolism of very-long chain fatty acids, biosynthesis of bile acids and other phospholipids (plasmalogens), and catabolism of dicarboxylic acids. Since Goldfischer et al. (1973) described an absence of peroxisomes in liver and kidney in the cerebrohepatorenal syndrome of Zellweger (CHRS), abnormalities of peroxisomes and peroxisomal functions have been recognized in several other conditions (Aubourg et al. 1986; Schutgens et al. 1986). In addition, Goldfischer et al. (1986) have

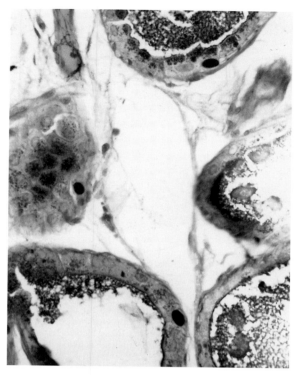

Fig. 16.31. Lafora body disease. Skin biopsy (axilla) showing the characteristic strongly PAS-positive inclusions in the subnuclear regions of the apocrine sweat gland epithelial cells.

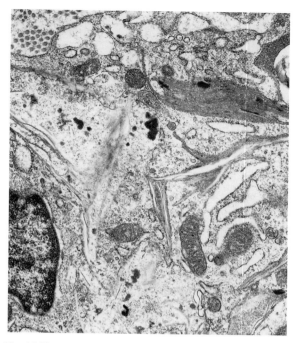

Fig. 16.32. Conjunctival biopsy, infantile neuroaxonal dystrophy. Electron micrograph showing angulate lysosomes in a macrophage. These appearances may be found in adrenoleucodystrophy, but also occur (as here) in patients who have a variety of other disorders. Such changes are non-specific. (× 17 400)

reported a patient who has the clinical, chemical and pathological features of CHRS, and, although peroxisomes were present, deficient activities of several peroxisomal enzymes possibly related to the cofactor flavin adenine dinucleotide were observed. They called this condition pseudo-Zellweger syndrome, in which a defect of peroxisomal thiolase has now been demonstrated. For a fuller description of the pathology of these and other peroxisomal disorders see Lake (1992).

A list of peroxisomal disorders and the state of liver peroxisomes are shown in Table 16.7. In CHRS, infantile Refsum's disease and neonatal adrenoleucodystrophy the liver progresses to an early micronodular cirrhosis. In the sinusoids and portal areas PAS-positive macrophages may be found and these stain palely with neutral fat stains.

The presence of peroxisomes and peroxisomal enzyme proteins can be assessed on paraffin sections using antibodies to the various proteins (Espeel et al. 1990). Peroxisomes are absent from the liver in CHRS and infantile Refsum's disease, and only a few small peroxisomes can be identified in neonatal adrenoleucodystrophy. These findings can be con-

Table 16.7. Peroxisomal disorders

Disorder	Peroxisomes in liver
Zellweger cerebrohepatorenal syndrome	Absent
Pseudo-Zellweger syndrome	Increased in number
Infantile Refsum's disease	Absent
Adult Refsum's disease	Present
Neonatal adrenoleucodystrophy	Very few small peroxisomes
X-linked adrenoleucodystrophy	Present
Hyperpipecolic acidaemia	Present
Rhizomelic chondroplasia punctata	Absent in most hepatocytes, rare large peroxisomes in a few hepatocytes
Cerebrotendinous xanthomatosis	Increased in number and size
Acatalasaemia	Present (in mice)
Primary hyperoxaluria type I	Present

firmed by electron histochemistry using a method for the demonstration of catalase activity (Fig. 16.33), and this method is useful to assess the shape and size

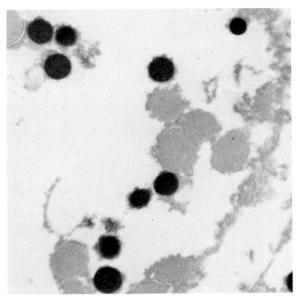
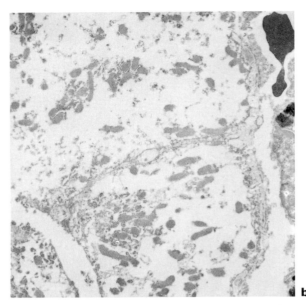

a   **b**

Fig. 16.33. Electron micrographs of liver stained to show peroxisomes by virtue of their catalase content. The dense reaction product indicates peroxidatic activity. **a** Normal liver. Nine peroxisomes are present in a hepatocyte together with unstained mitochondria. (× 12 000) **b** Infantile Refsum's disease. No peroxisomes can be identified in portions of several hepatocytes. A red blood cell (*top right*) is positive (haemoglobin peroxidase) and a portion of a neutrophil just below the red cell shows its myeloperoxidase activity. (× 4600)

of peroxisomes, which may give a clue as to whether a peroxisomal abnormality is present, because such abnormalities are a feature of peroxisomal malfunction (Roels 1991).

Trilaminar needle-like crystalline profiles can be found (Fig. 16.34), sometimes with difficulty, in lysosomes of hepatocytes and in Kupffer cells. These trilaminar profiles are also to be found in X-linked

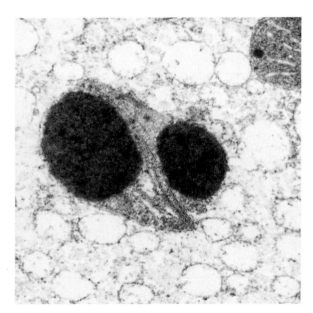
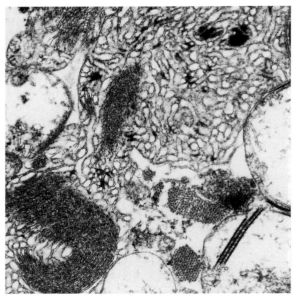

Fig. 16.34. Infantile Refsum's disease. Electron micrograph of a hepatocyte showing a lysosomal body in which trilaminar profiles are present. These are not always numerous and may require extensive searches. (× 48 000)

Fig. 16.35. Hereditary cardiomyopathy. Electron micrograph of a post-mortem sample of heart showing mitochondria with proliferation and compaction of cristae. (× 22 000)

adrenoleucodystrophy and are considered to represent the very-long-chain fatty acid content, but they also occur in other situations and may not all be of primary metabolic origin (Fig. 16.32) (Dingemans et al. 1983). The kidneys in CHRS show glomerular cystic changes, a feature also found in the pseudo-Zellweger syndrome, trisomy 13 and a variety of other conditions (Joshi and Kasznica 1984).

From the current clinical, biochemical and morphological data in this group of conditions, it is clear that there is overlap between them, and further delineation will be necessary as more patients are recognized.

Clues to diagnosis will have been primarily clinical and biochemical (very-long-chain fatty acids, bile acid analysis), and microscopy has little to offer apart from confirmation and further important descriptions of the pathology of these rare diseases. Post-mortem examination of the brain may reveal polymicrogyria and developmental abnormalities of the dentate and olivary nuclei.

Disorders of Mitochondria

Structural abnormalities of mitochondria may occur as a primary event or be secondary to an insult of some sort. Where there is known mitochondrial disease with a recognized enzyme defect, for example cytochrome oxidase deficiency, ornithine carbamoyl transferase deficiency or pyruvate dehydrogenase deficiency, there may be no change or only minor structural change. In other cases, where there is clear biochemical evidence for a mitochondrial defect (e.g. lactic acidosis), structural alterations may be prominent (Fig. 16.35). In muscle where mitochondrial DNA deletions or duplications can be documented, the same deletion may produce a different ultrastructure in the child compared with an adult. In mitochondrial cytopathy (Egger et al. 1981), the muscle mitochondria in the child usually exhibit proliferation of cristae and extreme variability in size, whereas in the adult mitochondria with paracrystalline inclusions are usually found. In alcoholic liver disease, bizarre mitochondria are present in the absence of any symptoms directly related to mitochondrial dysfunction. Thus the ultrastructural appearance of mitochondria may give no real clue to the underlying abnormality.

By light microscopy one of the more constant, but not exclusive, findings of mitochondrial disorders is the presence of neutral fat in the affected organ. Although the presence of neutral fat in liver is a very non-specific phenomenon. the occurrence in several organs (liver, kidney, muscle, heart) indicates a generalized defect of fatty acid oxidation (Hale and Bennett 1992) such as medium-chain CoA dehydrogenase (MCAD) deficiency. Cytochrome oxidase

deficiency of muscle can be severe (Di Mauro et al. 1980), reversible (Di Mauro et al. 1983) or comparatively mild with survival to 8 years (Jacobs et al. 1990). In other cases of cytochrome oxidase deficiency with liver disease, the defect in liver demonstrated by histochemical means is not always clear, and it may be difficult to distinguish between the primary deficiency and the secondary effect of severe liver disease using staining techniques alone. There may be patchy lobular staining with one lobule showing no activity adjacent to one with normal cytochrome oxidase activity. The situation is further complicated by the presence of tissue specific isoforms of cytochrome c oxidase (Kennaway et al. 1990). It is most important in all these disorders that the morphological appearance of the tissue submitted for biochemical analysis is evaluated so that sensible quantitative data are produced.

Conclusions

If the approach to the metabolic disorders outlined in the previous pages has been followed, any biopsy taken can be used for diagnosis by the most appropriate means. In different cases this will be by biochemical assay of an enzyme, by thin-layer chromatography of a lipid extract, by electron microscopy or light microscopy, or with histochemical techniques.

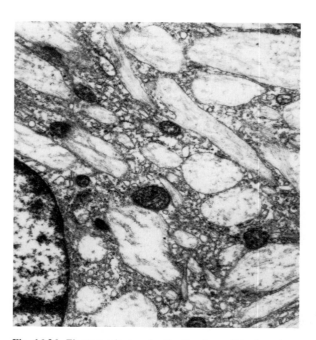

Fig. 16.36. Electron micrograph of a Gaucher cell in the spleen. The elongated membrane-bound storage bodies contain tubular inclusions of cerebroside. (× 15 000)

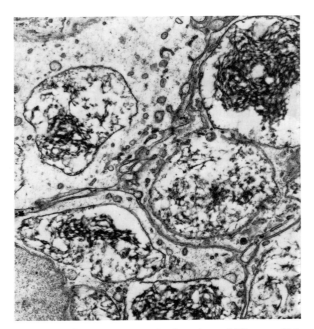

Fig. 16.37. Electron micrograph of portions of Niemann–Pick cells in a liver biopsy. The storage bodies are membrane-bound and contain lipid-like lamellae. Similar deposits are also present in hepatocytes. (× 15 000)

Electron microscopy of conventionally prepared tissue can help in showing which organelles are affected, and whether any deposited substance is membrane-bound. Most of the lysosomal storage disorders can be categorized on the basis of the appearance of the deposited substance. However, it is clear that what remains within the lysosome after the shrinkage and extraction of the stored substances caused by fixation, dehydration and embedding is something quite different from the original content (Figs. 16.36 and 16.37). However, the artefact induced is usually constant, and consequently its appearance is a useful marker of the disease.

References

Adachi M, Schneck L, Cara J, Volk BW (1973) Spongy degeneration of the central nervous system (van Bogaert and Bertrand type, Canavan's disease). Hum Pathol 4: 331

Adam G, Brereton RJ, Agrawal M, Lake BD (1988) Biliary atresia and meconium ileus associated with Niemann–Pick disease. Paediatr Gastroenterol Nutr 7: 128

Alder A (1939) Über konstitutionell bedingte Granulations – Veränderungen der Leukocyten. Dtsch Arch Klin Med 183: 372

Alshak NS, Cocjin J, Podesta L, van der Velde R, Makowka L, Rosenthal P, Geller SA (1994) Hepatocellular adenoma in glycogen storage disease type IV. Arch Pathol Lab Med 118: 88

Arsénio-Nunes ML, Goutières F (1978) Diagnosis of infantile neuroaxonal dystrophy by conjunctival biopsy. J Neurol Neurosurg Psychiatry 41: 511

Aubourg P, Scotto J, Rocchiccioli F, Feldmann-Pautrat J, Robain O (1986) Neonatal adrenoleukodystrophy. J Neurol Neurosurg Psychiatry 49: 77

Aula P, Autio S, Raivio KO, Rapola J, Thoden C-J, Koskila S-L, Yamashina I (1979) Salla disease. A new lysosomal storage disorder. Arch Neurol 36: 88

Aynsley-Green (1981) Hepatic glycogen synthetase deficiency. In: Randle PJ, Steiner DR, Whelan WJ (eds) Carbohydrate metabolism and its disorders. Academic Press London, p 139

Berkovic SF, Andermann F, Carpenter S, Wolfe LS (1986) Progressive myoclonus epilepsies: specific causes and diagnosis. N Engl J Med 315: 296

Bodian M, Lake BD (1963) The rectal approach to neuropathology. Br J Surg 50: 702

Boustany R-M, Kaye E, Alroy J (1990) Ultrastructural findings in skin from patients with Niemann–Pick disease type C. Pediatr Neurol 6: 177

Burchell A, Waddell ID (1990) Genetic deficiencies of the microsomal glucose-6-phosphatase system. In: Randle P, Bell J, Scott J (eds) Genetics and human nutrition. J Libby, London, p 93

Busard HLSM, Gabreëls-Festen AAWM, Renier WO, Gabreëls FJM, Stadhuoders AM (1987) Axilla skin biopsy. A reliable test for the diagnosis of Lafora's disease. Ann Neurol, 21: 599

Carpenter S, Karpati G (1981) Sweat gland duct cells in Lafora's disease: diagnosis by skin biopsy. Neurology (New York) 31: 1564

Casteels I, Taylor DSI, Lake BD, Spalton DJ, Bach G (1992) Mucolipidosis type IV. Presentation of a mild variant. Ophthalmic Paediatr Genet 13: 205

Ceuterick C, Martin JJ (1984) Diagnostic role of skin or conjunctival biopsies in neurological disorders. An update. J Neurol Sci 65: 179

Chow CW, Borg J, Billson V, Lake BD (1993) Fetal tissue involvement in the late infantile type of neuronal ceroid lipofuscinosis. Prenat Diagn 13: 833

Di Mauro S, Mendell JR, Sahenk Z, Bachman D, Scarpa A, Scholfield RM, Reiner C (1980) Fatal infantile mitochondrial myopathy and renal dysfunction due to cytochrome c oxidase deficiency. Neurology 30: 795

Di Mauro S, Nicholson JF, Hays AP, Eastwood AB, Papadimitriou A, Koenigsberger R, DeVivo DC (1983) Benign infantile mitochondrial myopathy due to reversible cytochrome c oxidase deficiency. Ann Neurol 14: 226

Dingemans KP, Mooi WJ, van den Bergh Weerman MA (1983) Angulate lysosomes. Ultrastruct Pathol 5: 113

Egger J, Lake BD, Wilson J (1981) Mitochondrial cytopathy. A multisystem disorder with ragged red fibres on muscle biopsy. Arch Dis Child 56: 741

Elleder M, Jirásek A (1983) International Symposium on Niemann–Pick disease. Eur J Pediatr 140: 90

Elleder M, Lojda Z (1973) New, rapid, simple and selective method for the demonstration of phospholipids. Histochemie 36: 149

Espeel M, Hashimoto T, De Craemer D, Roels F (1990) Immunocytochemical detection of peroxisomal β-oxidation enzymes in cryostat and paraffin sections of human post mortem liver. Histochem J 22: 57

Filipe MI, Lake BD (eds) (1990) Histochemistry in pathology, 2nd edn. Churchill Livingstone, Edinburgh

Gardiner RM (1992) Mapping the gene for juvenile onset neuronal ceroid lipofuscinosis to chromosome 16 by linkage analysis. Am J Med Genet 42: 539

Gasser C (1950) Discussion on Alder A, Konstitutionell bedingte Granulations-Veränderungen der Leukocyten und Knochen-Veränderungen. Schweiz Med Wochenschr 80: 1095

Gitzelmann, R, Spycher MA, Adank S, Steinmann B, Baerlocher K (1984) Anomalous eosinophil leukocytes in blood and bone marrow: a diagnostic marker for infantile G_{M1} gangliosidosis. Helv Paediatr Acta [Suppl] 50: 29 (abstract)

Goldfischer S, Moore CL, Johnson AB, Spiro AJ, Valsamis P, Wisniewski H, Ritch RH, Norton WT, Rapin I, Gartner LM (1973) Peroxisomal and mitochondrial defects in the cerebro-hepato-renal syndrome. Science 182: 62

Goldfischer S, Collins J, Rapin I, Neumann P, Neglia W, Spiro AJ, Ishii T, Roels F, Vamecq J, van Hoof F (1986) Pseudo-Zellweger syndrome: deficiencies in several peroxisomal oxidative activities. J Pediatr 108: 25

Hagberg B, Haltia M, Sourander P, Svennerholm L, Vanier M-T, Ljunggren C-G (1978) Neurovisceral storage disease simulating Niemann–Pick disease. A new form of oligosaccharidosis. Neuropaediatrie 9: 59

Hale DE, Bennett MJ (1992) Fatty acid oxidation disorders. A new class of metabolic diseases. J Pediatr 121: 1

Hall NA, Lake BD, Dewji NN, Patrick AD (1991) Lysosomal storage of subunit c of mitochondrial ATP synthase in Batten's disease (ceroid-lipofuscinosis). Biochem J 275 : 269

Haltia H, Palo J, Autio S (1975) Aspartylglycosaminuria: a generalized storage disease. Acta Neuropathol (Berl) 31: 234

Hansen HG (1972) Hematologic studies in mucopolysaccharidoses and mucolipidoses. Birth Defects 8: 115

Haust MD, Landing BH (1961) Histochemical studies in Hurler's disease. A new method for localization of acid mucopolysaccharide, and an analysis of lead acetate "fixation". J Histochem Cytochem 9: 79

Howat AJ, Bennett MJ, Variend S, Shaw J (1984) Deficiency of medium chain fatty acylcoenzyme A dehydrogenase presenting as the sudden infant death syndrome. Br Med J 288: 976

Jacobs JM, Harding BN, Lake BD, Payan J, Wilson J (1990) Peripheral neuropathy in Leigh's disease. Brain 113: 447

Jarvela I, Santavuori P, Puhakka L, Haltia M, Peltonen L (1992) Linkage map of the chromosomal region surrounding the infantile neuronal ceroid lipofuscinosis on 1p. Am J Med Genet 42: 546

Jenner FA, Pollitt RJ (1967) Large quantities of 2-acetamide-1-(beta-L-aspartamido)-1,2-dideoxyglucose in the urine of mentally retarded siblings. Biochem J 103: 48P

Jordans GHW (1953) The familial occurrence of fat containing vacuoles in leukocytes diagnosed in two brothers suffering from dystrophia musculorum progressiva (ERB). Acta Med Scand 145: 419

Joshi VV, Kasznica J (1984) Clinicopathologic spectrum of glomerulocystic kidneys. Report of two cases and a brief review of literature. Pediatr Pathol 2: 171

Judge MR, Hilaire N, Levade T, Salvayre R, Johnston DI, Winchester B, Atherton DA, Lake BD (1994) Neutral lipid storage disease. Case report and lipid studies. Br J Dermatol 130: 507

Kelly DA, Portmann B, Mowat AP, Sherlock S, Lake BD (1993) Niemann–Pick disease type C. Diagnosis and outcome in children with particular reference to liver disease. J Pediatr 123: 242

Kennaway NG, Carrero-Valenzuela RD, Ewart G, Balan VK, Lightowlers R, Zhang Y-Z, Powell BR, Capaldi RA, Buist NRM (1990) Isoforms of mammalian cytochrome c oxidase: correlation with human cytochrome c oxidase deficiency. Pediatr Res 28: 529

Kimura S (1991) Terminal axon pathology in infantile neuroaxonal dystrophy. Pediatr Neurol 7: 116

Kohn G, Sekeles E, Arron J, Ornoy A (1982) Mucolipidosis IV. Prenatal diagnosis by electron microscopy. Prenat Diagn 2: 301

Kornberg A (1977) Editorial. Arch Pathol Lab Med 101: 399

Lake BD (1971) Histochemical detection of the enzyme deficiency in blood films in Wolman's disease. J Clin Pathol 24: 617

Lake BD (1974) An improved method for the detection of β-galactosidase activity, and its application to G_{M1}-gangliosidosis and mucopolysaccharidosis. Histochem J 6: 211

Lake BD (1976) The differential diagnosis of the various forms of Batten disease by rectal biopsy. Birth Defects 12: 455

Lake BD (1977) Histochemical and ultrastructural studies in the diagnosis of inborn errors of metabolism. Records of the Adelaide Childrens Hospital 1: 337

Lake BD (1990) Blood, bone marrow, spleen and lymph nodes in metabolic disorders. In: Filipe MI, Lake BD (eds) Histochemistry in pathology, 2nd edn. Churchill Livingstone, Edinburgh, p 306

Lake BD (1992) Lysosomal and peroxisomal disorders. In: Adams JH, Duchen LW (eds) Greenfield's neuropathology. Edward Arnold, London, p 709

Lake BD, Ellis RB (1976) What do you think you are quantifying? An appraisal of histochemical methods in the measurement of the activities of lysosomal enzymes. Histochem J 8: 357

Lake BD, Goodwin HJ (1976) Lipids. In: Smith I, Seakins JWT (eds) Chromatographic and electrophoretic techniques, vol 1. Heinemann, London, p 345

Matalon R, Kaul R, Casanova J, Michals K, Johnson A, Rapin I, Gashkoff P, Deanching M (1989) Aspartoacylase deficiency. The enzyme defect in Canavan's disease. J Inherit Metab Dis 12 (suppl 2): 329

Muir H, Mittwoch V, Bitter T (1963) The diagnostic value of isolated urinary mucopolysaccharides and of lymphocytic inclusions in gargoylism. Arch Dis Child 38: 358

Neville BGR, Lake BD, Stephens R, Sanders MD (1973) A neurovisceral storage disease with vertical supra-nuclear ophthalmoplegia and its relationship to Niemann–Pick disease. A report of nine patients. Brain 96: 97

Pennock CA (1976) A review and selection of simple laboratory methods used for the study of glycosaminoglycan excretion and the diagnosis of the mucopolysaccharidoses. J Clin Pathol 29: 111

Pfeiffer RA, Kresse H, Baumer N, Sattinger E (1977) β-glucuronidase deficiency in a girl with unusual features. Eur J Pediatr 126: 155

Rampini S, Isler W, Baerlocker K, Bischoff A, Ulrich J, Plüss HJ (1970) Die Kombination von metachromatischer Leukodystrophie und Mucopolysaccharidose als selbstandiges Krankheitsbild (Mukosulfatidose). Helv Paediatr Acta 25: 436

Rapin I, Goldfischer S, Katzman R, Engel J, O'Brien JS (1978) The cherry-red spot–myoclonus syndrome. Ann Neurol 3: 234

Reynolds RD (1973) Sea-blue histiocytes. JAMA 226: 467 (letter)

Roberts GP (1977) Histochemical detection of sialic acid residues using periodate oxidation. Histochem J 9: 97

Roels F (1991) Peroxisomes. A personal account. VUB Press, Brussels

Schutgens RBH, Heymans HSA, Wanders RJA, van den Bosch H, Tager JM (1986) Peroxisomal disorders. A newly recognised group of genetic diseases. Eur J Pediatr 144: 430

Scriver CR, Beaudet AL, Sly WS, Valle D (eds) (1995) The metabolic basis of inherited disease, 7th edn. McGraw-Hill, New York

Spencer-Peet J, Norman ME, Lake BD, McNamara J, Patrick AD (1971) Hepatic glycogen storage disease. QJ Med 40: 95

Toppet M, Vamos Hurwitz E, Jonniau G, Cremer N, Tondeur M, Pelc S (1978) Farber's disease as a ceramidosis: clinical radiological and biochemical aspects. Acta Paediatr Scand 67: 113

Trend PStJ, Wiles CM, Spencer GT, Morgan-Hughes JA, Lake BD, Patrick AD (1985) Acid maltase deficiency in adults. Diagnosis and management in five cases. Brain 108: 845

Vanier MT, Wenger DA, Comly ME, Rousson R, Brady RO, Pentchev PG (1988) Niemann–Pick disease group C: clinical variability based on defective cholesterol esterification. Clin Genet 33: 331

Vanier MT, Rousson RM, Mandon G, Choiset A, Lake BD, Pentchev PG (1989) Diagnosis of Niemann–Pick disease type C on chorionic villus cells. Lancet i: 1014

Waddell ID, Burchell A (1993) Identification, purification and genetic deficiencies of the glucose-6-phosphatase system transport proteins. Eur J Pediatr 152 (suppl 1): S14

Whiteman P (1973) The quantitative determination of glycosaminoglycans in urine with Alcian blue 8GX. Biochem J 131: 351

17 · Embryonal Tumours

Colin L. Berry and Jean W. Keeling

In earlier editions of this book comments on incidence and death rates from neoplasia in infancy and childhood made it clear that these were remarkably constant despite variations of the kind described by Adelstein and White (1976). Examination of Table 17.1 and Fig. 17.1 shows that in general this relationship has remained constant until comparatively recently when, despite an increase in numbers in the age group, the death rate from neoplasia (and non-neoplastic deaths) has declined – a slowly improving trend.

Table 17.1. Deaths from malignant disease in children aged 1–15 years, 1983–1992

Year	Total in 0–14 year age group (million)	Total deaths in 0–14 year group (thousands)	Deaths from malignant disease		
			0–4 years	5–9 years	10–14 years
1983	9720.0	8980	140	126	146
1984	9576.7	8513	183	119	163
1985	9498.8	8717	132	137	141
1986	9421.2	8618	138	122	142
1987	9385.5	8515	139	121	121
1988	9408.5	8435	148	137	111
1989	9455.0	8061	166	128	88
1990	9567.0	7704	127	141	116
1991	9704.9	7316	134	157	107
1992	9840.0	6380	128	123	106

Haematological malignancies, including leukaemia, are the major variable component, and the overall picture is greatly influenced by their frequency and the outcome of their treatment (see p. 661). The role of irradiation in the genesis of these tumours is now thought to be less significant than before (Anonymous 1981), and recent suggestions of a paternal effect related to radiation (Gardiner et al. 1990) have not been supported by later studies (Parker et al. 1993). However, there have been real advances in our understanding of the neoplastic process in childhood. Some of these will be discussed in some detail, because they begin to suggest ideas for radical changes in therapy.

Aetiology

In childhood malignancies, the period of potential exposure to environmental carcinogens is generally short. Congenital tumours are well documented (more than 300 reported cases of non-leukaemic lesions) and the bulk of embryonic neoplasms occur in the first 4 years of life. Familial tumours and associations of tu-

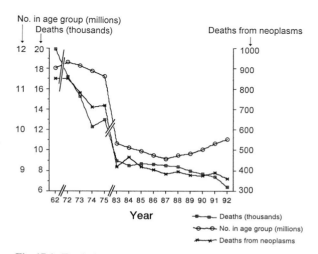

Fig 17.1. Totals in age group, non-tumour and tumour deaths, Lengland and Wales, 1962–92.

mours with other deviations from the normal pheno-type are sufficiently common to have allowed the application of the new techniques of genetics to well defined entities.

Comparison with studies in adults, where factors such as age, sex and race may be readily controlled but where climate, dietary and cultural factors, occupational changes, and variation of the intensity and duration of exposure to potential carcinogens are all independent variables, will illustrate the difficulties imposed on studies by prolonged extrauterine existence. It is evident that the massive variation in the frequency of different tumours in different adult populations (e.g. 300 × for carcinoma of the oesophagus), often thought to be attributable to environmental factors, is not seen in childhood malignancy. The constancy of tumour incidence rates in childhood led Innes (1972a) to suggest that the relatively constant incidence of a tumour (nephroblastoma) in different populations would allow the tumour to be used as an index of the degree of under-reporting of tumours in general.

In 1989 the outlines of the current views of pathogenesis of childhood tumours were in place and have now been shown to have a wide general relevance to the neoplastic process. It is worth reiterating that it was Ellsworth who, in 1969, first suggested that a germ cell mutation might be the first step in the development of bilateral retinoblastoma. In subsequent studies on retinoblastoma and neuroblastoma, and neuroblastoma and phaeochromocytoma, Knudson (1971) and Knudson and Strong (1972) suggested that these tumours arose in a manner consistent with a two-mutation model. According to this hypothesis two successive mutations are necessary in a somatic cell to produce a neoplasm. Hereditary cases would arise in individuals in whom one mutation has occurred in a germ cell and thus in all its progeny. One subsequent mutation in affected cells would then result in neoplasia.

In retinoblastoma data supportive of genetic influences of this type were provided by the work of Kitchin and Ellsworth (1974), who showed that the retinoblastoma "gene" had pleiotrophic effects, with an increase of second primary tumours, notably osteogenic sarcomas, in survivors of bilateral tumours. This effect was not seen in unilateral cases and provided evidence for increased tumour susceptibility in the group. Older data had shown that children with sporadic bilateral retinoblastoma are more likely to have a family history of consanguinity (Hemmes 1931) and to have affected offspring themselves.

Other oncogene changes may occur in embryonic tumours. The expression of N-*myc* is amplified in neuroblastoma, in both tumours and derived cell lines, and is apparently amplified to an increasing extent as the tumour becomes disseminated (Brodeur et al. 1984). Retinoic acid-induced differentiation in cultured neuroblastoma is accompanied by decreased levels of expression (Thiele et al. 1985). Thus an influence on both metastatic potential and differentiation can be invoked. N-*myc* is also amplified in retinoblastoma, and is found in both the hereditary and non-hereditary form (Lee et al. 1984). Its role is unclear but, again, an effect on differentiation, as opposed to proliferation, must be considered.

Many genetic abnormalities have been described in neuroblastoma, including double minutes, deletions of distal 1p and translocations on chromosomes 1 and 17. The suggestion of Innes (1970, 1972b) that human embryonic tumours are in Hardy–Weinberg equilibrium is interesting. This equilibrium, an important concept in population genetics, requires that, if genes are widely distributed in a randomly bred population, selection pressures (e.g. death) will have little effect on their frequency (see also Berry and Keeling 1975). Innes studied the relative frequencies of leukaemia and other childhood malignancies in children of British descent in Canada, England and Wales, and New Zealand, and found that despite differences in the incidence of some adult tumours, childhood malignancies occurred at a remarkably constant rate. When comparisons were made for two periods in the same continent the specific tumour proportions were found not to change. Data in some of the groups studied were scanty, as Innes has pointed out, but the stability of the relative rates argues against an active environmental component in these tumours.

Retinoblastoma

The frequency of retinoblastoma appears to be increasing in countries where reliable data are available (Holland and Finland), and this is thought by Warburg (1974) to be attributable to an increase in bilateral lesions. The increase cannot be explained by an increase in incidence in the progeny of those surviving a lesion in their own childhood. It is the commonest primary intraocular neoplasm of childhood, representing 3% of registered cases of malignant disease occurring in children under the age of 15 years in Great Britain (Lennox et al. 1975). The tumour may be unilateral or bilateral, the bilateral cases presenting, on average, much earlier than cases with unilateral tumours: at 8 months as against 25.7 months of age in the experience of Lennox et al.

(1975). The familial incidence of retinoblastoma has long been recognized (Sorsby 1962), and not surprisingly familial cases are diagnosed much earlier than sporadic ones.

The tumour is thought to be maintained by a mutation rate of around 4–6×10^6 (Briard-Guillemot et al. 1974; Czeizel and Gárdonyi 1974). Around 10% of cases are familial, but a family history is found more frequently with bilateral than with unilateral tumours (17.7% bilateral, 6.5% unilateral; Briard-Guillemot et al. 1974). The disease appears to be specifically associated with abnormalities of chromosome 13 and trisomy 21 (O'Grady et al. 1974; Orye et al. 1974).

Friend et al. (1986) reported the presence of a gene that predisposed to retinoblastoma and osteosarcoma, subsequently shown to be a tumour suppressor gene. The gene was recessive to the wild type allele and was situated at 13q14. The pattern suggested by Knudson was present in affected individuals, and further investigation has shown that the gene product was a tumour suppressor protein (RB1) and that retinoblastoma cells of both familial and non-familial tumours produced a form which functioned less effectively, than the normal protein in its role of sequestering transcription factor at particular stages of the cell cycle.

There are no differences in sex incidence in retinoblastoma, nor does sex seem to influence survival. The age at diagnosis influences survival rate, and a mortality rate of 6.9% was observed in children presenting at under 1 year of age, compared with 17.9% in children presenting after that time (Lennox et al. 1975). One factor that greatly influences survival is treatment in a specialized hospital, and it seems desirable that all children with retinoblastomas should be treated in such units (Bedford 1975). The finding of Lennox et al. (1975) that the survival rate was better in children with bilateral retinoblastoma was thought to be related to the younger age at diagnosis and to a higher incidence of treatment in specialized units.

Presentation and Histopathology

The tumour protrudes into the posterior chamber of the eye as solitary or multifocal papillary lesions with an irregular surface and pinkish-white in colour (Figs. 17.2 and 17.3). A high proportion of the tumours are sited peripherally. The appearance on direct ophthalmoscopic examination is usually diagnostic, and biopsy is contraindicated. The histological appearance of the tumour is one composed of small dark cells with little cytoplasm, often arranged in a ribbon-like configuration. True rosette formation occurs in about half these tumours (Fig. 17.4).

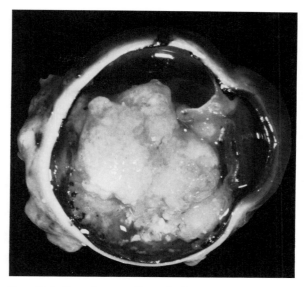

Fig. 17.2. Eye from a 7-month-old male with bilateral retinoblastoma. The globe is filled by tumour. ($\times 3.5$)

Necrosis and calcification are frequent findings. Extension of the tumour into the optic nerve may occur and should be sought histologically in enucleated specimens.

Invasion of the optic nerve and choroid by tumour is associated with poor prognosis, the volume of choroidal invasion probably being the most important factor (Redler and Ellsworth 1973). Histological differentiation in the tumour has been described as a useful prognostic feature (Brown 1966), but is probably not as important as choroidal infiltration. It has been suggested that survival without metastasis for 2 years after treatment of the tumour could be regarded as a cure, but there have been a number of reports of metastases occurring up to 8 years after presentation (Bedford 1975). Osteosarcoma of the orbit following radiotherapy for retinoblastoma has been reported (Lennox et al. 1975).

An extensive review of the tumour and its prognosis is given by Sang and Albert (1982).

Neuroblastoma

Neuroblastomas can arise from any neuroblast (Prasad 1975). These neoplastic neuroblasts are of neural crest origin and of varying degrees of cellular maturation, but most contain osmiophilic dense-core granules 500–900 nm in diameter in their cytoplasm.

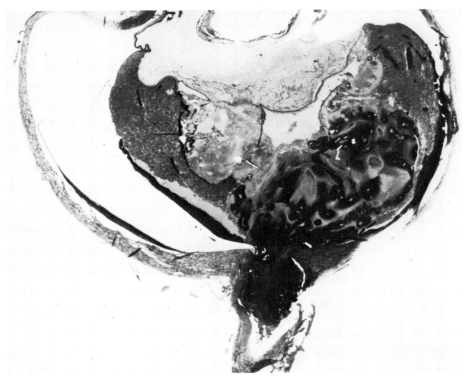

Fig. 17.3. Section through a necrotic tumour involving the optic nerve. (H & E, × 7.5)

The vast majority of these tumours arise from the autonomic nervous system, almost half in the adrenal gland and around 70% within the abdomen. They occur rarely in the peripheral nervous system and are generally considered to be the same nosological entity represented by the Askin tumour of the chest wall and primitive neurectodermal tumour of bone and soft tissue (Gonzalez-Crussi et al. 1984; Llombart-Bosch et al. 1988), which occur in older children and adolescents. These tumours are collectively known as primitive neuroectodermal tumours (PNET, Dehner 1986). Collectively, they have distinctive cytogenic and immunohistological characteristics (Pappo et al. 1993; Weidner and Tjoe 1994).

Microscopic aggregates of neuroblasts occur in the adrenal medulla of newborns and infants, and Beckwith and Perrin (1963) suggested that these lesions were related to the tumour neuroblastoma and that, because of their frequent occurrence (1 in 200 autopsies), the natural history of neuroblastoma was for involution to occur. They were supported in their assumption by the observation in such nodules of mitotic figures, peripheral invasion and absence of a capsule. Most paediatric pathologists have seen a number of similar cases with similar findings.

Turkel and Itabashi (1974) studied many human fetuses (10–30 weeks' gestation) and found neuroblastic nodules in every gland studied. These were greater than 60×60 μm in all instances and as much as 200×400 μm in one case. They pointed out that the migration pathways of neuroblasts from the paravertebral sympathetic ganglion could be traced via periadrenal sympathetic collections through the gland. This migration takes place mainly during weeks 6–7 of gestation, but it continues to a lesser extent throughout fetal life. Continuity of nodules with these pathways could be demonstrated. It seems likely that many in situ neuroblastomas are really normal developmental remnants rather than true neuroblastomas, and do not represent tumour-like lesions.

A well documented and singular aspect of neuroblastoma is its tendency to regress spontaneously, by maturation to ganglioneuroma, by haemorrhagic necrosis with a calcified and fibrous remnant, or by cytolysis (see Bolande 1971). Although a number of potential mechanisms have been proposed to explain these regressions, they are unsatisfactory in many ways. Extensive studies of the effects of nerve growth factor (NGF) on the developing nervous system have shown that it, and other neurotrophic

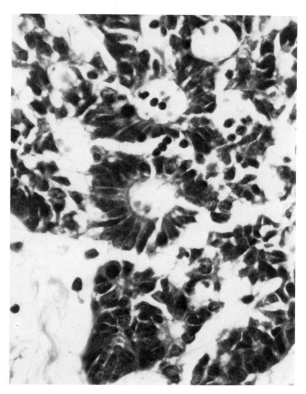

Fig. 17.4. Dark-staining tumour cells forming rosettes with well marked internal limiting membrane. (H & E, × 140)

factors, are necessary for the growth and maintenance of sympathetic and some sensory neurons. From a number of experiments it seems likely that NGF acts as an agent maintaining neuronal viability. Cultures of neuroblastoma show an ability to undergo the type of morphological development that occurs normally during growth and differentiation (Reynolds and Perez-Polo 1975). However, a role for NGF in the process of maturation in neuroblastoma is far from certain.

Presentation and Histopathology

Neuroblastoma is one of the commonest embryonal tumours, and Stiller (1993) reports an increase in incidence of this tumour in the UK over a 20 year period from 1971–1990. The age-standardized rate rose from 7.7 per million in 1971–1975 to 9.7 per million in 1986–1990. He found that the increase was similar in age groups < 1 year and 1–9 years, but observed a fall among children between 10 and 14 years, which is, in part at least, likely to be due to easier distinction between neuroblastoma and Ewing's sarcoma/PNET tumours. There are local differences within the UK; Birch (1988) recorded an increase in incidence in the Manchester Children's Tumour registry from 6.8 per million in 1954–1970 to 7.5 per million during 1971–1983, whereas in the adjacent West Midlands Region the rate has remained static at 7.2 per million (Huddart et al. 1993a).

Neuroblastoma is a tumour of early life, and some are clearly congenital (Voute et al. 1970; Andersen and Hariri 1983). The highest incidence is in the first year of life, and more than half of all cases present before the third birthday (Stiller 1993).

In infants, the usual presentation is with abdominal distension or mass, although some neuroblastomas are found incidentally during the investigation of unrelated illness. This is common for thoracic tumours, which are frequently identified on chest radiography.

International criteria for the diagnosis and staging of neuroblastoma have been agreed in an attempt to render national studies comparable and facilitate international collaborative studies (Brodeur et al. 1988). These criteria have been modified (Brodeur et al. 1993) in the light of the group's collective experience. They recommend the use of immunohistology to aid distinction from other PNETs, use needle-core biopsy rather than fine needle aspiration, and introduce an age limit of < 1 year at presentation for stage 4S. Diagnosis is based on histological examination of primary tumour or metastasis backed up by immunohistochemistry, cytogenetics and N-*myc* amplification in equivocal cases, or on bone marrow aspirate and/or trephine biopsy and elevation of serum or urinary catecholamines or their metabolites. The internationally agreed staging criteria set out in Table 17.2 are the basis for treatment.

Magnetic resonance imaging is the most useful imaging technique for staging of neuroblastomas (Ng and Kingston 1993). These authors found computed tomography with iliac crest biopsy the best alternative to magnetic resonance imaging; ultrasound revealed insufficient detail with thoracic and retroperitoneal tumours. None of the imaging techniques distinguished between enlarged reactive nodes and metastatic lesions, highlighting the need for thorough sampling of lymph nodes during surgery.

Treatment of neuroblastoma has not been as successful as that of other common childhood tumours, particularly lymphoblastic leukaemia and Wilms' tumour. Current therapeutic regimens combining surgery and high-dose continual chemotherapy have improved survival rates for those with large unresectable tumours, even if the primary tumour was intra-abdominal (Garaventor et al. 1993). The best prognostic factor remains age at presentation. Those < 1 year at presentation have better survival than

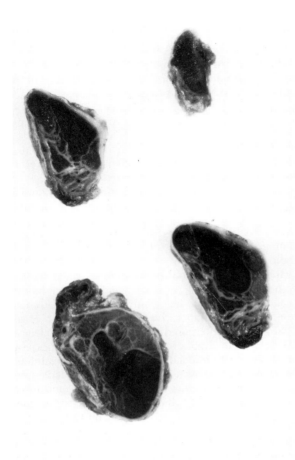

older infants and children. Other prognostic factors are tumour site and stage and the histological appearance of the tumour.

A neuroblastoma can arise from the adrenal medulla (Fig. 17.5) or from some part of the abdominal, thoracic, pelvic or cervical chains of sympathetic ganglia, pelvic tumours having the best prognosis, followed in declining order by those in the thorax (Fig. 17.6), the abdomen and neck, and the adrenals. Girls seem to do better than boys, and a greater incidence of histological maturation within the tumour has been reported in girls (Kinnier Wilson and Draper 1974).

Neuroblastomas extend locally and involve adjacent structures, subsequently metastasizing to lymph nodes. Distant spread is common, especially to bone, liver and skin (Fig. 17.7), with skull involvement a major feature in some instances (Fig. 17.8). However, the involvement of one distant site (liver, subcutaneous tissue or bone marrow) in the absence of radiological evidence of bone involvement does not necessarily carry a poor prognosis (Koop 1972).

Macroscopically, the tumour is usually soft, with areas of necrosis and haemorrhage. There is often extensive focal calcification, resulting in a gritty texture on cutting. Solid greyish-white areas may occur, which histologically contain considerable

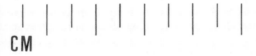

a

Fig. 17.5. a Slices of a small neuroblastoma in the adrenal, from a 6-month-old female with skin nodules and liver metastases at presentation. (× 75) **b** Tumour from a 6-month-old female, discovered incidentally after death from congenital heart disease.

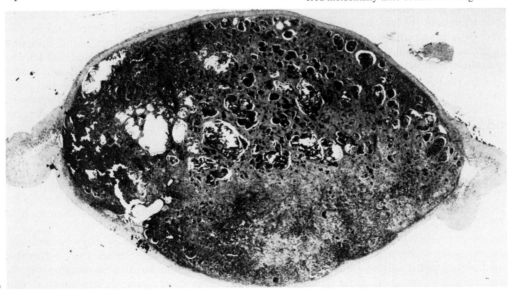

b

Table 17.2. Staging of neuroblastoma

Stage	Definition
1	Localized tumour with complete gross excision, with or without microscopic residual disease; separate ipsilateral lymph nodes negative for tumour microscopically
2A	Localized tumour with incomplete gross excision; ipsilateral non-adherent lymph nodes negative for tumour microscopically
2B	Localized tumour with or without complete gross excision, ipsilateral non-adherent lymph nodes positive for tumour Enlarged contralateral lymph nodes must be negative microscopically
3	Unresectable unilateral tumour infiltrating across the midline[a], with or without regional lymph node involvement; or localized unilateral tumour with contralateral regional lymph node involvement; or midline tumour with bilateral extension by infiltration or lymph node involvement
4	Any primary tumour with dissemination to distant lymph nodes, bone, bone marrow, liver, skin and/or other organs
4S	Localized primary tumour (stage 1, 2A or 2B); dissemination limited to skin, liver and/or bone marrow[b] in infants < 1 year of age

From Brodeur et al. (1993).

[a] The midline is the vertebral column. Tumours crossing the midline must infiltrate to or beyond the opposite side of the vertebral column.

[b] Marrow involvement in stage 4S should be minimal, i.e. < 10% of total nucleated cells malignant on bone marrow biopsy or aspirates. More extensive marrow involvement is stage 4. m-Iodobenzyl guanidine (MIBG) scan should be negative in the marrow.

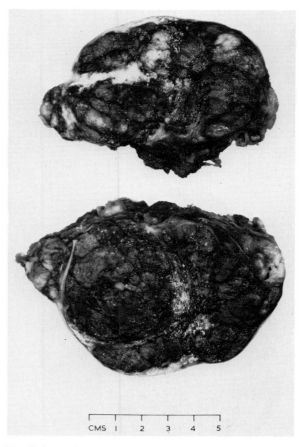

Fig. 17.6. Intrathoracic neuroblastoma from a 21-month-old male. The nodular appearance, with haemorrhages and flecks of calcification, is typical.

amounts of eosinophilic stroma resembling glia. Remnants of invaded or distorted local tissues may be seen.

Histologically, tumour cells are separated by fine vascular septa. Undifferentiated tumours are composed of cells like those of the primitive neural crest, and maturation results in the production of eosinophilic neurofibrillary processes and fibrillary stroma (Figs. 17.9 and 17.10). Rosette formation, consisting of an often ill-defined ring of cells around a central neurofibrillary core, is seen in some tumours. The lesion may shade imperceptibly into ganglioneuroblastoma by the formation of clumps of larger cells with abundant eosinophilic cytoplasm and well defined nucleoli, set in a dense fibrillary tangle (Fig. 17.11). Bizarre neurons are often present. Mature ganglioneuroblastomas often appear as solid tumours with a whorled cut surface and flecks of calcification (Fig. 17.12).

The presence of cellular differentiation within the tumour in the form of neurofibrillary process between tumour cells, and cytogical differentiation towards ganglion cells, are related to better outcome (Makinen 1972). Elaborate classification schemes that are difficult to use have been designed (Shimada et al. 1984), but the current trend is towards simpler schemes with clear definitions and less morphometry (Joshi et al. 1992). Joshi's group has correlated their classification with other prognostic markers (Joshi et al. 1993) and define three histological grades on the basis of mitotic rate and presence or absence of calcification. The often problematic decision about early neuroblast differentiation is thus avoided,

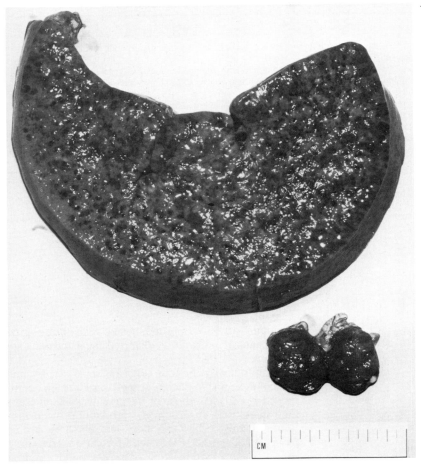

◀ **Fig. 17.7.** Neuroblastoma. Female aged 6 months, with abdominal distension produced by massive hepatomegaly due to diffuse infiltration by neuroblastoma. The small adrenal primary tumour is seen in the *inset*.

Fig. 17.8. Extensive skull metastasis of neuroblastoma. (Courtesy of Professor Zang Xue)

▼

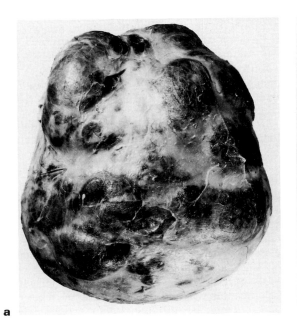

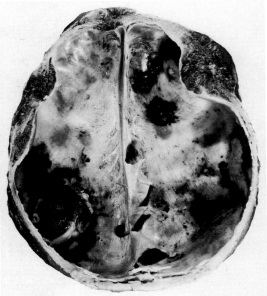

a

b

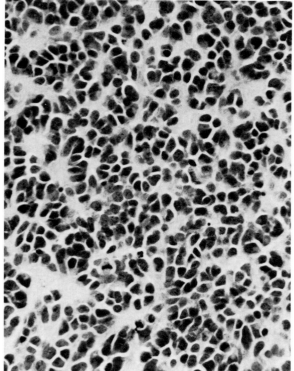

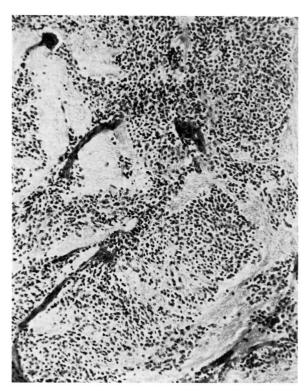

Fig. 17.9. Neuroblastoma. The tumour is composed of large darkly staining cells. The cells themselves show little differentiation but are separated by eosinophilic fibrillary material producing a loose rosettiform arrangement. (H & E, × 400)

Fig. 17.10. Neuroblastoma. Early differentiation results in the production of large amounts of fibrillary material, seen here separating islands of tumour cells. (H & E, × 150)

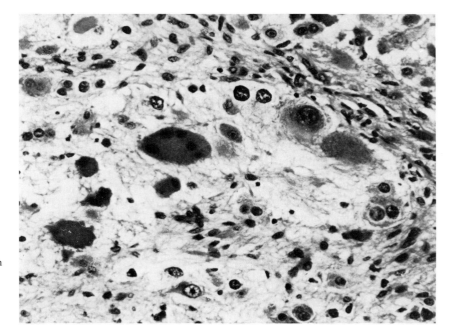

Fig. 17.11. Neuroblastoma. Differentiation within the tumour has produced large neuroblasts with abundant cytoplasm and multiple cytoplasmic processes. Some cells are multinucleate. Differentiation has also produced a mature intervening stroma.

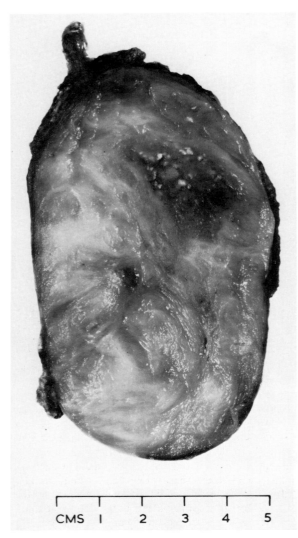

Fig. 17.12. Cut surface of ganglioneuroblastoma, resected at the age of 3 years 6 months (male child).

although secretogranin II expression may prove a useful marker of differentiation (Schmid et al. 1993).

Aneuploidy is associated with better outcome than diploidy in neuroblastoma, as is a single copy of N-*myc* gene (Huddart et al. 1993b; Joshi et al. 1993). Both MYCN (N-*myc*) amplification and chromosome 1p deletion can now be detected by in situ hybridization in tissue sections (Leong et al. 1993). The method is much quicker than Southern blotting and tissue culture/karyotype analysis. Infants with serum lactic dehydrogenase secretion of < 1500 IU/litre do better than those secreting higher amounts of the enzyme (Joshi et al. 1993).

Early Detection

Early detection of neuroblastoma by population screening using urinary catecholamine metabolites at age 6 months (Kaneko et al. 1990) and prenatal diagnosis by ultrasonography (Ho et al. 1993) identifies predominantly tumours with a good prognosis. This is not surprising, given the long recognized better prognosis of neuroblastomas presenting before 6 months of age. Rescreening at regular intervals until 3 years of age might detect more aggressive tumours at an earlier stage. Ho et al. (1993) describe seven of 11 tumours identified prenatally as in situ lesions. One effect of very early diagnosis may be to shed light on the behaviour of in situ tumours, enabling the likelihood of spontaneous regression to be calculated from changes in incidence. Although all the patients documented by Ho et al. survived, Newton et al. (1985) describe a fatality related to the development of fetal hydrops, a complication of either massive hepatomegaly or extensive placental involvement (Keeling 1993).

Currently, the staging system of Brodeur et al. (1993) is used for this tumour (Table 17.2).

Medulloblastoma

The important central nervous system tumour medulloblastoma arises in the posterior fossa. The parent cell is generally considered to be from the granular layer, a subpial layer of small cells present throughout the cortex at birth but disappearing by around 18 months of age. These cells may be bipotent, able to migrate inwards to become neurons in the definitive granular cell layer, but also to differentiate into neuroglia (Fujita 1967). In normal development, collections of cells morphologically similar to those of medulloblastoma were seen in 23 of 104 fetuses or neonates in which the posterior medullary velum was examined histologically, suggesting that collections of cells might become isolated at various sites on their normal migratory routes, with subsequent tumour formation.

Kadin et al. (1970) reported a case that supported the origin of these tumours from the cells of the fetal external granular layer. The spread of the tumour was studied in enough detail to show the transitional passage of the layer into true tumour formation. The case presented in the neonatal period, probably having arisen in intrauterine life, and showed irregular zones of proliferation with invasion of the molecular layer, which suggested malignant change. Electron microscopic findings (junctional complexes and cell processes containing microtubules) supported a neuro-epithelial origin for the neoplasm.

Medulloblastoma has been reported in siblings. Excluding cases without histological verification in both affected individuals, it has been reported in two pairs of identical twins, a half-brother and half-sister, two pairs of brothers, and two sisters. A striking feature of these reports is the similar age of onset of the tumour in the various sibships; in most instances there is very close approximation. There is a well established association of the tumour with the naevoid basal cell carcinoma syndrome (see Neblett et al. 1971), and prognosis is better in these children. Gorlin syndrome is found in 1%–2% of children with medullobastoma (Evans et al. 1991).

Medulloblastoma presents throughout childhood, with a maximum incidence between 2 and 4 years of age (Clausen et al. 1990).

Congenital medulloblastoma is rare; hydrocephalus resulting in dystocia is the usual mode of presentation (Poon et al. 1975). Intracranial tumours are recognized increasingly frequently during fetal life on ultrasound examination and may be associated with fetal hydrops. A predominance of females has been demonstrated in early-onset medulloblastoma, and association with the naevoid basal-cell carcinoma syndrome is also associated with early-onset.

A 12-year-old girl with medulloblastoma and multiple other cerebral tumours has also been reported (Bhangui et al. 1977). This was a curious combination of tumours: medulloblastoma, optic nerve glioma, pilocytic astrocytoma and ganglioglioma. Since the naevoid basal-cell carcinoma syndrome has been called the "fifth phacomatosis" the presence of optic nerve glioma is interesting. The author felt that this last lesion and the pilocytic astrocytoma might be two parts of the same tumour – they were in continuity in one area. With medulloblastoma and glial and neuronal tumour present in the same case there appears to be some support for the suggestion that bipolar differentiation of medulloblastoma may occur. A number of authors (e.g. Becker and Hinton 1983) consider that medulloblastoma should be regarded as one of a series of primitive neuroectodermal tumours, capable of very variable differentiation.

Presentation and Histopathology

This neoplasm, found in the posterior fossa of children, is over twice as common in males. Most examples in younger children are found in the midline, in the cerebellar vermis (Fig. 17.13); in the second decade they are seen in the hemisphere as well as the vermis. Although predominantly cerebellar, some

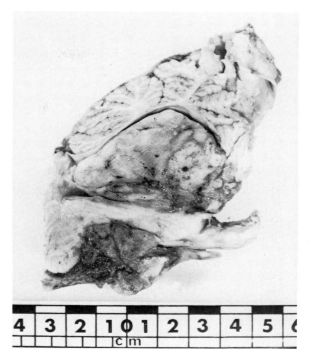

Fig. 17.13. Medulloblastoma of cerebellum extending around the medulla. (Courtesy of Professor J. Smith)

examples appear to arise in the medullary velum, and extension into the fourth ventricle with consequent hydrocephalus is common. On macroscopic examination they are described as purplish-grey at operation but grey after excision, with a granular cut surface. Metastasis via the cerebrospinal fluid is frequent, and in this case secondary deposits may be found in the walls of the ventricular system, in the depths of sulci, and scattered over the cord and cauda equina. Sometimes these meningeal deposits form thin grey sheets. Spread outside the CNS was found in only 6% of 112 autopsied cases in one study (Clausen et al. 1990).

Microscopic examination may show a fairly uniform picture of round or oval closely packed basophilic cells resembling the granular layer of the cerebellar cortex on cursory examination. However, closer examination indicates that the cells are somewhat larger than this type and mitoses are frequent. Sometimes the cells are grouped in trabeculae or whorls. Vascularity is variable, as is the presence of the characteristic pseudorosettes first described by Wright (1910) (Fig. 17.14). In these the carrot-like delicate processes are directed to a central focus, where they merge with one another, but there is no central lumen. It is exceedingly difficult to demonstrate neurofibrils in such foci; this is occasionally possible with very rare, somewhat similar, tumours

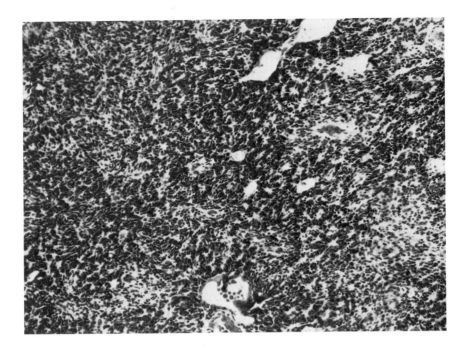

Fig. 17.14. Pseudorosette of medulloblastoma. (H & E, × 400) (Courtesy of Professor J. Smith)

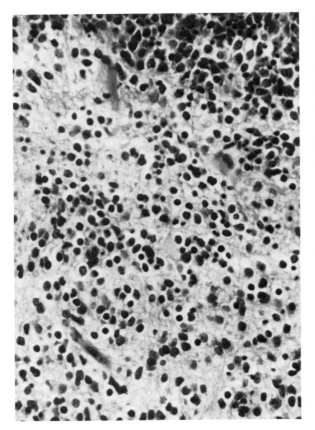

Fig. 17.15. Medulloblastoma differentiating to oligodendroglioma. (H & E, × 400)

that arise in the cerebrum and are more correctly classified as neuroblastomas.

In reports of large series, the occurrence of areas strongly suggestive of differentiation to oligoden-droglia in a minority of tumours is a consistent feature, and these areas are an integral part of the tumour (Fig. 17.15); differentiation to astrocytes and neurons was said to be rare, but glial fibrillary acidic protein (GAFP) staining identifies astrocytes in many tumours. Goldberg-Stern et al. (1991) found better survival if tumour astrocytes were GAFP positive.

Mitotic index (MI) has significant prognostic value. Gilbertson et al. (1992) found a stepwise asso-ciation with survival, with 42% 10 years survival in tumours with 0%–2% MI and no survival when it was > 3%. This group also found that tumours with > 50% c-$erb\beta2$ product expression had better survival.

The value of ploidy for prognosis in medulloblas-toma is unclear. Yasue et al. (1989) found aneuploidy to be related to better outcome, but Tait et al. (1993) could not demonstrate any difference in outcome between diploid and aneuploid tumours.

One particular feature of the local invasive proper-ties of these tumours has aroused controversy. This is the capacity of certain examples, occurring in the lateral lobes, and usually after the first decade, to excite a marked connective-tissue reaction in the lep-tomeninges. Rubenstein and Northfield (1964) re-ferred to these as desmoplastic medulloblastomas and could find no support for the thesis that some represented an independent entity, a circumscribed arach-noidal sarcoma, with a better prognosis.

Schofield et al. (1992) distinguish desmoplastic medulloblastoma in the lateral parts of the cerebellum as a separate group, which can usually be resected and has a better prognosis than medulloblastoma in general.

Nephroblastoma

Genesis

New data of general significance in embryonal tumours have come from the study of nephroblastoma, which occurs in sporadic, familial and syndrome-associated forms. Koufos et al. (1985) suggested that the development of homozygosity at a locus on chromosome 11 might explain the development of nephroblastoma, hepatoblastoma and rhabdomyosarcoma in the Beckwith-Wiedemann syndrome (BWS), and it is now established that this syndrome and the WAGR (Wilms' tumour, aniridia, genitourinary abnormalities and mental retardation) complex are associated with deletions at 11p13 or 11p15. Nephroblastoma results from a homozygous mutation of a gene located at chromosome 11p13 where loss of extended regions or of the whole chromosome may occur. Several other tumours, including rhabdomyosarcoma and hepatoblastoma, also show loss of heterozygosity at p, suggesting that loss of the same gene can produce different tumours depending on the cell lineage in which loss occurs. In the nephroblastomas occurring as part of BWS, deletions occur in bands 11p15.5. For retinoblastoma, similar changes occur at 13q14, a change which is also associated with a considerable increase in osteosarcomas in the survivors of the heritable form of the eye tumour (see p. 868). Loss of heterozygosity for 13q is also seen in sporadic cases of osteosarcoma, and the retinoblastoma gene is deleted in some of these tumours.

A gene product of the gene *WT1* is a transcription factor regulator which binds to DNA, but not all nephroblastomas show abnormalities of the *WT1* gene and a number of mechanisms of production of nephroblastoma must exist. Different modes of investigation of nephroblastoma have produced important data in this context by examining the phenomenon of imprinting.

Studies of imprinting have supplied important information about nephroblastoma, but have also illustrated some fundamental points about embryonal tumours. The epigenetic process of genomic imprint-

ing plays a role in development, allowing some homologous alleles to function differently in the conceptus depending on whether they come from the mother or the father (see Berry 1991). There is a clear functional difference between the activity of paternal and maternal chromosomes at several levels in development. This difference is manifested in haploid and diploid genomes, in single chromosome effects, at the level of part of a chromosome and at the single locus. A conceptus composed entirely of paternal chromosomes will form a complete hydatidiform mole, which usually arises as the result of duplication of a haploid chromosome set but sometimes occurs following dispermy with elimination of the maternal genomic contribution. Maternally derived diploid development gives rise to teratomata in the ovary; these tumours are frequently homozygous for centromeric chromosomal polymorphisms for which their host is heterozygous, suggesting that they are derived following the first meiotic division. The (mal)development of extraembryonic tissues in the paternally derived mole without evidence of fetal development and of embryonic development in the teratoma without evidence of extraembryonic tissue formation is evidence that the two genomes have different parts to play in early embryogenesis. However, in the genesis of embryonic tumours it is single gene effects that are of interest.

Single gene imprinting is probably related to differing methylation patterns in DNA. Vertebrate DNA contains much 5-methyl cytosine, which has the same relationship to cytosine that thymidine has to uracil; methylation has no effect on base pairing. 5-methyl cytosine is found in the CG sequence and is base-paired to exactly the same sequence in the opposite strand; there is thus a mechanism which makes certain that the pre-existing pattern of DNA methylation will be inherited. (In general inactive genes are more heavily methylated than active ones and activity is often associated with loss of methylation, but this level of control of DNA expression appears to be subsidiary to the role of growth regulating proteins.) The clearest examples of single gene level imprinting are seen in familial neoplastic disorders. Benign familial glomus tumours are transmitted as an autosomal dominant trait, but are only manifested in those who inherit the gene from their father (van der May et al. 1989). It appears that the maternal locus is inactivated in oogenesis and can only be reactivated during spermatogenesis. The genetics of retinoblastoma/osteogenic sarcoma suggest that the susceptibility to somatic mutation at the RB1 locus varies with the parental origin of the gene and the type of tissue. In the embryonic tumours of childhood the mechanism of development of the neoplasm appears to be that two mutant alleles of a putative tumour-suppress-ing gene are produced, the first by mutating one allele and the second by loss of the normally functioning allele, generally as a result of genetic recombination (although meiotic non-disjuncion may occur). This causes tumour tissue to become homozygous for markers located on the mutated chromosome, permitting identification of its origin. In familial cases the chromosome retained in the tumour is derived from the affected parent, but in sporadic tumours the somatic mutation thought to be the cause of the neoplasm should theoretically have an equal chance of occurring in the maternal or paternal gene. This is not the case for sporadic nephroblastoma or osteosarcoma, where it has been shown that the paternal chromosome is retained in the tumour and the maternal one is lost (Schroeder et al. 1987; Touchida et al. 1989). For retinoblastoma similar findings have been claimed but not all studies have confirmed this (Dryja et al. 1989). In the paper of Zhu et al. (1989), nine retinoblastomas from eight unrelated non-familial cases were studied using RB1-linked genetic markers. Six tumours retained the paternal allele and three the maternal; of the unilateral tumours only one retained the paternal allele. In contrast, tumours from four of the five bilaterally affected patients retained the paternal allele, suggesting either that the new germline RB1 mutations appear more readily in spermatogenesis than in oogenesis or that imprinting in the early embryo affects the chromosomal susceptibility to mutation.

Combining the data of the Zhu and Dryja groups gives 13 of 14 bilateral tumours retaining the paternal chromosome ($0.001 < P > 0.01$) with four of ten unilateral tumours doing the same – a non-significant difference.

The tendency for the first somatic mutation in Wilms' tumour to occur on the paternal chromosome is due to genomic imprinting; presumably the Wilms' locus is imprinted in embryonic kidney and the retinoblastoma locus in bone but not in retina.

Touchida et al. (1989) investigated the origin of chromosome 13 in osteosarcoma, studying a group of patients who were considered to have had somatic mutations, as none of them had had retinoblastoma. Of 13 sporadic osteosarcomas in which they found loss of heterozygosity for 13q markers, 12 retained the parental chromosome, and after eliminating three cases about which some doubt was evident they were left with a paternal : maternal retention ratio of 9 : 1. In nephroblastoma the cases associated with aniridia and genitourinary anomalies and the bilateral cases are probably caused by germinal mutation, and unilateral lesions by two somatic cell events. Schroeder et al. (1987) found that in all five of the cases of nephroblastoma that they studied the paternal region of 11p was retained.

The explanation of these observations is disputed (Reik and Surani 1989). We prefer the hypothesis which suggests, on the basis of observations on nephroblastoma, that the transforming gene is imprinted. Inactivation of the nephroblastoma gene product depresses the transforming gene and results in the development of a tumour. The maternal allele of the transforming gene is rendered inactive by methylation imprinting. (Increased methylation of paternal DNA would allow a greater frequency of mutation by deamination of 5-methylcytosine and is known to occur in transgenic mice.) Thus the combination of the inactive nephroblastoma gene and the transforming gene of the paternal chromosome results in a tumour.

However, another plausible hypothesis exists. Sapienza et al. (1989) suggest that only a small minority of cells in an embryo retain methylation differences between specific parental alleles. In these cells the maternal gene is likely to be relatively inactive because of increased methylation (an assertion based on their own data from work in the transgenic mouse). If the first mutation happens on a paternal chromosome opposite the relatively inactive maternal allele, this population will expand and a focus of tumour cells will appear in the target tissue. This focus represents an increased mass of cells in which the second mutation may occur, resulting in loss of the second allele. This hypothesis permits the attractive option that the remaining maternal allele need not be completely suppressed but may operate at a reduced level, which may vary at different stages of development. It is thus possible for the second hit not to happen, in which case "tumour like lesions … that have regressed" may be found in the affected tissue. These authors' nomenclature is not entirely satisfactory, but it is clear that evidence of focal abnormalities of development are found in association with nephroblastoma, and their so-called neuroblastoma in situ may represent such a focus.

The previously discussed reports of findings in BWS made clear that in many patients both copies of part of the short arm of chromosome 11 (11p15.5) come from the parental genome. Chimaeric mouse embryos containing cells partially disomic for the distal part of chromosome 7 also have features that resemble BWS and are abnormally large. The gene for insulin-like growth factor 2 (Igf-2) lies in this region in the mouse, and mouse chromosome 7 is homologous to human chromosome 11p15.5, as discussed by Little et al. (1991). In around 12%–13% of patients with BWS, nephroblastoma, rhabdomyosarcoma or hepatoblastoma occurs, and if there is loss of an 11p15.5 allele it is always a maternal one. The 11p15 trisomy found in a few patients with the syndrome always results from duplication of the paternal allele. There is tight linkage of familial BWS to 11p15.5, and the degree of homozygosity at 11p15.5 in sporadic probands is greater than that in the normal population, suggesting paternal isodisomy (two copies of the same allele from the father). The links between 11p15.5 and paternal duplication and BWS suggests that this region codes for a paternally active growth factor or a maternally active growth suppressor. An overabundance of Igf-2 messenger RNA is seen in the tumours of patients with BWS (Scott et al. 1985), which suggests that abnormal activity of the gene and abnormalities of the growth factor (or receptor) could be invoked as a mechanism for oncogenesis.

These concepts may seem far from those which might interest a practising pathologist. However, the demonstration by Haber et al. (1993) that the product of a zinc finger gene *WT1*, which is lost by mutational changes in nephroblastoma, will suppress the growth of a Wilms' tumour cell line indicates how precise knowledge of this kind may soon influence therapy and demand investigation of tumours with a greater degree of precision (in terms of their genetic constitution) than has been the case to date.

Pathology

Nephroblastoma is a common tumour of infancy, comprising around 18% of all malignant lesions in this age group. Forty per cent of cases present before 2 years of age and 85% before their fifth birthday; cases seldom occur after 12 years of age. Although the tumour is said to be rare in adults, there are more than 1500 cases in the literature (Klapproth 1959; Babain et al. 1980). The disease is rare in adolescence: in a report by Merton et al. (1976) two adolescents with Wilms' tumours are described, although one of these was apparently atypical. In many large series, presentation before the age of 2 years has been shown to be associated with a good prognosis, probably because of effects on the staging of the tumour at presentation (see Lemerle et al. 1976 for a bibliography).

Congenital tumours are rare, and most are congenital mesoblastic nephromas (Hilton and Keeling 1973) (see p. 500).

Of 30 patients with primary renal tumours presenting in the first year of life, Marsden and Lawler (1983) found 23 to be classic Wilms' tumours and four mesoblastic nephromas. Three lesions were the malignant rhabdoid tumours first described by Beckwith and Palmer (1978). However, since Wilms' tumours, like other embryonic tumours, may occasionally originate in intrauterine life, and as the bulk of cases occur between 2 and 4 years of age, it is interesting to note the results of a study comparable with that of Beckwith and Perrin on neuroblastoma,

conducted by Bove et al. (1969). Assuming that the tumour arises from metanephric blastema during embryonic and fetal life or in early infancy, they studied material from an autopsy series. Nodular renal blastema, defined as "the presence in the kidney of discrete nodules of primitive undifferentiated cells which were cytologically indistinguishable from nephroblastoma, which differed unequivocally, in both size and pattern, from the tubular metanephric structures which characterize normal development of nephrons from the metanephric blastema and which were unaccompanied by either intra–renal or extra–renal metastasis", was found to be associated with trisomy 18 and also to occur apart from this syndrome. Five of eight patients with trisomy 18 had nodular renal blastema (NRB), but multiple congenital abnormalities were associated with NRB in all instances. The lesion has been associated with nephroblastoma and hemihypertrophy (Mottu et al. 1981).

The lesions are usually sited under the cortex, but may be very extensive, causing nephromegaly (Mankad et al. 1974; de Chadarévian et al. 1977). They vary in size from 50 μm to 2 mm, and are discrete although not encapsulated. Ill-defined tubular structures may be present, but stomal or glomerular elements like those seen in Wilms' tumour are not found. Mitoses are extremely uncommon.

NRB is encountered in less than 1% of perinatal necropsies (Bove et al. 1969), but may be identified in 20%–44% of kidneys removed for nephroblastoma (Bennington and Beckwith 1975). It is more commonly found in younger infants (Heideman et al. 1985) and in those with bilateral or multifocal tumours (Tucker et al. 1986). The lesion has been carefully reviewed, with a clear redefinition of terminology by Beckwith (1993).

Wilms' tumour can often be bilateral, when a family history is sometimes obtained. However, it is seldom practicable to decide whether an apparently multicentric origin is a genuine phenomenon or represents metastatic spread, and some bilateral Wilms' tumours may represent nephroblastomatosis: Bové et al. stressed that, in five bilateral Wilms' tumours, subcapsular "focal development abnormalities" were particularly common. However, in only one instance did these lesions resemble NRB.

Associations of Wilms' tumour with aniridia, hemihypertrophy, hypospadias, cryptorchidism, microcephaly, pigmented and vascular naevi, and abnormalities of the pinna have all been reported (see Miller et al. 1964), but different anomalies have been reported with NRB, mainly those of the trisomy 18 syndrome. Further, NRB is commoner in females (presumably this is related to the predominance of females in trisomy 18), whereas there is a slight male preponderance in Wilms' tumour, which is marked in cases associated with aniridia.

Stambolis (1977) reported a case of Wilms' tumour in the right kidney, with bilateral nodular renal blastema and direct transformation of one such nodule into a benign epithelial "nephroblastoma" consisting of tubular and glomeruloid structures, with papillary areas. Mitoses were not seen. This suggests that there are three discrete entities: NRB, benign and malignant nephroblastoma. The interrelationship of the tumours is not presently explicable in mechanistic terms.

A study of Bennington and Beckwith (1975) found 12 cases of "persistent" metanephric blastema in 2452 consecutive paediatric autopsies (nine among 1035 cases of less than 3 months of age). This rate is much higher than the frequency of Wilms' tumours, suggesting that most instances of persistent blastema do not give rise to tumours.

De Chadarévian et al. (1977) have emphasized that massive bilateral nephroblastomatosis can be confused with Wilms' tumour. Describing four cases, all of which presented at under 2 years of age, they reported a negative family history in three cases, and one child whose relatives had urinary tract disease. Following chemotherapy, hypertension, which was present in three of the four cases, disappeared and the kidneys became smaller. Bové and McAdam (1976) have studied the kidneys of 69 patients with Wilms' tumours and found evidence of abnormalities of differentiation in many of them – adenomas, hamartomas, nodular blastema, cysts, dysplastic tubules, scar, etc. This list is one that pathologists might consider to include lesions found in kidneys in many conditions, and the study does not provide evidence for a general failure of control mechanisms in metanephric differentiation.

The report of Hughson et al. (1976) of two Wilms' tumour survivors who subsequently presented with benign tumours in the contralateral kidney is also of interest. These tumours were unlike many mesenchymal renal lesions in having a large striated muscle component. The authors suggested maturation of a metastatic lesion as a possible explanation but also pointed out that the lesions might have been benign from the outset.

Clinical Presentation

The commonest presenting feature of nephroblastoma is an abdominal mass giving rise to distention. Vague abdominal pain is common. Abdominal trauma may result in rupture of the tumour or haemorrhage into it, the resulting pain drawing attention to the presence of a renal mass. Haematuria is a much less common symptom of renal tumour in children than in adults, being present in less than a third of cases. Symptoms due to renin secretion by the tumour include hypertension, polydipsia and polyuria, and these may be the presenting features (Sheth et al. 1978). Removal of the tumour is often followed by the regression of symptoms, but these may recur with the appearance of metastases (Bradley and Drake 1949).

Examination of the Specimen

Pathological examination of paediatric renal tumours makes three critically important contributions to patient management. Firstly, diagnosis: up to 80% of tumours diagnosed on clinical and imaging criteria are not nephroblastoma (Webber et al. 1992). The second contribution relates to staging, which relies heavily on careful examination of the nephrectomy specimen (see Table 17.3). The third relates to histological appearance and the identification of both favourable

Table 17.3. Staging of nephroblastoma used by the National Wilms' Tumour Study (NWTS) (Beckwith 1994)

Stage	Definition
I	Limited to the kidney, completely resected Renal capsule not penetrated Renal sinus can be infiltrated, but not beyond the hilar plane of the kidney No biopsy or prior tumour spill
II	Extends beyond the kidney, but completely resected Specimen margin free of tumour Biopsy or controlled tumour spill at surgery Renal sinus or veins involved beyond the hilar plane, but resected completely
III	Residual tumour in the abdomen, peritoneal soilage, or involved nodes in the abdomen Involved specimen margin is presumptive evidence of residual tumour Tumour removed from vena cava piecemeal is presumed evidence of diffuse spill
IV	Haematogenous metastases, or involved nodes outside the abdomen
V	Bilateral renal tumours Bilateral disease should be "substaged" using the stage of the most advanced lesion

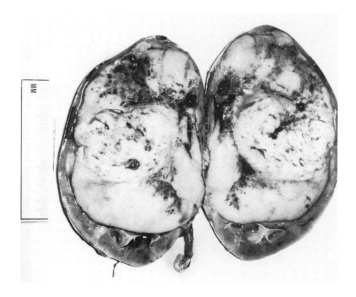

Fig. 17.16. Nephroblastoma. The kidney is almost completely replaced by an ovoid tumour mass, around which the remaining renal parenchyma is stretched. The edge of the tumour is well defined and areas of haemorrhagic necrosis are apparent on the cut surface.

and unfavourable features, which directly affect chemotherapy.

The nephrectomy specimen should reach the laboratory in a fresh unfixed state with the renal vein identified. It should not be incised or bisected by the surgeon. Lymph nodes away from the renal hilum should be sent separately from the tumour and their site of origin identified.

The surface of the specimen is examined and photographed. Areas of capsular thinning or permeation by tumour are carefully noted. Subsequent handling varies but is influenced by the friable nature of the tumour. Webber et al. (1992) incise an inked area of the tumour surface away from any thinning to remove fresh tissue for electron microscopy, cytogenetics and other biological studies and fix the specimen overnight before bisection. This is done to minimize contamination of the specimen by microscopic tumour fragments, which might alter tumour staging. Beckwith (1994) recommends bivalving the tumour, taking fresh samples from the bulging cut surface. He then makes further slices parallel to the first, photographs them and fixes the whole in refrigerated formalin overnight before taking blocks for histological examination. In his view, refrigeration improves cytological detail by retarding autolysis, but it also reduces the rate of permeation of fixative.

Our practice is to bisect the specimen to minimize distortion, avoiding problem areas in the capsule, to photograph and remove fresh samples from the bulging surface and to fix overnight before further dissection. Polaroid photographs are taken of cut surface to enable an accurate record of histological sampling to be kept.

When selecting blocks for histological examination, particular attention should be paid to the margins of the tumour and the renal hilum as these will influence staging. Any areas of unusual appearance in the tumour are sampled. The kidney is carefully inspected for foci suggestive of nephroblastomatosis, and appropriate samples obtained. All lymph nodes are sampled for histological examination. Enlarged nodes often display reactive changes and are uninvolved by tumour. A variety of benign lesions including epithelium/Tamm–Horsfall protein complexes, entrapped squamous epithelium, megakaryocytes and hyperplastic postcapillary venules can mimic metastatic nodal involvement (Weeks et al. 1990).

The tumour is usually larger than the kidney in which it arises when seen at nephrectomy. Tumour growth causes compression of surrounding renal tissue to form a fibrous pseudocapsule, dividing it from residual functioning kidney (Fig. 17.16). The surface of the involved kidney is frequently nodular, and the renal capsule is very thin and often fused with the pseudocapsule over convexities. On the cut surface, fibrous septa divide the tumour into nodules; some are cystic as the result of necrosis, or, rarely, because of the cystic or papillary configuration of the tumour. Focal haemorrhage is frequently present.

Histology

Nephroblastoma presents a wide variety of histological appearance because of divergent lines along which histological differentiation may occur. The typical picture is of islands of undifferentiated darkly

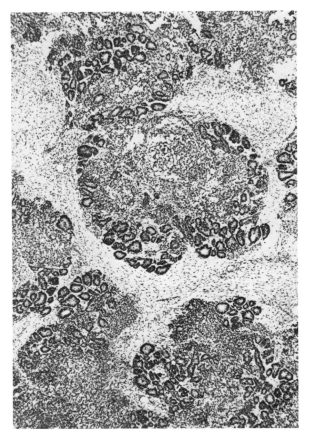

Fig. 17.17. Nephroblastoma. Islands of undifferentiated darkly staining blastema cells have peripheral tubular differentiation and are separated by strands of pale-staining tumour mesenchyme. (H & E, × 50)

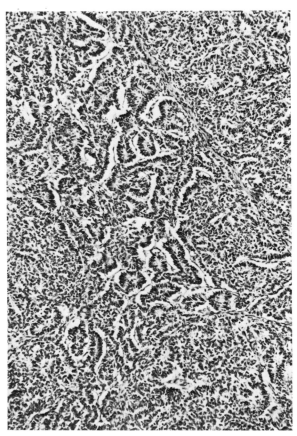

Fig.17.18. Nephroblastoma. Ribbon-like arrangement of blastema cells in double cords but without intervening lumen. These are the earliest stage of tubular differentiation. (H & E, × 120)

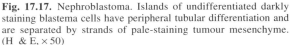

stained blastema cells with oval or slightly elongated nuclei and little cytoplasm, separated by bands of primitive mesenchyme – pale-staining elongated cells with a tendency towards a banded or whorled configuration. There is usually some tubular differentiation within areas of blastema. A wide variety of types of tubules are seen, recapitulating various stages of renal differentiation (Figs. 17.17–17.20). Glomerular differentiation is less common and seldom progresses further than a small knot of cells protruding into an epithelial lined space (Fig. 17.21).

Some tumours present an entirely blastematous appearance. This is sometimes diffuse and thus difficult to distinguish from other round blue cell tumour in young children. Immunohistochemistry and sometimes electron microscopy may assist in the accurate definition of the type. More often there is a serpentine pattern in which the cords of blastemal cells are separated by a vascular myxoid stroma.

Tubular epithelial differentiation is often very striking. Such a pattern rarely creates diagnostic difficulty. Differentiation within the mesenchyme component is less common, but smooth muscle, striated muscle and fatty tissue are recognized (Fig 17.22). Metaplastic tissues such as osteoid (Fig. 17.23), squameous epithelial nests and pilosebaceous structures are sometimes found. Where they comprise the major part of the tumour these are designated teratoid nephroblastomas. Differentiation within Wilms' tumour does not confer better prognosis for any given tumour stage than tumours without features of differentiation. They all fall into the "good" prognosis group.

The histological feature important in Wilms' tumour prognosis was designated "anaplasia" (Beckwith 1993), but the term has given rise to some confusion in that it is widely used in classifications of other tumours to mean undifferentiated. For Wilms' tumour this has a

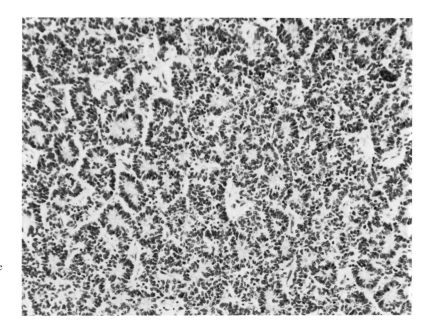

Fig. 17.19. Nephroblastoma. Incomplete tubular differentiation may produce "rosettes". The nuclei are more tapered than those of neuroblastoma. (H & E, × 140)

more specific definition and has been redesignated anaplastic nuclear change (Beckwith 1994). This is defined as marked nuclear enlargement with at least a three-fold increase in one nuclear axis and two-fold increase in the perpendicular axis, increased chromatin content in the enlarged nuclei manifested by normal or increased nuclear density, and multipolar or obviously polyploid mitotic figures (Beckwith 1994). For practical purposes anaplasia can be distinguished by microscopy at low magnification. This change is an adverse prognostic feature, except when it is a focal change defined as one or two discrete foci, bearing in mind the need to take at least one histological block of tumour per centimetre diameter, occurring within stage 1 nephroblastoma (Beckwith 1994).

Oncocytic change (eosinophilia of blastemal cell cytoplasm) is sometimes seen. Opinions about its significance vary, but Webber et al. (1992) suggest that it may be the result of ischaemia related to vascular permeation of the tumour. They found that it correlated with a high tumour stage and with worse prognosis.

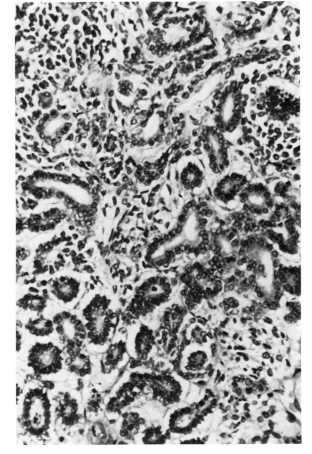

Fig. 17.20. Nephroblastoma. Tubular differentiation; undifferentiated blastema is present between tubules. The tubules have well defined lumina. (H & E, × 300)

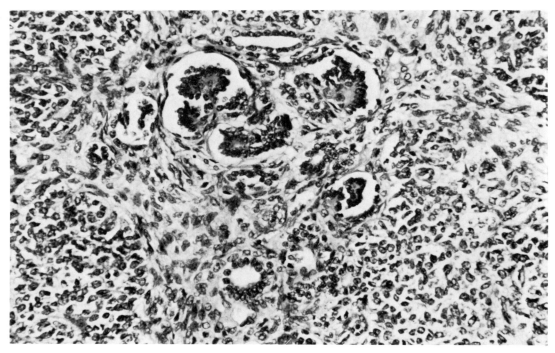

Fig. 17.21. Nephroblastoma. Glomerular differentiation does not proceed further than a clump of epithelial cells protruding into a space lined with a flattened cell layer. (H & E, × 300)

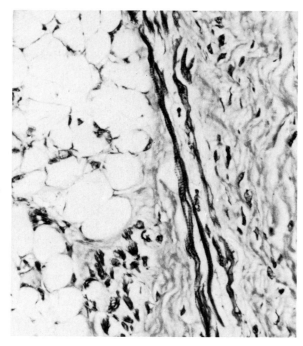

Fig. 17.22. Nephroblastoma. Differentiation with a nephroblastoma may produce mesenchymal tissues. Fatty tissue and strap-like muscle cells with well marked cross-striations and mature collagen are intimately mixed in this tumour. (H & E, × 400)

Cystic Variants of Wilms' Tumour

Views have changed about the origin of cystic renal tumours of childhood (Joshi 1979). Current thought suggests a spectrum of histological appearance, with differentiated cystic nephroma, (formerly often designated multilocular renal cyst) at the benign end of the spectrum and two grades of cystic partially differentiated nephroblastoma (Joshi and Beckwith 1989). Grade 1 has 50% more of mature elements within the septae between the cysts, and grade 2 has less than 50% of mature elements. Both have undifferentiated blastemal elements within them. In some cases there is a sizeable solid component. The prognosis of cystic lesions is better than that of classic nephroblastoma, putting them into an "extra good prognosis" group. Surgery is curative, and if the size of the lesion remits partial nephrectomy should be attempted. It is unfortunate that the most mature lesions have often attained such a large size, with consequent distortion of the kidney, that partial nephrectomy may not be possible.

Bilateral Wilms' Tumour

About 5% of children with Wilms' tumour have synchronic bilateral tumour, and a further 5% will

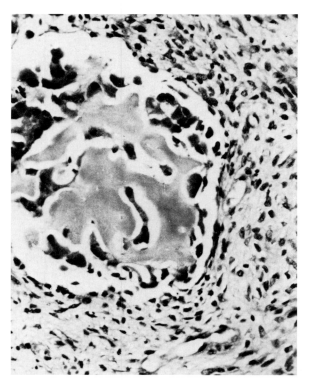

Fig. 17.23. Nephroblastoma. (Same tumour as in Fig. 17.22.) A circumscribed nodule of osteoid differentiation. (H & E, × 400)

develop a second tumour subsequently. Children with bilateral tumours have a higher incidence of malformations, and in particular overgrowth syndromes such as hemihypertrophy, BWS and Soto's syndrome. Bilateral tumour is associated with nephroblastomatosis. Treatment of bilateral tumour is often difficult, as treatment needs to be individualized for each child. When this is done the overall survival rate is about 70% (Shearer et al. 1993).

An interesting point about differentiation within this tumour is made by Fleming and Symes (1987), who have shown that ureteric bud-derived tubules may be found in nephroblastoma (Fig. 17.24). Further data suggest that active ureteric bud ampullae may occur in the tumour mass. Renin is also found, probably in an inactive form, in a large proportion of nephroblastomas (Lindop et al. 1984).

Metastasis

Tumour is found in both kidneys at presentation in between 4% and 13% of cases (Cochran and Froggatt 1967; Young and Williams 1969). It is possible, however, that the higher estimates are weighted by referrals to specialized units. Direct extension of the tumour occurs through the capsule to involve neighbouring viscera, into the hepatic vein and the inferior vena cava, and into the renal pelvis and down the ureter.

Lymphatic spread is commonly to hilar or para-aortic lymph nodes, although the porta hepatis and mediastinum may be involved. Haematogenous spread occurs most commonly to the lung. Solitary pulmonary metastases are not unusual, and have often been treated successfully by surgical excision. Hepatic metastases occur but are infrequent, whereas skeletal metastasis is rare and renal tumours in children that develop skeletal metastases are always of the bone-metastasizing (Lawler and Marsden 1979) or clear cell sarcoma (CCSK) type.

A comparison of the histological differentiation seen in metastatic nephroblastoma with the differentiation in the primary tumour (Banayan et al. 1971) showed more pronounced non-epithelial differentiation in metastases than in the primary tumour, where differentiation was mainly tubular. The authors considered that these changes were accelerated by radiotherapy.

Staging procedures for this tumour are shown in Table 17.3.

Extrarenal Tumours

Extrarenal Wilms' tumours are occasionally described. These seem to be of two types, one type arising in a line from the renal bed to the scrotum supposedly arising in residual embryonic renal tissue (Bhajekar et al. 1964; Akhtar et al. 1977; Aterman et al. 1979; Orlowski et al. 1980). Clusters of mature glomeruli and tubules have been present beneath the capsule of these tumours. The second type are nephroblastomas arising within teratomas. These have been described in the mediastinum (Moyson et al.1961) and the sacrococcygeal region (Ward and Dehner 1974) as well as in retroperitoneal tumours (Carney 1975). Whether one should regard renal differentiation in a teratoma as nephroblastoma rather than a distinctive form of maturation seems to be open to doubt; only one of the tumours described gave rise to metastases (Orlowski et al. 1980).

Fetal Rhabdomyomatous Nephroblastoma

Fetal rhabdomyomatous nephroblastoma, which occurs in infants and has a more favourable prognosis than Wilms' tumour, is described by Wigger (1976). The lesions are largely composed of bundles of immature striated muscle in a fibrous stroma, together with undifferentiated elements, fat, cartilage,

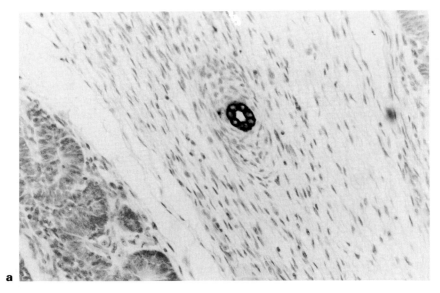

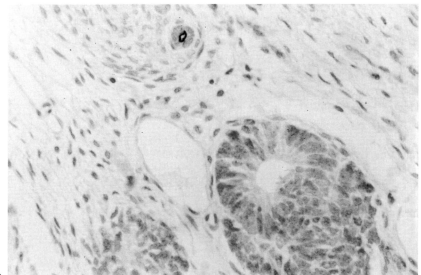

Fig. 17.24. Immunoperoxidase staining of ureteric duct with anti-high-molecular-weight-cytokeratin antibody. This protein is restricted to the collecting ducts and urothelium. (**a** × 110; **b** × 168) (Courtesy of Dr S. Fleming)

smooth muscle, and bone. We consider the tumour to be a variation of Wilms' tumour. Metastases were uncommon but death from local tumour extension occurred in a proportion of cases.

Complications of Therapy

Breatnach and Androulakakis (1983) have reported a 7-year-old girl with adenocarcinoma of the kidney following radiotherapy for nephroblastoma. Renal adenocarcinoma has previously been reported after radiotherapy for neuroblastoma and pelvic teratoma.

Rhabdomyosarcoma

The bulk of rhabdomyosarcomas (malignant tumours of striated muscle) occur in childhood, although no age is exempt. Of head and neck tumours, 80% occur in children aged 12 years or less (Dito and Batsakis 1962), most commonly in the orbital region or in the nose, mouth or pharynx. Bale et al. (1983) reported a total of 18 tumours in an eyelid or orbital group and found that all eyelid tumours were children under 1 year of age; one of these cases was clearly congenital. The majority of genitourinary tumours present before

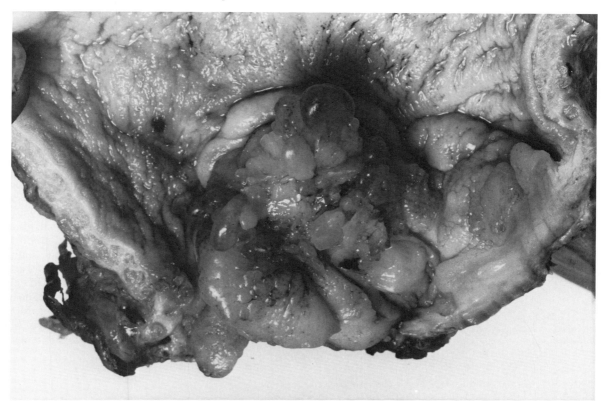

Fig. 17.25. From a 2-year-old boy presenting with strangury. Many polypoid masses are seen arising from a broad base in the trabeculated bladder.

the age of 4 years. There is an apparent male predominance (Legier 1961; Williams and Schistad 1964).

Li and Fraumeni (1969) reported an epidemiological study on the families of many of the 418 children dying of rhabdomyosarcoma in the USA between 1960 and 1964. In five families a second child was found to have had a soft-tissue sarcoma, the children affected being siblings (three) and cousins (two). The parents and grandparents of these children had a higher incidence than normal of carcinoma of various sites and of leukaemia, and the authors first suggested the existence of a familial cancer syndrome.

Systems of classification of rhabdomyosarcoma dependent on culture and experimental work are those of Horn and Enterline (1958), in which the lesion is divided into embryonal and botryoid, alveolar, and pleomorphic types, and of Ashton and Morgan (1965), which has three categories, embryonal sarcoma, non-striated embryonal rhabdomyosarcoma, and striated embryonal rhabdomyosarcoma. A more recent classification recognizes four histological types: classical, aggressive, leiomyomatous and pleomorphic (Tsokos et al. 1992).

Morales et al. (1972) have carried out an extensive ultrastructural study of human rhabdomyosarcoma, and have reviewed previous studies of this type. Their findings, which should be consulted by those attempting to confirm this diagnosis by electron microscopy, emphasize the importance of accurate identification of the fibres found in any tumour before assumptions are made about its origin. Their data suggest that the Ashton and Morgan system of classification, devised to deal with an experimentally induced tumour, will be of value in humans (see Clarke and O'Connell 1973).

Pathology

In the urogenital sinus area the tumour generally presents as a polypoid mass projecting into the vagina or bladder. The component lobules are greyish-white, opalescent and of varying size. The whole tumour is often of indeterminate origin, i.e. it has no distinct "base" (Figs. 17.25 and Fig. 17.26). Histologically, the polyps are usually covered by a layer of cuboidal

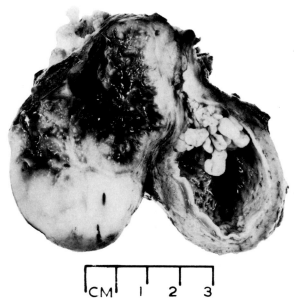

Fig. 17.26. From a 6-year-old. The tumour is infiltrating and ulcerated, with extensive secondary infection. The bladder wall is thickened.

or stratified squamous epithelium and may show areas of superficial ulceration. The polyps have an essentially myxomatous appearance, which may mislead the unwary, and the lesions, when solitary or infected, may be mistaken for inflammatory masses (Fig. 17.27). Examination of the cells in the zone immediately under the epithelium (Fig. 17.28) and of those scattered in the stroma will reveal a number with nuclear atypicality and eosinophilic cytoplasm, which may be arranged in strap-like forms showing cross-striation typical of muscle cells (Fig. 17.29). These are not essential for the diagnosis of rhabdomyosarcoma, as other cytological characteristics will permit the diagnosis to be made. Bale et al. (1983) found cross-striations in only 37 of 95 cases of juvenile rhabdomyosarcoma; longitudinal fibres were more frequent. Typical cytological findings include long spindle-shaped cells, with ovoid central nuclei, cells with cross-striation, or large bizarre "tadpole" cells with their nuclei at the expanded end. Immunohistochemical staining may assist diagnosis but there is no specific marker for this tumour. Most are desmin and muscle specific actin positive, but only well differentiated tumours are myoglobin posi-

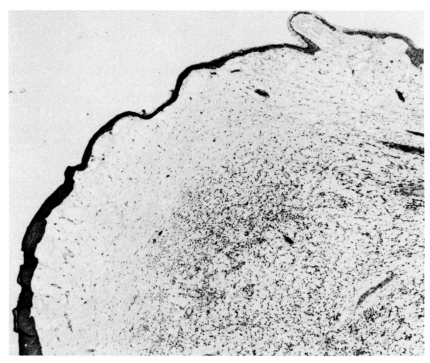

Fig. 17.27. Rhabdomyosarcoma. The botryoid polyps of rhabdomyosarcoma may be disarmingly hypocellular and the superficial part of the tumour very oedematous. Nuclei are well separated by a myxoid stroma. (H & E, × 40)

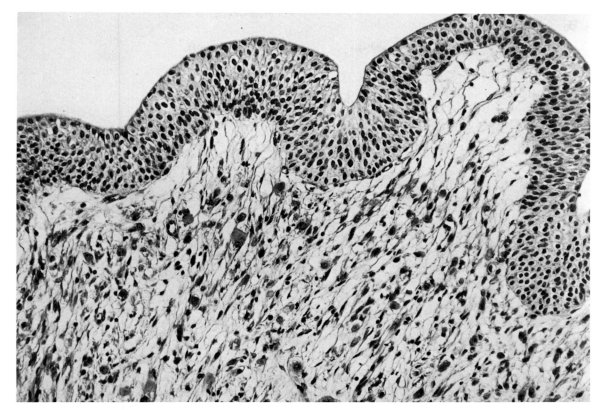

Fig. 17.28. Rhabdomyosarcoma of the bladder. Marked cellular pleomorphism in a loose zone beneath the transitional epithelium. Some cells have a densely eosinophilic cytoplasm. (H & E, × 250)

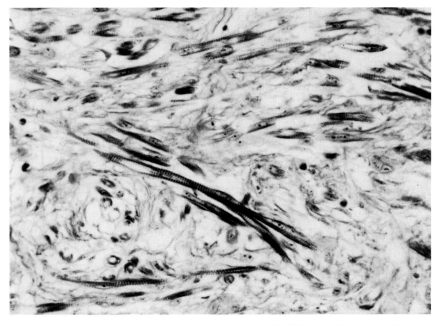

Fig. 17.29. Rhabdomyosarcoma. Cross-striations are seen in strap cells in this well differentiated urogenital sinus tumour. (PTAH, × 400)

tive, whereas some are positive for NSE (Malone 1993). About one-third of embryonal rhabdomyosarcomas were positive for 12E7, a monoclonal antibody to MIC2 gene product (Ramani et al. 1993), and alveolar rhabdomyosarcomas were unreactive.

Wijnaendts et al. (1994) have derived a scoring system for rhabodomyosarcoma based on the examination of 113 tumours. They found that a low nuclear cytoplasmic ratio, absence of necroses and absence of septae all correlate well with favourable clinical course. The same group (Wijnaendts et al. 1993) examined rhabdomyosarcomas by flow cytometry. Aneuploidy conferred better prognosis than diploidy. Tetraploid tumours formed an intermediate group.

Whether present in the head and neck or pelvis, the tumour spreads rapidly by local extension and involves the local lymph nodes. Blood-borne metastases are relatively uncommon in the normally short history of the disease. Nasopharyngeal tumours tend to involve bone early by local extension (Canalis et al. 1978).

Paratesticular rhabdomyosarcoma can be cured by radical surgery and radiotherapy or simple chemotherapy if they are non-infiltrating. Children with infiltrating tumours may survive if an aggressive surgical approach, i.e. retroperitoneal lymphadenectomy plus radiotherapy plus cyclic combined chemotherapy, is undertaken (Malek and Kelalis 1977).

Embryonal rhabdomyosarcoma of the botryoid type may also occur in the biliary tract. Taira et al. (1976) reviewed 20 verified cases and added a further case of their own. Most of these tumours occur in young children (average age at onset 3.9 years) and the prognosis is poor.

Hepatoblastoma

Hepatoblastoma is much less common than neuroblastoma or nephroblastoma, accounting for less than 5% of tumours in most series from children's hospitals, an effective incidence of around 1 per 100 000 of those under 15 years. Males are more frequently affected: a ratio of 1.5 : 1 was observed in 73 cases reviewed by Weinberg and Finegold (1983) and of 1.14 : 1 in 138 UK cases seen by us. Hepatoblastomas are tumours of early life, more than half present before the 2nd birthday, and some are undoubtedly congenital (13 of 138 in the UK series). There are apparently chromosomally related factors involved in the development of hepatoblastoma, but these (Table 17.4) are not as frequent as in nephroblastoma. Familial occurrence is reported but uncommon. A variety of chromosome abnormalities have been reported in children with hepatoblastoma, often in those with a predisposing syndrome (Table 17.5). A study of environmental

Table 17.4. Chromosome anomalies in children with hepatoblastoma

Abnormality	Reference
11p15.5 loss of heterozygosity	Koufos et al. 1985
i(8q)	Bardi et al. 1991
Trisomy 20 + double minutes	Mascarello et al. 1990
Trisomy 2	Bardi et al. 1992
11p15.5	Byrne and Smith 1993
p53 mutation at codon 249	Kar et al. 1993

Table 17.5. Associations of hepatoblastoma

Reference	No. of cases	No. of congenital tumours	Association
Ishak and Glunz 1967	35	1	Hemihypertrophy
Misugi et al. 1967	19	2	None recorded
Keeling 1971	40	2	Familial polyposis Bilateral talipes Meckel's diverticulum
Weinberg and Finegold 1983	27	2	Familial polyposis Pi M Z Cousin with "liver cancer"
Schmidt et al. 1985	24	–	Fetal alcohol syndrome Cleft lip and palate Cleft palate and macroglossia
Gauthier et al. 1986	26	–	Fetal alcohol syndrome
UK series (unpublished)	138	13	Beckwith syndrome Probable Beckwith syndrome (two cases) Familial polyposis coli Chromosome 2/4 translocation Wilms' tumour with Meckel's diverticulum

factors (Buckley et al. 1989) failed to find an association with recognized hepatotoxic substances such as exposure to alcohol, nitrosamines or maternal oestrogen therapy or hepatitis in utero.

The usual presentations are increasing girth or the palpation of an upper abdominal mass by the mother or other attendant. Abdominal radiography may confirm liver enlargement, and tumour calcification may be present. Computed tomography, inferior vena cavagram and hepatic arteriography are useful for localizing the tumour and distinguishing between a single tumour mass and multiple deposits (Clatworthy et al. 1974). A system to define the extent of pretreatment liver involvement by tumour based on a four-sector plan has been devised to monitor treatment response in a consistent fashion (MacKinlay and Pritchard 1992). Serum α-fetoprotein levels are usually elevated in infants with hepatoblastoma, and are a useful indication of recurrence in follow-up studies (Alpert et al. 1968). Chorionic gonadotrophin is produced less frequently by hepatoblastoma (Murphy et al. 1980), although the hormone may produce precocious puberty. (See Nakagawara et al. 1982 for a review.) Extreme thrombocytosis is common, probably due to thrombopoietin production by the tumour, and may be clinically useful in the child with an upper abdominal mass (Shafford and Pritchard 1993).

Current treatment protocols reserve primary surgery for stage I, easily resectable tumours. After biopsy, the rest are treated with combination chemotherapy; cisplatin and daunorubicin (Plado) is currently used. This has an improved survival at 18 months from 18% in 1965–1974 and 34% in 1975–1984 to 81% in 1991–1993 (SIOPEL 1 study).

Pathology

The tumour is more frequently seen in the right lobe than the left (Keeling 1971; Clatworthy et al. 1974), but in about one-third of cases both lobes are involved. Macroscopically, there is usually a firm, encapsulated, multinodular, brownish-tan tumour. Haemorrhages and cystic degeneration of necrotic areas are frequent findings (Fig. 17.30).

The histological appearance varies widely, making widespread sampling imperative. Areas resembling the fetal liver, with regular sized nuclei and very few mitoses, are the best differentiated cell type. This may be difficult to distinguish from normal liver in a biopsy. Haemopoiesis is usually prominent in fetal areas. A less differentiated appearance where cells resemble embryonal liver cells with less cytoplasm, mitotic figures and a sometimes tubular configuration

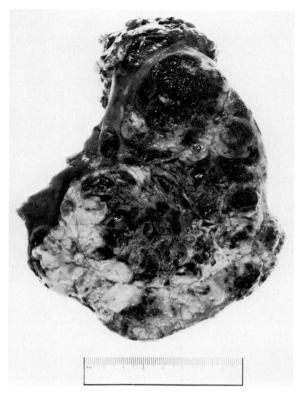

Fig. 17.30. Hepatoblastoma. Male of 6 months, presenting with abdominal distension. Hepatic lobectomy specimen, a massive lobulated tumour with extensive haemorrhage. (Reproduced from Keeling 1971, by courtesy of the Editor of the *Journal of Pathology*)

is seen (Fig. 17.31). Embryonal undifferentiated or anaplastic forms may be large celled or small celled. Other cell types may be present, including a spindle-cell mesenchymal component, large cells with marked nuclear pleomorphism indistinguishable from hepatocellular carcinoma, tubular differentiation (often seen within small-celled areas), and osteoid or, occasionally, osseous metaplasia (Figs. 17.32 and 17.33).

The overall configuration is usually in plates or narrow cords of cells. A macrotrabecular configuration (Gonzalez-Crussi et al. 1982) comprising cords of fetal or embryonal cells (usually the latter), about 20 cells thick and resembling hepatocellular carcinoma, is a marker of poor prognosis (Haas et al. 1989). In the authors' experience it is not a frequent finding.

Current classification systems are based on the histological grade of the least differentiated epithelial component rather than that of the predominant cell type present. The system used for the first SIOP study uses four groups: fetal, embryonal, macrotrabecular,

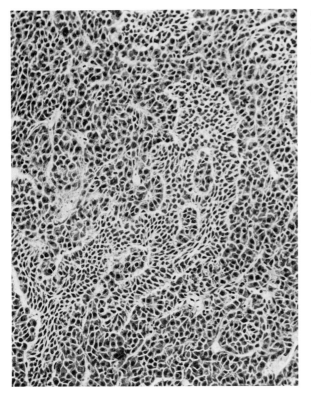

and small-cell undifferentiated. However, no classification system can be regarded as definitive at
present, and all histologic cell types are recorded so
that opportunities to modify the classification are not
lost.

Some studies show that infants with a pure fetal
histological type have a better prognosis (Weinberg
and Finegold 1983; Haas et al. 1989; Shafford et al.
1995), but this is not a universal finding (Schmidt et
al. 1985), although this diagnosis can be made with
certainty only in primary resection specimens,
which are likely to be the smaller localized
tumours. Because of this discrepancy, Schmidt et
al. (1993) have looked at DNA ploidy; they found
that diploid tumours had a better outcome than
hyperdiploid ones. Infants with diploid tumours
were younger – a factor related to better prognosis
in other embryonal tumours. Findings of the UK
retrospective childhood liver tumour study suggest
that "fetal-predominant" tumours may also have a
better prognosis.

Hepatoblastoma also stains positively with α-feto-
protein, but the best reaction is seen, not surprisingly,
in the best differentiated areas and its usefulness in
distinguishing primary liver tumour from other round

Fig. 17.31. Hepatoblastoma. Tumour cells resemble developing
hepatocytes and are arranged in a cord-like configuration. (H & E,
× 100) (Reproduced from Keeling 1971, by courtesy of the Editor
of the *Journal of Pathology*)

Fig. 17.32. Hepatoblastoma. A mixed cellular pattern. In the upper
part of the field pale-staining enlongated cells of tumour mesenchyme intervene between nodules of large r cells resembling
fetal hepatocytes. (H & E, × 365)

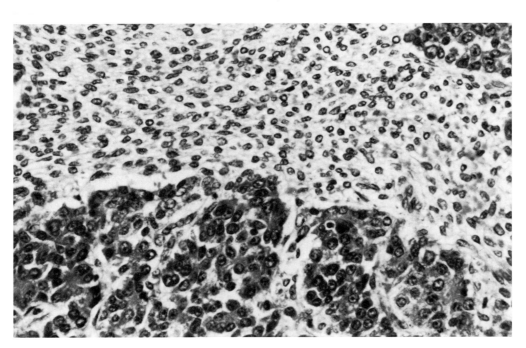

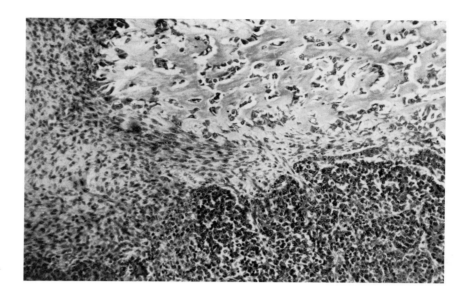

Fig. 17.33. Hepatoblastoma. An island of osteoid metaplasia is seen within tumour mesenchyme. (H & E, × 145)

blue cell tumours of infancy is limited. Some tumours show marked transferrin receptor staining (Sciot et al. 1990). Immunohistochemical demonstration of liver fatty acid-binding protein is another potential marker (Suzuki et al. 1990).

Examination of hepatoblastoma after chemotherapy usually shows extensive necrosis or haemorrhage, particularly within areas with embryonal histology. The fetal areas are more resistant to chemotherapy, although degenerative changes are often present. Osteoid often dominates the histological picture (Saxena et al. 1993), but whether this is therapy-induced metaplasia or a concentrating effect due to sensitivity of other tissue types to chemotherapy and their subsequent loss is not entirely clear.

The tumour spreads locally to involve other parts of the liver, to lymph nodes in the porta hepatis, and occasionally to the duodenum and pancreas. Metastatic spread is usually to the lungs, but involvement of the diaphragm and mediastinum and generalized intra-abdominal metastasis are quite common. Cerebral involvement and spread to other lymph node groups may occur (Keeling 1971). Resection of pulmonary metastases in stage I cases (where the tumour was initially completely resected) appears worthwhile (Feusner et al. 1993).

Most reviews of liver tumours in children distinguish the hepatoblastoma of the infant liver from hepatocellular carcinoma occurring in older children (Ishak and Gluntz 1967; Misugi et al. 1967; Keeling 1971). Ultrastructural differences between the two groups are described (Misugi et al. 1967; Ito and Johnson 1969). There do not appear to be behavioural differences between the various histological types of hepatoblastoma, and Misugi et al. (1967) and Keeling

(1971) consider them variations of the same embryonal tumour. Willis' (1962) division into hepatocellular, mixed and rhabdomyoblastic tumours is probably unjustified, because thorough examination of the tumour reveals mesenchymal elements in almost every case. All hepatoblastomas could be considered to be in Willis' mixed group, and rhabdomyosarcomatous tumours, occurring as they do in older children and taking their origin from the biliary tree, should be considered a distinct tumour entity (see also p. 305). An association between hepatoblastoma and polyposis coli has been noted by Kingston et al. (1983) in five children with the tumour, all of whom had mothers with polyposis. No related chromosomal abnormality has been detected.

Teratomas

The frequencies of individual sites of origin of these tumours in reported series is dependent on the age range of the population from which they were drawn. Claireaux and Keeling (1973) report the sites of origin of 104 teratomas seen at The Hospital for Sick Children, Great Ormond Street, London, from 1934 to 1971. At this hospital the upper age limit for new patients was 12 years and the majority of tumours arose in the sacrococcygeal region. Series in which the age range extends to 15 or 16 years have a larger proportion of ovarian tumours, many of which present just after puberty. The majority of testicular tumours also present later, 74% of patients with these

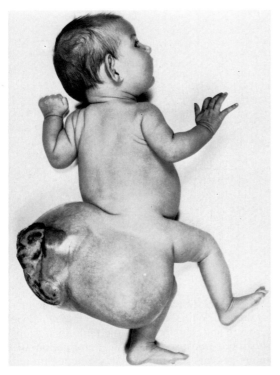

Fig. 17.34. Sacrococcygeal teratoma present at birth. A large ulcerated mass protrudes from the buttocks.

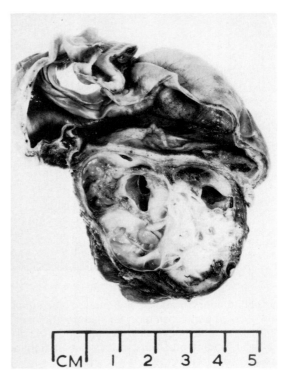

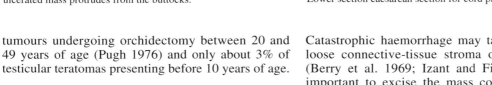

Fig. 17.35. Cystic mass arising from the sacrum in a male neonate. Lower section caesarean section for cord prolapse.

tumours undergoing orchidectomy between 20 and 49 years of age (Pugh 1976) and only about 3% of testicular teratomas presenting before 10 years of age.

Sacrococcygeal

Sacrococcygeal teratomas are tumours of the neonate and infant and are usually present at birth, when the tumour may be large enough to obstruct delivery (Heys et al. 1967). Some tumours precipitate heart failure and hydrops during the second half of pregnancy, resulting in intrauterine fetal death (Werb et al. 1992) or neonatal problems related to heart failure or intraoperative haemorrhage (Teitelbaum et al. 1994). Most tumours grow outwards from the sacrum (Fig. 17.34); an associated intrapelvic mass is sometimes observed, although intradural extension is unusual (Powell et al. 1993). Presentation after 1 year of age is associated with poor prognosis (60% recurrence, compared with 10% in infants who present before that time). The tumour is commoner in females in a ratio of 3 : 1. Immediate surgery is the treatment of choice in infants with teratoma, and observation and interval surgery are associated with an increased risk of occurrence (Berry et al. 1969).

Catastrophic haemorrhage may take place into the loose connective-tissue stroma of a large tumour (Berry et al. 1969; Izant and Filston 1975). It is important to excise the mass completely, and the coccyx should be taken en bloc with the tumour; failure to do this increase the likelihood of recurrence (Berry et al. 1969; Carney et al. 1972).

The tumours are usually partially cystic masses (Fig. 17.35). Histologically, the majority are composed of differentiated tissues (Fig. 17.36). Organoid differentiation is common (Fig. 17.37). Embryonic tissue is present in the tumours in between 13% and 27% of cases in large series and is frequently neural in type, often resembling a retinal anlage (Fig. 17.38), although mesenchymal and other developing structures are frequently seen (Fig. 17.39).

Sacrococcygeal teratomas that are histologically malignant on first resection or biopsy comprise between 11% and 27% of the cases in reported series. The most common histological type is a large-cell carcinoma; some are solid, but a papillary configuration is common and the malignant element may resemble endodermal sinus (Teilum) tumour (Figs. 17.40 and 17.41).

The high incidence of malignant change in some reports is probably a reflection of secondary referral

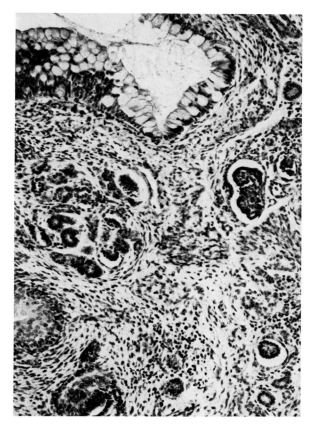

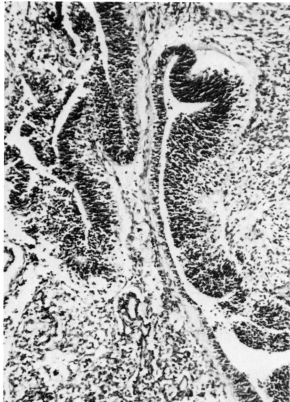

Fig. 17.36. Sacrococcygeal teratoma. A cyst lined with fully differentiated mucus-secreting columnar epithelium; mature renal tubules and glomeruli are present in a stroma of immature mesenchyme. (H & E, × 150) (Reproduced from Berry et al. 1969, by courtesy of the Editor of the *Journal of Pathology*)

Fig. 17.37. Sacrococcygeal teratoma. Organoid development; a developing tooth bud is present within its bony matrix. (H & E, × 10) (Reproduced from Berry et al. 1969, by courtesy of the Editor of the *Journal of Pathology*)

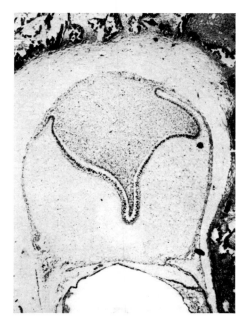

to specialist hospitals of cases treated originally elsewhere (Chretien et al. 1970). In series composed entirely of primary referrals, the incidence of malignancy is lower. Hawkins et al. (1993) reviewed the histology of apparently benign sacrococcygeal teratomas that subsequently recurred with malignant histological features. They found small foci of yolk sac tumour, which had been overlooked on internal examination. Routine use of immunohistochemistry for α-fetoprotein and human chorionic gonadotrophin might reduce the risk of missing this component in large tumours. In a review of sacrococcygeal anomalies of all types (including tumours) Bale (1984) gives a comprehensive and useful bibliography of these lesions.

Fig. 17.38. Sacrococcygeal teratoma in an infant born at 31 weeks' gestation. Embryonic neural tissue formed a major component of this tumour, here seen as retinal anlage. (H & E, × 150)

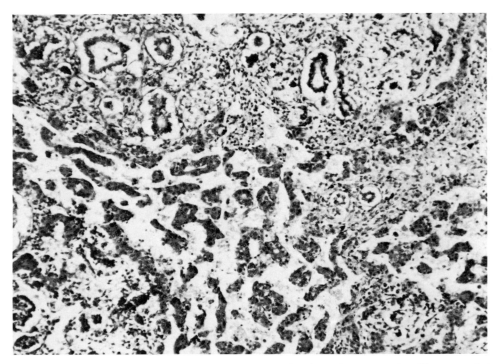

Fig. 17.39. Sacrococcygeal teratoma. (Same case as Fig. 17.38.) Hepatocytes forming rudimentary cords and immature tubular structures. (H & E, × 150)

Ovarian

Although a few ovarian teratomas are seen in infancy, many more are seen in older children and

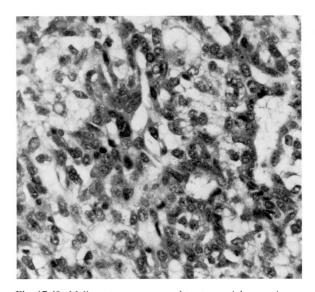

Fig. 17.40. Malignant sacrococcygeal teratoma. Adenocarcinoma with a tubular/papillary configuration. (H & E, × 150)

young adults. Histologically they are usually composed of differentiated tissues (Berry et al. 1969), but malignant ovarian teratomas are reported in children. Among the cases reported by Breen and Neubecker (1963), nine of 17 malignant ovarian teratomas occurred in girls before menarche, the youngest being 14 months of age. Chorion carcinoma was seen in several tumours from young patients; differentiation to papillary carcinoma, sarcoma and dysgerminoma was also seen. More than half these authors' young patients were dead within 1 year of presentation.

Testicular

Testicular teratomas do occur in infants and children but, as with ovarian tumours, much less commonly than in young adults. In children the tumours are usually Testicular Tumour Panel Grade TD (teratomas differentiated), and do not recur following surgical excision (Berry et al. 1969; Pugh 1976).

Mediastinal

Mediastinal teratomas are seen in both the infant and the older child. In some cases a thyroid origin is

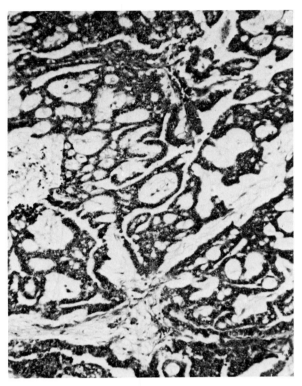

Fig. 17.41. Malignant sacrococcygeal teratoma. Solid adenocarcinoma. Some cells are mucus-secreting. (H & E, × 400)

obvious and in some a thymic origin is postulated, but in many cases the exact origin of the tumour is unclear. In infants the tumours are usually composed of differentiated tissues or a mixture of differentiated and embryonic elements, although the thyroid tumour reported by Heys et al. (1967), which obstructed delivery, had metastasized to the liver in utero.

In older children mediastinal teratomas may be malignant, with widespread metastases and rapid downhill course. These reported by Lakhoo et al. (1993) were all over 12 years at presentation and died within 6 months of surgery. Unusual histological appearances may be present, reminiscent of embryonal sarcoma with mesenchymal and tumular elements.

Occasionally a teratoma arises within the pericardial sac (Fig. 17.42) and gives rise to fetal hydrops with disproportionately excessive pericardial effusion and hydrops (Werb et al. 1992; Keeling 1994). These usually arise from the great vessels at the base of the heart (Claireaux 1951). The tumour may arise from the myocardium.

At Other Sites

Teratomas arising from the base of the skull may present as oral or intracranial masses (Fig. 17.43). Problems arise because of difficulty of excision rather than malignant change. Abdominal teratomas arising

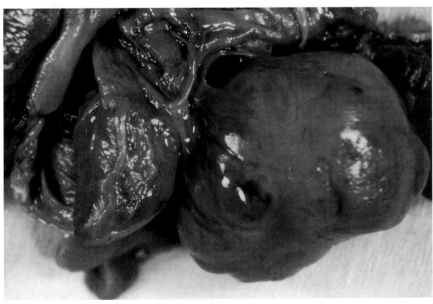

Fig. 17.42. Teratoma arising from the anterior surface of the heart in the region of the aortic and pulmonary artery origins. Fetal hydrops and pericardial effusion at 25 weeks' gestation (Keeling 1993).

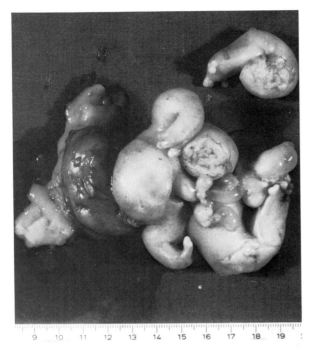

Fig. 17.43. Intracranial teratoma removed from the lateral ventricle of a 6-week-old child with hydrocephalus. One "limb" has been removed in the surgical resection.

from the stomach, retroperitoneal tissues (Berry et al. 1969) or liver (Yarborough and Evashnick 1956) are uncommon; they are usually well differentiated, although a malignant hepatic teratoma has been reported (Misugi and Reiner 1965).

Second Malignant Neoplasms in Children Surviving Embryonic Tumours

There are many reports of second malignant tumours in children, with Wilms' tumour and retinoblastoma being the commonest initial lesions, and osteosarcomas and chondrosarcomas the commonest second neoplasms. Many of the bone tumours in the report of Meadows et al. (1977) developed in areas previously irradiated, as did skin tumours (basal cell carcinomas) in the irradiated fields for medulloblastoma in individuals with the naevoid basal cell carcinoma syndrome. However, 33 of 102 second neoplasms were not associated with prior radiation. Twelve of these could be explained on the basis of a known

inherent susceptibility, but in the remaining 21 no predisposing cause was found. Associations between gliomas and leukaemia or lymphoma, and between the last two tumours and carcinoma of the colon, occurred with higher frequencies than would be expected by chance.

Penchansky and Krause (1982) reviewed the literature on acute leukaemia following radiotherapy or chemotherapy in childhood. Leukaemia was most common following treatment for Hodgkin's disease; cytogenetic abnormalities were found in more than 90% of cases – a far greater rate than in spontaneous acute leukaemia.

References

Adelstein AM, White C (1976) Population trends no. 3, p 9

Akhtar M, Kott E, Brooks B (1977) Extrarenal Wilms' tumour. Report of a case and review of literature. Cancer 40: 3087

Alpert ME, Uriel J, de Nechaud B (1968) Alpha-1-fetoglobulin in the diagnosis of human hepatoma. N Engl J Med 278: 984

Anonymous (1981) Imaging techniques in obstetrics. Lancet i: 923

Andersen HJ, Hariri J (1983) Congenital neuroblastoma in a fetus with multiple malformations. Virchows Arch A Pathol Anat 400: 219

Ashton N, Morgan G (1965) Embryonal sarcoma and embryonal rhabdomyosarcoma of the orbit. J Clin Pathol 18: 699

Aterman K, Grantmyre E, Gillis DA (1979) Extrarenal Wilms' tumour. J Invest Cell Pathol 2: 309

Babain RJ, Skinner DG, Waisman J (1980) Wilms' tumour in the adult patient. Diagnosis, management and review of the world medical literature. Cancer 45: 1713

Bale PM (1984) Sacrococcygeal development abnormalities and tumours in children. Perspect Pediatr Pathol 1: 9

Bale PM, Parsons RE, Stevens MM (1983) Diagnosis and behaviour of juvenile rhabdomyosarcoma. Hum Pathol 14: 596

Bannayan GA, Huvos AG. D'Angio GJ (1971) Effect of irradiation on the maturation of Wilms' tumour. Cancer 27: 812

Bardi G, Johansson B, Pandis N, Békássy AN, Kullendorf C-M, Hägerstrand I et al. (1991) i(8q) as the primary structural chromosome abnormality in a hepatoblastoma. Cancer Genet Cytogenet 51: 281

Bardi G, Johansson B, Pandis N, Heim S, Mandhal N, Békássy A, Hägerstrand I, Mitelman F (1992) Trisomy 2 as the sole chromosomal abnormality in hepatoblastoma. Genes Chromosome Cancer 4: 78

Becker LE, Hinton D (1983) Primitive neurectodermal tumours of the central nervous systems. Hum Pathol 14: 538

Beckwith JB (1993) Precursor lesions of Wilms' tumour: clinical and biological implications. Med Pediatr Oncol 21: 158

Beckwith JB (1994) Renal neoplasms in childhood. In: Sternberg SS (ed) Diagnostic surgical pathology, 2nd edn. Raven Press, New York, p 1741

Beckwith JB, Palmer NF (1978) Histopathology and prognosis of Wilms' tumour. Results from the First National Wilms' Tumour Study. Cancer 41: 1937

Beckwith JB, Perrin EV (1963) In-situ neuroblastomas: a contribution to the natural history of neural crest tumours. Arch Pathol 43: 1089

Bedford MA (1975) Treatment of retinoblastoma. Adv Ophthalmol

31: 2

Bennington JL, Beckwith JB (1975) Tumours of the kidney, renal pelvis and ureter. In: Atlas of tumour pathology, 2nd ser, Fasc 12. Armed Forces Institute of Pathology, Washington DC, p 33

Berry CL (1991) Embryonal tumours and genetic imprinting. Virchows Arch A Pathol Anat 419: 449

Berry CL, Keeling JW (1975) Genetic aspects of childhood cancer. In: Symington T, Carter RL (eds) Scientific foundations of oncology. Heinemann Medical, London

Berry, CL, Keeling JW, Hilton C (1969) Teratoma in infancy and childhood: a review of 91 cases. J Pathol 98: 241

Bhajekar AB, Joseph M, Bjat HS (1964) Unattached nephroblastoma. Br J Urol 36: 189

Bhangui GR, Roy S, Tandon PN (1977) Multiple primary tumours of the brain including a medulloblastoma in the cerebellum. Cancer 39: 292

Birch JM (1988) United Kingdom: Manchester Children's Tumour 1954–70 and 1971–83. In: Parkin DM, Stiller CA et al. (eds) International incidence of childhood cancer. IARC Scientific Publications no. 87. IARC, Lyon, p 299

Bolande RP (1971) Benignity of neonatal tumours and concept of cancer repression in early life. Am J Dis Child 122: 12

Bové KE, McAdam AJ (1976) The nephroblastomatosis complex and its relationship to Wilms' tumour. A clinicopathological treatise. Perspect Pediatr Pathol 3: 185

Bové KE, Koffler H, McAdam AJ (1969) Nodular renal blastoma, definition and possible significance. Cancer 24: 323

Bradley, JE, Drake ME (1949) The effect of preoperative roentgen-ray therapy on arterial hypertension in embryoma (kidney). J Pediatr 35: 710

Breatnach F, Androulakakis PA (1983) Renal papillary adenocarcinoma following treatment for Wilms' tumour. Cancer 52: 520

Breen JL, Neubecker RD (1963) Malignant teratoma of the ovary. An analysis of 17 cases. Obstet Gynecol 21: 699

Briard-Guillemot ML, Nonaiti-Pellie C, Feingold J, Frezal J (1974) Étude génétique du retinoblastome. Humangenetik 24: 271

Brodeur GM, Seeger RC, Schwab M, Yarmus HE, Bishop JM (1984) Amplification of N-myc in untreated human blastomas correlates with advanced disease stage. Science 224: 1121

Brodeur GM, Seeger RC, Barrett A et al. (1988) International Criteria for diagnosis, staging and response to treatment in patients with neuroblastoma. J Clin Oncol 6: 1874

Brodeur GM, Pritchard J, Berthold F, Carlsen NLT, Castel V et al. (1993) Revisions of the International Criteria for neuroblastoma diagnosis, staging, and response to treatment. J Clin Oncol 11: 1466

Brown DH (1966) The clinico-pathology of retinoblastoma. Am J Ophthalmol 61: 508

Buckley JD, Sather H, Ruccione K, Rogers PCJ, Haas JE, Henderson BE, Hammond GD (1989) A case–control study of risk factors for hepatoblastoma. Cancer 64: 1169

Byrne JA, Smith PJ (1993) The 11p15.5 ribonucleotide reductase M 1 subunit. Hum Genet 41: 275

Canalis RF, Jenkins HA, Hemenway WG, Lincoln C (1978) Nasopharyngeal rhabdomyosarcoma. Arch Otolaryngol 104: 122

Carney JA (1975) Wilms' tumour and renal cell carcinoma in retroperitoneal teratoma. Cancer 35: 1179

Carney JA, Thompson DP, Johnson CL, Lynn HB (1972) Teratomas in children: clinical and pathologic aspects. J Pediatr Surg 7: 271

Chretien PB, Milam JD, Foote FW, Miller TW (1970) Embryonal adenocarcinomas (a type of malignant teratoma) of the sacrococcygeal region. Clinical and pathologic aspects of 21 cases. Cancer 26: 522

Claireaux AE (1951) An intraperitoneal teratoma in a newborn infant. J Pathol Bacteriol 63: 743

Claireaux AE, Keeling JW (1973) Teratomas in children. Arch Dis Child 48: 159 (abstract)

Clarke MA, O'Connell KJ (1973) An ultrastructural study of embryonal rhabdomyosarcoma (sarcoma botryoides) of the bladder. J Urol 109: 897

Clatworthy HW, Schiller M, Grosfeld JL (1974) Primary liver tumours in infancy and childhood. Arch Surg 109: 143

Clausen N, Garwics S, Glomstein A, Jonmundsson G, Kruus S, Yssimg M (1990) Medulloblastoma in Nordic children. 1. Acta Paediatr Scand Suppl 371: 5

Cochran W, Froggatt P (1967) Bilateral nephroblastoma in two sisters. J Urol 97: 216

Czeizel A, Gárdonyi J (1974) Retinoblastoma in Hungary 1960–1968. Humangenetik 22: 153

de Chadarévian JP, Fletcher BD, Chatten J, Rabinovitch HH (1977) Massive infantile nephroblastomatosis. A clinical, radiological, and pathological analysis of four cases. Cancer 39: 2294

Dehner L (1986) Peripheral and central primitive neuroectodermal tumours. A nosologic concept seeking a consensus. Arch Pathol Lab Med 110: 997

Dito WR, Batsakis JG (1962) Rhabdomyosarcoma of the head and neck. Arch Surg 84: 582

Dryja TP, Mukai S, Petersen R, Rappaport JM, Walton D, Yandeell DW (1989) Parental origin of mutations of the retinoblastoma gene. Nature 339: 556

Ellsworth RM (1969) The practical management of retinoblastoma. Trans Am Ophthalmol Soc 67: 462

Evans DGR, Farndon PA, Burnell LD, Gattarmaneni HR, Birch JM (1991) The incidence of Gorlin syndrome in 173 consecutive cases of medulloblastoma. Br J Cancer 64: 959

Feusner JH, Krailo MD, Haas JE, Campbell JR, Lloyd DA, Ablin AR (1993) Treatment of pulmonary metastases of initial stage I hepatoblastoma in childhood. Report from the Children's Cancer Group. Cancer 71: 859

Fleming S, Symes CE (1987) The distribution of cytokeratin antigens in the kidney and in renal tumours. Histopathology 2: 157

Friend SH, Bernards R, Rogelj S, Weinberg RA, Rapaport JM, Albert DM, Dryja TP (1986) A human DNA segment with properties of the gene that predisposes to retinoblastoma and osteosarcoma. Nature 323: 643

Fujita S (1967) Quantitative analysis of cell proliferation and differentiation in the cortex of the post-natal mouse cerebellum. J Cell Biol 22: 277

Garaventor A, de Bernardi B, Pianca C, Donfrancesco A, Cordero di Montezemolo L et al. (1993) Localized but unresectable neuroblastoma: treatment and outcome of 145 cases. J Clin Oncol 11: 1770

Gardiner MJ, Snee MP, Hall AJ, Powell CA, Downes S, Terrell JD (1990) Results of a case–control study of leukaemia and lymphoma among young people near Sellafield nuclear plant in West Cumbria. Br Med J 423: 9

Gauthier F, Valayer J, Thai BL, Sinico H, Kalifa C (1986) Hepatoblastoma and hepatocarcinoma in children: analysis of a series of 29 cases. J Pediatr Surg 21: 424

Gilbertson RJ, Jaros EB, Perry RH, Pearson ADJ (1992) Prognostic factors in medulloblastoma. Lancet 340: 480 (letter)

Goldberg-Stern H, Gadoth N, Stern S, Cohen IJ, Zaizov R, Sandbank U (1991) The prognostic significance of glial fibrillary acidic protein staining in medulloblastoma. Cancer 68: 568

Gonzalez-Crussi F, Upton MP, Maurer HS (1982) Hepatoblastoma: attempt at characterization of histologic subtypes. Am J Surg Pathol 6: 599

Gonzalez-Crussi F, Wolfson SL, Misugi K, Nakajima T (1984) Peripheral neurectodermal tumours of the chest wall in childhood. Cancer 54: 2519

Haas JE, Muczynski KA, Krailo M, Ablin A, land V, Vietti TJ, Hammond GD (1989) Histopathology and prognosis in childhood hepatoblastoma and hepatocarcinoma. Cancer 64: 1082

Haber DA, Park S, Maheswaran S, Englert C, Re GG, Hazen-Martin DJ, Sens DA, Garvin AJ (1993) WT-1 mediated growth suppression of Wilms tumour cells expressing a WT-1 splicing variant. Science 262: 2057

Hawkins E, Issacs H, Cushing B, Rogers P (1993) Occult malignancy in neonatal sacrococcygeal teratomas. Am J Pediatr Hematol Oncol 15: 406

Heideman RL, Haase GM, Foley CL, Wilson HL, Bailey WC (1985) Nephroblastomatosis and Wilms' tumour. Clinical experience and management of seven patients. Cancer 55: 1446

Hemmes GD (1931) Untersuchungen nach dem Vorkommen von Glioma retinae bei Verwandten von mit dieser Krankheit Behafteten. Klin Monatsbl Augenheikd 86: 331

Heys RF, Murray CP, Kohler HG (1967) Obstructed labour due to foetal tumours: cervical and coccygeal teratoma. Two case reports. Gynaecologia 164: 43

Hilton C, Keeling JW (1973) Neonatal renal tumours. Br J Urol 46: 157

Ho PT, Estroff JA, Kozakewich H, Shamberger RC, Lillehei CW et al. (1993) Prenatal detection of neuroblastoma: a ten-year experience from the Dana-Farber Cancer Institute and Children's Hospital. Pediatrics 92: 358

Horn RC Jr, Enterline HR (1958) Rhabdomyosarcoma: clinicopathological study and classification of 39 cases. Cancer 11: 181

Huddart SN, Muir KP, Parkes S, Mann JR, Stevens MCG et al. (1993a) Neuroblastoma: a 32-year population-based study – implications for screening. Med Pediatr Oncol 21: 96

Huddart SN, Muir KR, Parkes SE, Mann JR et al. (1993b) Retrospective study of prognostic value of DNA ploidy and proliferative activity in neuroblastoma. J Clin Pathol 46: 1101

Hughson MD, Hennigar GR, Othersen HB (1976) Cytodifferentiated renal tumours occurring with Wilms' tumours on the opposite kidneys. Am J Clin Pathol 66: 376

Innes MD (1970) Possible genetic basis of childhood neoplasia. Med J Aust 2: 187

Innes MD (1972a) Nephroblastoma, possible index tumour of childhood. Med J Aust 1: 18

Innes MD (1972b) Hereditary theory of childhood oncogenesis. Oncology 26: 474

Ishak KG, Gluntz PR (1967) Hepatoblastoma and hepatocellular carcinoma in infancy and childhood. Cancer 20: 396

Ito J, Johnson WW (1969) Hepatoblastoma and hepatoma in infancy and childhood. Light and electron microscopic studies. Arch Pathol 87: 259

Izant RJ, Filston HC (1975) Sacrococcygeal teratomas. Analysis of forty-three cases. Am J Surg 130: 617

Joshi VV (1979) Cystic partially differentiated nephroblastoma: an entity in the spectrum of infantile renal neoplasia. In: Rosenberg HS, Bolande RP (eds) Perspectives of pediatric pathology. 5. Masson, New York, p 217

Joshi VV, Beckwith JB (1989) Multilocular cyst of the kidney (cystic nephroma) and cystic, partially differentiated nephroblastoma: terminology and criteria for diagnosis. Cancer 64: 466

Joshi VV, Cantor AB, Altshuler G, Larkin, Neill JSA et al. (1992) Age-linked prognostic categorization based on a new histologic grading system of neuroblastomas: a clinicopathologic study of 211 cases from the Pediatric Oncology Group. Cancer 69: 2197

Joshi VV, Cantor AB, Brodeur GM, Look AT, Shuster JJ et al. (1993) Correlation between morphologic and other prognostic markers of neuroblastoma: a study of histologic grade, DNA index, N-myc gene copy number, and lactic dehydrogenase in patients in the pediatric oncology group. Cancer 71: 3173

Kadin ME, Rubenstein LJ, Nelson JS (1970) Neonatal cerebellar medulloblastoma originating from the fetal external granular layer. J Neuropathol Exp Neurol 29: 583

Kaneko Y, Kanda N, Maseki N et al. (1990) Current urinary mass screening for catecholamine metabolites at 6 months of age may be detecting only a small portion of high risk neuroblastomas: a chromosome and N-myc amplification study. J Clin Oncol 8: 2005

Kar S, Jaffe R, Carri RI (1993) Mutation at coda 249 of p53 gene in human hepatoblastoma. Hepatology 18: 566

Keeling JW (1971) Liver tumours in infancy and childhood. J Pathol 103: 69

Keeling JW (1993) Fetal hydrops. In: Keeling JW (ed) Fetal and neonatal pathology, 2nd edn. Springer-Verlag, London, p 253

Keeling JW (1994) Fetal pathology. Churchill Livingstone, Edinburgh, p 88

Kingston JE, Herbert A, Draper GJ, Mann JR (1983) Association between hepatoblastoma and polyposis coli. Arch Dis Child 58: 959

Kinnier Wilson LM, Draper GJ (1974) Neuroblastoma, its natural history and prognosis: a study of 487 cases. Br Med J iii: 301

Kitchin FD, Ellsworth RM (1974) Pleiotrophic effects of the gene for retinoblastoma. J Med Genet 11: 244

Klapproth H (1959) Wilms' tumour – a report of 45 cases and an analysis of 1351 cases reported in the world literature. J Urol 81: 633

Knudson AG Jr (1971) Mutation and cancer statistical study of retinoblastoma. Proc Natl Acad Sci USA 68: 820

Knudson AG Jr, Strong LC (1972) Mutation and cancer neuroblastoma and phaeochromocytoma. Am J Hum Genet 24: 514

Koop CE (1972) The neuroblastoma. In: Rickham PP, Hecker WC, Prevot J (eds) Progress in paediatric surgery. Urban and Schwarzenberg, Munich

Koufos A, Hansen MF, Copeland NG, Jenkins NA, Lampkin BC, Cavence WK (1985) Loss of heterozygosity in three embryontal tumours suggests a common pathogenetic mechanism. Nature 316: 330

Lakhoo K, Boyle M, Drake DP (1993) Mediastinal teratomas: review of 15 pediatric cases. J Pediatr Surg 28: 1161

Lawler W, Marsden HB (1979) Bone metastases in children presenting with renal tumours. J Clin Pathol 32: 608

Lee W-H, Murphree AL, Benedict WF (1984) Expression and amplification of the N-myc gene in primary retinoblastoma. Nature 309: 458

Leiger JF (1961) Botryoid sarcoma and rhabdomyosarcoma of the bladder: review of the literature and report of three cases. J Urol 86: 583

Lemerle J, Tournade MF, Gerard Marchant R, Flamant R, Sarrazin D, Flamant F, Lemerle M, Junt S, Zucker J-M, Schwisguth O (1976) Wilms' tumour: natural history and prognostic factors. A retrospective study of 248 cases treated at the Institut Gustave-Roussy 1952–1967. Cancer 37: 2557

Lennox EL, Draper GJ, Sanders BM (1975) Retinoblastoma: a study of natural history and prognosis of 268 cases. Br Med J iii: 731

Leong PK, Thorner P, Yeger H, Ng K, Zhang Z et al. (1993) Detection of MYCN gene amplification and deletions of chromosome 1p in neuroblastoma by in situ hybridization using routine histologic sections. Lab Invest 69: 43

Li EP, Fraumeni JF Jr (1969) Rhabdomyosarcoma in children: epidemiology study and identification of a familial cancer syndrome. J Natl Cancer Inst 43: 1365

Lindop G, Gleming S, Gibson AAM (1984) Immunocytochemical localisation of renin in nephroblastoma. J Clin Pathol 37: 738

Little M, van Heyyningen V, Hastie N (1991) Dads and disomy and disease. Nature 351: 609

Llombart-Bosch A, Lacombe MJ, Peydro-Olaya A, Perez-Bacete M, Contesso G (1988) Malignant peripheral neurectodermal tumours of bone other than Askin's neoplasm: characterisation of 14 new cases with immunocytochemistry and electron microscopy. Virchows Ach A Pathol Anat 412: 421

MacKinlay GA, Pritchard J (1992) A common language for childhood liver tumours. Pediatr Surg 7: 325

Makinen J (1972) Microscopic patterns as a guide to prognosis of neuroblastoma in childhood. Cancer 29: 1637

Malek RS, Kelalis PP (1979) Paratesticular rhabdomyosarcoma in childhood. J Urol 118: 450

Malone M (1993) Soft tissue tumours in childhood. Histopathology 23: 203

Mankad VN, Gray GF, Miller DR (1974) Bilateral nephroblastomasis and Klippel Trenaunay syndrome. Cancer 33: 1462

Marsden HB, Lawler W (1983) Primary renal tumours in the first year of life. Virchows Arch A Pathol Anat 399: 1

Mascarello JT, Jones MC, Kadota RP, Krous HF (1990) Hepatoblastoma characterized by trisomy 20 and double minutes. Cancer Genet Cytogenet 47: 243

Meadows AT, D'Angio GJ, Mike V, Banfi A, Harris C, Jenkin RDT, Schwartz A (1977) Patterns of second malignant neoplasms in children. Cancer 40: 1903

Merton DF, Yang SS, Bernstein J (1976) Wilms' tumour in adolescence. Cancer 37: 1532

Miller RW, Fraumeni JF Jr, Manning MD (1964) Association of Wilms' tumour with aniridia, hemihypertrophy and other congenital malformations. N Engl J Med 270: 922

Misugi K, Reiner CB (1965) A malignant true teratoma of liver in childhood. Arch Pathol 80: 409

Misugi K, Okajima H, Misugi N, Newton WA Jr (1967) Classification of primary malignant tumours of liver in infancy and childhood. Cancer 20: 1760

Morales AR, Fine G, Horn RC Jr (1972) Rhabdomyosarcoma: an ultrastructural appraisal. Pathol Annu 7: 81

Mottu D, Wyss M, Cox J, Paunoer L (1981) Nephroblastomatose et Tumeur de Wilms associées à une hemihypertrophie. Helv Paediatr Acta 46: 87

Moyson F, Maurus-Desmarex R, Gompel C (1961) Tumeur de Wilms mediastinale? Acta Chir Belg [Suppl] 2: 118

Murphy ASK, Vawter GS, Lee ABH, Jockin H, Filler RM (1980) Hormonal bioassay of gonadotrophin-producing hepatoblastoma. Arch Pathol Lab Med 104: 513

Nakagawara A, Ikeda K, Hayashida Y, Tsuneyoshi M, Enjoji M, Kawaoi A (1982) Immunocytochemical identification of human chorionic gonadotrophin and alfa-fetaprotein-producing cells of hepatoblastoma associated with precocious puberty. Virchows Arch A Pathol Anat 398: 45

Neblett CR, Waltz TA, Anderson DE (1971) Neurological involvement in the naevoid basal cell carcinoma syndrome. J Neurosurg 35: 577

Newton ER, Louis F, Dalton ME, Feingold M (1985) Fetal neuroblastoma and catecholamine-induced maternal hypertension. Obstet Gynecol 65: 495

Ng YY, Kingston JE (1993) The role of radiology in the staging of neuroblastoma. Clin Radiol 47: 226

O'Grady RB, Rothstein TB, Romano PE (1974) D-group deletion syndromes and retinoblastoma. Am J Ophthalmol 77: 40

Orlowski JP, Levin HS, Dyment PG (1980) Intrascrotal Wilms' tumour developing in a heterotopic renal anlage of probable mesonephric origin. J Pediatr Surg 15: 679

Orye E, Delbebe MJ, Vandenbale B (1974) Retinoblastoma and long arm deletion of chromosome 13: attempts to define the deleted segment. Clin Genet 5: 457

Pappo AS, Douglass EC, Meyer WH, Marina N, Parham DM (1993) Use of HBA 71 and anti-beta 2-microglobulin to distinguish peripheral neuroepithelioma from neuroblastoma. Hum Pathol 24: 880

Parker L, Craft AM, Smith J, Dickinson H, Wakeford R, Binks K, McElvenney D, Scoot L, Slovak A (1993) Geographical distribution of preconceptual radiation doses to fathers employed at the Sellafield nuclear installation, West Cumbria. Br Med J 307: 966

Penchansky L, Krause JR (1982) Acute leukemia following a malignant teratoma in a child with Klinefelter's syndrome. Case report and review of secondary leukemias in children following treatment of a primary neoplasm. Cancer 50: 684

Poon CCS, Lim SM, Hwang WS (1975) Congenital medulloblastoma. Singapore Med J 16: 230

Powell RW, Weber ED, Manci EA (1993) Intradural extension of a sacrococcygeal teratoma. J Pediatr Surg 28: 770

Prasad KN (1975) Differentiation of neuroblastoma cells in culture. Biol Rev 50: 129

Pugh R (1976) Pathology of the testis. Blackwell Scientific, Oxford, p 153, 205

Ramani P, Rampling D, Link M (1993) Immunocytochemical study of 12E7 in small round-cell tumours of childhood: an assessment of its sensitivity and specificity. Histopathology 23: 557

Redler LD, Ellsworth RM (1973 Prognosis importance of choroidal invasion of retinoblastoma. Arch Ophthalmol 90: 294

Reik W, Surani MA (1989) Genomic imprinting and embryonal tumours. Nature 338: 112

Reynolds CP, Perez-Polo JR (1975) Human neuroblastoma: glial induced morphological differentiation. Neurosci Lett 1: 91

Rubenstein LJ, Northfield DWC (1964) The medulloblastoma and the so-called arachnoid cerebellar sarcoma. Brain 87: 379

Sang DN, Albert DM (1982) Retinoblastoma: clinical and histopathological features. Hum Pathol 13: 133

Sapienza C, Tran TH, Paquette J, McGowan R, Peterson A (1989) A methylation mouse model for mammalian genome imprinting. Prog Nucleic Acids Re Mol Biol 36: 145

Saxena R, Leake JL, Shafford EA, Davenport M, Mowat AP, Pritchard J, Mieli-Vergani G, Howard ER, Spitz L, Malone M et al. (1993) Chemotherapy effects on hepatoblastoma. A histological study. Am J Surg Pathol 17: 1266

Schmid KW, Dockhorn-Dworniczak B, Fahrenkamp A, Kirchmair R et al. (1993) Chromogranin A, secretogranin II and vasoactive intestinal peptide in phaeochromocytomas and ganglioneuromas. Histopathology 22: 527

Schmidt D, Harms D, Lang W (1985) Primary malignant hepatic tumours in childhood. Virchows Archiv A Pathol Anat 407: 387

Schofield DE, Yunis EJ, Geyer JR, Albright AL, Berger MS, Taylor SR (1992) DNA content and other prognostic features in childhood medulloblastoma. Cancer 69: 1307

Schroeder WT, Chao LY, Dao DD, Strong LC, Pathak S, Riccardi V, Lewis HH, Saunders GF (1987) Non-random loss of maternal chromosome 11 alleles in Wilms tumours. Am J Hum Genet 40: 413

Sciot R, van Eyken P, Desmet VJ (1990) Transferrin receptor expression in benign tumours and in hepatoblastoma of the liver. Histopathology 16: 59

Scott J, Cowell J, Robertson ME, Priestly LM, Wadely R, Hopkins B, Pritchard J, Bell GI, Rall LB, Graham CF, Knott TJ (1985) Insulin-like growth factor-II gene expression in Wilms tumour and embryonic tissues. Nature 317: 260

Shafford EA, Pritchard J (1993) Extreme thrombocytosis as a diagnostic clue to hepatoblastoma. Arch Dis Child 69: 171 (letter)

Shearer P, Parham DM, Fontanesi J, Kumar M, Lobe TE, Fairclough D, Douglass EC, Wilimas J (1993) Bilateral Wilms' tumour. Review of outcome, associated abnormalities, and late efforts in 36 pediatric patients treated at a single institution. Cancer 72: 1422

Sheth KJ, Tang TT, Blaedel ME, Good TA (1979) Polydipsia, polyria, and hypertension associated with renin-secreting Wilms' tumour. J Pediatr 92: 921

Shimada H, Chatten J, Newton WA Jr, Sachs N, Hamoudi AB, Chiba HT, Marsden HB, Misugi K (1984) Histopathologic prognostic factors in neuroblastic tumours: definition of subtypes of ganglioneuroblastoma and an age linked classification of neuroblastomas. J Natl Cancer Inst 73: 405

Sorsby A (1962) Bilateral retinoblastoma. Br Med J ii: 580

Stambolis C (1977) Benign epithelial nephroblastoma, a contribution to its histogenesis. Virchows Arch A Pathol Anat 376: 267

Stiller CA (1993) Trends in neuroblastoma in Great Britain: incidence and mortality, 1971–1990. Eur J Cancer 29A: 1008

Suzuki T, Watanabe K, Ono T (1990) Immunohistochemical

demonstration of liver fatty acid-binding protein in human hepatocellular malignancies. J Pathol 161: 79

Taira Y, Nakayama I, Moriuchi A, Takajara O, Ito T, Tsuchiya R, Hirano T, Natsushita T (1976) Sarcoma botryoides arising from the biliary tract of children – a case report with review of the literature. Acta Pathol Jpn 26: 709

Tait DM, Eeles RA, Carter R, Ashley S, Ormerod MG (1993) Ploidy and proliferative index in medulloblastoma: useful prognostic factors? Eur J Cancer 29A: 1383

Teitelbaum D, Teich S, Cassidy S, Karp M et al. (1994) Highly vascularized sacrococcygeal teratoma: description of this atypical variant and its operative management. J Pediatr Surg 29: 98

Thiele CJ, Patrick Reynolds C, Israel MA (1985) Decreased expression of N-myc precedes retionoic acid-induced morphological differentiation of human neuroblastoma. Nature 313: 404

Touchida J, Ishizaki K, Sasaki S, Nakamura Y, Ikenaga M, Kato M, Sugimot M, Kotoura Y, Yamamuro T (1989) Preferential mutation of paternally derived RB gene as the initial event in sporadic osteosarcoma. Nature 338: 156

Tsokos M, Webber BL, Parham D et al. (1992) Rhabdomyosarcoma: a new classification scheme related to prognosis. Arch Pathol Lab Med 116: 847

Tucker OP, McGill CW, Pokorny WJ, Fernbach DJ, Harberg FJ (1986) Bilateral Wilms' tumour. J Pediatr Surg 21: 1110

Turkel S B, Itabashi HH (1974) The natural history of neuroblastic cells in the fetal adrenal gland. Am J Pathol 76: 225

van der May AGL, Maaswinkel-Mooy PD, Cornelisse CJ, Schmidt PH, van der Kamp JJP (1989) Genomic imprinting in hereditary glomus tumours: evidence for new genetic theory. Lancet ii: 1291

Voute PA, Wadman SK, Van Putten WJ (1970) Congenital neuroblastoma. Symptoms in the mother during pregnancy. Clin Pediatr 9: 206

Warburg M (1974) Retinoblastoma. In: Glodberg MF (ed) Genetic and metabolic eye disease. Little Brown, Boston

Ward S, Dehner LP (1974) Sacrococcygeal teratoma with nephroblastoma – a variant of extragonadal teratoma in childhood. Cancer 33: 1355

Webber BL, Parham DM, Drake LG, Wilimas JA (1992) Renal

tumors in childhood. Pathol Annu 1: 191

Weeks DA, Beckwith JB, Mierau GW (1990) Benign nodal lesions mimicking metastases from pediatric renal neoplasms. A report of the National Wilms' Tumour Study Pathology Center. Hum Pathol 21: 1239

Weidner N, Tjoe J (1994) Immunohistochemical profile of monoclonal antibody O13: antibody that recognizes glycoprotein p30/32[MIC2] and is useful in diagnosing Ewing's sarcoma and peripheral neuroepithelioma. Am J Surg Pathol 18: 486

Weinberg AG, Finegold MJ (1983) Primary hepatic tumours of childhood. Hum Pathol 14: 512

Werb P, Scurry J, Östör A, Fortune D, Attwood H (1992) Survey of congenital tumours in perinatal necropsies. Pathology 24: 247

Wigger HJ (1976) Fetal rhabdomyomatous nephroblastoma – a variant of Wilms' tumour. Hum Pathol 7: 613

Wijnaendts LCD, van der Linden JC, van Diest PJ, van Unnik AJM, Delemarre JFM, Voute PA, Meijer CJLM (1993) Prognostic importance of DNA flow cytometric variables in rhabdomyosarcomas. J Clin Pathol 46: 948

Wijnaendts LCD, van der Linden JC, van Unnik AJM, Delemarre JFM, Voute PA, Meijer CJLM (1994) Histopathological features and grading in rhabdomyosarcomas of childhood. Histopathology 24: 303

Williams DI, Schistad G (1964) Lower urinary tract tumours in children. Br J Urol 36: 51

Willis RA (1962) The pathology of the tumours of children. Oliver and Boyd, Edinburgh, p 57

Wright JH (1910) Neurocytoma or neuroblastoma, a kind of tumour not generally recognized. J Exp Med 12: 556

Yarborough SM, Evashnick G (1956) Case of teratoma of the liver with 14 years post-operative survival. Cancer 9: 848

Yasue M, Tomita T, Engelhard H, Gonzalez-Crussi F, McLone DG, Bauer KD (1989) Prognostic importance of DNA ploidy in medulloblastoma of childhood. J Neurosurg 70: 385

Young DG, Williams DI (1969) Malignant renal tumours in infancy and childhood. Br J Hosp Med 8: 74

Zhu X, Dunn JM, Phillips RA, Goddard AD, Paton KE, Becker A, Gallie B (1989) Preferential germline mutation of the paternal allele in retinoblastoma. Nature 340: 312

18 · Sudden Unexpected Infant Death

J.W. Keeling

Introduction

Sudden unexpected infant death (SUD) is a problem that regularly confronts any pathologist who performs necropsy examination on behalf of the coroner, procurator fiscal or medical examiner. Many of these deaths will remain unexplained even when all have been investigated in a thorough systematic way, and a wide variety of pathological abnormalities will be encountered (Byard and Cohle 1994). Routine examination of such infant deaths will include microbiological investigations as well as whole-body radiography, dissection of all viscera, including the brain, and histological examination of major organs. Samples of body fluids may also yield useful information. Recent experience suggests that in certain cases fresh frozen samples for possible toxicological examination should be kept until every aspect of the case has been considered, including a multidisciplinary case conference or review.

Sudden infant death syndrome (SIDS) is a conclusion reached only after perusal of a clinical history that yields no clues and a thorough, but negative, autopsy. Beckwith's (1970) definition, "the death of an infant or young child, which is unexpected by history and in whom a thorough necropsy examination fails to reveal the cause of death", is succint and has been useful in practice, although it introduces certain questions. How sudden is "sudden"? "Unexpected" by whom? What is a "thorough necropsy examination"? Some would now insist on negative death scene investigations: 20 years on, efforts to improve on this definition (Willinger et al. 1991) have put particular emphasis on examination of the circumstances surrounding the death.

The SIDS concept has been useful in two ways: it has removed blame and perhaps prevented excessive feelings of guilt in parents whose infants might previously have been certified as dying from asphyxia or inhalation of vomit, and it has removed a need for pathologists to fabricate a cause of death. (Many will be aware that "bronchopneumonia", "viral pneumonia" and similar terms were widely used, and made accurate assessment of the number of unexplained deaths impossible.) However, it is important not to stop thinking about a problem once it has been categorized, and the term "SIDS" may have outlived its usefulness: no-one dies from syndromes. I agree with Gilbert-Barness and Barness (1993) that its use should be discouraged and "sudden (unexplained) infant death" substituted, adding appropriate qualification(s) to encompass historical features and minor pathological findings.

Age at Death

The infant period extends from birth to the second birthday, and pathological findings in SUD are related both to age at death and to antecedent history. In the first month of life sudden death is not very common. Many of the infants who die suddenly at this time have ductus-dependent congenital heart disease, particulary mitral and aortic valve stenosis or atresia (hypoplastic left heart syndrome), but they will not always have a history suggestive of cardiac pathology. Both β-haemolytic streptococcal infection and echoviral infection are rapidly progressive in young babies and, although prior illness may be recognized, death occurs before a specific diagnosis is reached. In some deaths in this age group there is evidence of hypoxic cerebral injury of antepartum or intrapartum origin, but an immediate cause of death may not be apparent. Siderophages may be prominent in the lung, suggesting recurrent hypoxic episodes of presumed central origin.

Sudden deaths in infants over 1 year of age are infrequent, and the majority will be explained by investigation and autopsy. Most natural deaths in this age group result from infection. The possibility of accidental asphyxiation from foreign body inhalation should be borne in mind, and laryngoscopic examination before commencing dissection is useful.

The majority of SUDs occur in the age group 1 month to 1 year, peaking at 12–16 weeks, so that a clear majority occurs at 6 months or less. In this group the majority of deaths will be unexplained (SIDS), even though the number of unexplained deaths has fallen. In Scotland a fall of 40% has been observed in the 3 years since 1989 (Gibson 1992). A similar decrease has been observed in the rest of the UK, the Netherlands and New Zealand.

Particular care is required in the investigation of deaths in this age group. Emery and Taylor (1986) suggest that up to 20% may be non-natural deaths, about half being accidents, and that a thorough family and social history contribute important information. Properly conducted death scene investigations are thought to be essential by some workers (Bass et al. 1986; Byard et al. 1994).

Perimortem Events

Another way of looking at sudden infant deaths is to consider the perimortem circumstances. As with age at death, examination of perimortem events defines three groups (Berry and Keeling 1989):

1. Instantaneous death
   a) Cause obvious: accident or trauma
   b) Cause not apparent:
      i) Cardiac: malformations, coronary arteritis, myocarditis, cardiomyopathy, dysrhythmia
      ii) Respiratory: foreign body, laryngeal cyst
2. Rapid death: recognized illness
   a) Respiratory infections
   b) CNS infections
   c) Gastroenteritis
   d) Other infections
   e) Reye's syndrome
   f) CNS haemorrhage
   g) Congenital adrenal hyperplasia
3. Found dead in cot
   a) Congenital heart disease
   b) Respiratory infections

c) CNS infections
d) Septicaemia (e.g. meningococcal)
e) Intoxications
f) Seizure disorders
g) Suffocation and non-accidental injury
h) Unexplained (90%)

Infants who are observed to die without antecedent history make up a small group comprising both non-natural and natural deaths. The former are clearly defined by circumstances. The latter are likely to have upper respiratory pathology or cardiac abnormalities. The second group comprises those infants who are found dead in their cots. More than 80% of deaths in this group will be unexplained. The last group includes infants who die suddenly or collapse and subsequently die without regaining consciousness but have a history of illness, which is often nonspecific or minor. Many of these babies exhibit signs of significant disease, which constitute a cause of death.

Lack of History

The lack or paucity of clinical history in the majority of sudden infant deaths has exercised both clinicians and pathologists who are involved in this field. There are several possible explanations, all of which apply to some SUDs and deserve consideration by the pathologist before necropsy is begun. These include:

1. Rapid progression of illness during normal household sleeping hours, e.g. septicaemia, meningitis
2. Insidious onset of symptoms so that changes in infant health go unnoticed, e.g. total anomalous pulmonary venous drainage
3. Seriousness of symptoms not appreciated by carers, e.g. respiratory tract infection
4. Deliberately misleading history, e.g. non-accidental injury (NAI)
5. No significant symptoms (see Gilbert et al. 1990)

Investigation of Sudden Infant Death

Necropsy examination of infants dying unexpectedly is usually undertaken on behalf of the coroner, procurator fiscal or public examiner. There is a pressing need to distinguish between natural and non-natural death. This distinction is usually made on the basis of external examination and gross dissection of the organs. There follows a more detailed examination, which is open-ended in terms of the number of investigations that may be carried out. It is important to identify investigations that yield useful information at reasonable cost, and a standing arrangement whereby some microbiological samples are obtained in casualty or on arrival in the mortuary is worth considering (Wigglesworth et al. 1987). Other, similar, guidelines for the investigation of SUD are published by the Royal College of Pathologists (1993) and Valdés-Dapena et al. (1993).

It is important that a consistent approach to the investigation of SUD is adopted and that the same investigations are done in every case. Pathologists who are *not* prepared to spend considerable amounts of time on these cases should not undertake them. When a second SUD occurs in a family – or in a family which has suffered an unexplained neonatal death – it is important to involve a paediatric pathologist at the outset. Detailed time-consuming investigations are almost inevitable in these circumstances, and special expertise is necessary.

The diagnosis of NAI requires a high index of suspicion on the part of the pathologist. Despite the wide publicity given to child abuse in both the medical and the lay press, clinicians may accept the parent's account of accidental injury at face value and omit essential investigations. Parents may attempt to pass off NAI as a cot death (Macauley and Mason 1977).

Necropsy Investigations

Studies Within 12 Hours of Death

In many instances children found dead or moribund are taken to accident and emergency departments after discovery. Many have a routine for dealing with these cases, which may include sampling of cerebrospinal fluid, radiography and other investigations. It is important that the pathologist be informed of these procedures and receive copies of any reports.

Where practical, heart blood should be taken for culture in addition to cerebrospinal fluid, and a search for respiratory or enteropathic viruses and bacteria made on postnasal and rectal swabs.

Routine whole body radiographs are recommended in the investigation of SUD. Should there be the slightest suspicion of child abuse, a radiological skeletal survey is essential before the necropsy examination is begun. An informed radiologist's opinion on the adequacy of the views obtained is important, and a report prior to autopsy is desirable: it may help in deciding on the approach to examining a particular region and which bones to remove for histological examination (Fig. 18.1).

Standard Necropsy Study

A thorough external examination must be made, with measurement of weight and length and assessment of nutritional status. It is necessary to look for bruises, abrasions and burns, and to pay particular attention to their distribution, also noting the general standard of cleanliness and extent of any nappy rash. Photographs of skin lesions and sketches of their distribution are useful adjuncts to the written report and are helpful in court. The mouth and tongue should be carefully examined for laceration or abrasions, and the conjunctivae inspected for petechial haemorrhages.

Vitreous humour can be a useful source of a reliable measurement of glucose if taken within 12 h; sodium and urea determination may help in assessing dehydration (the globe can be easily refilled with water after aspiration at the outer canthus with a fine needle). This examination is contraindicated when NAI is suspected, and instead the eyes should be removed for examination after fixation and histological examination, particularly if abnormalities have been seen on ophthalmoscopic examination during life.

Examination of viscera follows the method described in Chapter 1. Organ weights are recorded. Evidence of trauma as well as disease is sought. Cardiac dissection follows an established pattern to detect congenital heart disease. It is important to investigate the cardiac conduction system when there has been a previous sudden infant death, but such investigation is seldom fruitful unless electrophysiological studies have been carried out or structural defects of the heart exist. Samples of liver and urine are useful for toxicology and investigation of genetic metabolic disease (GMD).

The amount and appearance of gastric contents should be carefully noted. A sample can be kept frozen short-term. Evidence of rib fractures should be sought after evisceration of the thorax, because anterior and lateral fractures are difficult to visualize radiologically (Fig. 18.2), as is damage to the costochondral junction. The brain should always be fixed before examination. This is the only way to ensure constant sampling for evaluation of appropriateness of myelination and other features dependent on postnatal maturation, in utero ischaemic injury and accurate evaluation of any traumatic injury.

Routine samples for histological evaluation are:

1. Respiratory tract
   a) Epiglottis
   b) Larynx
   c) Trachea
   d) Main bronchii
   e) Lungs – four major lobes

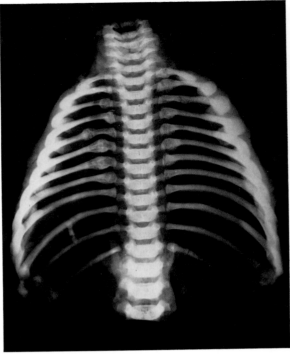

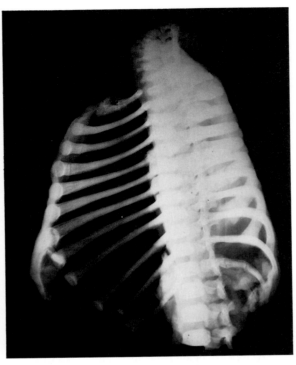

Fig. 18.1. Rib cage with multiple fractures of the ribs on both sides. Fractures of ribs 6–8 have the most prominent callus formation, and the fracture line is obliterated, suggesting that these are of longer duration than the fractures on the left.

Fig. 18.2. (Same case as in Fig. 18.1.) This view shows recent fracture of rib 1.

2. Cardiovascular system
   a) Left atrium–ventricle
   b) Interventricular septum (with related left and right ventricles)
3. Alimentary system
   a) Salivary glands
   b) Duodenum/head of pancreas
   c) Jejunum
   d) Ileum (with Peyer's patch)
   e) Liver
4. Reticuloendothelial system
   a) Thymus
   b) Spleen
   c) Mesenteric node
5. Endocrine system
   a) Adrenal
   b) Thyroid – with trachea
6. Renal tract
   a) Kidneys – one block of each
7. Central nervous system
   a) Meninges – with inferior surface of cerebellum
   b) Frontal lobe – with centrum semiovale
   c) Corpus callosum, head of caudate and ependyma

8. Skeletal system
   a) Costochondral junction (rib 5 or 6)
   b) Psoas muscle, longitudinal and transverse sections
9. Frozen sections for fat
   a) Liver
   b) Kidney
   c) Heart
   d) Skeletal muscle

In cot deaths, the respiratory tract is a frequent site of significant pathology and requires extensive sampling: the laryngeal block should include the vocal cord (Fig. 18.3).

Histological examination of bruises and other skin lesions should be made, for evidence of vital reaction and assessment of the age of the lesion. Fractures should be removed en bloc with generous margins; specimens of bone are also needed from sites away from the injury, to exclude bone disease and leukaemia. The appearance of the costochondral junction is a useful marker of duration and severity of prexisting illness (Sinclair-Smith et al. 1976). The

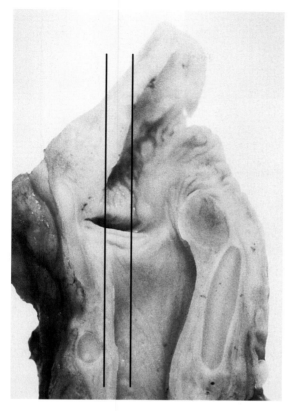

Fig. 18.3. A vertical block through the middle of the vocal cord is an informative and easily reproducible sample.

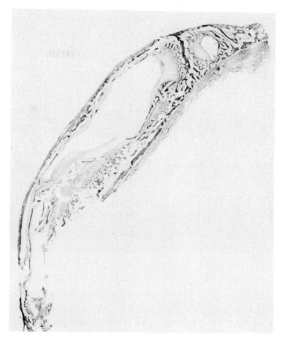

Fig. 18.4. Organizing cephalohaematoma from the parietal bone in SUD. Its presence raised suspicion of non-accidental injury. (Reproduced from Keeling 1987)

extracellular matrix of the cartilage is normal (Byard et al. 1993).

Fibroblast cultures for metabolic studies and storage of fibroblast lines are justified when there are features in the history or necropsy suggestive of metabolic disease or where there has been a previous unexpected death. However, defects of lipid metabolism are readily overlooked, and it is worthwhile including routine lipid stains on liver and kidney in all cases.

Necropsy Findings

Inappropriate Interpretation of Incidental Findings

The presence of gastric contents is a common finding in infant deaths of all causes. The mere act of moving a baby after death when sphincters are lax is sufficient to eject gastric contents into the œsophagus and pharynx. Attempts at resuscitation, whether by parents or health care professionals, are likely to displace gastric contents into large airways and intrapulmonary bronchi, where it is readily seen in histological sections, often with focal bacterial overgrowth. In the past, this has been interpreted as aspiration and therefore the cause of asphyxial death. It has been the cause of much parental anguish. Before a diagnosis of gastric aspiration is seriously entertained, there must be evidence of vital reaction to the inhaled material. It is more convincing if there is evidence of previous aspiration, and particularly if there is clinical evidence of neuromuscular dysfunction.

Residual changes of birth injury, usually minor and inconsequential, are encountered among infant deaths. An organizing cephalohaematoma gives rise to irregular hard swelling, usually over the parietal bone (Fig. 18.4), and may arouse suspicion about NAI. Most are not accompanied by fracture of the underlying bone. Cephalohaematomas are not an indication of difficult delivery. The majority occur in spontaneous vertex deliveries. When a fracture coexists with cephalohaematoma, it is single and linear, running from the sagittal suture line down towards

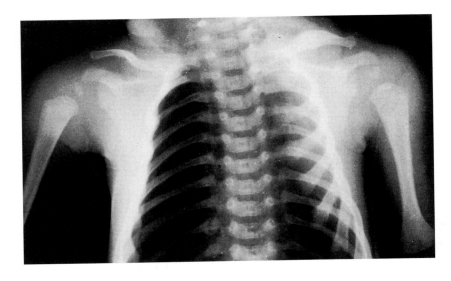

Fig. 18.5. Callus round a fracture of the right clavicle results in thickening of the bone. SUD at 8 weeks; fracture consistent with birth injury.

the ear. Other birth injuries to recognize are fracture of the clavicle (Fig. 18.5) and of long bones. Clavicular fracture is more likely in large babies (does the mother have diabetes?), and femoral fractures usually complicate breech delivery in preterm deliveries or when there is postural deformity (it may be necessary to see obstetric or neonatal case notes). These injuries will usually have been recognized in the neonatal period and show signs of healing appropriate to the age of the baby.

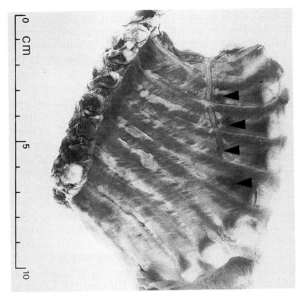

Fig. 18.6. SUD at 12 weeks. Resuscitation at home and in the casualty department. Fractures of ribs 3–6 are accompanied by minimal subperiostial haemorrhage, suggesting infliction after death.

Brown or yellow staining of the dura lining the middle or posterior fossa is sometimes seen as the result of organization of a small subdural haemorrhage, an inconsequential birth injury. The stage of organization should be consistent with the infant's postnatal age, and the extent of the lesion small (1–2 cm diameter). Occasionally, ribs are fractured during attempts to resuscitate the baby. Such fractures usually involve several ribs in a linear fashion (Fig. 18.6) and are accompanied by minimal subperiosteal haemorrhage. The perpetrator is usually aware of inflicting injury during attempted resuscitation.

Explosive desquamation of bronchial and bronchiolar epithelium has been described in cot deaths (Bodian and Heslop 1960) and interpreted as the result of infection. Most pathologists now regard this as post-mortem artefact. Another inconsequential pulmonary finding is an isolated granuloma, probably the result of a single minor gastric aspiration (Valdés-Dapena et al. 1993).

Explained Infant Deaths

Accidental Deaths

Fatal accidental injuries are uncommon in young infants but undoubtedly occur. It is important that a clear, preferably corroborated, account of the accident is available before necropsy is begun. The injuries should fit the explanation given. Major incidents, such as road traffic accidents (RTAs) rarely pose a problem for the pathologist. Of more difficulty are asphyxial deaths involving beds or cradles and bedding (Moore et al. 1993). When clothing has become caught and

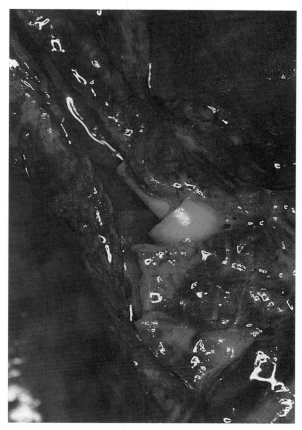

Fig. 18.7. Opened upper airway. A small plastic toy component is lodged in the right main bronchi.

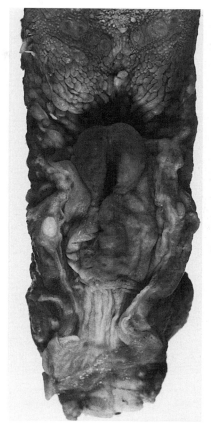

Fig. 18.8. *H. influenzae* epiglottitis. There is marked swelling, with obstruction of the laryngeal inlet.

acted as a ligature, fine cutaneous petechial haemorrhages are frequently found distributed cranial to the line of constriction.

Deaths of infants taken into bed with parents can be difficult to evaluate. Ingestion of alcohol or recreational drugs by parents should be investigated, and toxicological investigations should be performed on the baby.

Asphyxia due to laryngeal impaction of food or a foreign body is more common in infants who have achieved some degree of mobility (Fig. 18.7), but the possibility of objects being "fed" to babies by young siblings should not be forgotten.

Natural Deaths

Explanations for death are more likely to be found in infants whose death is instantaneous or rapidly follows a recognized illness than among the much larger group of infants who are found dead in their cots. Although a wide variety of diseases may be encountered, respiratory and cardiac pathology are particularly important in this context.

Respiratory Pathology. Epiglottitis is less common in infants than in older children but does occur in this age group. Respiratory obstruction of acute onset is usual. The epiglottis is red and swollen, clearly obstructing the laryngeal inlet (Fig. 18.8).

The best sample for bacteriological examination is tissue fluid from the epiglottis. The whole syringe should be despatched for culture.

Laryngeal cyst is an uncommon cause of upper airways obstruction (Fig. 18.9), and laryngeal papillomas are a further cause (Fig. 18.10). Lower respiratory infection, particulary viral bronchiolitis, is a well recognized cause of sudden death in infants. Apnoeic episodes are frequent in bronchiolitis, and infants require hospital admission when the diagnosis is made. Bronchopneumonia is also encountered in sudden deaths occurring in symptomatic infants. The

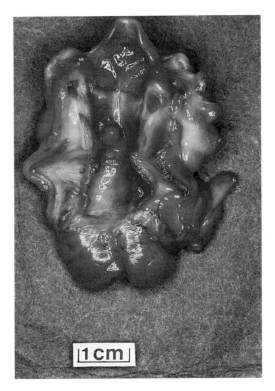

Fig. 18.9. Male aged 16 weeks: respiratory symptoms for 4 weeks, followed by sudden death. There are mucus-filled cysts below the vocal cords.

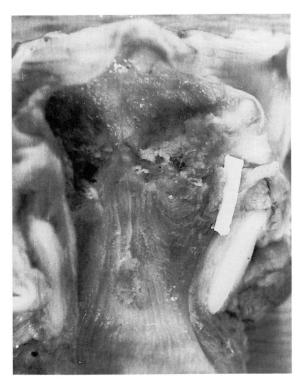

Fig. 18.10. Laryngeal papilloma (*R*). The dark area (*L*) is the result of laser diathermy of a similar lesion.

rapidity of progression of respiratory infection in babies should not be underestimated.

Cardiac Pathology. Congenital structural malformations are the commonest form of cardiac abnormality encountered among sudden infant deaths. They are not, however, representative of congenital heart disease (CHD) in general; some types are more commonly encountered in these circumstances. In infants <1 month of age, ductus-dependent lesions are usual, particularly variants of hypoplastic left heart. In older infants, aortic valve stenosis, total anomalous venous drainage and subendocardial fibroelastosis are the usual lesions (Valdés-Dapena 1983; James et al. 1994).

Cardiac conduction system abnormalities are also encountered in SUD. They can occur in anatomically normal hearts or may accompany structural defects, such as large ventricular septal defects. Involvement of conduction tissue in the fibrosing edge of a (previously closing) ventricular septal defect, producing sequential heart block and then sudden death, is recorded (Smith and Ho 1994).

Anomalous origin of the coronary arteries is associated with SUD. When the left coronary artery arises from the pulmonary artery (Lalu et al. 1992), subendocardial fibroelastosis of the left ventricle is usual, as well as fibrosis or infarction of the myocardium. When both coronary arteries arise from the same aortic sinus, sudden death appears to be related to the course of the anomalous vessel when it runs between the aorta and pulmonary trunk or with the interventricular septum (Herrmann et al. 1992). Lipsett et al. (1994) describe a range of coronary artery anomalies. Half of their 35 cases died suddenly.

Myocarditis is a cause of sudden deaths in both the neonatal and the postneonatal periods (De Sa 1985; Smith et al. 1992). Affected babies are usually symptomatic, but symptoms may be of short duration (< 12 h) and non-specific. Myocarditis can also occur as part of a generalized infective illness. It is important to remember that the heart is often grossly normal, although pallor, hypertrophy, congestion and endocardial fibrosis are described (Smith et al. 1992). Histological changes are often focal, so that generous sampling (both ventricles and the interventricular septum) are recommended (Smith et al. 1992).

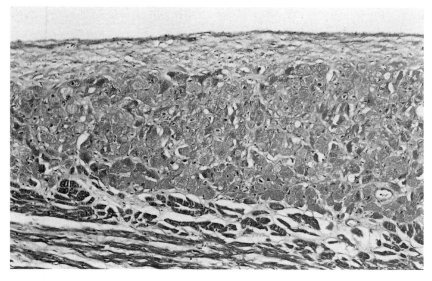

Fig. 18.11. Histiocytoid cardiomyopathy: myocytes beneath a thickened endocardium are enlarged with foamy cytoplasm. (Courtesy: Professor P.J. Berry , Bristol)

Histiocytoid cardiomyopathy has been described in SUD (Suarez et al. 1987). Although sometimes recognized at necropsy as pale yellowish foci in the myocardium, diagnosis is usually made histologically (Fig. 18.11). It is seen in both normal and malformed hearts. Rhabdomyomas are also described in SUD, although perhaps more often recognized as a fetal or neonatal cause of arrhythmia and heart failure. Fibromas, usually protruding into a ventricular chamber (Fig. 18.12), are another cardiac cause of sudden death in early life.

Other Causes of Death. Most other pathology encountered in SUD is infectious. Septicaemia and/or meningitis, particularly due to group B β-haemolytic streptococcal infection, is not rare in neonates, and this and meningococcal infection after this period may be rapidly fatal, producing little macroscopic change. In infants, the petechial rash of *N. meningitidis* may be sparse, and adrenal haemorrhage is neither common nor specific to this infection.

Non-accidental injury

Most fatal non-accidental injuries (NAIs) occur in the infant age group, and parents may offer a story of sudden collapse and attempted resuscitation or cot death.

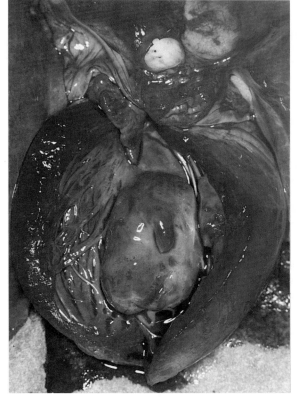

Fig. 18.12. Sudden death in a female aged 2 months. A fibroma arising from the interventricular septum protrudes into the right ventricular cavity.

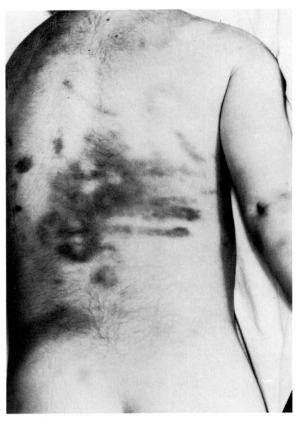

Fig. 18.13. Bruising of the back. The situation and linear characteristics of the bruising make accidental injury unlikely.

Table 18.1. Types of injury in abused children

	Smith and Hanson (1974)	Lauer et al. (1974)	Cameron et al. (1966)
Number of cases	134	130	29
Died	21	6	29
Permanent damage	20	NK	NK
Battered previously	72	57	26
Battered sibling	31	NA	7
Bruises	110	92	Most
Burns or scalds	23	16	?
Skull fractures	37	29	20
Subdural haemorrhage	30	11	20
Abdominal injury	26	3	7
Long-bone fractures	71	19	11
Rib fractures	20	19	14

NA, not assessed; NK, not known.

External Findings. Evidence of poor hygiene in the form of dirty ears and flexures, dirty uncut nails and extensive nappy rash may be present. This is not invariable and some infants appear to have been well cared for. Body weight is often low; this is often ascribed to neglect, but in view of the frequency of rib fractures (present in almost half the cases seen by Cameron et al. 1966), unwillingness to feed because of pain is likely.

Serious congenital defect is more frequent among abused children (7.5% of Smith and Hanson's 1974 cases, compared with 1.5% in the general population).

Bruises are the commonest form of injury (Table 18.1). The bruises of non-accidental injury are characteristically flat without any overlying skin abrasion, but their distribution betrays their origin (Roberton et al. 1982). Bruises made by gripping tightly so as to shake the infant show a single large discolouration corresponding to the thumb, which can be matched with a line of smaller bruises caused by finger tips a few inches away. Characteristic sites of bruising are the face, particularly over the eye, the zygomatic arch, or the mandible, with smaller bruises on the opposite side. Finger bruises matching a thumb mark over the mandible may merge into one indistinct bruise on the neck (Cooper 1975). Sets of bruises can be matched by colour, and bruises of different ages are often present.

When the trunk has been gripped tightly in shaking there will usually be a large bruise on either side of the midline, usually one higher than the other, with matching fingertip bruises on the opposite side of the trunk. A hand imprint may be visible on the buttock from slapping. Striking the body with a hard object may leave an impression with a pattern that can be matched to the object (Fig. 18.13); sharp edges or protruberances will cause superimposed abrasions. Fingertip bruises may be seen on the limbs, particularly around the elbow and knee, if the infant has been grasped and thrown into its cot or against a hard object (Cameron 1972).

The difference in distribution of bruises resulting from accidents and those deliberately inflicted are documented in children of different ages by Roberton et al. (1982). They found that accidental injury commonly resulted in lower leg bruising and was most frequently seen in 4- and 5-year-olds, whereas non-accidental injuries were most frequently seen on the face or head and between 10 months and 3 years of age.

Human bites are usually identified as two crescentic rows of small bruises that become confluent. They can be distinguished from self-inflicted bites by the inaccessibility of site and disparity of size (Sims et al. 1973). They can be matched to the dentition by forensic dental experts.

Burns and scalds are commonly inflicted injuries. Serious thermal injury was present in almost one-fifth of cases seen by Smith and Hanson (1974) and 12.5% of those seen by Lauer et al. (1974). Minor burns

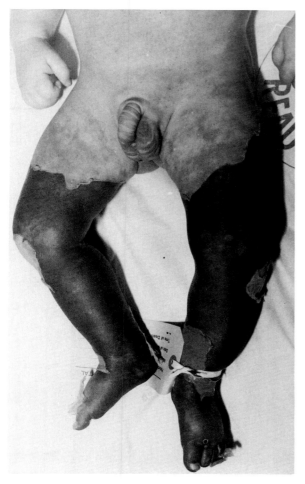

Fig. 18.14. Dip scalds in an infant. Most of the epidermis has detached. Petechial haemorrhages are present over the trunk and lower limbs. (Courtesy of the Chief Constable, Oxfordshire)

were present in other cases. Burns of the buttock and perineum caused by placing the child on a hot surface are described by Smith and Hanson (1974) and Keen et al. (1975), who pointed out that burned and scalded children tended to be older than the rest of their battered children; they advise caution in accepting an accidental explanation of such injury in older children. The dorsum of the hand, buttocks, legs and feet are sites of non-accidental thermal injury observed by Hobbs (1986). The proffered explanation of pulling a pan of hot liquid off a high surface should be rejected if the submental region and axilla are spared from injury. "Dip" scalds to hands and feet are unlikely to be accidental in the absence of splash scalds further up the limbs (Keen et al. 1975) (Fig. 18.14).

Yeoh et al. (1994) looked for differences between accidental and non-accidental scald injuries from bathwater among children admitted to a burns unit. They found that forced injuries were severe, symmetrical and had a clearer distinction from adjacent normal skin. They drew attention to the presence of associated injuries and an implausible history.

Circular burns from cigarettes are sometimes seen, and lesions of different ages may be found; this type of injury suggests premeditated insult (Simpson 1973).

Bruising of the scalp is often difficult to demonstrate at necropsy, when the telltale tenderness on palpation of the scalp, which makes such lesions apparent clinically, is lacking. Deep bruising is more easily seen after reflection of the scalp.

Bruising and abrasions of the gums may be the result of thrusting a bottle or fist into the mouth of a crying infant. A torn frenulum is regarded as pathognomonic of non-accidental injury (Cameron et al. 1966).

Black eyes are a common form of injury. These are caused by a fist or hard object being thrust into the orbit. The history is usually of an accident, but this is much more likely to cause supraorbital bruising unless there is concomitant fracture of the roof of the orbit. Bilateral orbital bruises do not result from a single accident (Cooper 1975). Bruising of the ear may be present, often accompanied by petechial haemorrhages in the surrounding skin.

Petechial haemorrhages may be present in the conjunctivae. Ocular manifestations range from transient retinal haemorrhages accompanying subdural haematoma to subhyaloid, vitreous and gross retinal haemorrhages (Fig. 18.15) and retinal detachment leading to extensive scarring and optic atrophy producing blindness (Mushin 1971).

Visceral Injury. Visceral injuries result from direct blows to the abdomen. Surface bruising may be absent in cases of serious, even fatal, visceral injury. Rupture of the liver is frequently fatal. Perforation of the small bowel, particularly the duodenum because of its relative immobility, and tearing of the mesentery are also seen (Fig. 18.16). Liver damage was seen in 19% and injury of the duodenum, pancreas or mesentery in 15% of fatal cases recorded by Camps (1969). A high incidence of liver injury in fatal cases is reported by several authors (Cameron et al. 1966; Smith and Hanson 1974). Rupture of the heart may occur in cases in which the chest is jumped on (C.L. Berry, personal communication).

Cranial Trauma. Intracranial haemorrhage and cerebral injury may be the result of blunt trauma to the head or the effect of violent shaking when the head is unsupported. Natural disease, other than complications of prematurity, arteriovenous malformations or

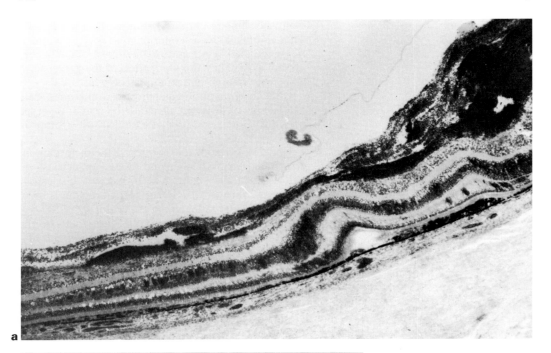

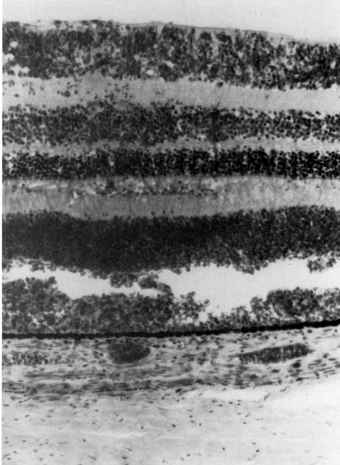

Fig. 18.15. Vitreous (**a**) and subhyaloid (**b**) bleeding after repeated blows to the eye in an 18-month-old boy. (H&E, **a** × 30, **b** × 120) (Courtesy of Professor C.L. Berry)

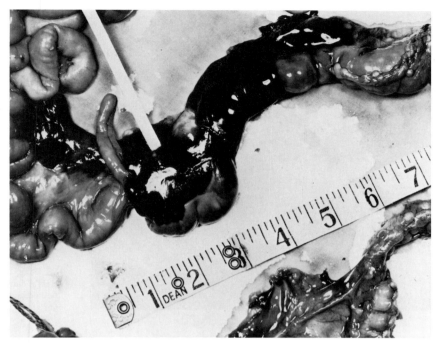

Fig. 18.16. Mesenteric haemorrhage following deliberate injury.

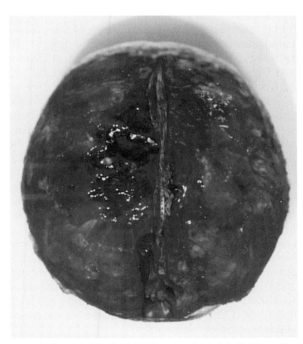

Fig. 18.17. Four-month-old infant, interior of skull. There is a thin confluent layer of subdural haemorrhage over both sides of the skull vault and blood clots on the right side close to the falx.

tumour, is unlikely to be the cause of serious intracranial haemorrhage in the first year of life (Billmire and Myers 1985).

Direct trauma to the head is often accompanied by skull fractures (see below) but, because of the pliability of infant skull bones, fractures are not always present. Extradural and subdural haemorrhage are often localized beneath a fracture site.

Intracranial haemorrhage is found in infants in the absence of skull fractures. Acceleration–deceleration injury results from violent shaking. There is extensive subdural haemorrhage with both fluid blood and blood clot on the surface of the cerebrum. Subdural haemorrhage caused by shaking is usually bilateral (Fig. 18.17) (Caffey 1974; Benstead 1983). The brain rapidly becomes oedematous, with ischaemic injury in survivors. Cerebral ischaemic injury can be seen in histological sections within days of injury (Table 18.2). After several weeks, macroscopic lesions are apparent (Fig. 18.18).

Fractures. Fractures are the commonest injury after bruises (see Carty 1993 for review). Characteristically, multiple fractures of different ages are present. The presence of a predisposing disorder to account for multiple fractures must be offered in

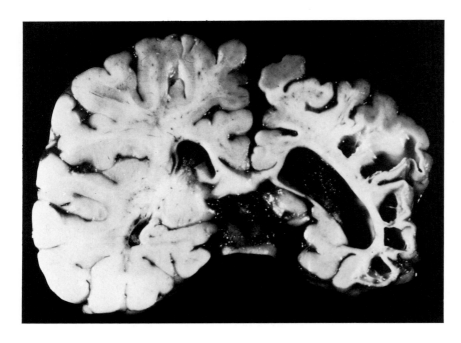

Fig. 18.18. Severe longstanding cerebral damage in a repeatedly injured child. From a female aged 15 months.

Table 18.2. Timing of histological changes following ischaemic injury in the fetal and neonatal brain

Change	Timing
Macrophages	
Microglial proliferation	3 h to 3 days
Macrophages	4–5 days
Macrophages with phagocytosis	4–6 days
Astrocytes	
Astrocyte proliferation	12 h to 4 days
Astrocytes, cytoplasmic processes	3–11 days
Astrocyte fibrillary gliosis	6 days
Capillaries	
Endothelial swelling	1–3 days
Endothelial reduplication	5 days
Other	
Coagulation necrosis	3 h
Retraction balls	3 h
Neuronal karyorrhexis	12–48 hours
Mineralization	8–14 days
Cysts	14–42 days

From Squier (1993) with permission of the author and publisher.

court. It is useful to remember that copper deficiency is likely only in particular clinical circumstances and has non-skeletal manifestations such as hypopigmentation, prominent scalp veins and hepatosplenomegaly as well as osteoporosis (Shaw 1988). Normal plasma copper and caeruloplasmin levels will exclude the diagnosis. Mild osteogenesis imperfecta is another proffered explanation for fractures. Here, fractures are not seen until the toddler stage and usually in the diaphysis of long bones. Wormian bones are almost invariably present in the skull. Dentinogenesis imperfecta may be found in erupted teeth (Carty 1988).

The pathologist may be asked to give an opinion on the age of a fracture on histological appearances. It is important to remember that the rate of healing is age dependent and very rapid in babies (Chapman 1992), and that repeated injury provokes exuberant callus formation. A comprehensive review of the radiological dating of fractures is that of O'Connor and Cohen (1987). The skull is the commonest site of fracture; skull fractures were present in 29% of Smith and Hanson's (1974) cases and 22.3% of the patients described by Lauer et al. (1974). Long-bone fractures are next in frequency, all long bones being affected with almost equal frequency. Ribs are the third most frequent site of fracture (Table 18.1). Recent fractures can be seen radiologically. Callus formation around the fracture, seen radiologically from about the eighth day, can be of considerable help in dating fractures. The periostium is not so firmly attached to the bone in infants as in adults, and shearing injury may be followed by subperiosteal bleeding, with subperiosteal new bone formation producing a "double contour" of long bones (Silverman 1953). Traumatic fragmentation of the metaphysis of long bones with subsequent joint deformity has been described (Caffey 1957). Bones of the wrists, hands and feet are rarely damaged.

Skull fractures resulting from accidental injury are usually single, linear and involve the parietal bone. Those resulting from abuse are more likely to be multiple or complex, depressed and non-parietal, or involve several bones. Fractures having a width greater than 3 mm and growing fractures suggest abuse (Hobbs 1984).

Helfer et al. (1977) documented the injuries in 246 children under 5 years of age who had fallen from beds, sofas or hospital examination couches. Only seven had serious injuries: three skull fractures, three fractured clavicles, and one humeral fracture. No child had serious intracranial haemorrhage or other life-threatening injury. Levene and Bonfield (1991) reviewed 781 accidental injuries to children on hospital wards. Most were falls from a height, slipping or forceful contact with ward furniture. Only three injuries were serious. These studies are useful when examining the relationship between proffered history and observed injuries.

Other Forms of Abuse. Poisoning as a form of non-accidental injury should not be overlooked. The drug may be anything to which the parent has access: fenformin, diuretics and common salt have been reported in this connection, in addition to the commonly used sedatives and tranquillizers (Rogers et al. 1976). Rogers et al. called attention to bizarre symptoms, signs and biochemical values and the frequency of neurological symptoms at presentation. There were two deaths among their six cases, and three had a dead sibling. The episodic nature of the illness, with recurrence on returning home or following access by the mother to the child in hospital, and suspicious injury or illness in siblings are points to seek out; suspicions are confirmed by isolation of the poison.

Alcohol intoxication in children is usually accidental and self-administered. Forced alcohol administration as a form of child abuse is described by Grubbauer and Schwarz (1980).

Nixon and Pearn (1977) describe immersion in the bath as a form of child abuse. In one of their cases the child had been injured previously and in another the child died later with skull fractures. They distinguish non-accidental immersion from accidental drowning in the bath in that abused children are older, of all social classes, likely to be handicapped, the eldest in the family, in the bath alone and at an odd time of day, and with a high proportion of personality defects in the parents. Accidental drowning, however, is usually a cause of death in the youngest of a large family of low social class (several being bathed together in the evening), together with a high incidence of family crises.

Imposed upper airways obstruction may present as a cyanotic attack, unprovoked collapse or sudden unexpected death. Multiple episodes are usual, and one-third of siblings may have experienced similar episodes (Samuels et al. 1992).

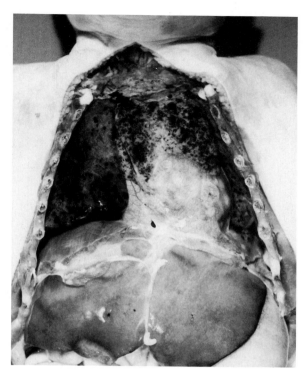

Fig. 18.19. SUD. Many petechiae are present within the thymus and beneath the pleura of both lungs. The liver is enlarged and acutely congested.

Findings in Cot Deaths

Although cot deaths are, by definition, unexplained, there are nevertheless abnormalities present at necropsy. These comprise evidence of minor disease and other findings, which may shed light on the mechanisms by which death occurs in these babies, and must be explained by theories about causation. A cogent argument for investigating all deaths in the infant age group in a standard fashion, whether they are hospital or home deaths, is an awareness of patterns in the occurrence of minor pathological abnormalities.

Molz et al. (1992) found an excess of minor anomalies such as hernias, ectopias, adrenal neuroblastomas and angiomas among unexplained deaths, compared with explained ones.

The most consistent findings in SIDS cases are within the thorax (Fig. 18.19). The thymus is normal, or slightly reduced, in size and there are petechial haemorrhages in its thoracic, but rarely its cervical, part (Beckwith 1988). The lungs are bulky and fill the chest. They are firm and do not collapse with finger pressure. Petechial haemorrhages beneath the visceral

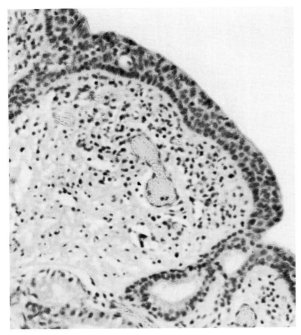

Fig. 18.20. SUD at 16 weeks. Parainfluenza virus isolated; metaplasia of upper airways epithelium with round-cell infiltration of adjacent connective tissue.

pleura, and indeed throughout the lungs, are a frequent finding. When the lungs are sliced they maintain their shape, and blood-tinged fluid exudes from the surface on pressure. There may be 1–2 ml of serous fluid in the pericardial sac. Petechiae are often present along the course of the coronary arteries. They are occasionally widespread beneath the epicardium.

The epithelium of larynx, trachea and main bronchi is often congested and may be deep purple and thickened. A little clear or slightly turbid fluid is often present in the peritoneal cavity. Peyer's patches are often prominent, and mesenteric lymph nodes are enlarged.

The brain is swollen, with flattening of the tops of gyri. Occasionally, brain swelling is more severe, with protrusion of cerebellar tonsils through the foramen magnum. Leptomeninges are usually congested. It is rarely possible to distinguish between meningitis and massive congestion in these infants on naked-eye examination. A diagnosis of meningitis depends on organism isolation and histological evidence of inflammation. The appearance of pus and diffuse venous thrombosis takes several days to develop. Venous sinus thrombosis is occasionally seen in dehydrated infants.

On histological examination, the thymus may be normal, or may show a minor cortical lymphocyte

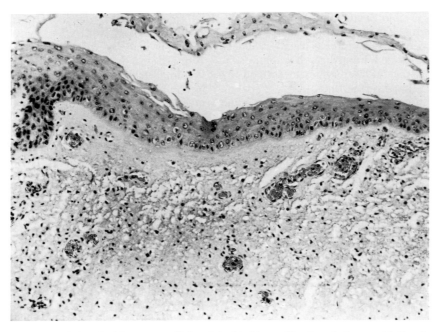

Fig. 18.21. A 12-week-old male infant, "cold, runny nose", found dead in his cot. Vocal cords: intact epithelium basement membrane thickening with eosinophilic amorphous material beneath the basement membrane and scanty round-cell infiltration of underlying structures. (H&E, × 180)

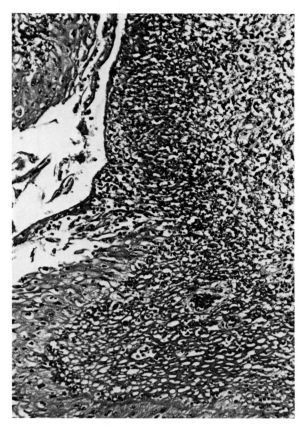

Fig. 18.22. A 16-week-old female infant, "perfectly well", unexpectedly found dead. Extensive inflammatory cell infiltration of vocal cords and larynx, with epithelial destruction and fibrin deposition. (Martin's scarlet blue, × 240)

depletion with reduction in cortical width and the appearance of histiocytes within the cortex, the "starry-sky" appearance of the thymus. In some cases large numbers of histiocytes are present in the cortex, usually associated with a marked reduction in cortical width.

In the upper airways, round-cell or mixed inflammatory cell infiltration is frequently present in the nasal septum, epiglottis, larynx and trachea, decreasing in severity in the lower parts of the airways. This may be accompanied by epithelial changes; ulceration and regeneration may both be present, particularly in respiratory syncytial virus and parainfluenza virus infection (Fig. 18.20).

Histological abnormalities of the vocal cords are a frequent findings in SIDS, and range from basement membrane thickening with minor round-cell infiltration of the epithelium and deeper structures (Fig. 18.21) to ulceration of the epithelium with underlying necrosis and acute inflammatory cell infiltration (Fig.

18.22). Shatz et al. (1991) have suggested that laryngeal membrane thickening is pathognomonic of cot death, but although it is most frequent in these deaths, it may also be present in "explained" infant deaths.

The commonest finding on histological examination of the lungs is oedema. There is diffuse interstitial oedema and an alveolar exudate which may be focal or confluent (Herbert and Andrews 1979). The alveolar walls are diffusely thickened, with a slight increase in round cells within the walls.

Peribronchial and peribronchiolar round-cell infiltration are often present and sometimes extensive, although inflammatory exudate within the airways is scanty. Lymphoid aggregates, some with well formed germinal centres, are seen and have been interpreted as evidence of past respiratory infection (Emery and Dinsdale 1974).

In the heart, minor subendocardial fibroelastic thickening is sometimes present, usually in the left ventricle, although its significance is not clear. Focal interstitial round-cell infiltration of the myocardium is often seen. Fu et al. (1994) report a paucity of nerve fibres in the atrioventricular node and bundle of His in five of seven cases using an immunohistological technique. They did not examine the whole of the conduction system.

Within the liver, small foci of erythropoiesis are often present. Fatty infiltration of hepatocytes, particularly around portal tracts, is a common finding. More extensive steatosis (Fig. 18.23) raises the possibility of a defect of fatty acid metabolism (Howat et al. 1985); fatty infiltration of myocardium and kidney should be sought as corroborative evidence and attempts made to reach a specific diagnosis either biochemically or using specific genetic markers.

Lipid depletion from the definitive adrenal cortex is common. Pérez-Platz et al. (1994) found focal lipid depletion in 92% of their cases. Iron deposition is often present, but this is merely the sequel of normal postnatal degeneration of the fetal cortex.

Histological abnormalities in the brain include focal ischaemia (Takashima et al. 1978a), brain stem gliosis (Takashima et al. 1978b) and rosettes of ependymal cells beneath the ventricular lining (Fig. 18.24). Displaced ependyma may be accompanied by gliosis and is the result of past ischaemic insult or low-grade infection.

Focal round-cell infiltration around epithelial tubules with intranuclear cytomegalovirus inclusions is present in the parotid and kidney of some infants.

Pathogenesis of Unexplained Infant Death

Theories concerning the aetiology of cot death are legion (see reviews by Valdés-Dapena 1967, 1977,

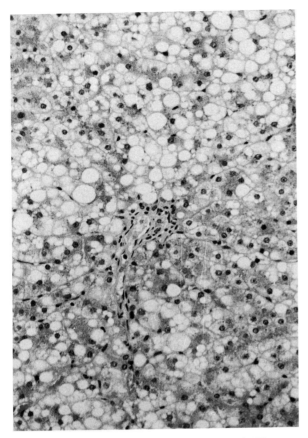

Fig. 18.23. SUD at 8 weeks. Massive hepatic steatosis. There was extensive fatty change in the heart and kidneys. Probable defect of fatty acid metabolism.

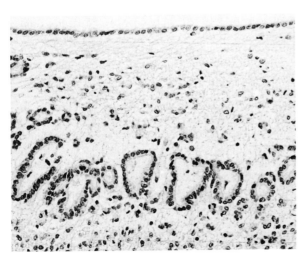

Fig. 18.24. SUD at 12 weeks. Linear arrangement of rosettes of ependymal cells below the ependymal lining of a lateral ventricle.

1980; Krous 1984; Limerick 1992), but it seems certain that there is no single cause for death in these infants, although the mode of dying may be the same in many cases. When it was usual practice to take the infant into its parents' bed, many of these deaths were ascribed to overlying. "Status thymolymphaticus" was a fashionable theory, but it became apparent that the enlarged thymus, supposed to cause death by extrinsic respiratory obstruction, was the norm.

Finding petechial haemorrhages in thoracic viscera has given rise to a number of hypotheses for SIDS involving upper airways obstruction. The suggestion that these infants have a narrower larynx than normal, making them more vulnerable to obstruction by secretions during upper respiratory infections, has been disproved by careful dissection (Beckwith 1970). Choanal atresia has also been discounted by systematic observation of the posterior nares. Accidental smothering by pillows and bed clothes is unlikely in normal circumstances (Woolley 1945), as is the possibility that a healthy infant may suffocate by lying prone; even a neonate is capable of adjusting his or her head to maintain an adequate airway. The possibility of non-accidental suffocation cannot be discounted if a soft object such as a pillow is used, but it is unlikely that this accounts for many deaths.

Several theories such as epidural haemorrhage, adrenal insufficiency, congenital leukaemia and absence of hypoplasia of the parathyroid glands can be refuted by careful necropsy examination; furthermore, it is evident from embryological considerations (see p. 628) that significant parathyroid abnormality is unlikely to occur in the presence of a normal thymus.

The possibility of cows' milk protein hypersensitivity (Parish et al. 1960; Coombs and McLaughlan 1982) has attracted a lot of attention, and gained support from the low incidence of breast feeding observed in some epidemiological studies (Carpenter 1972). Other studies have not demonstrated any difference in feeding practice between SIDS infants and the control group when social class (Fedrick 1974) or standards of housing (Watson et al. 1981) are taken into account. There has been a large increase in the number of mothers breast feeding over the past 15 years, which has not been accompanied by a comparable decrease in unexplained infant deaths. Evidence for cows' milk protein hypersensitivity from immunological studies has been conflicting. Turner et al. (1975) found elevated levels of IgE antibodies to bovine β-lactoglobulin, housedust mite and *Aspergillus fumigatus* in SIDS victims, but Clark et al. (1979) and Mirchandani et al. (1984) did not.

Unspecified immunological abnormality has been put forward as a possible cause of sudden infant death, but Warnasuriya et al. (1980) found evidence of atopy in half the parents of infants dying unexpectedly and a similar frequency among parents of controls. Immunohistological studies of mast cells and eosinophil numbers and distribution in SIDS support the theory of antigenically provoked terminal events (Howat et al. 1994). This group is currently pursuing a number of related studies.

A relationship between infant immunization programmes was proposed after reports of unexpected deaths following diphtheria–pertussis–tetanus immunization (Stewart 1979). No association between triple vaccine and unexpected infant death has been demonstrated (Taylor and Emery 1982; Bernier et al. 1984; Knowelden et al. 1984).

A role for viral infection in the aetiology of some unexpected deaths has been supported by increasingly successful viral isolation, particularly from the respiratory tract (Uren et al. 1980), and histological evidence of inflammation in the respiratory tract (Scott et al. 1978). The viral isolates in SUD are often as prevalent in the community at the same time, but Williams et al. (1984) found a higher incidence of respiratory syncytial virus (RSV) in infants over the age of 3 months who died suddenly than in younger unexpected deaths or the local community as a whole. An allergic response to a second encounter with RSV protein was suggested as a possible mechanism for death in infants who clearly did not have an overwhelming respiratory infection (Gardner et al. 1970), but the apnoea-provoking potential of minor respiratory infections is well recognized (Mitchell et al. 1983; Williams et al. 1984). Viral nucleic acids have been demonstrated more often in SIDS cases than controls by in situ hybridization (An et al. 1993). This method may be useful in the investigation of the role of viral proteins as antigens. Localization of α-interferon in brain stem nuclei in SIDS is further support for a causal role for infection (Howatson 1992) and suggests a possible mechanism.

A role for bacterial toxins has been suggested (Morris et al. 1987). This theory relates the age distribution of deaths to the decline in passively transferred maternal antibody, viral respiratory infection and postnatal parental smoking as factors that modify nasopharyngeal bacterial carriage. Drucker et al. (1991) have demonstrated sinergy between staphylococcal and *E. coli* toxins and an excess of *E. coli* nasopharyngeal carriage in SIDS victims. Blackwell et al. (1992) suggest that Lewis [a] antigen, which is expressed in the buccal epithelial cells of Lewis non-secretors, may act as a receptor site for *Staphylococcus aureus*, enhancing the possibility of toxin absorption. High endotoxin core antigen levels in younger cot deaths may point to unusually early or severe exposure to endotoxin (Oppenheim et al. 1994).

Clostridium botulinum or its toxin have been found in the intestine or spleen in SUD (Arnon et al. 1978; Sonnabend et al. 1985). Nigro et al. (1983) reported *Legionella pneumophila* in infants and children without pneumonia and speculate that it may cause some cot deaths.

James (1968) postulated that remodelling of the cardiac conducting system may result in an unstable conduction system so that minor disturbances could give rise to arrhythmias and atrioventricular block. This suggestion has prompted ECG studies on the relatives of SIDS victims and screening programmes of infants in the neonatal period. Kukolich et al. (1977), in a controlled study of 108 subjects from the immediate family of 26 cot deaths, found no difference in the length of the Q–T interval between family members and controls. Southall et al. (1977) obtained ECG recordings on 2030 selected infants in the neonatal period, and found arrhythmias or other conduction abnormalities in 35 (1.8%). Abnormalities persisted for periods from 1 week to more than 28 weeks, although only one infant required treatment. The same group (Keeton et al. 1977) described six "near miss" SIDS cases who had abnormalities of the conducting system; these were interpreted as evidence of a relationship between conduction system abnormalities and cot death.

Most unexpected deaths occur during sleep, and Steinschneider's (1972) suggestion that an exaggeration of the episodes of apnoea that normally occur during sleep in both infants and adults might play a part in sudden infant death has resulted in a number of investigations into the regulation of respiration in infants and neonates and the mechanisms of production of apnoea at this age. Shannon et al. (1977) investigated ventilation and response to carbon dioxide in "aborted" SIDS infants and controls, and found that hypoventilation occurred during quiet sleep and that the response to carbon dioxide was impaired. Three of these infants later died during sleep at home. Milner et al. (1977) looked at the response of neonates and infants to total airway obstruction. They observed periodic respiration and were able to inhibit respiratory efforts on 15 occasions in preterm infants but not in full-term babies. They suggest that this mechanism of respiratory inhibition might be important in the production of SIDS, not only among preterm infants but also in those who have upper respiratory tract infections. Apnoeic episodes are described during both lower and upper respiratory tract infections in infants (Mitchell et al. 1983). Kelly et al. (1980) demonstrated an increase in periodic breathing in siblings of SIDS victims compared with controls.

Prolonged apnoea has been produced in newborn lambs by the introduction of "foreign" fluid into the larynx (Johnson et al. 1972). Respiration was abolished if water, an acid solution, or cows' milk was introduced into the entrance of the larynx in tracheostomized lambs, but ewes' milk or amniotic fluid had no effect on respiration. Reflex inhibition of respiration, initiated by laryngeal chemoreceptors, was abolished by superior laryngeal nerve section. Inhibition was age-dependent and did not occur in older animals. It is tempting to speculate that the regurgitation of acid gastric contents in the human infant might produce a similar effect.

A number of studies have looked for evidence of chronic or repeated hypoxia. Naeye (1973) found smooth-muscle hypertrophy and hyperplasia in the media of small pulmonary arteries of SIDS victims compared with non-hypoxic controls. He suggested that the most likely mechanism is repeated apnoeic episodes or chronic alveolar hypoventilation (see also Williams et al. 1979). Kendeel and Ferris (1977) were unable to demonstrate any difference between the media of small pulmonary arteries and arterioles compared with non-hypoxic and acutely hypoxic controls.

The status of the other potential markers of chronic hypoxaemia is still contentious. An increase in the proportion of brown fat in periadrenal adipose tissue has been described in chronic hypoxaemic states in adults (Teplitz and Lim 1974), although Heaton (1972) found great variability from site to site in the same individual. Naeye (1974) describes a higher percentage of brown fat (cells with a reticular infrastructure) in the periadrenal fat of SIDS cases and infants with cyanotic congenital heart disease than in non-hypoxic controls. Emery and Dinsdale (1978) could not confirm this finding.

The role of the carotid body as a chemoreceptor that maintains the oxygen tension of systemic arterial blood is well documented. An increase in the weight and volume of the carotid bodies of humans and a variety of animals living at high altitudes and of laboratory animals living in conditions simulating such a habitat have been described (Arias-Stella 1969; Laidler and Kay 1975). If infants who die unexpectedly have been chronically hypoxic, one would expect an increase in both variables. Dinsdale et al. (1977) estimated volumes of carotid bodies in SIDS victims and controls and found wide variation in both groups. They found that carotid body volumes were increased in only a few unexplained deaths over 1 year of age. Naeye (1976) found, somewhat surprisingly, that the carotid bodies of SIDS victims were smaller than those of controls. Elevated vitreous hypoxanthine levels in the vitreous humour of cot death babies are described (Rognum et al. 1988) and interpreted as evidence of chronic hypoxia. Subsequently Carpenter et al. (1993) investigated the

effect of increasing death-to-autopsy interval on cerebrospinal fluid and vitreous hypoxanthine levels, and after suitable correction for this time interval were not able to confirm Rognum's findings.

A variety of cerebral lesions have been described in infants dying unexpectedly. Gadston and Emery (1976) describe the perivascular accumulation of fat-laden macrophages in the corpus callosum, which they attribute to hypoxia-induced demyelination. However, Esiri et al. (1990), who compared SIDS cases with chronically hypoxic and non-hypoxic controls, also looked at the postconceptional age of the three groups and concluded that such changes were part of normal developmental processes.

Takashima et al. (1978a) describe an increase in subcortical or periventricular leucomalacia in SIDS victims and in infants with congenital heart disease. They found that the site of the lesion was age dependent, and suggested that the lesions were hypoxic in origin. Such damage may be the result of acute rather than chronic hypoxia. Similar periventricular lesions are clearly related to documented discrete hypoxic episodes in neonates.

Naeye (1976) found an abnormal proliferation of astroglial fibres in the brain stems of 14 of 28 infants dying unexpectedly who were compared with non-hypoxic controls. Increased gliosis in the respiratory control area of the brain stem has been identified in SIDS victims (Takashima et al. 1978b). Chigr et al. (1992) describe an increased density of neurotensin binding sites in SIDS, constituting an immature pattern in their experience. This might be expected to compromise both cardiorespiratory and arousal control.

Defects of fatty acid metabolism, particularly medium-chain acyl-coenzyme A dehydrogenase deficiency, can present as unexpected infant death (Howat et al. 1985; Anonymous 1986). Panlobular fatty change was found in 14 of 200 consecutive unexpected deaths (Howat et al. 1985), and enzyme estimation successfully undertaken on frozen liver from some of their cases enabled the specific defect to be identified. Fatty infiltration of heart and kidney was also present. Subsequent studies have not demonstrated such high levels of β-oxidation defects in sudden unexpected death (Holton et al. 1991). Lundemose et al. (1994) suggest that the incidence of β-oxidation defect in SIDS is no greater than in the general population. The author's experience is that fatal cases of β-oxidation defect (particularly MCAD) are older than typical cot deaths and have a significant (though short) history of illness and often a family history of infant death.

The roles of chronic carbon monoxide poisoning (Cleary 1984) and overheating (Staton 1984) in the pathogenesis of cot death have been vigorously disputed (Sturner 1985). However, work from Bristol identifies overwrapping and viral infection as independent risk factors for SIDS (Fleming et al. 1990). Heat stress, via increased energy consumption, can produce direct rapid effects on the respiratory centre and may thus be an important factor in cot death (Fleming et al. 1993). If changes in composition of surfactant contribute to some cot deaths (Morley et al. 1982), they clearly do not act in the same manner as in hyaline membrane disease in neonates. This change may be secondary to bacterial phospholipase A2 activity (James et al. 1990).

Although the incidence of hypernatremic dehydration has fallen as a cause of unexpected infant death (Sunderland and Emery 1979; Arneil et al. 1985), minor dehydration is still common, particularly in infants with evidence of gastrointestinal or respiratory tract infection (Herbert and Andrews 1979) in cases I have investigated.

Richardson (1990) postulated that cot deaths were due to toxic gases released as a result of microbial contamination and subsequent breakdown of the plastic covering of cot mattresses. The suggestion caused a great deal of public anxiety, was very carefully investigated (Department of Health 1991a; Kelley et al. 1992) and has been shown to be without foundation.

Prone sleeping position had been shown to be associated with cot death (Fleming et al. 1990). This sleeping position was advocated as a way of minimizing the probably fictitious hazard of inhalation of gastric contents. Subsequent parental advice, the Back to Sleep Campaign, (Department of Health 1991b) has reduced cot deaths by about 50% in the UK, after similar reductions had been described in the Netherlands (de Jonge et al. 1993), New Zealand (Mitchell et al. 1992) and the USA. The mechanism of the protective effect of supine sleeping position is not understood. One possibility is easier arousal in the supine position. The importance of the head's surface area in temperature control in infants should not be forgotten; covers over the face are easier to repel then those encroaching on the back of the head.

From the vast number of theories of the aetiology of SIDS, it is clear that we are far from solving the problem. However, as evidence from epidemiological studies accumulates and pathological changes are documented in many organs it seems very unlikely that there is any one cause of cot death. It is probable, furthermore, that in any individual case many different factors are involved, including minor illness, the internal and external environment, developmental processes and past insults. In future, we may be able to recognize more of the factors involved and so understand their complex and potentially fatal interrelationships.

References

An SF, Gould S, Keeling JW, Fleming KA (1993) Role of respiratory viral infection in SIDS: detection of viral nucleic acid by in situ hybridization. J Pathol 171: 271

Anonymous (1986) Sudden infant death and inherited disorders of fat oxidation. Lancet ii: 1073

Arias-Stella J (1969) Human carotid body at high altitudes. Am J Pathol 55: 82a

Arneil GC, Gibson AAM, McIntoch H, Brooke H et al. (1985) National post-perinatal infant mortality and cot death study, Scotland 1981–82. Lancet i: 740

Arnon SS, Midura TF, Damus K, Wood RM, Chin J (1978) Intestinal infection and toxin production by *Clostridium botulinum* as one cause of sudden infant death syndrome. Lancet i: 1273

Bass M, Kravath RE, Glass L (1986) Death-scene investigation in sudden infant death. N Engl J Med 315: 100

Beckwith JB (1970) Introduction: discussion of terminology. In: Bergmann AB, Beckwith JB, Ray CG (eds) Sudden infant death syndrome. University of Washington Press, Washington DC, p 18

Beckwith JB (1988) Intrathoracic petechial hemorrhages: a clue to the mechanism of sudden infant death syndrome? Ann NY Acad Sci 533: 37

Benstead JG (1983) Shaking as a culpable cause of subdural haemorrhage in infants. Med Sci Law 23: 242

Bernier RH, Dondero TJ, Lammer E (1984) DTP immunization and SIDS. J Pediatr 105: 169

Berry PJ, Keeling JW (1989) The investigation of sudden unexpected death in infancy. In: Anthony PP, McSween RNM (eds) Recent advances in histopathology, Churchill Livingstone, Edinburgh, p 251

Billmire ME, Myers P (1985) Serious head injury in infants: accident or abuse? Pediatrics 75: 340

Blackwell CC, Saadi AT, Raza MW, Stewart J, Weir DM (1992) Susceptibility to infection in relation to SIDS. J Clin Pathol 45 (suppl): 20

Bodian M, Heslop B (1960) Sudden infant death syndrome. In: Siim J-C (ed) Proceedings of the Eighth International Congress of Paediatrics, Basel, 1956. Williams and Wilkins, Copenhagen, p 91

Byard RW, Cohle SD (1994) Sudden death in infancy, childhood and adolescence. Cambridge University Press, Cambridge

Byard RW, Foster BK, Byers S (1993) Immunohistochemical characterisation of the costochondral junction in SIDS. J Clin Pathol 46: 108

Byard RW, Carmichael E, Beal S (1994) How useful is postmortem examination in sudden infant death syndrome? Pediatr Pathol 14: 817

Caffey J (1957) Some traumatic lesions in growing bones other than fractures and dislocations: clinical and radiological features. Br J Radiol 30: 225

Caffey J (1974) The whiplash shaken infant syndrome: manual shaking by the extremities with whiplash-induced intracranial and intraocular bleedings, linked with residual permanent brain damage and mental retardation. Pediatrics 54: 396

Cameron JM (1972) The battered baby syndrome. Practitioner 209: 302

Cameron JM, Johnson HRM, Camps FE (1966) The battered child syndrome. Med Sci Law 6: 2

Camps FE (1969) Injuries sustained by children from violence. In: Recent advances in forensic pathology. Churchill Livingstone, Edinburgh, chap 6

Carpenter RG (1972) Epidemiology. In: Camps FE, Carpenter RG (eds) Sudden and unexpected deaths in infancy. Wright, Bristol, p 7

Carpenter KH, Bonham JR, Worthy E, Variend S (1993) Vitreous humour and cerebrospinal fluid hypoxanthine concentration as a marker of pre-mortem hypoxia in SIDS. J Clin Pathol 46: 650

Carty H (1988) Brittle or battered. Arch Dis Child 63: 350

Carty HML (1993) Fractures caused by child abuse. J Bone Joint Surg (Br) 75-B: 849

Chapman S (1992) The radiological dating of injuries. Arch Dis Child 67: 1063

Chigr F, Jordan D, Najimi M, Denoroy L et al. (1992) Quantitative autoradiographic study of somatostatin and neurotensin binding sites in medulla oblongata of SIDS. Neurochem Int 20: 113

Clark JW, Yunginger JW, Bonnes PA, Ray CG, Saltzstein SL (1979) Serum IgE antibodies in sudden infant death syndrome. J Pediatr 95: 85

Cleary J (1984) Carbon monoxide and cot death. Lancet ii: 1403

Coombs RRA, McLaughlan P (1982) The enigma of cot death: is the modified-anaphylaxis hypothesis an explanation for some cases? Lancet i: 1399

Cooper C (1975) The doctor's dilemma – a paediatrician's view. In: Franklin AW (ed) Concerning child abuse. Churchill Livingstone, Edinburgh, p 21

Department of Health (1991a) Sudden infant death syndrome (SIDS). Report of the expert working group enquiring into the hypothesis that toxic gases evolved from chemicals in cot mattress covers and cot mattresses are a cause of SIDS. HMSO, London

Department of Health (1991b) Reducing the risk of cot death. Report of the Chief Medical Officer's Expert Group on the sleeping position of infants and cot death. HMSO, London

De Sa DJ (1985) Isolated myocarditis in the first year. Arch Dis Child 60: 484

Dinsdale F, Emery JL, Gadston DR (1977) The carotid body – a quantitative assessment in children. Histopathology 1: 179

Drucker DB, Aluyi HS, Morris JA, Telford DR, Gibbs A (1991) Lethal synergistic action of toxins of bacteria isolated from sudden infant death syndrome. J Clin Pathol 45: 799

Emery JL, Dinsdale F (1974) Increased incidence of lymphoreticular aggregates in lungs of children found unexpectedly dead. Arch Dis Child 49: 107

Emery JL, Dinsdale F (1978) Structure of peri-adrenal brown fat in childhood in both expected and cot deaths. Arch Dis Child 53: 154

Emery JL, Taylor EM (1986) Investigation of SIDS. N Engl J Med 315: 1676

Esiri MM, Urry P, Keeling J (1990) Lipid-containing cells in the brain in sudden infant death syndrome. Dev Med Child Neurol 32: 319

Fedrick J (1974) Sudden unexpected death in infants in the Oxford record linkage area. Br J Prev Soc Med 28: 164

Fleming PJ, Gilbert R, Azaz Y, Berry PJ et al. (1990) Interaction between bedding and sleeping position in the sudden infant death syndrome: a population based case–control study. Br Med J 301: 85

Fleming PJ, Azaz Y, Wigfield R (1992) Development of thermoregulation in infancy: possible implications for SIDS. J Clin Pathol 45 (Suppl): 17

Fleming PJ, Levine MR, Azaz Y, Wigfield R, Stewart AJ (1993) Interactions between thermoregulation and the control of respiration in infants: possible relationship to sudden infant death. Acta Paediatr (Suppl) 389: 57

Fu C, Jasani B, Vujanic GM, Leadbeatter S et al. (1994) The immunocytochemical demonstration of a relative lack of nerve fibres in the atrioventricular node and bundle of His in the sudden infant death syndrome (SIDS). Forensic Sci Int 66: 175

Gadston DR, Emery JL (1976) Fatty change in perinatal and unexpected death. Arch Dis Child 51: 42

Gardner PS, McQuilin J, Court SDM (1970) Speculation on pathogenesis in death from respiratory syncytial virus infection. Br Med J i: 327

Gibson AAM (1992) Current epidemiology of SIDS. J Clin Pathol (Suppl) 45: 7

Gilbert-Barness EF, Barness LA (1993) Sudden infant death syndrome: is it a cause of death? Arch Pathol Lab Med 117: 1246

Gilbert RE, Fleming PJ, Azaz Y, Rudd PT (1990) Signs of illness preceding sudden unexpected death in infants. Br Med J 300: 1237

Grubbauer HM, Schwarz R (1980) Peritoneal dialysis in alcohol intoxication in a child. Arch Toxicol (Berl) 43: 317

Heaton JM (1972) The distribution of brown adipose tissue in the human. J Anat 112: 35

Helfer RE, Slovis TL, Black M (1977) Injuries resulting when small children fall out of bed. Pediatrics 60: 533

Herbert A, Andrews PS (1979) The pathology of cot deaths. J Pathol 128: 39

Herrmann MA, Dousa MK, Edwards WD (1992) Sudden infant death with anomalous origin of the left coronary artery. Am J Forensic Med Pathol 13: 191

Hobbs CJ (1984) Skull fracture and the diagnosis of abuse. Arch Dis Child 59: 246

Hobbs CJ (1986) When are burns not accidental? Arch Dis Child 61: 357

Holten JB, Allen JT, Green CA, Partington S, Gilbert RE, Berry PJ (1991) Inherited metabolic diseases in the sudden infant death syndrome. Arch Dis Child 66: 1315

Howat AJ, Bennett MJ, Variend S, Shaw L, Engel PC (1985) Defects of metabolism of fatty acids in sudden infant death syndrome. Br Med J 290: 1771

Howat WJ, Moore IE, Judd M, Roche WR (1994) Pulmonary immunopathology of sudden infant death syndrome. Lancet 343: 1390

Howatson AG (1992) Viral infection and α interferon in SIDS. J Clin Pathol 45 (suppl): 25

James TN (1968) Sudden death in babies: new observation in the heart. Am J Cardio 22: 479

James D, Berry PJ, Fleming P, Hathaway M (1990) Surfactant abnormality and the sudden infant death syndrome – a primary or secondary phenomenon? Arch Dis Child 65: 774

James CL, Keeling JW, Smith NM, Byard, RW (1994) Total anomalous pulmonary venous drainage associated with fatal outcome in infancy and early children: an autopsy study of 52 cases. Pediatr Pathol 14: 665

Johnson P, Robinson JS, Salisbury D (1972) The onset and control of breathing after birth in foetal and neonatal physiology. Cambridge University Press, Cambridge

de Jonge GA, Burgmeijer RJF, Engelberts AC, Hoogenboezem J et al. (1993) Sleeping position for infants and cot death in the Netherlands 1985–91. Arch Dis Child 69: 660

Keen JH, Lendrum J, Wolmon B (1975) Inflicted burns and scalds in children. Br Med J iv: 268

Keeton BR, Southall E, Rutter N, Anderson RG et al. (1977) Cardiac conduction disorders in six infants with "near miss" sudden infantile deaths. Br Med J ii: 600

Kelly J, Allsopp D, Hawksworth DL (1992) Sudden infant death syndrome (SIDS) and the toxic gas hypothesis: microbiological studies of cot mattresses. Hum Exp Toxicol 11: 347

Kelly DH, Walker AM, Cahen L, Shannon DC (1980) Periodic breathing in siblings of sudden infant death syndrome victims. Pediatrics 66: 515

Kendeel SR, Ferris JAJ (1977) Apparent hypoxic changes in pulmonary arterioles and small arteries in infancy. J Clin Pathol 30: 481

Knowelden J, Keeling J, Nicholl JP (1984) A multicentre study of post-neonatal mortality. Medical Care Research Unit, University of Sheffield

Krous HF (1984) Sudden infant death syndrome: pathology and pathophysiology. Pathol Annu 19: 1

Kukolich MK, Telsey A, Olt J, Motulsky AG (1977) Sudden infant death syndrome: normal QT interval on ECGs of relatives. Pediatrics 60: 51

Laidler P, Kay JM (1975) A quantitative morphological study of the carotid bodies of rates living at a stimulated altitude of 4300 metres. J Pathol 117: 183

Lalu K, Karhunen PJ, Rautiainen P (1992) Sudden and unexpected death of a 6-month-old baby with silent heart failure due to anomalous origin of the left coronary artery from the pulmonary artery. Am J Forensic Med Pathol 13: 196

Lauer B, Brock ET, Grossman M (1974) Battered child syndrome: review of 130 patients with controls. Paediatrics 54: 67

Levene S, Bonfield G (1991) Accidents on hospital wards. Arch Dis Child 66: 1047

Limerick SR (1992) Sudden infant death in historical perspective. J Clin Pathol 45 (suppl): 3

Lipsett J, Cohle SD, Berry PJ, Byard RW (1994) Anomalous coronary arteries: a multicenter pediatric autopsy study. Pediatr Pathol 14: 287

Lundemose JB, Gregersen N, Kolvraa S, Norgaard-Pedersen B et al. (1993) The frequency of a disease-causing point mutation in the gene coding for medium-chain acyl-CoA dehydrogenase in sudden infant death syndrome. Acta Paediatr 82: 544

Macauley RAA, Mason JK (1977) Violence in the home. In: Mason JK (ed) The pathology of violent injury. Arnold, London, p 218

Milner AD, Saunders RA, Hopkin IE (1977) Apnoea induced by airflow obstruction. Arch Dis Child 52: 379

Mirchandani HG, Michandani IH, House D (1984) Sudden infant death syndrome: measurement of total and specific serum immunoglobulin E (IgE). J Forensic Sci 29: 425

Mitchell K, Barclay RPC, Railton R, Fisher J, Conely J (1983) Frequency and severity of apnoea in lower respiratory tract infection in infancy. Arch Dis Child 58: 497

Mitchell EA, Taylor BJ, Ford RPK et al. (1992) Four modifiable and other major risk factors for cot death: the New Zealand study. J Paediatr Child Health 28: 3

Molz G, Brodzinowski A, Bär W, Vonlanthen B (1992) Morphologic variations in 180 cases of sudden infant death and 180 controls. Am J Forensic Med Pathol 13: 186

Moore L, Bourne AJ, Beal S, Byard RW, Collett M (1993) An association between suspended rocking cradles and infant death? Med J Aust 159: 215

Morris JA, Haran D, Smith A (1987) Hypothesis: common bacterial toxins are a possible cause of the sudden infant death syndrome. Med Hypotheses 22: 211

Mushin AS (1971) Ocular damage in the battered baby syndrome. Br Med J iii: 402

Naeye RL (1973) Pulmonary artery abnormalities in the sudden infant-death syndrome. N Engl J Med 289: 1167

Naeye RL (1974) SIDS – evidence of antecedent chronic hypoxia and hypoxemia in SIDS 1974. In: Robinson RR (ed) Proceedings of the Frances E. Camps International Symposium on sudden and unexpected deaths in infancy. Canadian Foundation for the Study of Infant Deaths, Toronto, p 1

Naeye RL (1976) Brain-stem and adrenal abnormalities in the sudden-infant-death syndrome. Am J Clin Pathol 66: 526

Nigro G, Castellani PM, Mozzotti FM, Midulla IVM (1983) Legionellosis and cot deaths. Lancet ii: 1034

Nixon J, Pearn J (1977) Non-accidental immersion in bathwater: another aspect of child abuse. Br Med J i: 271

O'Connor JF, Cohen J (1987) Dating fractures. In: Kleinman PK (ed) Diagnostic imaging of child abuse. Williams and Wilkins, Baltimore, p 103

Oppenheim BA, Barclay GR, Morris J, Knox F et al. (1994) Antibodies to endotoxin core in sudden infant death syndrome. Arch Dis Child 70: 95

Parish WE, Barrett AM, Coombs RRA, Gunther M, Camps FE (1960) Hypersensitivity to milk and sudden death in infancy. Lancet ii: 1106

Pérez-Platz U, Saeger W, Dhom G, Bajanowski T (1994) The pathology of the adrenal glands in sudden infant death syndrome (SIDS). Int J Legal Med 106: 244

Richardson BA (1990) Cot mattress biodeterioration and SIDS. Lancet 335: 670

Roberton DM, Barbor P, Hull D (1982) Unusual injury? Recent injury in normal children and children with suspected non-accidental injury. Br Med J 285: 1399

Rogers D, Tripp J, Bentovim A, Robinson A, Berry D, Goulding R (1976) Nonaccidental poisoning: an extended syndrome of child abuse. Br Med J i: 793

Rognum TO, Saugstad OD, Oyasaeter S, Olaisen B (1988) Elevated levels of hypoxanthine in vitreous humour indicate prolonged cerebral hypoxia in victims of sudden infant death. Pediatrics 82: 615

Royal College of Pathologists (1993) Guidelines for post mortem reports

Samuels MP, McGloughin W, Jacobsen RR, Poets CF, Southall DP (1992) Fourteen cases of imposed upper airway obstruction. Arch Dis Child 67: 162

Scott DJ, Gardner PS, McQuilin J, Stanton AN, Downham MAPS (1978) Respiratory viruses and cot death. Br Med J ii: 12

Shannon DC, Kelly DH, O'Connell K (1977) Abnormal regulations of ventilation in infants at risk for sudden-infant-death syndrome. N Engl J Med 297: 747

Shatz A, Hiss J, Arensburg B (1991) Basement-membrane thickening of the vocal cords in sudden infant death syndrome. Laryngoscope 101: 484

Shaw JCL (1988) Copper deficiency and non-accidental injury. Arch Dis Child 63: 448

Silverman FN (1953) The roentgen manifestations of unrecognized skeletal trauma in infants. AJR Am J Roentgenol 69: 413

Simpson K (1973) Child abuse – the battered baby. In: Mant AK (ed) Modern trends in forensic medicine, vol 3. Butterworths, London, chap 2

Sims BG, Grant JH, Cameron JM (1973) Bite marks in the "battered baby syndrome". Med Sci law 13: 207

Sinclair-Smith C, Dinsdale F, Emery J (1976) Evidence of duration and type of illness in children found unexpectedly dead. Arch Dis Child 51: 424

Smith SM, Hanson R (1974) 134 battered children: a medical and psychological study. Br Med J ii: 666

Smith NM, Ho SY (1994) Heart block and sudden death associated with fibrosis of the conduction system at the margin of a ventricular septal defect. Pediatr Cardiol 15: 139

Smith NM, Bourne J, Clapton WK, Byard RW (1992) The spectrum of presentation at autopsy of myocarditis in infancy and childhood. Pathology 24: 129

Sonnabend OAR, Sonnabend WFF, Krech U, Molz G, Sigrist T (1985) Continuous microbiological and pathological study of 70 sudden and unexpected infant deaths: toxigenic intestinal Clostridium botulinum infection in 9 cases of sudden infant death syndrome. Lancet i: 237

Southall DP, Orrell MJ, Talbot JF, Brinton RJ et al. (1977) Study of cardiac arrhythmias and other forms of conduction abnormality in newborn infants. Br Med J ii: 597

Squier MV (1993) Acquired diseases of the nervous system. In: Keeling JW (ed) Fetal and neonatal pathology, 2nd edn. Springer-Verlag, London, p 571

Stanton AN (1984) Overheating and cot death. Lancet ii: 1199

Steinschneider A (1972) Prolonged apnoea and sudden infant death syndrome: clinical and laboratory observations. Pediatrics 50: 646

Stewart GT (1979) Deaths of infants after triple vaccine. Lancet i: 354

Sturner WQ (1985) Unlikely explanations of cot deaths. Lancet i: 457

Suarez V, Fuggle WJ, Cameron AH, French TA, Hollingworth T (1987) Foamy myocardial transformation of infancy: an inherited disease. J Clin Pathol 40: 329

Sunderland R, Emery JL (1979) Apparent disappearance of hypernatraemic dehydration from infant deaths in Sheffield. Br Med J 11: 575

Takashima S, Armstrong D, Becker LE, Huber J (1978a) Cerebral white matter lesions in sudden infant death syndrome. Pediatrics 62: 155

Takashima S, Armstrong D, Becker L, Bryan C (1978b) Cerebral hypoperfusion in the sudden infant death syndrome? Brainstem gliosis and vasculature. Ann Neurol 4: 257

Taylor EM, Emery JL (1982) Immunisation and cot deaths. Lancet ii: 721

Teplitz C, Lim YC (1974) The diagnostic significance of diffuse brown adipose tissue (B.A.T.). Transformation of adult periadrenal fat: a morphologic indicator of severe chronic hypoxemia. Lab Invest 30: 390

Turner KJ, Baldo BA, Hilton JMN (1975) IgE antibodies to *Dermatophagoides pteronyssinus* (house-dust mite), *Aspergillus fumigatus,* and β-lactoglobulin in sudden infant death syndrome. Br Med J i: 357

Uren EC, Williams AL, Jack I, Rees JW (1980) Association of respiratory virus infections with sudden infant death syndrome. Med J Aust 1: 417

Valdés-Dapena MA (1967) Sudden and unexpected death in infancy: a review of the world literature 1954–1966. Pediatr 39: 123

Valdés-zDapena MA (1977) Sudden unexplained infant death, 1970 through 1975: an evolution in understanding. Pathol Annu 12: 117

Valdés-Dapena MA (1980) Sudden infant death syndrome: a review of the medical literature 1974–1979. Pediatr 66: 597

Valdés-Dapena MA (1983) The morphology of the sudden infant death syndrome: an overview. In: Tildon JT, Roeder LM, Steinschneider A (eds) Sudden infant death syndrome. Academic Press, New York, p 169

Valdés-Dapena M, McFeeley PA, Hoffman HJ, Damus KH, Franciosi RR et al. (1993) Histopathology atlas for the sudden infant death syndrome. Armed Forces Institute of Pathology, Washington DC

Warnasuriya N, Downham MAPS, Skelton A, Turner MW, Soothill JF (1980) Atopy in parents of children dying with sudden infant death syndrome. Arch Dis Child 55: 876

Watson E, Gardner A, Carpenter RG (1981) An epidemiological and sociological study of unexpected death in infancy in nine areas of Southern England. Med Sci law 21: 78

Wigglesworth JS, Keeling JW, Rushton DT, Berry PJ (1987) Pathological investigations in cases of sudden infant death. J Clin Pathol 40: 1481

Williams A, Vawter G, Reid L (1979) Increased muscularity of the pulmonary circulation in victims of sudden infant death syndrome. Pediatrics 63: 18

Williams AL, Uren EC, Bretherton L (1984) Respiratory viruses and sudden infant death. Br Med J 288: 1491

Willinger M, James LS, Catz C (1991) Defining the sudden infant death syndrome (SIDS). Pediatr Pathol 11: 677

Woolley PV (1945) Mechanical suffocation during infancy. Relation to total problem of sudden death. J Pediatr 26: 572

Yeoh C, Nixon JW, Dickson W, Kemp A, Sibert JR (1994) Patterns of scald injuries. Arch Dis Child 71: 156

Index